Human
Nutrition

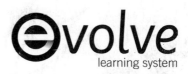

learning system

Evolve Learning Resources for Students and Lecturers:

Think outside the book...evolve

Commissioning Editor: Mairi McCubbin
Development Editor: Catherine Jackson
Project Manager: Alan Nicholson
Designer: Charles Gray
Illustration Manager: Gillian Richards

Human Nutrition

TWELFTH EDITION

Edited by

Catherine A Geissler BDS MS PhD RNutr
Emerita Professor of Human Nutrition, Nutritional Sciences Division, King's College London;
Director, Health Sciences and Practice Subject Centre, Higher Education Academy, London, UK

Hilary J Powers BSc PhD RNutr
Professor of Nutritional Biochemistry and Head of Human Nutrition Unit, Faculty of Medicine, Dentistry and
Health Sciences, University of Sheffield, Sheffield, UK

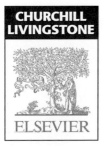

CHURCHILL
LIVINGSTONE

ELSEVIER

EDINBURGH LONDON NEW YORK OXFORD PHILADELPHIA ST LOUIS SYDNEY TORONTO 2011

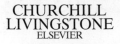

CHURCHILL
LIVINGSTONE
ELSEVIER

First edition 1959
Second edition 1963
Third edition 1966
Fourth Edition 1969
Fifth Edition 1972
Sixth Edition 1975

Seventh Edition 1979
Eighth Edition 1986
Ninth Edition 1993
Tenth Edition 2000
Eleventh Edition 2005
Twelfth Edition 2011

ISBN 978 0 7020 3118 2
Reprinted 2011, 2012

British Library Cataloguing in Publication Data
A catalogue record for this book is available from the British Library

Library of Congress Cataloging in Publication Data
A catalog record for this book is available from the Library of Congress

Notices

Knowledge and best practice in this field are constantly changing. As new research and experience broaden our understanding, changes in research methods, professional practices, or medical treatment may become necessary.

Practitioners and researchers must always rely on their own experience and knowledge in evaluating and using any information, methods, compounds, or experiments described herein. In using such information or methods they should be mindful of their own safety and the safety of others, including parties for whom they have a professional responsibility.

With respect to any drug or pharmaceutical products identified, readers are advised to check the most current information provided (i) on procedures featured or (ii) by the manufacturer of each product to be administered, to verify the recommended dose or formula, the method and duration of administration, and contraindications. It is the responsibility of practitioners, relying on their own experience and knowledge of their patients, to make diagnoses, to determine dosages and the best treatment for each individual patient, and to take all appropriate safety precautions.

To the fullest extent of the law, neither the Publisher nor the authors, contributors, or editors, assume any liability for any injury and/or damage to persons or property as a matter of products liability, negligence or otherwise, or from any use or operation of any methods, products, instructions, or ideas contained in the material herein.

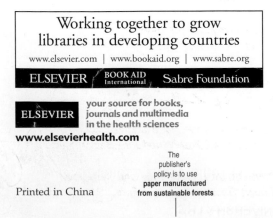

Working together to grow
libraries in developing countries

www.elsevier.com | www.bookaid.org | www.sabre.org

ELSEVIER | BOOK AID International | Sabre Foundation

ELSEVIER your source for books, journals and multimedia in the health sciences

www.elsevierhealth.com

The publisher's policy is to use paper manufactured from sustainable forests

Printed in China

Contents

Contributors

Arne Astrup MD DrMedSci
Head of Department, Professor, Department
of Human Nutrition, Faculty of Life Sciences,
University of Copenhagen, Copenhagen,
Denmark

Margo Barker PhD
Lecturer, Human Nutrition Unit, University of
Sheffield, Sheffield, UK

Christopher J Bates MA DPhil
Retired. Formerly Head of Micronutrient Status
Research, MRC Human Nutrition Research, Elsie
Widdowson Laboratory, Cambridge, UK

David A Bender BSc PhD RNutr
Professor of Nutritional Biochemistry, University
College London, London, UK

Aubrey Blumsohn MBBCh PhD MSc FRCPath
Consultant in Clinical Biochemistry,
Sheffield Teaching Hospitals NHS Trust,
Sheffield, UK

Barry Bogin MA PhD
Professor of Biological Anthropology, School of
Sport, Exercise and Health Sciences,
Loughborough University, Leicestershire, UK

Eric Brunner PhD FFPH
Reader in Epidemiology, Department of
Epidemiology and Public Health, University
College London, London, UK

Brunella Capaldo MD
Senior Investigator in Endocrinology and
Metabolic Disease, Federico II University, Naples,
Italy

Marc J Cohen PhD
Senior Researcher, Oxfam America, Washington
DC, USA

Zafra Cooper DPhil DipClinPsych
Principal Clinical Research Fellow Department of
Psychiatry, University of Oxford, Oxford, UK

Maureen Duggan MD MSc FRCP FRCPCH DCH DTM&H
Formerly Visiting Lecturer, Human Nutrition
Unit, University of Sheffield; formerly Senior
Lecturer in Paediatrics, University of Sheffield,
and Professor of Paediatrics, Mbarara University,
Uganda

Abdul G Dulloo PhD
Lecturer and Researcher, Department of Medicine,
Division of Physiology, University of Fribourg,
Switzerland

C G Fairburn DM FRCPsych FMedSci
Welcome Principal Research Fellow and Professor
of Psychiatry, Department of Psychiatry,
University of Oxford, Oxford, UK

Fiona A Ford MSc
Research Dietitian, Centre for Pregnancy
Nutrition, University of Sheffield, Sheffield, UK

Robert Fraser MD FRCOG
Reader in Obstetrics and Gynaecology, University of Sheffield, Sheffield, UK

Salah Gariballa MBBS MD FRCP
Professor of Medicine and Clinical Nutrition, faculty of Medicine and Health Sciences, United Arab Emirates University, Al-Ain, United Arab Emirates

Catherine A Geissler BDS MS PhD RNutr
Emerita Professor of Human Nutrition, Nutritional Sciences Division, King's College London; Director, Health Sciences and Practice Subject Centre, Higher Education Academy, London, UK

Michael H Gordon MA DPhil
Professor of Food Chemistry, School of Chemistry, Food and Pharmacy, University of Reading, Reading, UK

George Grimble BSc PhD
Reader in Clinical Nutrition, Department of Food and Nutritional Sciences, University of Reading, UK; Principal Teaching Fellow, UCL Centre for Gastroenterology and Nutrition, Windeyer Institute, London, UK

Bridget A Holmes BSc PhD RPHNutr
Senior Nutritional Epidemiologist, Danone Research, Global Nutrition Department, Palaiseau Cedex, France

J O Hunter MA MD FRCP FACG AGAF
Consultant Physician, Addenbrooke's Hospital, Cambridge; Visiting Professor of Medicine, Cranfield University, Bedfordshire, Swindon, UK

Ross Hunter MRCP BSc
Research Fellow, Nutritional Sciences Division, King's College London, London, UK

John M Kearney BSc PhD
Lecturer and Researcher in Nutritional Epidemiology, School of Biological Sciences, Dublin Institute of Technology (DIT), Dublin, Ireland

Timothy J Key BVMS MSc DPhil RPHNutr
Professor of Epidemiology and Deputy Director, Cancer Epidemiology Unit, University of Oxford, Oxford, UK

Jenny L Lee BSc MSc PGDip
Senior Gastroenterology Dietitian, Department of Nutrition and Dietetics, Addenbrookes Hospital, Cambridge, UK

Jim Mann CNZM DM PhD FRACP FRSNZ
Professor in Human Nutrition and Medicine, Department of Human Nutrition, University of Otago, Dunedin, New Zealand

D Joe Millward DSc PhD RPHN
Professor of Human Nutrition, University of Surrey, Guildford, Surrey, UK

Anne M Minihane BSc PhD
Reader in Integrative Nutrition, Hugh Sinclair Nutrition Group, Department of Food and Nutritional Sciences University of Reading, Reading, UK

Jane B Morgan MSc PhD
Formerly Reader in Childhood Nutrition, University of Surrey, Surrey, UK

Annhild Mosdøl MSc PhD
Associate Professor, Akershus University College, Faculty of Health, Nutrition and Management, Lillestrøm, Norway

Paula Moynihan PhD BSc
Professor of Nutrition and Oral Health, Institute for Ageing and Health, School of Dental Sciences, Newcastle University, Newcastle-upon-Tyne, UK

Sue Pedersen MD FRCPC
Specialist in Endocrinology and Metabolism, Department of Human Nutrition, Faculty of Life Sciences, University of Copenhagen, Copenhagen, Denmark

Timothy J Peters DSc PhD FRCP FRCPE FRCPath
Honorary Senior Research Fellow, Institute of Archaeology and Antiquity, University of Birmingham, Birmingham, UK

Elizabeth M E Poskitt MB BChir FRCP FRCPCH
Retired Paediatrician, previously Senior
Lecturer, Public Health Nutrition Group, London
School of Hygiene and Tropical Medicine,
London, UK

Hilary J Powers BSc PhD RNutr
Professor of Nutritional Biochemistry and Head of
Human Nutrition Unit, Faculty of Medicine,
Dentistry and Health Sciences, University of
Sheffield, Sheffield, UK

Victor R Preedy DSc PhD FIBiol FRCPath
Professor of Nutritional Biochemistry, Nutritional
Sciences Division, King's College London,
London, UK

Gabriele Riccardi MD
Professor of Endocrinology and Metabolic
Disease, Chief of the Diabetes Unit, Federico II
University, Naples, Italy

Angela A Rivellese MD
Associate Professor of Internal Medicine, Federico
II University, Naples, Italy

Tom Sanders DSc PhD
Professor of Nutrition and Dietetics, Nutritional
Sciences Division, King's College London,
London, UK

Wim H M Saris PhD MD
Professor of Human Nutrition, Department of
Human Biology, Maastricht University Medical
Centre, Maastricht, The Netherlands

Paul Sharp BSc PhD
Senior Lecturer, Nutritional Sciences Division,
King's College London, London, UK

Yves Schutz MPH PhD
Institute of Physiology, Faculty of Medicine,
University of Lausanne, Switzerland

Mario Siervo MD MSc RPHN
Research Scientist, MRC Human Nutrition
Research, Cambridge, UK

Elizabeth A Spencer MMedSci PhD RPHNutr
Nutritional Epidemiologist, Cancer
Epidemiology Unit, University of Oxford,
Oxford, UK

Stephen Strobel MD PhD FRCP FRCPCH
Honorary Professor of Paediatrics and Clinical
Immunology, UCL Institute of Child Health, and
Great Ormond Street Hospital NHS Trust,
University College London, London, UK

David I Thurnham BSc PhD
Howard Professor of Human Nutrition
(Emeritus), University of Ulster, Coleraine, UK

Paul Trayhurn DPhil DSc FRSE
Emeritus Professor of Nutritional Biology, Obesity
Biology Unit, University of Liverpool, Liverpool,
UK; and Honorary Professor, University of
Buckingham, Buckingham, UK

Luc J C Van Loon PhD
Associate Professor, Department of Human
Movement Sciences, Maastricht University
Medical Centre, Maastricht, The Netherlands

Christine M Williams BSc PhD
Pro-Vice Chancellor (Enterprise), University of
Reading, Reading, UK

I Stuart Wood BSc PhD
Lecturer, Obesity Biology Research Unit, School of
Clinical Sciences, University of Liverpool,
Liverpool, UK

Parveen Yaqoob MA DPhil
Professor of Nutritional Physiology, School of
Chemistry, Food Biosciences and Pharmacy,
University of Reading, Reading, UK

Preface

Publication of the 11th edition of the textbook *Human Nutrition* in 2005 constituted an important shift in content and format from previous editions of this classic textbook (formerly *Human Nutrition and Dietetics*). Central to the changes inherent in the 11th edition was an appreciation of the tremendous expansion in the broad discipline of human nutrition, to embrace subdisciplines as diverse as nutritional genomics and the evolution of thinking about food and nutrition security. The success of the 11th edition was evident from the demand for reprinting in years subsequent to 2005, which encouraged the editors to believe that a need was being met. Even so, the subject of human nutrition continues to evolve, and, with the overall aim of keeping the readership abreast of important new developments in this broad field, the 12th edition has been produced.

The successful format of the 11th edition of this textbook has been largely retained. The book comprises six parts, each considering a particular aspect of human nutrition. Part one considers the chemical characteristics of foods and nutrients and patterns of their consumption across the globe. Part two is concerned with the physiology of food digestion and nutrient absorption and examines the main features of fat, protein, carbohydrate and alcohol metabolism, and the regulation of energy balance. Part three is a comprehensive consideration of micronutrients, including dietary sources and functional effects of inadequate and excessive intakes. Dietary requirements for different age groups of the population are considered in part four, together with specific consideration of the needs of vegetarians and those people involved in sports and exercise. The evidence base for a link between energy and nutrient intake and disease risk is examined critically in part five , the largest section of the book. This section also considers how diet and genotype can interact to modulate disease risk. The final part six of the book deals with the broad discipline of public health nutrition, including the principles of nutritional epidemiology, the assessment of nutritional status, consideration of factors affecting food supply, and the development of food and nutrition policies worldwide. All of the constituent chapters have been updated since the 11th edition, the great majority by the original authors.

Additional to the material presented in the textbook, the 12th edition of *Human Nutrition* includes an accompanying on-line resource (*evolve*). This offers the reader a more in-depth consideration of some important aspects of the material in each chapter, as well as providing links to other useful websites.

This 12th edition of *Human Nutrition* is intended to provide an authoritative, comprehensive resource for students of human nutrition and other health sciences, and a concise source of information for all working in nutrition and related fields. An understanding of the many facets of human nutrition has never been more important to human health and well-being.

The editors sincerely thank the authors for contributing their expertise to this new edition.

London and Sheffield,
2010

Catherine Geissler
Hilary Powers

PART 1

Food and nutrients

Chapter 1

Food and nutrient patterns

John Kearney and Catherine Geissler*

CHAPTER CONTENTS

OBJECTIVES

By the end of this chapter you should be able to:

- identify the main sources of nutrients in Western diets
- understand the social, psychological, geographic and economic factors determining food choices and diet patterns
- appreciate the similarities and variability in food and nutrient patterns in different population groups and countries
- be aware of changing trends over time including novel foods.

1.1 INTRODUCTION

This chapter examines food and nutrient patterns in the context of the major foods and food products in the Western diet and their nutritional

*Updated and modified from the previous edition chapter written by John Kearney, Jane Thomas and Lawrence Haddad

importance. Taking the UK as an example of a country with a typical Western diet, it considers the main food groups and identifies the main sources of nutrients in the Western diet. It also outlines the main contributors to the nutrient and non-nutrient content of the UK diet. Another important aspect of this chapter is the exploration of the variations in dietary patterns in terms of the causes of variation such as availability (geographic, trade, demand) as well as economics, food beliefs and cultural differences. Examples of variations in dietary patterns in population subgroups such as vegetarians, and those defined by religion and region (national and international) are also outlined. This should enable the reader to appreciate the similarities and variability in different population groups and to clarify the social, psychological and geographical factors influencing food intake patterns. The variability in the consumption of foods, nutrients and non-nutrients, in terms of time (secular trends) and place (geographical differences – between developing and developed countries as well as between different developed countries), is described. This highlights the ability of different diets (foods consumed) to provide optimal nutrient intake. The wide diversity in the quantities of foods consumed between different countries and the changes with nutritional transition will serve to illustrate this.

In summary, in this chapter the major food groups in the diet are examined in terms of their nutrient and non-nutrient contribution, their variability between countries and between subgroups in the population, as well as changing trends in food intake patterns, including novel foods, over time.

1.2 MAJOR FOOD GROUPS IN THE WESTERN DIET

Western diets are composed of several food groups collectively providing the nutritional needs of the body. The particular food groups in the Western diet that provide all the nutrients and non-nutrients for optimum health include: cereals and cereal products (e.g. bread); vegetables and fruit; roots and tubers; milk and other dairy products; meats, fish, eggs and other sources of protein; fats and oils. A typical pattern of the Western diet may be illustrated in terms of the food intake patterns for British adults (Table 1.1). How these patterns vary between countries (i.e. geographically) is discussed below in Section 1.3, while changes over time are discussed in Section 1.4. The non-nutrients discussed in this

chapter are those believed to have a potentially beneficial effect on human health. They include both dietary fibre and phytoprotectants such as flavonoids and phytoestrogens. Other non-nutrients in foods such as contaminants, allergens and food additives do not have specific nutritional benefits and are not discussed here (see Ch. 2).

NUTRITIONAL IMPORTANCE OF FOOD GROUPS IN THE WESTERN DIET

For a fuller version of this section see Section *evolve* 1.2 🖱. For main food sources of macronutrients, vitamins, minerals and dietary fibre in UK adults see Tables *evolve* 1–4 🖱.

Cereals and cereal products

Cereals represent the most important plant foods in the human diet for their contribution to energy and carbohydrate intake and many micronutrients. They are all seeds from domesticated members of the grass family. Their contribution to energy intake varies markedly between developing and developed countries. In developing countries such as those in Africa and parts of Asia, cereals contribute as much as 70% of energy intake. By contrast, in developed countries, such as the UK, they provide approximately 30% of the energy intake. In the UK, cereals also provide about 10% of fat, 25% of protein and 50% of available carbohydrates. They also make a significant contribution to dietary fibre as non-starch polysaccharides (NSP). The major cereals in the human diet are wheat and rice followed by maize, barley, oats and rye.

Cereals are the staple foods in almost all populations. Carbohydrates form the major part of the cereal grain and consequently these are often referred to as carbohydrate foods.

Vegetables and fruit

These include a wide range of plant families and consist of any edible portion of the plant including roots, leaves, stems, buds, flowers and fruits. The leaves, stems, buds, flowers and some fruits (tomatoes, cucumbers, marrows and pumpkins) are commonly classified as vegetables while the fruits that are sweet are classified as fruits. Root crops are usually classified separately for human consumption rather than botanically. Vegetables and fruits are primarily seen as sources of vitamins and are important contributors to the intake of dietary fibre. Fruits tend to be high in potassium and low in sodium. Although quite low in B vitamins (with the

Table 1.1	Food intakes in grams/day among British adults (n = 1724)		
FOOD GROUP	FOODS	MEN (n = 833) G/DAY	WOMEN (n = 891) G/DAY
Cereal	Bread	126	81
	Pasta, rice, miscellaneous cereals including pizza	57	62
	Breakfast cereals	40	27
	Biscuits, buns, cakes, pastries and fruit pies	47	29
	Puddings (including dairy desserts and ice-cream)	27	19
Dairy	Milk (whole, semi-skimmed and skimmed)	229	192
	Other milk & cream	7.3	8.1
	Cheese	18	14
	Yoghurt and fromage frais	22	24
Vegetables and Fruit	Vegetables & vegetable dishes (excluding potatoes)	162	132
	Potatoes	121	93
	Fruit (excluding fruit juices)	122	103
	Fruit juice	55	47
Meat, Fish etc	Meat, meat dishes & meat products	184	124
	Fish and shellfish	42	31
	Eggs and egg dishes	20	16
	Savoury snacks	8.3	6.4
	Nuts	2.4	1.7
Other	Sugars, preserves and sweet spreads	22	11
	Confectionery	12	11
	Soft drinks, not low-calorie	68	100
	Soft drinks, low-calorie	55	100
	Fats and oils	17	10

Data from NDNS, Henderson et al (2002).

exception of folates, for which leafy vegetables are rich sources), they are the most important source of vitamin C. Also, fruits and vegetables are important sources of such non-nutrients as the phytoprotectants, carotenoids and anthocyanins (flavonoids in berries).

Roots and tubers

Roots and tubers are the underground organs of many plants and could be included in the vegetable and fruit group. However, due to differences in their nutrient composition and the important role they play in the Western diet (especially the potato) they are discussed separately.

Root crops: Most roots have a high water content and tend to be rich in carbohydrates as free sugars, with small amounts of starch in mature organs. They are generally low in dietary fibre, protein and micronutrients.

Tubers: Tubers are not true roots but rather underground stems that store large quantities of carbohydrate, usually starch. The potato is a stem tuber native to the Andes and was brought into Europe in the seventeenth century. The nutrient composition of the potato varies according to variety but all contain large amounts of starch (Table 1.2). They also contain significant amounts of vitamin C and their high levels of consumption make them an important source of this vitamin.

Meat and meat products

Meat has comprised an important part of the human diet for a large part of our history and still is the centrepiece of most meals in developed countries. In many developing countries, non-animal-based sources of protein such as legumes are still dominant. In the USA and the UK the most important meat sources are pigs, sheep and cattle. In other regions such as India, the Middle East and Africa, goat and camel are the main meats consumed. Other meat sources include wild animals such as rabbits, deer for venison, and poultry (chicken, ducks, turkey and geese). In the UK poultry (chicken) has now become the most popular meat source. Apart from the muscle, other parts of the animal collectively described as offal are also

Table 1.2	Contribution to energy and selected nutrient intakes from potatoes, all other vegetables and total fruits		
	POTATOES	OTHER VEGETABLES	TOTAL FRUITS
Energy (MJ)	6.8	3.1	4.0
Protein (g)	4.2	4.9	1.9
Carbohydrate (g)	10.2	4.2	6.8
Dietary fibre (g)	14.7	23.3	11.2
Iron (mg)	6.2	9.2	3.0
Carotenoids (mg)	0	79.0	2.8
Vitamin C (mg)	13.8	19.0	44.8
Folates (mg)	13.8	18.3	6.3

Data from Ministry of Agriculture, Fisheries and Food (1994) The Dietary and Nutritional Survey of British Adults – Further Analysis. HMSO, London.

consumed. The liver, kidneys, brain and pancreas (sweetbreads) are the most commonly consumed organs. Meat products such as sausages, pork pies etc. count for almost half of total meat consumption. Conventionally viewed as protein foods, meats as a whole are a major source of protein of high biological value. In developed countries such as the UK, where meat consumption is relatively high, it provides the main source of protein. Meats are also an important source of fat in the diet.

Fish

While fish catches worldwide are on the increase according to the Food and Agriculture Organization (FAO), fish stocks are being depleted due to over-fishing. The main fish consumed are white fish, oily fish and sea-food invertebrates. Fish are an important source of good quality protein and are low in fat, except for the oily fish, which provide a very good source of long-chain polyunsaturated fatty acids (PUFA). Fish are also a major source of iodine, which has been accumulated from their environment. Also, they may be an important source of calcium (in fish with fine bones) and vitamin D. The importance of vitamin D in health has, of late, been a very active area of nutrition research and good dietary sources are most important in supplementing that provided from non-dietary sources (i.e. exposure of skin to UV B in sunlight and supplements).

Eggs

The most widely consumed eggs in the UK are hens' eggs. The proteins found in eggs contain the amino acids essential for the chick embryos' complete development. Because of this it was considered the 'reference protein' for biological evaluation of other protein sources in terms of their amino acid patterns. Lipids found in eggs are rich in phospholipids and cholesterol. The fatty acid profile shows a high proportion of polyunsaturated fatty acids relative to saturated fatty acids (high P:S ratio).

Milk and other dairy products

Cows provide the bulk of all milk consumed in the UK, with goat and sheep making only a minor contribution to overall milk consumption. Milk is an excellent source of many nutrients. The major protein in milk is casein, comprising up to 80% of the protein in cow's milk. Other proteins include lactalbumin, and immunoglobulins, which are responsible for the transfer of maternal immunity of the young animal for a short period following birth. Milk from ruminant animals, such as the cow, contains a large proportion of short chain fatty acids produced from the fermentation of carbohydrates in the rumen. Milk and its products are excellent sources of many inorganic nutrients especially calcium and certain vitamins, both fat-soluble and water-soluble. Other dairy products include:

- cheese, which contains, in a concentrated form, many of milk's nutrients; and
- yoghurt, which is produced from the culturing of a mixture of milk and cream products with the lactic-acid-producing bacteria *Lactobacillus bulgaricus* and *Streptococcus thermophilus* and other bacterial cultures (e.g. *Lactobacillus acidophilus*, *Bifidobacteria*).

The contribution of dairy products to the UK diet, and to that of many other northern European countries, is very important. They can be an important source of calcium and riboflavin, especially in children and adolescents.

Fats and oils

These are distinguished by their physical characteristics, with fats being solid at room temperature (due to a high relative concentration of saturated fatty acids) while oils are liquid and usually of plant origin, either from the flesh of the fruit (olive oil) or from the seed (sunflower and linseed). They have a higher concentration of unsaturated fatty acids. Lipids that are isolated from animal products tend to be solid fats (e.g. butter, lard and suet). In recent years there has been increased consumption of margarine made from highly unsaturated fats such as sunflower due to the beneficial effects on serum cholesterol. In many countries, including the UK, margarines are required by legislation to be fortified with vitamins A and D so that they are nutritionally equivalent to butter.

FOOD SOURCES OF NUTRIENTS AND HEALTH-RELATED NON-NUTRIENTS

The importance of specific foods as sources of macro- and micronutrients for particular populations depends not only on the level of the nutrient in the food or food product (and its availability to the body), but also on the extent to which the food is consumed (the quantity and the proportion of the population that consumes that food). The way the food is consumed (raw, cooked or processed) will also influence its nutritional importance. Thus, it is important to distinguish between the nutritional importance of various foods generally and 'the main contributors' from food sources to nutrient intakes of a particular population. Such information is obtained from individual dietary surveys including diet histories or food records (see Ch. 31). One such survey was the Diet and Nutrition Survey of British Adults (DNSBA conducted in 1986/7) commissioned by the former Ministry of Agriculture, Fisheries and Food (now FSA and DEFRA) and the Department of Health. This has been followed up by the more recent adult survey among UK adults (NDNS) in 2000/1. The main food sources of carbohydrates in the UK are cereal products and potatoes. Biscuits, cakes and snacks also make a sizeable contribution. Important contributors to protein and fat intakes are meat, fish and eggs as well as dairy products, while vegetables and fruit make important contributions to a considerable number of the micronutrients (vitamins and minerals), dietary fibre and other non-nutrients (the phytoprotectants).

Dietary fibre

Fibre (total fibre) in the diet has a new definition based upon dietary fibre (indigestible carbohydrate and lignin, which are intrinsic and intact in plants) and functional fibre (isolated non-digestible carbohydrates that have beneficial physiological effects) (see Ch. 6). Previous definitions were based upon methods of analysis. The main contributors to fibre in the diet of British adults are cereal products and potatoes.

Phytoprotectants

Epidemiological studies indicate that a diet rich in fruits and vegetables has health benefits particularly related to protection against certain chronic diseases such as cancer. Experimental studies are being conducted to help establish causality and to elicit mechanisms for these observations, and this currently focuses on the antioxidant potential of certain nutrients and non-nutrients. The term 'phyto' originates from a Greek word meaning plant. Also known as phytochemicals and bioactive compounds, they are derived from foods of plant origin and, while not regarded as nutrients, they may be beneficial to health (e.g. reduce risk of certain cancers and cardiovascular disease, and of age-related blindness). Fruits, vegetables, grains, legumes, nuts and teas are rich sources of phytonutrients. Phytoprotectants are extremely varied in their chemical composition, the plants in which they are found and their putative beneficial effects. There are tens of thousands of phytonutrients in plants that have not yet been tested. The best way to benefit from these phytonutrients is to increase consumption of plant foods. Indeed, variety in colour appears to be important. (A more detailed description of phytoprotectants and their effects is given in Ch. 13.) Some of the common classes of phytonutrients include: flavonoids (polyphenols) including isoflavones (phytoestrogens), inositol phosphates (phytates), lignans (phytoestrogens), isothiocyanates, indoles, phenols and sulphides and thiols.

Polyphenols: Polyphenolic compounds are natural components of a wide variety of plants; they are also known as secondary plant metabolites. Much of the total antioxidant activity of fruits and vegetables is related to their phenolic content. Research suggests that many flavonoids are more potent antioxidants than vitamins C and E. Chlorogenic acid and caffeic acid are important phenolic compounds in our diet. The interest in these compounds is increasing because phenolic compounds have antioxidant activity in vitro. It has recently been shown that chlorogenic acid and caffeic acid are absorbed in humans, which increases the possibility that they might affect health. Food sources rich in polyphenols include onion, apple, tea, red wine, red grapes, grape juice, strawberries, raspberries, blueberries, cranberries, and certain nuts. The average polyphenol/flavonoid intake in the USA has not been determined with precision, as there is presently no US national food database for these compounds. USDA scientists and their colleagues are in the process of developing a database for foods rich in polyphenols. It has been estimated that in the Dutch diet a subset of flavonoids (flavonols and flavones) provides 23 mg per day. Polyphenols can be classified as non-flavonoids and flavonoids.

The flavonoids quercetin and catechins are the most extensively studied polyphenols in terms of their absorption and metabolism. The flavonol quercetin belongs to the group of flavonoids, one of the large groups of secondary plant metabolites occurring widely throughout the plant kingdom. Experimental studies in animals suggest that dietary quercetin, at relatively high doses, could inhibit the initiation and development of tumours in humans. These results are supported by in vitro studies showing that quercetin inhibits the growth of isolated human tumour cell lines. Furthermore, quercetin, the most commonly consumed flavonoid, is reported to exhibit antioxidant activity. A relationship has been reported between quercetin intake and reduced risk of cancer and coronary heart disease in a Finnish population. Further studies on epidemiology, mechanisms and interventions are needed before firm conclusions on the health-protective effects of quercetin can be drawn. Examples of other beneficial effects from phytoprotectants include lycopene, in tomatoes, which may decrease risk of developing prostate cancer, and lutein, found in dark green leafy vegetables, which is believed to reduce age-related blindness. Table 1.3 summarises some types of flavonoid and non-flavonoid polyphenols.

CONTRIBUTION OF MACRONUTRIENTS TO ENERGY NEEDS

Energy is required for the body to function, in particular to maintain basal metabolic rate and also for physical activity and for thermogenesis (see Ch. 5). The energy needs of the body are served by the contribution of the three macronutrients: carbohydrate, fat and protein. Alcohol is the other energy

Table 1.3	Examples of significant sources of non-flavonoid and flavonoid polyphenols
SOURCES	
Non-flavonoids	
Ellagic acid	Strawberries, blueberries, raspberries
Coumarins	Citrus fruits, some herbs
Flavonoids	
Anthocyanins	Berry fruits
Catechins	Tea, wine
Flavanones	Citrus fruits
Flavones	Fruits and vegetables
Flavonols	Fruits, vegetables, tea, wine
Isoflavones	Soya beans

source. Carbohydrate and fat are the primary fuel sources and for this purpose they can be largely used interchangeably. To a large extent the body can synthesise de novo the specific carbohydrates and lipids it needs, with the exception of the requirement for small amounts of carbohydrate and n-6 and n-3 fatty acids. Thus a mixture of macronutrients is required as a source of fuel to meet the energy requirements of the body. Defining the optimal mix of energy sources to optimise health and promote longevity is not easy. There are no clinical trials that compare various macronutrient combinations with longevity in humans.

Patterns of consumption of the macronutrients have changed radically from those of our ancient ancestors, for whom the relative contribution to energy has been estimated as 34% protein, 45% carbohydrate and 21% fat, contrasting to that of a typical current Western diet of 12% protein, 46% carbohydrate and 42% fat. Differences also exist in the energy contribution of these macronutrients between countries; developing countries have a much higher energy contribution from carbohydrates relative to fat than developed countries, where fat constitutes well over a third of energy intake. The acceptable (i.e. healthy) macronutrient distribution ranges (AMDR) are 10–15% of energy for protein, 25–30% of energy for fat and 45–65% of energy for carbohydrate. The recommendations (dietary reference values – DRV) for total fat are 33% of total energy or 35% of food energy. Considerable debate exists on the importance of total fat (quantity versus the qualitative composition of the fat) in relation to cardiovascular disease and certain cancers (see Ch. 7).

1.3 VARIATIONS IN DIETARY PATTERNS

EXAMPLES OF VARIATIONS IN DIET

For further details see Section *evolve* 1.3(a) 🖱.

Developing versus developed countries

Diets in the developing world are very different from those in the rich countries, although there is evidence of convergence between the two. The diets of the former tend to be characterised by lower total calorie intake, more calories from cereals and roots and tubers, less diversity in terms of food groups consumed, fewer animal source foods (and less fat), less processed food and less food away from home. Many of these differences are explained by socio-economic factors, but there is considerable variation in consumption patterns even accounting for such factors (as an example, see Section *evolve* 33.4(c) on South Korea's attempts to promote a 'traditional' diet 🖱).

Europe and the USA

For further details see also Section *evolve* 1.3(b) 🖱.

Differences in European diets can be examined from two main sources: a questionnaire-based survey carried out by the World Health Organization (WHO) Regional Office for Europe; and food supply data published by the Food and Agriculture Organization of the United Nations (FAO). Table 1.4 shows the total energy and macronutrient energy intakes in 13 EU member countries. For the comparative consumption of selected foods by men in selected European countries see Table *evolve* 1.5 🖱.

Both the WHO dietary intake and the FAO food available for consumption data show that fruit and vegetable intake is higher in southern European countries than it is in northern, western, central and eastern European countries. Indeed, large variations were found, with up to a five-fold variation in mean vegetable intakes from 100 g/day in Norway and Iceland to 370–500 g/day in Greece. Such a marked north–south variation in vegetable intakes is not as clear for fruit intakes, although wide inter-country variations do exist. For example, both sets of data indicate that people in Spain eat twice as much fruit and vegetables as people in the UK and three times as much as people in Kazakhstan (see Table *evolve* 1.6 🖱).

Whereas the intakes of polyunsaturated fatty acids (PUFA) are generally similar for countries in the north and south of Europe, the intakes of

Table 1.4	Mean energy intake and macronutrient energy intakes in 13 EU member states			
COUNTRY	ENERGY (MJ/DAY)	% ENERGY		
		CARBOHYDRATE	PROTEIN	FAT
Northern Europe				
Belgium	13.2	38.7	14.3	41.8
Denmark	10.2	43.5	14.5	37.0
Finland	9.0	47.7	16.1	33.8
France	8.6	38.2	17.4	38.9
Germany	9.6	39.2	15.1	40.7
Ireland	9.4	47.8	14.8	35.2
Netherlands	9.7	43.6	15.4	37.5
Sweden	8.8	46.0	15.0	36.5
UK	8.6	42.3	14.7	38.4
Southern Europe				
Greece	7.6	44.0	14.2	40.3
Italy	8.7	47.5	16.9	32.6
Portugal	9.7	49.1	18.0	28.5
Spain	8.9	40.2	19.6	38.0

Source: British Journal of Nutrition (1999) Food-based dietary guidelines – a staged approach. Volume 81, Supplement Number 2.

monounsaturated (MUFA) and saturated fatty acids (SFA) differ markedly. The intakes of SFA as % energy are higher in northern European countries, ranging from 14 to 18% energy compared with 9–13% in southern European countries, while intakes of monounsaturated fatty acids (MUFA) as % energy are higher in southern European countries (12–20%) compared with 11–15% in northern European countries. This difference in MUFA intake may be directly attributed to the higher consumption of olive oil in the southern countries of Europe. For % energy from fats and fatty acid categories in selected European countries see Tables *evolve* 1.7 and *evolve* 1.8 .

One specific diet survey, the SENECA (Survey in Europe on Nutrition and the Elderly) project, examined cross-cultural variations in intakes of food groups among elderly Europeans (Schroll et al 1997) in four European countries (Denmark, the Netherlands, Switzerland and Spain). The dietary pattern followed a typical Western diet, with all participants from all four countries consuming milk, grain products and vegetables and virtually all consuming meat and fruit. Fewer participants consumed fish, eggs and sugar. While variation was found between these food groups, the main variation seen between countries was in the types of foods comprising the food groups and with which meals the foods are consumed.

Variation within the UK

The UK National Expenditure and Food Survey (EFS) (DEFRA, 2008) enables comparison of different patterns according to socioeconomic group and region (see Tables *evolve* 1.9A-B and *evolve* 1.10A-B). There is considerable variation between countries in the UK and more specifically across regions of England with the lowest and highest levels of consumption of particular foods. For example, the highest consumption of fruit is in England and the lowest in Northern Ireland and Scotland whereas the highest consumption of meat products, confectionery and sugar and preserves is in Wales and the lowest in England. The low levels of vegetable and fruit consumption recorded in Northern Ireland and Scotland are the result of a number of historical and economic factors, and this observation is clearly linked to the current high levels of cardiovascular disease.

A number of important variations are also evident in relation to income and employment status. Non-pensioner households with the lowest head of household income (quintile 1 or bottom 20%) per week consumed lower amounts of fresh fruits and fresh vegetables (excluding potatoes), skimmed milk, cheese, fruit juices, breakfast cereals and alcoholic drinks than those earning the most (quintile 5 or top 20%). However, they consumed more liquid whole milk, eggs, fats and oils, sugar and preserves, fresh potatoes, frozen and canned vegetables and bread compared to the top income households.

For further details about economic and regional variation in food consumption in the UK see Section *evolve* 1.3(c) .

FACTORS IN DIETARY VARIATIONS

So far in this chapter we have considered foods and the nutritional contribution of food groups. But of course, in practice, people do not eat 'food groups' any more than they eat 'nutrients'. They choose foods to eat which usually contain ingredients from a number of the groups, for example pizza, apple pie, beef stew. Food groupings are useful tools for nutritionists, especially in relation to public nutrition policy, but they are not entirely satisfactory in picturing the way in which people eat. The way that people think about foods and how they group them together when making choices about what to eat may be very different from nutritionists' view of food groups.

Of all the animal and plant species that could be safely consumed, humans choose from a relatively narrow range of species. Those which may be considered a delicacy by some groups are rejected as inedible by others. Individuals' food choice at any given time will be influenced not only by what they consider to constitute 'food' and whether it is available (either physically accessible or affordable) but also by what is appropriate according to a variety of sociocultural factors, ideas, beliefs and attitudes as well as psychological factors and their level of hunger or satiety.

This section describes the main factors in dietary variation for developed and developing countries (Fig. 1.1).

Biological and physiological factors

Human physiology places few restrictions on food choice. Clearly the quantity of food consumed is limited to some extent by the capacity of the

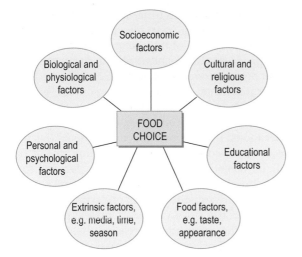

Fig. 1.1 The main factors determining dietary variation.

gastrointestinal tract, which results in the necessity to feed regularly, at least once a day and preferably more often. The quality of the diet is also limited, for example, by the fact that humans are monogastric, which renders plants with a very high fibre content impossible to digest.

Although factors such as age, gender, pregnancy, lactation and activity patterns all affect nutritional requirements, humans are unable to perceive their specific needs and act in response. No convincing evidence has been produced by studies that have attempted to demonstrate 'gustatory sensibility' (the innate ability of an individual to select foods that meet variations in nutritional status with regard to specific nutrients). However, studies with infants fed solely on milk have shown an innate ability to regulate energy intake in early life by adjusting the quantity of milk consumed in response to the level of dilution in order to maintain energy intake (Fomon et al 1969). This ability appears to decline when the diet becomes more varied, and is easily overridden by other factors influencing the timing of eating and the amount and types of food consumed in later life. Nonetheless the familiar experience of a decrease in pleasantness in association with increasing consumption of a particular food serves to limit the amount of that food which is eaten (Rolls 1986). This innate mechanism (sensory specific satiety) serves to ensure that humans eat a varied diet and are therefore more likely to meet their requirements for all nutrients. While this may have served humans well from a survival point of view in earlier times, it is

potentially more problematic when surrounded by a huge variety of different, highly palatable, food items.

Humans experience general and non-specific feelings of hunger or satiety as a result of complex physiological processes which are not fully understood but involve an integrated set of feedback mechanisms.

In recent years there has been growing interest in the possible identification of gene-related determinants of nutritional behaviour. It has been proposed that these might be modulated through sensory sensitivity to specific chemical substances and reflected in taste preferences. However, it appears that while biology determines humans' nutritional needs, it does not substantially affect food choices. For further information on hunger and satiety see Section *evolve* 1.3(d) .

Economic factors

Access to food is a primary determinant of food choice and dietary variation. The availability of food will be influenced by (a) geography, season and factors such as food preservation and distribution systems which affect physical availability and (b) the ability of the individual to acquire what is available. These two elements are closely interlinked and the relative importance of either will depend on the situation.

In remote rural areas, with poorly developed food markets, decisions about what to produce have an important effect on what is consumed, both at the village and at household level. In these cases, decisions about production and consumption cannot be treated as entirely separate. Where markets are stronger, physical access to foods becomes less important and economic constraints assume a greater role. About 20% of the world's 6 billion population participate in the cash economy and about 90% of the world's food consumption occurs where it is produced. In towns and cities people depend almost entirely on purchased foods, while in rural populations people consume around 60% of the food they produce (McMichael 2001).

In situations where food must be purchased, there are two key aspects of the relationship between income and food consumption patterns. The first relates to the overall level of expenditure on food, the second to the types of food consumed. As income levels increase, families spend more on food, although as a proportion of overall expenditure food is likely to decline in importance (called Engels's law). This may occur within a fairly narrow range in an industrialised country, such as the UK, where expenditure may range from 15% to 29% of reported expenditure between high income and low income households. However, in developing countries the differences may be far more dramatic, ranging between 15 and 80% of household expenditure.

One important outcome of this is the increased vulnerability of low income groups to changes in the price of foodstuffs and other necessities. This may be particularly important to the urban poor in less industrialised countries. If a diet which requires a high level of expenditure is barely adequate nutritionally, then any increase in price which leads to the purchase of reduced quantities of food may have serious nutritional consequences. Income may also be very unreliable. People are likely to be casually employed, or receive small amounts of cash intermittently as a result of different activities, and there is usually only enough money to buy small quantities of food at a time. Low income families have few opportunities to accumulate savings. As a result it is not possible to take advantage of the economies which are possible through bulk purchase. The urban poor may also be disadvantaged in the range and quality of foodstuffs available to them as well as the price they pay for food.

The cost of utilities – fuel, water, clothing, transport, rent – also affects food choices. The budgets of low income households leave very little room for manoeuvre and often food is the most flexible element of expenditure. If the price of cooking fuel increases, disposable income goes down and food purchases are affected. This may result in a change in the types of food purchased and a reduction in the amount of food eaten. Some or all of the family members may go without meals. It is commonly a priority to maintain the diet of the 'breadwinner', while women and children are particularly adversely affected by any shortfall.

The second area where income has a marked influence on food intake is in relation to the type of foods eaten. It is an internationally observed phenomenon that, as income levels rise, people diversify away from a reliance on cereals and roots/tubers and begin to purchase more animal source foods, fruits and vegetables. In the UK more affluent households eat more fruit and vegetables, polyunsaturated margarine, low fat products and carcass meat. In contrast, low income families eat less fruit and more of the cheaper cuts of meat and meat products such as meat pies and sausages. The use of high fat foods such as these contributes to the observation that, in a European context, energy-dense diets tend to cost less (Darmon et al 2004). Prices of one food can affect the consumption of other foods. If two foods are complements (i.e. they are eaten in combination), a price increase in one will, in the short run, lead to a lower demand for it and a lower demand for its complement. For two foods that are substitutes (e.g. one type of cereal for another), if the price of one increases, people will switch to the substitute, increasing the demand for it. These food prices can be dramatically affected by food policies that subsidise the consumption and production of certain foods, typically not based on nutritional goals (see Ch. 33).

Food prices are not the only prices that affect food consumption and diets. Financial needs and the availability of paid employment may cause men and women to work outside the home. As a result, less food will be prepared at home and more food will be consumed away from home. This has an effect on the types of food that are eaten. Only certain foods are 'portable' and suitable for advance preparation and consumption elsewhere, especially in the absence of refrigeration. Food choices become increasingly influenced by the types of food produced by others and available at times and in places convenient to the work schedule. The tendency to consume food away from home increases in urban areas, associated with a greater concentration of food vendors and restaurants.

Cultural and religious factors

The human is basically an omnivore who has to learn what to eat, and what is learned is strongly influenced by culture and religion. This includes learning what is acceptable or not acceptable as food and appropriate foods for different occasions and different types of people according to age, gender and social status. Rules about the preparation of food and how it is eaten may also be culturally determined. Food has many important social uses and although the food items associated with these uses may vary from society to society and change over time, these 'non-nutritional' functions persist.

Communication

An invitation to share food or drink, in a range of different settings, is widely used to initiate and maintain personal relationships. The actual foods and drinks that are consumed will vary according to the nature of those relationships and are hence imbued with layers of social meaning. What may be considered appropriate when the setting is a casual encounter between old friends will probably be very different from what might be served on a more formal occasion with people who are less well known and whom the host might want to impress. Food can be used as a means of demonstrating status and prestige. Arrangements for feeding guests at a wedding celebration may well be designed to reflect the status of the bride's father rather than being a response to the perceived hunger and nutritional needs of the guests. In addition to cementing relationships through hospitality and demonstrating social status, food is widely used to reward, punish or influence the behaviour of others. This may range from the use of sweets by parents to reward children for good behaviour to, in the wider world, the giving/withholding of food aid to particular countries, depending on whether the politics of the regime in power are acceptable to the donor government.

Identity

As part of the socialisation process, children grow up learning the conventions of their social, gender and age group concerning appropriate food choices and the manner in which such foods should be prepared and consumed. In some parts of the world, notably northern India and Pakistan, such conventions may have a marked impact on the diets of women and children, particularly girls, as a result of restrictions on the amount and types of foods which are considered suitable. More generally, the selection of foods that are deemed as inappropriate for a particular situation may have social consequences. The saying 'Tell me what you eat, and I will tell you who you are' is attributed to Brillat-Savarin and encapsulates this phenomenon. People's choice of food identifies them in various aspects of social background and may demonstrate whether they do or do not 'fit in' with another social group. The existence of clearly defined 'food rules' may play an important role in reinforcing 'in-group' identity. This may assume considerable importance in the context of religion, where such rules operate to set those with particular beliefs apart from others who do not share their beliefs.

Ethics and religion

Food may play a very special role in the 'living out' of an individual's beliefs. Since food is ultimately incorporated into the body, food choices become part of who we are in a very real sense and as food must be eaten every day it serves as a constant reminder of what we believe. In recent years vegetarianism and veganism have become increasingly popular in the UK (see Ch. 17) and for many people this choice has been based on ethical concerns about the exploitation of farm animals. In contrast to ethical considerations, which operate primarily on an individual level, religious food rules serve not only to enhance the spiritual life of the individual but also to enhance allegiance to a community of believers.

An individual may use the restriction of food choice or fasting as a means to enhance personal spiritual growth through the rejection of worldliness, or use foods in rituals associated with communication with God/supernatural forces. Following specified food rules can also be used to express separateness from non-believers and enhance feelings of identity and belongingness with co-religionists. The 2001 UK census showed a culturally diverse population. While the eating habits of the majority, white Christian population are relatively unaffected by their religious affiliation, nearly 3% of the population are Muslim (1591000) whose religion requires the following of particular food rules, as is the case for the next largest groups, Hindus (559000), Sikhs (336000) and Jews (267000).

Some dietary restrictions are based on direct injunctions from the holy texts of the religions concerned, while others have their origins in the commemoration of particular events in religious history. For example, the prohibition against pork in Judaism is firmly based on Leviticus 11:4, whereas the eating of matzahs by Jewish people at Passover commemorates the deliverance from Egypt, when their ancestors had no time to allow the bread to rise.

Such rules may affect different aspects of food choice. This includes the items which are considered acceptable as food. For example, those that are acceptable to Muslims are described as 'halal' and those that are forbidden, such as pork and alcohol, as 'haram'. Certain foods may be proscribed on particular days – Roman Catholics should not eat meat on Fridays during Lent. The time of day at which food is eaten may also be restricted – Buddhist monks should not eat after midday. Rules may include the preparation of food. Ritual slaughter is important in rendering meat acceptable to both Muslims (halal) and Jews (kosher). In addition, meat and dairy products must be kept separate and no food prepared on the Sabbath in Jewish households. Fasting is important to the followers of many religions and may take different forms, varying in length and the extent of restriction. In the case of the Ramadan fast for Muslims, no food or drink should be taken between sunrise and sunset for one month. In the Greek Orthodox Church it is expected that during the 40 days of Lent, which precede Easter, the faithful will abstain from all animal foods. In contrast, Hindus may 'fast' once or twice a week throughout the year, restricting themselves to 'pure' foods.

To prevent and treat illness

Later chapters of this book will examine in detail the scientific basis for our understanding of nutritional requirements and how dietary intake can affect health. However, popular beliefs about the links between diet, health and disease are shaped by their cultural context and consequently vary in different parts of the world. Not only do ideas vary geographically, but they also change over time. The history of medicine (using the term broadly) is not characterised by a linear succession in which old systems of thought are exchanged wholesale for new ones. We can see this clearly in relation to diet. Despite an enormous growth in the understanding of physiology and the origins of disease, popular advice in the early nineteenth century in England was still based on the dietetic works of Hippocrates and ideas about the effects of diet on humoral balance attributed to Galen and Avicenna. The concept of 'balance' as a key to health is central to these and in relation to diet focuses particularly on the 'heating' and 'cooling' effects attributed to foods. Individuals by nature of their age, gender and other characteristics are perceived to have a basic tendency towards the hot or cold end of a spectrum and in order to be healthy should select foods which counteract these tendencies and bring them back into a neutral position. Foods are classified as inherently 'heating' or 'cooling' regardless of the actual temperature of the food at the moment

when it is eaten, although the same food may be classified differently in different cultures. In addition, some conditions and diseases are associated with an excess of 'cold' or 'heat' and treatment should include foods with the opposite characteristic to restore health. It is usually considered to be particularly important for women to avoid imbalances during menstruation, pregnancy and lactation. Young children are also considered to be more vulnerable to imbalance and this may affect the foods that parents consider it appropriate to feed them. These ideas about the heating and cooling effects of foods are found in the classical health systems of the Indian subcontinent (Ayurvedic-Hindu and Unani-Islamic, medicine) as well as in traditional Chinese medicine, and are still widely practised in these communities. In addition, this approach was carried by the Spaniards (under the influence of Islamic medicine) to Central and South America. In some instances these beliefs may, in practice, support an improvement in diet for an individual, but in others they may restrict the diet and increase the risk of nutritional inadequacy.

Personal and psychological factors

Personal factors, including emotions, personality, self-esteem and self-efficacy, as well as beliefs and attitudes play an important role in shaping eating habits.

Food becomes associated with emotion from the very start of life, when feeding provides a pleasurable experience of comfort, security and well-being as well as satiety. Throughout childhood, humans learn to associate particular foods with feelings related to the circumstances in which they were eaten. Thus positive feelings of pleasure may be associated with foods given as a reward, or eaten on special occasions with much-loved people whilst negative feelings may be felt with foods used as a punishment or which had to be eaten because of financial hardship. These associations are woven together and colour an individual's response to food and situations in later life (Birch et al 1980).

As a result, a response to stress, loneliness and anxiety may be to eat and to choose particular foods that provide comfort through positive associations. Food may be used as a means of feeling secure, and the hoarding of food is often seen as a response to past experiences of food insecurity. All of these elements may play a part in promoting eating habits which lead to overweight and obesity for some individuals. In addition, parents' desire to show love, to spare their children any deprivation which they themselves experienced when growing up, or to deal with guilt that they do not spend enough 'quality time' with their children, may result in overfeeding them.

Food also provides a useful vehicle for demonstrating emotions such as anger and protest and may elicit very powerful feelings in the bystanders. The refusal to eat is a particularly powerful weapon – whether that is in the context of a child refusing to eat because they are angry or attention-seeking or a politically motivated hunger striker.

Even very young children have been shown to associate particular personality characteristics with different body sizes (thin – mean and sneaky, overweight – stupid and lazy) and the media are often criticised for reinforcing these stereotypes. But the evidence linking personality type to food preferences is not at all clear, although some work has suggested that introverts may have more food dislikes than extroverts.

The impact of 'self-esteem' and 'locus of control' on an individual's eating habits is of particular interest in relation to weight control, but is not clearly established. Some studies have pointed to the higher prevalence of overweight and obesity in relatively deprived population groups in North America and Europe, where self-esteem and people's perception of their ability to exert control over their lives may be low. Consequently some health promotion programmes incorporate activities designed to increase self-esteem and 'empower' participants.

Attitude and belief factors

Traditional approaches to understanding health beliefs that underpin eating behaviour have focused on three particular aspects: awareness of risks (relevance and seriousness), beliefs that dietary advice is effective and beliefs that the benefits of adopting a particular eating habit outweigh the costs (both social and financial).

Perceptions of risk
People find it very difficult to assess the relative risk of different diet-related health threats, particularly in the face of almost weekly 'food scares'. In addition, food safety concerns have become more pronounced in the past decade, partly as a result of the

loss of trust in governments' ability to regulate food supply ('mad cow disease' is the leading example), the new possibilities afforded by new technologies (e.g. biotechnology and genetically modified foods) and partly by the longer food chains, many of which originate in areas that may be out of reach of domestic food safety agencies. These risk perceptions are powerful drivers of food choice and are influenced by trust in government, the food industry and scientists and also by the accuracy of the information contained in food labels and in media reporting.

Perceptions of effectiveness of dietary advice
Two factors in particular may contribute to public uncertainty. Coverage of nutritional topics in the popular media is frequently adversarial, where a topic is debated by two 'experts' with opposing views. This may serve to confuse people. In addition, the most widespread and serious nutritional problems in Western countries are often themselves complex, multifactorial and develop over long time periods. Consequently dietary advice may change as scientific understanding unfolds. In addition, dietary change in relation to these health problems does not necessarily result in a clearly visible 'quick-fix' to the problem (as giving vitamin C to someone with scurvy would) producing convincing evidence of the effectiveness of change.

Belief that benefits outweigh the costs
Because eating is a social activity, making changes may involve social costs as well as financial ones. Perceptions of the behaviour that is considered to be the 'norm' in an individual's particular social group and the extent to which they feel bound to comply with that 'norm' and able, if necessary, to go against that norm, may be important determinants of food choice.

Educational factors

Within most societies people who have more knowledge about nutrition tend to have better diets. However, it is clear that just giving people more information about food and health does not necessarily result in a change to healthier eating habits. For many the practical difficulties of implementing change (access to affordable, healthy food) and the social barriers to changing eating patterns (lack of support from family, friends and neighbours) will result in apparently insurmountable difficulties when the benefits of making changes are weighed up against the costs.

Food factors

Taste and appearance

People are generally cautious when encountering foods for the first time (neophobic) and repeated exposure and consumption of a range of different foods in early childhood plays an important part in establishing a varied diet in later life.

A range of senses (vision, smell, hearing, etc.) contribute to our perception of the appearance, texture and flavour of foods. Whether or not we like those aspects of the food when it is presented to us will depend in part on our expectations of how that food should be, our memories of past experiences with that food, and the context in which the food is served. Finally our level of hunger will determine whether we accept and consume the food item.

Vision plays a critical role in food acceptance. Although colour is probably the most important visual aspect, other attributes such as gloss (on fruit), translucency (of jelly), size, shape and appearance of surface texture (of vegetables and baked goods) are all visual attributes which make a major contribution to the consumer's perception of the quality and appeal of a food item.

There are four basic taste qualities, salty, sweet, sour and bitter, and the experience of taste is also influenced by the smell of food (Cardello 1996). A further taste, umami, was identified in Japan in 1908, provided by glutamate, which is abundant in plants and animal proteins, and 5'-ribonucleotides, including 5'-inosinate (mainly in meat), 5'-guanylate (in plants), and 5'-adenylate (abundant in fish and shellfish) (Yamaguchi & Ninomiya 2000). It appears that infants have an innate preference for sweet tastes. A preference for salty foods does not appear until later in the first year of life and is more susceptible to modification by experience. People learn to like a certain level of saltiness. Taste/food *aversions* are strongly influenced by conditioning – particularly when consumption of a particular food has been followed by illness. Conditioning of taste/food *preferences* seems to be based on a more subtle mixture of positive associations with exposure, other flavours and satiety. Ageing is often associated with marked loss in sensitivity to taste, which is an important contributory factor to a decline in the enjoyment of food by older people.

The appeal of different textures may also vary throughout life. A crisp and crunchy apple may be much more attractive to a teenager than to an elderly person who has lost all their teeth. Furthermore, the role of texture in food acceptance is highly product dependent. In the case of meat, celery and mashed potato, for example, perception of texture makes a major contribution to the overall acceptability of the food. Socially and culturally learned expectations also play an important part in evaluating texture.

Awareness of the sensory attributes of food which appeal to consumers is clearly of major importance to food manufacturers. Insights into how the senses interact in the experience of eating can also have implications for product formulation; for example, consumers of a fruit drink with a deeper colour will report a stronger fruit taste. Foods are also made tastier through the use of fats, sugars and salts, all items that in modest excess can lead to health problems such as diabetes, hypertension and some forms of heart disease and cancer.

Extrinsic factors

Huge amounts of money are spent each year marketing foods in rich and middle income countries. In the UK the top ten food and drink companies spent over £130 million on advertising in 2000. Advertising is a very powerful influence on food choice, especially for highly processed and packaged foods. Some groups of the population may be much more susceptible to this influence and there has been particular concern about the impact on children. In experimental situations, young children clearly have high levels of recall of advertisements and are more likely to request advertised products. The extent to which this results in increased consumption will depend on the relationship with the parent or food provider and the extent to which that person is resistant to 'pester power'. Once children are older and have more money to spend they are clearly in a position to make their own purchases. Advertising also contributes to the creation of social norms – projecting images about what 'people do' and offering images of people who the audience might want to identify with. This has been the focus of extensive debate in relation to the contribution that media images make to the development of eating disorders, particularly anorexia nervosa, in young girls.

The types of foods that are advertised are often high in fat and simple sugars and the emphasis on the promotion of these types of foods in contrast to the low level of marketing of fruit and vegetables is also considered to have a distorting effect on food habits. In less affluent countries it is also the nature of the foods that are promoted (expensive and nutrient-poor) and the distortion that consumption of these may cause to already overstretched food budgets that raises ethical questions, when Western food companies are involved.

Seasonality

In parts of the world where food markets are not well integrated, local physical availability is a key determinant of food consumption. In rich countries, there are fewer and fewer seasonal food items as foods are sourced from all corners of the globe.

1.4 CHANGING DIETARY PATTERNS

CHANGING DIETARY PATTERNS – MIGRATION

The large-scale rural–urban and international migration seen around the world in the second half of the twentieth century has been accompanied by major changes in eating habits as people have adapted to the demands of their new environments. As people move from the countryside to the city they are forced to enter into a cash economy, while at the same time often having few employment-related skills. Lack of cash may severely limit access to food and food choice. Income generation may also often involve several jobs spread over long working hours. This has particular implications for women in relation to food preparation and child care. Facilities for cooking are often limited and living conditions poor.

Access to familiar foods, economic factors and food preparation facilities may also contribute to changes in the eating habits of international migrants. But the eating habits of the host community will also have an impact, depending on the extent to which the migrants are exposed to these and the strength of individual factors which may affect their resistance to change (Table 1.5). The dietary changes that are made first usually involve the adoption of foods that are convenient, affordable and do not clash with religious or cultural beliefs. The adoption of ready-to-eat breakfast cereals and the decline in cooking traditional foods at breakfast has been widely observed in migrants to the USA and UK. Breakfast is also a meal with

Table 1.5	Factors associated with changes in international migrants' eating habits
1.	Food availability: • physical • economic • time and cooking facilities
2.	Exposure: • length of stay • social contacts • education and language skills • mass media
3.	Individual: • age • religious beliefs • beliefs about diet and health

less social significance, whereas traditional dishes and foods are more often retained at evening meals when family members gather to eat. The presence of children in a family can accelerate the incorporation of non-traditional foods and eating patterns and the gradual development of eating patterns that incorporate elements of both the traditional and new food environments.

For further details see Section *evolve* 1.4(a) 🖱.

CHANGING PATTERNS – SUPPLY AND DEMAND

In response to changing lifestyle and popular demand (initially among more affluent, more industrialised Western countries and subsequently the growing middle classes in developing countries) global food supply systems have been transformed, through changes in agriculture, food technology and transport in the past fifty years.

These trends are linked to two major developments in relation to patterns of diet and health on a global basis. The first of these is the demographic transition – the shift from high fertility and high mortality to low fertility and low mortality which has been associated with increased industrialisation. The second is the epidemiological transition, the shift from a pattern of high levels of infectious diseases associated with unreliable food supply, malnutrition and poor environmental sanitation to a high prevalence of chronic degenerative diseases associated with urban-industrial lifestyles. These two changes underpin the so-called 'nutrition transition' (Popkin 2002).

At one time, nutrition-related non-communicable diseases (NR-NCDs) were referred to as 'diseases of affluence', more commonly found in industrialised Western countries than the developing world. However, it has long been recognised that this name was misleading in higher income countries, where these diseases were in fact more common in lower income groups, associated with lifestyle and dietary differences. It has also become apparent that NR-NCDs are emerging increasingly among lower and middle income groups in less affluent countries. This shift from a high prevalence of undernutrition to a situation where NR-NCDs predominate is referred to as the 'nutrition transition'.

The dietary changes associated with the nutrition transition are outlined below and commented on in relation to global trends in the following sections of this chapter.

Against a background of urbanisation, economic growth, technological changes for work, leisure and food processing, mass media growth, the changes in dietary and activity patterns can be summarised in three stages:

1. Receding famine pattern characterised by: diet – starchy, low variety, low fat, high fibre; labour intensive work/leisure
2. Degenerative disease pattern characterised by: increased fat, sugar, processed foods; shift in technology of work and leisure
3. Behavioural change pattern characterised by: reduced fat, increased fruit and vegetables, carbohydrate, fibre; increased activity (Popkin 2002).

Although lifestyle and other factors clearly lie behind these changes in eating habits (Fig. 1.2) there are other aspects of the 'globalisation' process that need to be recognised as having a powerful part to play in shaping food choice. Throughout history foods have 'migrated' and been incorporated into the diets of people thousands of miles away – the tomato and potato, originally from America, transformed the cuisines of Europe. These dietary changes have sometimes had huge social consequences, as in the case of sugar and the slave trade or the development of the Irish dependence on the potato and the subsequent impact of the potato famine. What is different about the changes in the past 50 years is the pace and scale of change. This is in part due to the application of marketing techniques to mould changes in taste. Most cuisines

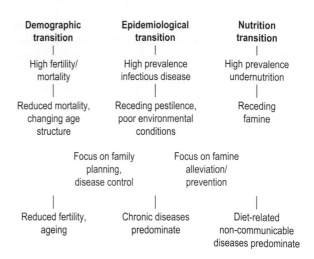

Fig. 1.2 The demographic, epidemiological and nutrition transitions. *(Modified from Popkin 2002, with permission.)*

have traditionally included 'fast foods' but the spread of the hamburger has been achieved through systematic and sophisticated marketing strategies. For a case study on the hamburger in Hong Kong see Section *evolve* 1.4(b) 🖥. The current phase of globalisation is also marked by concentration at regional, national and international levels. This applies throughout the food chain including production, processing and retailing. Decisions in all these areas affect the choices that people can exercise about what they actually eat. A relatively small number of companies dominate the world food markets, affecting every aspect of the route from farm to consumer. Supermarkets place contracts with distant suppliers to enable previously seasonal foods to be available all year round. The UK's food manufacturing sector is also highly concentrated. In 1995, three companies (Unilever, Cadbury Schweppes and Associated British Foods) dominated UK food manufacturing, and half the world's top 100 food sector companies are US-owned. Estimates suggest that the global food industry will come to be dominated by up to 200 groups who account for approximately two-thirds of sales. In the classical market economy, many suppliers compete for the attention of the consumer, responding to what the consumer wants. It has been suggested that in the evolving hypermarket economy, sophisticated systems of contracts and specifications and tight managerial control enable the retailer rather than the primary food producer or consumer to control the entire supply chain. Selection of foods which are *acceptable* to an individual increasingly takes place in a context where *availability* is substantially influenced by the food industry and food retailers.

EXAMPLES OF VARIATION IN DIETS OVER TIME

For more detailed information see Section *evolve* 1.4(c) 🖱.

Worldwide

On a worldwide basis the consumption of meat, milk, and eggs varies widely among countries, reflecting differences in food production resources, production systems, income, and cultural factors. Per capita consumption is much higher in developed countries but the current rapid increase in many developing countries is projected to continue. Total meat consumption in developing countries is projected to more than double between the years 2000 and 2020, whereas in developed countries it is projected to increase no more and, in some cases, by less than population growth. Because most of the world's population is in developing countries, which are experiencing the most rapid growth rates, global demand for meat is projected to increase by more than 60% of 2000 consumption by 2020. Thus, diets in developing countries are changing with rising incomes. The share of staples, such as cereals, roots and tubers, is declining, while that of meat, dairy products and oil crops is rising. Between 1964–6 and 1997–9, per capita meat consumption in developing countries rose by 150% and that of milk and dairy products by 60% (see Ch. 32).

Table 1.6 outlines world trends in the supply of vegetables and indicates the regional and temporal variations in the per capita availability of vegetables per year over the past few decades. In 2000, the global annual average per capita vegetable supply was 102 kg, with the highest level in Asia (116 kg), and the lowest levels in South America (48 kg) and Africa (52 kg).

Diets in developing countries are changing rapidly; as incomes grow, populations urbanise and age, and food choice options change. The latter occurs due to transformations in technology (such as global positioning systems and other information and communications technology) and food distribution systems (such as a reduction in the

Table 1.6	Supply of vegetables per capita, by region, 1979 and 2000 (kg per capita per year)	
REGION	1979	2000
World	66.1	101.9
Developed countries	107.4	112.8
Developing countries	51.1	98.8
Africa	45.4	52.1
North and Central America	88.7	98.3
South America	43.2	47.8
Asia	56.6	116.2
Europe	110.9	112.5
Oceania	71.8	98.7

numbers of wholesalers and retailers and longer food chain linkages). The transition in diets is happening most rapidly in China (see Ch. 33 and Table 1.7, and in middle income, urbanising countries such as Brazil, Mexico, Indonesia and Nigeria. The diet transition is causing a relative shift in the causes of disease away from those related to undernutrition only, towards those related to both under- and overnutrition – the nutrition transition.

Europe

As trade and cultural links within the European Union (EU) have strengthened over time, the consumption patterns of the first 15 EU members (EU-15) have been converging. A new study from FAO's Global Perspectives Studies Group, based on Food Balance Sheets (FBS), shows that the diets of the UK and Sweden were much more similar to the USA in the 1960s, but are now more similar to the EU average. Similarly Mediterranean diets have moved more towards the EU mainstream although variations persist. There has been little convergence of diets between the EU average and the USA; they are still relatively distinct, with the latter consuming much higher levels of added sugars.

Examples of temporal changes in a southern European country may be seen in Italy. In the early 1960s the diet consumed in the rural population of southern Italy was based mainly on cereals, fresh vegetables and olive oil. It was low in animal fat, protein and cholesterol and high in fibre. Since then, there has been a progressive move towards a higher nutrient density with fat intake increasing from 28% energy at that time to 36% in the 1980s. For trends in cereals consumption in selected

Table 1.7	Trends in the dietary supply of fat				
REGION	SUPPLY OF FAT (G PER CAPITA PER DAY)				% INCREASE FROM
	1967–69	1977–79	1987–89	1997–99	1978–79 TO 1997–99
North Africa	441	58	65	64	10
Sub-Saharan Africa	41	43	41	45	5
North America	117	125	138	143	14
Latin America and the Caribbean	54	65	73	79	22
China	24	27	48	79	193
East and Southeast Asia	28	32	44	52	63
South Asia	29	32	39	45	41
European Community	117	128	143	148	16
Eastern Europe	90	111	116	104	26
Near East	51	62	73	70	13
Oceania	102	102	113	113	11
World	53	57	67	73	28

Note: Sub-Saharan Africa excludes South Africa.
Source: SCN 2004 The Fifth Report on the World Nutrition Situation. UN Standing Committee on Nutrition, Geneva.

European countries between 1972 and 1997, see Figure *evolve* 1.1 🖐.

The UK

Consistent survey-based estimates of diets are available only for the rich countries. In the UK, the National Food Survey (NFS) reveals 50-year trends in food intakes from 1940 to 1990 (MAFF 1991). This has been followed by the Expenditure and Food Surveys, the results of which have been published by DEFRA since 2002.

World War II and its aftermath had a significant effect on the UK diet. During the war years and in the early post-war years dietary habits were shaped by the prevailing scarcity and restriction of many foods at that time. While many foods such as fruits and meat were restricted others such as foods rich in starch including potatoes and wholemeal brown bread (known as national bread) were increased. From 1954, consumers were able to return to their pre-war diets, higher in butter, sugar, fresh meat and white bread. It was not until the 1980s that the brown and wholemeal breads considered as healthier foods become more popular again. The 50-year trend shows a marked decline in total bread consumption. While brown bread declined sharply it was only partly replaced by white bread. This decline in bread consumption has continued, with a 5% decline in the purchase of bread between 2003/4 and 2006. The decline of white bread within this category has been even sharper, at 25%.

Recent changes in the pattern of consumption of milk products in the UK are reflected in a lower proportion of the population consuming full fat milk and more consuming semi-skimmed and skimmed milk. The purchase of whole milk declined by 19% between 2003/4 and 2006. These changes may have resulted from dietary guidelines recommending a reduction in total fat and more specifically saturated fat intake (see Section *evolve* 33.4(a) 🖐). Thus, there is now a substantial demand for low fat and skimmed milk. In addition, butter has been partly replaced by margarines and low fat spreads. These changes are most evident from the early 1980s when lower fat products became readily available. The decreasing consumption has also been accompanied by an increase in vegetable oils.

The main temporal changes in meat consumption between 1940 and 1990 were the rise in consumption of beef, lamb and pork in the early 1950s and the subsequent decline in lamb consumption. This has been accompanied by a huge rise in the consumption of chicken, which was rarely consumed 50 years ago in the UK and has now become the most common form of dietary protein. Overall, fish consumption trends show little change from a low intake level although data from 2006 reveal a modest increase of 9% in the purchase of fish. Taken together, fruit and vegetable consumption did not change appreciably in the 50 years to the late 1990s in the UK. Vegetables declined slightly but this was offset by the increase in fruit consumption. There was a decline in intakes of brassica vegetables including cabbage, cauliflower and Brussels sprouts as well as the traditional root vegetables. On the other hand, there has been an increase in salad vegetables and frozen vegetables. The consumption of frozen vegetables increased by a factor of 6 since 1965, of which frozen peas are the single largest contributor accounting for 25% of all frozen vegetables consumed. The sizeable increase in the consumption of the fruit group since the 1970s may be attributed to fruit juice (now accounting for 75% of fruit products) as well as the increasing year-round availability of fresh fruit. Apples are the most commonly consumed fruit followed by bananas and oranges. The changes in consumption of specific fruit and vegetables between 1975 and 1995 may be seen in Figure *evolve* 1.2 .

More recent data from the Expenditure and Food Survey (EFS) (report on Family Spending in 2005/6, produced by the ONS (Office for National Statistics) and published by DEFRA (www.statistics.gov.uk), indicate healthier trends in food purchases over the last several years. People in the UK are buying more fruit and vegetables, with quantities of fresh and processed fruit purchased having risen by 10% between 2003/4 and 2006, and increases of 5.8% in the quantities of vegetables purchased. Household expenditure also rose for cheese, eggs and milk, with a continuing switch from whole milk to semi-skimmed milk. The survey also found that people are buying less confectionery and soft drinks, and indicates a decline in purchases of alcoholic drinks, both for the household and in pubs and restaurants.

NOVEL FOODS

'Novel foods' are foods or food ingredients that do not have a significant history of consumption in the European Union before 1997 (see also Section *evolve* 1.4(d)). A novel food may be defined as: (1) a substance, including a microorganism, that does not have a history of safe use as a food; (2) a food that has been manufactured, prepared, preserved or packaged by a process that (i) has not been previously applied to that food, and (ii) causes the food to undergo a major change; (3) a food that is derived from a plant, animal or microorganism that has been genetically modified such that (i) the plant, animal or microorganism exhibits characteristics that were not previously observed in that plant, animal or microorganism, (ii) the plant, animal or microorganism no longer exhibits characteristics that were previously observed in that plant, animal

or microorganism, or (iii) one or more characteristics of the plant, animal or microorganism no longer fall within the anticipated range for that plant, animal or microorganism.

Most of these products are crop plants (e.g. corn, canola (rape), potatoes and soya bean) that have been genetically modified to improve agronomic characteristics such as crop yield, hardiness and uniformity, insect and virus resistance, and herbicide tolerance. Tomatoes that express delayed ripening characteristics have also been assessed and approved. A few of the products have been modified to intentionally change the composition, e.g. canola oil with increased levels of lauric acid. In the UK, the Food Standards Agency has a research programme on the safety of novel foods, with specific emphasis on GM foods. However, other novel foods, including 'functional foods', also fall within the scope of this programme.

Genetically modified foods

Genetically modified foods (GM foods) have ingredients in them that have been modified by a technique called gene technology (see Ch. 32 for further details). This technology allows food producers to alter certain characteristics of a food crop by introducing genetic material and proteins from another source. An example of this is a corn plant with a gene that makes it resistant to insect attack. With this technology it is possible to speed up the breeding of new and 'improved' crop varieties and to introduce completely new genetic information, for example from bacteria or animals into plants. Currently, only genetically modified soya beans and maize have been approved within the EU market. However, several others have been notified to the Commission as being substantially equivalent to traditional varieties according to the 1997 Novel Food Directive. In the USA more than 50 new recombinant-DNA (r-DNA) derived foods have been evaluated successfully by the Food and Drug Administration. The USA is the market leader in the total area occupied by genetically modified crops at 68%, while in Europe the figure is close to zero. For almost a decade genetically modified foods such as corn, soya beans, canola and tomatoes have been part of the American diet. This is not the case in Europe. It may well be that recent food safety issues such as the BSE outbreak in Europe and the way they were dealt with, or more importantly perceived to be inadequately dealt with, and the decided lack of trust in government sources with respect to information on food safety have resulted in the slower adoption of GM foods in Europe. (See also Section *evolve* 1.4(e)).

Functional foods

Consuming a nutritionally balanced diet was formerly considered as eating an adequate diet to avoid deficiency. But among developed countries, consuming a nutritionally balanced diet has come to mean consuming an optimal diet for promoting health as well as reducing the risk of diet-related chronic diseases. Optimal nutrition focuses on optimising the quality of the diet in terms of its quantity of nutrients and non-nutrients that favour the maintenance of health. This is where functional foods may have an important role to play since they are considered to have a specific role in relation to disease or the promotion of health. Indeed, a functional food is one claiming to have additional benefits other than nutritional value, for example a margarine that contains a cholesterol-lowering ingredient.

A functional food may be a natural food in which one of the components has been naturally enhanced through special growing conditions, a food to which a component has been added to provide benefits, a food from which a component has been removed so that the food has less adverse health effects (e.g. the reduction of saturated fatty acids), a food in which the nature of one or more components has been chemically modified to improve health (e.g. the hydrolysed protein in infant formulas to reduce the likelihood of allergenicity) or a food in which the bioavailability of one or more components has been increased to provide greater absorption of a beneficial component. A recent and comprehensive review of the role of functional foods in health is published in a recent supplement to the British Journal of Nutrition, including their possible future role (Westrate et al 2002). (See also Section *evolve* 1.4(f)).

KEY POINTS

- The typical Western diet is characterised by a diet relatively high in fat and low in carbohydrates when compared to the typical diet of most developing countries.
- While nutrient intakes and even broad food groups may not differ dramatically between developed countries (for example in Europe) the foods that contribute to these nutrient intakes do differ markedly. Despite some recent convergence within the EU, there is no single 'Western diet', or even European diet. The European diet differs considerably in the foods that compose it. Factors in dietary variations include those that are: physiological, such as age, gender, pregnancy, lactation, activity; economic; cultural and religious; psychological; beliefs and perceptions, such as risk, benefit; educational; related to food characteristics such as taste, appearance, texture; and extrinsic, such as advertising.
- Diets in developing countries are changing rapidly, driven by urbanisation, food distribution and retail technology, increased trade, income growth and food price policies. Rather than transition from undernutrition through health to overnutrition, many countries are moving to a situation of a double burden of malnutrition. This double burden is characterised by many people in a given population not getting enough food in terms of quality and quantity coexisting with many who are in danger of chronic disease due to excess calorie, fat, sugar or salt consumption.
- While nutrient intakes have remained remarkably consistent in the last 50 years or so (in the UK) there have been certain notable changes in food consumption patterns, e.g. the partial replacement of butter by low fat spreads and vegetable-based margarines, the partial replacement of full fat milk by low fat and skimmed milk, an increase in fruit juice consumption, a decrease in certain vegetables (e.g. swedes, turnips and Brussels sprouts), which have been replaced by salad vegetables and mushrooms. This changing pattern in food intakes is also evident in other countries.
- The most important sources of dietary fibre in the British diet are cereal products and vegetables (including potatoes) and fruits.
- Novel foods, including genetically modified and functional foods, are increasing in the Western diet with increasing emphasis on an optimal diet for promoting health as well as reducing the risk of diet-related chronic diseases. The rigorous safety evaluations that these foods must undergo should increase their consumer acceptance.

References

Birch LL, Zimmerman S, Hind H: The effect of social-affective context on pre-school children's food preferences, *Child Development* 51:856–861, 1980.

Cardello A: The role of human senses in food acceptance. In Meiselman HL, MacFie HJH, editors: *Food choice, acceptance and consumption*, London, 1996, Blackie Academic & Professional, pp 1–82.

Darmon N, Briend A, Drewnowski A: Energy-dense diets are associated with lower diet costs: a community study of French adults, *Public Health Nutrition* 7(1):21–27, 2004.

Fomon SJ, Filer LJ, Thomas LN, et al: Relationship between formula concentration and rate of growth in normal children, *Journal of Nutrition* 198:241–243, 1969.

Henderson L, Gregory J, Swan G: *National Diet and Nutrition Survey: adults aged 19 to 64 years. Volume 1: Types and quantities of foods consumed*, London, 2002, The Stationery Office.

McMichael P: The impact of globalisation, free trade and technology on food and nutrition in the new millennium, *Proceedings of the Nutrition Society* 60:215–220, 2001.

Office for National Statistics: *Expenditure and Food Survey 2001–2002*, London, 2002, The Stationery Office.

Popkin BM (Special Editor): The Bellagio Conference on the Nutrition Transition and its implications for health in the developing world, *Public Heath Nutrition (Special Issue)* 5(1A):1–280, 2002.

Rolls BJ: Sensory-specific satiety, *Nutrition Reviews* 44:93–101, 1986.

Schroll K, Moreiras-Varela O, Schlettwein-Gsell D, et al: Cross-cultural variations and changes in food-group intake among elderly women in Europe: results from the survey in Europe on nutrition and the elderly a concerted action: (SENECA), *American Journal of Clinical Nutrition* 65(suppl):1282S–1289S, 1997.

Weststrate JA, van Poppel G, Verschuren PM: Functional foods, trends and future, *British Journal of Nutrition* 88(suppl 2):S233–S235, 2002.

Yamaguchi S, Ninomiya K: Umami and food palatability, *Journal of Nutrition* 130:921S–926S, 2000.

Further reading

Fieldhouse P: *Food and nutrition: customs and culture*, London, 1995, Chapman & Hall.

Gibney MJ: Nutrition, physical activity and health status in Europe: an overview, *Public Health Nutrition (Special Issue)* 2(3A):329–334, 1999.

Lang T: Diet, health and globalisation: five keyquestions, *Proceedings of the Nutrition Society* 58:335–343, 1999.

MacClancy J, Henry CJ, Macbeth H, editors: *Consuming the inedible: neglected dimensions of food choice, Anthropology of Food and Nutrition*, Oxford, 2007, Berghahn Books.

Millstone E, Lang T: The Atlas of Food: Who eats what, where and why, ed 2, Earthscan Atlas Series, 2008.

Meiselman HL, Macfie HJH, editors: *Food choice, acceptance and consumption*, London, 1996, Blackie Academic and Professional.

Paul AA, Southgate DAT: *McCance and Widdowson's The composition of foods*, ed 4, London, 1978, HMSO.

Roberfroid MD. Defining functional foods. In Gibson G, Williams C, editors. *Functional foods*, Cambridge, UK, 2000, Woodhead Publishing.

Shepherd R, Raats M, editors: *The psychology of food choice. Frontiers in Nutritional Science no 3*, Wallingford, UK, 2006, CABI.

Vaughan JG, Geissler CA: The New Oxford Book of Food Plants, ed 2, Oxford, 2009, Oxford University Press.

EVOLVE CONTENTS (available online at: evolve.elsevier.com/Geissler/nutrition)

Chapter 2

Food and nutrient structure

Michael H Gordon

CHAPTER CONTENTS

OBJECTIVES

By the end of this chapter you should be able to:
- describe the main structures of the macronutrients
- characterise the effects of food processing on nutrient content
- describe the main types of natural toxins, pollutants and pathogenic agents
- identify the classes and functions of phytoprotectants.

2.1 INTRODUCTION

Humans have found that a wide range of plant varieties, animals, and some microbial sources can be consumed as food. Originally, food raw materials were selected on the basis of materials that could be consumed without harmful effects, and it was subsequently found that processing of foods by heat could improve the texture, and in some cases inactivate harmful components within the food. As understanding of the composition of foods has developed, it has become convenient to classify food components into macronutrients, which are present as bulk components of foods, and micronutrients, which are present at lower levels. Energy is mainly derived from the macronutrients, which comprise carbohydrates, fat, proteins and alcohol, but both macronutrients and micronutrients provide dietary components that are essential for normal physiological processes. This chapter informs readers about the chemical structures, properties and functions of a wide range of food components including nutrients and toxic

DOI: 10.1016/B978-0-7020-3118-2.00002-4

substances. The effects of processing and storage on these components are discussed.

2.2 CHEMICAL CHARACTERISTICS OF MACRONUTRIENTS

CARBOHYDRATES

Carbohydrates are mainly important as a source of energy (16 kJ/g or 3.8 kcal/g) in the human diet, being converted to glycogen or fat as energy stores. Carbohydrates include simple sugars, such as glucose, fructose and sucrose, plus polymers of sugars, which are termed polysaccharides, of which starch is the most important dietary component. Other polysaccharides include glycogen and cellulose. Many properties of sugars and polysaccharides are very different, but the molecular formula of all carbohydrates approximates to $(CH_2O)_n$, and the presence of carbon and water in this structure is why the class gained its name. Carbohydrates are synthesised in plants from carbon dioxide and water during photosynthesis.

Sugars

Monosaccharides are the building blocks for oligosaccharides and polysaccharides. Monosaccharides and some oligosaccharides occur as sweet components in foods, with glucose and fructose being the most common monosaccharides, and lactose and sucrose being examples of oligosaccharides that are sweet and are classed as sugars. Oligosaccharides contain from 2 to 10 monosaccharide units linked together. The sweetness found in the monosaccharides disappears in the higher molecular weight oligosaccharides. Polysaccharides have very different properties from sugars, since they are non-sweet and their solubility in water is normally very low. They are commonly of significance as thickeners or gelling agents in foods.

Glucose occurs in fruits and vegetables, but it is also formed by the hydrolysis of oligosaccharides and polysaccharides during digestion in the small intestine.

Fructose occurs together with glucose in fruits and vegetables and in some sweet foods such as honey. Hydrolysis of sucrose in the small intestine is also a source of fructose.

The chemical structures of monosaccharides comprise chains of between four and six carbon atoms with multiple hydroxyl substituents. Each monosaccharide contains a carbonyl group along the chain, and this may either be at the end of the chain, in which case it corresponds to an aldehyde, e.g. glucose, or it may be away from the end of the chain, in which case it corresponds to a ketone group as in fructose. The chemical structures can be represented in several ways. The Fischer projection formula is often used to show sugar structures. Figures 2.1 and 2.2 show the orientation of the hydrogen atoms and hydroxyl groups relative to carbon atoms (which are not drawn but which are present at each point where four bonds meet). The ends of the carbon skeleton are behind the plane of the paper with the substituents above the plane of the paper (Fig. 2.1).

In solution, monosaccharides exist as the open chain form shown in Figure 2.1 in equilibrium with ring forms (Fig. 2.2), which develop when one of the hydroxyl groups forms an intramolecular bond with the carbonyl carbon atom. Since six-membered rings are most stable, glucose exists in solution as an equilibrium between the open chain form (2%) and the six-membered ring forms termed glucopyranose (98%). When the open chain form of a sugar closes to form a ring, the hydroxyl group at carbon-1 may either be in an axial position in the chair structure as in α-glucopyranose or in an

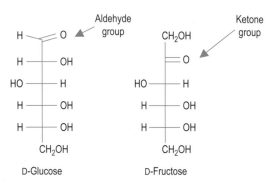

Fig. 2.1 Common sugar structures.

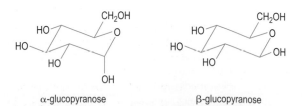

Fig. 2.2 The ring forms of glucose and fructose.

equatorial position as in β-glucopyranose. These isomers are termed anomers.

Monosaccharide units may be linked together by an acetal or glycosidic link which is formed when the carbonyl group of one monosaccharide unit links to a hydroxyl group on a second monosaccharide unit. Molecules comprising a small number of monosaccharide units are termed oligosaccharides, with sucrose, maltose and lactose being common disaccharides, comprising two monosaccharide units. Raffinose and stachyose are examples of tri- and tetrasaccharides that occur in foods.

Sucrose is well known as the most common sugar used in domestic kitchens and added to processed foods. It is refined on an industrial scale from sugar cane and sugar beet. Hydrolysis of sucrose during digestion provides glucose and fructose.

Lactose is present in cow's milk at about 4.7% of the milk, which corresponds to nearly 40% of the dry matter in milk. Its concentration in human milk is even higher at about 6.8% of the milk or nearly 60% of the dry matter in the milk. Hydrolysis of lactose forms galactose and glucose.

Polysaccharides

Polysaccharides contain large numbers of monosaccharide units linked together. Polysaccharides include starch, glycogen and cellulose, which are all polymers of glucose. They vary in whether the monosaccharide units are linked by α- or β-linkages, and whether they are linear or branched. These structural features are important since many enzymes including those of significance for digestion of the polysaccharides are selective in terms of which type of linkage is cleaved in the presence of the enzyme.

Starch, which is an important polysaccharide in plant foods including potatoes and bread, is a mixture of two polymers, amylose and amylopectin. Amylose contains glucose units linked by α-linkages between carbon-1 and carbon-4 of successive monosaccharide units, and these linkages cause the molecule to be linear. Amylopectin contains some α-1:6 linkages as well as α-1:4 linkages, and the α-1:6 linkages cause the polysaccharide to be branched. Starches from different plants differ in properties due to variations in the ratio of amylose to amylopectin present.

Glycogen is the form in which animals store carbohydrates, and this is similar to amylopectin in having both α-1:4 and α-1:6 linkages between

glucose molecules, although there are rather more α-1:6-linkages than in amylopectin.

Cellulose is a polymer of glucose with β-1:4 linkages between the glucose units. As a consequence of this structure, cellulose is non-digestible because humans lack enzymes that are capable of hydrolysing polymers of glucose linked by β-glycosidic bonds. In contrast, starch is split by amylases, which are secreted by the salivary glands and by the small intestine, so that starch is initially hydrolysed to disaccharides which can be hydrolysed to monosaccharides for absorption.

Pectins are important polysaccharides for the food industry. They occur in fruits and vegetables including apples and carrots, but they are important for their gelling properties in acid foods with a high sugar content such as jam. Pectins are polymers mainly comprising α-1:4 linked galacturonic acid with some other sugars. The degree of esterification of the polysaccharide has a major effect on the gelling properties.

FATS

Fats are components of foods that are extractable with organic solvents such as hexane or diethyl ether, but are insoluble in water. Dietary fats are converted to energy (37 kJ/g or 8.8 kcal/g), but they are also sources of essential fatty acids. Dietary fatty acids or metabolites are incorporated into phospholipids in cell membranes to provide the membrane structure. Essential fatty acids are converted into prostaglandins and other biologically active compounds described as eicosanoids, which control biochemical reactions within cells.

Fats comprise several classes of chemical compounds, which are termed lipids. The bulk of the fats in food (often >95% of the fat) are triacylglycerols, which are often referred to by the more traditional name of triglycerides. These molecules consist of three fatty acid residues esterified to a glycerol backbone (see Fig. *evolve* 2.1). The properties of triacylglycerols depend on the structures of the constituent fatty acid residues. The structure of fatty acids consists of a chain of carbon atoms with the required number of hydrogen atoms attached and a carboxylic acid residue at one end of the chain. The most common fatty acids have a chain of 16 or 18 carbon atoms, but fatty acids with between 4 and 22 carbon atoms occur in food lipids. Fatty acids with even numbers of carbon atoms occur almost exclusively because of the

Structure	**Class**
$CH_3-(CH_2)_4-CH=CH-CH_2-CH=CH-(CH_2)_7\ COOH$	Polyunsaturated (Linoleic acid, 18:2 n-6)
$CH_3-(CH_2)_7-CH=CH-(CH_2)_7\ COOH$	Monounsaturated (Oleic acid, 18:1 n-9)
$CH_3-(CH_2)_{16}\ COOH$	Saturated (Stearic acid, 18:0)

Fig. 2.3 Fatty acid structures.

biosynthetic pathway by which they are formed in plants and animals. Fatty acids may be classified according to the number of carbon–carbon double bonds as saturated with 0, monounsaturated with 1, and polyunsaturated with 2–6 (Fig. 2.3; Fig. *evolve* 2.2).

In polyunsaturated fatty acids, each of the carbon–carbon double bonds is separated from the next double bond by a methylene (CH_2) group. This allows a convenient short-hand nomenclature to be used for fatty acid structures, with the number of carbon atoms in the fatty acid chain followed by a colon, the number of double bonds and then the position of the double bond nearest the methyl end of the fatty acid chain. The number of carbons (x) from the methyl end of the molecule is indicated by n-x. Hence linoleic acid may be represented as 18:2 (n-6). An alternative nomenclature is to denote the position of the double bond by ω, so that linoleic acid is denoted as 18:2 ω6.

The most common fatty acids in food lipids are oleic acid (18:1 n-9), palmitic acid (16:0), stearic acid (18:0), linoleic acid (18:2 n-6) and α-linolenic acid (18:3 n-3). The nutritionally important polyunsaturated fatty acids eicosapentaenoic acid (EPA) (20:5 n-3) and docosahexaenoic acid (DHA) (22:6 n-3) are present in fish oil. Linoleic and linolenic acids are important dietary components because humans lack the enzymes required to introduce double bonds into fatty acids at the n-6 or n-3 positions, but metabolism of linoleic and linolenic acids allows the biosynthesis of metabolites including arachidonic acid (20:4 n-6) and eicosapentaenoic acid (20:5 n-3) by desaturation and chain elongation. Although longer-chain metabolites may be formed from 18:3 n-3, the process is not very efficient and the consumption of EPA and DHA (22:6 n-3), which occur in fish oils, has been found to be beneficial in reducing inflammation and risk factors for

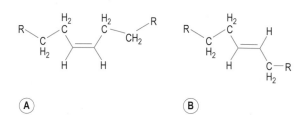

Fig. 2.4 Distribution of atoms at a carbon–carbon double bond: (a) *cis* and (b) *trans* configuration.

coronary heart disease including plasma triacylglycerol levels.

The substituents at carbon–carbon double bonds of fatty acids may be on the same side of the bond (*cis*) or on the opposite side of the double bond (*trans*), as shown in Figure 2.4. The configuration of the double bonds in natural plant lipids is exclusively *cis*, although small amounts of *trans*-unsaturated fatty acids are found in animal fats, such as milk fat, due to formation by hydrogenation of polyunsaturated fatty acids in the rumen of the animal. *Trans* fatty acids are also sometimes found in processed foods because fats containing these fatty acids can be prepared from liquid oils by an industrial process known as hydrogenation and these fats have the correct melting properties for use in foods such as margarine. However, because of concern about the health effects of excessive levels of intake of *trans* fatty acids, manufacturers in western Europe normally use other methods of preparing fats that do not form *trans* fatty acids. Low levels of *trans* fatty acids are consumed in foods containing animal products such as butter, or are present at very low levels in vegetable oils as a consequence of the heating that the oil is subjected to during refining. Although *cis* and *trans* unsaturated fatty acids are similar in chemical structure (Fig. 2.4), the different stereochemistry has important consequences. Polyunsaturated fatty acids containing one or more *trans* double bonds cannot act as essential fatty acids. Excessive dietary intake of *trans* unsaturated fatty acids may lead to increased risk of cardiovascular disease.

Phospholipids, the second major lipid class in foods besides triacylglycerols, are important structural components in biological membranes, and consequently are present in plants and animals consumed as food. The main phospholipids are phosphatidylcholine, phosphatidylethanolamine, phosphatidylserine, phosphatidylinositol and phosphatidic acid. These are acylglycerol derivatives with fatty acids at positions 1 and 2 of the glycerol molecule, with a phosphoric acid derivative at carbon-3 (see Fig. *evolve* 2.3). Phospholipids are added to many foods as they act as emulsifiers, helping to stabilise emulsions such as mayonnaise.

Sterols occur as minor lipid components in biological membranes. Animal tissues contain almost exclusively cholesterol (see Fig. *evolve* 2.4), whereas plant tissues contain a mixture of sterols, termed phytosterols, with β-sitosterol being a major component. Other phytosterols include campesterol and stigmasterol. Sterols are extracted with edible oils and fats from plant tissues, and they commonly occur at <1% concentration in edible oils such as sunflower oil. Their solubility in oils is limited but much higher levels of sterols have been incorporated into some functional foods by esterification of the sterols with fatty acids to form steryl esters. A functional food may be defined as a food having health-promoting benefits and/or disease-preventing properties over and above its usual nutritional value. In the case of foods containing steryl esters, the effect is to reduce blood serum cholesterol levels.

Other lipids occur as minor components in foods. These include glycolipids, sphingolipids, mono- and diacylglycerols and fat-soluble vitamins.

PROTEINS

Proteins are nitrogen-containing macromolecules that occur in major amounts in foods. Dietary proteins provide energy (17 kJ/g or 4.06 kcal/g), but they are also sources of amino acids which are essential for the synthesis of a wide variety of proteins with important functions, including carriers of vitamins, oxygen and carbon dioxide plus enzymes and structural proteins (Table 2.1). Proteins

Table 2.1 Amino acid composition of selected proteins (%)

AMINO ACID	BOVINE SERUM ALBUMIN	CASEIN	GELATIN	WHOLE EGG	PORK	BEEF
Alanine	6.3	3.1	11.0	5.4	15.3	20.0
Arginine	5.9	3.3	8.8	6.1	–	–
Aspartic acid	10.9	7.6	6.7	10.7	5.0	0.5
Cystine (0.5)	6.0	0.3	0.0	1.8	–	–
Glutamic acid	16.5	24.5	11.4	12.0	7.1	8.2
Glycine	1.8	1.9	27.5	3.0	10.0	4.2
Histidine	4.0	3.8	0.8	2.4	9.3	7.3
Hydroxyproline	0.0	0.0	14.1	0.0	–	–
Isoleucine	2.6	5.6	1.7	5.6	3.8	3.6
Leucine	12.3	9.2	3.3	8.3	9.8	6.8
Lysine	12.8	8.9	4.5	6.3	15.6	11.0
Methionine	0.8	1.8	0.9	3.2	2.5	3.6
Phenylalanine	6.6	5.3	2.2	5.1	1.9	2.4
Proline	4.8	13.5	16.4	3.8	2.3	–
Serine	4.2	5.3	4.2	7.9	10.8	13.4
Threonine	5.8	4.4	2.2	5.1	1.8	2.0
Tryptophan	–	–	–	1.8	–	–
Tyrosine	5.1	5.7	0.3	4.0	2.0	3.3
Valine	5.9	6.8	2.6	7.6	1.1	5.3
1-methylhistidine	–	–	–	–	1.8	8.5

Data from Deman J M (1999) Principles of food chemistry, 3rd edn; Aspen, Gaithersburg, MD; and Francis F J (2000) Encyclopedia of food science and technology, 2nd edn, John Wiley & Sons Inc., New York.

comprise polymers of amino acids with molecular weights varying from about 5000 up to several million. Twenty amino acids occur in most proteins (Fig. 2.5), but additional amino acids, namely hydroxyproline and hydroxylysine, occur in some animal proteins such as gelatin (see Fig. *evolve* 2.5). In proteins, the amino acids are linked together by peptide linkages, which are formed when the carboxylic acid group of one amino acid condenses with the amine group of a second amino acid with the elimination of water.

Most amino acids have the chemical structure $H_2N–C(R)H–COOH$, with variation in chemical structure arising from the nature of the substituent R, which may correspond to an aromatic or aliphatic residue or to a hydrogen atom in the case of glycine. In the case of proline, the amino acid contains a secondary amine group in a ring instead of a primary amine group. The common amino acids comprise alanine, arginine, asparagine, aspartic acid, cysteine, glutamine, glutamic acid, glycine, histidine, isoleucine, leucine, lysine, methionine, phenylalanine, proline, serine, threonine, tryptophan, tyrosine and valine. These amino acids provide the common polypeptide backbone of proteins, with the identity of the amino acids determining the substituents along the polypeptide chain of the protein. The amino acid sequence of a protein is described as the primary structure of the protein.

Plants can synthesise all the amino acids they need from inorganic nutrients, but animals cannot synthesise the amine group. Animals must consume plants in order to introduce amino acids for protein synthesis, but they are able to synthesise some amino acids by transamination in which an amine group is shifted from one amino acid to another. Transaminases act with pyridoxal phosphate as a coenzyme to catalyse this reaction. However, isoleucine, leucine, lysine, methionine, phenylalanine, threonine, tryptophan and valine cannot be synthesised in this way and these amino acids are described as essential amino acids, because they can only be introduced into the body by eating foods that contain these amino acids. The adult human body can maintain nitrogen equilibrium on a mixture of these amino acids as the sole source of nitrogen. If one or more of the essential amino acids is omitted from the diet, an adult would go into negative nitrogen balance. In the case of infants, histidine is also needed for growth.

The secondary structure of a protein is the conformation that the protein adopts along the long

Amino acid	Abbreviation	Side chain (R)
Alanine	Ala	CH_3-
Arginine	Arg	H_2N / HN $>-N(H)-CH_2-CH_2-CH_2-$
Aspartic acid	Asp	$HOOC-CH_2-$
Cysteine	Cys	$HSCH_2-$
Glutamic acid	Glu	$HOOC-CH_2-CH_2-$
Glycine	Gly	$H-$
Histidine	His	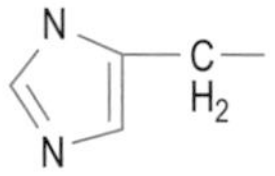 imidazole ring $-CH_2-$
Isoleucine	Ile	$CH_3-CH_2-CH(CH_3)-$
Leucine	Leu	$(H_3C)_2CH-CH_2-$
Lysine	Lys	$H_3N^+ -CH_2-CH_2-CH_2-CH_2-$
Methionine	Met	$H_3C-S-CH_2-CH_2-$
Phenylalanine	Phe	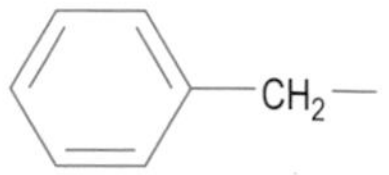 phenyl $-CH_2-$
Serine	Ser	$HOCH_2-$
Threonine	Thr	$H_3C-CH(OH)-$
Tryptophan	Trp	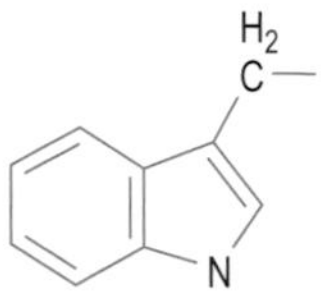 indole $-CH_2-$
Tyrosine	Tyr	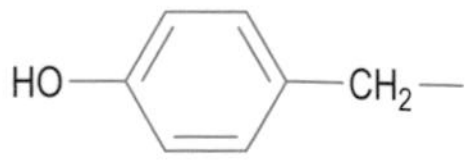 $HO-$ phenyl $-CH_2-$
Valine	Val	$(H_3C)_2CH-$
Proline	Pro	Formula 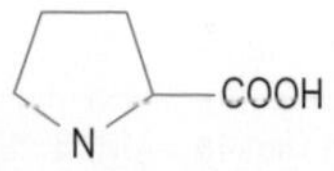 (pyrrolidine ring $-COOH$)

Fig. 2.5 Amino acid structures.

axis. The native protein adopts a certain conformation, which is energetically favourable. The precise conformation of a protein depends on the polarity, hydrophobicity and steric hindrance of the side-chains of the amino acids in the protein. The α-helix is a conformation that is adopted by many proteins. It has 3.6 amino acid residues per turn with a separation of 0.54 nm between successive coils of the helix (Fig. 2.6). The α-helix is stabilised by hydrogen-bonding between the backbone carbonyl of one residue and the backbone NH of the fourth residue along the chain.

The β-pleated sheet is another common secondary protein structure (Fig. 2.7). The sheet is formed from several individual β-strands, which are at a distance from each other along the primary protein sequence. The individual strands are aligned next to each other in such a way that the peptide carbonyl oxygens hydrogen-bond with neighbouring NH groups. The atoms of the α-carbons alternate above and below the plane of the main chain of the polypeptide.

The tertiary structure of a protein is established when the chains are folded over into compact structures stabilised by hydrogen bonds, disulphide bridges and van der Waals forces. The quaternary structure of proteins is the non-covalent association of subunits of proteins due to hydrogen bonds and van der Waals forces. The full protein structure (see Figs *evolve* 2.6, 2.7) is thus characterised by the amino acid sequence, the conformation along the y axis, the folding and the association of subunits.

Denaturation of proteins is the loss of structure that commonly occurs on heating proteins in solution. It can also be caused by salts, pH, surface effects or freezing. No covalent bonds are broken, but the change in properties can be very large. Minor degrees of denaturation may be reversible when the denaturing agent is removed but if denaturation has proceeded further it is commonly irreversible. Enzymes lose activity on denaturation, and the texture of foods may change due to a reduction in protein solubility on denaturation. Thus, the change in eggs on boiling, or the toughening of fish on frozen storage, are examples of changes in food texture due to protein denaturation.

ALCOHOL

Alcohol, which is more fully described as ethanol, C_2H_5OH, is formed by the fermentation of sugars during manufacture of beer, wines and spirits. Beer, wines, fortified wines and spirits contain ethanol at concentrations of about 30, 100, 150 and 300 g/l. Ethanol is fully miscible with water and fat. It is absorbed rapidly and metabolised in the liver to yield energy (29.7 kJ/g or 7.1 kcal/g). Many organic molecules are more soluble in aqueous ethanol solutions than in water and the presence of alcohol in a beverage may increase the bioavailability of minor components such as flavonoids from red wine.

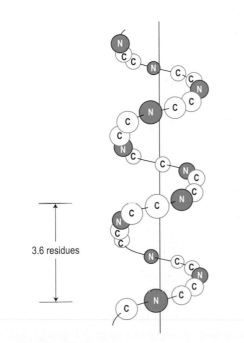

3.6 residues

Fig. 2.6 The α-helix structure.

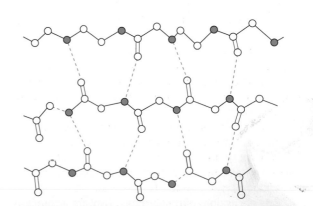

Fig. 2.7 The β-pleated sheet structure.

SUMMARY OF RELATIONSHIP BETWEEN STRUCTURE AND FUNCTION

Fats provide a major contribution to the sensory quality of food, and they are also the richest energy source in foods. They are present at high levels in some foods such as butter and margarine, where the fat content is about 80%. Liquid oils provide foods with an oily texture, but semi-solid fats are important in foods such as chocolate, where the melting of the fat as it warms in the mouth is an important contributor to the sensory quality of the product. Fats are important in foods as carriers of the fat-soluble vitamins A, D, E and K, and they are also important as carriers of oil-soluble flavour compounds. Some liquid oils such as sunflower oil are rich in the essential polyunsaturated fatty acid linoleic acid (18:2 n-6), and some liquid oils also contain α-linolenic acid (18:3 n-3). Fish oils are the main source of the fatty acids eicosapentaenoic acid (20:5 n-3) and docosahexaenoic acid (22:6 n-3), which are considered as beneficial dietary components.

Proteins may be soluble or insoluble in water. If they are soluble they may be important as enzymes and they may contribute to a viscous texture in liquid foods, but when they are insoluble they are normally more important in determining the texture of foods such as meat. Proteins are sources of the essential amino acids isoleucine, leucine, lysine, methionine, phenylalanine, threonine, tryptophan and valine.

Carbohydrates vary in properties from low molecular weight components that contribute sweetness through to high molecular polysaccharides such as starch that may be important for food texture. If the carbohydrates are not hydrolysed in the small intestine, they are normally important as dietary fibre. Table 2.2 provides the typical values for protein, fat and carbohydrate content of selected foods.

KEY POINTS

- Carbohydrates include sugars and polysaccharides. They are important as an energy source or as dietary fibre.
- Sugars are mainly monosaccharides (e.g. glucose) or disaccharides (e.g. sucrose).
- Polysaccharides include thickeners (e.g. starch), gelling agents (e.g. pectin) and dietary fibre (e.g. cellulose).
- Fats are mainly triacylglycerols. They are a source of the essential fatty acids linoleic acid and

Table 2.2 Typical values for protein, fat and carbohydrate content of selected foods (% of wet weight)

FOOD	PROTEIN	FAT	CARBOHYDRATE
Apple	0.4	0.1	11.8
Runner beans: raw	1.6	0.4	3.2
Runner beans: boiled	1.2	0.5	2.3
Beef	22.5	4.3	0.0
White bread	7.9	1.6	46.1
Hard cheese	24.9	34.5	0.1
Roast chicken	27.3	7.5	0
Baked cod	21.4	1.2	Trace
Sweetcorn	4.2	2.3	19.6
Egg	9.0	Trace	Trace
Haddock, steamed	20.9	0.6	0
Whole milk	3.3	3.9	4.5
Peas	5.8	0.7	13.8
Pork	21.8	4.0	0.0
Potatoes, new boiled	1.5	0.3	17.8
Rice: white, raw	7.3	3.6	85.8
Rice: cooked	2.6	1.3	30.9
Sardines, canned, drained	21.5	9.6	0
White wheat flour	9.4	1.3	77.7

From: Food Standards Agency (2002) McCance and Widdowson's The composition of foods. Sixth Summary Edition. Royal Society of Chemistry, Cambridge. Data from the Composition of Foods 6th Summary Edition Crown copyright material is reproduced with the permission of the Controller of HMSO and Queen's Printer for Scotland.

linolenic acid, which are utilised for eicosanoid synthesis.
- Fish oils contain EPA and DHA, which have beneficial effects in reducing inflammation and risk of cardiovascular disease.
- Proteins are macromolecules comprising chains of amino acids linked by a peptide bond.
- The essential amino acids are isoleucine, leucine, lysine, methionine, phenylalanine, threonine, tryptophan and valine.

2.3 EFFECTS OF FOOD PROCESSING AND STORAGE

TYPES OF FOOD PROCESSING

Foods are processed either to improve their palatability or to extend their lifetime before deterioration reduces sensory or microbial quality to a level where they can no longer be consumed. The methods vary in the temperatures used and in the contact with water or oil as heat transfer media. Other variables that affect the rate of destruction of nutrients are the presence of oxygen, light and the pH of the aqueous phase.

Cooking processes such as roasting animals on a fire or boiling in a pot have been used for thousands of years. Preservation processes such as salting or drying in air have also been applied for hundreds of years. Modern industrial processes have been developed to maintain or improve flavour, texture, and nutritional or other quality aspects. Preservation techniques have been improved so as to improve the shelf life of products, whilst maintaining optimal quality. Common processing methods include baking, frying, boiling and microwaving. Losses of vitamin C during the processing of small cylinders of potato fell in the order boiling > frying > baking > microwaving (Han et al 2004).

Baking

Baking involves cooking cakes, pastry, potatoes or fruit in a dry oven at temperatures in the range 170–230°C. The surface of the food reaches the oven temperature, but in most foods, e.g. potatoes or fruit, the high water content limits the internal temperature to 100°C or less. Some loss of nutrients, e.g. vitamin C, may occur from the surface layer, but the bulk of the nutrients are retained. The loss of thiamin has been widely studied. In the mildly acid environment of many fermented products, including bread, most thiamin is retained but if the pH rises above 6, most of the vitamin can be lost. Some of the amino acid lysine can be destroyed by baking due to the browning reactions between proteins and carbohydrates that contribute to the brown colour and aroma of baked products. Average losses of lysine during bread-making were reported to be about 15%.

Frying

Frying involves cooking in oil at temperatures in the range 160–200°C. Oil gives better heat transfer than air, so cooking times tend to be shorter than for baking. Losses of nutrients especially vitamin C may occur, but the food absorbs some oil which in the case of vegetable oils contains vitamin E. Plant foods rich in water such as potatoes tend to absorb more fat than meat does, because the fat is sucked into channels near the surface as the water is lost

by evaporation. In potatoes, 80% of the ascorbic acid was converted to dehydroascorbic acid (DHA) during frying for 5 minutes at 180°C, with no residual ascorbic acid being detectable (Davey et al 2000). However, DHA is readily reduced by glutathione in cells, and this change should not reduce the bioavailability of ascorbic acid from fried foods. Longer frying periods can cause irreversible losses of ascorbic acid due to oxidation. Frying of meat causes losses of thiamin and riboflavin, with reductions of up to 72% and 55% respectively during the frying of chicken (Al-Khalifa & Dawood 1993).

Grilling

Grilling involves the application of dry heat by radiation from a heating element. Grilling of beef caused losses of 34% vitamin A, 14% vitamin E, 74% thiamin, 49% riboflavin, and 40% nicotinic acid (Gerber et al 2009). With high temperatures being reached by the surface of the food during grilling, small concentrations of toxic compounds, e.g. heterocyclic amines, are formed.

Boiling

Boiling involves cooking in water at about 100°C. It is commonly applied to vegetables and starch-rich foods such as rice or potatoes. Plant cell walls soften, and starch-rich foods absorb water and swell. Water-soluble vitamins such as vitamin C, thiamin, riboflavin and minerals leach out of the food and losses increase with the amount of added water and also if the food is over-cooked. Mashing of boiled potatoes increases losses of vitamin C by oxidation due to the increased exposure to oxygen. Immersing small amounts of vegetables into rapidly boiling water minimises loss of vitamin C by rapid denaturation of enzymes that catalyse oxidation of ascorbic acid. Losses of vitamin C during the boiling of spinach were 60%, compared to 46% through steaming and 58% through pressure cooking (Rumm-Kreuter & Demmel 1990). Boiling of beef led to losses of 100% thiamin and 83% riboflavin (Gerber et al 2009).

Microwaving

Microwaving involves shorter cooking times than other processing methods, and the fact that the food is heated internally rather than from the surface explains the reduced losses of vitamin C when this method is used. Other methods, such as baking, have higher temperatures on the surface, where exposure to oxygen is greater and oxidation more severe, or, in the case of boiling, allow losses by leaching into the processing water. Retention of thiamine and riboflavin in vegetables processed by microwave cooking is also higher than in vegetables that are boiled in water (Orzaez-Villanueva et al 2000).

Canning

Canning is a traditional food preservation technique. The times and temperatures applied in canning must be sufficient to ensure that all pathogens are inactivated or destroyed. The most heat-resistant pathogen normally found in canned food is *Clostridium botulinum*. Heating for 2.5 minutes at 121°C is sufficient to destroy *C. botulinum* spores. For foods with a pH < 4.5, a less severe heat treatment may be applied because *C. botulinum* spores are less heat stable and will not grow under these conditions. The amount of oxygen available in the headspace of canned food is small and this limits losses of vitamin C by oxidation. Losses of well over 50% vitamin C are typical for canned vegetables, but losses are much less for most fruits due to the stabilising effects of low pH. About 60% of the vitamin C content of green peas remains after the canning process, but about half of the remaining vitamin C is lost when the product is reheated before serving (Ang & Livingstone 1974).

Pasteurisation

Pasteurisation is a mild heat treatment applied to foods to reduce the number of spoilage organisms present and kill the pathogenic organisms, but it does not render the food sterile. Although commonly associated with milk, it is applied to a wide variety of foods. The process involves a temperature–time combination sufficient to kill enough organisms to achieve reduction to an acceptable number, but without unacceptable changes in the flavour or nutrients of the food. For heat treating milk, either a high-temperature/short time process, which involves a temperature of 71.7°C for 15 seconds, or a low-temperature/longer-time process, which involves holding the milk at 62.8°C for 30 minutes, is applied. The milk must then be cooled rapidly to <10°C. These conditions are sufficient to destroy tuberculosis organisms and other more sensitive pathogenic organisms in the milk. For liquid egg, the pasteurisation conditions require heating at 64.4°C for 2.5 minutes prior to cooling to below 3.3°C.

Fermentation

Fermentation is defined as the action of microorganisms or enzymes on food raw materials to cause biochemical changes. Fermentation is widely used as a processing method for improving the nutritional quality, digestibility, safety or flavour of food. Fermentation is a relatively low-energy process that can improve product life and reduce the need for refrigeration. Foods such as beer, cheese, mushrooms, bread, yoghurt, soy sauce, pepperoni, tempeh and many others are produced by fermentation. Lactic acid bacteria which convert carbohydrates to lactic acid, thereby lowering the pH, and which also produce flavour compounds, are important in many fermented foods including fermented milk, cheese, meat and cereal products.

Storage of foods

Storage of foods may cause deterioration by aerial oxidation or by enzyme action, which can lead to losses of nutrients and textural changes. Microorganisms may multiply in some foods, e.g. milk and yoghurt, unless the storage temperature is kept below 6°C, but dry foods can be kept at higher temperatures because microorganisms will not grow in foods with a water activity below 0.6. In intermediate water foods (jam, dried and salted meats and fish, cakes, dried figs etc.) where the water activity is 0.70–0.90, mould and yeast spores, or pathogenic bacteria, can survive and then they can grow if the moisture content accidentally rises. The effect of water on microbiological changes is often discussed with reference to the water activity, a_w, where a_w is the ratio of the vapour pressure of water in a food to the saturated vapour pressure of water at the same temperature.

Refrigeration

Refrigeration slows down changes in stored foods. A temperature below 5°C is recommended to retard the growth of microorganisms but chemical or enzymatic changes can still occur slowly at these temperatures. Leafy vegetables, e.g. spinach, are very vulnerable to vitamin C loss during storage, but reducing the storage temperature from 20°C to 4°C significantly reduces losses (Favell 1998).

Freezing

Freezing slows down all chemical and enzymatic changes, but these processes can progress slowly even at −20°C, which is about the temperature in domestic freezers. Blanching, which involves heating briefly in hot water or steam, is commonly applied to vegetables prior to freezing in industrial processes in order to inactivate enzymes such as lipoxygenase that catalyse biochemical deterioration during frozen storage. Vitamin C is mainly lost at the blanching stage, both due to thermal degradation and due to leaching into the blanching medium. Losses of 10–40% vitamin C throughout the freezing process are typical, but the extent of losses depends on exposure to air during the process and the type of blanching process that is used. Losses are generally lower for steam blanching than for water blanching (Favell 1998).

Drying or dehydration

Drying or dehydration is the removal of water, and is traditionally achieved by leaving commodities in the sun. The larger the surface area the faster the drying process but the application of vacuum and heat accelerates the drying process. Drying reduces the activity of enzymes and also inhibits the growth of microorganisms. Industrially, dehydration is applied more widely to potatoes than to fruit and vegetables, and losses of about 75% of the vitamin C can occur. Vitamin C is commonly added to dehydrated potatoes, because of the importance of potatoes as a dietary source of vitamin C.

Freeze–drying

Freeze-drying is a process where water is removed under vacuum by sublimation from the frozen state of a food. Freeze-dried foods can normally be rehydrated to dissolve rapidly in water or to recover the original texture more closely than foods dried at higher temperatures. Thus freeze-drying is commonly applied in the manufacture of instant coffee powder because the powder has good solubility in water.

Salting

Salting is an effective method of preserving foods, e.g. meat, because the water activity is reduced. Salting in combination with smoking and drying was the main preservation method for centuries prior to the twentieth century. Salt-preserved products such as ham and bacon are still important in our diet but canning, refrigeration and freezing have become more common preservation techniques.

Irradiation

Irradiation is a physical method of processing food using ionising radiation. The radiation generates free radicals, which can react with the DNA of living insects and microorganisms. For food irradiation, maximum irradiation doses of 10 kGy are allowed, although lower doses are often used. Irradiation is permitted in Europe for fruits, vegetables, cereals, fish, shellfish and poultry, but the main application is herbs and spices, where chemical treatment is often required if irradiation is not used. Low irradiation doses, <1 kGy, inhibit sprouting, sterilise insects and delay ripening. At 1–3 kGy, the numbers of some spoilage microorganisms are reduced, but viruses and spores of sporulating bacteria such as *Clostridium botulinum* are not affected by food irradiation. Thiamin is the most sensitive of the water-soluble vitamins. More than 50% of the thiamin in chicken can be lost by an irradiation dose of 10 kGy at 10°C. Vitamin E is also sensitive to irradiation, with significant losses of vitamin E in irradiated cereals. However, although foods containing vitamins E and A are susceptible to irradiation, the main food sources of these vitamins are not irradiated. Losses of nutrients by irradiation are often no greater than losses by thermal processing methods. Irradiation of selected foods, especially herbs and spices, is a very safe procedure and it would be much more widely applied if consumer concern about the effects of radiation on human tissues was not carried over into prejudice against irradiated foods, where no radiation is retained by the food.

High–pressure processing

When high pressures up to 1000 MPa (10^4bar) are applied to packages of food that are submerged in a liquid, the pressure is distributed instantly and uniformly throughout the food. The high pressure causes destruction of microorganisms and inactivation of some enzymes, although a combination of heating and high pressure is often applied. The process has the potential for providing products with improved flavour, good retention of nutrients, and changed texture compared to products that are processed by heat alone. Fruit juices processed by high pressure processing are now sold in Europe and other products processed by this technique including jams, fruit jellies, sauces, fruit yoghurts and salad dressings are on sale in Japan. Losses of ascorbic acid from vegetable juice increase in the order high pressure processing < pasteurisation < sterilisation.

ADDITIVES

The use of additives in food in the UK is strictly controlled by legislation. The legislation aims to protect the health of the consumer and to prevent fraud. Additives are allowed for specific functions (antioxidant, colour etc.) and are restricted to those listed in the regulations. In some cases additives may be allowed for use in selected foods and at limited levels. Prior to being included in the regulations, the technical need for an additive is assessed by the Food Advisory Committee. If a technical need is demonstrated, the Committee on Toxicity of Chemicals in Food, Consumer Products and the Environment is consulted before the additive is included in the legislation.

Preservatives

Preservatives are substances added to foods to inhibit microbial spoilage. Common foods including meats, cheeses, baked goods, fruit juices and soft drinks are likely to include preservatives. Even if sterile foods are produced initially by thermal processing, infection with bacteria, fungi and yeasts can occur in these foods, which are often not consumed at one sitting, and preservatives are required to extend the shelf life of the products. Sorbic acid, benzoic acid, sulphites, thiabendazole, nitrites and biphenyl are amongst the substances approved for use as food preservatives (see Fig. *evolve* 2.8). Some food preservatives including benzoates and sulphur dioxide have been identified as causing sensitising or allergic reactions including chronic urticaria and asthma in susceptible individuals. Nitrites and nitrates, which are used in cured meats and some cheeses, have caused some concern because secondary amines may react with nitrite derivatives to form N-nitroso compounds that are possibly carcinogenic. However, nitrites are formed naturally in saliva within the body and nitrates are ingested in vegetables and water, so it is considered that the possibility of N-nitrosated compounds being formed in treated foods is of little consequence compared with other sources of these compounds. Sulphur dioxide is not used in foods containing thiamin because it brings about the destruction of the vitamin in the food.

Flavours

Flavours added to food may be natural components derived from raw materials such as spices by physical processes such as extraction or distillation. A range of essential oils, including clove oil and orange oil, are isolated by these processes and they are widely used for flavouring foods. Other flavour compounds are synthesised by controlled chemical synthesis, by transformations using living biological systems, by enzyme-catalysed synthesis or by the reaction flavour approach which mimics established food-cooking techniques. Synthetic flavour compounds include vanillin, menthol, methyl salicylate, benzaldehyde, maltol, ethyl maltol and cinnamaldehyde (see Fig. *evolve* 2.9).

Colours

The classes of natural or nature-identical colourings used for food include carotenoids, chlorophyll, anthocyanins and betalaines. Besides these, some synthetic compounds are allowed for addition to food. Synthetic food colours can be classified as azo (e.g. sunset yellow FCF), azo-pyrazolone (e.g. tartrazine), triarylmethane (e.g. green S), xanthene (e.g. erythrosine), quinoline (e.g. quinoline yellow) or indigoid compounds (e.g. indigo carmine) (see Fig. *evolve* 2.10). Most of the allowed synthetic food colours are water-soluble. Some food colours have been found to cause allergic responses in susceptible individuals. Most concern has been expressed about tartrazine. It has been estimated that about 100 000 people in the USA are sensitive to tartrazine. Symptoms of the allergic response include urticaria, swelling, often of the face and lips, runny nose and occasionally asthma. The Food Standards Agency has asked food manufacturers to impose a voluntary ban on tartrazine, quinoline yellow, sunset yellow, carmoisine, ponceau 4R and allura red because of concern that they make children hyperactive and inattentive.

Sweeteners

Consumers are very interested in low calorie food and beverage products. Since the sugars present are significant contributors to the calorific content of many foods, the food industry has developed a range of zero or low calorie sweeteners. Aspartame, saccharin, acesulfame K and cyclamates are high potency sweeteners (see Fig. *evolve* 2.11). Aspartame is used widely in foods because it is the sweetener that most closely mimics the taste of sucrose. It consists of two amino acids, aspartic acid and phenylalanine, and it is 180 times sweeter than sucrose. Aspartame is quite stable in acid foods but it is less stable in the neutral pH range found in baked foods. People with phenylketonuria, a rare inherited disorder, must avoid foods containing aspartame because they do not metabolise phenylalanine effectively.

Saccharin is a very stable, highly water-soluble and cheap food additive, but although it is a high potency sweetener, some consumers are sensitive to its bitter and metallic off-tastes. Although concerns about the safety of saccharin were raised following a Canadian study in the 1970s in which bladder tumours were found in the second generation of rats fed saccharin, there is no evidence that saccharin has caused cancer in humans. Some studies have suggested that it was the sodium component of sodium saccharin that caused the bladder tumours in rats at the high level of consumption, and there is no evidence that similar effects occur in humans at realistic consumption levels. Acesulfame K is structurally related to saccharin and suffers from similar taste defects. Although it is not as stable as saccharin, it is used together with other sweeteners especially aspartame in foods such as diet cola drinks. Cyclamates are sodium or calcium salts of cyclamic acid. The taste is considered better than that of saccharin, but the concentration is limited to 400 mg/L in soft drinks, and the Food Standards Agency has recommended that young children should not consume more than three beakers of dilutable soft drinks to avoid exceeding the acceptable daily intake (ADI). Weak biological effects for the main metabolite of cyclamate, cyclohexylamine, have limited the ADI to 11.0 mg/kg.

Sucralose was developed as a non-nutritive sweetener in the 1970s. It is a trichlorinated derivative of sucrose with excellent flavour and stability.

Sugar alcohols including sorbitol, mannitol and xylitol have comparable sweetness and about the same calorific content as sucrose, but are absorbed more slowly from the digestive tract and do not raise postprandial blood sugar and insulin levels; thus they are suitable for sweetening diabetic foods.

Processing aids

Processing aids are substances used to facilitate food processing by acting as chelating agents, enzymes, antifoaming agents, catalysts, solvents, lubricants or propellants. They are not consumed as food ingredients by themselves, and are used during food processing without the intention that they should be present in the final product. Residues of the processing aids may be present in the finished product and it is a legal requirement that they do not present any risk to human health. Chymosin, which was developed as a replacement for rennet, the milk clotting enzyme traditionally used in cheese manufacture, was classified as a processing aid.

Genetically modified organisms (GMOs)

GMOs are plants, animals or microorganisms which have had DNA inserted into them by means other than the natural processes of combination of an egg and a sperm or natural bacterial conjugation (see Ch. 32.6). The use of GMOs in food has been the subject of intense debate in recent years. GMOs have a number of potential benefits including improved nutritional attributes, e.g. reduction of anti-nutritive and allergenic factors, and increase of the vitamin A content in rice to reduce blindness in South-east Asia. Tomato puree produced from GM tomatoes was widely accepted for several years in the UK but it is no longer available. Advantages claimed for the product included better flavour, consistency and lower price than the non-GM alternative. However, concerns about antibiotic resistance, transferring allergenic components between plant species, and environmental concerns about the risks of GM crops to the agricultural environment have prevented widespread acceptance of GM foods by consumers.

2.4 TOXIC COMPONENTS FORMED BY PROCESSING

The processing of foods is essential to inactivate microorganisms and to allow flavour and texture development. However, processing may lead to losses of nutrients, and it may also lead to the formation of toxic components under certain conditions. A wide range of chemical reactions occur at high temperatures, such as those that occur during frying or grilling of food. The following compounds are examples of toxic products that may be formed.

3-MONOCHLOROPROPANE-1,3-DIOL (3-MCPD)

3-Monochloropropane-1,3-diol (3-MCPD) (see Fig. *evolve* 2.12 🖱) is an example of a chemical that may form in foods by the reaction of chloride with lipids. It has been shown to be a carcinogen by laboratory animal studies. 3-MCPD can be formed as a result of industrial processing of foods such as hydrolysed vegetable protein or soy sauce but it may also form during domestic cooking of foods or it may transfer into foods from packaging material. The European Commission's Scientific Committee on Food (SCF) has proposed a tolerable daily intake of 2 mg/kg body weight.

ACRYLAMIDE (2-PROPENAMIDE)

Acrylamide (2-propenamide) (see Fig. *evolve* 2.13 🖱) is found in fried and baked goods at levels up to 3 mg/kg. Highest levels are found in crisps, crispbread, chips and fried potatoes. The WHO classifies acrylamide as a probable human carcinogen based on experiments on laboratory animals and effects on humans exposed to high levels through industrial exposure. However, there is a lack of scientific information about the nature and extent of uptake from foods, and it is not known whether there is a relationship between the consumption of acrylamide in foods and cancer in humans. The Maillard reaction between the amino acid asparagine, which occurs in potatoes and cereals, and glucose is thought to be an important route for the formation of acrylamide.

POLYCYCLIC AROMATIC HYDROCARBONS (PAHS)

Polycyclic aromatic hydrocarbons (PAHs) are a group of about 250 related compounds that are present in wood smoke and are detected at low levels in charred meat and in foods exposed to smoke. PAHs are chemically very stable and they are widespread in the environment, since they do not degrade easily. Consequently, a variety of food products that are not smoked, including vegetable oils and fish, contain detectable levels of PAHs. Many PAHs are carcinogenic to animals, and carcinogenic effects have been demonstrated in humans following occupational exposure to high levels of PAHs. Benzo(a)pyrene (BaP), benz(a)anthracene (BaA) and dibenz(ah)anthracene (DBahA) are PAHs about which there is most concern as potential carcinogens. Research by the Food Standards Agency showed that the average dietary intake of BaP, BaA and DBahA in the UK was less than 3 ng/kg body weight per day in 2000, and this was 2–5 times less than in 1979.

KEY POINTS

- Foods are processed either to improve their palatability or to extend their shelf life, especially by the destruction of microorganisms.
- Food processing operations applied to foods include baking, frying, grilling, boiling, microwave cooking, canning, pasteurisation, irradiation, freeze-drying, drying and high pressure processing.
- Losses of water-soluble vitamins may occur by leaching into processing water. Vitamins may also be lost by reaction with oxygen or by thermal degradation. Vitamin C and thiamin are particularly susceptible to degradation.
- Frying or grilling of foods may lead to the formation of toxic components in some products.
- Temperatures below 6°C prevent the growth of microorganisms.
- Food additives include preservatives, processing aids, flavours, colours, sweeteners.

2.5 NATURAL FOOD TOXINS

Many natural substances are harmful to health when consumed in foods at a sufficient dose. For example, fat-soluble vitamins cause toxic effects when excessive amounts are consumed, and at a high level of intake these can be fatal. However, toxins are substances that cause harmful effects when foods are consumed at levels comparable to those which may be eaten by consumers. These may be natural products that accumulate in foods during processing or storage or they may be introduced into plants or animals that are subsequently consumed as foods. Some toxins, e.g.

polychlorinated biphenyls, are cumulative but other toxins, e.g. glycoalkaloids, are completely harmless when consumed repeatedly at sub-toxic doses. Food components may cause toxic effects within hours, days or weeks of consumption of the food or they may have mutagenic or carcinogenic effects in which an inheritable change in the genetic information of a cell may lead to cancer or other disease states over a period of years. When there is evidence from animal experiments that food components are toxic, regulatory authorities normally allow the components to be present in foods when the maximum amount consumed is 100 times less than the minimum amount shown to have an adverse effect in animals with due allowance for the body weight of the animal. Close monitoring of foods by government agencies helps to prevent chemical toxins reaching levels at which harmful effects occur, and pathogenic bacteria are much more common causes of human disease than chemical toxins.

NATURAL PLANT TOXINS

Glycoalkaloids

Solanine is the main glycoalkaloid, which commonly occurs with other glycoalkaloids including chaconine at low levels in potatoes. However, high levels of solanine may be found in green potatoes, since conditions which lead to an increase in chlorophyll content also cause increases in solanine levels (see Fig. *evolve* 2.14 🖱).

Glycoalkaloid levels of over 200 mg/kg fresh weight may lead to harmful effects. Solanine acts by inhibiting the enzyme cholinesterase, which catalyses hydrolysis of acetylcholine to acetate and choline. The action of this enzyme is essential for the repolarisation of neurons following transmission of a nerve impulse. Increased gastric pain followed by nausea, vomiting and respiration difficulties, which may cause death, have been reported in individuals following consumption of potatoes with high levels of glycoalkaloids. Cholinesterase activity recovers within a few hours following ingestion of low doses of glycoalkaloids, so there are no ill-effects from repeat ingestion of small doses.

Lathyrus

Lathyrism is a disease caused by consumption of vetch peas, chickpeas, or garbanzos, which have the systematic name *Lathyrus sativus*. The illness occurs in two forms, which are osteolathyrism and neurolathyrism. Osteolathyrism is characterised by skeletal deformities and weakness in aortic and connective tissue. The toxic constituent of *L. sativus*, which causes osteolathyrism, is β-L-glutamylaminopropionitrile, which inhibits cross-linking of collagen, thereby affecting the structure of connective tissue and bone. Osteolathyrism mainly occurs in animals, but the second form of lathyrism, neurolathyrism, affects humans, especially young men, following long-term consumption of the peas. Neurolathyrism involves damage to the central nervous system, which causes paralysis of the legs, with general weakness and muscle rigidity developing. The disease mainly occurs in some areas of India, where *L. sativus* grows despite its cultivation being banned. The toxic component is β-N-oxalyl-L-a,b-diaminopropionic acid (see Fig. *evolve* 2.15 🖱).

MARINE TOXINS

The neurotoxin tetrodotoxin (see Fig. *evolve* 2.16 🖱) occurs in some organs of the puffer fish, which is a culinary delicacy in Japan. Great skill is required by the chef to separate the muscles and testes, which are free of the toxin, from the liver, ovaries, skin and intestines. Tetrodotoxin is fatal above a dose of 1.5–4.0 mg, whereas the concentration may exceed 30 mg/100 g in the liver and ovaries. The toxin blocks movement of sodium ions across the membranes of nerve fibres, inhibiting transmission of nerve impulses, which causes distressing symptoms that develop into total paralysis and respiratory failure causing death within 6–24 hours. There is no known antidote to the poison, and fatalities continue to occur regularly. Japanese regulatory authorities require chefs to be licensed for cooking the puffer fish, and this has helped to reduce the number of fatalities in recent years.

Paralytic shellfish poisoning is caused by consumption of shellfish such as clams or mussels that have fed on dinoflagellate algae, which reach high concentrations in red tides that develop in seawater. The algal bloom is common in coastal waters close to Europe, North America, Japan and South Africa. The algae, especially *Gonylaux* sp., produce a toxin, saxitoxin (see Fig. *evolve* 2.17 🖱), that accumulates in the flesh of the shellfish. Most shellfish break down or excrete the toxin within 3 weeks after ingestion ceases, but some species of clams may retain the toxin for several months. Saxitoxin is considered to be fatal at a dose of about 4 mg, with symptoms including numbness of lips, hands and feet that develop into vomiting, coma and death. A dose of 1 mg causes mild intoxication.

FUNGAL TOXINS

Mycotoxins

Many species of fungi produce metabolites that are toxic. Mycotoxins are produced by filamentous fungi. Epidemics due to the consumption of rye that had been stored in damp conditions were common in the Middle Ages. The grain was contaminated by the fungus *Claviceps purpurea*, known as ergot, and ergot poisoning was manifested either as gangrenous or convulsive ergotism. Gangrenous ergotism caused severe pain, inflammation and blackening of limbs, and loss of toes and fingers. Convulsive ergotism caused numbness, blindness, paralysis and convulsions.

The main pharmacologically active compounds in ergot are a series of alkaloid derivatives of lysergic acid (see Fig. *evolve* 2.18). The most important alkaloids are ergotamine, ergonovine and ergotoxin. Some of these alkaloids have found applications in medicine for treatment of migraine.

Greater care over the harvesting and storage of grain has reduced the occurrence of ergot in grain very considerably, but a restricted outbreak occurred in France as recently as 1951. However, concern over the presence of mycotoxins in mouldy food has developed since the 1960s, when it was found that metabolites produced by the fungus *Aspergillus flavus* (aflatoxins) were toxic to animals. Aflatoxins occur in mouldy grain, soya beans or nuts and are carcinogenic at very low levels of intake. Toxin-producing fungi usually produce only two or three aflatoxins under a given set of conditions, but fourteen chemically related toxins have been identified. Aflatoxins are a series of bis-furan polycyclic compounds, which vary in the structure of at least one ring or substituent.

Aflatoxin B_1 is one of the most potent chemical carcinogens known (see Fig. *evolve* 2.19). A high incidence of liver cancer is induced in rats by feeding diets containing 15 mg/kg aflatoxin B_1. There have been many reports of animals suffering from toxic effects following the consumption of mouldy feeds. In 1960, over 100000 turkeys died in England with extensive necrosis of the liver after consuming mouldy feed. Cattle consuming feed contaminated by aflatoxins excrete milk containing aflatoxin M_1. Aflatoxins may also be transmitted to humans via animals in meat or eggs. When food has been contaminated with mycotoxins, the toxins remain in the food even after the mould has been removed or has died. Aflatoxins and many other mycotoxins are quite stable during normal food processing operations.

Most toxins from other fungi are much less potent than the aflatoxins. Some mushrooms are toxic but sometimes they can be rendered edible by cooking, and only a few species are lethal if consumed. *Amanita muscaria* is a fleshy fungus that grows widely in temperate areas of the world. It causes hallucinogenic effects, and has commonly been used as a narcotic or intoxicant. The compounds responsible for the toxic effects are a series of isoxazoles, including muscimol.

POLLUTANTS (for extended version see Section *evolve* 2.5 'pollutants')

Pesticides are used to control weeds or insects that would otherwise reduce crop production or cause post-harvest losses. Several hundred pesticides, which correspond to several chemical classes, are used in agriculture. The use of pesticides has made a major contribution to food production and preservation. Pesticides are designed to kill or adversely affect living organisms, and consequently there is in principle a risk to health. Maximum residue levels of many pesticides in foods such as fruit, vegetables and other plant and animal products are specified in the legal regulations.

Antibiotics

Antibiotics used to treat animals may remain as residues in meat. There is concern that this may lead to the development of antibiotic resistance in humans, although it is only one of the mechanisms for the development of antibiotic-resistant organisms in humans.

Hormones

Hormones are used in the rearing of animals in some countries because they act as active growth promoters. Although a total ban exists on the use of hormones in raising cattle in the EU, a black market exists and there is evidence that between 35 and 55 illegal hormones are used in the EU. The levels of hormone residues found in beef are below the Maximum Residue Limit set by the FAO/WHO Expert Committee of Food Additives.

Heavy metals

Heavy metals have received attention as widespread environmental contaminants and as accidental food contaminants. They enter the environment as a consequence of industrial pollution and they enter the food chain in various ways. The two metals of main concern are mercury and cadmium.

Polychlorinated and polybrominated biphenyls (PCBs and PBBs)

PCBs and PBBs are mixtures of inert molecules, which have been used as electrical insulators and fire retardants. They are resistant to chemical and biological breakdown and as a consequence of their stability, they have become widespread environmental contaminants, which are a potential hazard to human health. PCBs are frequently found at mg/kg levels in fish, poultry, milk and eggs.

Radioactive fallout

Radioactive isotopes, or radionuclides, are atoms that are unstable and emit energy as radiation when they decay to more stable atoms. Some radionuclides such as carbon-14, uranium-238 and radon-222 occur naturally in the environment due to the effects of cosmic radiation or due to their creation in prehistoric times. However, fallout from nuclear power stations and the use of radioactive materials in industry, medicine and research have led to increases in the levels of radionuclides in the environment. When living tissue is exposed to ionising radiation it will absorb some of the radiation's energy and may become damaged, with the development of cancer.

PATHOGENIC AGENTS

Pathogenic agents are a very common cause of food poisoning. Organisms may be associated with endogenous animal infections transmissible to humans (zoonoses) by consumption of meat or fish. This group includes bacterial, viral, fungal, helminthic and protozoan species. The second group of organisms are species that are exogenous contaminants of food, which may cause infections in humans. This group includes common food poisoning organisms such as *Salmonella*, *Staphylococcus* and *Clostridium botulinum*.

Seafood poisoning

Bacterial decomposition of fish that is stored at unacceptably high temperatures or for excessive time is the main cause of seafood poisoning. Seafood poisoning is often called scombroid poisoning because fish of the *Scombroidea* species including mackerel and tuna are widely consumed. However, fish from other species including sardines and herring may also cause outbreaks. Consumption of contaminated fish may cause symptoms to appear within about 2 hours of the fish being eaten. The main symptoms include pain, vomiting and diarrhoea. Seafood poisoning has been attributed to the formation of histamine by bacterial decomposition of the amino acid histidine in fish. However, pure histamine has low oral toxicity, and it appears that other components in the fish such as putrescine and cadaverine are important in allowing the toxicity of histamine to be manifested.

Food poisoning organisms

Salmonella

Salmonella is one of the most common intestinal infections in the UK. In recent years, there have been about 30000 reported cases per year. The most common organism involved is *S. enteritidis* followed by *S. typhimurium* but the known number of strains of the bacterium is over 2300. Eggs are the most common vehicle for the transmission of salmonellosis. The common contamination of eggs is due to the fact that hens lay eggs through a passageway called the vent, which is an exit shared by their intestines, where *Salmonella* is commonly present. Other foods of animal origin including unpasteurised milk, poultry and cheese are also possible sources. The organism is readily inactivated by cooking, but cross-contamination of cooked food by uncooked food is a common pathway for contamination of food in domestic kitchens. Symptoms normally follow ingestion of contaminated food within 6–48 hours. *Salmonella* causes diarrhoea, often with fever and abdominal cramps. The onset may be sudden and there may be nausea and vomiting initially.

Campylobacters

Campylobacters are the leading cause of bacterial diarrhoea in humans. Campylobacteriosis commonly affects babies and young children. The WHO estimates that 1% of the population of western Europe is infected by *Campylobacter* spp. each year. The illness is a gastrointestinal infection caused by *C. jejuni* or *C. coli*. Symptoms may show themselves as bloody diarrhoea, fever, nausea and abdominal cramps. The illness normally lasts 2–10 days but some symptoms may persist for several months. The disease is usually self-limiting, so antibiotic treatment is not normally required except in serious cases. Campylobacters occur widely in the intestinal tract of many animals, especially chickens and turkeys. During slaughtering and preparation of raw bird, a large number of birds may become contaminated, and therefore undercooked poultry meat and offal are a major source of infection. Raw milk and poorly treated water supplies are also causes of campylobacter infections.

Verocytotoxin–producing *Escherichia coli*

Verocytotoxin-producing *Escherichia coli* is an uncommon but important pathogen because serious infections particularly in children may result. The illness was first recognised in the early 1980s. Infection may produce mild diarrhoea or a severe or fatal illness. Cattle are the main source of infection, with most cases being associated with the consumption of undercooked beef burgers and similar meat or raw milk. The infective dose appears to be very low, probably less than 10 cells. A temperature of 70°C for 2 minutes is sufficient to destroy the organism in meat.

Listeria monocytogenes

Listeria monocytogenes is a potentially dangerous foodborne pathogen. The bacterium occurs in cheese. Hard cheeses do not support the multiplication of the bacterium and numbers less than 20/g do not present a hazard to health in hard cheese. However, the bacterium can multiply in soft cheeses at refrigeration temperatures, and the occurrence of the bacterium in cheese should be minimised by the use of Hazard Analysis Critical Control Point (HACCP) systems throughout the whole food chain. *L. monocytogenes* causes very serious illness including meningitis and septicaemia. The mortality rate can be as high as 30%, with pregnant women, infants, the elderly and people who are immune suppressed being most vulnerable.

Clostridium welchii

Clostridium welchii is a common source of food poisoning, normally from meat that has been cooked and then stored at insufficiently low temperatures. The organism is anaerobic and spores that survive cooking may develop vegetative forms that multiply in the gut and produce an enterotoxin. Symptoms, which include diarrhoea and abdominal pain, normally occur within 8 to 24 hours following consumption of the food.

Staphylococcus aureus

Staphylococcus aureus is a potentially pathogenic organism that is carried by large numbers of the population. Foods may be contaminated by carriers, and ingestion of contaminated food may be followed within 2–4 hours by vomiting and diarrhoea, which may be severe and may lead to collapse due to dehydration.

Clostridium botulinum

Clostridium botulinum is an organism found in soils, which may contaminate canned meats and meat pastes. The organism forms heat-resistant spores, which may develop vegetative forms anaerobically if not inactivated by heat. The vegetative forms of the organism produce a toxin that is extremely potent at very low levels. Difficulty in swallowing may develop into paralysis and death. Cases of botulism are rare, since the food industry uses nitrites to prevent anaerobic growth in processed meats.

VIRAL INFECTIONS

Viruses have no cellular structure and possess only one type of nucleic acid (either RNA or DNA) wrapped in a protein coat. Consequently they cannot multiply in foods, but food handlers with dirty hands or dirty utensils may allow foods to become contaminated by viruses, which can subsequently multiply in the intestinal tract by using the host cells' mechanism for replication. Viral infections often have much longer incubation periods of up to several weeks compared to several hours for bacterial infections.

Hepatitis A is a member of the genus *Enterovirus*, which causes symptoms of anorexia, fever, malaise, nausea and vomiting followed after a few days by symptoms of liver damage. Exposure to the virus is limited in the developed world due to good public hygiene and sanitation. In Delhi in 1955–6, 36 000 cases occurred in a waterborne epidemic of infectious hepatitis after the main water supply had been contaminated with sewage due to flooding. However, smaller numbers of cases have been caused by infected foods such as shellfish or fruit or by infected food handlers.

Poliomyelitis is another enterovirus that can be transmitted by contaminated food such as milk. However, it is now virtually eradicated in developed countries. Norwalk-like viruses, which have not been fully characterised, may cause gastroenteritis with an incubation period of 15–50 hours followed by diarrhoea and vomiting.

PRIONS

A prion protein is a small protein molecule that occurs mainly in the brain cell membrane. It differs in conformation from most proteins since it occurs mainly in a β-sheet flattened form, which is heat resistant and protease resistant. Prions are believed to be the infectious agent causing humans to develop new variant Creutzfeldt–Jakob disease (vCJD). Cases of this disease were first reported in the early 1990s. Although CJD had been known as a rare disease that occurred worldwide since the 1920s, vCJD affected younger people than the earlier form, and there were unusual clinical features. This disease is believed to have developed in humans following consumption of meat from cattle affected by BSE (bovine spongiform encephalopathy), which is a fatal brain disease that affected large numbers of cattle in the UK in the 1980s and 1990s. The disease in cattle was reduced after 1993 by the removal of meat and bonemeal from cattle feed concentrates and by the slaughter of large numbers of animals. vCJD presents as psychiatric disorders including anxiety, depression and withdrawal but it develops over a period of months into forgetfulness and memory disturbance. A cerebellar syndrome develops with gait and limb ataxia and eventually death. The annual number of deaths identified as being due to vCJD in the UK reached 28 in the year 2000, but small reductions in the annual number of deaths have been recorded since that year.

HELMINTHS AND NEMATODES

Helminths and nematodes are flatworms and roundworms which develop as parasites in humans following the consumption of contaminated water or food, especially meat or raw salads. Liver flukes, *Fasciola hepatica*, and tapeworms of the genus *Taenia* are the most common helminths. The liver fluke develops as a leaf-like animal in humans, sheep or cattle. It grows up to 2.5 cm long by 1 cm wide and establishes itself in the bile duct after entering and feeding on the liver. When mature the liver fluke produces eggs, which are excreted in the faeces. Symptoms include fever, tiredness and loss of appetite with pain and discomfort in the liver region of the abdomen.

Tapeworms include *Taenia solium*, which occurs in pork, and *T. saginata*, which is associated with beef. The mature tapeworm develops in the human intestine, and may cause severe symptoms in the young and in individuals weakened by other diseases. Effects may include nausea, abdominal pain, gut irritation, anaemia and a nervous disorder resembling epilepsy. If gut damage allows eggs to be released in the stomach, the resulting bladder worms may invade the central nervous system with fatal consequences.

Trichinella spiralis is a nematode (roundworm) that causes trichinosis in humans with symptoms of discomfort, fever and even death. Consumption of raw or poorly cooked infected pork products is the normal source of foodborne illness.

KEY POINTS

- Natural plant toxins, marine toxins, fungal toxins and pollutants may contaminate food, but they rarely occur at levels which are harmful to health in foods sold in western Europe.
- Growth of pathogenic organisms including bacteria, yeasts and moulds may cause food poisoning.
- Processing of foods, e.g. heat treatment under selected conditions, reduces the levels of many pathogenic organisms, so that the foods may be consumed safely. Cross-contamination of cooked products by unprocessed products during domestic storage, or storage at higher temperatures or for longer times than recommended by manufacturers, are common causes of food poisoning incidents.
- Under certain conditions, processing of foods may cause the formation of potentially toxic compounds, although effects in humans have rarely been demonstrated.

2.6 PHYTOPROTECTANTS

There is strong evidence that a diet rich in fruits and vegetables can reduce heart disease and probably some cancers in the human population. However, identification of the individual components of the diet which may confer this protection is still a matter of intense study. Plants and plant extracts have been used for centuries in the treatment of chronic ailments. Foods and herbs to which the highest anticancer activity has been assigned include garlic, soya beans, cabbage, ginger, liquorice and the umbelliferous vegetables (carrots, celery, parsley and parsnips). Onions, flax, citrus, turmeric, cruciferous vegetables (broccoli, Brussels sprouts, cabbage and cauliflower), solanaceous vegetables (tomatoes and peppers), brown rice and whole wheat possess moderate levels of anticancer activity (Steinmetz & Potter 1991). Research has identified an array of phytochemicals including organosulphur compounds, carotenoids, terpenes and polyphenols including flavonoids and phytoestrogens that have been shown to produce beneficial physiological effects.

Phytoprotectants may inhibit tumour development by scavenging chemical carcinogens to prevent them binding to electron-rich sources in the cell including DNA, RNA and proteins. They may also act by their effect on phase I enzymes involved in activation of environmental and chemical carcinogens or phase II enzymes involved in detoxification pathways.

Organosulphur Compounds

Organosulphur compounds present in garlic represent some of the more efficient phase I and II enzyme modulators. Diallyl sulphide (DAS), diallyl disulphide (DADS), triallyl sulphide and diallyl polysulphides are lipid-soluble components in garlic, and S-allylcysteine (SAC) and S-allylmercaptocysteine (SAMC) are among the water-soluble components that are considered important. DAS and DADS from garlic, and isothiocyanates, which occur in cabbage, broccoli and cauliflower, have been shown to inhibit chemically induced cancers in animals. Sulforaphane, an isothiocyanate found in broccoli, is a potent inducer of phase II enzymes.

Carotenoids

Carotenoids (see Fig. *evolve* 2.22 🖱) are a class of structurally related compounds, which are strongly coloured red or orange, and which are found in foods that are coloured red, orange or green including tomatoes, carrots and spinach. Carotenoids comprise molecules with hydrocarbon structures including α-, β-, and γ-carotene and lycopene as well as molecules with one or more polar substituents attached to the hydrocarbon backbone including astaxanthin, zeaxanthin, lutein and β-cryptoxanthin. Some of the most common carotenoids act as provitamin A, being converted to vitamin A by β-carotene-15, 15′-oxygenase in the intestinal mucosa. Provitamin A activity is restricted to carotenoids such as β-carotene in which at least half of the molecule shares the ring and chain structure of vitamin A. The role of carotenoids in cancer prevention is uncertain (see Section 11.1, under 'Vitamin A and carotene in cancer prevention').

Carotenoids also have antioxidant properties and may contribute to a reduced risk of coronary heart disease by protecting low density lipoproteins against oxidation. Lycopene does not have provitamin A activity but it has been the subject of much research because it may provide some protection against prostate cancer in men. Processed tomato products are a good source of lycopene.

Polyphenols

Polyphenols are defined as classes of plant components, the structure of which includes more than one aromatic ring and several phenolic hydroxyl groups. The term was originally restricted to vegetable tannins, which are water-soluble compounds having molecular weights between 500 and 3000, and which have the ability to precipitate proteins. The theaflavins and thearubigins, which contribute the colour to black tea, are examples of tannins. In recent years, the use of the term polyphenols has been extended to include lower molecular weight compounds containing at least one aromatic ring and one or more hydroxyl groups. Flavonoids comprise the most important group of low molecular weight polyphenols.

Flavonoids

Flavonoids are phenolic compounds that occur widely in plant tissues, mainly as glycosides. All flavonoids have a C_6–C_3–C_6 structure in which a six-carbon aromatic ring is linked by a three-carbon bridging unit to a second aromatic ring (see Fig. *evolve* 2.23). The nature of the central C_3 unit defines the class of flavonoid. The classes include: the anthocyanins, which contribute the red, purple or black colours to fruits such as strawberries, plums and blackcurrants; the flavonols, which occur widely in vegetables including onions, broccoli and beans; flavanols, which occur in green tea; flavones, which often accompany flavonols; and proanthocyanidins, which occur in cocoa, cider and wine.

The position of the benzenoid substituent on the C-ring divides the flavonoid class into flavonoids (2-position) and isoflavonoids (3-position). Isoflavones in soya products are of current nutritional interest because of their oestrogenic structure (see Fig. *evolve* 2.23). Other flavonoids are of interest as bioactive dietary components because of effects on cell-signalling, cognitive function or other effects. They also have antioxidant properties.

PHYTOESTROGENS

Phytoestrogens include any plant substance or metabolite that induces biological responses in vertebrates and can mimic or modulate the actions of endogenous oestrogens, usually by binding to oestrogen receptors (UK Food Standards Agency Committee on Toxicity 2002). Most of the work investigating the properties of phytoestrogens has been on isoflavones, with a little work on prenylated flavonoids, coumestrol or lignans. Phytoestrogens mimic or block the action of the human hormone oestrogen, although they are much less potent. They are of interest because they may have benefits for prevention of certain cancers, as well as heart disease and osteoporosis in postmenopausal women. However, there are possible links to fertility problems in animals, which raises concerns that similar effects could occur in humans, particularly babies fed soya-based infant formulas.

Isoflavones are present in several legumes but soya beans are the primary human dietary source. The three main isoflavones are genistein, daidzein and glycitein, which are mainly present as the glycosides genistin, daidzin and glycitin. Isoflavones also occur as malonyl or acetyl esters but these derivatives are commonly hydrolysed during the processing of soya products such as tofu (Song et al 1998).

Metabolites of isoflavones such as equol, a bioactive metabolite of daidzcin, and glucuronide and sulphate conjugates are formed by metabolism in the intestine and the liver.

KEY POINTS

- Phytoprotectants include organosulphur compounds, flavonoids, carotenoids and phytoestrogens.
- Phytoprotectants may be important in contributing to a reduction in cardiovascular disease or cancer by various mechanisms. These include inhibition of cancer by their effect on phase I enzymes that are involved in activation of environmental and chemical carcinogens or phase II enzymes that are involved in detoxification pathways.

References

Al-Khalifa AS, Dawood AA: Effects of cooking methods on thiamine and riboflavin contents of chicken meat, *Food Chemistry* 48(1):69–74, 1993.

Ang CYW, Livingstone GE: Nutritive losses in the home storage and preparation of raw fruits and vegetables. In White PL, Selvey N, editors: *Nutritional qualities of fresh fruit and vegetables,* Mount Kisco, 1974, Futura Publishing, pp 121–132

Davey MW, Van Montague M, Inze D, et al: Plant L-ascorbic acid chemistry, metabolism, bioavailability and effects of processing, *Journal of the Science of Food and Agriculture* 80:825–860, 2000.

Favell DJ: A comparison of the vitamin C content of fresh and frozen vegetables, *Food Chemistry* 62:59–64, 1998.

Gerber N, Scheeder MRL, Wenk C: The influence of cooking and fat trimming on the actual nutrient intake from meat, *Meat Science* 81:148–154, 2009.

Han JS, Kozukue N, Young K-S, et al: Distribution of ascorbic acid in potato tubers and in home processed and commercial potato foods, *Journal of Agricultural and Food Chemistry* 52:6516–6521, 2004.

Orzaez-Villanueva, et al: Modification of vitamins B1 and B2 by culinary processes, *Food Chemistry* 71(1):417–421, 2000.

Rumm-Kreuter D, Demmel I: Comparison of vitamin losses in vegetables due to various cooking methods, *Journal of*

Nutrition Science and Vitaminology 36:S7–S15, 1990.

Song T, Barua K, Buseman G, Murphy P: Soy isoflavone analysis, *American Journal of Clinical Nutrition* 68:1474S–1479S, 1998.

Steinmetz KA, Potter JD: Vegetables, fruit and cancer I. Epidemiology, *Cancer Causes and Control* 2:325–357, 1991.

UK Food Standards Agency Committee on Toxicity: Draft report

of the COT Working Group on phytoestrogens, October 2002. 2002. Online. Available: http://www.food.gov.uk/multimedia/pdfs/phytoestrogenreport.pdf

Further reading

Ballantine B, Marrs T, Syversen T: *General and applied toxicology*, ed 2, Basingstoke, 2000, Macmillan.

Coultate TP: *Food: The chemistry of its components*, ed 5, London, 2008, RSC.

Deshpande SS: *Handbook of food toxicology*, New York, 2002, Marcel Dekker.

Ryley J, Kajda P: Vitamins in thermal processing, *Food Chemistry* 49:119–129, 1994.

Shahidi F, editor: *Antinutrients and phytochemicals in food*, Washington, 1997, American Chemical Society.

Shibamoto T, Bjeldanes LF: Introduction to food toxicology, San Diego, 1993, Academic Press.

EVOLVE CONTENTS (available online at: evolve.elsevier.com/Geissler/nutrition)

PART 2

Body composition and macronutrient metabolism

Chapter 3

The physiology of nutrient digestion and absorption

George Grimble

CHAPTER CONTENTS

OBJECTIVES

By the end of this chapter you should be able to:
■ explain the most important functions of the various parts of the gastrointestinal tract
■ describe the main actions of digestive enzymes and the neural and hormonal regulators of digestion
■ discuss the main features of absorption and secretion of specific nutrients, water and electrolytes
■ appreciate that luminal factors play a role in the regulation of food intake

3.1 INTRODUCTION

The major components of the diet are starches, sugars, fats and proteins. These have to be hydrolysed to their constituent smaller molecules for absorption and metabolism. Starches and sugars are absorbed as monosaccharides; fats are absorbed as free fatty acids and glycerol (plus a small amount of intact triacylglycerol); proteins are absorbed as their constituent amino acids and small peptides. These are the processes of digestion and absorption that occur in the gastrointestinal tract.

The gastrointestinal tract is 'zoned' not only in terms of anatomy, but also in terms of digestion and absorption, metabolism and neural control. Anatomically, nutrient absorption can be described by reference to its linear distribution along the intestine; specialised compartments with different digestive and absorptive functions follow each other. Digestive and absorptive mechanisms are very effective because many are duplicated. This means

© 2010 Elsevier Ltd/Inc/BV
DOI: 10.1016/B978-0-7020-3118-2.00003-6

that impairment of one process by disease does not necessarily lead to complete malabsorption of a particular nutrient. The digestive and absorptive capacity of the human intestine closely matches the metabolic mass of each individual, just as it matches the metabolic mass of species, from shrew to whale, which have been compared in this way. Clearly, an excessively large intestine would be inefficient because at the extreme, its maintenance cost may exceed the energy value of food ingested.

Conversely, inefficient digestion also carries penalties. The most rapid period of intestinal growth occurs after birth and if part of the intestine of a neonate is removed by surgery because of gastrointestinal disease, some adaptation of remaining digestive and absorptive capacity can occur but it is not great. As a result, intravenous nutrition may become necessary. Animal studies suggest that the excess capacity of the intestine or 'safety margin' (i.e. capacity/dietary load) is approximately 2.

The gastrointestinal tract has a very active maintenance metabolism and meets its energy requirements from substrates in arterial blood and directly from food itself. An eating-related activity such as chewing uses 1–2% of the energy content of food. About one half of dietary protein is utilised to meet the amino acid requirements of the gut but only 10% of dietary glucose is metabolised during passage into the portal circulation. Eating leads to increased blood-flow around the intestine and to increased transmembrane transport of substrates, water and ions, all of which are energy consuming processes.

It has now become clear that intestinal function is modulated by more than 100 gastrointestinal peptide hormones and an enteric nervous system (ENS) that has as many neurons as the spinal cord. Individual neurons are independent of the central nervous system (CNS) but the ENS communicates with the CNS via sympathetic and parasympathetic pathways. This autonomic system controls functions such as contraction, secretion, motility and mucosal immune defences and is influenced by central mechanisms which may set the threshold of autonomic phenomena such as appetite and satiety. To conclude, therefore, the gut is not an inert digestive tube but is a dynamic organ in which, each day, solid foodstuffs of amazing variety perform the trick of disappearing and reappearing as soluble nutrients in the circulation. See also Chapters 23 and 26 and Figure *evolve* 3.1 🔋.

3.2 THE STRUCTURE AND FUNCTION OF THE GASTROINTESTINAL TRACT

The gastrointestinal tract is 7–10 metres long, stretching from mouth to anus and, together with the liver comprises about 3% of adult body-weight. It is divided into zones that accomplish different digestive and absorptive tasks. The first zone, the mouth and pharynx, leads to the oesophagus, a pipe that enters the stomach via the oesophageal sphincter. Exit from the stomach is governed by the pyloric sphincter, which allows food to pass into the small intestine (duodenum, jejunum and ileum). This is 2.8–8.5 metres long and is longer in men than in women, who have lower average metabolic mass. The duodenum (20–30 cm long, 5 cm diameter) leads to the jejunum and ileum, which respectively comprise the upper two-fifths and lower three-fifths of the small bowel. There is no strict anatomical differentiation between these zones but the lumen narrows towards the terminal ileum and this reduction in volume per segment length reflects the decreasing luminal fluid loads along the small bowel. Similarly, the jejunal wall is thicker and villi are longer and this correlates with the amount of substrate absorbed in each region. Some of these regional differences are summarised in Table 3.1. The small intestine, also called small bowel, enters the large bowel via the ileocaecal valve which, like the oesophageal sphincter, prevents back-flow or reflux of luminal contents. Zones within the colon are defined as the caecum, transverse and distal colon which terminates in the rectum and anus (see Figures *evolve* 3.2 A, B & C 🔋).

Chewing reduces the particle size of food and increases the surface area available for digestive enzyme action. In addition, it will release the intracellular contents of meat and plants. Some enzymes are secreted with saliva. The stomach is a muscular sac which not only physically reduces the particle-size of food, but also forms a barrier to ingress of bacteria into the gastrointestinal tract. There is considerable release of enzymes that break down (hydrolyse) lipid and protein. The thin emulsion of food which enters the small bowel from the stomach is neutralised by duodenal bicarbonate secretions and further digested by enzymes secreted by the pancreas. This process is aided by detergent bile salts released by the gall bladder. During passage along the jejunum, a large amount of water (9 litres) is secreted and reabsorbed with the products of

Table 3.1	Regional anatomy of the intestine and sites of nutrient absorption					
REGION	FUNCTIONS PERFORMED	MUCOSAL SURFACE	NUTRIENTS DIGESTED	NUTRIENTS ABSORBED	MAJOR SITE OF ABSORPTION	ELECTROLYTES ABSORBED
Mouth	Grinding food to smaller particle size Moistening food (saliva) Initial digestion by lipase and alpha amylase Initiation of satiety mechanisms	Small folds	Small amount of protein Starch	Small amounts of glucose, peptides and amino acids	No	No
Stomach	Intestinal defence (e.g. acid secretion) Homogenising food to smaller particle size Moistening food (gastric secretions) Further enzyme digestion Gastric emptying meters delivery of nutrients to the small intestine Feedback of satiety messages	Rugae and pits	Protein, lipid	Insignificant amounts	No	No
Small intestine	Completion of digestion by pancreatic enzymes Absorption of digestion products of carbohydrate, protein and fat Absorption of water and electrolytes Absorption of minerals and micronutrients Feedback of satiety messages	Rugae, villi and microvilli	Protein, lipid, carbohydrate	Amino acids, peptides, fatty acids, glucose, fructose, glycerol, galactose and vitamins	Carbohydrate, fat protein, water, electrolytes	Sodium, potassium, calcium, magnesium, chloride, phosphate
Colon	Final salvage of water and electrolytes Mucin breakdown Conversion of bilirubin to urobilinogen Cholesterol catabolism Organic acid production ('acetate buffer')	Rugae and pits	Dietary fibre – digested by bacteria and fermented to short-chain fatty acids	Acetate, propionate and butyrate and dicarboxylic acids	Short-chain fatty acids, water, electrolytes	Magnesium and calcium in form of soaps with fatty acids

luminal and brush-border digestion. Efficient reabsorption means that only 60–120 ml of fluid pass the ileocaecal valve each hour, carrying undigested material into the caecum to be metabolised by the numerous bacteria that have established a stable environment there. Colonic fermentation generates short chain fatty acids (SCFA) that stimulate absorption of salts and water to produce a formed stool which is passed per rectum. It is a sobering thought that the bacteria excreted each day outnumber the cells in the human body.

Figure 3.1 shows the anatomy of the gastrointestinal tract, Table 3.1 and Figure *evolve* 3.2 C 🖱 the main processes that occur in each region.

The intestinal wall also has zoned anatomy (Figure 3.2), the absorptive surface of which is amplified by three structures:

1. Folds or ridges (rugae) in the intestinal wall increase absorptive area.
2. Villi, finger-like projections 0.5–1.0 mm long covered with mucosal absorptive cells

the water-insoluble products of fat digestion and transformation from the enterocytes to the thoracic duct.

Blood is supplied abundantly (500 ml/min) to the intestine by numerous small arteries that branch from the arch of the mesenteric artery. This blood drains, via the portal vein, to the liver, which regulates the supply of nutrients to the periphery through the hepatic vein into the vena cava. Only one-quarter of this blood supplies the submucosa, muscularis and serosa, the remainder goes to the mucosal layer, which has very active metabolism and needs a good oxygen supply, and where absorbed nutrients are quickly diluted out and removed to the portal vein, thus preventing any high osmotic loads developing. In some respects, the intestine behaves like a 'pre-liver' because it:

1. metabolises considerable amounts of dietary glucose and amino acids,
2. transforms and degrades dietary arginine and nucleotides respectively
3. detoxifies drugs and dietary toxins through the action of mucosal cytochrome P-450 enzymes and the UDP glucosyltransferases and sulphotransferases,
4. extrudes toxins through the action of the p-glycoprotein (multi-drug resistance) transporter back into the gut lumen.

The gut is therefore a formidable barrier to dietary carcinogens and the rapid turnover of enterocytes may explain why tumours of the small intestine are much rarer than those in the large bowel.

Alterations in intestinal motility can increase absorptive capacity by increasing the contact time between nutrients and the absorptive mucosal surface. Motility disorders often cause nutrient malabsorption; their importance can be judged from the depth of the muscular zone of the intestine and the size of the enteric nervous system (see Figure 3.2), in which regular nerve plexuses control motility at a local level whilst also responding to signals generated by the presence of luminal nutrients in the lumen.

The intestine also has several lines of defence against ingress of bacteria:

1. The concentration of gastric acid in fasting is about 0.1M HCl (pH 1.0), forming an effective bactericidal barrier.
2. The gastric mucosal surface is very hydrophobic and damaging agents have

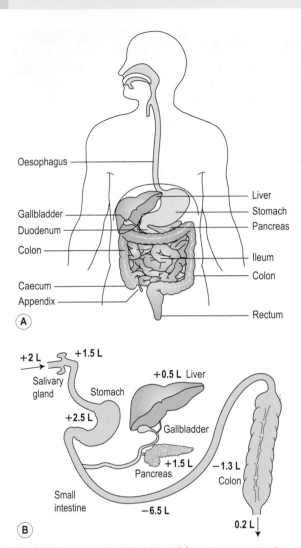

Fig. 3.1 The gastrointestinal tract (a) and movement of fluid through different regions (b). L, litres. *(The daily amounts and sites of fluid secretion and absorption in humans are from the data reported by Ma & Verkman (1999) Journal of Physiology (London) 517: 317–326)*

(enterocytes) further increase the absorptive capacity of mammals with higher continuous metabolic rates.

3. Enterocytes have further finger-like projections on their luminal surface, known as microvilli, and these define the brush-border membrane.

These features increase the absorptive area of the human intestine to 200 m². Each villus is supplied by an arteriole and is drained by a venule and a lacteal. The venules drain into the hepatic portal vein and carry water-soluble nutrients, while the lacteals are part of the lymphatic system and carry

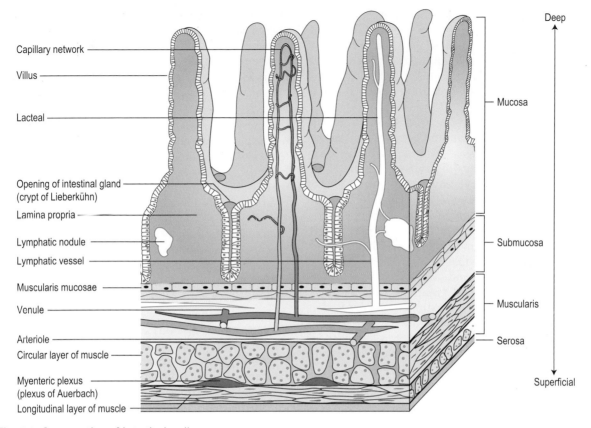

Fig. 3.2 Cross-section of intestinal wall. *(Redrawn with permission from Tortora G, Anagnostakos N P (1990) Principles of anatomy and physiology (figure 24–18, p760) Harper and Row, New York)*

limited ability to wet it and thus cause local injury.

3. Goblet cells secrete an adherent sticky film of mucus that has a low viscosity surface layer. Bacteria will therefore be swept off this fragile outer layer by peristaltic waves in the gut. The mucus layer is thickest in the stomach and colon, which have highest luminal concentrations of bacteria.

4. About one-third of cells in the intestine comprise the gut-associated lymphatic tissue (GALT), which secretes IgA into the gut lumen.

3.3 PROCESSES OF DIGESTION

DIGESTIVE PROCESSES IN THE MOUTH

Chewing both grinds the food and also mixes it with saliva, which contains α-amylase and proteolytic enzymes that initiate digestion of dietary starch and protein and hence development of taste during chewing. In addition, these enzymes maintain periodontal health.

Salivary amylase, for example, binds to specific oral streptococci that maintain the microbial ecology of the mouth and also binds to tooth enamel, thus controlling attachment of bacteria. Furthermore, saliva not only lubricates food and aids in formation of the bolus to be swallowed, but also protects the mucosal surface of the pharynx and oesophagus. Bicarbonate in saliva neutralises acid that refluxes back up the oesophagus (a surprisingly common event) and thus protects the oesophageal mucosa, the growth of which is stimulated by salivary epidermal growth factor (EGF). Lipid digestion also begins in the mouth, initiated by lipase secreted by the tongue (lingual lipase).

The efficiency of chewing varies through the lifecycle. Infants can efficiently eat only milk and puréed food before they develop teeth, and up to three quarters of the elderly population in UK have few teeth because of a lifetime of dental neglect or periodontal disease. The link between tooth loss in the elderly and poor nutrition is complex. Fitting dentures does not always improve nutritional status because dentures require a symmetrical bite if they are not to become displaced and not all people can achieve this because the normal bite is often asymmetrical.

Swallowing transfers a food bolus from the mouth to the oesophagus, and involves contraction and relaxation of at least 14 groups of muscles in about 10 seconds in healthy subjects (Figure *evolve* 3.3). A 'normal' swallow is present in 80% of young people but in only 16% of those over 70 years old. Whilst an abnormal swallow does not necessarily predispose to swallowing problems (i.e. adaptation has occurred), these nevertheless affect 30–60% of elderly people in care. The swallowing complex is initiated and distributed by neurons within the dorsal and ventrolateral medullas, respectively and may be impaired by stroke. Recovery of adequate swallowing after a stroke (and tube-feeding if swallowing is not re-established) remains a major nutritional challenge in care of elderly people (see Chapter 16).

DIGESTIVE PROCESSES IN THE STOMACH

Control of gastric secretion

The gastric lumen is an environment hostile to the mucosal surface; gastric juice is chemically very corrosive (typically pH 1.0), containing aggressive proteolytic enzymes, the action of which is regularly augmented with hot foods, detergent bile reflux or alcohol. The first line of defence against attack is the gastric mucus, which is multi-layered. The gastric glands secrete acid through narrow channels in mucus (5–7 μm wide) that guide acid into the gastric lumen and protect the mucosal cells. The total thickness of mucus varies throughout the length of the gastrointestinal tract (Figure *evolve* 3.4) but in the stomach it is nearly 0.3 mm thick and is half firmly and half loosely adherent (Atuma et al 2001).

The surface of the mucosa is covered with gastric pits or crypts that are lined with four types of cells.

1. G Cells secrete the hormone gastrin (which stimulates acid secretion).
2. Parietal cells secrete hydrochloric acid
3. Chief cells secrete pepsinogen, the inactive precursor of pepsin

4. Mucous cells secrete the glycoprotein mucin the composition and mechanical properties of which vary with site. These cells are found at the neck of the pit.

The bulk of the gastric contents is typically at pH 3.0 increasing progressively to 5.0 within the strongly adherent mucus layer. At the outlet to the gastric crypt, pH falls to 4.6 and then to pH 3.0 at the base of the crypt. By contrast, the intracellular pH of cells lining the crypt is neutral or slightly alkaline in the deepest parietal cells. This pH gradient is maintained by the directional secretion of H^+ into the gastric lumen and formation of $HCO3^-$ which neutralises acid and so protects mucosal cells. Parietal cells carry receptors for three agents that stimulate acid secretion: acetylcholine, gastrin and histamine.

Following a meal, gastric secretory activity follows three well-defined phases:

1. The 'cephalic phase' of eating (sight, aroma and anticipation of food) stimulates the parasympathetic intestinal nervous system via the vagus nerve, with acetylcholine release near parietal- and G-cells leading to acid and gastrin secretion.
2. The 'gastric phase' is defined by increased acid and pepsinogen secretion in response to stretching of mechanoreceptors by food ingestion. This stimulates gastrin release which increases secretions.
3. The 'intestinal phase' occurs towards the end of liquidisation of food in the stomach.

Receptors in other parts of the intestine inhibit gastric emptying through neural and hormonal pathways. This is known as the 'pyloric brake'. Each of these phases has a counterpart that controls appetite and eating behaviour (see 'Control of the rate of gastric emptying', below).

Digestive properties of gastric juice

Both dietary lipid (triacylglycerol) and protein are hydrolysed by enzymes secreted in the gastric juice; salivary amylase action continues in the centre of the food bolus until mixing with gastric acid causes its pH to fall low enough to inactivate amylase. During passage from plate to stomach, food lipid will have been reduced to an emulsion of droplets 10–100 μm in size. Gastric lipase, secreted by the gastric mucosa, has little activity at low concentrations of lipid substrate concentration. Its activity increases dramatically when the triacylglycerol concentration is high enough to form a reverse emulsion of lipid in water micelles. Gastric lipase binds to the surface of the micelle and will hydrolyse triacylglycerol to release free fatty acids that generate osmotic pressure within the micelle and lead to budding of new, smaller micelles. Even though only 10–30% of dietary triacylglycerol is hydrolysed by gastric lipase, this is sufficient to emulsify dietary fat very considerably (Figure *evolve* 3.5 🐭). The process is self-limiting as these fatty acid-rich buds inhibit surface-bound lipase. Proteins are relatively resistant to enzymic hydrolysis until their structure has been denatured by heat (e.g. in cooking) or extreme pH. Gastric acid achieves considerable denaturation of many dietary proteins, but some resist digestion in the stomach. Up to 75% of ingested lactoferrin, an iron-binding transferrin-like protein in human milk, survives passage through the stomach intact.

Pepsins which initiate the process of protein digestion are secreted as pepsinogens: inactive precursors or zymogens. Pepsinogen is inactive because it contains a peptide sequence that blocks the active site. At low pH, this peptide unwinds and is cleaved off by the active site of the enzyme itself, thus resulting in active pepsin which may then activate other pepsinogens.

There are eight pepsins, which can be assigned to four families; pepsin A, pepsin B, pepsin C (or gastricsin) and chymosin (which is expressed in the neonate but not the adult). The active site of the enzymes is a deep cleft that can accommodate at least seven amino acid residues of the substrate protein. Hydrolysis occurs mainly, but not exclusively, at the carboxyl side of the aromatic amino acids, tyrosine, phenylalanine and tryptophan, resulting in formation of (relatively large) soluble oligopeptides and some free amino acids. Free amino acids in the gastric lumen activate a receptor that leads to further stimulation of gastrin secretion, so dietary protein stimulates gastric secretion.

Pepsins are activated by acid and have an acid pH optimum but do not necessarily operate at acid pH. Meal-induced acid secretion is rapidly buffered by food so that the pH of the bulk-phase of the stomach lumen rises from pH 1.5 to pH 4.5 within 15 minutes of the end of a meal. Secreted zymogens are activated at the sub-mucosal layer by gastric acid secretion whereas hydrolysis of bulk phase dietary proteins, which have been acid denatured by contact with the mucosal surface, occurs at a relatively high luminal pH.

Control of the rate of gastric emptying

Gastric emptying matches not only the amount of food eaten during a meal, but also nutrients present in the food and the progress made in liquidising it within the stomach. Simple fluids like water will empty at a rate proportional to gastric volume, whereas nutrients will empty at a rate that depends on their energy density and potency in altering the duodenal brake.

Furthermore, fat that reaches the ileum exerts a profound inhibitory effect on gastric motility, known as the 'ileal brake'. After a meal, the two parts of the stomach show different motility responses:

1. Upper stomach (fundus, upper body) – slow, sustained contractions that generate pressure
2. Lower stomach (lower body, antrum) – powerful peristaltic contractions towards the pyloric sphincter.

These combined movements, together with hydrolysis of lipids and proteins, lead to liquidisation of food, which is released into the duodenum in spurts. The upper stomach acts as a 'pressure pump'. In the lower stomach, solid food larger than 1–2 mm is recycled through the 'antral mill' until it has reached a size small enough to pass the pyloric sphincter.

Gastric emptying is controlled by neural or hormonal signals arising in response to nutrients in other parts of the gut. For example, the proximal and distal small bowel detect lipids and inhibit gastric motility; the effect is strongest with free fatty acids with a chain length >10 carbon atoms. There seem to be four types of sensor:

1. Luminal lipid stimulates release of the regulatory peptide hormones cholecystokinin (CCK), neurotensin, peptide YY (PYY) and glucagon-like peptides (GLP) (Figure *evolve* 3.6 🐭). CCK has local effects on motility.
2. CCK stimulates afferent nerve pathways in the intestine that inhibit gastric activity
3. Chylomicrons, which are the products of lipid digestion packaged for export to lymph (see 'Digestion and Absorption of Fat', below) are also sensed by an as yet unknown mechanism.

4. Short-chain fatty acids which reflux back into the ileum are sensed and signal the release of PYY, which inhibits gastric motility.

In this way, nutrient overload in the intestinal lumen is sensed and motility is inhibited so permitting more time before the remainder of the meal is released. Even at rest, the stomach is never quiescent since rhythmic waves of polarisation and depolarisation of gastric smooth muscle occur every 20 seconds, controlled by a pacemaker. Abnormalities in this pacemaker are associated with abnormal gastric emptying (e.g. 'dumping syndrome'). Slow emptying can be treated by prokinetic drugs and a new treatment for dumping is to give 1–2 g of oleic acid before a meal to stimulate maximum inhibition of gastric motility by both the duodenal and ileal brakes.

Gastric emptying is also slowed by increased blood glucose concentration and is accelerated by insulin injection, which reduces blood glucose concentration. This is an example of a feedback mechanism that balances the amount of nutrient presented for absorption by the small intestine, with the amount already absorbed. Another way in which gastric emptying is controlled is through inhibition of eating.

Gastric distension is a very powerful inhibitory signal that increases feelings of fullness and satisfaction (satiety) and hence counters the stimulatory afferent signals produced by eating tasty food. When the former signal predominates, eating is reduced and the stomach will, on balance, empty.

DIGESTIVE PROCESSES IN THE SMALL INTESTINE

Intestinal secretions and their control

Gastrin secreted by the stomach stimulates the secretion of enzymes by acinar cells in the pancreas. As the meal is released by the pylorus, acid-sensing cells in the duodenal mucosa release the hormone secretin, which stimulates water and bicarbonate secretion by pancreatic duct cells. This in turn flushes the pancreatic enzymes into the duodenum via the pancreatic duct. A second hormone, cholecystokinin, is also released and elicits two responses: 1) The acinar cells of the pancreas release large quantities of pancreatic enzymes as inactive zymogens; 2) The gall-bladder contracts powerfully and squirts bile into the duodenum through the common bile duct.

Although digestion will increase luminal osmolality and mucosal water secretion, the absorption of the products of digestion reduces osmolality and the water will be reabsorbed. This is an impressive process; it is estimated that 7.5 litres of water are secreted and absorbed in this way, every day.

Digestive function of intestinal secretions

The pancreas secretes digestive enzymes in the form of inactive precursors (zymogens), and this may amount to up to 30% of the protein passing through the gastrointestinal tract with the meal. If these pancreatic enzymes were completely hydrolysed and the amino acids absorbed, a large amount of protein would need to be synthesised each day in order to digest 80–90 g of dietary protein. There is evidence that patients with an ileostomy (surgical fistula that drains ileal contents) do indeed excrete that amount of partially digested protein.

However, there is also evidence that pancreatic enzymes are absorbed intact and recycled in an enteropancreatic circulation that is analogous to the enterohepatic circulation of bile salts (Rothman et al 2002). Compelling arguments for this view are that pancreatic enzymes can be detected in the circulation and that the pancreas does not have the capacity to synthesise such a large amount of secretory enzymes each day. The mechanism of the proposed selective intestinal absorption of pancreatic enzymes is unknown.

Various pancreatic enzymes hydrolyse proteins (proteases), lipids (lipase, phospholipase), starch (amylase) and nucleic acids (ribonuclease, deoxyribonuclease) together with esterases and two specific proteases, gelatinase and elastase. These enzymes carry out luminal digestion of more highly polymerised substrates of >10 units (e.g. larger maltodextrins) whereas brush border hydrolases favour shorter oligomers (e.g. maltose, maltotriose).

Proteases

The pancreatic proteases are either endopeptidases (trypsin, chymotrypsin and elastase) that cleave internal amino acid bonds or they are carboxypeptidases (A & B) that will sequentially cleave amino acids from the C-terminal of oligopeptides. The endopeptidases have specificities for bonds adjacent to dibasic amino acids (trypsin), hydrophobic amino acids (chymotrypsin) or small neutral amino acids (elastase). The combined actions of these enzymes will reduce dietary proteins to a mixture of free amino acids and peptides with a chain-length of 2–8 amino acids.

Like gastric pepsins, pancreatic proteases are secreted as inactive zymogens.

Enteropeptidase (sometimes known as enterokinase), a glycoprotein bound to the enterocyte brush-border, converts trypsinogen to trypsin by cleavage of a peptide sequence that blocks the active site of trypsin. Active trypsin which is released cannot catalyse further activation of trypsinogen, but does activate the zymogens of the other major proteases to yield chymotrypsin, elastase, carboxypeptidase A and carboxypeptidase B. The highest concentration of enteropeptidase is found in the duodenum and decreases distally; and its level of expression on the membrane depends on the luminal presence of pancreatic enzymes, amino acids or glucose.

Amylase

Both salivary and pancreatic α-amylases are most active at neutral pH and act as endoglucosidases that have an absolute specificity for α-1,4 glucose linkages with two adjacent α-1,4 linkages. Therefore, amylase will not cleave other glucose polymers such as α-glucans (oats), cellulose (plants) or dextran (dental plaque) or lactose or sucrose. The end products of starch digestion are maltose, maltotriose and the α-1,6 branched limit dextrins. No free glucose is released. Further digestion of the branched limit dextrins can only occur at the brush-border (catalysed by isomaltose or glucoamylase). The chain-length of the linear, α-1,4 linked dextrins in the lumen after a starch meal depends on the extent to which α-amylase digestion has gone to completion, but is probably in the range 5–10 glucose units.

Lipases

There are three pancreatic lipases. Pancreatic triacylglycerol lipase (PL) is the most abundant and important in adult life; pancreatic lipase-related proteins 1 and 2 (PLRP-1, PLRP-2) are expressed pre- and perinatally but not in adulthood. PL has a preference for triacylglycerols rather than phospholipids. It is inhibited by bile salts but this inhibition is relieved by the colipase, another pancreatic protein, which binds to the C-terminal of the enzyme and helps it to bind to the lipid droplet surface. The N-terminal of the enzyme has a 'lid'

sequence, a highly mobile structure which, upon lipid binding, will swing aside to reveal the active site and thus allow lipid hydrolysis to occur. Fat digestion comprises the following steps:

1. Partial digestion and emulsification in the stomach.
2. Mixing of tricylglycerols, diacylglycerols, monoacylglycerols and fatty acids with detergent (bile salts), cholesterol and phospholipid to form mixed micelles that have a hydrophobic core and hydrophilic outer surface. Their small size and high surface area results in efficient hydrolysis.
3. Binding of colipase and lipase to the surface of these micelles leads to release of free fatty acids and retinol.
4. Osmotic pressures generated within the micelle by triacylglycerol hydrolysis cause budding of monoacylglycerol- and fatty-acid-rich micelles from the surface of these structures. These easily penetrate the unstirred water layer adjacent to the absorptive surface of the enterocyte.

Regulation of small intestinal motility

The pattern of intestinal motility depends critically on whether the subject is fasted, fed or post-prandial. A typical peristaltic wave or migrating motor complex (MMC) will occur 4–6 hours after a meal and is a complex entity, comprising four phases that cycle continuously:

1. Phase I – inactivity (30–40 minutes)
2. Phase II – irregular pressure spike activity (30–40 min).
3. Phase III – intense repetitive high amplitude contractions (4–6 minutes)
4. Phase IV – irregular activity.

This cycle moves down the intestine at 4–6 cm/min before slowing in the terminal ileum and does not occur until 4–6 hours after a meal. Feeding initiates irregular activity throughout the small intestine, which resembles phase II of the MMC. It leads to greatly reduced rates of intestinal contraction and rate of movement, and this lengthens transit time in the bowel. The absorption of nutrients from the lumen of the small intestine is increased by the way in which the mucosa repeatedly dips into the chyme, minimising the diffusion barrier to absorption. At the same time, villous contractions help lymph and blood flow to carry away absorbed nutrients. These repetitive segmenting contractions are interspersed with erratic motile patterns that move chyme forwards rapidly by 10–30 cm before segmenting contractions recommence.

These responses are nutrient dependent. Lipid has particularly potent effects because it generates strong clustered contractions that enhance emulsification. In summary, fasting motility sweeps debris, shed cells and bacteria down the intestine whereas fed motility enhances digestion and absorption of nutrients. The transition between fasting and fed patterns is modulated by the presence of nutrients in the lumen. During a meal, a small portion of chyme (the head of the meal) will be rapidly swept down to the distal ileum, where the presence of digested fat evokes the ileal brake leading to a marked reduction in transit rate. In addition, the passage of food into the small bowel stimulates colonic segmental movement, known as the 'gastrocolonic reflex' (Figure *evolve* 3.7A). This reflex is partially controlled by the cephalic phase of eating and leads to increased churning of colonic contents that increases absorption of nutrients, water and electrolytes from the colon and will eventually lead to defecation (Figure *evolve* 3.7B). The short-chain fatty acids produced by bacterial fermentation in the colon not only stimulate water absorption, but if they reflux back through the ileocaecal valve into the ileum will simultaneously inhibit gastric emptying and stimulate peristalsis in the terminal ileum. The net effect is to sweep colonic bacteria from the distal small bowel.

Nasogastric tube feeding is associated with diarrhoea. One cause is that the slow rate of nutrient infusion (4.2–6.3 kJ/min) is insufficient to trigger a normal postprandial slowing of intestinal transit. It does, however, maintain colonic water secretion and hence provokes diarrhoea.

3.4 THE ABSORPTION AND SECRETION OF NUTRIENTS

Absorbed nutrients must cross four barriers to reach the bloodstream (Schultz 1998, Pacha 2000):

1. The mucus layer – a diffusion barrier which is rather thin in the small intestine.
2. The enterocyte apical membrane – a lipid bilayer, which requires transport proteins for water-soluble molecules
3. The enterocyte – a metabolic barrier which may metabolise the nutrient.
4. The basolateral membrane – a lipid bilayer which again requires transport proteins for water-soluble molecules.

In addition to transport proteins, absorption is enhanced by metabolic compartmentation or zonation within the enterocytes, which prevents excessive metabolism (e.g. only 10% of absorbed glucose).

The classification of transporters is shown in Figure *evolve* 3.8 and main intestinal transporters are listed in Table *evolve* 3.1 . Although different transporters carry very different substrates, they share many common structural features. They have regions of hydrophobic amino acids that can fold into helices which, when grouped together like the staves of a barrel, span the membrane and form a 'pore' through which substrates can be transported. Parts of the protein (bearing a sugar-polymer) are outside the membrane and can act as a signalling receptor to allow other compounds to control the rate of transport of the main substrate. Alternatively, a transport protein may be linked to another regulatory protein that can chaperone the transporter into the membrane and thus modulate transport capacity. Transport may be either passive, allowing the transported nutrient to come to equilibrium across the membrane, or active, permitting a higher concentration to be achieved on one side of the membrane than on the other.

PASSIVE TRANSPORTERS

These comprise facilitated transporters and ionchannels, which permit the transfer of a solute across the membrane in either direction. Transport therefore takes place down a concentration gradient (so-called 'downhill transport'). Net accumulation of the transported material in the cell can occur as a result of either onward metabolism to a compound that does not cross the membrane (e.g. vitamin B6 is accumulated intracellularly by phosphorylation to pyridoxal phosphate) or by binding to cytosolic proteins (e.g. ferritin, which binds iron).

ACTIVE TRANSPORTERS

These transport solutes against a concentration gradient, linked to either direct ATP utilisation (P-type transporters) or co-transport of an ion down its concentration gradient (symporters, which transport two solutes in parallel) (Figures *evolve* 3.8 and 3.9).

Direct utilisation of ATP involves phosphorylation of the transport protein, which permits it to transport one or more solute molecules in one direction only; solute transport causes dephosphorylation of the protein, so closing the pore.

Symporters commonly utilise a sodium ion gradient across the membrane, although some systems use a hydrogen ion gradient. The ionic gradient is generated by membrane ATPases that pump ions across the membrane. Intestinal absorption of glucose and some amino acids is by sodium-linked symporters.

DIGESTION AND ABSORPTION OF CARBOHYDRATES

The main dietary carbohydrates are starch, lactose and sucrose, as well as smaller amounts of glucose, sugar alcohols and fructose. Carbohydrates are only absorbed as monosaccharides, so starch assimilation proceeds in two phases.

Starch is hydrolysed by pancreatic amylase (and to some extent also by salivary amylase) to yield a mixture of glucose oligomers with a chain length in the range 5–10 glucose 20 units. These are further hydrolysed by the brush-border glucosidases to glucose. In addition some maltose and isomaltose is formed. Disaccharides are hydrolysed to their constituent monosaccharides by disaccharidases on the brush border of the enterocytes: lactase, trehalase and a bifunctional enzyme, sucrase/isomaltase.

Glucose and galactose are taken up by the same active (sodium-linked) transporter (SGLT1) (Figure *evolve* 3.10), while fructose, some other monosaccharides and sugar alcohols are carried by passive transporters. This means that only a proportion of fructose and sugar alcohols can be absorbed, and after a large dose much may remain in the lumen, leading to osmotic diarrhoea.

However, although SGLT1 has high affinity for glucose, it has a low transport capacity. There is a second glucose transporter, GLUT2, in the enterocyte that is only inserted into the membrane in response to glucose absorption via SGLT1. This process is controlled by insulin and dietary amino acids, mediated by protein kinase C activation. This leads to a great increase in transport capacity in response to dietary load.

Starch assimilation provides a good example of the distribution of digestive and absorptive function. It can be inferred that this occurs mainly in the duodenum, upper jejunum and proximal ileum because 1) they have the highest mucosal expression of sucrase-isomaltase and the sodium glucose-linked transporter (SGLT1); 2) rapid appearance of blood glucose after a starch meal fits with this site of absorption; 3) removal of the distal small intestine hardly affects glucose assimilation. By contrast, most fat and fat-soluble vitamin assimilation occurs in the ileum, which has the highest transport capacity. Surgical removal of the ileum may therefore leave the patient at risk of essential fatty acid and fat-soluble vitamin deficiency.

DIGESTION AND ABSORPTION OF PROTEIN

The endopeptidases of gastric and pancreatic juice hydrolyse proteins to yield oligopeptides; aminopeptidases secreted by the intestinal mucosa and pancreatic carboxypeptidases then remove terminal amino acids sequentially from these oligopeptides, yielding free amino acids and di- and tripeptides. Early studies indicated the presence of amino acid transport systems with the following characteristics:

1. Stereospecific – L-amino acids are transported very much faster than D-amino acids
2. Very specific so that only a small number of chemically related amino acids are transported by any one carrier system
3. Duplicated – some amino acids are transported by more than one carrier system.

Some are sodium-linked, others are not. The main amino acid transport systems are shown in Table *evolve* 3.1 . The naming system is complex because it developed piecemeal: 1) system A (Alanine) is a sodium symporter for small neutral aliphatic amino acids; 2) system ASC (i.e. Alanine, Serine and Cysteine) is also a sodium-symporter; 3) system L (Leucine) is not sodium-dependent and carries branched chain and aromatic amino acids; 4) system y+ is not sodium-dependent and carries dibasic amino acids; 5) system XAG is a sodium symporter and carries dicarboxylic (acidic) amino acids.

Di- and tripeptides are transported by separate systems from free amino acids. Patients with genetic defects of system ASC (cystinuria), which prevents intestinal absorption of arginine, lysine and cysteine, or system L (Hartnup disease), which prevents the absorption of aromatic and branched-chain amino acids, still absorb enough of the essential amino acids as small peptides to maintain nitrogen balance.

Di- and tripeptides are taken up into the enterocyte by peptide transporters (PEPT1 and PEPT2), hydrogen ion symporters that take advantage of the acid micro-climate of the submucosal space. Unlike the amino acid transporters, PEPT1 and PEPT2 are:

1. Stereospecifically promiscuous – they will transport cyclic peptides, D-peptides, and cis-peptides.
2. Non-specific – they will transport most, if not all, of the theoretically possible 400 dipeptides and 8000 tripeptides, in addition to beta-lactam antibiotics (e.g. penicillin) and valaciclovir, an anti-herpes drug that has no peptide bond.

The absorbed di- and tripeptides are hydrolysed by intracellular peptidases, and the resultant amino acids, together with those absorbed from the lumen as free amino acids, are secreted into the villous microcirculation.

Some relatively large peptides (large enough to elicit antibody formation) enter the bloodstream intact, either by passing between cells or by uptake into mucosal cells. These are normally trapped by the gut-associated lymphoid tissue, but can enter the systemic circulation – this is the basis of food allergy (see Ch. 26).

DIGESTION AND ABSORPTION OF FAT

The process of fat digestion is one of progressive emulsification of dietary lipids and hydrolysis of triacylglycerol to free fatty acids and monoacylglycerols. The final product of fat digestion is the mixed micelle, which buds smaller micelles (as a result of the osmotic action of the free fatty acids), which are transferred across the enterocyte brush border membrane. Short chain fatty acids enter the villus microcirculation, but most of the fatty acids are re-esterified to triacylglycerol in the mucosal cell then are packaged into chylomicrons and secreted into the lacteals, and then into the lymphatic system (see Ch. 7).

Cholesterol and fat soluble vitamins are absorbed dissolved in the hydrophobic core of the micelles. Much of the cholesterol destined for chylomicrons is esterified in the enterocyte, and competition between cholesterol and other sterols and stanols for the acyltransferase probably explains why these compounds reduce cholesterol absorption, and hence have a hypocholesterolaemic action.

There is still lively debate about how fatty acids can cross the enterocyte apical membrane. The classic view is that, being lipophilic, they can dissolve in the membrane and traverse it, by a 'flip-flop' mechanism, as protonated, uncharged fatty acids. This process of permeation is rapid, about 1000 times greater than for water and more than a million times faster that that of glucose. Protonation of fatty acids in the acidic microenvironment adjacent to the brush-border membrane will promote permeation, whilst ionisation of free fatty acids by the higher intracellular pH or incorporation into TAG inside the enterocyte would prevent back-diffusion of fatty acids. The second proposed route of uptake is via membrane-bound transport proteins. Candidates include CD36 (fatty acid translocase) and FATP4 (fatty acid transporter protein 4) and their importance is currently being investigated by use of 'knock-out' mice. Most evidence for the significance of the FATP family has come from other organs such as muscle, heart and adipose tissue. The true situation in the intestine may differ because there may be parallel transport systems of low (FATP) and high (permeation) capacity to cope with feast and famine in the gut lumen. This type of dual transport has been shown for amino acid and glucose uptake. The situation is summarised in Figure evolve 3.11A .

Within the enterocyte, fatty acids are transferred by intracellular fatty acid binding proteins (FABP) to the nascent lipid droplet where they are re-esterified to triacylglycerol. This lipid droplet enters the endoplasmic reticulum together with cholesterol, phospholipids, fat soluble vitamins and apolipoproteins before moving to the Golgi apparatus where the chylomicron matures. Buds from the Golgi apparatus fuse with the enterocyte lateral membrane leading to exocytosis and the release of chylomicrons into the lymphatic system.

The rate limiting step in this process is transfer of lipid from the endoplasmic reticulum to the Golgi apparatus and triacylglycerol from excess dietary lipid may either be oxidised or temporarily stored within the endoplasmic reticulum. Components of chylomicrons (e.g. apoprotein A-IV) that enter the circulation can inhibit gastric emptying. This suggests that the intestinal motility is a key factor in controlling nutrient absorption because it is controlled by every stage of lipid digestion, absorption and repackaging.

The rate of movement of dietary fat into lymph depends on its fatty acid composition. Olive oil appears to be most rapidly absorbed, and cocoa butter and menhaden oil are most slowly absorbed. In malabsorption syndromes such as cystic fibrosis, medium chain triglycerides (MCT, chain length of 8–10 carbon atoms) are used because their shorter chain length and greater water solubility results in uptake into the portal circulation and hence a faster overall rate of macronutrient uptake.

The colonic microflora produce short-chain fatty acids (SCFA), acetate, propionate and butyrate, by fermentation of resistant starch (see Chapter 6 and Figure *evolve* 3.11B) and non-starch polysaccharides. The presence of SCFA in the colonic lumen is of interest because butyrate is a preferential fuel for the colonic mucosa, and promotes colonocyte differentiation. It may thus have a significant role in preventing colon cancer. Absorption of SCFA can occur by diffusion across the colonocyte membrane, and they are also transported by a membrane transporter that co-transports Na^+ or K^+. Water uptake is stimulated by SCFA absorption and this is likely to be one of the major mechanisms for water and electrolyte salvage in the large intestine.

ABSORPTION OF VITAMINS

The fat-soluble vitamins A, D, E and K, and carotenoids (see Chapter 11) are absorbed dissolved in lipid micelles together with the products of fat digestion. Esters of vitamin A (retinyl esters) are hydrolysed in the duodenum by either pancreatic lipase or enterocyte brush-border phospholipase B. There is some evidence that there is a membrane transporter for retinol, then inside the cell, cellular retinol binding proteins (CRBP) bind retinol and channel it for resynthesis of retinyl-esters by lecithin: retinol acyl transferase (LRAT) or acyl-CoA: retinol acyltransferase (ARAT).

The water-soluble vitamins (see Chapter 10) are absorbed by specific transport proteins. Vitamin C is present in the intestinal lumen as both reduced ascorbic acid and oxidised dehydro-ascorbic acid. Ascorbic acid is absorbed by a sodium-dependent transporter (SVCT1), while dehydroascorbic acid is absorbed by the sodium-independent glucose transporters GLUT1 and GLUT3. Phosphorylated derivatives of vitamins B_1, B_2 and B_6 are dephosphorylated in the intestinal lumen, absorbed by

facilitated (passive) transporters, then trapped inside the cells by rephosphorylation (see Chapter 10). Vitamin B_{12} is absorbed bound to intrinsic factor, a glycoprotein that is secreted by the parietal cells of the gastric mucosa (see Chapter 10).

WATER AND ELECTROLYTES

The human small intestine absorbs 6.5–7.5 litres of water each day (Figure *evolve* 3.12). This comes from several sources, as indicated in Figure 3.1. How this gets across the membrane is still a mystery because the lipid bilayer that surrounds each cell is impermeable to water, and the intestinal mucosal surface is rather hydrophobic. Before describing several hypotheses of water movement across the mucosa, it is worth summarising the known characteristics of the process. Water absorption is proportional to the amount of substrate and electrolyte that moves across the membrane; approximately 2 Na^+ ions and 210 water molecules accompany each molecule of glucose absorbed. The direction of water movement is governed by solute movement. The mechanisms for secretion and reabsorption of water and electrolytes by the intestine are very efficient. Under normal circumstances, daily secretion of Na^+ and K^+ by the gut is equivalent to a half and two-thirds of these electrolytes present in the human body's extracellular space, respectively. In cholera, excessive secretion of chloride into the colon is accompanied by water secretion and diarrhoea, leading to dehydration and eventually death, unless treated. Therefore, stimulation of water uptake by glucose (and sodium) is the basis of oral rehydration therapy for the treatment of diarrhoea, which is the most important cause of infant death worldwide (Duquette et al 2001, Schultz 2007).

The hypotheses for water transport are broadly reviewed by Spring (1999). The intestinal mucosa acts as a semipermeable membrane through which water flows in either direction in response to differences in osmotic pressure. Luminal nutrient digestion renders the bulk phase hypertonic and water moves from the intestinal fluid into the gut lumen. Nutrient absorption, however, renders it more hypotonic such that water is absorbed along with these solutes. In this way, the luminal contents are adjusted to near isotonicity throughout the small bowel.

1. Simple osmosis across the apical and basolateral membranes may account for some

water uptake. The osmolality gradient is small (3–30 mosmol/kg) and this model would mean that enterocytes replaced their entire fluid volume every few seconds.

2. Water may move between the enterocytes, through the so-called 'tight-junctions', by osmotic flow because enterocytes have absorbed Na^+ (not water) and secreted this into the lateral intercellular space as a hyperosmolar fluid. This is the most popular hypothesis.

3. Specific transporters may move significant amounts of water across the enterocyte membranes. This means that enterocytes will still replace their intracellular water volume every few seconds. These membranes are termed 'aquaporins' and are very versatile. Their structure is similar to that of other transporters except that the hydrophobic inner surface of the transmembrane-pore is lined with some hydrophilic amino acids which will selectively allow passage of water (Sui et al 2001). The aquaporins are versatile and can also transport other small molecules such as urea, CO_2, NH_3 and glycerol in addition to water (Sasaki 2008).

The colon acts as an organ of water and electrolyte salvage, but its capacity is limited. Rapid infusion of 500 ml or more of water into the colon will provoke diarrhoea through reflex defecation and this is the basis of rectally-administered enemas.

Sugar alcohols used as sweeteners, such as xylitol, lactitol and sorbitol, are poorly absorbed and will enter the colon with sufficient water to maintain luminal isotonicity before fermentation and the absorption of SCFA, water and Na^+. If the colonic fermentation capacity is exceeded then osmotic diarrhoea ensues because the excess water cannot be absorbed.

Clinically the synthetic disaccharide lactulose (which is not hydrolysed in the small intestine) and the sugar alcohol lactitol are used as laxatives. Other causes of osmotic diarrhoea include dietary fibre such as guar gum, probiotics such as fructose oligosaccharide and beans that contain large quantities of stachyose, all of which are good substrates for bacterial fermentation. The laxative threshold (at which gastointestinal symptoms are unacceptable) for most readily fermentable non-absorbed carbohydrates is about 70 g/day, but most people will notice the effects of 40 g/day.

Most minerals are absorbed by carrier-mediated diffusion, and are then accumulated by binding to intracellular binding proteins, followed by sodium-dependent transport from the enterocyte into the villous microcirculation. Genetic defects of either the intracellular binding proteins or the active transport systems at the basal membrane of the enterocyte can result in mineral deficiency despite an apparently adequate intake. As discussed in Chapter 11, the enterocyte calcium binding protein is induced by vitamin D, and vitamin D deficiency results in much reduced absorption of calcium.

3.5 THE ROLE OF THE GASTROINTESTINAL TRACT IN THE REGULATION OF FEEDING

As discussed in Chapter 5, there are both long-term and short-term mechanisms to regulate food intake and energy expenditure so as to maintain energy balance. Short-term control of appetite is regulated by the gastrointestinal tract as well as by the metabolic response to ingested nutrients. There are three ways in which the gastrointestinal tract provides regulatory feedback signals. These signals arise from direct effects of absorbed nutrients in the circulation, from neural signals from the gut and liver and from hormonal signals (Karra et al 2009).

Although the existence of more than 100 gastrointestinal peptide hormones complicates this, one investigative approach has been to predict the properties of an ideal short-term 'satiety hormone' and a 'hunger hormone'. These would be secreted in response to feeding or during a short-term fast, and have receptors in both the gut and the central nervous system that will result in a decrease in the size of a single meal or a move to acquire food, respectively (Figure *evolve* 3.13A). Several hormones secreted by the gastrointestinal tract meet these criteria.

Cholecystokinin (CCK), secreted by the duodenum (which also stimulates secretion of bile and pancreatic juice, and regulates intestinal motility) and peptide YY (PYY) appear to signal the presence of nutrients in the gut lumen and this will lead to decreased voluntary food intake. Ghrelin is secreted by the stomach during the fasting period and increases appetite and food intake. Leptin is mainly secreted by adipose tissue and its main function is to regulate long-term food intake and energy expenditure in response to the state of fat reserves (see Chapter 5 and Figure *evolve* 3.13B).

THE MOUTH

The taste of food, as well as the smell before eating, stimulates secretion of gastric juice and intestinal motility. There are five families of receptors on the tongue, for sweet, salty or meaty/savoury (umami) flavours, which are generally pleasurable, and for sour or bitter tastes, which are generally aversive. In addition the tongue can sense the fatty acids liberated from triacylglycerols by lingual lipase. Combinations of taste and sensation may have additive effects, for example sugar mixed with fat is particularly pleasurable, and salt may be useful in masking bitter flavours that are taste-aversive. The importance of taste in controlling sensations of hunger and satiety is seen in patients receiving long-term tube-feeding who experience constant feelings of hunger although nutritionally replete.

The taste of food provides a strong signal to stimulate eating. However, this process operates only when there are sensations of hunger and is suppressed when sensations of satiety become strong. This is known as sensory-specific or conditioned satiety. It is thought that a dominant factor in this process is the action of dopamine on the hypothalamus in response to absorbed fat.

THE STOMACH

During eating, food stretches the stomach and induces a complex series of signals that lead to cessation of eating. The importance of this can be illustrated by taking a glass of water with a meal to induce feelings of satiety whilst eating, but not afterwards. Conversely, in rats in which gastric contents are continuously removed during the meal through a fistula ('sham feeding'), the amount of food eaten at each meal is greatly increased. The mechanism is due to gastric stretch, not pressure, and works through direct inhibition of the stimulating effect of pleasurable tastes on eating. Signals from taste receptors in the mouth and from gastric stretch receptors are integrated in the parabrachial nucleus of the pons in the brain stem so that one signal will down-regulate the other (Figure *evolve* 3.14 ▇).

THE SMALL INTESTINE

In addition to stretch receptors, the intestinal mucosa possesses an abundance of receptors for acid and for fatty acids and glucose and amino acids, which will provide information about the contents of the lumen that the brain stem will integrate and use to control eating behaviour. Cholecystokinin, released in response to luminal fat, leads to powerful inhibition of eating.

Absorbed nutrients are also potent signals that modulate eating behaviour. For example, in adequately nourished subjects, the intravenous infusion of lipid stimulates dopamine activity (which acts as a feeding inhibitor) and increases satiety ratings, feelings of fullness and reduces the desire to select particular foodstuffs. In contrast, studies in the hospital population (which experiences 40–50% malnutrition) have shown that fortification of hospital food with fat actually stimulates energy intake. This mechanism thus depends on sensations of hunger that are related to nutritional status. However, these mechanisms can be overridden centrally. An example of this would be the inability to resist the unexpected offer of a plate of strawberries and cream after a particularly heavy meal.

KEY POINTS

- The gastrointestinal tract provides a linear sequence of events resulting in the hydrolysis of dietary carbohydrates, triacylglycerols and proteins, and the absorption of the products of digestion.
- Salivary and gastric secretions are stimulated before eating, then the presence of food in the mouth and stomach stimulates further secretion.
- Gastric emptying is controlled by both the amount of food eaten during a meal, and nutrients present in the food and the progress made in liquidising it within the stomach.

- Pancreatic and intestinal secretion are stimulated by hormones secreted in response to the presence of food in the stomach.
- The monosaccharides resulting from carbohydrate digestion, and free amino acids from protein digestion, are absorbed into the hepatic portal vein, and the liver regulates the entry into the peripheral circulation of the products of digestion.
- Amylases in saliva and pancreatic juice catalyse hydrolysis of starch to disaccharides and limit dextrins; disaccharides are hydrolysed by intestinal brush-border enzymes, and monosaccharides are

- absorbed by active transport (glucose and galactose) or passive transport (other monosaccharides and sugar alcohols).
- Lipases secreted by the tongue, in gastric juice and pancreatic juice catalyse the progressive hydrolysis of triacylglycerol until dietary lipid is emulsified into micelles small enough to be absorbed across the small intestinal lumen. Most absorbed fatty acids are re-esterified in the mucosal cells and absorbed into the lymphatic system in chylomicrons, but medium-chain fatty acids are absorbed into the hepatic portal vein.
- Proteolytic enzymes are secreted as inactive zymogens. Pepsinogen in the gastric juice is activated by gastric acid and autocatalysis;

trypsinogen in the pancreatic juice is activated by intestinal enteropeptidase. Trypsin then activates the other intestinal zymogens.
- Protein digestion begins with the action of endopeptidases, which hydrolyse proteins at specific sites within the molecule, resulting in the formation of a large number of oligopeptides. Exopeptidases then remove amino and carboxy terminal amino acids, resulting in free amino acids and di- and tripeptides.
- Free amino acids are absorbed by a variety of group-specific transporters; di- and tripeptides are absorbed by a specific transporter with wide substrate tolerance, and hydrolysed within the intestinal mucosal cells.

References

Atuma C, Strugala V, Allen A, Holm L: The adherent gastrointestinal mucus gel layer: thickness and physical state in vivo, *American Journal of Physiology (Gastrointest and Liver Physiology)* 280(5):G922–G929, 2001.

Duquette PP, Bissonnette P, Lapointe JY: Local osmotic gradients drive the water flux associated with Na$^+$/glucose cotransport, *Proceedings of the National Academy of Sciences of the U S A* 98:3796–3801, 2001.

Karra E, Chandarana K, Batterham RL: The role of peptide YY in appetite regulation and obesity, *Journal of Physiology (Lond)* 587:19–25, 2009.

Pacha J: Development of intestinal transport function in mammals, *Physiological Reviews* 80(4):1633–1667, 2000.

Rothman S, Liebow C, Isenman L: Conservation of digestive enzymes, *Physiological Reviews* 82(1):1–18, 2002.

Sasaki S: Introduction for Special issue for Aquaporin: Expanding the world of aquaporins: new members and new functions, *Pflügers Archiv* 456:647–649, 2008.

Schultz SG: A century of (epithelial) transport physiology: from vitalism to molecular cloning, *American Journal of Physiology (Cell Physiology)* 274(1):C13–C23, 1998.

Schultz SG: From a pump handle to oral rehydration therapy: a model of translational research, *Advances in Physiological Education* 31:288–293, 2007.

Spring KR: Epithelial fluid transport – a century of investigation, *News in Physiological Sciences* 14:92–98, 1999.

Sui H, Han BG, Lee JK, Walian P, Jap BK: Structural basis of water-specific transport through the AQP1 water channel, *Nature* 414:872–878, 2001.

Further reading

Havel PJ: Peripheral signals conveying metabolic information to the brain: short-term and long-term regulation of food intake and energy homeostasis, *Experimental Biology and Medicine (Maywood)* 226(11):963–977, 2001.

Lowe ME: Molecular mechanisms of rat and human pancreatic triglyceride lipases, *Journal of Nutrition* 127(4):549–557, 1997.

Stevens CE, Hume ID: Contributions of microbes in vertebrate gastrointestinal tract to production and conservation of nutrients, *Physiological Review* 78(2):393–427, 1998.

Website

Bowen R. Colorado State University. Fundamental Physiology and Anatomy of the Digestive System. http://arbl.cvmbs.colostate.edu/hbooks/pathphys/digestion/basics/index.html#top

Chapter 4

Body size and composition

Mario Siervo*

CHAPTER CONTENTS

OBJECTIVES

By the end of this chapter you should be able to:
- define terms for components of body composition
- describe their relative size and variation
- describe their main characteristics and functions
- summarise the use of composition information in nutrition
- describe the main methods for measurement of body fat, fat-free mass, lean body mass, body water and blood fractions.

*Updated and modified from the previous edition chapter written by John Garrow

4.1 INTRODUCTION

Nutrients in the diet are essential to provide the elements from which the human body is built, the energy on which all metabolic activity depends, and cofactors (vitamins and trace elements) which cannot be synthesised within the body. This chapter is concerned with composition of the body, and the information that this gives us about the quality of the diet, lifestyle and disease status. For example, normal growth in children is impaired without an adequate intake of protein and energy, normal fat stores depend on balancing energy input and output, synthesis of essential components such as haemoglobin or thyroid hormone depends respectively on an adequate intake of iron, or iodine, and important physiological functions such as vision and bone development depend on adequate intake of vitamin A and vitamin D.

4.2 BODY COMPOSITION AND FUNCTION

FAT-FREE MASS OR LEAN BODY MASS: DEFINITIONS

The science of body composition started probably more than 2000 years ago, when Archimedes gave his name to the principle stating that any object wholly or partially immerged in a fluid is buoyed up by a force equal to the weight of the fluid displaced by the object, and the weight of the displaced fluid is directly proportional to the volume of the displaced fluid. This principle has been applied thousands of years later to calculate body density and derive fat mass. However, the earliest measurements of body composition in living human subjects were made to discover if overweight individuals contained an unusually large amount of fat or of muscle (see 'Body fat', below). The approach used was to measure average body density, since fat has a density of 0.900 g/cm^3 and a typical mixture of non-fat tissues has a density of 1.100 g/cm^3. Therefore density, and other measurements that have been calibrated against density, like skinfold thickness, yield estimates of *fat* and *fat-free mass*, which together make up total body weight.

Computer scanning methods recognise tissues, such as adipose tissue, by the amount of X-radiation they absorb. Adipose tissue is not pure fat, but approximately 79% fat, 3% protein and 18% water.

Tissue other than adipose tissue is not totally fat-free, since there is lipid in cell membranes to increase membrane fluidity, in nervous tissue to efficiently conduct electric signals and in muscular tissue to act as an energetic reservoir. Therefore scanning methods measure *adipose tissue* and *lean body mass*, which together make up total body weight. The terms fat-free mass and lean body mass are often used interchangeably, but this is not correct as it may have implications for the interpretation of body composition analysis.

HUMAN CADAVER ANALYSIS

Our understanding of body composition in human subjects is based on the chemical analyses of six cadavers (five male and one female), performed between 1945 and 1956. First the fat in these bodies was separated by dissection and extraction with an ether-chloroform mixture, so what remained was fat-free mass. The fat-free body in adults has a fairly constant composition with respect to its water, protein and potassium content. Table 4.1 summarises these results. On average, fat-free tissue contains about 72.5% water, 20.5% protein and 69 mmolK/kg. In Section 4.4 there is further discussion about the methods by which estimates of whole body density, or water, or potassium, combined with the data in Table 4.1, can be used to calculate the fat-free mass of living people. The Visible Man project, a scientific initiative coordinated by the National Institutes of Health (NIH, USA), has used advanced imaging techniques (magnetic resonance imaging) to obtain transverse sections of the human body from three human cadavers to provide detailed and high-resolution images of the anatomical and topographical features of tissues and organs.

The concept of a fat-free mass of constant composition is a great help in estimating fat-free mass in living people, but Table 4.1 also shows that this assumption is an over-simplification. For example, skin and brain have very different chemical compositions. Skin has a very high protein content and low water content (30.0% and 69.4%, respectively) and very little K (23.7 mmol/kg). By contrast, brain has a very low protein and high water content (10.7% and 77.4%, respectively) and a high concentration of K (84.6 mmol/kg). This is because brain has a lot of intracellular water, which contains K, whereas skin has little water, and most of that is extracellular. This detailed information about the

Table 4.1	The contribution of water and protein to the fat–free weight of adult bodies and in some organs				
	WATER (g/kg)	PROTEIN (g/kg)	REMAINDER (g/kg)	POTASSIUM (mmol/kg)	K:N RATIO
Fat-free whole bodies					
Age (years)					
25	728	195	77	71.5	2.29
35	775	165	60	–	–
42	733	192	75	73.0	2.38
46	674	234	92	66.5	1.78
48	730	206	64	–	–
60	704	238	58	66.6	1.75
Mean	724	205	71	69.4	2.05
Selected organs					
Skin	694	300	6	23.7	0.45
Heart	827	143	30	66.5	2.90
Liver	711	176	113	75.0	2.66
Kidneys	810	153	37	57.0	2.33
Brain	774	107	119	84.6	4.96
Muscle	792	192	16	91.2	2.99

Data compiled from various sources.

chemical composition of individual tissues and organs can only be obtained by chemical analysis of autopsy or biopsy samples. In addition, different physiological (growth, pregnancy, lactation) and pathological conditions (kidney failure, muscular disorders, lipodistrophy) can challenge these assumptions and complicate even more the assessment of the chemical properties of bodily tissues.

WATER AND ELECTROLYTES: INTRACELLULAR AND EXTRACELLULAR

Using the data from cadaver analyses we can construct a diagram of the components of the body of a typical normal young adult who weighs 70 kg: this is shown in Figure 4.1. We call it the Reference Man.

For the sake of simplicity we will use rounded numbers, and assume a fat content of 12 kg (17%), so the fat-free mass is 58 kg. By far the largest component of fat-free mass is water (42 kg), which is 72.5% of fat-free weight. Approximately 70% of this water (28 kg) is inside cells, i.e. intracellular fluid (ICF), and the remaining 30% (14 kg) is extracellular, i.e. extracellular fluid (ECF).

The total amount of water in the body, and the partition of body water between ICF and ECF, is

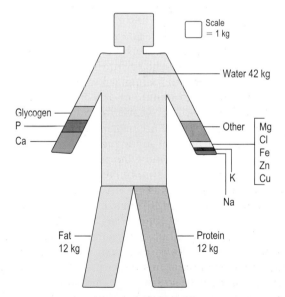

Fig. 4.1 Diagrammatic representation of the body composition of a normal adult male weighing 70 kg. The contributions of the components to body weight are represented by their area in the diagram: only fat, protein and glycogen contribute to the energy stores of the body.

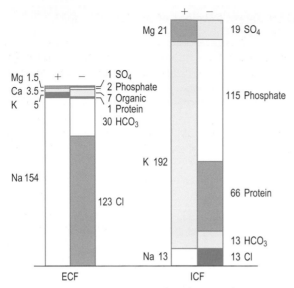

Fig. 4.2 Electrolyte composition (mEq/kg water) of extracellular fluid (ECF) and intracellular fluid (ICF).

closely regulated. Body stores of protein, energy, vitamins and minerals ensure survival for many weeks without dietary intake, but deprivation of water causes death in a few days by multi-organ failure due to electrolyte disorders (see 'Changes in hydration: diarrhoea, oedema, kwashiorkor, heart or kidney failure', below).

The electrolyte composition of ICF and ECF is shown in Figure 4.2. The principal cation in ICF is K, with a small amount of Na and Mg. The principal cation in ECF is Na, and Cl is the principal anion. The total electrical charge of anions and cations is exactly balanced in ICF and in ECF. The total concentration of ions is greater in ICF than ECF, because ICF contains polyvalent cations, particularly proteins, but the osmolality (determined by the concentration of molecules, rather than ions) of the two fluids is identical.

Methods by which we can measure the total amount of water in a living subject, and the proportion of this water that is extracellular, are described in 'Total body water (TBW)', below.

BONE: COMPOSITION, TYPES, DENSITY, GROWTH AND TURNOVER

Bone contains a matrix of fibrillar collagen that gives it tensile strength. Packed in an orderly manner around the collagen fibres is the mineral that gives the bone rigidity. This mineral is a complex crystalline calcium phosphate, called hydroxyapatite. Finally the bone is covered by a vascular fibrous sheath, the periosteum. An adult body contains approximately 1 kg of Ca, of which 99% is in bone. The skeleton also contains approximately 500 g of P, and more than half the collagen in the body, the remaining collagen being in skin, tendons and fascial sheaths.

Every bone has a dense outer osseous layer which is filled inside by spongy bone arranged with trabeculae of different direction and strength, depending on the stress to which the bone is subjected. The spaces between the trabeculae are filled with bone marrow which is highly vascular, and in which new blood cells are made.

Bone has two main functions: to provide a rigid frame for the body and protect certain organs from injury, to afford attachments for muscles and their tendons and to act as the main reservoir of calcium, magnesium and phosphate to maintain the balance of these electrolytes. The shape of the bone depends on its function. For example, the bones of the skull, shoulder blade and pelvis are flat, and have dense outer layers separated by a small amount of spongy bone. They provide protection to the brain, chest and pelvic organs, respectively, as well as attachment for muscles. The long bones of the limbs are designed to resist twisting and bending stresses, for which their design is appropriate. The shaft of the long bones is a thick-walled tube of dense bone that has expanded ends to bear the articular surfaces of the shoulder, elbow, wrist, hip, knee or ankle joints, and to provide anchorage for the powerful muscles that move these joints.

Bone density (g/cm^3) is determined by the quantity of bone per unit volume. This in turn depends on the balance of activity between osteoblasts (cells that stimulate new bone formation) and osteoclasts (cells that cause resorption of bone). Factors that influence this balance are discussed in Chapter 24. It has become possible to measure the bone mineral content of selected bones since the development of quantitative radiological scanning techniques (see 'Body fat', below). Normally bone density reaches a maximum around the age of 30 years, and then declines. Peak bone density is greater in men than in women, so women are more liable than men to develop osteoporosis in later life. This is a condition in which the quantity of bone per unit volume is decreased, so the trabeculae become thinner and weaker, and the dense cortical bone becomes porous. (This should not be confused with osteomalacia (or rickets, in children), which is a defect of bone mineralisation, and causes deformities because the bones are unduly pliable.) Osteoporosis is a common and important disorder in the elderly, since it predisposes to fractures, especially of the vertebrae, femoral neck and forearm. (See Section 24.3 for further information.)

Bone growth does not progress at an equal rate in all parts of the skeleton. The brain (and therefore also the skull that encloses it) is proportionately very large in the fetus, but after birth the limbs grow more rapidly in both length and strength. At birth there are no ossification centres for the wrist bones, or for the ends of the humerus, radius, ulna or fibula. This is of importance for nutritional assessment, since a child who is chronically undernourished will show delayed development of these ossification centres. If the undernutrition is severe and prolonged the normal growth of long bones will not occur, and adult height will be stunted. Normal changes in body size and composition throughout the lifespan are described further in Section 4.3. The proportion of body weight as adipose tissue, muscle bone and skin is shown in Table *evolve* 4.1.

The constituents of bone are not static: both the protein and mineral in bone are constantly exchanging with the amino acid and mineral metabolic pools in the body. Whereas most body proteins turn over with a half-life of days or weeks, the turnover of collagen is very slow. Enzymic hydrolysis of collagen yields a mixture of amino acids that have a low nutritional value, because, in the synthesis of collagen, proline is hydroxylated, and hydroxyproline cannot be used to synthesise new protein. The turnover rate of collagen can be estimated from the urinary excretion of hydroxyproline, which is typically about 20 mg per day in an adult. This is very little compared with the 10 g of urea nitrogen excreted daily from the catabolism of all the other body proteins in an adult on a normal diet.

Bone calcium also exchanges with calcium in other organs, especially kidney and gut. These fluxes are controlled by the action of parathyroid hormone, 1,25-dihydroxycholecalciferol (vitamin D, see Ch. 11) and calcitonin. It is essential for normal muscular and neurological function that plasma Ca is maintained in the range of 2.25–2.60 mmol/l. Disorders of bone metabolism are described further in Chapter 24.

MUSCLE: TYPES, GROWTH, REPAIR, FUNCTION

In a typical adult, skeletal muscle accounts for approximately 40% of body weight, and another 10% is smooth muscle. The water, protein and potassium content of muscle is shown in Table 4.1. Since muscle makes up so much of fat-free weight, the composition of muscle is similar to that of the average of all fat-free tissues. However, skeletal muscle differs markedly from other tissues in an important respect: resting muscle has a lower energy consumption per unit weight than tissues such as heart, liver, kidneys or brain, but during vigorous physical exercise the energy consumption in muscle greatly exceeds the total of all other body tissues. Organs can be ranked according to their energy expenditure per unit of body mass (kg) and in proportion to their relative contribution to resting energy expenditure (REE). Humans can be considered at the top of the phylogenetic evolutionary ladder and the brain is one of the most expensive organs, energetically speaking, as it consumes 1008 kJ/kg/day. The kidneys and the heart have the highest metabolic rate (1848 kJ/kg/day for both) followed by the liver (840 kJ/kg/day), skeletal muscle (55 kJ/kg/day) and adipose tissue (19 kJ/kg/day).

There are three types of muscle: skeletal, smooth and cardiac. Skeletal muscle consists of bundles of individual muscle fibres, each of which ranges from 10 to 80 μm in diameter. In most muscles these fibres extend the whole length of the muscle. Each fibre is activated by a single nerve ending, situated near the middle of the fibre. Each fibre contains several hundred to several thousand myofibrils. Each myofibril contains about 1500 myosin filaments and 3000 actin filaments arranged longitudinally with an overlapping zone between the two types of filament that shows as a darker band on electron micrographs, which causes a striated appearance on the whole muscle. When the muscle contracts the overlap between the actin and myosin fibres increases, and thus the two ends of the muscle, and the bones to which these ends are attached, are pulled towards each other. During muscle relaxation the actin and myosin units slide apart, but even at full relaxation they retain a degree of overlap.

Smooth muscle also consists of actin and myosin units sliding together and apart, but the muscle fibres are far smaller. Smooth muscle fibres are 2–5 μm in diameter, and only 50–200 μm in length, whereas the diameter of skeletal muscle fibres is up to 20 times greater, and they are thousands of times longer. Smooth muscle does not move joints, but lies in the walls of blood vessels, gut, bile ducts, ureters and uterus. Contraction and relaxation of the smooth muscle in the walls of these organs alters the diameter of the tubes, or may be organised in peristaltic waves so as to move forwards the contents of the tube.

Cardiac muscle, as its name implies, forms the chambers of the heart. Unlike skeletal muscle it is not organised as bundles of individually innervated muscle fibres, but is a syncytium of cells fused end-to-end in a latticework. The electrical potential that causes one cell to contract readily passes to adjacent cells, and the whole mass of muscle contracts and relaxes synchronously. Thus contraction expels the blood within the chamber through an exit valve, and then as it relaxes the chamber refills by permitting blood to flow in through an entry valve.

In skeletal muscle, physiologists distinguish two types of muscle cell: red and white fibres. In birds, for example, muscles in the breast are designed for the rapid movement required for flight, and breast muscle is white. However, the legs of birds contain mainly red muscle, since legs are required to sustain posture for long periods, but not to move as quickly as wings. In human subjects there is a less marked difference between the fibre types of muscles in different parts of the body, and most muscles in human beings contain a mixture of red and white fibres. The effect of different types of physical training on the size and proportions of red and white fibres is considered in Chapter 18, and fuel selection in muscle in Chapter 5.

BLOOD: SERUM, PLASMA, RBC, WBC, NORMAL VALUES, CELL TURNOVER

Blood consists of plasma and cells – red blood cells (RBC), white blood cells (WBC) and platelets. It is primarily a medium for the transport of oxygen, nutrients and hormones to the tissues, and for the removal of carbon dioxide and other waste products from tissues. In a typical adult the volume of blood is approximately 5 litres, of which about 55% is plasma and 45% the volume of packed cells (the haematocrit). If a sample of blood is withdrawn from a peripheral vein and put in a glass test tube it will solidify as a web of fibrin forms. The fibrin then contracts and squeezes together the trapped cells, so after a few minutes there is a firm dark red mass at the bottom of the tube (a blood clot) and a clear yellowish supernatant fluid (serum). Serum is plasma from which the proteins involved in blood clotting have been removed. If we wish to obtain a sample of plasma it is necessary to put the fresh blood sample into a tube with an anticoagulant, and then to separate the cells by centrifugation.

If blood did not contain red cells (RBC) it would be able to transport only 0.3 ml of oxygen dissolved in 100 ml of plasma. This would be quite inadequate to meet the oxygen requirements of the body tissues, even under conditions of basal metabolism. RBCs are packets of haemoglobin in a rather tough bi-concave cell wall which is freely permeable to oxygen, so the presence of RBCs enables 100 ml of blood to transport up to 20 ml of oxygen.

Red blood cells develop in the bone marrow from stem cells to the reticulocyte stage in about 3 days. The reticulocyte is so called because, on staining, remnants of nucleic acid appear as a blue network in the cytoplasm. This is the most immature form of red cell normally seen in the peripheral circulation, but normally 99% of red blood cells are fully mature, with no nucleic acid or nucleus. The mature red blood cells survive in the circulation for about 120 days, after which they are destroyed in the reticuloendothelial system. The haemoglobin is broken down to bilirubin, and the iron is recycled for the synthesis of new haemoglobin for new red blood cells.

White cells are approximately a thousand times less numerous than red cells in the blood. The commonest type of white blood cell is the polymorph, or neutrophil granulocyte, which, like RBCs, is formed in bone marrow. The neutrophil count increases rapidly in response to infection or tissue injury. Neutrophils survive in the peripheral circulation for a very short time: their half-life is estimated at 6 to 8 hours. The next commonest white blood cell is the lymphocyte, which is formed in lymphoid tissue. This cell is involved in immune responses. The remaining white blood cells (monocytes, basophil and eosinophil granulocytes) occur still more rarely. Platelets are very small cells that are involved in blood clotting and the repair of damaged blood vessels.

BODY FAT: SUBCUTANEOUS, INTRA-ABDOMINAL AND INTRA-ORGAN, AND BROWN FAT

Body fat has become unfashionable: in modern affluent communities it is desirable to be slim, but to our ancestors, and to those now living in subsistence economies, body fat is a valuable store of energy during times of famine, and a thermal insulator when the environment is cold. These valuable characteristics of fat still exist, but in affluent countries (and increasingly in developing countries) the need for protection from famine and cold is less often required, and excessive fatness is increasingly common.

The typical adult illustrated in Figure 4.1 contains 12 kg of fat, which is 17% of body weight. This degree of fatness is within the healthy range. Usually 90% of this fat is in a layer under the skin (subcutaneous fat), but there is also fat within the abdominal cavity (visceral fat), and a small amount is in the fascial planes between muscles (extramyocellular fat). Not all of body fat is available as an energy store: even in the bodies of people who have died of starvation there is still about 2 kg of fat remaining, which reinforces the concept of essentiality of body fat. A reserve of 10 kg of fat contains 375 MJ (90 000 kcal), equivalent to about 4 weeks of normal energy requirements assuming a total energy expenditure of ~3000 kcal/day. In fact, people of normal weight on total starvation survive for about 10 weeks, because energy expenditure decreases. In severely obese people the fat stores may reach 80 kg: such people can survive a year of starvation, but this is not appropriate treatment for severe obesity. See Chapters 5 and 20 for further discussion of this topic.

The distribution of body fat differs between men and women, and this has metabolic significance. At puberty, women tend to store fat around breast, hip and thigh regions, whereas men tend to accumulate fat in and on the abdomen. If adults become obese they may deposit the excess fat in female (or gynoid) pattern, or the male (android) pattern (see Fig. *evolve* 4.1 🖰). This pattern is determined by the action of sex hormones which are probably linked to the genetic background: even when excess fat is lost the characteristic pattern is preserved. In vitro measurement of rates of lipolysis in biopsies of adipose tissue have shown similar basal rates of lipolysis in femoral and abdominal adipose tissue in non-pregnant women. However, lipolysis in femoral fat increases during lactation. It seems that femoral fat is conserved in the non-pregnant woman, but made available as an energy source in later stages of pregnancy and lactation.

It has been observed that obesity, and particularly fat deposited in the abdominal cavity (and hence associated with the android body shape), strongly predisposes to diabetes mellitus and heart disease. This is probably because the intra-abdominal fat is much more sensitive to lipolytic stimuli than subcutaneous fat, and this intra-abdominal lipolysis causes a rapid increase in the free fatty acid flow into the liver via the portal vein. This in turn predisposes to hyperinsulinaemia, hyperlipidaemia and hypertension. For further discussion of the risk factors associated with abdominal obesity see Chapter 20.

Body fat is synthesised by, and stored in, fat cells, or adipocytes. Adipocytes from subcutaneous white fat can be sampled by needle biopsy and studied in the laboratory. They have a nucleus in a thin rind of cytoplasm surrounding a large fat globule (see Fig. *evolve* 4.2 🖰). A typical adipocyte in a biopsy sample from a normal-weight person contains about 0.6 µg of fat. If we assume that the 12 kg of fat in the man in Figure 4.1 is stored in adipocytes of this size we can calculate that he has 2.0×10^{10} fat cells in his body. If a biopsy sample is taken from an obese adult with, say, 60 kg of body fat, the average adipocyte is not five times the normal size, but only about 50% larger than normal, so there must be more adipocytes than normal in obese people. This reasoning led to the hypothesis that if a child became obese before a certain age then proliferation of adipocytes was stimulated, and the child would be predisposed to obesity in later life.

We now know the hypothesis is not true, because new adipocytes can develop at any age if the amount of fat to be stored increases. However, the idea stimulated research into the metabolic activity of adipocytes, which has yielded valuable information. We now know that white adipose tissue has two important functions related to energy balance and reproductive function. Aromatase is an enzyme in adipose tissue that catalyses the conversion of androstenedione to oestrogen, and in postmenopausal women it is the only route of oestrogen production. This probably explains the association between obesity and abnormalities of sex steroid hormones, especially in conditions such as polycystic ovarian syndrome.

There has been intense research into the product of the *ob* gene, which is lacking in the obese mutant mouse. This is the hormone leptin. It was discovered in 1994, it is produced by adipocytes, and it is involved in the control of both food intake and energy expenditure. Obese mice are deficient in leptin and infertile, so there was great excitement when it was shown that administration of leptin cured both obesity and infertility in these animals. Unfortunately studies on obese human subjects showed that they had abnormally high, rather than low, leptin concentrations (leptin resistance), and therapeutically the administration of leptin has not realised early expectations. However, a very small number of obese subjects may have very low levels of leptin due to a congenital disorder impairing the secretion of leptin. The phenotype of these subjects is characterised by childhood obesity, excessive eating and other endocrinological abnormalities (hypothyroidism, hypogonadism, puberty failure, hyperinsulinemia). Replacement therapy with recombinant leptin improves most of the metabolic disorders and it reduces dramatically their energy intake.

Unlike the white fat cell, the brown fat cell has small fat droplets in a cytoplasm rich in mitochondria in which heat can be generated (see Fig. *evolve* 4.2 🖱). It is important to small mammals to be able to generate heat to maintain body temperature in cold environments. Hypothermia is particularly a problem in newborn mammals (including human babies) because their small body mass does not generate enough heat by normal metabolic processes to maintain body temperature, so some extra thermogenic source is required. A defect in thermogenesis is the cause of obesity in some animal models, so it was thought that defective brown fat might be a cause of human obesity. However, obese human beings have a higher (not lower) total heat production than lean people, and in mammals weighing more than 6 kg the heat generated in normal metabolism is sufficient to maintain body temperature in normal environments, so there is no need for additional thermogenesis.

4.3 CHANGES IN BODY SIZE AND COMPOSITION

THROUGHOUT THE LIFESPAN – NORMAL GROWTH AND COMPOSITION

On the first day after fertilisation the human embryo is a single cell, approximately 0.15 mm in diameter. After 2 months of intrauterine life it is about 30 mm long with recognisable head, trunk and limbs; at that stage the head accounts for half the total body length. By the end of normal gestation, at 9 months, the fetus is 500 mm in length and weighs about

3.5 kg: the head is then one-quarter of total length. After two decades of extrauterine life the average adult weighs about 70 kg, is 1.7–1.8 m tall, of which the head accounts for only one-eighth of total stature.

Changes in the ratio of head size to that of the whole body during growth are associated with changes in the chemical composition of the tissues. The embryo contains a very high percentage of water, but with maturation the proportion of water decreases, and there is a shift in the distribution of water from extracellular (with sodium, Na^+, as the chief cation) to intracellular (with potassium, K^+, as the chief cation). As the proportion of water decreases, protein and electrolytes, as a proportion of body weight, increase. Fat is deposited mainly during the last trimester of pregnancy and the first year of extrauterine life. These changes are shown in Table 4.2.

During childhood and adolescence the proportion of water in the body, and the proportion of extracellular to intracellular water, continues to decrease. Increase in total body K, Ca and P in fat-free tissue reflects the increase in intracellular water and growth in the skeleton. Fat-free mass remains fairly constant in both men and women between the ages of 20 and 65 years, but then decreases by about 15% in the next two decades (see Fig. *evolve* 4.3). Throughout adult life there is a trend for fat mass to increase in both men and women, but the increase is more rapid in postmenopausal women. Changes in body composition with age are shown in Table *evolve* 4.2 🖱 and changes in tissue protein content with age in Table *evolve* 4.3 🖱.

EFFECTS OF DIET AND EXERCISE ON BODY SIZE AND COMPOSITION

The laws of thermodynamics require that if over a given period the energy intake of an individual is 10 MJ (2400 kcal) less than energy output, then the energy stored in the body must be reduced by 10 MJ. That is invariably true. However, a decrease of 10 MJ in energy stores may be achieved by losing 0.27 kg of fat, or 2.4 kg of fat-free tissue, or (more probably) an intermediate amount of weight made up from a mixture of lean and fat tissue. But it does not follow that if the individual increases his energy output by 10 MJ (for example by exercising) and does not change his energy intake, the above losses will be achieved. As weight is lost, resting energy expenditure also decreases, so for a given energy

Table 4.2   Effect of growth, malnutrition and obesity on the composition of the body and of fat-free tissue

	FETUS, 20–25 WEEKS	PREMATURE BABY	FULL-TERM BABY	INFANT (1 YEAR)	ADULT MAN	MALNOURISHED INFANT	OBESE MAN
Body weight (kg)	0.3	1.5	3.5	20	70	5	100
Water (%)	88	83	69	62	60	74	47
Protein (%)	9.5	11.5	12	14	17	14	13
Fat (%)	0.5	3.5	16	20	17	10	35
Remainder (%)	2	2	3	4	6	2	5
Fat-free weight (kg)	0.30	1.45	2.94	8.0	58	4.5	65
Water (%)	88	85	82	76	72	82	73
Protein (%)	9.4	11.9	14.4	18	21	15	21
Na (mmol/kg)	100	100	82	81	80	88	02
K (mmol/kg)	43	50	53	60	66	48	64
Ca (g/kg)	4.2	7.0	9.6	14.5	22.4	9.0	20
Mg (g/kg)	0.18	0.24	0.26	3.5	0.5	0.25	0.5
P (g/kg)	3.0	3.8	5.6	9.0	12.0	5.0	12.0

Data compiled from various sources.

intake the energy deficit, and hence the rate of weight loss, also decreases, a process called metabolic adaptation. This effect is quite small: about 70 kJ (16 kcal)/day/kg weight lost in men, and about 50 kJ (12 kcal)/day/kg weight lost in women.

A larger rate of weight loss was observed in a study of 108 obese women whose average starting weight was 100.8 kg (SD 23.6) (see Fig. *evolve* 4.4 📖). On a diet supplying 3.4 MJ (800 kcal)/day their average weight loss in 3 weeks was 5.0 kg, but it was significantly faster (330 g/day) during the first week than during the next 2 weeks (210 g/day). This is because during the first week on a diet, glycogen (and its associated water, see Chapter 6) is lost, with an energy density of 4.2 MJ/kg, but by the second week the tissue lost is a mixture of 75% fat and 25% fat-free mass (FFM), which has an energy density of 30 MJ (7000 kcal)/kg. Very low carbohydrate diets cause rapid initial weight loss because they cause early loss of glycogen and the attached water (glycogen: water ratio is ~ 1:3).

During total starvation weight loss is even more rapid, partly because the energy deficit is greater, and partly because a higher proportion of the weight loss is FFM (to provide amino acids for glucose synthesis; see Section 6.3, under 'Gluconeogenesis – the synthesis of glucose from non-carbohydrate precursors' and Section 8.4, under 'The metabolism of amino acid carbon skeletons'). Severely obese patients lose 300 to 500 g/day on

prolonged starvation, but about 50% of the weight lost is FFM. Total starvation ceased to be an acceptable treatment for gross obesity because several patients died unexpectedly, due to damage to heart muscle, mostly related to altered electrolytes movements, abnormal acid–base homeostasis and decreased protein synthesis.

The interaction between diet, exercise and muscle bulk is controversial. There is no doubt that strenuous isometric exercise causes muscle hypertrophy, and immobilisation causes atrophy of muscle (see Ch. 18). It is also true that exercise increases energy expenditure, so it is plausible that in obese people a combination of a low energy intake and exercise should achieve more fat loss, and less loss of FFM, than diet alone. A meta-analysis of 28 publications reporting trials on overweight subjects (BMI 25–29) showed that aerobic exercise without dietary restriction caused a weight loss of 3 kg in 30 weeks in men, and 1.4 kg in 12 weeks in women, but had no effect on FFM. A more recent systematic review, including 26 cohorts undergoing dietary and behavioural treatment and 29 studies evaluating the effects of bariatric surgery on body composition, has instead observed that the level of negative energy balance is a determinant of FFM loss. In addition, in three randomised controlled trials on obese subjects there was a protective effect of exercise on FFM loss during weight reduction. In summary, a combination of diet and exercise seems to have a protective effect on body composition by preserving fat free mass. However, more studies are needed to confirm these results, particularly in obese subjects.

The effect of diet and exercise on bone density is even more controversial. Studies have shown that calcium supplementation in the diet increases bone density, but bone density is high in African and other countries where people have a low calcium intake but a high level of physical activity. Bone density is clearly affected by diet, exercise and no doubt genetic and other factors not yet clarified. For further discussion see Chapter 24.

CHANGES IN HYDRATION: DIARRHOEA, OEDEMA, KWASHIORKOR, HEART OR KIDNEY FAILURE

In the previous section it has been assumed that there will be no change in the hydration of the body with diet and exercise, but if there is a change in hydration during changes in these factors, there will be weight changes that bear no simple relationship to energy balance.

Total body water is regulated to maintain an osmotic pressure in body fluids of 285 mosmol/kg. If the tonicity of these fluids increases then water intake is stimulated by thirst, and water losses are reduced by secretion of more concentrated urine. If the tonicity decreases, dilute urine is secreted to remove the excess water. Urine osmolality can vary from 50 to 1200 mmol/kg. This regulatory mechanism may be overwhelmed, and dehydration may occur if water losses are very high, as in severe diarrhoea, or with sweat loss in high ambient temperature or during prolonged vigorous exercise. Dehydration may also occur with abuse of diuretic drugs to achieve weight loss, or during the recovery phase of diabetic coma. In severe untreated diabetes mellitus (due to infection, or interruption of insulin administration in a diabetic), the patient becomes dehydrated by two mechanisms. First, the excretion of large amounts of glucose in urine causes an osmotic diuresis and hence excessive loss of water. Second, ketosis is associated with vomiting and further water loss, and potassium leaches out of cells. Treatment of this condition with insulin only makes the dehydration even worse because correction of the acidosis allows potassium to re-enter the cells and causes a catastrophic reduction in extracellular fluids (including blood volume). In the management of diabetic coma the replacement of fluids

(as well as insulin) is essential, and potassium must be replaced judiciously to avoid the dangers of either hyper- or hypokalaemia (see Ch. 21).

The opposite problem of water excess, indicated by oedema, is much more common than dehydration. The commonest cause in elderly people is congestive heart failure: the heart is unable to pump blood out as fast as it returns from the veins, the veins become engorged and leak fluid into the tissues. A similar situation may arise when the glomeruli in the kidney leak albumin into the urine or the liver is unable to synthesise enough albumin, so the plasma oncotic pressure decreases and fluid passes from the vascular system into the extracellular spaces.

Oedema is also a feature of certain types of malnutrition. In prolonged starvation hepatic albumin synthesis is reduced, on which the oncotic pressure of plasma mainly depends, and oedema is a striking feature of kwashiorkor (see Ch. 28). It is particularly important to understand the fluid and electrolyte metabolism of malnourished children who may appear to be dehydrated when in fact they are overhydrated. A marasmic child does not show obvious oedema, but is terribly wasted with wrinkled skin covering an emaciated body. Such children often have vomiting and diarrhoea, so the temptation is to rehydrate the child with intravenous fluid, but this is much more likely to kill the child than save it because an aggressive rehydration therapy would impose a strong haemodynamic load on a weak cardiac muscle causing heart failure. Measurements of total body water (see 'Total body water (TBW)', below) in such children show that water accounts for too large a proportion of body weight: the limbs are thin and the skin wrinkled because almost all the muscle and fat has been lost, not because the child is dehydrated.

4.4 USE OF SIZE AND COMPOSITION DATA IN NUTRITION

FOR ASSESSMENT OF NUTRITIONAL STATUS: OBESITY, THINNESS, MUSCLE WASTING, STUNTING, OSTEOPOROSIS, ANAEMIA

Clinical nutrition is about understanding the relationship between diet and health and about the correction of nutritional disorders in diseased states to re-establish a normal health. To learn more about these relationships we need reliable measures of health and of diet in either individuals or communities. We may define health in terms of longevity, development limited only by genetic potential, and freedom from disease and disability. All these are measurable with reasonable accuracy, but the weakest link is in reliably measuring habitual diet in free-living people. Chapter 31 discusses methods for assessing diet and body composition, many of which are satisfactory for assessing if an individual has been taking a suitable diet, or if the diet has supplied too little, or too much, of certain nutrients. For example, a simple measurement of weight and height, and perhaps also waist circumference, is adequate to identify those individuals who are obese, too thin, or stunted in growth. But simple anthropometry will not tell us if a malnourished infant is overhydrated or underhydrated (see 'Changes in hydration: diarrhoea, oedema, kwashiorkor, heart or kidney failure', above). Unless we could measure body composition accurately we would have not learnt that total starvation, or treatment with supra-physiological doses of thyroid hormones, is not an appropriate treatment for severe obesity, although it causes spectacular weight loss: the problem is that the weight lost includes too much lean tissue and too little fat. We would not know the extent and severity of tissue potassium depletion in a comatose diabetic, or a child with kwashiorkor, if we could not measure total body potassium; in such cases serum potassium concentrations are seriously misleading. We could not compare the relative effects of exercise and diet on the progress of osteoporosis if we could not measure bone density.

Many of the methods for measuring body composition discussed in Section 4.5 are research tools that cannot be used in normal clinical practice, but they serve as reference methods against which to calibrate simpler methods. For example, skinfold thickness has been calibrated against body density to give a measure of body fat.

FOR STANDARDISATION OF METABOLIC RATE/DRUG DOSAGE/RENAL CLEARANCE

Many physiological measurements give results that are related to body size or composition. For example, glomerular filtration rate is higher in large people than in small people, because they have larger kidneys, although someone who weighs 120 kg does not have kidneys twice as large as someone who weighs 60 kg. Autopsy data showed that kidney weight is well correlated with body surface area, which was typically 1.73 m^2 in normal young men in 1930. So now glomerular filtration rates are 'corrected' to a surface area of 1.73 m^2. Energy physiologists had a similar problem, and unfortunately chose the same (inappropriate) solution. It is said that obese people have a lower resting metabolic rate than lean people, and this is a cause of their obesity. Consider Figure 4.1: this person weighs 70 kg and contains 12 kg of fat and 48 kg of FFM. Suppose he becomes obese and gains 40 kg, of which 30 kg is fat and 10 kg is FFM. His resting metabolic rate (RMR) will increase by a factor of 58/48 (1.21) because RMR is proportional to FFM, and his FFM has increased by 1.21. But his weight has increased by 110/70 (1.57) and his surface area by 2.25/1.80 (1.25). If his obese metabolic rate is compared with baseline values in absolute terms it has *increased* by 21%, if 'corrected' for FFM it is unchanged, if 'corrected' for surface area it has *decreased* by 1.21/1.25 (23%), and if 'corrected' for body weight it has *decreased* by 1.21/1.57 (223%). The correct calculation depends on the question to be answered. If the question is 'What is the relationship of energy requirements for weight maintenance after weight gain compared with baseline?' the change should be expressed in absolute values (i.e. 121%). If the question is 'What is the change in metabolism per unit weight of FFM?' the answer is that it has not changed. There is no justification for 'correcting' metabolic rates by either surface area or body weight because they would give an erroneous estimate of energy metabolism owing to the confounding effect of non-energy generating compartments (water) included in the correction.

There are situations in which it is necessary to adjust for body size or composition. This particularly applies to calculating doses of drugs given to small children, such as in cancer therapy and dialysis.

4.5 MEASUREMENT AND INTERPRETATION OF BODY COMPOSITION

ANTHROPOMETRY

Measurements of body composition may be made to assess current nutritional status, or serial measurements may be made to assess change in status. These two purposes require different levels of precision in measurement. For example, if an observer is asked to determine which of two people is more obese a simple measurement of skinfold thickness would serve to rank the subjects correctly. However, if they returned 2 weeks later having lost some weight, and wanted to know which of them had lost more fat, a repeat of the skinfold measurements would not be adequate, because the error of an estimation of fat from skinfolds is large compared with the amount of fat that people lose in 2 weeks. Furthermore, many anthropometric measurements are subject to observer bias. If the observer believes subject A should have lost more fat than B, then a measurement of a skinfold, or circumference, or diameter, may support that prejudice because the observer (consciously or unconsciously) pulls the tape a little tighter on A than on B. (For detailed discussion of the techniques of anthropometry see Section 31.3.)

For sensitivity, precision and objectivity, body weight is the best and most reliable of all anthropometric measurements. Do not trust the slimming club leader who says: 'Your weight has slightly increased since last week, but my measurements show that your fat has decreased, so you must have gained lean tissue'. It is far more likely that the measurement of fat is inaccurate.

In adults the easiest anthropometric measure of fatness is to measure weight (W, kg) and height (H, m) and calculate W/H^2. The normal range in adults is between 20 and 25 kg/m^2. This measurement was suggested by the Belgian astronomer Quetelet in 1869, and so is known as Quetelet's index. However, in the USA the same index was proposed in 1972 by Keys, and named body mass index (BMI). The application of this index in the study of obesity and undernutrition is discussed in more detail in Chapters 20 and 31. In growing children the normal range of BMI changes with age, so age-specific standards must be used. See Ellis (2000) and Jebb & Wells (2005) for a more detailed overview of this method.

Skinfold thickness and mid-upper arm circumference (MUAC)

In adults the percentage body fat can be estimated by measuring, with special calipers, the sum of thickness of the skinfolds over the biceps, triceps, subscapular and supra-iliac sites. For a given skinfold thickness the corresponding fat content varies with age and gender: Table 4.3 shows the relationship of skinfold to percentage body fat. Accurate measurement of skinfold thickness requires good technique, which is described in Chapter 31.

Table 4.3   Percentage body fat in men and women related to the sum of four skinfolds (biceps, triceps, subscapular and suprailiac)

SKINFOLD (MM)	MEN, AGE (YEARS)				WOMEN, AGE (YEARS)			
	17–29	*30–39*	*40–49*	*50+*	*17–29*	*30–39*	*40–49*	*50+*
20	8.1	12.2	12.2	12.6	14.1	17.0	19.8	21.4
30	12.9	16.2	17.7	18.6	19.5	21.8	24.5	26.6
40	16.4	19.2	21.4	22.9	23.4	25.5	28.2	30.3
50	19.0	21.5	24.6	26.5	26.5	28.2	31.0	33.4
60	21.2	23.5	27.1	29.2	29.1	30.6	33.2	35.7
70	23.1	25.1	29.3	31.6	31.2	32.5	35.0	37.7
80	24.8	26.6	31.2	33.8	33.1	34.3	36.7	39.6
90	26.2	27.8	33.0	35.8	34.8	35.8	38.3	41.2
100	27.6	29.0	34.4	37.4	36.4	37.25	39.7	42.6
110	28.8	30.1	35.8	39.0	37.8	38.6	41.0	42.9
120	30.0	31.1	37.0	40.4	39.0	39.6	42.0	45.1
130	31.0	31.9	38.2	41.8	40.2	40.6	43.0	46.2
140	32.0	32.7	39.2	43.0	41.3	41.6	44.0	47.2
150	32.9	33.5	40.2	44.1	42.3	42.6	45.0	48.2
160	33.7	34.3	41.2	45.1	43.3	43.6	45.8	49.2
170	34.5	34.8	42.0	46.1	44.1	44.4	46.6	50.0

Source: from data reported by Durnin & Womersley (1974).

Mid-upper arm circumference is a useful tool for assessing the nutritional status of both adults and children in famine conditions. The technique of measurement and calculation is given in Chapter 31.

It has been recognised in the last decade that intra-abdominal fat has a greater influence on the risk of heart disease and diabetes than an equal weight of fat in subcutaneous sites (see Chs 19 and 21). Attempts have therefore been made to estimate intra-abdominal fat by measurements of waist circumference, or sagittal diameter. However, these measurements are difficult to make accurately, and computerised scanning techniques, such as computer assisted tomography or magnetic resonance imaging, are now generally used to assess intra-abdominal fat. See Ellis (2000) and Jebb & Wells (2005) for a more detailed overview of this method.

BODY FAT

There is no 'best' method for measuring body composition in living subjects: every method has errors, and some methods require expensive laboratory equipment that would be impossible to use in the field, for example during famine relief. The first three methods described below estimate FFM and so, by subtraction from total body weight, fat mass (FM). They all require expensive laboratory equipment and cooperative subjects. They are used (preferably in combination) to provide reference values with which simpler methods can be compared and calibrated. They all depend on an assumption, based on the data in Table 4.1, that the fat-free body has a constant density, water content and potassium content.

Body density

Human fat at body temperature has a density of 0.900 g/cm^3. The remainder of the body (the fat-free mass) is a mixture of water, protein, bone mineral, glycogen, and minor components such as nucleic acids and electrolytes. This mixture has a density of approximately 1.100 g/cm^3 (Keys & Brozek 1953). Therefore if we know the average density of all the tissues of the body we can calculate the ratio of fat to fat-free mass: for example, if the average density was 1.00 g/cm^3 then that person must be 50% fat and 50% FFM. The body shown in Figure 4.1 weighs 70 kg and has 12 kg fat, so his fat content is 17% and his total body density would be 1.06 g/cm^3.

It is easy to measure the weight of a subject accurately, but difficult to measure tissue volume with similar accuracy. For example, the 70 kg subject who is 50% fat will have a volume of 70 litres, but if he had only 17% fat his volume would be 66.05 litres. The usual method for measuring body volume is to compare body weight in air and totally immersed in water: the decrease in weight on immersion shows the volume of water displaced. However, some of the water is displaced by air trapped in the subject's lungs and gut, and if allowance is not made for this the fat content of the subject will be overestimated. It is difficult to measure this trapped air, so other methods for measuring FFM that do not require total immersion have been developed, such as air displacement plethysmography, commonly known as 'Bod Pod', which is gradually replacing the hydrodensitometric method. A further development of this technique is a smaller device, using the same principle, called Pea-Pod, to measure body density in infants (Garrow et al 1979, McCrory et al 1995, Fields et al 2002, Ma et al 2004).

Total body water (TBW)

The total amount of water in the body can be measured quite accurately by isotope dilution. The subject is given a known dose of water labelled with deuterium (^2H), the stable heavy isotope of hydrogen, and this is allowed to equilibrate with total body water, which takes about 3 hours. Then the dilution of ^2H in a sample representative of body water, such as blood plasma, is measured, and TBW is calculated. Fat (by definition) does not contain any water. If we assume that the fat-free tissues contain 73% of water, then FFM is TBW/0.73. By subtraction of FFM from body weight, the weight of fat in the body is estimated.

The limitations of this approach are that it requires a high-precision isotope-ratio mass spectrometer with a competent operator to measure the concentration of ^2H in the equilibrated body water sample, and that in many conditions the assumption that FFM is 73% water is not valid. In patients with oedema caused by heart or kidney disease, in severely obese people, and in severely malnourished people, the assumption that FFM is TBW/0.73 will overestimate FFM and hence underestimate fat. In dehydrated subjects the same assumption will overestimate fat.

It is possible to measure subcompartments of total body water using a similar dilution principle.

Instead of using deuterated water as a tracer, a tracer that distributes only in the vascular space (such as radiolabelled red cells) can be used to measure blood volume. Various compounds (such as thiocyanate, sodium bromide, sodium sulphate or inulin) that distribute in the extracellular water can be used to measure the volume of extracellular water. These measurements are rarely made in clinical practice. The situation in which it is dangerous to life to have an excessive volume of extracellular water is congestive heart failure, leading to over-filling of the venous circulation, pulmonary oedema and death. In this case central venous pressure is easier, quicker and more relevant to measure.

Total body potassium (TBK)

All potassium (K), including that in the human body, contains a natural radioactive isotope (^{40}K), so each gram of K emits three gamma rays per second. This radiation is of high energy (1.46 MeV) so most of it emerges from the tissues and can be counted by high sensitivity detectors. However, this level of radiation is low compared with the normal background, which arises mainly from cosmic rays, so the subject being measured, and the detectors, must be screened by a massive shield of lead and steel. With this cumbersome and expensive 'whole body counter' it is possible to measure total body potassium and, assuming a constant K content in FFM, to calculate FFM, and hence fat mass.

The value of this technique is mainly that the errors in estimates of body composition by TBK and TBW arising from oedema or dehydration are in opposite directions. With oedema TBK overestimates fat, while TBW underestimates fat; with dehydration the converse applies. However, the practical inconvenience and the limited availability of whole body counters means that this method is very rarely used today.

A 'gold standard' for measurement of fat and fat-free mass

For research purposes it is useful to have a best, or 'gold standard', estimate of fat and FFM in living subjects against which simpler methods can be compared. The two-compartment models regard body weight as the sum of fat and FFM, and make assumptions about density, water or potassium content for FFM. If the assumptions are wrong, then the estimate is wrong. To try to avoid this source of

error the four-compartment models measure water (see 'Total body water (TBW)', above) and bone mineral by DEXA (see 'Dual-energy X-ray absorptiometry (DEXA)', below) and density (see 'Body density', above). Knowing the water and bone mineral content of the body, the remainder must be either fat or non-mineral, non-water FFM, which means essentially protein and glycogen. Thus by combining the results of three measurements (water, density and bone mineral) it is not necessary to assume that FFM has a density of 1.100 or a water content of 73% (Wang et al 1992). The relation of body weight to body fat, measured by these three methods, is shown in Figure *evolve* 4.5 🖥️. Over a wide range of weight (42–132 kg) and fat (9–75 kg) the relationship is linear ($r = 0.960$) with a slope of 1.27. This shows that for every 1 kg extra fat by which an obese woman exceeds a normal-weight control, body weight is (on average) increased by 1.27 kg. The excess weight is not pure fat, but about 75% fat and 25% a mixture of water and protein.

Dual–energy X-ray absorptiometry (DEXA)

Unlike the methods discussed so far, this technique measures three compartments of the body: fat, lean soft tissue and bone mineral. The analysis is based on an X-ray image composed of individual pixels, rather than shades of grey on a conventional X-ray film, just as digital photography differs from conventional film photography. The X-ray source produces rays of two defined energies: 100 and 140 keV (Hologic), 38 and 70 keV (Lunar), or 49 and 80 keV (Norland) in the three commercially available instruments. These pairs of beams are scanned across the area of interest in the subject (which may be the whole body) and the energy spectrum of the emerging beam is analysed. When the beam passes through material of high opacity to X-rays (such as bone mineral) the emerging energy is severely attenuated, but especially the lower energy beam. When the tissue being irradiated is fat there will be very little attenuation of either beam, and if the tissue is lean soft tissue the attenuation will be intermediate. At each instant the energy emerging is recorded in a pixel relating to that particular beam position, and the information stored in all the pixels is integrated by the computer to provide an estimate of the composition of the tissue scanned. An important check on the validity of DEXA analyses is that the computer makes an independent estimate of total body weight (by summing estimated fat, soft tissue and bone), and this estimate can be compared with body weight obtained by simple weighing.

The technique was originally devised to measure bone mineral density, which can be done by comparing the energy spectrum in pixels derived from an instant when the beam went through bone with adjacent pixels in which the beam has just missed the bony structure. However, the newer instruments analyse the energy spectrum in pixels where the tissue is a mixture of lean soft tissue and fat and, since the attenuation coefficient of both of these is known, the ratio of lean tissue to fat can be calculated. For a more detailed review of the technique see Genton et al 2002.

It is important to note that the 'fat' determined by the methods previously discussed is not the same as the 'adipose tissue' determined by DEXA. With the DEXA technique what is being measured is the ability of a particular core of tissue to absorb X-rays of two energies. If this attenuation matches the values assigned to 'fat' then the computer reports the tissue as fat, but if that tissue was dissected out it would be mainly fat, but also contain some protein and water, because the adipose cells that contain fat also contain some protein and water. By contrast, methods that depend on measuring body density or water would include the water component of adipose tissue as 'fat-free mass', because it is not fat. It would help if authors would use the terms 'fat' and 'fat-free mass' to describe results that are obtained by methods that measure the chemical composition of the tissue, and 'adipose tissue' and 'lean body mass' to describe results that are obtained by measuring the X-ray absorption of tissues. Unfortunately many authors use the terms interchangeably.

The DEXA method has been described in some detail because it has become one of the most common methods for measuring body composition in living subjects. The scan can be performed in 5–10 minutes, which is much quicker and less demanding on the subject than measurements of density, water or potassium. It is much more accurate and independent of operator bias than any technique depending on anthropometry. The radiation dose to the subject is very low, about equivalent to one day of background radiation. It measures bone mineral, which can otherwise only be measured by CT scan, which is more expensive and involves a higher radiation dose. Perhaps the most important advantage over all other methods (except CAT and MRI scan) is that it permits analysis of specific regions of the body, in particular the adipose tissue within the abdominal cavity, and the muscle mass in the limbs.

Computer imaging

Undoubtedly the development of better techniques for computer analysis of X-ray imaging has led to the most important advances in the measurement of human body composition in the last decade. In conventional radiography a wide parallel beam of X-rays (or gamma rays) is passed through the tissues of a subject, and from the rays that emerge on the other side an image is formed on a sheet of photographic film. Where the tissue is relatively opaque to the X-rays (as in bone) the film is little exposed, and therefore remains clear when the film is developed. Where the tissue is easily penetrated by X-rays (as in lung) the film is dark, and where there is tissue of intermediate density (such as muscle) there are various shades of grey.

In computed tomography (CT) the X-rays are emitted in a narrow beam from a source that travels in a semi-circle round the subject, and the energy emerging from the body is recorded by a detector which is mounted diametrically opposite the X-ray source. A computer is programmed to analyse the constantly changing output of the detector, and from this information it constructs a picture of the 'slice' of body that has been scanned. Since fat, water, lean tissue and bone have different absorption characteristics, the computer shows on a video screen a picture of the distribution of these tissues, as if the subject had been cut through at the level of the scan. If serial scans are performed at different levels of the body from head to foot it is possible to build up data on the total volume of different types of tissue, and how these tissues are distributed in different sections of the body. An alternative technique is to use helical computed tomography, in which the radiation source rotates around the supine patient, who lies on a table that travels at a constant speed. Thus the scan, instead of being in a series of parallel slices, is made in a continuous spiral. This technique reduces errors arising from respiratory movements in the subject.

CT scanning has proved very valuable in showing the size and position of abnormal tissue (such as tumours) in the body, but it is expensive and involves a rather high dose of radiation, so it is not suitable for routine estimation of body composition in normal subjects.

Magnetic resonance imaging (MRI) is a relatively new application in body composition research and its application is constantly growing. MRI utilises the different electromagnetic properties of tissues to reconstruct high-quality images of the organs inside the body. More specifically this technique exploits the physical properties of the water molecule which carries an asymmetric charge. If a body is placed in a strong magnetic field some hydrogen nuclei will change their orientation in the field but they will flip back when the magnetic field is switched off. The return to the their original state will release energy which is then captured, integrated and converged into images which show the differences in energy state and level of hydration of the tissues. The potential applications of MRI are large in body composition research owing to the high resolution of the images and to the non-radioactive nature of the radiations. The procedure is very expensive but the information on tissue distribution and anatomo-morphological characteristics of organs can give precious insights into the relationship between body composition and nutritional status in health and disease (Ross, 2003).

Neutron activation

If a person is irradiated with a beam of fast neutrons, some elements (notably nitrogen, calcium, chlorine, sodium, carbon and some of the trace elements) form very short-lived radioactive isotopes. The radiation from these isotopes can be detected, and hence the body content of these elements can be calculated. By this method it is possible to measure, for example, total body calcium. This is an extremely expensive procedure, and involves a significant radiation dose to the subject, so it is only applicable to some very specialised research protocols.

Electrical conductivity

Fat is an electrical (as well as a thermal) insulator, but the FFM is a tissue bathed in an electrolyte solution, and therefore is a good conductor. If a small electric current is passed from the hand to the foot of two subjects of the same weight and height, but with different proportions of fat to FFM, the voltage drop will be greater in the fatter than in the leaner subject, because the higher fat content in the fatter subject offers more resistance to the electric current. Obviously, there are many problems to be overcome before this difference in electrical conductivity between the two hypothetical subjects can reliably be converted into estimates of FFM.

Heitmann (1990) validated estimates of FFM obtained with a commercial 'bio-impedance analyser' (BIA) against a four-compartment model using total body water, total body potassium, weight and height. The standard deviation of the difference between the two methods was 4.36 kg.

There are now several commercial BIA instruments; some require the operator to attach electrodes to the hands and feet (tetrapolar method) of the subject while others have electrodes in the baseplates of a stand-on machine (leg-to-leg method).

A weakness of whole-body BIA is that it measures the average impedance of an ill-defined electrical path through the arm, trunk and leg. The cross-sectional area of the limbs is much less than that of the trunk, so the limbs make a disproportionately great contribution to overall impedance and, other things being equal, subjects with long limbs will have a greater impedance, and therefore a smaller estimated FFM, than subjects with shorter limbs. Recent innovations include the development of the method to estimate segmental body composition by assessing electrical conductivity of the limb and truncal sections separately. Also, the frequency of the alternating current affects the ability of the current to penetrate from extracellular to intracellular water. Multi-frequency devices have been developed to measure the specific resistance offered by the extracellular fluid (low frequencies) and intracellular fluid compartments (high frequencies). See Kyle et al (2004a,b) for a more detailed overview of this method.

4.6 ESTIMATING CHANGE IN BODY COMPOSITION

Body composition measurements may be made to find out if a given patient, or population, has an abnormal amount of some component, such as fat or bone mineral. The techniques described above will usually provide a reliable answer to this question.

The estimate of changes in body compartments is a different matter and therefore the accuracy, the precision and the technical features of the different body composition methods discussed above have to be taken into account to maximise the likelihood of detecting significant clinical changes after an intervention. Different techniques differ in their capacity to measure changes in body composition and the integration of this capacity with the precision of the method, the sample size and the biological variation of the outcome will give an estimate of the likelihood to detect significant differences. For example, a bigger sample size will increase the chance to detect significant changes whereas a decrease in precision or an increase in the biological variation will decrease the sensitivity.

The choice of the best method is very much based on the nature of the primary outcome of interest. If, for example, it is important to measure in individuals the composition of changes in body fat, an evaluation of the characteristics of the body composition techniques available in the study, the sample size, the biological variability of fat mass in that particular population and the time interval between measurements are objective factors which have to be considered for a rational selection of the method to be used in the intervention. The four-compartment model of body composition is currently considered the best method to estimate changes in fat mass as it eliminates most of the assumptions made by the individual techniques. The alternative is to perform metabolic balance studies to measure the total intake and output of the element of interest – for example N balance for protein, and Ca balance for bone mineral.

KEY POINTS

- There are remarkably few data on the chemical composition of the body from analysis of cadavers; a healthy adult male contains about 60% water, 17% protein and 17% fat.
- Total body water, the partition between intracellular and extracellular water, and its electrolyte composition are normally tightly regulated.
- The skeleton accounts for 14% of total body weight. Bone contains 99% of total body calcium, which acts as a reservoir to maintain an appropriate plasma concentration of calcium. Bone turnover can be estimated from the urinary excretion of hydroxyproline.
- Skeletal muscle accounts for 40% of body weight, and smooth muscle 10%, but resting muscle accounts for only 22% of basal metabolic rate.
- Total blood volume is about 5 litres, of which 55% is plasma and 45% packed cells.
- In a lean male fat amounts to 17% of body weight, of which about 80% can be considered to be energy reserves.
- Fat reserves are in white adipose tissue. White adipocytes contain about 80% triacylglycerol, as a single central droplet surrounded by a thin layer of cytoplasm containing the nucleus.
- Males tend to accumulate fat in the abdomen, while women accumulate subcutaneous fat stores around the breast, hip and thigh. In obesity, people may accumulate fat in the male or female pattern; this is probably genetically determined. Abdominal adipose tissue is more closely related to diabetes and heart disease than is total body fat.

- In addition to being a storage organ, adipose tissue has endocrine functions concerned with fertility and regulation of food intake and energy balance.
- Brown adipose tissue cells contain small droplets of triacylglycerol in a cytoplasm rich in mitochondria. Its main function is thermogenesis, especially in infants.
- Body composition changes throughout life. The water content of the body decreases, and the content of protein and fat increases, through gestation, infancy and into adolescence.
- Fat-free mass remains relatively constant from age 20 to 65, but then decreases; fat mass increases throughout adult life.
- Food restriction and starvation result in loss of fat-free mass as well as adipose tissue.
- Excessive water losses can lead to dehydration.
- A variety of conditions can lead to excessive accumulation of body water, resulting in oedema. Even severely wasted undernourished people may be oedematous.
- Assessment of body composition can be used to assess current nutritional status; serial measurements assess changes in status.
- Most of the methods available to assess body composition are research methods that are not suitable for use in the field or clinic; they are used to validate simpler methods that are applicable to field and clinic use.
- The two most common methods of assessing body fat are skinfold thickness and (becoming increasingly applicable outside research laboratories) dual-energy X-ray absorptiometry (DEXA) and air displacement plethysmography.

References

Durnin JVGA, Womersley J: Body fat assessed from total body density and its estimation from skinfold thickness: measurements on 481 men and women aged from 16 to 72 years, *British Journal of Nutrition* 23:77–97, 1974.

Ellis K: Human body composition: in vivo methods, *Physiological Reviews* 80:649–680, 2000.

Fields DA, Goran MI, McCrory MA: Body-composition assessment via air-displacement plethysmography in adults and children: a review, *American Journal of Clinical Nutrition* 75:453–467, 2002.

Garrow JS, Stalley S, Diethelm R, et al: A new method for measuring body density of obese adults, *British Journal of Nutrition* 42:173–183, 1979.

Genton L, Hans D, Kyle UG, et al: Dual-energy X-ray absorptiometry and body composition: differences between devices and comparison with reference methods, *Nutrition* 18:66–70, 2002.

Heitmann BL: Evaluation of body fat estimated from body mass index, skinfolds and impedance: a comparative study, *European Journal of Clinical Nutrition* 44:831–837, 1990.

Jebb SAJ, Wells JCK: Measuring body composition in adults and children. In Kopelman P, Caterson I, Dietz W, editors: *Clinical obesity in adults and children*, 2005, Oxford, Blackwell, pp 12–28.

Keys A, Brozek J: Body fat in adult man, *Physiological Reviews* 33:245–325, 1953.

Kyle UG, Bosaeus I, De Lorenzo AD, et al: Bioelectrical impedance analysis – part I: review of principles and methods, *Clinical Nutrition* 23:1226–1243, 2004a.

Kyle UG, Bosaeus I, De Lorenzo AD, et al: Bioelectrical impedance analysis – part II: utilization in clinical practice, *Clinical Nutrition* 23:1430–1453, 2004b.

Ma G, Yao M, Liu Y, et al: Validation of a new paediatric air phlethysmography for assessing body composition in infants, *American Journal of Clinical Nutrition* 79:653–660, 2004.

McCrory MA, Gomez TD, Bernauer EM, et al: Evaluation of a new air displacement plethysmography for measuring human body composition, *Medical Science in Sports and Exercise* 27:1686–1691, 1995.

Ross R: Advances in the application of imaging methods in applied and clinical physiology, *Acta Diabetologica* 40:S45-S50, 2003.

Wang Z, Pierson R Jr, Heymsfield S: The five-level model: a new approach to organizing body-composition research, *American Journal of Clinical Nutrition* 56:19–28, 1992.

Further reading

Brodie D, Moscrip V, Hutcheon R: Body composition measurement: a review of hydrodensitometry, anthropometry and impedance methods, *Nutrition* 14:296–310, 1998.

Chaston TB, Dixon JB, O'Brien PE: Changes in fat free mass during significant weight loss: a systematic review, *International Journal of Obesity and Related Metabolic Disorders* 31:743–750 2007.

Demerath EW, Guo SS, Chumlea WC, et al: Comparison of percent body fat estimates using air displacement plethysmography and hydrodensitometry in adults and children, *International Journal of Obesity and Related Metabolic Disorders* 26:389–397, 2002.

Norgan NG: Laboratory and field measurements of body composition, *Public Health Nutrition* 8:1108–1122, 2005.

Rogalla P, Meii N, Hoksch B, et al: Low-dose spiral computed tomography for measuring abdominal fat volume and distribution in a clinical setting, *European Journal of Clinical Nutrition* 52:597–602, 1998.

Chapter 5

Energy balance and body weight regulation

Abdul G Dulloo and Yves Schutz

CHAPTER CONTENTS

© 2010 Elsevier Ltd/Inc/BV
DOI: 10.1016/B978-0-7020-3118-2.00005-X

OBJECTIVES

By the end of this chapter you should be able to:
- Define types and units of energy
- Understand the concept of metabolisable energy intake
- Describe the main factors affecting energy intake
- Describe the assessment of energy needs and approximate values throughout the life cycle
- Explain the components of energy expenditure, their relative size and variability
- Describe the classic and modern methods of measurement of energy expenditure and their validity for different purposes
- Identify the main types of signals in relation to hunger and satiety
- Describe the changes in energy expenditure that occur in response to undernutrition and overnutrition
- Summarise the components of models of energy intake and energy expenditure.

5.1 INTRODUCTION

Understanding how body weight is regulated is still challenging for human research today. It is likely that long-term constancy of body weight is achieved through a highly complex network of regulatory systems through which changes in food intake, body composition and energy expenditure are interlinked. Failure of this regulation leads either to obesity and its co-morbidities or to protein-energy malnutrition and cachexia in disease states such as anorexia, cancer and infections. Between these disorders attributed to 'failure of regulation' lie those due to chronic undernutrition because of poverty, war and famine. Achieving energy balance and weight homeostasis is central to the quality of life. An understanding of how they are achieved requires an appreciation of the following:

- the basic concepts and principles about the flux of energy transformations through which body weight is regulated,
- an appraisal of factors affecting food intake and energy expenditure, which represent the entry and exit in this flux of energy transformations,
- the methods for assessing energy expenditure and energy requirements, and
- a number of models that have been proposed to explain the regulation of body weight and body composition in humans.

5.2 BASIC CONCEPTS AND PRINCIPLES IN HUMAN ENERGETICS

ENERGY BALANCE AND THE LAWS OF THERMODYNAMICS

Energy represents the capacity of a system to perform work. It can appear in various forms – light, chemical, mechanical, electrical – all of which can be completely converted to heat. According to the first law of thermodynamics, energy cannot be created or destroyed but can only be transformed from one form into another. Biological systems, like machines, depend on the transformation of some form of energy in order to perform work. Whereas plants depend on light energy captured from the sun to synthesise molecules like carbohydrates, proteins and fats, animals meet their energy needs from chemical energy stored in plants or in other animals. The chemical energy obtained from foods (plant or animal in origin) is used to perform a variety of work, such as in the synthesis of new macromolecules (chemical work), in muscular contraction (mechanical work) or in the maintenance of ionic gradients across membranes (electrical work). Overall energy balance is given by the following equation:

$$\text{Energy intake} = \text{Energy expenditure} + \Delta \text{Energy stores}$$

Thus, if the total energy contained in the body (as fat, protein and glycogen) is not altered (i.e. Δ Energy stores = 0), then energy expenditure must be equal to energy intake, when the individual is said to be in a state of energy balance. If the intake and expenditure of energy are not equal, then a change in body energy content will occur, with negative energy balance resulting in the utilisation of the body's energy stores (glycogen, fat and protein) or positive energy balance resulting in an increase in body energy stores, primarily as fat. There are, however, interrelationships between energy intake and energy expenditure. Voluntary energy intake may rise with intense physical activity (lumberjacks eat more than clerks), energy expenditure may increase in response to increased food intake, and both energy intake and expenditure can be influenced by changes in body energy stores (body fat depletion may lead to increased hunger and reduced energy expenditure).

The second law of thermodynamics, in biological terms, makes a subtle distinction between the potential energy of food, useful work and heat. It states that when food is utilised in the body, whether for muscle contraction, synthesis of new tissues or maintenance of electrolyte equilibrium across membranes, these processes must be accompanied inevitably by a loss of heat. In thermodynamic terms, some energy is degraded, and such heat energy, which is no longer available for work, is termed 'entropy'. In other words, the conversion of available food energy is not a perfectly efficient process, and about 75% of the chemical energy contained in foods may be ultimately dissipated as heat because of the inefficiency of intermediary metabolism in transforming food energy into a form (e.g. adenosine triphosphate, ATP) which can be used for useful work, whether it be the internal work required to maintain structure and function or external physical work.

UNITS OF ENERGY

Since all the energy used by the body at rest is ultimately lost as heat, and physical (external) work will also be eventually degraded as heat, the energy that is consumed, stored and expended is expressed as its heat equivalent. The calorie was originally adopted as the unit of energy in nutrition; it is defined as the amount of heat required to raise the temperature of 1 gram of water by 1°C (from 14.5 to 15.5°C); nutritionally the kilocalorie (= 1000 calories) is used . With the introduction of the SI system, energy is expressed as joules (J). One joule is the energy used when a mass of 1 kilogram (kg) is moved through 1 metre (m) by a force of 1 newton (N). Because one joule is a very small unit of energy,

it is more convenient to use kilojoules (kJ), or megajoules (MJ) in nutrition. Rates of energy expenditure (often referred to as metabolic rate) are expressed in kJ or MJ per unit time (kJ/min or MJ/day), which correspond to 10^3 J and 10^6 J, respectively. The conversion of calorie to joules is: 1 calorie = 4.18 J, or 1 kilocalorie (kcal) = 4.18 kilojoules (kJ).

SOURCES OF ENERGY AND MACRONUTRIENT BALANCE

The macronutrients (carbohydrate, fat, protein and alcohol) are the sources of energy, so it makes sense to consider energy balance and macronutrient balance together. There is a strong relationship between energy balance and macronutrient balance, and the sum of individual substrate balance (expressed as energy) must be equivalent to the overall energy balance. Thus, it follows that:

$$\text{exogenous carbohydrate} - \text{carbohydrate oxidation} = \text{carbohydrate balance}$$

$$\text{exogenous protein} - \text{protein oxidation} = \text{protein balance}$$

$$\text{exogenous lipid} - \text{lipid oxidation} = \text{lipid balance}$$

$$\text{total energy intake} - \text{total oxidation} = \text{energy balance}$$

Unlike the size of the fat stores, which can increase very considerably, there is a limited capacity for storing protein in fat-free mass and carbohydrate as glycogen in liver and muscles (Table 5.1). It is therefore not surprising that protein and glucose tend to be oxidised more readily than fat, and that alcohol, which is not stored in the body, is oxidised rapidly (sparing fat).

Acute substrate imbalance, resulting from acute changes in either substrate intake (in absolute or relative value) or substrate oxidation, or both, is of paramount importance for our understanding of short term, day-to-day body weight changes.

Figure 5.1 demonstrates that large weight changes over the short term necessarily involve storage of a low energy density substrate such as glycogen, which is stored with water in tissues and has an energy density about nine times lower than fat (triglycerides) stored in adipose tissue.

In positive balance, lipids stored in adipose tissue can originate from dietary (exogenous) lipids or from nonlipid precursors, mainly from CHOs

Table 5.1	Macronutrient storage in the body, its energy density and its degree of autoregulation				
SUBSTRATE	FORM OF STORAGE	POOL SIZE	TISSUES	ENERGY DENSITY (kJ/g)	AUTOREGULATION
Carbohydrate	Glycogen	Small	Liver, Muscle	~4	Accurate
Fat	Triglycerides	Moderate-large (unlimited)	Adipose tissue	~33	Poor
Protein	Protein	Moderate (limited)	Lean tissue	~4	Accurate

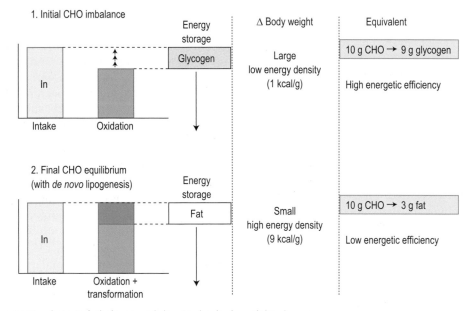

Fig. 5.1 Short-term substrate imbalance and day-to-day body weight changes.

but also from ethanol, that is, from substrates, which produce acetyl-CoA (during their catabolism), and are therefore susceptible to be converted to fatty acids in the intermediary metabolism. This process is known as de novo lipogenesis (DNL). The conversion of CHO into fat is a high energy-requiring process as compared to the direct storage of exogenous fat as body fat. About 25% of the energy content of CHOs is converted into heat, whereas the deposition of dietary triglycerides into adipose tissue requires only about 2% energy. Therefore, DNL from CHO would theoretically constitute a protective factor inhibiting the increase in body fat stores.

In summary, fat-free mass (FFM) is a large compartment (about 80% of body weight in non-obese men) that is capable of dynamically utilising glucose and fatty acids released from adipose

tissue and other tissues. In the size-limited, labile glycogen-water pool (which belongs to FFM compartment) exogenous CHO is stored (muscles and liver) and quickly released on demand thanks to a fast glycogen turnover (Figure 5.2).

Carbohydrates may be transformed into fat (by net de novo lipogenesis) involving a spilling-over process in case of continuous metabolic CHO overload. This occurs only when the glycogen stores are becoming full. By contrast, the adipose (fat) mass is a relatively smaller compartment than FFM (about 20% of body weight in non-obese men) but larger than the glycogen-water pool. Fat mass is capable of utilising mostly glucose from the circulation and not typically fatty acids. The turnover of fat mass is very slow compared with the glycogen–water pool. Today we believe that it is also a site of de novo lipogenesis.

Fig. 5.2 Dietary fat and carbohydrate (CHO) turnover.

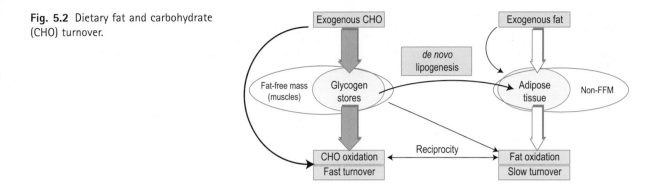

5.3 ENERGY INTAKE

ENERGY VALUE OF FOODS AND ATWATER FACTORS

The traditional way of measuring the energy content of foostuffs is to use a 'bomb calorimeter' in which the heat produced when a sample of food is combusted (in presence of oxygen) is measured. When the food is combusted, it is completely oxidised to water, carbon dioxide and oxides of other elements such as sulphur and nitrogen. The total heat liberated (expressed in kilocalories or kilojoules) represents the gross energy value or heat of combustion of the food. The heat of combustion differs between carbohydrates, proteins, and fats. There are also important differences within each category of macronutrient. The gross energy yield of sucrose, for example, is 16.5 kJ/g, whereas starch yields 17.7 kJ/g. The energy yield of butterfat is 38.5 kJ/g and of lard 39.6 kJ/g. These values have been rounded off to give 17.3 kJ/g for carbohydrates rich in starch and poor in sugar, 39.3 kJ/g for average fat and 23.6 kJ/g for mixtures of animal and vegetable proteins. The heat of combustion of alcohol is 29 kJ/g.

The gross energy value of foodstuffs, however, does not represent the energy actually available to body, since no potentially oxidisable substrate can be considered available until it is presented to the cell for oxidation. None of the foodstuffs is completely absorbed; some energy therefore never enters the body and is excreted in faeces. Digestibility of the major foodstuffs, however is high; on average 97% of ingested carbohydrates, 95% of fats, and 92% of proteins are absorbed from the intestinal lumen (see Ch. 3). There is a difference between the true and apparent digestibility – the latter includes energy which is excreted in the faeces from

sources such as bacteria in the gut and enzyme secretions.

In the body, the tissues are able to oxidise carbohydrate and fat completely to carbon dioxide and water, but the oxidation of protein is not complete, and results in the formation of urea and other nitrogenous compounds which are excreted in the urine. Determination of both the heat of combustion and the nitrogen content of urine indicates that approximately 33.0 kJ/g of urine nitrogen is equivalent to 5.3 kJ/g of protein since 1 g urinary N arises from ~ 6.25 g protein. This energy represents metabolic loss and must be subtracted from the 'digestible' energy of protein. From these considerations, the 'Atwater factors' for available energy (or metabolisable energy) of the three macronutrients have been derived (Fig. 5.3). It is the metabolisable energy value that is quoted in food composition tables (Southgate & Durnin 1970). It is important to remember that these factors make allowance for the energy in the food lost in faeces and urine. They are physiological approximations based on experiments on a limited number of subjects on one kind of diet.

PATTERNS OF FOOD INTAKE

Human beings eat food in a discontinuous manner, even under conditions of nibbling, and the amount of food eaten can range from zero to up to 21MJ/day in highly active individuals or during acute episodes of hyperphagia. This contrasts with energy expenditure, which is continuous irrespective of the conditions encountered. This irregularity of food behaviour occurs both within-day and between-days, which explains why there is a 2–3 times greater coefficient of variation for energy intake (15–20%) than for energy expenditure (5–8%). It also explains the difficulty in assessing food intake

| Gross energy (kcal/g) | | | |
| Heat of combustion | | | |
Source	Prot.	CHO	Lip.
Animal	5.65	3.90	9.5
Vegetable	5.80	4.20	9.3

Fig. 5.3 Physiological energy value of yielding nutrients obtained in humans consuming a mixed American diet early in the 20th Century.

Coefficient of apparent digestibility		
	Animal	Vegetable
Protein	97	85
CHO	98	97
Lipid	95	90

→ Energy in faeces

Digestible energy (kcal/g)			
Source	Prot.	CHO	Lip.
Animal	5.48	3.82	9.03
Vegetable	4.93	4.07	8.37

→ Energy in urine
7.9 kcal/g N
1.25 kcal/g protein
oxidised

Metabolisable energy (kcal/g)			
Source	Prot.	CHO	Lip.
Animal	4.23	3.82	9.03
Vegetable	3.68	4.07	8.37
Mixed American diet (%)			
Animal	61%	5%	92%
Vegetable	39%	95%	8%
Atwater factors			
	4.0	4.0	9.0

(4.01)   (4.06)   (8.98)

in order to obtain a representative picture of 'habitual' food (energy) intake. The physiological control of food intake is highly complex (see section 5.6 below). There is a wide variety of food behaviour. This makes it extremely difficult to interpret data on food intake, the measurement of which has plagued nutritionists for more than a century. The various methods used to assess energy intake are described in Chapter 31. Some factors leading to underestimation or overestimation of energy intake, and hence leading to a bias in energy balance, are shown in Figure 5.4.

FACTORS AFFECTING PATTERNS OF FOOD INTAKE AND ENERGY INTAKE

Since the ultimate function of energy intake is the provision of energy for metabolic processes and performance of work, body size and physical activity are important factors influencing energy intake.

However, eating is a pleasure which fulfils not only nutritional but also social, cultural, emotional and psychological needs. The increasing buying power in industrialised society, combined with the intense marketing from food companies, has led to a progressive change in eating behaviour over the past two decades. Food technologists are constantly inventing new foods and flavours, which may not be compatible with sound nutritional guidelines. Many processed foods and snacks are rich in refined sugars and fats, and their high energy density and palatability are conducive to overeating. Apart from snacking and quick eating, a non-exhaustive list of the exogenous factors contributing to a poor control of food intake is given in Table 5.2. Among these factors, it has long been known that the nutrient composition of the diet has marked effects on food intake. Diets which are either very low or very high in protein, as well as those with an unbalanced amino acid mixture, tend to depress food intake.

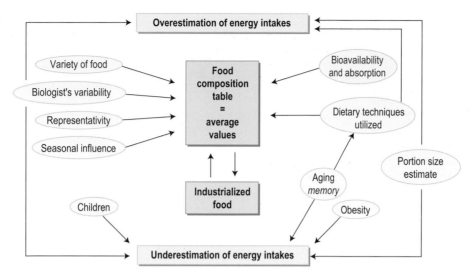

Fig. 5.4 Factors contributing to underestimation or overestimation of energy intake.

Table 5.2	Exogenous factors, typically encountered in affluent societies, contributing to a poor control of food intake in humans

1. Large food diversity and high palatability diets
2. Profuse availability of food
3. Television watching (reduced activity, pressure of food advertising)
4. Snacking rather than meal eating
5. Fast rate of eating ('fast foods')
6. High-energy density diets (e.g. high-fat diet)
7. Eating outside home and unsociable eating
8. Technological developments, less activity
9. Reduced physical activity level
10. Urbanization: more access to energy-dense food, less need to walk

Similarly, low-fat diets cause a reduction in food intake, in part because they are bland and difficult to swallow, and also because of their low energy density; the total bulk may limit energy intake through greater gastric distension and delayed gastric emptying. Furthermore, carbohydrates, and specifically glucose, have been directly implicated in the control of food intake, and it is well established that low blood glucose (hypoglycaemia) stimulates hunger and feeding. By contrast, high-fat diets, in addition to adding palatability to foods, have high energy density and low bulk, which leads to diminished gastric distension and gastric emptying, so retarding the feeling of fullness and the cessation of eating.

5.4 ENERGY EXPENDITURE

COMPONENTS OF TOTAL DAILY ENERGY EXPENDITURE

It is customary to consider energy expenditure as being made up of three components: the energy spent for basal metabolism (or basal metabolic rate), the energy spent on physical activity, and the increase in resting energy expenditure in response to a variety of stimuli (including food, cold, stress and drugs). These three components are depicted in Figure 5.5 model A, and are described below.

Basal metabolic rate (BMR)

This is the largest component of energy expenditure for most individuals. Typically in developed countries, BMR accounts for 60–75% of daily energy expenditure, and reflects the energy needed for the work of vital functions (maintaining electrolyte equilibrium across cell membranes, cell and protein turnover, respiratory and cardiovascular functions, etc.). By far the most important determinant of BMR is body size, and in particular the fat-free mass of the body, which is influenced by weight, height, gender and age. On average, men have greater fat-free mass and BMR than women of the same age, weight and height, and older people have lower fat-free mass and BMR than young adults. Most, but not all, of the differences in BMR

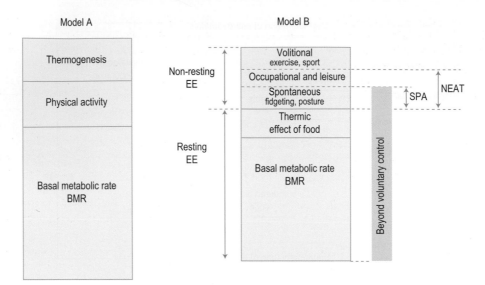

Fig. 5.5 Components of energy expenditure.

between these groups disappear when BMR is expressed as a function of fat-free-mass. This is not surprising since fat-free mass contains tissues and organs which have high metabolic activities such as liver, kidneys, heart, and to a lesser extent the resting muscles. In contrast, the contribution of adipose tissue to BMR is small. BMR can vary up to ±10% between individuals of the same age, gender, body weight and FFM, suggesting that genetic factors are also important. Day-to-day intra-individual variability in BMR is low in men (coefficient of variation of 1–3%) but is larger in women because of changes in BMR over the menstrual cycle. In both women and men, BMR is greater than the metabolic rate during sleep by 5–15%, the difference between BMR and sleeping metabolic rate being explained by the effect of arousal. BMR is known to be depressed during starvation. Although this is to a large extent explained by the loss in body weight and lean tissue, the fall of BMR is often reported to be lower than predicted from the reduction in body weight or FFM. During rapid overfeeding, the evidence that BMR is increased is equivocal, and when it is found to be increased, it is within 5–10% of the excess energy intake.

Energy expenditure due to physical activity

The energy spent on physical activity depends on the type and intensity of the physical activity and on the time spent in different activities. Physical activity is often considered to be synonymous with 'muscular work' which has a strict definition in physics – force × distance, when external work is performed on the environment. During muscular work (muscle contraction), the muscle produces 3–4 times more heat than mechanical energy, so that useful work costs more than muscle work. There is a wide variation in the energy cost of any activity both within and between individuals. The latter variation is due to differences in body size and in the speed and dexterity with which an activity is performed. In order to adjust for differences in body size, the energy cost of physical activities is expressed as multiples of BMR. These generally range from 1–5 for most activities, but can reach values between 10 and 14 during intense exercise. In terms of daily energy expenditure, physical activity can represent up to 70% of daily energy expenditure in an individual involved in heavy manual work or competition athletics. For most people in industrialised societies, however, the contribution of physical activity to daily energy expenditure is relatively small (10–15%). In a hospitalised patient in bed, it is even lower.

Energy expenditure in response to various thermogenic stimuli

This component of energy expenditure – often referred to as 'thermogenesis' – is best described by the various forms in which it can exist. These have been described by Miller (1982) as follows:

1. Isometric thermogenesis: This is due to increased muscle tension; no physical work is done. The differences in energy expenditure in a person who is lying, sitting or standing are due mainly to changes in muscle tone.

2. Dynamic thermogenesis: The term 'negative work' is used to describe heat production of stretched muscle, with heat being again produced without any work. For example, when someone goes down a ladder, heat production increases but no work is done. In the physical sense of work, contracting muscles produce heat because of their inefficiency, but tensed and stretched muscles are simply thermogenic.

3. Psychological thermogenesis: The psychological state may affect energy expenditure, as anxiety, anticipation and stress stimulate adrenaline (epinephrine) secretion, leading to increased heat production. A two-fold difference can be found in the energy cost of sitting at ease and sitting playing chess, a difference that cannot entirely be attributed to muscular movement. The best evidence comes from a study on pilots whose energy expenditure (assessed from heart rate measurements) increased when they were under air traffic control, with the rise being inversely related to their level of experience.

4. Cold-induced thermogenesis: Human beings rarely need to increase heat production for the purpose of thermal regulation because they are able to seek an equitable environment or wear suitable clothing. At low temperatures, resting metabolic rate (and hence heat production) increases. For example, normal weight women maintained in identical clothing in a room calorimeter increased their 24h heat production by about 7% when the temperature in the calorimeter room was lowered from 28 to 22°C. It is customary to distinguish between two forms of cold-induced thermogenesis – shivering and non-shivering thermogenesis. Shivering is rythmic muscle contraction. Non-shivering thermogenesis is increased heat production not associated with muscle contraction, and is due to increased sympathetic nervous system activity, particularly in brown adipose tissue (BAT) in small mammals. Non-shivering thermogenesis is inversely correlated with body size, age and ambient temperature and has been demonstrated in adult human beings chronically exposed to extreme temperatures. Although several lines of evidence are consistent with an important role for the sympathetic nervous system (SNS) in the regulation of thermogenesis in humans, the importance of BAT as a site of adaptive thermogenesis in adults has proved elusive. However, recent morphological and scanning studies have raised the possibility that BAT in humans may not be as rare as once believed. Indeed the use of fluorodeoxyglucose positron emission tomography (FDG-PET) scans have visualised areas of uptake that correspond to BAT, with main depots occurring primarily in the supraclavicular and neck regions, with some additional locations in the axillary and paravertebral regions, of normal individuals. These BAT-like depots express uncoupling protein 1 (UCP1) – the unique identifying characteristic of BAT (Virtanen et al 2009). Furthermore, the demonstrations that the activity of these BAT-like depots (as assessed by uptake of FDG) is stimulated by acute exposure to mild cold and inhibited by β-adrenoceptor blockade are in line with a tissue that is under direct sympathetic neural control. These findings have regenerated interest into approaches to activate BAT for obesity management.

5. Diet-induced thermogenesis: Heat production increases following the consumption of a meal, and this thermic effect of food was classically termed 'specific dynamic action'. Heat production also increases on a high plane of nutrition, the so-called 'luxusconsumption'. These two forms of thermogenesis related to food have been regrouped under the term 'diet-induced thermogenesis' or DIT, and are often divided into an obligatory component (related to the energy costs of absorption and metabolic processing of nutrients or the energy cost of tissue synthesis during overfeeding) and a facultative component which in part results from the sensory aspects of foods (smell and taste) and in part from stimulation of the sympathetic nervous system.

6. Drug-induced thermogenesis: The consumption of caffeine, nicotine and alcohol may form an integral part of daily life for many people, and all three of these drugs stimulate

thermogenesis. A cup of coffee (containing 60–80 mg caffeine) can increase BMR by 5–10% over an hour or two. Oral intake of 100 mg caffeine every two hours during the day or smoking of a packet of 20 cigarettes increases energy expenditure by 5% and 15%, respectively. Furthermore the thermogenic effect of nicotine is potentiated by caffeine. The cessation of elevated thermogenesis induced by nicotine or nicotine and caffeine may be a factor that contributes to the average weight gain of 7 kg after cessation of smoking.

Spontaneous physical activity and non-exercise activity thermogenesis

Another way to look at the components of energy expenditure is shown in Figure 5.5 model B, where energy expenditure is divided into resting and non-resting expenditure, but also into voluntary and involuntary energy expenditure. Resting energy expenditure comprises all measurements of energy expenditure made at rest – BMR and the thermic effect of food – and which are beyond voluntary control. Non-resting energy expenditure is divided into voluntary and involuntary physical activities. The voluntary physical activity comprises volitional activities such as exercise and sports as well as occupational activities (going to work and performing work duties) and leisure activities (e.g. gardening). The involuntary physical activity comprises spontaneous and subconscious fidgeting and posture maintenance, and is referred to as spontaneous physical activity (SPA). SPA is an important component of 'non-exercise activity thermogenesis' or NEAT – the latter being defined as as the energy expended for all physical activities other than volitional exercise and sports activities (Levine et al. 1999, 2005). The potential importance of variations in SPA and NEAT in body weight regulation is discussed below (in section 5.7).

FUEL METABOLISM AT THE LEVEL OF ORGANS AND TISSUES

The energy supplied by the diet is in the form of macronutrients (also called substrates or metabolic fuels): carbohydrates, proteins and fat. These macromolecules cannot be directly utilised by the tissues as such but must be first broken down into smaller molecules: carbohydrates into monosaccharides (see Ch. 6), triacylglycerols into free fatty acids (see Ch. 7) and proteins into amino acids (see Ch. 8). Ethanol (alcohol), not considered a macronutrient, also constitutes a source of energy utilised by the body (see Ch. 9) The major substrates, which circulate in the blood and are taken up by the tissues to serve as fuels, are shown in Table 5.3. The amount stored in the tissues, the level of exogenous supply and the metabolic state of the individual determine the relative importance of the utilisation of each fuel, with synthesis and utilisation of body reserves controlled by hormones.

Metabolic rate at the level of organs and tissues

The heat production of individual tissues and organs can be calculated from the oxygen consumption by measuring blood flow and the arteriovenous

Table 5.3	Substances which circulate in the blood and are used to supply energy (from Elia 2000)
FUEL	**SOURCE**
Glucose	Dietary carbohydrate; Glycogen stores; Gluconeogenesis in liver and kidney from lactate, amino acids and glycerol
Free fatty acids (FFA)	Dietary fats; Triglyceride stores (especially in adipose tissue); Synthesized from carbohydrate in liver and adipose tissue, especially after feeding on low-fat diets
Amino acids	Dietary protein; Tissue protein stores; Synthesized from carbohydrates
Ketone bodies (*acetoacetate, 3-hydroxybutyrate*)	Produced from FFA and some amino acids in liver
Glycerol	Produced from triglyceride breakdown
Lactate	Anaerobic glycolysis
Acetate	Gut fermentation of carbohydrates; Produced from FFA in liver and muscle, and from ethanol in liver
Ethanol	Dietary intake; Gut fermentation
Fructose	Dietary sucrose
Galactose	Dietary intake, especially as milk lactose

difference in oxygen concentration across tissues and organs. Normalised for body mass, adipose tissue has the lowest metabolic rate (approx. 18.8 kJ/kg/day for subcutaneous abdominal adipose tissue). Note that there are regional differences in the lipolytic activity of different anatomical sites of adipose tissue with the intra-abdominal depot having the greatest metabolic activity and gluteal fat the lowest. In a non-obese subject, adipose tissue contributes 3–5% of the total resting energy expenditure, although it represents 20–30% of body weight. The majority of the heat production (about 60%) comes from active organs such as the liver, kidney, heart and brain, although they account for only 5–6% of total body weight (Table 5.4). The heat production of muscle per unit mass (42–63 kJ/kg) is 15–40 times lower than that of metabolically active organs, but because of its large size (more than half of the total fat-free mass) it contributes about 20% of total heat production.

The heat production or metabolic rate per kg of organ seems to change little during growth and development. However, the metabolic rate per kg body weight (or per kg fat-free mass) is much greater in young children than in adults. The reduction of metabolic rate with increasing age is mostly due to a change in a proportion of different tissues, and to a lesser extent to a reduction in the metabolic rate per kg of individual (Elia 2000). The larger proportion of metabolically active tissues (brain, liver, heart, kidneys) in infants and children explains their higher metabolic rates compared with adults when expressed in relation to fat-free

mass). The contribution of different tissues to body weight and BMR in a 'reference male' is shown in Table 5.4.

Fuels used by different tissues and fuel selection

The main fuels available to tissues are glucose, triacylglycerol, free fatty acids and ketone bodies; Table 5.5 shows the fuels that can be used by different tissues. Red blood cells are wholly reliant on anaerobic metabolism of glucose, releasing lactate, and the brain is largely reliant on glucose; it cannot utilise fatty acids, but in prolonged fasting and starvation ketone bodies can meet about 20% of its energy needs. Other tissues can utilise a variety of fuels, depending on their availability in the circulation, and hormonal control.

MEASUREMENT OF ENERGY EXPENDITURE

Principles of energy expenditure measurement

The energy expended by an individual can be assessed by two different techniques: direct and indirect calorimetry. Direct calorimetry is the direct measurement of heat output; indirect calorimetry depends on the fact that the heat released by metabolic processes can be calculated from the rate of oxygen consumption ($\dot{V}O_2$). This is because energy expenditure to maintain electrochemical

Table 5.4	Contribution of different tissues and organs to basal metabolic rate (BMR) of a reference man (from Elia 2000)				
	WEIGHT OF TISSUE		**ORGAN/TISSUE METABOLIC RATE**		
	Kg	*% body weight*	*MJ/kg/day*	*MJ/day*	*% BMR (7.03 MJ/day)*
Liver	1.8	2.6	0.84	1.51	21
Brain	1.4	2.0	1.00	1.41	20
Heart	0.33	0.5	1.84	0.61	9
Kidney	0.31	0.4	1.84	0.57	8
Muscle	28.0	40	0.054	1.52	22
Adipose tissue	15	21.4	0.019	0.28	4
Miscellaneous by difference, *e.g.* skin, intestine, bone	23.16	33.1	0.049	1.13	16
Whole body	70	100	0.1	7.03	100

Table 5.5	Important fuels utilized by various tissues (from Elia 2000)
Brain	Glucose, ketone bodies
Muscle	Glucose, NEFA, ketone bodies (starvation), acetate (after alcohol ingestion), triacylglycerol, branched-chain amino acids
Liver	Amino acids, fatty acids including short chain fatty acids, glucose, alcohol
Kidney	
Cortex	Glucose, NEFA, ketone bodies
Medulla	Glucose (glycolysis)
Brown adipose tissue	Mainly NEFA
White adipose tissue	Glucose, ? NEFA
Gastrointestinal tract	
Small intestine	Glutamine, ketone bodies (starvation), a variety of other fuels in smaller amounts
Large intestine	Short-chain fatty acids, glutamine, glucose, and other fuels in smaller amounts
Red blood cells	Glucose (glycolysis)
Lymphocytes/macrophages	Glutamine, glucose, ? NEFA/ketones

gradients, support biosynthetic processes, and generate muscular contraction utilises ATP (adenosine triphosphate), which is formed by oxidative phosphorylation, directly linked to the oxidation of substrates and reduction of oxygen to water. It is the rate of ATP utilisation that determines the rate of substrate oxidation and therefore oxygen consumption.

The energy expenditure per mole of ATP formed can be calculated from the heat of combustion of 1 mole of substrate, divided by the total number of moles of ATP generated in its oxidation. Each mole of ATP formed is accompanied by the release of about the same amount of heat (~ 75 kJ/mol ATP) during the oxidation of carbohydrates, fats or proteins and the consumption of 1 litre of oxygen can be assumed to be equivalent to 20.3 kJ energy expenditure, regardless of the substrate being oxidised. Direct calorimetry consists of the measurement of heat dissipated by the body through radiation, convection, conduction, and evaporation.

Under conditions of thermal equilibrium in a subject at rest and in postabsorptive conditions, heat production, measured by indirect calorimetry, is identical to heat dissipation, measured by direct calorimetry. This is an obvious confirmation of the first law of thermodynamics, which states that the energy released is ultimately transformed into heat (and external work during exercise), and validates the use of indirect calorimetry.

Energy metabolism and nutrient utilisation

Open-circuit indirect calorimeters permit measurement of oxygen consumption and carbon dioxide production both at rest, when a ventilated hood is placed over the subject, and over 24 hours, by confining the subject to a respiration chamber (fitted with furniture, bed, washbasin, TV, etc.) and analysing O_2 and CO_2 in the air entering and leaving the chamber. Descriptions of available equipment and techniques are given by Murgatroyd et al (1993).

Metabolic rate (M), which corresponds to energy expenditure, can be calculated from oxygen consumption ($\dot{V}O_2$, in litres at standard temperature (0°C), pressure (760 mmHg) and dry (STPD) per minute, according to the Weir formula as follows:

$$M\,(kJ/min) = 20.3 \times \dot{V}O_2$$

The value of 20.3 is a mean value (in kJ/L) of the energy equivalent for the consumption of 1 litre (STPD) of oxygen (see Table 5.6) and is practically independent of the respiratory quotient (RQ) because the error involved is less than 1%. To estimate the contribution of the three macronutrients (carbohydrates, fats, and proteins) to metabolic rate, three measurements must be carried out: oxygen consumption ($\dot{V}O_2$), carbon dioxide production ($\dot{V}CO_2$) and urinary nitrogen excretion (N). Metabolic rate is then:

$$M = a\,\dot{V}O_2 + b\,\dot{V}CO_2 - cN$$

The factors a, b, and c (which are the coefficients of regression) depend on the respective constants for the amount of O_2 used and the amount of CO_2 produced during oxidation of the three classes of nutrients (Table 5.6). An example of such a formula is given below.

$$M = 16.18\,\dot{V}O_2 + 5.02\,\dot{V}CO_2 - 5.99\,N$$

where M is in kilojoules, $\dot{V}O_2$ and $\dot{V}CO_2$ are in litres STPD, and N is in grams, per unit time. As an example, if $\dot{V}O_2 = 600$ L per day, $\dot{V}CO_2 = 500$ L per

Table 5.6 Energy yields from oxidation of substrates (from Livesey & Elia 1988)

Substrates	O_2 consumed*	CO_2 produced*	RQ	HEAT RELEASED kJ/g	ENERGY EQUIVALENT kJ/LO$_2$	kJ/LO$_2$
Starch	0.829	0.829	1.00	17.6	21.2	21.2
Saccharose	0.786	0.786	1.00	16.6	21.1	21.1
Glucose	0.746	0.746	1.00	15.6	21.0	21.0
Lipid	2.019	1.427	0.71	39.6	19.6	27.7
Protein	1.010	0.844	0.83	19.7	19.5	23.3
Lactic acid	0.746	0.746	1.00	15.1	20.3	20.3

RQ = respiratory quotient
*in litres per gram of substrate oxidized

day (respiratory quotient or RQ = 0.83), and N = 12 g per day, then M = 12016 kJ per day.

Indirect calorimetry also allows calculation of the nutrient oxidation rates in the whole body. An index of protein oxidation is obtained from the total amount of nitrogen excreted in the urine during the test period. Because 1 g urinary nitrogen arises from approximately 6.25 g protein, the protein oxidation rate (P in grams per minute) is given by the equation:

$$P = 6.25 \, N$$

An index of carbohydrate oxidation (c) and of fat oxidation (f) is given below:

$$c - 4.59 \, \dot{V}O_2 - 3.25 \, \dot{V}O_2 - 3.68 \, n$$

$$f - 1.69 \, \dot{V}O_2 - 1.69 \, \dot{V}CO_2 - 1.72 \, n$$

Assessment of BMR and energy cost of activity

The measurement of BMR is made under standardised conditions – i.e. in an awake subject lying in the supine position, in a state of physical and mental rest in a comfortably warm environment, and in the morning in the post-absorptive state, usually 10–12 hours after the last meal. Under these conditions, the expired air (collected in a Douglas bag over a certain period of time, or coming from a ventilated hood system at a constant flow rate) is analysed for changes in O_2 and CO_2 concentrations. The energy cost of activities is measured by a portable indirect calorimeter. Nowadays, new technologies have permitted the development of small size (< 1 kg) computerised calorimeters, fixed to the trunk and connected to a comfortable face mask, which

Table 5.7 Non-calorimetric methods for estimating energy expenditure or physical activity in humans

Physiological measurements
Pulmonary ventilation volume
Heart rate
Electromyography
Energy intake / body composition

Human observations and records
Time and motion studies
Activity diary
Activity recall (*i.e.* questionnaire and interview)

Kinematic recordings
Radar
Cine photography
Mechanical activity meters (i.e. accelerometers, pedometers, global positioning system)

Isotope dilution methods
Doubly labelled water ($^2H_2^{18}O$) or triple labeled water ($^2H^3H^{18}O$)
Bicarbonate method

continuously measure pulmonary ventilation. Breath-to-breath analysis can be performed on systems which allow to track the minute-by-minute profile of energy expenditure up to the time when steady state is reached.

Assessment of energy expenditure in free-living conditions

Various indirect methods have been used to assess total energy expenditure in humans under natural conditions of life. As shown in Table 5.7 they have been based either on physiological measurements, human observations and records, on kinematic recordings, or more recently on isotopic dilution techniques. Early studies estimated energy expenditure using an activity diary, but today the most commonly employed non-calorimetric methods are the heart rate and the doubly labelled water technique.

Ambulatory heart rate, accelerometry and global positioning system (GPS)

As far back as 1914, the pioneer American investigators Benedict and Talbot suggested that in infants 'heart rate may be considered a very fair index of energy metabolism'. The method involves establishing individual regression lines between heart rate and energy expenditure within a range of activities that bracket the habitual heart rate observed in normal life. By monitoring heart rate minute-by-minute throughout the day, using portable heart rate integrators, a frequency histogram can be obtained giving the number of minutes spent at each heart rate. By referring this value to the individual regression line, the energy expenditure at a given heart rate can be calculated and integrated throughout the day. Unfortunately, the relationship between heart rate and energy expenditure is not linear within the sedentary range of measurements. This is primarily due to the confounding effects of variations in stroke volume, which substantially increase in a non-linear fashion up to 40% of the maximal aerobic capacity. As a result, the measurement of cardiac output (i.e. heart rate × stroke volume) would predict energy expenditure with more accuracy and precision than heart rate itself, but the non-invasive monitoring of cardiac output in free-living conditions is not yet possible. In addition, a variety of confounding factors (such as eating meals, variations in posture, and cigarette smoking) affect heart rate more than than energy expenditure. The development of respiration chambers has allowed the validation of the heart rate method for estimating energy expenditure (Schutz et al 1981). At the group level, the average accuracy in 4 studies involving 8 to 22 subjects ranged from 1 to 3%. However, the standard deviation of the error is much greater, suggesting that the heart rate method is much less reliable for an individual than for a group.

Humans move in a bipedal mode so that each anteroposterior displacement (step by step) involves, even at a constant speed, an acceleration and deceleration of the body.

Acceleration requires energy, the latter also depending upon the body mass moved (Force = acceleration × mass). Accelerometer–based systems, typically fixed to the upper body, are being increasingly used by researchers and clinicians in the quantification of both physical activity and physical inactivity under free-living conditions among very young to very old people. Note that self-report questionnaire, mechanical pedometer step counts and doubly labelled water (see below) assess different things. The latter is considered the gold standard for measuring energy expenditure. These methods cannot be easily compared to each other due to differences in temporal factors, outcome calculation, etc. Today, several miniaturised accelerometers are on the market with widely different technical characteristics (sampling rate, monitoring duration and 'hidden' algorithms to calculate energy expenditure from the acceleration signals combined with the anthropometric parameters of the subject). The advantages of accelerometers are that they a) are non-invasive, b) provide objective measurement of physical activity (displacement), c) detail profile of activity level and activity-inactivity durations, as well as step counts assessment, d) are reasonably inexpensive and d) allow identification and classification of the nature of movements performed using advanced raw signal analysis (e.g. neural networks). Future technological improvements will provide models for accurate energy expenditure predictions.

The global positioning system (GPS) consists of a network of satellites in orbit around the earth, initially developed for the American army for tracking the position of soldiers anywhere on earth. The principle is based on geometric trilateration, which requires a minimum of 4 satellites to get a single punctual positioning in 3 dimensions. Accurate assessment of change in position and hence speed of displacement on earth (geolocalisation), using miniature receivers worn by the subject, allows us to accurately measure the distance travelled as well as the intensity of work, correlated with the velocity of displacement (from zero movements to fast running speeds).

Used in combination with accelerometry, it offers great potential in the objective measurement and study of daily outdoor physical activity and the relationship of numerous environmental attributes to human behaviour (Schutz & Terrier 2005).

Doubly labelled water

The stable (nonradioactive) isotope method for estimating energy expenditure using doubly labelled water ($^2H_2$ and ^{18}O) can simultaneously provide an estimation of total body water (and hence body composition) and of water intake (and hence milk intake in studies of infants), as well as an estimate of energy expenditure. The method is based on the difference in the rates of turnover of ^2H_2O and $H_2^{18}O$ in body water, which is used to estimate the CO_2 production rate and hence the rate of energy expenditure. Briefly, a subject is given a single oral dose of $^2H_2^{18}O$ so that body water is labelled by both isotopes. After equilibrium is reached, ^{18}O will be lost as both $C^{18}O_2$ and $H_2^{18}O$, because of the rapid exchange of ^{18}O between water and carbon dioxide. The loss of the isotope as water is determined by measuring the rate of disappearance of ^2H_2O. The rate of CO_2 production is calculated from the difference in rates of loss of the oxygen and hydrogen labels. The disappearance rates can be measured in urine, blood or saliva for a period equivalent to 2 to 3 biological half-lives, i.e. about one week in adults. Under controlled conditions, studies have compared the energy expenditure obtained by using the doubly labelled water method with that measured by indirect calorimetry in a respiration chamber or with a ventilated hood system. These studies have demonstrated that the error at the group level ranged from 2 to 5%. However, greater errors are expected for a given individual. The accuracy and precision of the doubly labelled water method in free-living conditions is probably not constant and depends on the physiologic and nutritional state of the subject as well as the environmental conditions.

ESTIMATIONS OF ENERGY REQUIREMENTS

The energy requirement of an individual is defined by the World Health Organization (WHO) as 'the level of energy intake that will balance energy expenditure when the individual has a body size and composition, and a level of physical activity, consistent with long-term good health' (FAO/WHO/UNU 1985). The energy requirement should also allow the maintenance of economically necessary and socially desirable physical activity. In children and pregnant or lactating women, the energy requirement includes the energy needs associated with the deposition of tissues or the secretion of milk at rates consistent with good health. There are two approaches to assess the energy requirement of people of different age, sex, and physical activity:

1. assessment of food intake followed by the calculation of energy intake
2. assessment of total energy expenditure.

The energy needs of a group represent, in contrast to protein and micronutrient needs, the average value of the individuals making up that group. When possible, energy requirements should be based on estimates of energy expenditure rather than on energy intake. The term 'requirements' refers to the 'habitual' or 'usual' requirements over a certain period. From one day to the next, individuals are not expected to maintain energy balance precisely, and hence energy intake and energy expenditure measurements may not give the same values. Because the variability of energy intake is greater than the variability of expenditure, the habitual energy requirements can be best determined from expenditure rather than intake measurements. In addition, it is difficult to measure energy intake accurately without influencing the subject's ingestive behaviour.

In the estimation of daily energy expenditure by the so-called 'factorial' approach, the BMR is first calculated (Durnin 1991, Ainsworth et al 1993). The physical activities are broken down into occupational activities (work) and discretionary (i.e. desirable) activities. Occupational activities include salaried and non-salaried chores (such as housework). The energy expenditure for occupational activities will depend on the type of occupation, the time spent in performing the work and the physical characteristics of the individual. These activities are classified into light ($1.7 \times$ BMR), moderate ($2.2 \times$ BMR for women and $2.7 \times$ BMR for men) and heavy ($2.8 \times$ BMR for women and $3.8 \times$ BMR for men). Discretionary activities include socially desirable activities (such as the exploratory activities of children and the participation in tasks implying social improvement), exercise for physical and cardiovascular fitness, and optional household tasks. In addition, the BMR is used to estimate the energy cost of sleeping. Finally, the residual time during which there is no clear definition of activity has been taken as BMR $\times$ 1.4. To calculate energy requirements by this factorial method, using an activity diary, see the CD Energy Balance Programme.

Once the separate components of energy expenditure (sleep, physical activity and residual time) have been calculated, the total energy requirement can be calculated by summation. It should be realised that when the energy expenditure is calculated over 24 hours and categorised into 'light', 'moderate' and 'heavy' work, the value expressed in multiples of BMR is obviously much lower than that calculated during a working task. For example, a group with occupational work classified as 'moderate' activity will have an energy requirement calculated over 24 hours of 1.78 × BMR in men and 1.64 × BMR in women because it includes sleeping hours and residual time, whereas during the actual performance of the given task, the energy expended will be 2.7 × BMR for men and 2.2 × BMR for women.

The rate of total energy expenditure (TEE), directly assessed in a respiration chamber or by doubly labelled water, can be expressed as a multiple of some baseline values such as BMR. This approach has been used by an international expert committee (James & Schofield 1990) for calculating the energy requirement in the 'factorial' method. The ratio of TEE and BMR provides a rough index of

physical activity (referred to as 'physical activity level' or PAL) but the contribution of the thermic effect of foods represents a small confounding factor. Since the energy cost of a given activity is proportional to body weight, especially for weight-bearing activities, the absolute energy expenditure during weight-bearing activity will be linearly related to body weight. In non-obese subjects the ratio TEE/BMR ranged from 1.64 to 1.98, based on doubly labelled water measurements of energy expenditure. In the confined condition of a respiratory chamber (without prescribed exercise on a treadmill or bicycle, etc.) the ratio is 1.3 to 1.35, indicating that small discontinuous activities of daily life (washing, moving around, studying, watching TV, etc.) increase basal energy expenditure by one-third.

Body weight and body composition (fat-free tissues) constitute two major parameters affecting total energy expenditure. Prentice et al (1996) studied 319 women and men from roughly 60 to 160 kg (Figure 5.6). The results showed that: 1) for identical body weights, resting and total energy

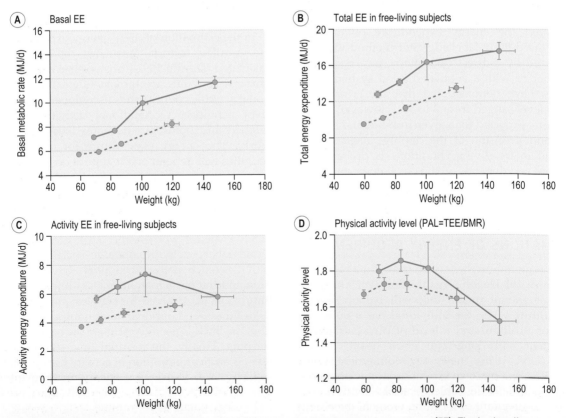

Fig. 5.6 The effect of body weight and gender on various components of energy expenditure (EE). The broken lines represent data for women, while the solid lines represent men.

expenditure are substantially larger in men than in women; 2) conversely, for identical energy expenditure (and hence energy requirement, say 8 MJ/d resting EE and 13 MJ/d total EE), the differences in body weight range at least between 20 and 40 kg, respectively, in favour of women. This is partly explained by a greater physical activity level (PAL) by more than one unit in men together with a larger fat-free mass. Note that PAL tails off between 80 and 90 kg in both genders and then diminishes progressively. At morbid body weights (about 120 kg or above), this is partly explained by the suppressive mechanical effect of excess mass to carry on spontaneous physical activity.

5.5 TIMESCALE OF ENERGY BALANCE AND BODY WEIGHT VARIABILITY

Any regulated function varies within limits that are largely determined by the limits for survival. These are clearly much narrower for body temperature and blood pH than for body weight and body fat. Because large variations in body fat can be observed both between and within individuals, it could therefore be argued that body weight is a poorly regulated variable. By contrast, the fact that, in many individuals, body weight remains relatively constant over years and decades in spite of large day-to-day variations in the amount of food consumed might instead suggest that body weight is precisely regulated in these individuals. But, constancy of body weight per se is not evidence for regulation. In fact, a critical feature of any regulated system is that disturbance of the regulated variable results in compensatory responses that tend to attenuate the disturbance and to restore the system to its 'set' or 'preferred' value. The direct application of this approach to test whether body weight is regulated in human beings is difficult because of ethical and practical considerations, but observations on adults recovering from food shortages during post-war famine or from experimental starvation indicate that a return to normal body weight is eventually achieved. Conversely, excess weight gained during experimental overeating or during pregnancy is subsequently lost, and most individuals return to their initial body weight. There is therefore little doubt that regulation of body weight occurs (albeit with varying degrees of precision), although the time-scale over which it occurs is not clear. In this context, it is important to emphasise

three cardinal features of energy balance and weight regulation:

1. Human beings do not balance energy intake and energy expenditure on a day-to-day basis nor is positive energy balance one day spontaneously compensated by negative energy balance the next day. Near equality of intake and expenditure most often appears over 1–2 weeks. Longer measurements are difficult to conduct and impractical because of cumulative errors, but there is no doubt that over months and years, total energy intake and expenditure must be very close in any individual whose body weight and body composition have remained relatively constant.

2. This matching of long-term energy intake and energy expenditure must be extremely precise since a theoretical error of only 1% between input and output of energy, if persistent, will lead to a gain or loss of about 10 kg per decade. But this does not occur for most individuals, whose weight remains constant with a few kg over several decades.

3. Even in adults who apparently maintain a stable body weight over months, years and decades, there is in reality no 'absolute' constancy of body weight. Instead, body weight tends to fluctuate or oscillate around a constant mean value, with small or large deviations from a 'set' or 'preferred' value being triggered by events that are seasonal and/or cultural (week-end parties, holiday seasons), psychological (stress, depression, anxiety or emotions) and pathophysiological (ranging from minor health perturbations to serious diseases). According to Garrow (1974), very short-term day-to-day changes in body weight have a standard deviation of about 0.5% of body weight, while longitudinal observations over periods of between 10 and 30 years indicate that individuals experience slow trends and reversal of body weight amounting to between 7 and 20% of mean weight. In the town of Framingham, in the USA, after 10 examinations spanning 18 years among both men and women, the average peak-to-peak fluctuation in body weight was 10 kg (Gordon & Kannel 1973). Figure *evolve* 5.1 shows the day-to-day variation in body weight over a 4-year period in a non-obese male aged 33 years 🖱.

5.6 CONTROL OF FOOD INTAKE

HUNGER AND SATIETY

Research into the control of energy intake is very difficult, primarily because habitual intake is not easy to measure (see section 5.3) and because the intake of foods is altered by the experiments themselves. Because of these difficulties, much of the work carried out in human beings has been concerned with short-term hunger and appetite studies or with short-term satiety and satiation. It is important to differentiate between these terms. Hunger may be defined as 'a demand for energy (e.g. after starvation), while appetite refers to 'a demand for a particular food'. In rodents kept in cages and fed ad lib on standard laboratory chow, energy intake is controlled mainly by the sensations of hunger and satiety. If (like human beings) the laboratory rat has access to a variety of palatable foods rather than to a monotonous diet, it may be stimulated to eat by appetite rather than by hunger. The physiological mechanisms which control energy intake in the rat certainly exist in humans. If a person is deprived of food, s/he becomes hungry, and if s/he has eaten a lot, s/he becomes satiated. Satiation refers to processes involved in the termination of a meal, and is studied by providing individuals with test meals and measuring the amount consumed when the food is freely available. Satiety refers to the inhibition of further intake of a food and meal after eating has ended. However lifestyle factors ensure that appetite is a powerful but poorly controlled stimulus to eat even when not hungry. Thus, the total energy ingested in a day is determined by the interaction of many exogenous and endogenous factors.

PSYCHOSOCIAL FACTORS AND SENSORY SPECIFIC SATIETY

It is common experience that feeding patterns are influenced strongly by psychological, economic and social factors. Even though subjects may feel satiated by one particular food, they will continue to eat when a new food is presented – a phenomenon that is referred to as 'sensory specific satiety'. Conversely, when subjects are presented with a monotonous diet, their intakes are usually low. In many parts of the third world, the major part of energy intake derives from one staple food, which, together with low fat intakes, constitutes a bland and monotonous diet, so that even when supplies are adequate, obesity is rarely seen. These observations suggest that when the psychosocial incentives to eat are removed, human beings (like the laboratory rat fed chow diet) can control food intake quite precisely.

HUNGER–SATIETY CONTROL CENTRES IN THE BRAIN

Much of our understanding about centres in the brain that are involved with the control of food intake derives from studies conducted in laboratory animals. As a result of numerous experiments involving ablation, electrical and chemical stimulation of specific areas in the brain, it has been proposed that 'centres' in the hypothalamus are involved in the control of feeding behaviour. People with damage in the hypothalamus, due to trauma or tumour, often show abnormalities in feeding behaviour and weight regulation. Two subpopulations of hypothalamic neurons, whose activations have opposing effects on food intake, have been identified (for details see Section *evolve* 5.6(a)).

HUNGER–SATIETY SIGNALS FROM THE PERIPHERY

The sensations of hunger and satiety result from the central integration of numerous signals originating from a variety of peripheral tissues and organs, including the gastrointestinal tract, liver, adipose tissue and perhaps also skeletal muscle. The putative hunger–satiety signalling systems that have generated the most interest are outlined below (for further detail see Section *evolve* 5.6(b)).

Signals from the gastrointestinal tract

The progression of food through the stomach and small intestine initiates a number of sequential peripheral satiety signals from stretch- and mechanoreceptors or from chemoreceptors that respond to the products of digestion (sugars, fatty acids, amino acids and peptides), which are transmitted via the vagus to the hind-brain for integration. By this pathway the properties of food regulate food intake in the short term by limiting the size of a single meal and may also affect energy intake in a subsequent meal. Among endocrine signals from the gut that are believed to exert important influences on food intake are:

- cholecystokinin (CCK), released from the small intestine into the circulation in response to food, reduces meal size
- gastric inhibitory peptide (GIP), glucagon-like peptide-1 (GLP-1) and the PYY, the peptide YY(3–36), released after food consumption, reduce appetite
- ghrelin, secreted by the stomach, increases after food deprivation and decreases after food consumption. Ghrelin is the only known circulating factor to increase hunger.

Aminostatic or protein–static signals

A link between fluctuations in serum amino acids and food intake was proposed nearly 50 years ago. Dietary protein induces satiety in the short term, and consumption of low-protein diets leads to increased appetite for protein-containing foods. The aminostatic theory states that food intake is determined by the level of plasma amino acids, possibly related to the regulation of lean body mass, which is rigorously defended against experimental or dietary manipulation.

Glucostatic and glycogenostatic signals

A glucostatic theory for the regulation of feeding behaviour was proposed by Mayer, also some 50 years ago. It proposes that there are chemoreceptors in the hypothalamic satiety centre which are sensitive to the arteriovenous difference in glucose or to the availability and utilisation of glucose. Flatt later (1995) proposed that the control of food intake, via the prevention of hypoglycaemia and maintainance of adequate glycogen levels, primarily serves the maintenance of the carbohydrate balance (see Nutrient Balance Model, below).

Lipostatic or adipostat signals

A lipostatic theory of food intake control, first proposed by Kennedy in the early 1950s, postulates that substances released from the fat stores function as satiety signals. Body fat is thus maintained at a set value, and any deviation from this value is detected by the the hypothalamus via a circulating metabolite related to the size of the fat stores, eliciting compensatory changes in energy intake. The lipostatic hypothesis provides the most plausible explanation of long-term regulation of the fat stores. A major advance came in 1995 following the

cloning of the *ob* gene, whose protein product (leptin) is primarily produced by adipocytes. Leptin is released into the circulation and acts on hypothalamic receptors to induce satiety. Rare people with mutations causing complete leptin deficiency show marked hyperphagia and severe obesity – which can be reversed by administration of small doses of leptin. However leptin is elevated in the obese, leading to the hypothesis that resistance to the action of leptin is a factor in obesity, but as blood leptin concentration varies widely in individuals with the same degree of obesity, subpopulations might have relative leptin deficiency.

Insulin also has a role as an adiposity signal as it stimulates leptin release from adipose tissue and leads to postprandial increase in circulating leptin, and also circulates at levels proportional to body fat content.

Impact of peripheral signals on brain higher centres

Although the classic signals from the periphery, such as leptin, insulin, gut hormones and circulating nutrients themselves, act mainly on a few areas of the brain such as specific areas of the hypothalamus and brain stem, recent studies suggest that these metabolic signals have a much broader influence on brain function (Zheng & Berthoud 2008). Leptin and gut hormones do not only act on the 'energy balance' control circuits in the hypothalamus and brain stem, but also on cortico-limbic systems involved in cognitive, reward and executive brain functions important for ingestive and exercise behaviour, particularly in our modern environment.

INTEGRATED MODELS OF FOOD INTAKE CONTROL

(For more detail see Section *evolve* 5.6(c) 🖱)

The various signals from the periphery can be integrated in a model (see Figure *evolve* 5.2 🖱) in which the control of food intake is considered in three phases:

- short-term (hour to hour) blood glucose homeostasis by dampening episodes of hypoglycaemia or hyperglycaemia
- medium-term (day-to-day) maintenance of adequate hepatic stores of glycogen

- long-term (weeks, months or years) maintenance of the body's fat and protein compartments, i.e. fat mass and fat-free mass.

Nutrient balance model

The long-term stability of body weight and body composition requires not only that energy expenditure is equal to energy intake, but also that the composition of the fuel mix which is oxidised follows that which is ingested. Since, as shown in Table 5.1, the protein and carbohydrate stores in the body are limited, they tend to be modulated by an autoregulatory process, allowing an increase in their own oxidation in response to an increase in their exogenous supply. In contrast, the stores of fat are not well regulated by fat oxidation since an increase in dietary fat does not promote its oxidation. Hence, (unlike carbohydrate and protein) fat balance is not precisely regulated. The size of carbohydrate stores exerts negative feedback on total energy intake, so that high-fat diets (containing little carbohydrate) will promote excess energy intake to reach an appropriate level of carbohydrate intake. This energy imbalance would persist until the fat stores build up sufficiently to provide a greater supply for fat oxidation. When the higher fat oxidation matches the higher intake, the individual would then be both in fat balance and in energy balance, but at a higher percentage of body fat.

This nutrient-balance theory, which centres upon the need to maintain specific carbohydrate (glycogen) stores as a determinant of appetite, has been challenged by Stubbs (1998). In people fed a very low carbohydrate (high fat) diet to deplete the glycogen stores, appetite did not increase, and fat oxidation increased to meet energy needs. The complex relationships between fat and other constituents of foods in the control of appetite cannot be ignored. Several reviews have appeared on the control of human appetite and the regulation of macronutrient balance (Blundell 1996, Stubbs 1998).

5.7 AUTOREGULATORY ADJUSTMENTS IN ENERGY EXPENDITURE

Whatever mechanisms operate for the control of food intake, this control is not by itself sufficient to explain long-term regulation of body weight and body composition. There is also ample evidence that autoregulatory adjustments in energy expenditure play an important role in correcting deviations in body weight and body composition (for a fuller version of this topic see Section *evolve* 5.7).

THE DYNAMIC EQUILIBRIUM MODEL

There is a built-in stabilising mechanism in the overall homeostatic system for body weight regulation. Any imbalance between energy intake and energy requirements would result in a change in body weight, which, in turn, will alter the maintenance energy requirements in a direction that will tend to counter the original imbalance and hence be stabilising. There is a built-in negative feedback and the system thus exhibits dynamic equilibrium. For example, an increase in body weight will ultimately increase metabolic rate, which will then produce a negative energy balance and hence a subsequent decline in body weight.

INTERINDIVIDUAL VARIABILITY IN ADAPTIVE THERMOGENESIS

The most striking feature of virtually all experiments of overfeeding is the wide range of individual variability in the amount of weight gained per unit of excess energy consumed. These differences in the efficiency of weight gain are mostly attributed to (a) variability in the ability to convert excess calories to heat, i.e. in diet-induced thermogenesis (DIT), and (b) differences in body composition for the same change in body weight. In addition to the control of food intake, changes in efficiency of energy utilisation (via adaptive thermogenesis) play an important role in the regulation of body weight and composition. The magnitude of adaptive changes in thermogenesis is strongly influenced by the genetic make-up of the individual.

ADAPTIVE THERMOGENESIS AT REST AND DURING MOVEMENT

The component(s) of energy expenditure that could be contributing to adaptive thermogenesis in the regulation of body weight and body composition are difficult to quantify. Resting energy expenditure is measured as basal metabolic rate (BMR) or as thermic effect of foods (Figure 5.5, model B). Changes in the thermic effect of food (as % of energy ingested) or resting energy expenditure (after adjusting for changes in fat-free mass and fat mass) can be quantified, and reflect changes in metabolic efficiency and hence in adaptive thermogenesis (Dulloo et al 2004). But changes in heat production in non-resting energy expenditure – the most variable component of energy expenditure – are more difficult to quantify. The efficiency of muscular contraction during exercise is low (~ 25%), but that of spontaneous physical activity (SPA) – including fidgeting, muscle tone and posture maintenance, and other low-level physical activities of everyday life – is even lower since these essentially involuntary activities comprise a larger proportion of isometric work which is simply thermogenic – actual work done on the environment during SPA is very small compared to the total energy spent on such activities. As SPA is essentially subconscious and hence beyond voluntary control, a change in the level or amount of SPA in a direction that defends body weight also constitutes an autoregulatory change in energy expenditure.

In subjects confined to a metabolic chamber, the 24h energy expenditure attributed to SPA (as assessed by radar systems) was found to vary between 400 and 3000 kJ/day, and to be a predictor of subsequent weight gain. Levine et al (1999) found that more than 60% of the increase in total daily energy expenditure in response to overfeeding was associated with SPA, an important component of non-exercise-activity thermogenesis (NEAT), and that inter-individual variability in SPA expenditure was the most significant predictor of the resistance or susceptibility to obesity.

Levine et al (2005) have demonstrated that obese participants spent 2 hours longer per day sitting than lean participants. This difference is not altered after weight gain in lean individuals or weight loss in obese individuals, indicating that increased sedentariness is not secondary to the increased body mass in the obese subjects, and that SPA and NEAT might be biologically determined.

Adaptive thermogenesis is often separated into resting and non-resting, but this separation is artificial. For example, energy expenditure during sleep, which is generally nested under 'resting' energy expenditure, also comprises a 'non-resting' component due to spontaneous movement (or SPA) occurring during sleep, the frequency of which seems to be highly variable between individuals. Relatively low-intensity exercise can lead to potentiation of the thermic effect of food and the effect of physical activity on energy expenditure can persist well after the period of the physical activity. Any changes in metabolic efficiency in resting or non-resting state that would tend to attenuate energy imbalance or to restore body weight and body composition towards its 'set' or 'preferred' value constitute adaptive changes in thermogenesis.

MODEL OF ADAPTIVE THERMOGENESIS IN BODY COMPOSITION REGULATION

The available evidence suggests the existence of two distinct control systems underlying adaptive thermogenesis (Dulloo et al 2002). One control system responds rapidly to attenuate the impact of changes in food intake on changes in body weight; it is suppressed during starvation and increased during overfeeding. The other control system has a much slower time-course since it operates as a feedback loop between the size of the fat stores and thermogenesis. Its suppression reduces the rate of fuel utilisation during starvation, and its sustained suppression until body fat is recovered during refeeding accelerates the replenishment of the fat stores, while its activation opposes the maintenance of excess fat and hence restores body fat to its 'set' or 'preferred' level.

Throughout much of evolutionary history, we have been faced with periodic food shortages, specific nutrient deficiencies and sometimes food abundance, and it is conceivable that specialised mechanisms for energy conservation (via enhanced metabolic efficiency), but also for energy wastage (via decreased metabolic efficiency), have evolved to the extent that these autoregulatory control systems constitute key control systems in the regulation of body weight and composition. In societies where food is plentiful all year round and physical activity demands are low, subtle variations between individuals in adaptive thermogenesis can, over the long term, be important in determining constancy of body weight in some and in provoking the drift towards obesity in others.

5.8 INTEGRATING ENERGY INTAKE AND ENERGY EXPENDITURE

(For a fuller version of this section see evolve 5.8 📖).

To achieve long-term constancy of body weight, compensatory adjustments occur in both energy intake and energy expenditure, so that unravelling the importance of one or other is difficult, if not impossible. Models of body weight regulation have primarily focused on physiologically induced autoregulatory adjustments in energy intake and in energy expenditure, i.e those beyond voluntary control. However there is certainly some degree of cognitive control, as pointed out by Garrow (1974), when clothes no longer fit, and changes occur in appearance, exercise tolerance and general well-being. In many individuals the importance of cognitive (conscious) controls over food intake and energy expenditure can be as important as non-conscious physiological regulations.

KEY POINTS

- Energy in foods is provided by the macronutrients (carbohydrate, proteins, fats) and alcohol. In the transformation of the chemical energy in food (i.e. gross energy) to energy available for the body (i.e. metabolisable energy), 5–10% is lost through faeces and urine. The metabolisable energy is on average 16 kJ/g of carbohydrate, 17 kJ/g of protein, 37 kJ/g of fat and 29 kJ/g of alcohol.

- Energy balance is the difference between metabolisable energy intake and total energy expenditure. It is strongly related to macronutrient balance, and the sum of individual substrate balances, expressed as energy, must be equivalent to the overall energy balance.

- The matching between energy intake and expenditure is poor over the short term, but (in most people) it is accurate over the long term. Because day-to-day variability in energy intake is much greater than that of energy expenditure, the habitual energy requirement is best determined from total energy expenditure.

- The mechanisms underlying long-term energy balance and weight regulation are unknown, but involve both involuntary controls as well as conscious alterations in lifestyle to correct unwanted changes in body weight.

- Modern lifestyles have led to considerable changes in the kind and amount of food eaten and in the amount of time spent on physical activity, leading to an environment where the matching between energy intake and energy expenditure is more difficult to achieve.

- A high-fat (energy-dense) diet promotes weight gain because it promotes increased energy intake. However, there is a large inter-individual variability in susceptibility to overconsume high-fat diets and in the ability to oxidise excess fat; part of this variability is genetically determined.

- Undernutrition leads to a decrease in energy expenditure, in part because of the loss in body weight (and metabolically active tissues) and in part because of energy conservation resulting from increased efficiency of metabolism.

- Overnutrition leads to gain in body weight which is often less than predicted because of compensatory increases in energy expenditure – the magnitude of which is determined the composition of the diet, the proportion of lean to fat tissue in the extra weight gained and the capacity of the individual to burn off excess calories through diet-induced thermogenesis.

References

Ainsworth BE, Haskell WL, Leon AS, et al: Compendium of physical activities: classification of energy costs of human physical activities, *Medicine and Science in Sports and Exercise* 25:71–80, 1993.

Blundell JE, Lawton CL, Cotton JR, Macdiarmid JI: Control of human appetite: implications for the intake of dietary fat, *Annual Review of Nutrition* 16:285–319, 1996.

Bouchard C, Tremblay A, Després JP, et al: The response to long-term overfeeding in identical twins, *New England Journal of Medicine* 322:1477–1482, 1990.

Dulloo AG, Seydoux J, Jacquet J: Adaptive thermogenesis and uncoupling proteins: a re-appraisal of their roles in fat metabolism and energy balance, *Physiology and Behaviour* 83:587–602, 2004.

Dulloo AG, Jacquet J, Girardier L: Poststarvation hyperphagia and body fat overshooting in humans: a role for feedback signals from lean and fat tissues, *American Journal of Clinical Nutrition* 65:717–723, 1997.

Dulloo AG, Jacquet J, Montani JP: Pathways from weight fluctuations to metabolic diseases: focus on maladaptive thermogenesis during catch-up fat, *International Journal of Obesity* 26(Suppl 2):S46–S57, 2002.

Durnin JVGA: Practical estimates of energy requirements, *Journal of Nutrition* 121:1907–1913, 1991.

Elia M: Fuel of the tissues. In *Human nutrition and dietetics,* 10th edition, edited by Garrow JS, James WPT, Ralph A, Edinburgh, 2000, Churchill Livingstone, chapter 4, pp 37–59.

Fantino M: 1994. Contrôle physiologique de la prise alimentaire. In *Traité de nutrition clinique de l'adulte,* edited by Basdevant A, Laville M, Lerebours E, Paris, 1994, Médecine-Sciences.

FAO/WHO/UNU: Energy and protein requirements, WHO Technical Report Series No. 724, Geneva, 1985, World Health Organization.

Flatt JP: Diet, lifestyle and weight maintenance, *American Journal of Clinical Nutrition* 62:820–836, 1995.

Garrow JS: *Energy balance and Obesity in Man,* Amsterdam, 1974, North-Holland publishing company.

Gordon T, Kannel WB: The effects of overweight on cardiovascular disease, *Geriatrics* 28:80–88, 1973.

Hainer V, Stunkard AJ, Kunesova M, Parizkova J, Stich V, Allison DB: A twin study of weight loss and metabolic efficiency, *Internationmal Journal of Obesity* 25:533–537, 2001.

James WPT, Schofield EC: *Human energy requirements. A manual for planners and nutritionists,* Published by arrangement with the Food and Agricultural Organization of the United Nations, Oxford, 1990, Oxford University Press, pp 25–34.

Keys A, Brozek J, Hanschel A, Mickelson O, Taylor HL: *The biology of human starvation,* Minneapolis, 1950, University of Minnesota Press.

Leibel RL, Rosenbaum M, Hirsch J: Changes in energy expenditure resulting from altered body weight, *New England Journal of Medicine* 332:621–628, 1995.

Levine JA, Eberhardt NL, Jensen MD: Role of nonexercise activity thermogenesis in resistance to fat gain in humans, *Science* 283:212–214, 1999.

Levine JA, Lanningham-Foster LM, McCrady SK, et al: Interindividual variation in posture allocation: possible role in human obesity, *Science* 307:584–586, 2005.

Livesey G, Elia M: Estimation of energy expenditure, net carbohydrate utilisation and net fat oxidation and synthesis by indirect calorimetry: evaluation of errors with special reference to the detailed composition of fuels, *American Journal of Clinical Nutrition* 47:608–628, 1988.

Miller DS: Factors affecting energy expenditure, *Proceedings of the Nutrition Society* 41:193–202, 1982.

Miller DS, Mumford P, Stock MJ: Gluttony 2. Thermogenesis in overeating man, *American Journal of Clinical Nutrition* 20:1223–1229, 1967.

Murgatroyd PR, Shetty PS, Prentice AM: Techniques for the measurement of human energy expenditure: a practical guide, *International Journal of Obesity* 17:549–568, 1993.

Prentice AM, Black AE, Coward WA, Cole TJ: Energy expenditure in overweight and obese adults in affluent societies: an analysis of 319 doubly-labelled water measurements, *Eur J Clin Nutr* 50:93–97, 1996.

Schutz Y: Macronutrients and energy balance in obesity, *Metabolism* 44(Suppl 3):7–11, 1995.

Schutz Y, Garrow JS: Energy and substrate balance, and weight regulation. In *Human nutrition and dietetics,* 10th edition, edited by Garrow JS, James WPT, Ralph A, Edinburgh, 2000, Churchill Livingstone, chapter 9, pp 137–148.

Schutz Y, Bray GA, Margen S: Effect of a meal on the oxygen consumption-heart rate relationship, *Am J Clin Nutr* 34:965–966, 1981.

Schutz Y, Terrier P: How useful is satellite positioning system (GPS) to track gait parameters? A review, *J Neuroeng Rehabil* 2:28, 2005.

Southgate DAT, Durnin JVGA: Calorie conversion factors. An experimental reassessment of the factors used in the calculation of the energy value of human diets, *British Journal of Nutrition* 24:517–535, 1970.

Stubbs FJ: Appetite, feeding behaviour and energy balance in humans, *Proceedings of the Nutrition Society* 57:341–356, 1998.

Virtanen KA, Lidell ME, Orava J, et al: Functional brown adipose tissue in healthy adults, *N Engl J Med* 360:1518–1525, 2009.

Zheng H, Berthoud HR: Neural systems controlling the drive to eat: mind versus metabolism, *Physiology* 23:75–83, 2008.

Further reading

Blundell JE, Finlayson G, Halford JCG: Eating behavior. In Kopelman PG, Cateson ID, Dietz WH, editors:

Clinical obesity in adults and children, ed 3, Chichester, UK, 2009, Wiley-Blackwell, pp. 134–150.

Stock MJ: Gluttony and thermogenesis revisited, *International Journal of Obesity* 23:1105–1117, 1999.

Chapter 6

Carbohydrate metabolism

David A Bender*

CHAPTER CONTENTS

---

*Updated and modified from the previous edition chapter
written by Nils-George Asp and David A Bender

© 2010 Elsevier Ltd/Inc/BV
DOI: 10.1016/B978-0-7020-3118-2.00006-1

OBJECTIVES

By the end of this chapter you should be able to:
- classify the dietary carbohydrates
- explain the importance of the glycaemic index
- describe the main functions of glycaemic and non-glycaemic carbohydrates
- describe the main types of dietary fibre (non-starch polysaccharides, resistant starch, resistant oligosaccharides), and their effects on health, including intestinal bacterial fermentation and effects on digestion and absorption of other nutrients.
- describe the pathway of glycolysis, and how it can operate under aerobic or anaerobic conditions
- describe the Cori cycle of anaerobic glycolysis and gluconeogenesis
- describe the metabolic importance of pyruvate and the principal factors that determine its metabolic fate
- describe the complete oxidation of acetyl CoA through the citric acid cycle
- describe the role of glycogen as a carbohydrate reserve and explain how its synthesis and utilisation are regulated
- explain the importance of gluconeogenesis and describe the pathway
- explain how carbohydrate utilisation in tissues is controlled by hormones and by the products of fatty acid metabolism
- describe the main factors involved in the control of carbohydrate metabolism in muscle
- explain the metabolic effects of a high intake of fructose

6.1 INTRODUCTION

Carbohydrates are not essential nutrients since there is no absolute requirement for a dietary intake, as long as there is an adequate intake of protein to permit de novo synthesis of glucose, and of fat as an energy source. Red blood cells are wholly dependent on (anaerobic) glycolysis and so have an absolute requirement for glucose. The central nervous system is largely dependent on glucose, but can meet a proportion of its energy needs from ketone bodies (see Section 7.4). A very low carbohydrate diet, however, results in chronically increased production and plasma concentrations of the ketone bodies (ketosis) and absence of glycogen stores, with adverse effects on high-intensity work by muscles. Other possible adverse effects of diets very low in carbohydrates are bone mineral loss, hypercholesterolaemia and increased risk of urolithiasis.

Based on the rate of carbohydrate utilisation by the brain, the average requirement of carbohydrate has been estimated to be 100 g/day (20% of energy intake). As little 10% of energy intake from carbohydrate (50 g/day) will prevent ketosis but there are advantages of higher intakes of carbohydrate, not least in reducing the proportion of energy provided by fat. However, when carbohydrate provides more than about 80% of energy, it is difficult to consume sufficient bulk of food to meet energy requirements.

The main role of dietary carbohydrate is as a metabolic fuel; in average Western diets carbohydrates provide about 40–45% of energy intake; in developing countries, where fat is scarce, 75% or more of energy may come from carbohydrates. It is considered desirable that carbohydrate should provide at least 50% of energy intake. Dietary carbohydrates can affect satiety, insulin secretion and glucose homeostasis, lipid metabolism, gut function and intestinal microflora, so that the amount (and type) of carbohydrate consumed will be important with respect to body weight control, type 2 diabetes mellitus, cardiovascular disease and cancer.

6.2 THE CLASSIFICATION OF DIETARY CARBOHYDRATES

As shown in Table 6.1, dietary carbohydrates can be divided into three groups: sugars

Table 6.1   Classification of main food carbohydrates

CLASS (DP^a)	SUBGROUP	COMPONENTS	MONOMERS	DIGESTIBILITY^b
Sugars (1–2)	Monosaccharides	Glucose		1
		Galactose		1
		Fructose		1
	Disaccharides	Sucrose	Glu, Fru	1
		Lactose	Glu, Gal	1 (2)
		Trehalose	Glu	1
Oligosaccharides (3–9)	Malto-oligosaccharides	Maltodextrins	Glu	1
	Other oligosaccharides	α-Galactosides	Gal, Glu	2
		Fructo-oligosaccharides	Fru, Glu	2
Polysaccharides (>9)	Starch	Amylose	Glu	1 (2)
		Amylopectin	Glu	1 (2)
		Modified starch	Glu	1 2
	Non-starch polysaccharides	Cellulose	Glu	2
		Hemicelluloses	Variable	2
		Pectins	Uronic acids	2
		Hydrocolloids, e.g. gums and mucilages	Variable	2

^{a}DP, Degree of polymerisation.
^{b}Denotes digestibility in the small intestine: 1 digestible, 2 indigestible, 1 2 partly digestible, 1 (2) mainly digestible.
Adapted from Asp N-G 1996 Dietary carbohydrates: classification by chemistry and physiology. Food Chemistry 57: 9–14.

(mono- and disaccharides), oligosaccharides (with 3–9 monomer units) and polysaccharides (with 10 or more monomer units). Polysaccharides can be further divided into starch and non-starch polysaccharides.

There are two different ways of determining the carbohydrate content of foods. The older method (still used in the US FDA food composition tables) is carbohydrate 'by difference'. Carbohydrate is calculated as the difference between the total mass of the food and the measured content of water, fat, protein and minerals. More accurate determination of available carbohydrate (as used in UK tables of food composition since the 1920s) measures sugars and starches specifically. Measurement of carbohydrate by difference not only compounds the errors in determining the other components of the food, but includes indigestible carbohydrates (oligosaccharides and non-starch polysaccharides) and non-carbohydrate material, and overestimates both the carbohydrate content and energy yield of the food.

SUGARS AND SUGAR ALCOHOLS

Sugars can be considered in two groups: those that are free in solution (sometimes called extrinsic sugars) and those that are contained within cell walls in plant foods (known as intrinsic sugars).

Extrinsic sugars will include both sugars naturally present in fruit juice, etc. and those added in manufacture and at the table. Intrinsic sugars will have a lower availability than extrinsic sugars because the cellulose of plant cell walls is not digested. However, what is measured analytically is the total sugar content of the food, after more or less complete disruption of cell walls, and this is what is reported in nutrition labelling.

Lactose in milk is an extrinsic sugar, but unlike other sugars is not associated with dental caries, so extrinsic sugars can be further divided into non-milk extrinsic sugars and lactose in milk. The general consensus is that non-milk extrinsic sugars should not account for more than about 10% of energy intake (compared with an average in UK of about 14%). This is because (added) sugars will dilute the nutrient density of foods, and can be readily over-consumed, leading to positive energy balance, overweight and obesity. In populations in which the intake of non-milk extrinsic sugars is 6–10% of energy intake, the incidence of dental caries is significantly lower than when the intake is above 10% of energy intake. However, the frequency with which sugary solutions are consumed is more important than the total amount of sugar consumed.

Fruits also provide fructose, and small amounts of pentose (5-carbon) and other sugars, as well as sugar alcohols (polyols). Fructose is 40% sweeter-tasting than sucrose, and 75% sweeter than glucose. High-fructose syrups prepared by hydrolysis of corn starch and isomerisation of some of the glucose to fructose are now widely used in food manufacture, and have been associated with increased synthesis of fatty acids and the development of hyperlipidaemia and obesity.

Various sugar alcohols are 50–100% as sweet as sucrose; they are poorly absorbed, so have an energy yield about half that of sugars, and provoke a lower insulin response. They are useful in food manufacture, especially foods for energy-restricted diets, because, unlike intense (artificial) sweeteners, they provide bulk with a lower energy yield than sucrose. However, relatively large intakes may cause gastrointestinal upset because of bacterial fermentation in the large intestine.

GLYCAEMIC AND NON–GLYCAEMIC CARBOHYDRATES

Nutritionally, carbohydrates can be classified in two broad categories:

1. Those that are digested in, and absorbed from, the small intestine, and so provide carbohydrate for metabolism; these are glycaemic carbohydrates – they increase the blood concentration of glucose. This group includes sugars, much dietary starch and dextrins (glucose oligosaccharides resulting from starch digestion).
2. Those that are not digested in the small intestine, but pass into the large intestine, providing substrates for the colonic microflora; these are non-glycaemic carbohydrates – they do not increase the blood concentration of glucose. This group includes non-starch polysaccharides, most oligosaccharides and a proportion of starch that is resistant to digestion.

GLYCAEMIC CARBOHYDRATES, THE GLYCAEMIC INDEX AND GLYCAEMIC LOAD

The main glycaemic carbohydrates are glucose and fructose (monosaccharides), sucrose and lactose (disaccharides), starch and dextrins, and small amounts of other disaccharides (maltose, isomaltose, lactose and trehalose).

The concept of the glycaemic index (GI) of foods was originally introduced to simplify exchanges between carbohydrate foods in the control of diabetes mellitus. The GI of a carbohydrate-containing food is the extent to which it raises the blood concentration of glucose compared with an equivalent amount of a reference carbohydrate. It is calculated from the area under the blood glucose response curve after the consumption of a portion of the food containing 50 g of carbohydrate, divided by the blood glucose response after either 50 g of glucose or a standard food (commonly white bread) containing 50 g of carbohydrate.

Carbohydrate foods with a high GI generally provoke a higher secretion of insulin than those with a low GI, and both the GI of, and insulin response to, dietary carbohydrates are important in the maintenance of glycaemic control in diabetes mellitus (see Section 21.5). However, amino acids from protein digestion also stimulate insulin secretion, and foods with a low GI may nevertheless provoke a relatively large insulin response. Protein and fat influence the glycaemic response to a meal, as does the amount of liquid taken with the meal.

A food with a low GI but a high carbohydrate content will have a greater effect on blood glucose and insulin secretion than a food with a high GI but a low carbohydrate content. The glycaemic load is the product of the GI of a food × the amount of carbohydrate in a normal portion.

The GI of a food is influenced by a number of factors: the nature of the different mono- and disaccharides present; the nature of the starch (the relative amounts of amylose and amylopectin); cooking and processing, which affect both the extent of disruption of plant cell walls and the degree of gelatinisation of starch. Intact kernels in cereal products hinder starch digestion so lowering the GI. A proportion of the starch and intrinsic sugars in foods may be enclosed by plant cell walls, which are composed of indigestible non-starch polysaccharides, and so is protected against digestion. Other factors lowering the GI are viscous solutions of non-starch polysaccharides (which hinder diffusion), organic acids (which inhibit gastric emptying and interact with starch) and amylase inhibitors. Food factors that affect the glycaemic index are listed in Table 6.2.

Uncooked starch is resistant to amylase action, because it is present as small, insoluble, partly crystalline granules. The process of cooking swells the starch granules, resulting in a gel on which amylase can act. The swelling and solubilisation of starch by

Table 6.2	Food factors influencing the glycaemic index of foods	
STRUCTURAL PROPERTIES	PROPERTIES OF THE STARCH	OTHER FACTORS
Gross structure, e.g. whole cereal grains	Degree of gelatinisation	Soluble, viscous types of dietary fibre, e.g. guar gum, pectin
Cellular structures, e.g. leguminous seeds	Amylose/ amylopectin ratio	Organic acids, e.g. lactate, propionate
Starch granular structure	Crystallinity Retrogradation, i.e. recrystallisation	Amylase inhibitors Disaccharidase inhibitors

cooking is gelatinisation. Thus, uncooked starches have very low GI, which increases with the degree of gelatinisation, but falls again as foods stale and the starch undergoes retrogradation (crystallisation). Because of the high activity of amylase in the small intestine, fully gelatinised starch may have a GI as high as glucose.

The concentration of blood glucose is determined by three main factors: the rate of intestinal absorption, the net liver uptake or output, and peripheral glucose uptake, which in turn depends upon insulin secretion and the sensitivity of tissues to insulin. With a constant dietary carbohydrate load, there is a range of blood glucose responses between individuals, from low responses through what is defined as 'impaired glucose tolerance, IGT' and 'diabetes' (see Ch. 21, Section 21.3).

The aim of dietary treatment of diabetes mellitus is to avoid both hyperglycaemia and an excessive postprandial rise in blood glucose, which will lead to a large insulin response, with the possibility of reactive hypoglycaemia. A stable blood glucose concentration is also advantageous in relation to satiety and mood, and epidemiological studies suggest that a low glycaemic load may help to reduce the risk of developing type 2 diabetes and cardiovascular disease.

The glycaemic response to one meal may influence the response to the next. Improved glucose tolerance has been reported at lunch-time after a low GI breakfast, and in the morning after a late evening meal with low GI. The colonic fermentation of non-starch polysaccharides may be partly responsible for this.

Some intervention studies, mainly in people with diabetes, but also in non-diabetic people, have demonstrated a reduction in both total and LDL-cholesterol (and an increase in HDL cholesterol) with low GI diets.

CARBOHYDRATE INTAKE AND OBESITY

Although the average requirement for carbohydrate is only about 10% of energy intake, the consensus is that ideally carbohydrates should provide 50–75% of energy intake, with (non-milk extrinsic) sugars providing no more than 10%. The benefit of increasing starch intake is that it will replace fat, and so help to achieve the goal of 30–35% of energy coming from fat. This is likely to be beneficial in terms of reducing the prevalence of obesity, since it is easier to over-consume a high fat food than one that is isocaloric but high in starch.

High carbohydrate meals lead to greater short-term satiety than low carbohydrate meals. This is mainly an effect of the bulk of starch and non-starch polysaccharides; sugars, especially in free solution, have a low satiety value, and it is easy to overconsume them.

The extent to which there is de novo lipogenesis from carbohydrates is unclear. There is clear evidence that fructose (including that derived from sucrose) leads to increased fatty acid synthesis and hypertriglyceridaemia. An intake of other carbohydrates in excess of energy requirements will indeed lead to obesity, but this may be more a matter of increased utilisation of carbohydrate, and hence decreased utilisation of lipids, so sparing adipose tissue fat reserves, than lipogenesis from glucose.

There seems to be no difference between the efficacy of isocaloric low-fat and low-carbohydrate diets for weight reduction. Very low carbohydrate diets (providing only 20 g of carbohydrate per day in the early stage) are effective for weight reduction, but much of their effectiveness is the result of nausea and hence loss of appetite caused by ketosis.

NON–GLYCAEMIC CARBOHYDRATES: NON–STARCH POLYSACCHARIDES, OLIGOSACCHARIDES AND DIETARY FIBRE

For many years the non-glycaemic carbohydrates were regarded as having no nutritional importance, simply providing bulk in the diet. As discussed below, their importance to health is now widely recognised.

Dietary fibre was originally defined as the remnants of plant cell walls that resist digestion in the human small intestine. This definition excludes resistant starch and resistant oligosaccharides (non-cell-wall material), but includes non-carbohydrate materials such as lignin. A more accurate approach is to measure the different individual non-starch polysaccharides and oligosaccharides present in the food. This gives numerical values that are lower than dietary fibre.

There are three classes of non-digestible carbohydrate: non-starch polysaccharides (NSP), resistant starch (RS) and resistant oligosaccharides. In the large intestine, all are substrates for anaerobic fermentation by the intestinal microflora, leading to increased bacterial cell mass and metabolites that affect both the colon and peripheral metabolism.

NSP consists of cellulose, a glucose polymer, which is the main component of plant cell walls, and a variety of other polysaccharides of differing monomer composition, molecular size and structure – hemicellulose, pectins, gums, mucilages. NSP can also be classified according to the main monomeric constituents, e.g. fructans (fructose oligosaccharides), galactans (galactose oligosaccharides).

The physicochemical properties of NSPs vary widely, as do their physiological effects. Viscous solutions of NSP affect digestion and reduce the rate of absorption from the small intestine, attenuating postprandial rises in blood glucose and lipids. Insoluble NSPs are relatively resistant to fermentation and bind water in the distal large bowel, providing faecal bulk.

RS is starch that escapes digestion in the small intestine, and may be a substantial fraction of the total carbohydrate delivered to the colon. Four types of RS can be defined, depending on why they resist digestion:

1. physically enclosed starch within intact cell walls (RS1)
2. ungelatinised starch granules, as in green bananas and high-amylose corn starch (RS2)
3. retrograded starch: as gelatinised starch cools, a proportion undergoes crystallisation (retrogradation) to a form that is again resistant to amylase action – this is part of the process of staling of starchy foods (RS3)
4. chemically modified starches used as food additives may be partially resistant (RS4).

Foods with a low GI also often have a high content of RS, e.g. beans, but in bread and corn flakes, there is a substantial RS content in spite of a high GI for the digestible starch.

Resistant oligosaccharides include polymers of fructose (fructo-oligosaccharides, from onions and artichokes, as well as added inulin and oligofructose), and galactose-containing oligosaccharides from legumes.

6.3 FUNCTIONS OF GLYCAEMIC CARBOHYDRATES

The most obvious function of glycaemic carbohydrates is as an energy source, yielding 16 kJ (4 kcal)/g. In the fed state, most tissues metabolise glucose as their main metabolic fuel. In addition, liver and muscle synthesise the polysaccharide glycogen in the fed state, as a reserve of carbohydrate for use in the fasting state between meals. Carbohydrate metabolism is discussed in section 6.5.

AMINO ACID SYNTHESIS FROM CARBOHYDRATES

The carbon skeletons of the non-essential amino acids (Ch. 8, Fig. 8.1) are derived from intermediates of carbohydrate metabolism. As shown in Figure 6.1, several amino acids are synthesised from pyruvate, the end-product of glycolysis, and others are synthesised from intermediates of the citric acid cycle.

SYNTHESIS OF OTHER SUGARS WITH SPECIFIC FUNCTIONS

The main carbohydrate entering the bloodstream from carbohydrate digestion is glucose, with small amounts of fructose and galactose, and traces of other monosaccharides. A number of sugars are required for specific purposes, and these can all be synthesised from glucose. Glycerol phosphate, which is required for esterification of fatty acids to triacylglycerol and phospholipids, arises from dihydroxyacetone phosphate, an intermediate in glycolysis.

There is a requirement for relatively large amounts of two pentoses, ribose for synthesis of RNA and deoxyribose for synthesis of DNA. In addition, ribose is required for the synthesis of ATP and GTP, as well as the coenzymes NAD and NADP. In addition, its sugar alcohol, ribitol, is

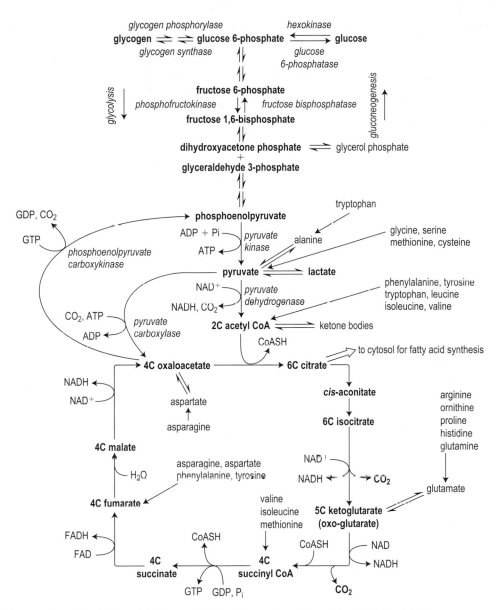

Fig. 6.1 Pathways of carbohydrate metabolism, and interactions with amino acid and lipid metabolism.

required for the synthesis of the flavin coenzymes derived from vitamin B₂, riboflavin. Ribose is an intermediate in, and can be a product of, the pentose phosphate pathway of glucose metabolism (see 'The pentose phosphate pathway – an alternative to glycolysis', below, and Fig. *evolve* 6.3 🖰); deoxyribose and ribitol are synthesised by reduction of ribose.

Glucuronic acid is required for the conjugation of bile salts, steroid hormone metabolites and the metabolites of a variety of xenobiotics, including compounds ingested in the diet and taken as drugs, in order to render them water-soluble for excretion in bile or urine. It is synthesised from glucose, by the oxidation of uridine diphosphate glucose. In animals for which vitamin C is not a dietary essential, glucuronic acid is metabolised onwards to ascorbate; in human beings and other animals for which ascorbate is a dietary essential, glucuronic acid is metabolised to yield the pentose sugar xylulose and its alcohol xylitol, which is further metabolised via the pentose phosphate pathway. Genetic lack of the enzyme that reduces xylulose to xylitol results in the harmless condition of pentosuria – urinary excretion of relatively large amounts of xylulose. Xylulose is a reducing sugar, and gives a positive result when urine is tested with copper reagents for monitoring glycaemic control in diabetes mellitus, although it does not react with glucose oxidase, which is the basis of dip-stick tests for glucose.

Carbohydrates with special functions

The amino sugar glucosamine is synthesised from fructose 6-phosphate (an intermediate in glycolysis, see 'Glycolysis – the (anaerobic) metabolism of glucose', below), and is the precursor for synthesis of other amino sugars, including N-acetyl-glucosamine, N-acetyl-galactosamine and the 9-carbon sialic acid N-acetyl-neuraminic acid. These amino sugars are important for the synthesis of glycoproteins, glycosaminoglycans and glycolipids.

Glycoproteins

Glycoproteins are proteins esterified to one or more oligosaccharides containing various sugars and amino sugars; the carbohydrate content of different glycoproteins ranges between 1 and 85% of the mass. They include albumin and other serum proteins, collagen in connective tissue, mucins secreted to protect the intestinal mucosa, immunoglobulins, peptide hormones and enzymes. In addition, glycoproteins at cell surfaces are important in cell recognition, including the major blood group determinants.

Lectins are proteins that recognise, and bind to, cell surface glycoproteins, and may cause cell agglutination. A number of lectins occur in legumes and other foods, and if not denatured by adequate cooking can cause severe intestinal disorder by binding to intestinal mucosal cell surface glycoproteins.

Glycosaminoglycans and proteoglycans

Glycosaminoglycans are unbranched polysaccharides made up of repeating disaccharide units; one component of the disaccharide is an amino sugar (glucosamine or galactosamine), and the other is normally glucuronic acid. Most glycosaminoglycans are also sulphated, and apart from hyaluronic acid they all occur as proteoglycans, linked to proteins. Major glycosaminoglycans include:

- hyaluronic acid, in synovial fluid, cartilage and loose connective tissue
- chondroitin sulphates, in cartilage and at the sites of calcification in bone
- keratan and dermatan sulphates, which also occur in cartilage and have a critical role in maintaining the transparency of the cornea
- heparin, a proteoglycan secreted by the liver that acts as an anticoagulant.

A number of proteoglycans are found at the outer surface of cell membranes, where they may function as receptors and mediators of cell–cell communication.

Glycolipids

Glycolipids are found in cell membranes, especially in the nervous system. The major glycolipids consist of a fatty acid esterified to sphingosine with covalently bound glucose, galactose, N-acetyl-neuraminic acid and other amino sugars. Like glycoproteins and proteoglycans, they act as receptors and cell-surface recognition compounds.

6.4 FUNCTIONS AND HEALTH BENEFITS OF NON-GLYCAEMIC CARBOHYDRATES

Non-glycaemic carbohydrates (non-starch polysaccharides, resistant starch and oligosaccharides) may influence digestion and absorption in the small intestine, and provide faecal bulk and substrates for the microflora in the large intestine. The importance of fermentation products, mainly short-chain fatty acids, for the function and health of the colon, as well as effects on host metabolism, is increasingly being recognised.

Insoluble, especially lignified, NSPs, as in wheat bran, are largely resistant to fermentation. They have laxative effects due to binding water in the distal colon. Fermented carbohydrates also contribute to the faecal bulk through an increased bacterial mass. The increase in faecal mass ranges from 1 g per gram of ingested pectin to 6 g per gram of wheat bran NSP.

FERMENTATION IN THE LARGE INTESTINE

Carbohydrates that are not digested in the small intestine are substrates for anaerobic fermentation by the colonic microflora. The rate, extent and site of fermentation in the colon are dependent on both the substrate and host factors – the molecular structure and physical form of the carbohydrates, the bacterial flora and intestinal transit time. The main products of fermentation are short-chain fatty acids (acetate, propionate and butyrate) and gases (carbon dioxide, hydrogen and methane).

The decrease in pH of the colon contents resulting from the formation of these short-chain fatty acids may reduce the formation of bile salt metabolites that have been implicated in carcinogenesis. A low pH may also promote colonic absorption of calcium. Butyrate is a major source of energy for colonocytes with effects on cell differentiation and apoptosis that may be protective against cancer. Acetate and propionate are absorbed and metabolised in the liver and other tissues, and may have effects on carbohydrate and lipid metabolism. Propionate inhibits liver cholesterol synthesis in experimental animals, and is a substrate for gluconeogenesis, but its importance in human beings is not clear. Resistant starch and oat bran yield more butyrate than other substrates. Depending on the extent of fermentation and the mixture of short-chain fatty acids produced, fermentation of non-glycaemic carbohydrates results in an energy yield of 4–8 kJ (1–2 kcal)/g.

The intestinal microflora contains several hundred different species, some of which are beneficial, while others are potentially pathogenic. The name prebiotics has been coined for non-glycaemic carbohydrates that stimulate the growth and/or activity of bacteria in the colon that have the potential to improve host health, and out-compete pathogens and prevent them from colonising the large intestine. Fructo-oligosaccharides (inulin and shorter oligosaccharides), as well as other oligosaccharides (galacto-oligosaccharides, resistant malto-oligosaccharides and resistant starch), have prebiotic effects in increasing the growth of *Bifidobacteria* and *Lactobacillus* spp. One of the advantages of breastfeeding infants over formula feeding is that breast milk contains a variety of oligosaccharides that stimulate the growth of *Bifidobacteria* spp. – the so-called bifidus factor.

Oligosaccharides and unabsorbed sugar alcohols are fermented rapidly in the proximal colon, and gas formation can lead to abdominal discomfort and flatulence if the intake exceeds some 20 g/day. Resistant starch is fermented more slowly and does not cause flatulence. Lactose may also cause intolerance in some people with low intestinal lactase activity if the intake exceeds 5–10 g/day.

Otherwise, unabsorbed lactose can also be regarded as a prebiotic carbohydrate with potentially beneficial effects in stimulating what is perceived as a 'healthy' intestinal microflora.

EFFECTS OF NON–STARCH POLYSACCHARIDES AND OLIGOSACCHARIDES IN THE UPPER GASTROINTESTINAL TRACT

Some oligosaccharides inhibit amylase, and have been marketed as slimming aids (so-called 'starch blockers'), although there is little evidence of efficacy. Viscous solutions of NSP have a high water-binding capacity, and may inhibit gastric emptying, and also have beneficial effects on both lipid and carbohydrate metabolism.

Total and LDL blood cholesterol are reduced by viscous solutions of NSP, such as pectins, gums and mucilages – especially guar gum, which is a galactomannan. These effects are related to reduced absorption of cholesterol and bile salts, helping to lower the body pool of cholesterol. Fasting triacylglycerol levels are generally not affected, but attenuation of the postprandial rise in triacylglycerol may be important. Resistant starch and oligosaccharides affect lipid metabolism in experimental animals, but there is little evidence in human beings.

Viscous solutions of NSP also attenuate the postprandial rise in blood glucose and insulin responses, and thus lower the glycaemic index of foods. They act by forming diffusion barriers due to increased viscosity of the intestinal contents, hindering both amylase action in the lumen and the absorption of monosaccharides. Inhibition of gastric emptying may also contribute.

Foods rich in NSP inhibit the absorption of iron, zinc and calcium. However, this is due to phytate (inositol hexaphosphate) associated with the NSP in cereal bran and legumes, and can be abolished by the degradation of phytate (e.g. by the action of phytase from yeast in breadmaking, and phytase secreted in the small intestine). There is no evidence that the NSP per se inhibits mineral absorption.

NON–STARCH POLYSACCHARIDES AND CHRONIC DISEASES

There is good epidemiological evidence that high intakes of NSP may be protective against cancer, cardiovascular disease and type 2 diabetes. However, it is difficult to disentangle the effects of

NSP from the effects of phytonutrients present in the fruits, vegetables and whole grain cereals that are the sources of NSP, or the reduction in fat intake that is implied by a diet rich in carbohydrate and NSP.

A high intake of NSP increases faecal bulk, both as a result of the water-binding capacity of polysaccharides that are not fermented, and also as a result of the increase in bacterial mass that results from providing additional fermentable substrates. This increased faecal bulk enhances peristalsis and reduces straining on defecation, and so reducing the risk of developing diverticular disease of the colon and haemorrhoids.

A high intake of NSP may reduce the risk of colorectal and other cancers by dilution of the intestinal contents (and reduced intestinal transit time), so reducing exposure to, and absorption of, dietary carcinogens. In addition, many potential carcinogens will bind to cellulose and other NSP, so preventing their absorption. When there is plenty of fermentable carbohydrate available, intestinal bacteria will use all the available amino acids for synthesis of bacterial proteins and biomass; when the bacteria have limited carbohydrate available for fermentation they also ferment amino acids, yielding a variety of potentially carcinogenic (and foul smelling) end-products.

Perhaps more importantly, the butyrate produced by fermentation of NSP and RS is the preferred fuel for colon enterocytes. It regulates cell growth and induces proliferation and apoptosis, so providing protection against colorectal cancer.

There is evidence from both epidemiological and intervention studies that NSP may be an important factor in combating obesity. This is mainly the effect on satiety of the greater bulk of food consumed, but the products of bacterial fermentation may also affect satiety.

A number of epidemiological studies have shown a lower risk of coronary heart disease (CHD) with increased intake of whole grain cereals and fruit and vegetables. Viscous solutions of NSP, such as pectin, guar gum and oat α-glucans, lower serum cholesterol, but it is not known to what extent the protective effects of whole grain cereals and fruits are due to NSP rather than other protective compounds in these foods.

There is epidemiological evidence for a protective effect of NSP and resistant starch against type 2 diabetes. There are two factors involved here. A diet high in NSP and RS is associated with lower incidence of obesity, and obesity (especially abdominal obesity) is a major risk factor in the development of insulin resistance and type 2 diabetes. In addition, viscous solutions of NSP slow absorption and reduce the glycaemic index of foods. Intervention trials show a beneficial effect of viscous NSP, while prospective studies show a beneficial effect of whole grain cereals.

CARBOHYDRATE MALABSORPTION AND DISACCHARIDE INTOLERANCE

High intakes of sugar alcohols and fructose may cause gastrointestinal upset, since they are only slowly absorbed in the small intestine and after a relatively large intake a significant amount may enter the colon, to undergo rapid fermentation, producing relatively large volumes of gases and increasing the osmolality of the intestinal contents, so causing osmotic diarrhoea.

Malabsorption of sugars as a result of lack of disaccharidase activity may also cause excessive delivery of readily fermentable substrate to the colon, leading to abdominal bloating, cramps and watery diarrhoea. Genetic lack of lactase (alactasia) is rare, but can lead to severe diarrhoea and consequent malnutrition in affected infants (breast milk and most infant milk formula contains about 7% lactose, providing half the energy). Genetic lack of sucrase is also rare, causing diarrhoea and malnutrition when sucrose is introduced into the diet. Lack of sucrase is relatively common among the Inuit, but only became a problem as sucrose-containing foods and beverages were introduced – there are no sources of sucrose in the traditional Inuit diet.

In most ethnic groups, apart from people of northern European origin, intestinal lactase is lost gradually through late adolescence and early adult life. Some, but not all, people with low lactase activity experience gastrointestinal symptoms due to fermentation of unabsorbed lactose in the colon. Most adults can drink 1–200 ml of milk (containing 5–10 g of lactose) without symptoms. In yoghurt much of the lactose has been fermented to lactic acid, and cheese is almost lactose-free. These products are therefore normally well tolerated.

6.5 THE METABOLISM OF GLYCAEMIC CARBOHYDRATES

Figure 6.1 shows an overview of carbohydrate metabolism. The first stage is glycolysis, which results in the cleavage of glucose to yield 2 mol of the 3-carbon compound pyruvate and a net yield of 7 × ATP under aerobic conditions. Glycolysis is (indirectly) reversible, so that glucose can be synthesised from non-carbohydrate precursors that yield pyruvate (see 'Gluconeogenesis', below). Glycolysis can also occur under anaerobic conditions, when there is a net yield of only 2 × ATP per glucose; anaerobic glycolysis is important in muscle under conditions of maximum exertion, and in red blood cells at all times.

Pyruvate arising from glycolysis enters the mitochondria and is oxidised and decarboxylated to yield 2.5 × ATP per pyruvate (and hence 5 per glucose) and acetyl CoA, which may undergo one of two fates:

- complete oxidation in the citric acid cycle, yielding 10 × ATP per acetyl CoA (and hence 20 per glucose);
- utilisation for synthesis of fatty acids and cholesterol (and hence other steroid hormones and the bile acids).

GLYCOLYSIS – THE (ANAEROBIC) METABOLISM OF GLUCOSE

Glycolysis occurs in the cytosol; overall it results in cleavage of the 6-carbon glucose molecule into two 3-carbon units. The key steps in the pathway are:

- two phosphorylation reactions to form fructose bisphosphate
- cleavage of fructose bisphosphate to yield two molecules of triose (3-carbon sugar) phosphate
- two steps in which phosphate is transferred from a substrate onto ADP, forming ATP (4 × ATP formed per glucose)
- one step in which NAD$^+$ is reduced to NADH (2 mol of NADH formed per glucose)
- formation of 2 mol of pyruvate per mol of glucose metabolised.

The immediate substrate for glycolysis is glucose 6-phosphate; this may arise from two sources:

- by phosphorylation of glucose, at the expense of ATP, catalysed by hexokinase (and by glucokinase in the liver in the fed state)
- by phosphorolysis of glycogen in liver and muscle to yield glucose 1-phosphate, catalysed by glycogen phosphorylase, using inorganic

phosphate as the phosphate donor. Glucose 1-phosphate is readily isomerised to glucose 6-phosphate.

The pathway of glycolysis is shown in Figure *evolve* 6.1 . Although the aim of glucose oxidation is to form ATP from the phosphorylation of ADP, there is a modest cost of ATP to initiate the metabolism of glucose. The pathway involves two steps in which ATP is used, one to form glucose 6-phosphate when glucose is the substrate, and the other to form fructose bisphosphate.

Glucose 6-phosphate is isomerised to fructose 6-phosphate, which is then phosphorylated to fructose bisphosphate. The formation of fructose bisphosphate, catalysed by phosphofructokinase, is the main regulatory step in glucose metabolism. Fructose bisphosphate is then cleaved into two 3-carbon compounds, dihydroxyacetone phosphate and glyceraldehyde 3-phosphate, which are interconvertible. The onward metabolism of these 3-carbon sugars is linked to both the reduction of NAD$^+$ to NADH and direct (substrate-level) phosphorylation of ADP to form ATP. The result is the formation of 2 mol of pyruvate from each mol of glucose.

As discussed below in 'Gluconeogenesis', the reverse of the glycolytic pathway is important as a means of glucose synthesis the process of gluconeogenesis. Most of the reactions of glycolysis are readily reversible, but at three points (the reactions catalysed by hexokinase, phosphofructokinase and pyruvate kinase) there are separate enzymes involved in glycolysis and gluconeogenesis.

The glycolytic pathway also provides a route for the metabolism of fructose, galactose (which is phosphorylated to galactose 1-phosphate and isomerised to glucose 1-phosphate) and glycerol. Some fructose is phosphorylated directly to fructose 6-phosphate by hexokinase, but most is phosphorylated to fructose 1-phosphate by fructokinase. Fructose 1-phosphate is then cleaved to dihydroxyacetone phosphate and glyceraldehyde, which is phosphorylated to glyceraldehyde 3-phosphate by triose kinase. The metabolism of galactose and fructose occurs in the intestinal mucosa and liver, so little fructose or galactose reaches the peripheral circulation. Ethanol inhibits the metabolism of galactose, leading to increased plasma levels and galactosuria.

Glycerol, arising from the hydrolysis of triacylglycerols, can be phosphorylated and oxidised to dihydroxyacetone phosphate. Glycerol phosphate, which is important for triacylglycerol synthesis, is formed from dihydroxyacetone phosphate.

Glycolysis under aerobic conditions

Glycolysis occurs in the cytosol, but the oxidation of NADH, linked to phosphorylation of ADP to form ATP, occurs inside the mitochondria. The mitochondrial inner membrane is impermeable to NAD, and two substrate shuttles are used to oxidise cytosolic NADH, transport reduced substrates into the mitochondrion and reoxidise them at the expense of mitochondrial coenzymes. These are then reoxidised by the electron transport chain, linked to phosphorylation of ADP to ATP. The two substrate shuttles operate as follows:

1. The malate–aspartate shuttle involves reduction of oxaloacetate by NADH in the cytosol to form malate, which enters the mitochondria and is reduced back to oxaloacetate (forming NADH). Oxaloacetate is then transaminated to aspartate for export back into the cytosol.
2. The glycerol phosphate shuttle involves the reduction of dihydroxyacetone phosphate by NADH in the cytosol to form glycerol 3-phosphate, which enters the mitochondria and is oxidised back to dihydroxyacetone phosphate (reducing FAD). Dihydroxyacetone phosphate is then exported back into the cytosol.

Glycolysis under anaerobic conditions – the Cori cycle

In red blood cells, which lack mitochondria, the NADH formed in glycolysis cannot be reoxidised aerobically. Similarly, under conditions of maximum exertion, for example in sprinting, the rate at which oxygen can be taken up into muscle is not great enough to allow for the reoxidation of all the NADH that is formed. In order to maintain glycolysis and the formation of ATP, NADH is oxidised to NAD^+ by the reduction of pyruvate to lactate, catalysed by lactate dehydrogenase.

The resultant lactate is exported from the muscle and red blood cells, and taken up by the liver, where it is used for the resynthesis of glucose. This is the Cori cycle (see Fig. *evolve* 6.2), an inter-organ cycle of glycolysis in muscle and gluconeogenesis in liver. The synthesis of glucose from lactate is an ATP (and GTP)-requiring process.

The 'oxygen debt' after strenuous physical activity is due to an increased rate of energy-yielding metabolism to provide the ATP and GTP that are required for gluconeogenesis from lactate. While most of the lactate will be used for gluconeogenesis, a proportion will have to undergo oxidation to CO_2 in order to provide the ATP and GTP required.

Lactate may also be taken up by other tissues, where oxygen availability is not a limiting factor, such as the heart. Here it is oxidised to pyruvate, which is then a substrate for complete oxidation to carbon dioxide and water, via the citric acid cycle (see 'Oxidation of acetyl CoA', below).

Many tumours have a poor blood supply and hence a low capacity for oxidative metabolism, so that much of their energy-yielding metabolism is anaerobic. Lactate produced by the tumours is exported to the liver for gluconeogenesis. The energy cost of this increased cycling of glucose between anaerobic glycolysis in the tumour and gluconeogenesis in the liver may account for much of the weight loss (cachexia) that is seen in patients with advanced cancer.

THE PENTOSE PHOSPHATE PATHWAY – AN ALTERNATIVE TO GLYCOLYSIS

There is an alternative pathway for the conversion of glucose 6-phosphate to fructose 6-phosphate, the pentose phosphate pathway (sometimes known as the hexose monophosphate shunt), shown in Figure *evolve* 6.3 .

Overall, the pathway produces 2 mol of fructose 6-phosphate, 1 mol of glyceraldehyde 3-phosphate and 3 mol of carbon dioxide from 3 mol of glucose 6-phosphate, linked to the reduction of 6 mol of $NADP^+$ to NADPH. The sequence of reactions is as follows:

- 3 mol of glucose is oxidised to yield 3 mol of the 5-carbon sugar ribulose 5-phosphate + 3 mol of carbon dioxide
- 2 mol of ribulose 5-phosphate is isomerised to yield 2 mol of xylulose 5-phosphate
- 1 mol of ribulose 5-phosphate is isomerised to ribose 5-phosphate
- 1 mol of xylulose 5-phosphate reacts with the ribose 5-phosphate, yielding (ultimately) fructose 6-phosphate and erythrose 4-phosphate
- The other mol of xylulose-5-phosphate reacts with the erythrose 4-phosphate, yielding

fructose 6-phosphate and glyceraldehyde 3-phosphate.

This is also the pathway for the synthesis of ribose for nucleotide synthesis, and the source of about half the NADPH required for fatty acid synthesis. Tissues that synthesise large amounts of fatty acids have a high activity of the pentose phosphate pathway. It is also important in the respiratory burst of macrophages that are activated in response to infection.

The pentose phosphate pathway in red blood cells – favism

NADPH is required in red blood cells to maintain an adequate pool of reduced glutathione, which is used to remove hydrogen peroxide.

The tripeptide glutathione (γ-glutamyl-cysteinyl-glycine) is the reducing agent for glutathione peroxidase, which reduces H_2O_2 to H_2O and O_2. Oxidised glutathione (GSSG) is reduced back to GSH by glutathione reductase, which uses NADPH as the reducing agent. Glutathione reductase is a flavin-dependent enzyme, and its activity in red blood cells can be used as an index of vitamin B_2 status (see Ch. 10, Section 10.2).

Partial or total lack of glucose 6-phosphate dehydrogenase (and hence impaired activity of the pentose phosphate pathway) is the cause of favism, an acute haemolytic anaemia with fever and haemoglobinuria. It is precipitated in genetically susceptible people by the consumption of broad beans (fava beans) and a variety of drugs, all of which, like the toxins in fava beans, undergo redox cycling, producing hydrogen peroxide. Infection can also precipitate an attack, because of the increased production of oxygen radicals as part of the macrophage respiratory burst. Favism is one of the commonest genetic defects; an estimated 200 million people worldwide are affected. It is an X-linked condition, and female carriers are resistant to malaria; this advantage presumably explains why defects in the gene are so widespread.

Because of the low activity of the pentose phosphate pathway in affected people, there is a lack of NADPH in red blood cells, and hence an impaired ability to remove hydrogen peroxide, which causes oxidative damage to the cell membrane lipids, leading to a haemolytic crisis. Other tissues are unaffected because there are mitochondrial enzymes that can provide a supply of NADPH; red blood cells have no mitochondria.

THE METABOLISM OF PYRUVATE

Pyruvate arising from glycolysis can be metabolised in four different ways, depending on the metabolic state of the body:

- Reduction to lactate under anaerobic conditions (see 'Glycolysis under anaerobic conditions – the Cori cycle', above).
- Transamination to alanine; this provides a pathway for the indirect utilisation of muscle glycogen as a source of blood glucose in the fasting state, the glucose-alanine cycle (see 'Glycogen utilisation' below).
- As a substrate for gluconeogenesis (see 'Gluconeogenesis', below). This also provides a pathway for gluconeogenesis from pyruvate arising from amino acids (see Fig. 6.1).
- Oxidation to acetyl CoA, followed by complete oxidation to carbon dioxide and water through the citric acid cycle (see 'Oxidation of acetyl CoA – the citric acid cycle', below).

The oxidation of pyruvate to acetyl CoA

The first step in the complete oxidation of pyruvate is a reaction in which carbon dioxide is lost, and the resulting 2-carbon intermediate is oxidised to acetate, linked to the reduction of NAD^+ to NADH. Since 2 mol of pyruvate are formed from each mol of glucose, this step represents the formation of 2 mol of NADH, equivalent to $5 \times$ ATP, for each mol of glucose metabolised. The acetate is released from the enzyme esterified to coenzyme A, as acetyl CoA. The reaction sequence is shown in Figure *evolve* 6.4 .

The decarboxylation and oxidation of pyruvate to form acetyl CoA requires the coenzyme thiamin diphosphate, which is formed from vitamin B_1 (see Section 10.1). In thiamin deficiency this reaction is impaired, and deficient subjects have impaired glucose metabolism. Especially after a test dose of glucose or moderate exercise they develop high blood concentrations of pyruvate and lactate. In some cases this may be severe enough to cause life-threatening acidosis.

OXIDATION OF ACETYL COA – THE CITRIC ACID CYCLE

The acetate of acetyl CoA undergoes a stepwise oxidation to carbon dioxide and water in a cyclic pathway, the citric acid cycle or tricarboxylic acid cycle (TCA), shown in Figure 6.1. This pathway is sometimes known as the Krebs cycle, after its discoverer, Sir Hans Krebs. For each mol of acetyl CoA oxidised in this pathway, there is a yield of 10 ATP equivalents, and hence 20 per glucose (see also Figs *evolve* 6.5 and *evolve* 6.6 📖).

The first step in the cycle is reaction of the 4-carbon compound, oxaloacetate, with acetyl CoA to form a 6-carbon compound, citric acid. There is then a series of reactions in which two carbon atoms are lost as carbon dioxide, followed by oxidation and other reactions, eventually reforming oxaloacetate. The CoA of acetyl CoA is released, and is available for further formation of acetyl CoA from pyruvate.

The citric acid cycle is also involved in the oxidation of acetyl CoA arising from other sources:

- β-oxidation of fatty acids
- cleavage of ketone bodies in muscle and other tissues
- oxidation of alcohol
- acetate entering from the gut as a result of bacterial fermentation of NSP
- those amino acids that give rise to acetyl CoA or acetoacetate (the ketogenic amino acids).

Citrate is isomerised to isocitrate, followed by two reactions involving both oxidation (linked to reduction of NAD$^+$ to NADH) and decarboxylation, yielding α-ketoglutarate, then the 4-carbon succinyl moiety of succinyl CoA. Succinyl CoA loses its CoA to yield succinate in a reaction linked to phosphorylation of either GDP or ADP. The GTP-linked reaction occurs only in tissues that are capable of gluconeogenesis, and serves to control the rate of removal of oxaloacetate from the cycle for glucose synthesis.

The sequence of reactions between succinate and oxaloacetate is chemically the same as that involved in the β-oxidation of fatty acids. Oxidation of succinate yields fumarate, linked to the reduction of a flavin. Addition of water across the carbon–carbon double bond of fumarate yields malate, which is oxidised in a reaction linked to reduction of NAD$^+$, yielding oxaloacetate.

The citric acid cycle as pathway for metabolic interconversion

In addition to its role in oxidation of acetyl CoA, the citric acid cycle is an important central metabolic pathway, providing the link between carbohydrate, fat and amino acid metabolism. Many of the intermediates can be used for the synthesis of other compounds:

1. α-Ketoglutarate and oxaloacetate can give rise to the amino acids glutamate and aspartate respectively (and from these a variety of other non-essential amino acids).
2. Oxaloacetate is the precursor for glucose synthesis in the fasting state (see 'Gluconeogenesis', below).
3. Citrate formed in the mitochondria is exported to the cytosol to provide acetyl CoA for fatty acid synthesis.

If oxaloacetate is removed from the cycle for gluconeogenesis, it must be replaced, since if there is not enough oxaloacetate available to form citrate, the rate of acetyl CoA metabolism, and hence the rate of formation of ATP, will slow down. A variety of amino acids give rise to citric acid cycle intermediates, so replenishing the cycle and permitting the removal of oxaloacetate for gluconeogenesis. In addition, the reaction of pyruvate carboxylase can be a major source of oxaloacetate to maintain citric acid cycle activity.

The removal of oxaloacetate for gluconeogenesis is controlled. The decarboxylation and phosphorylation of oxaloacetate to form phosphoenolpyruvate as a substrate for gluconeogenesis uses GTP as the phosphate donor. In tissues such as liver and kidney, which are active in gluconeogenesis, the major source of GTP in mitochondria is the reaction of succinyl CoA → succinate. If so much oxaloacetate were withdrawn that the rate of cycle activity fell, there would be inadequate GTP to permit further removal of oxaloacetate. In tissues such as brain and heart, which do not carry out gluconeogenesis, this reaction is linked to phosphorylation of ADP rather than GDP (see Fig. *evolve* 6.7 📖).

GLYCOGEN AS A CARBOHYDRATE RESERVE

The main carbohydrate reserve in the body is glycogen: some 50–120 g in the liver (depending on whether the person is in the fed or fasting state) and 350–400 g in muscle. Other tissues contain small amounts of glycogen to meet their short-term needs.

Glycogen is a branched polymer of glucose, with essentially the same structure as amylopectin (see Section 2.2), except that it is more highly branched, with a $1 \rightarrow 6$ bond about every tenth glucose. The branched structure of glycogen means that it binds a considerable amount of water within the molecule. In the early stages of food restriction there is depletion of muscle and liver glycogen, with the release and excretion of this bound water. This leads to an initial rate of weight loss that is very much greater than can be accounted for by catabolism of adipose tissue, and, of course, it cannot be sustained – once glycogen has been depleted the rapid loss of water (and weight) will cease.

Glycogen synthesis

In the fed state, glycogen is synthesised from glucose in both liver and muscle. The reaction is a stepwise addition of glucose units onto the glycogen that is already present. The pathway is shown in Figure *evolve* 6.8 .

Glycogen synthesis involves the intermediate formation of UDP-glucose (uridine diphosphate glucose) by reaction between glucose 1-phosphate and UTP (uridine triphosphate). As each glucose unit is added to the growing glycogen chain, so UDP is released, and must be rephosphorylated to UTP by reaction with ATP. There is thus a significant cost of ATP in the synthesis of glycogen: 2 mol of ATP is converted to ADP + phosphate for each glucose unit added, and overall the energy cost of glycogen synthesis may account for 5% of the energy yield of the carbohydrate stored.

Glycogen synthetase forms only the $\alpha1 \rightarrow 4$ links that form the straight chains of glycogen. The branch points are introduced by the transfer of 6–10 glucose units in a chain from carbon-4 to carbon-6 of the glucose unit at the branch point.

Glycogen utilisation

In the fasting state, glycogen is broken down by the removal of glucose units one at a time from the many ends of the molecule. The reaction is a phosphorolysis – cleavage of the glycoside link between two glucose molecules by the introduction of phosphate. The product is glucose 1-phosphate, which is then isomerised to glucose 6-phosphate. In the liver glucose 6-phosphatase catalyses the hydrolysis of glucose 6-phosphate to free glucose, which is exported for use by the brain and red blood cells.

Muscle cannot release free glucose from the breakdown of glycogen, since it lacks glucose 6-phosphatase. However, muscle glycogen can be an indirect source of blood glucose in the fasting state. Glucose 6-phosphate from muscle glycogen undergoes glycolysis to pyruvate, which is then transaminated to alanine. Alanine is exported from muscle, and taken up by the liver for use as a substrate for gluconeogenesis (see 'Gluconeogenesis', below).

Glycogen phosphorylase stops cleaving $\alpha1 \rightarrow 4$ links four glucose residues from a branch point, and a debranching enzyme catalyses the transfer of a three glucosyl unit from one chain to the free end of another chain. The $\alpha1 \rightarrow 6$ link is then hydrolysed by a glucosidase, releasing glucose.

The branched structure of glycogen means that there are a great many end points at which glycogen phosphorylase can act; in response to stimulation by adrenaline (epinephrine) there can be a very rapid release of glucose 1-phosphate from glycogen.

GLUCONEOGENESIS – THE SYNTHESIS OF GLUCOSE FROM NON–CARBOHYDRATE PRECURSORS

The pathway of gluconeogenesis is essentially the reverse of the pathway of glycolysis (see 'Glycolysis – the (anaerobic) metabolism of glucose', above). However, at three steps there are separate enzymes involved in the breakdown of glucose (glycolysis) and gluconeogenesis. The reactions of pyruvate kinase, phosphofructokinase and hexokinase cannot readily be reversed (i.e. they have equilibria that are strongly in the direction of the formation of pyruvate, fructose bisphosphate and glucose 6-phosphate respectively).

There are therefore separate enzymes, under distinct metabolic control, for the reverse of each of these reactions in gluconeogenesis:

1. Pyruvate is converted to phosphoenolpyruvate for glucose synthesis by a two-step reaction, with the intermediate formation of oxaloacetate. Pyruvate is carboxylated to oxaloacetate in an ATP-dependent reaction in which the vitamin biotin is the coenzyme. This reaction of pyruvate carboxylase can also be used to replenish oxaloacetate in the citric acid cycle when intermediates have been withdrawn for use in other pathways. Oxaloacetate then undergoes a phosphorylation reaction, in which it also loses carbon dioxide, to form phosphoenolpyruvate. The phosphate donor for this reaction is GTP. The only source of GTP

in mitochondria is the reaction of succinyl CoA → succinate; this provides a link between citric acid cycle activity and gluconeogenesis, preventing excessive withdrawal of oxaloacetate for gluconeogenesis if citric acid cycle activity would be impaired.

2. Fructose bisphosphate is hydrolysed to fructose 6-phosphate by a simple hydrolysis reaction catalysed by the enzyme fructose bisphosphatase.

3. Glucose 6-phosphate is hydrolysed to free glucose and phosphate by the action of glucose 6-phosphatase.

The other reactions of glycolysis are readily reversible, and the overall direction of metabolism, either glycolysis or gluconeogenesis, depends mainly on the relative activities of phosphofructokinase and fructose bisphosphatase.

Many of the products of amino acid metabolism can also be used for gluconeogenesis, since they are sources of pyruvate or intermediates in the citric acid cycle, and hence provide increased oxaloacetate. The requirement for gluconeogenesis from amino acids in order to maintain a supply of glucose for the nervous system and red blood cells explains why there is a considerable loss of muscle in prolonged fasting or starvation, even if there are apparently adequate reserves of adipose tissue to meet energy needs.

Substrates that give rise to acetyl CoA directly (alcohol, fatty acids, ketone bodies and ketogenic amino acids) cannot be substrates for gluconeogenesis since the two carbons added in the reaction to yield citrate are lost in the citric acid cycle, and acetyl CoA cannot provide an increase in the pool of oxaloacetate to act as a precursor for gluconeogenesis. However, the glycerol that arises from the hydrolysis of triacylglycerol in the fasting state can be a substrate for gluconeogenesis, since it is interconvertible with dihydroxyacetone phosphate, an intermediate in glycolysis.

6.6 THE CONTROL OF CARBOHYDRATE METABOLISM AND INTEGRATION WITH LIPID AND PROTEIN METABOLISM

Energy expenditure is relatively constant throughout the day, but most food intake normally occurs in two or three meals. There is therefore a need for metabolic regulation to ensure that there is a more or less constant supply of metabolic fuel to tissues, regardless of the variation in intake.

There is a particular need to regulate carbohydrate metabolism since the nervous system is largely reliant on glucose as its metabolic fuel, and red blood cells are entirely so. The plasma concentration of glucose is maintained between 3 and 5.5 mmol/l in the fasting state. If it falls below about 2 mmol/l there is loss of consciousness – hypoglycaemic coma. An excessively high concentration in the fed state can cause hyperglycaemic coma, and prolonged moderate hyperglycaemia leads to the complications of poorly controlled diabetes mellitus (see Ch. 21).

The plasma concentration of glucose is maintained in short-term fasting by the use of glycogen, and by releasing free fatty acids from adipose tissues, and later ketone bodies from the liver, which are preferentially used by muscle, so sparing such glucose as is available for tissues that require it. However, the total body content of glycogen would be exhausted within 12–18 hours of fasting if there were no other source of glucose, and in more prolonged fasting gluconeogenesis from amino acids and the glycerol of triacylglycerol is important. The regulation of blood glucose is achieved largely by changes in the rates of glycolysis and gluconeogenesis, as well as changes in the rates of glycogen synthesis and break-down. Both hormonal control (mainly insulin and glucagon) and regulation of carbohydrate metabolism by intermediates of fatty acid metabolism are important.

HORMONAL CONTROL OF CARBOHYDRATE METABOLISM IN THE FED STATE

During the 3–4 hours after a meal, there is an ample supply of metabolic fuel entering the circulation from the gut. Glucose from carbohydrate digestion and amino acids from protein digestion are absorbed into the portal circulation, and to a considerable extent the liver controls the amounts that enter the peripheral circulation. Under these conditions, when there is a plentiful supply of glucose, it is the main metabolic fuel for most tissues, and after a meal the RQ (respiratory quotient: the ratio of the volume of carbon dioxide formed to oxygen consumed in metabolism) is close to 1.0, indicating that it is mainly glucose that is being oxidised.

The increased concentration of glucose and amino acids in the portal blood stimulates the β-cells of the pancreas to secrete insulin, and suppresses the secretion of glucagon by the α-cells of the pancreas. Insulin has five main actions:

1. Increased uptake of glucose into muscle and adipose tissue. This is effected by recruitment to the cell surface of glucose transporters that are in intracellular vesicles in the fasting state.
2. Stimulation of the synthesis of glycogen from glucose in both liver and muscle, by activation of glycogen synthetase, and parallel inhibition of glycogen phosphorylase.
3. Stimulation of fatty acid synthesis in adipose tissue by activation of acetyl CoA carboxylase and parallel inactivation of hormone-sensitive lipase.
4. Stimulation of amino acid uptake into tissues, leading to an increased rate of protein synthesis.
5. Induction of lipoprotein lipase in muscle and adipose tissue, so permitting the uptake of fatty acids from triacylglycerol in chylomicrons and very low density lipoprotein.

In the liver, glucose uptake is by carrier-mediated diffusion and metabolic trapping as glucose 6-phosphate, independent of insulin. The uptake of glucose into the liver increases very significantly as the concentration of glucose in the hepatic portal vein increases, and the liver has a major role in controlling the amount of glucose that reaches peripheral tissues after a meal. There are two isoenzymes that catalyse the formation of glucose 6-phosphate in liver:

1. Hexokinase has a K_m of approximately 0.15 mmol/l. This enzyme is saturated, and therefore acting at its V_{max}, under all conditions. It acts mainly to ensure an adequate uptake of glucose into the liver to meet the demands for liver metabolism.
2. Glucokinase has a K_m of approximately 20 mmol/l. This enzyme will have very low activity in the fasting state, when the concentration of glucose in the portal blood is between 3 and 4 mmol/l. However, after a meal the portal concentration of glucose may well reach 20 mmol/l or higher, and under these conditions glucokinase has significant activity, and there is increased formation of glucose 6-phosphate in the liver. Most of this will be used for synthesis of glycogen, although some may also be used for synthesis of fatty

acids that will be exported in very low density lipoprotein.

HORMONAL CONTROL OF CARBOHYDRATE METABOLISM IN THE FASTING STATE

In the fasting state or the post-absorptive state, (beginning about 4–5 hours after a meal, when the products of digestion have been absorbed) metabolic fuels enter the circulation from the reserves of glycogen, triacylglycerol and protein laid down in the fed state. Because the brain is largely dependent on glucose, and red blood cells are entirely so, those tissues that can utilise other fuels do so, in order to spare glucose for the brain and red blood cells.

As the concentration of glucose and amino acids in the portal blood falls, so the secretion of insulin by the β-cells of the pancreas decreases and the secretion of glucagon by the α-cells increases. Glucagon has two main actions:

● stimulation of the breakdown of liver glycogen to glucose 1-phosphate, resulting in the release of glucose into the circulation
● stimulation of the synthesis of glucose from amino acids in liver and kidney (gluconeogenesis, see Section 6.3, under 'Gluconeogenesis').

At the same time, the reduced secretion of insulin results in:

● a reduced rate of glucose uptake into muscle
● a reduced rate of protein synthesis, so that the amino acids arising from protein catabolism are available for gluconeogenesis
● relief of the inhibition of hormone-sensitive lipase in adipose tissue, leading to release of non-esterified fatty acids.

Three further hormones are important for glucose homeostasis. Adrenaline (epinephrine) stimulates glycogenolysis and gluconeogenesis, as well as lipolysis, making fatty acids available as an alternative fuel. Cortisol and growth hormone stimulate gluconeogenesis and lipolysis, and also inhibit glucose uptake, with a resulting blood glucose elevating effect.

CONTROL OF GLYCOGEN SYNTHESIS AND UTILISATION

In response to insulin (secreted in the fed state) there is increased synthesis of glycogen, and inactivation of glycogen phosphorylase. In response to glucagon (secreted in the fasting state) or adrenaline (secreted in response to fear or fright) there is inactivation of glycogen synthase, and activation of glycogen phosphorylase, permitting utilisation of glycogen reserves. Both effects are mediated by protein phosphorylation and dephosphorylation:

- In response to glucagon or adrenaline, protein kinase is activated, and catalyses phosphorylation of both glycogen synthase, resulting in loss of activity, and glycogen phosphorylase, resulting in activation of the inactive enzyme
- In response to insulin, phosphoprotein phosphatase is activated, and catalyses dephosphorylation of both phosphorylated glycogen synthase, restoring its activity, and phosphorylated glycogen phosphorylase, resulting in loss of activity.

Intracellular metabolites can override this hormonal regulation. Inactive glycogen synthase is allosterically activated by high concentrations of its substrate, glucose 6-phosphate. Active glycogen phosphorylase is allosterically inhibited by ATP, glucose and glucose 6-phosphate, all of which signal that there is an ample supply of glucose available. (See also Fig. *evolve* 6.9 🖱).

CONTROL OF GLYCOLYSIS – THE REGULATION OF PHOSPHOFRUCTOKINASE

The reaction catalysed by phosphofructokinase in glycolysis, the phosphorylation of fructose 6-phosphate to fructose 1,6-bisphosphate, is essentially irreversible. In gluconeogenesis the hydrolysis of fructose 1,6-bisphosphate is catalysed by a separate enzyme, fructose bisphosphatase. Regulation of the activities of these two enzymes determines whether the overall metabolic flux is in the direction of glycolysis or gluconeogenesis.

Inhibition of phosphofructokinase leads to an accumulation of glucose 6-phosphate in the cell; this inhibits hexokinase, which has an inhibitory binding site for its product. The result is a decreased rate of entry of glucose into the glycolytic pathway.

Phosphofructokinase is inhibited by ATP binding at a regulatory site that is distinct from the substrate-binding site for ATP. This is end-product inhibition, since ATP can be considered to be an end-product of glycolysis.

When there is a requirement for increased glycolysis, and hence increased ATP production, this inhibition is relieved, and there may be a 1000-fold or higher increase in glycolytic flux in response to increased demand for ATP. However, there is less than a 10% change in the intracellular concentration of ATP, which would not have a significant effect on the activity of the enzyme. What happens is that, as the concentration of ADP begins to increase, so adenylate kinase catalyses the reaction:

$$2 \times ADP \rightarrow ATP + AMP$$

AMP acts as an intracellular signal that energy reserves are low and ATP formation must be increased. It binds to phosphofructokinase and reverses the inhibition caused by ATP. It also binds to fructose 1,6-bisphosphatase, reducing its activity.

Phosphoenolpyruvate, which is synthesised in increased amounts for gluconeogenesis, and citrate, which accumulates in the cytosol when fatty acids are to be synthesised, also inhibit phosphofructokinase.

Substrate cycling

It would seem sensible that the activities of opposing enzymes such as phosphofructokinase and fructose 1,6-bisphosphatase should be regulated in such a way that one is active and the other inactive at any time. If both were active at the same time then there would be cycling between fructose 6-phosphate and fructose 1,6-bisphosphate, with hydrolysis of ATP – a so-called futile cycle.

What is observed is that both enzymes are indeed active to some extent at the same time, although the activity of one is greater than the other, so there is a net metabolic flux. One function of such substrate cycling is thermogenesis – hydrolysis of ATP for heat production.

Substrate cycling also provides a means of increasing the sensitivity and speed of metabolic regulation. The increased rate of glycolysis in response to need for ATP for muscle contraction would imply a more or less instantaneous 1000-fold increase in phosphofructokinase activity if phosphofructokinase were inactive and fructose 1,6-bisphosphatase active. If there is moderate activity of phosphofructokinase, but greater activity of fructose 1,6-bisphosphatase, so that the metabolic flux is in the direction of gluconeogenesis, then a more modest increase in phosphofructokinase activity and decrease in fructose 1,6-bisphosphatase activity will achieve the same reversal of the direction of flux.

CONTROL OF THE UTILISATION OF PYRUVATE

Pyruvate is at a metabolic crossroads, and in the liver and kidney it can either undergo decarboxylation to acetyl CoA, and hence oxidation in the citric acid cycle, or be carboxylated to provide oxaloacetate for gluconeogenesis. Its metabolic fate is largely determined by the oxidation of fatty acids.

Pyruvate dehydrogenase is inhibited by acetyl CoA, and an increase in the NADH: NAD⁺ ratio in the mitochondrion. The concentration of acetyl CoA will be high when β-oxidation of fatty acids is occurring, and there is no need to utilise pyruvate as a metabolic fuel. Similarly, the NADH: NAD⁺ ratio will be high when there is an adequate amount of metabolic fuel being oxidised in the mitochondrion, so that again pyruvate is not required as a source of acetyl CoA. Under these conditions it will mainly be carboxylated to oxaloacetate for gluconeogenesis.

The regulation of pyruvate dehydrogenase is by phosphorylation. Pyruvate dehydrogenase kinase is activated by acetyl CoA and NADH, and catalyses the phosphorylation of the enzyme to an inactive form. Pyruvate dehydrogenase phosphatase acts continually to dephosphorylate the inactive enzyme, so restoring its activity, and maintaining sensitivity to changes in the concentrations of acetyl CoA and NADH.

CONTROL OF GLUCOSE UTILISATION IN MUSCLE

Muscle can use a variety of fuels: plasma glucose; its own reserves of glycogen; triacylglycerol from plasma lipoproteins; plasma non-esterified fatty acids; plasma ketone bodies; triacylglycerol from adipose tissue reserves within the muscle. The selection of metabolic fuel depends on the intensity of work being performed and whether the individual is in the fed or fasting state. (See also Ch. 18.)

The effect of work intensity on muscle fuel selection

Skeletal muscle contains two types of fibre:

1. Type I (red muscle) fibres. These are also known as slow-twitch muscle fibres. They are relatively rich in mitochondria and myoglobin (hence their colour), and have a high rate of citric acid cycle metabolism, with a low rate of glycolysis. These are the fibres used mainly in prolonged, moderate work.
2. Type II (white muscle) fibres. These are also known as fast-twitch fibres. They are relatively poor in mitochondria and myoglobin, and have a high rate of glycolysis and large glycogen reserves. Type IIA fibres also have a high rate of aerobic (citric acid cycle) metabolism, while type IIB have a low rate of citric acid cycle activity, and are mainly glycolytic. White muscle fibres are used mainly in high intensity work of short duration (e.g. sprinting and weight-lifting).

Intense physical activity requires rapid generation of ATP, usually for a relatively short time. When substrates and oxygen cannot enter the muscle at an adequate rate to meet the demand for aerobic metabolism, muscle depends on anaerobic glycolysis of its glycogen reserves. As discussed above in 'Glycolysis under anaerobic conditions – the Cori cycle', this leads to the release of lactate into the bloodstream, which is used as a substrate for gluconeogenesis in the liver, mainly after the exercise has finished. Less intense physical activity is often referred to as aerobic exercise, because it involves mainly red muscle fibres (and type IIA white fibres), and there is less accumulation of lactate.

The increased rate of glycolysis for exercise is achieved in three ways:

1. As ADP begins to accumulate in muscle, it undergoes the reaction catalysed by adenylate kinase: $2 \times ADP \rightarrow ATP + AMP$. AMP activates phosphofructokinase, so increasing the rate of glycolysis.
2. Nerve stimulation of muscle results in an increased cytosolic concentration of calcium ions, and hence activation of calmodulin. Calcium–calmodulin activates glycogen phosphorylase, increasing the rate of formation of glucose 1-phosphate, so providing substrate for glycolysis.

3. Adrenaline, released from the adrenal glands in response to fear or fright, acts on cell surface receptors, leading to the formation of cAMP, which leads to increased activity of protein kinase and increased activity of glycogen phosphorylase.

In prolonged aerobic exercise at a relatively high intensity (e.g. cross-country or marathon running), muscle glycogen and endogenous triacylglycerol are the major fuels with a gradual switch from glucose to fatty acid oxidation, with a modest contribution from plasma non-esterified fatty acids and glucose. As the exercise continues, and muscle glycogen and triacylglycerol begin to be depleted, so plasma non-esterified fatty acids become more important.

Muscle fuel utilisation in the fed and fasting states

Glucose is the main fuel for muscle in the fed state, but in the fasting state glucose is spared for use by the brain and red blood cells; glycogen, fatty acids and ketone bodies are now the main fuels for muscle. There are four mechanisms involved in the control of glucose utilisation by muscle:

1. The uptake of glucose into muscle is dependent on insulin. This means that in the fasting state, when insulin secretion is low, there will be little uptake of glucose into muscle.
2. The activity of glycogen phosphorylase is increased in response to glucagon in the fasting state and the resultant glucose 6-phosphate inhibits hexokinase and hence the utilisation of glucose.
3. The activity of pyruvate dehydrogenase is reduced in response to increasing

concentrations of NADH and acetyl CoA. This means that the oxidation of fatty acids and ketone bodies will inhibit the decarboxylation of pyruvate. Under these conditions the pyruvate that is formed from muscle glycogen by glycolysis will be transaminated to alanine, which is used for gluconeogenesis in the liver.
4. ATP inhibits both pyruvate kinase and phosphofructokinase. This means that under conditions where the supply of ATP is more than adequate to meet requirements, the metabolism of glucose is inhibited.

SPECIFIC FEATURES OF DIETARY FRUCTOSE METABOLISM

Fructose does not stimulate the secretion of insulin or leptin, nor does it suppress the secretion of ghrelin, so it does not suppress appetite in the same way that glucose does. This means that a high intake of fructose may be a contributing factor in positive energy balance and the development of obesity.

High intake of fructose causes increased plasma concentrations of triacylglycerol. Hepatic fructose metabolism begins with phosphorylation by fructokinase to fructose 1-P, which then enters the glycolytic pathway at the level of triose phosphate. Fructose thus bypasses phosphofructokinase, which is the major control point for glycolysis, so that more enters the pathway than is required for energy-yielding metabolism. The resultant acetyl CoA is used for lipogenesis, and will lead to obesity.

Fructose also increases the turnover of purines, resulting in an increased rate of production of uric acid, and high intakes may be a factor in the aetiology of gout.

KEY POINTS

- Carbohydrates, and especially starch, provide the main energy source in the diet, and after a meal it is mainly carbohydrate that provides metabolic fuel to all tissues.
- Dietary carbohydrates can be classified as glycaemic (sugars, starches and dextrins) or non-glycaemic (non-starch polysaccharides, oligosaccharides and resistant starch).
- The glycaemic index of a food is the extent to which it raises blood glucose compared with an equivalent amount of a reference carbohydrate.

Low GI foods may confer benefits in metabolic control of diabetes and may help to reduce risk factors for chronic diseases.
- Non-glycaemic carbohydrates (including resistant starch) are not digested in the small intestine, but provide substrate for fermentation by the colonic microflora. They also have a prebiotic action, promoting the growth of Lactobacillus and Bifidobacteria spp., which inhibit the growth of pathogenic bacteria.

- Fermentation products, notably the short-chain fatty acids acetate, propionate and butyrate, are important sources of energy for the colonic epithelial cells and may influence peripheral metabolism. Butyrate regulates the proliferation and apoptosis of colon enterocytes, and may protect against colorectal cancer.
- Non-glycaemic carbohydrates increase faecal bulk through water binding by unfermented carbohydrate and through an increased microbial mass.
- Glucose is the precursor for synthesis of ribose, deoxyribose, glucuronic acid, and the carbohydrate moieties of complex carbohydrates, including glycoproteins and glycolipids, which have important structural and cell signalling and recognition functions.
- The main monosaccharides are all metabolised by the same pathway, glycolysis, leading to the formation of pyruvate. Fructose bypasses a main control point in glycolysis.
- Glycolysis can operate either aerobically or anaerobically; under anaerobic conditions lactate is formed and is used in the liver for resynthesis of glucose.
- Under aerobic conditions pyruvate arising from glycolysis is oxidised to acetyl CoA, which can either be a precursor for fatty acid synthesis or undergo complete oxidation in the citric acid cycle.

- Pyruvate and intermediates of the citric acid cycle can be used for synthesis of non-essential amino acids, and can also be formed by the metabolism of amino acids.
- A net increase in citric acid cycle intermediates permits utilisation of oxaloacetate for gluconeogenesis to maintain a supply of glucose in the fasting state and starvation. Acetyl CoA arising from fatty acids and ketone bodies cannot provide a source of oxaloacetate for gluconeogenesis.
- The main storage carbohydrate in the body is glycogen in liver and muscle; its synthesis in the fed state and utilisation in the fasting state are regulated by insulin and glucagon.
- In the fasting state glucose is spared for the brain and red blood cells by regulation of its uptake into, and utilisation by, muscle and other tissues. This is achieved by both hormonal control and also inhibition of glucose metabolism by products of fatty acid and ketone body metabolism.
- The plasma concentration of glucose is regulated within strict limits; failure of this regulation, and poor glycaemic control, leads to the complications of diabetes mellitus.
- Fructose bypasses the main regulatory step of glycolysis and leads to increased synthesis of fatty acids, and elevated plasma triacylglycerol concentrations.

Further reading

Bender DA: *Introduction to nutrition and metabolism,* 4th edn. Boca Raton, 2008, CRC Press.

Bosscher D, van Loo J, Franck A: Inulin and oligofructose as prebiotics in the prevention of intestinal infections and disease, *Nutrition Research Reviews* 19:216–226, 2006.

Champ M, et al: Advances in dietary fibre characterisation: 1) definition of dietary fibre, physiological relevance, health benefits and analytical aspects, *Nutrition Research Reviews* 26:71–82, 2003a.

Champ M, et al: Advances in dietary fibre characterisation: 2) consumption, chemistry,

physiology and measurement of resistant starch: implications for health and food labeling, *Nutrition Research Reviews* 16:143–161, 2003b.

Frayn KN: *Metabolic regulation: a human perspective,* 2nd edn. Oxford, 2003, Blackwell Science.

Gibson GR, et al: Dietary modulation of the human colonic microbiota: updating the concept of prebiotics, *Nutrition Research Reviews* 17:259–275, 2004.

Joint FAO/WHO Expert Consultation: Carbohydrates in human nutrition. Food and Agriculture Organization. World Health Organization. FAO Food and Nutrition Paper 66. Rome 1998. Available at ftp://ftp.fao.org/es/esn/nutrition/carboweb/

carbo.pdf. The scientific background papers for a proposed update of this expert consultation are published in European Journal of Clinical Nutrition 61: supplement 1, 2007.

Livesey G: Health potential of polyols as sugar replacers, with emphasis on low glycaemic properties, *Nutrition Research Reviews* 16:163–191, 2003.

McClenaghan NH: Determining the relationship between dietary carbohydrate intake and insulin resistance, *Nutrition Research Reviews* 18:222–240, 2005.

Mittendorfer B, Klein S: Physiological factors that regulate the use of endogenous fat and carbohydrate fuels during endurance exercise, *Nutrition Research Reviews* 16:97–108, 2003.

National Academy of Sciences: *Dietary reference intakes for energy, carbohydrates, fiber, fat, protein and amino acids (macronutrients)*, USA, 2002, The National Academy of Sciences.

Chapter 7

Fat metabolism

Parveen Yaqoob, Anne Marie Minihane and Christine Williams

CHAPTER CONTENTS

© 2010 Elsevier Ltd/Inc/BV
DOI: 10.1016/B978-0-7020-3118-2.00007-3

OBJECTIVES

By the end of this chapter you should be able to:

- relate fat structure with function
- describe main features of metabolism of fat in the fed and fasted states
- explain time-frame and location of fat metabolism following a meal containing fat
- understand the main regulatory features of fat metabolism
- explain the relationship between fat, carbohydrate and protein metabolism.

7.1 INTRODUCTION

The major form of dietary fat is triacylglycerol (Fig. 7.1), which comprises approximately 90–95% of the total with cholesterol and phospholipids being the other main components. Fat is a major contributor to total energy intakes in most Western diets, supplying 35–40% of food energy through consumption of 80–100 g of fat per day. Because a gram of fat (9 kcal/g) yields more than twice as much metabolisable energy as a gram of either carbohydrate or protein (4 kcal/g), altering the fat content of a food can profoundly affect its energy density. All fat sources contain mixtures of saturated, monounsaturated and polyunsaturated fatty acids, although the proportions vary depending on the source (see Ch. 2). The fatty acids present in dietary lipids mostly contain even numbers of carbon atoms and the most abundant have 16 or 18 carbon atoms. Dietary lipids are digested in the lumen of the small intestine and the digestion products are packaged into lipoproteins in intestinal epithelial cells before delivery to the bloodstream, where they become available for uptake by tissues (see Ch. 3).

Fats play diverse roles in human nutrition. They are important as a source of energy, both for immediate utilisation by the body and in laying down a storage depot (adipose tissue) for later utilisation when food intake is reduced. Dietary fats act as a vehicle for the ingestion and absorption of fat-soluble vitamins (see Ch. 11). Two fatty acids, linoleic acid and α-linolenic acid, cannot be synthesised in mammalian tissues and are essential in the diet. Lack of essential fatty acids in animals leads to typical scaling of the skin, growth retardation and impaired reproduction. Similar skin symptoms have been described in humans, for example infants fed artificial milk formula lacking essential fatty

acids and in patients on long-term intravenous nutrition which lack essential fatty acids but essential fatty acid deficiency is rarely observed in human beings consuming mixed diets. Essential and non-essential fatty acids are integral components of cell membrane phospholipids, and play important structural and functional roles in the cell. Following cell stimulation, long-chain (C20 and C22) polyunsaturated fatty acids in membrane phospholipids are the precursors of prostaglandins and other eicosanoids, compounds that have local hormone effects. Cholesterol is also an essential component of cell membranes and is the precursor for synthesis of adrenocorticoid and sex hormones.

Because most Western diets contain relatively large amounts of fat, the regulation of fat storage in the fed state is essential to ensure that circulating triacylglycerols do not exceed optimal limits and that dietary fat is stored in adipose tissue. Raised fasting and postprandial concentrations of triacylglycerols are recognised risk factors for coronary heart disease, so that a good understanding of the processes through which their concentrations in the circulation are regulated is important. Conversely, in the fasted state the mobilisation of adipose tissue fat stores is central to the maintenance of tissue and cellular energy homeostasis, prevents excessive catabolism of protein stores and aids in the regulation of blood glucose concentrations. In addition, the balance in the type of fats in the diet (whether saturated or unsaturated) can influence circulating cholesterol concentrations (see Ch. 19) both in terms of the pro-atherogenic LDL cholesterol and anti-atherogenic HDL cholesterol. Because of the importance of understanding relationships between dietary fats and chronic disease, this chapter focuses on the transport of fats in the body as exogenous (dietary) and endogenous (hepatic) lipoproteins (Section 7.3) and the regulation of fatty acid metabolism at the cellular and whole body level in fed and fasted states (Sections 7.4 and 7.5). However, emphasis on adverse effects of excess fat intake can obscure the essential structural and functional roles that fats play in the body (Section 7.2) and this chapter also considers the role of fat as a precursor for the synthesis of specialist molecules (Section 7.2 under 'Specific functions in membranes').

7.2 FUNCTIONS OF DIETARY FAT

Fats perform a range of essential functions within the body, including the provision of energy,

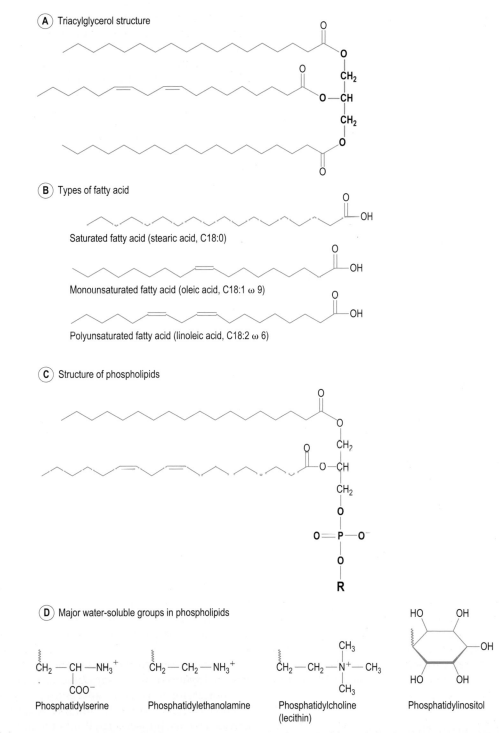

A Triacylglycerol structure

B Types of fatty acid

Saturated fatty acid (stearic acid, C18:0)

Monounsaturated fatty acid (oleic acid, C18:1 ω 9)

Polyunsaturated fatty acid (linoleic acid, C18:2 ω 6)

C Structure of phospholipids

D Major water-soluble groups in phospholipids

Phosphatidylserine

Phosphatidylethanolamine

Phosphatidylcholine
(lecithin)

Phosphatidylinositol

Fig. 7.1 Structure of triacylglycerol (TAG) and phospholipids. Triacylglycerol (a) consists of a glycerol backbone esterified to three fatty acids (b). In phospholipids (c) carbon-3 of glycerol is esterified to phosphate, and to one of a number of water-soluble bases shown in (d).

structural and specific functional roles in cell membranes and hormone-like activities.

ENERGY STORAGE

Due to its energy density, fat, (Fig. 7.1), is the nutrient of choice to act as a long-term fuel reserve for the organism. The majority of fat is stored as triacylglycerols. Although some fat reserve is also found in other cells in the body, such as liver and muscle cells, (where excessive accumulation has pathological consequences), the majority of fat is stored in specially adapted adipose tissue cells, adipocytes (see Section 4.2). Although there is a relationship between the fatty acid composition of the adipose tissue and long-term dietary intake (e.g. an individual eating polyunsaturated fatty acids will have a greater proportion in their adipose tissue), fatty acids stored in the adipocyte as triacylglycerol tend to be more saturated than the fatty acids in cell membrane phospholipids.

Following a meal, ingested fat which is not required by the body tissues for immediate use is transported to the adipose tissue in lipoproteins (Section 7.3). The fatty acids are hydrolysed from the triacylglycerols in circulating lipoproteins by the enzyme lipoprotein lipase (LPL), taken up by the adipose tissue and re-esterified into triacylglycerols. When dietary energy is limited (e.g. after an overnight fast), the fat is mobilised and fatty acids are released from the adipocyte into the circulation, bound to serum albumin. This tightly controlled dynamic process is regulated by the concentration of metabolites (glucose, fatty acids, triacylglycerols) in the blood and by hormones (insulin, glucagon, adrenaline), which are themselves responsive to diet (Section 7.5).

In addition to its role as an energy reserve, subcutaneous adipose tissue is important in the maintenance of body temperature, whereas internal fat (visceral fat) protects the vital organs such as the kidney and spleen. Accumulation of excessive visceral fat (abdominal obesity), is a risk factor for heart disease and diabetes and is linked with insulin resistance (see Ch. 20).

STRUCTURAL FUNCTIONS: AS COMPONENTS OF CELL MEMBRANES

Fats form an integral part of cell membranes, which form a barrier between the cell and the external environment. Intracellular membranes compartmentalise different areas within the cell. The basic structural unit of most biological membranes is phospholipids, which, like triacylglycerols, have fatty acids esterified at carbons-1 and -2 of glycerol. Carbon-3 is esterified to a phosphate group, which in turn is esterified to one of a variety of bases (choline, ethanolamine, serine, inositol); this contributes to the amphiphilic nature of membrane lipids providing both hydrophobic (fat-soluble) and hydrophilic (water-soluble) regions. In mammalian tissues the most common base is choline, and phosphatidylcholine is the main membrane phospholipid (Fig. 7.1).

Lipids based on a sphingosine rather than a glycerol backbone (sphingolipids) are also widespread in membranes, and are particularly abundant in the brain and nervous system (see Fig. *evolve* 7.1). In sphingomyelin the amino group of the long unsaturated hydrocarbon chain of sphingosine is linked to a fatty acid and the hydroxyl group is esterified to phosphoryl choline, yielding a molecule with a similar conformation to phosphatidylcholine. Glycolipids contain carbohydrate (see Section 6.2, under 'Glycolipids'). They consist of a sphingomyelin backbone and a fatty acid unit bound to the amino group, with one or more sugars attached to the hydroxyl group. The simplest is cerebroside, which contains a single sugar, either glucose or galactose.

In the membrane, phospholipids and sphingolipids arrange themselves in a lipid bilayer with the hydrophobic fatty acid tails facing inwards and the hydrophilic head interacting with the aqueous environment of the cytosol (at the inner face) and the extracellular fluid at the outer face (see Fig. *evolve* 7.2). The chain length and degree of unsaturation of the fatty acids within the bilayer have a large impact on the physical properties of the membrane, altering membrane fluidity and therefore function. Dietary fatty acid intake affects membrane composition to a limited extent. The presence of lipid-soluble antioxidants such as α-tocopherol within the membrane serves to minimise oxidation of the unsaturated fatty acids.

Cholesterol, which is almost entirely absent from plant tissues, is the most common sterol found in animal tissues. It inserts itself into the lipid bilayer, where its hydrophobic interactions with fatty acids are essential to maintain membrane structure and fluidity. On a diet rich in polyunsaturated fatty acids, an increase in the cholesterol to phospholipid ratio serves to maintain membrane fluidity.

In addition to lipids, membranes contain a variety of proteins: enzymes, receptors or transporters (see Fig. *evolve* 7.2). The protein content is variable and reflects the function of the cell.

SPECIFIC FUNCTIONS IN MEMBRANES

In addition to their relatively non-specific function in membrane structure, membrane lipids have a wide variety of specific roles such as a lung (pulmonary) surfactant, in cell signalling and as precursors of a diverse range of the metabolically active eicosanoids.

Pulmonary surfactant

Each time we exhale, our lungs are prevented from collapsing by a protein–lipid mixture known as pulmonary surfactant. It contains about 85% lipid, dominated by a single compound, dipalmitoyl-phosphatidylcholine. Surfactant forms a solid film on the alveolar surface as we breathe out, reducing the surface tension and preventing lung collapse. Its importance is evident in newborn infants with acute respiratory distress, an often fatal condition, resulting from an inability to synthesise pulmonary surfactant, leading to respiratory dysfunction.

Cell signalling

Various lipids are involved in cell signalling and the conversion of extracellular signals into intracellular ones. The discovery of the phosphatidylinositol cycle indicated that membrane inositol phospholipids are important mediators of hormone and neurotransmitter action (see Fig. *evolve* 7.3). The binding of a hormone to membrane receptor proteins activates the enzyme phospholipase C, which hydrolyses the phosphatidylinositol molecule to diacylglycerol and inositol-1,4,5-triphosphate (IP_3). Both products activate protein kinases and act as secondary messengers involved in regulation of cellular processes such as smooth muscle contraction, glycogen metabolism (see Section 6.3, under 'Glycogen as a carbohydrate reserve') and cell proliferation and differentiation.

In addition to inositol phospholipids, sphingolipids are important modulators of membrane receptor activity in all stages of the cell cycle, including apoptosis (cell death) and in inflammation. Intact membrane sphingolipids act as ligands for receptors on nearby cells, and modulate the activity of receptors and membrane-associated proteins in the same cell. Hydrolysis of sphingolipids can give rise to a variety of second messengers, such as ceramide, lactosylceramide, glycosylceramide and sphingosine, via the sphingomyelin cycle (see Fig. *evolve* 7.4). Ceramide is the best known of the sphingoid signalling molecules. Activation of membrane-bound sphingomyelinase releases ceramide from membrane sphingolipids. Ceramide activates protein kinases involved in various metabolic processes within the cell, including cell growth and death, and inflammatory responses (see Fig. *evolve* 7.4).

The eicosanoids

See also Sections *evolve* 7.2(a) and *evolve* 7.2(b) .

Membrane unsaturated fatty acids, in particular the C20 and C22 PUFA, are the precursors of a variety of hormone-like compounds known collectively as eicosanoids, which mediate a variety of cellular functions including smooth muscle contraction and blood clotting. They act locally to their site of synthesis and are metabolised very rapidly. It is largely this role of fatty acids as precursors of eicosanoids that underlies the essentiality of linoleic and α-linolenic acids, since these two fatty acids, which cannot be synthesised in the body, are the precursors of the C20 and C22 PUFA.

The main precursor for the synthesis of eicosanoids is arachidonic acid (C20:4 n-6), which can be released from membrane phospholipids by phospholipase A following an appropriate stimulus, and metabolised by lipoxygenases or by cyclo-oxygenase, as illustrated in Figure *evolve* 7.5 . Metabolism by lipoxygenases gives rise to leukotrienes, lipoxins and hydroxy fatty acids, while metabolism by cyclo-oxygenase gives rise to prostaglandins and thromboxanes.

The range of biological activities of the eicosanoids is enormous and varies from tissue to tissue. For examples of the known activities of selected eicosanoids, refer to Section *evolve* 7.2(b) .

Although arachidonic acid is regarded as the main precursor of eicosanoids, a separate family of eicosanoids is derived from the 20-carbon n-3 polyunsaturated fatty acid EPA (see Fig. *evolve* 7.5). Oily fish and fish oils are rich sources of dietary EPA, which is readily incorporated into biological membranes and can replace arachidonic acid to some degree. This has two consequences. First, the replacement of arachidonic acid in the membranes of eicosanoid-synthesising cells by EPA results in a decrease in the production of arachidonic-acid-derived eicosanoids. Second, there appears to be production of selected EPA-derived eicosanoids.

The physiological significance of the n-3 polyunsaturated fatty-acid-derived eicosanoids is relatively poorly understood. Some studies have demonstrated that the EPA-derived eicosanoids are less potent than those derived from arachidonic acid. For example, leukotriene C_4, derived from arachidonic acid, is a chemotactic factor with approximately 10-fold higher activity than leukotriene C_5, which is derived from EPA. This type of observation has formed the basis of suggestions that the n-3 polyunsaturated fatty acids possess anti-inflammatory and immunomodulatory properties. However, the full range of biological activities of these compounds has not yet been investigated.

7.3 PLASMA LIPOPROTEINS

As triacylglycerols, cholesterol and phospholipids are not water-soluble, they cannot be transported free in the blood; transport of these largely hydrophobic compounds occurs using specialised structures known as lipoproteins. Lipoproteins are particles in the circulation whose function is to 'shuttle' lipids to tissues where they are needed. They have a hydrophobic core of triacylglycerols and cholesterol esters and a hydrophilic surface consisting of phospholipids and free cholesterol,

which interacts with the aqueous environment of the blood and lymph (see Fig. *evolve* 7.6). Free cholesterol is amphiphilic, as the free hydroxyl group gives the molecule some hydrophilic properties. Lipoproteins also contain specific proteins, apolipoproteins which, in addition to being essential for maintaining the structure and the solubility of the particle, determine how the lipoprotein is metabolised. Apolipoproteins recognise and interact with specific receptors on the cell surface, and the receptor–lipoprotein complex is internalised into the cell by the process of endocytosis. Apolipoproteins also determine the activities of a range of proteins, including hydrolysing enzymes (lipases), and lipid transfer proteins which are involved in all stages of lipoprotein metabolism (Table 7.1). Five main series of apolipoproteins have been identified: apoA (1, 2, 4, 5), apoB (B48 and B100), apoC (1, 2, 3), apoE and apo(a). However, other classes have been recognised recently (apoD, apoF, apoH and apoL), although as yet no functions have been assigned to them. (See Section *evolve* 7.3(a) for notes on genetic polymorphisms of the apolipoproteins.)

LIPOPROTEIN CLASSES AND THEIR APOLIPOPROTEINS

In order to aid description, lipoproteins have traditionally been classified according to their density into four main subgroups: chylomicrons, very-low-density lipoproteins (VLDL), low-density lipoproteins (LDL) and high-density lipoproteins (HDL).

Table 7.1 Major classes of plasma lipoproteins

	CHYLOMICRONS	VLDL	IDL	LDL	HDL
Density (g/ml)	<0.95	<1.006	1.006–1.019	1.020–1.063	1.064–1.210
Diameter (nm)	75–1200	30–80	25–35	18–25	5–12
M_r (10^3 kDa)	400	10–80	5–10	2.3	0.175–0.36
% protein	1.5–2.5	5–10	15–20	20–25	40–55
% phospholipids	7–9	15–20	22	15–20	20–35
% free cholesterol	1–3	5–10	8	7–10	3–4
% triacylglycerol	84–89	50–65	22	7–10	3–5
% cholesteryl esters	3–5	10–15	30	35–40	12
Electrophoretic mobility	At origin	Pre-β	Between pre-β and β	Pre-β	α
Major apolipoproteins	A-I, A-II, B-48, C-I, C-I, C-II, C-III, E	B-100, C-I, C-II, C-III, E	B-100, C-III, E	B-100	A-I, A-II, B-48, C-I, C-I, C-III, D, E
Turnover in plasma	4–5 min	1–3 h	1–3 h	45%/day	4 days

Recent research has focused on a fifth category of lipoproteins, lipoprotein (a) (Lp(a)), due to its strong independent association with the development of atherosclerosis.

Chylomicrons formed in the gut, and VLDL formed in the liver, are the main transporters of triacylglycerols to the tissues and are referred to as triacylglycerol-rich lipoproteins (TRL). They are the least dense of the lipoproteins as they contain the lowest protein:lipid ratio. ApoB48 and apoB100 represent the main protein component of chylomicrons and VLDL respectively, with both proteins encoded. A gener by the same gene; apoB48 represents the N-terminal domain (48%) of apoB100. Only one molecule of apoB protein is present per lipoprotein particle. ApoE and apoC are smaller apolipoproteins, which are passed from one particle to another, and the transfer of these molecules from HDL is an important mediator of triacylglycerol metabolism. An increased secretion or delayed clearance of TRL is a significant risk factor for coronary heart disease (see Ch. 19)

The smaller, denser LDL and HDL are involved in the transport of cholesterol to and from the cells, with about 70% of total cholesterol present in LDL. LDL is derived from the metabolism of VLDL in the circulation and therefore also contains apoB100 as its main apolipoprotein. HDL, which is originally synthesised in the gut and the liver, is responsible for the removal of excess cholesterol from peripheral tissues and its return to the liver, a process called reverse cholesterol transport. These particles are relatively small, contain a high protein:lipid ratio (50:50), and are therefore more dense than chylomicrons, VLDL or LDL. ApoA1 and A2 are the main proteins of HDL.

Lipoprotein(a) is a small, cholesterol-ester-rich, LDL-like particle containing apo(a) as its characteristic protein. Assembly of Lp(a) appears to occur extracellularly, with apo(a) receiving cholesterol from circulating LDL. Lp(a) is thought to be highly variable within populations, with levels largely genetically determined by a very polymorphic (variable) apo(a) gene. Recent evidence suggests that this particle is highly atherogenic.

Although it is useful from a descriptive point of view to divide lipoproteins into five main classes, it must be remembered that lipoproteins are a heterogeneous and dynamic group of particles, with apolipoproteins and lipids continuously moving between them.

THE EXOGENOUS AND ENDOGENOUS LIPOPROTEIN PATHWAYS

The exogenous lipoprotein pathway, as the name suggests, distributes fat entering the circulation from outside, i.e. dietary fat. In contrast, the endogenous pathway distributes fat either synthesised or stored in the liver. These two pathways are shown in Figure 7.2.

The exogenous lipoprotein pathway

As described in Chapter 3, dietary fat is packaged into chylomicrons in the enterocytes of the small intestine, which are secreted into the lymphatic system and enter the circulation via the thoracic duct. They pass through the lungs and heart relatively unchanged and subsequently rapidly acquire apoC2. This apolipoprotein is essential for interaction of chylomicrons with lipoprotein lipase (LPL). Unlike LDL, which can be taken up by cells intact, chylomicrons are too large to move through the capillary wall, so cells cannot take them up directly. Adipocytes, muscle and mammary cells synthesise and secrete LPL, which hydrolyses the triacylglycerols in chylomicrons, and the released fatty acids are subsequently taken up by the tissues.

The released fatty acids rapidly cross the endothelium into the interstitial space, enter the cell and are immediately re-esterified in order to maintain a concentration gradient. In adipose tissue and mammary gland the fatty acids are stored as triacylglycerol as an energy reserve and to provide milk fatty acids, whereas in the muscle the fat is used as an immediate source of fuel to provide ATP for muscle contraction.

The process of chylomicron hydrolysis is rapid, with 50% of chylomicron triacylglycerol being removed within the first 2–3 minutes of entry into the bloodstream. Following a number of cycles through the tissues and the eventual removal of a large fraction of the triacylglycerol and a portion of cholesterol, and the surface phospholipids and apolipoproteins (to HDL), a smaller, more cholesterol ester-enriched particle remains. This contains the original apoB48 and the majority of the fat-soluble vitamins. ApoE is acquired from HDL and the liver cell takes up the chylomicron remnant by a receptor-mediated by interaction with the LDL-receptor (LDL-R, also known as the apoB/apoE receptor) or the LDL-R related protein (LRP).

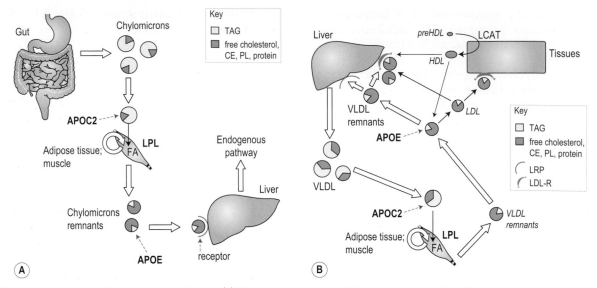

Fig. 7.2 Pathways of lipoprotein metabolism. (a) Exogenous pathway of lipoprotein metabolism. Chylomicrons may pass through the tissue capillary beds several times where they are hydrolysed by lipoprotein lipase (LPL), resulting in a chylomicron remnant which has lost a large portion of its original TAG content (see Fig. *evolve* 7.14). The resultant particle is taken up by the liver by receptor-mediated endocytosis. (b) Endogenous pathway of lipoprotein metabolism. VLDL may pass through the tissue capillary beds several times where they are hydrolysed by lipoprotein lipase, resulting in a VLDL remnant which has lost a large portion of its original TAG content (see Fig. *evolve* 7.14). The remnant particle has two possible metabolic fates: (a) it can be further hydrolysed to LDL, which is the main transporter of cholesterol to the target tissue; (b) the remnant particle is taken up by the liver by receptor-mediated endocytosis. Excess tissue cholesterol is returned to the liver by reverse cholesterol transport mediated by HDL and lecithin cholesterol acyltransferase. *Abbreviations*: LDL-R, LDL receptor; LRP, LDL-R-related protein; LPL, lipoprotein lipase; CE, cholesterol esters; PL, phospholipids; LCAT, lecithin-cholesterol acyltransferase.

The endogenous lipoprotein pathway: VLDL metabolism

VLDL distributes triacylglycerols from the liver to the tissues via the endogenous lipoprotein pathway. The sources of fatty acids for liver triacylglycerol synthesis include fatty acids returned to the liver by chylomicron remnants, LDL or HDL, fatty acids delivered bound to albumin, and fatty acids formed by de novo lipogenesis in the liver. This latter source is thought to be small on a typical Western diet, but may become more significant on a high-carbohydrate diet. ApoB100 is the main structural and functional protein of VLDL. Upon secretion into the bloodstream VLDL acquires apoC2 from HDL, then VLDL triacylglycerols are hydrolysed by LPL and the fatty acids are accumulated by tissues in a similar manner to those from chylomicrons. However, chylomicrons are thought to provide a better substrate for LPL and are hydrolysed preferentially when both particles are present in the postprandial (fed) state.

VLDL remnants, known as intermediate density lipoproteins (IDL), have two metabolic fates. Approximately 40–50% are taken up by the liver by receptor-mediated endocytosis; the remaining 50–60% lose all surface components except for a layer of phospholipids, free cholesterol and apoB100 and become LDL, the major carrier of cholesterol in the blood.

The endogenous lipoprotein pathway: LDL metabolism

The role of LDL is to transport cholesterol to the peripheral tissues and regulate de novo synthesis of cholesterol at these sites. On arrival at the cell surface, the apoB100 component of LDL is recognised by the LDL-receptor. Following internalisation of the LDL-receptor complex, the vesicle fuses with lysosomes, which contain a variety of degradative enzymes. The apoB100 protein is hydrolysed to free amino acids and the cholesterol esters to free cholesterol. The majority of the LDL-receptor is returned to the cell surface unaltered. The released cholesterol can be used immediately for incorporation into cell membranes or synthesis of steroid hormones. Alternatively, the cholesterol can be re-esterified and stored within the cell. Cellular cholesterol is derived from both extracellular sources (LDL) and synthesised in the cell. The process of cellular cholesterol metabolism is tightly regulated.

The physiological importance of the LDL-receptor in cholesterol homeostasis is demonstrated in the condition familial hypercholesterolaemia (FH), in which there is an absence or deficiency of functional LDL-receptors. Marked elevations in circulating LDL levels are evident, which leads to deposition of cholesterol in a variety of tissues, including the artery walls, thus contributing to atherogenesis.

A number of additional receptors which recognise LDL, one class of which is known as the scavenger receptors, have been identified. These receptors, which are present in large numbers on the surface of macrophages, do not bind to native LDL, but only LDL that has been chemically modified, e.g. oxidised. Unlike the LDL-receptor, scavenger receptors are not subject to downregulation and therefore macrophages can take up LDL indefinitely until they become lipid laden, when they are known as foam cells. This process forms the basis of the lipid accumulation which occurs in the development of atherosclerosis and the process is accelerated in people with high circulating LDL levels (see Ch. 19).

Reverse cholesterol transport: HDL metabolism

Excessive accumulation of cholesterol in tissues is toxic as cells cannot break down cholesterol and in the artery wall this leads to the development of atherosclerosis. This excess cholesterol is transported in HDL back to the liver, where it can be excreted in the bile, or be transported to other cells via the VLDL–LDL pathway. More than 40% of individuals who have a myocardial infarction (heart attack) have low HDL levels.

Pre-β-HDL is synthesised in the intestine and liver and secreted into the bloodstream as a discoidal pre-HDL particle containing apoA1 and a small amount of phospholipid. The emerging HDL particles gather some surface material (phospholipids and free cholesterol) released following the

hydrolysis of chylomicrons and VLDL by LPL. Nascent HDL particles bind to cell surface receptors and avidly absorb cholesterol from the cell membrane. Lecithin-cholesterol acyltransferase (LCAT) present in HDL esterifies the cholesterol, allowing it to move to the core of the particle and freeing up space on the surface for more cholesterol. LCAT, which is activated by apoA1, ensures a unidirectional movement of cholesterol from the cell to the HDL particle. Gradually the HDL accumulates cholesterol and becomes a mature spherical α-HDL particle (HDL_2).

Subsequent movement of this excess cholesterol in HDL back to the liver is mediated by either a direct or an indirect pathway. In the direct pathway, HDL itself takes the cholesterol to the liver, although quantitatively this is not the most important route. The majority of cholesterol delivery is achieved via the indirect route, where HDL transfers its cholesterol to chylomicrons and VLDL remnants, which subsequently transport the cholesterol to the liver. In addition to its role in reverse cholesterol transport, HDL may also have some additional benefits with respect to the development of atherosclerosis. For example, it inhibits the movement of macrophages (cells which accumulate cholesterol) into the artery wall, it is important for maintaining endothelial (cells lining the blood vessels) health and it inhibits LDL oxidation.

GENETIC AND DIETARY REGULATION OF LIPOPROTEIN METABOLISM

The concentration and composition of circulating lipoproteins is influenced by both genetic and environmental factors, including diet.

Genetic factors influencing circulating lipoprotein concentrations

Rare but major gene defects, such as familial hypercholesterolaemia (FH), cause large increases in lipoprotein concentrations resulting in high risk of premature myocardial infarction. More common variants (known as single nucleotide polymorphisms (SNPs)) in genes encoding for apolipoproteins, lipases, lipoprotein receptors and fatty acid transport proteins, have lesser impact on the concentration and composition of circulating lipoproteins, but contribute to a moderately increased risk of coronary heart disease. Overall, greater than 50% of the variation in fasting and postprandial lipoprotein concentrations is genetically determined. The adverse impact of these lesser gene defects on lipoprotein concentrations can vary according to background diet. A collection of lipoprotein abnormalities termed the atherogenic lipoprotein phenotype (ALP) (raised triglycerides, reduced levels of HDL cholesterol and a high proportion of LDL in the small, dense atherogenic form), is becoming increasingly common and is linked with the metabolic syndrome and central obesity (see Ch. 20, Section 20.3). The ALP, which increases risk of coronary heart disease 3–4-fold, is thought to arise due to complex interactions between diet, adiposity and a number of SNPs in genes encoding for proteins which regulate lipoprotein metabolism and insulin function.

Familial Hypercholesterolaemia (FH) (Type II$_a$ Hyperlipidaemia)

Familial hypercholesterolaemia is an autosomal recessive disorder first characterised by the pioneering studies of Goldstein and Brown (Goldstein et al 1983). The condition is characterised by a deficiency or complete absence of functional LDL receptors on the cell surface (Thompson 1990). As a result, the uptake of cholesterol into the liver and other tissue is impaired, resulting in markedly elevated levels in the circulation. Heterozygotes typically have circulating cholesterol levels two- to three-fold higher than normal. Homozygotes have almost no receptors for LDL and have up to 10-fold higher cholesterol than the levels in 'normal' individuals. Untreated, more than 85% of FH males will suffer a myocardial infarction before the age of 60 and many before the age of 40. The condition is usually treated by following a reduced total fat, saturated fat and cholesterol diet together with a combined drug therapy of resins (which sequester bile acid) and statins (which inhibit HMG-CoA reductase, the main enzyme involved in cholesterol synthesis). Such a combined treatment can reduce LDL cholesterol by up to 50%.

Familial defective apolipoproteinaemia

A number of dyslipidaemias are due to an inherited defect in a particular apolipoprotein. Familial defective apoB 100 (FDB) results in defective lipoprotein clearance and increased atherogenesis. It is clinically indistinguishable from heterozygous familial hypercholesterolaemia. An altered apoB100 struc-

ture results in decreased binding of the LDL particle to its receptor and subsequent increases in LDL cholesterol levels.

Familial defective apolipoprotein E is characterised by a low affinity of apoE for lipoprotein receptors, resulting in the accumulation of chylomicron and VLDL remnants in the circulation.

Atherogenic lipoprotein phenotype and the metabolic syndrome

The importance of hypertriacylglycerolaemia as a risk factor for coronary heart disease is now well established (Havel et al 1993, Castelli 1986). In addition to the ability of TRL to directly infiltrate and transport cholesterol in the developing atherosclerotic plaque, raised circulating triacylglycerols have been implicated as a major metabolic component of the atherogenic lipoprotein phenotype (ALP). As described above this is a term frequently used to describe a collection of pro-atherogenic lipoprotein abnormalities which constitute the main dyslipidaemia of the metabolic syndrome (Assmann & Schulte 1992, Austin et al 1990, Ruotolo & Howard 2002). The ALP lipid profile, which occurs in up to 25% of middle-aged males, is associated with a three-fold increased risk of coronary heart disease. It is characterised by a moderate fasting hypertriacylglycerolaemia (1.5–4.0 mmol/l), exaggerated postprandial triacylglycerol levels (Sethi et al 1993), low HDL cholesterol levels (<1.1 mmol/l) and a predominance of the potentially atherogenic small dense LDL-3 particle (>40% of total LDL).

When levels of TRL are high in the circulation there is a net transfer of triacylglycerol from these particles to LDL and HDL in exchange for cholesterol ester (Fig. *evolve* 7.15 🖱). This system of 'neutral lipid exchange' is catalysed by cholesterol ester transfer protein (CETP). The cholesterol-enriched TRLs have an increased capacity to transport cholesterol into the artery wall. In addition, the triacylglycerol-enriched LDL and HDL make ideal substrates for hepatic lipase (HL), which hydrolyses the relevant particle into small dense LDL-3 and HDL-3. HDL-3 is rapidly removed from the circulation, thereby reducing circulating levels of the protective HDL cholesterol. LDL-3 has greater atherogenic potential than larger LDL particles due to the fact that it is less readily removed from the circulation by hepatic LDL receptors, remains in circulation longer than normal LDL particles and is more prone to oxidation and uptake into macrophages in the arterial wall.

Diet and other environmental factors influencing lipoprotein concentration

Numerous environmental factors (diet, exercise, alcohol consumption and prescribed drug use) influence both fasting and postprandial lipid levels. The use of pharmacological therapies such as statins and fibrates reduces total and LDL cholesterol, and reduces triacylglycerols and increases HDL cholesterol, respectively. The evidence suggests a J- or U-shaped relationship between alcohol consumption and coronary heart disease with light to moderate consumption (1–4 units per day, up to 20g and 30g of alcohol per day in women and men) associated with a reduced risk (see also Ch. 9). Numerous mechanisms have been proposed to explain this protective effect, including a beneficial impact on thrombosis, inflammation or insulin sensitivity. However, increases in HDL cholesterol concentration due to an in increase in apoA1 and A2 are thought to be in large part responsible for the cardioprotective actions of moderate alcohol consumption. A beneficial impact of aerobic exercise on all lipoprotein classes has been reported with the greatest effect evident for triacylglycerols and HDL cholesterol levels, which is likely to be in part attributable to the known effect of exercise on insulin sensitivity, as well as increased utilisation of circulating triacylglycerols as oxidative substrates in skeletal muscle.

The amount and composition of dietary fat is arguably the most important dietary factor determining blood lipid metabolism.

The replacement of saturated fat, in particular lauric acid (C12:0), myristic acid (C14:0) and palmitic acid (C16:0), with polyunsaturated fat is associated with a reduction in LDL cholesterol. In 2003, Mensink and co-workers produced a meta-analysis of 60 studies published between 1970 and 1998, involving a total of 1672 participants, with intervention periods ranging from 13–91 days. The results of the meta-analysis were summarised by a series of predictive equations which indicated that the replacement of 1% of dietary energy from saturated fat by carbohydrate, monounsaturated fat or polyunsaturated fat would be associated with a decrease in LDL cholesterol of 0.036, 0.042 and 0.057 mmol/l respectively. However it must be noted that replacement of SFA also decreases the

beneficial HDL cholesterol. Large replacements of SFA with carbohydrate should be avoided because although this will reduce LDL cholesterol it will also result in significant increases in triacylglycerol levels. The consumption of soluble dietary fibre and plant sterols/stanols is associated with a significant reduction in LDL cholesterol which is attributable to the reduced absorption of dietary cholesterol and reabsorption of cholesterol in the form of bile salts. The n-3 polyunsaturated fatty acids eicosapentaenoic acid (EPA) and docosahexaenoic acid (DHA) are highly effective hypotriacylglycerolaemic agents. Intakes of 3–4 g per day decrease fasting and postprandial triacylglycerol by 20–35% (Minihane et al 2000), through reducing the production and secretion of triacylglycerol by the liver and improving LPL-mediated TRL clearance.

7.4 THE ROUTES OF INTRACELLULAR FAT METABOLISM

FATTY ACID UPTAKE AND ACTIVATION

Fatty acids can be oxidised to form ATP by many tissues. They are delivered to tissues either in the form of non-esterified fatty acids (NEFAs), bound to serum albumin, or by the hydrolysis of the triacylglycerol component of circulating lipoproteins. The mechanism by which NEFAs are taken up by cells has often been controversial, but it is possible that both carrier-mediated transport and diffusion are involved. The proteins implicated in fatty acid transport are fatty acid binding proteins (FABPs), fatty acid translocase (FAT) and the fatty acid transport protein (FATP). In addition to their roles in fatty acid uptake by cells, FABPs are also important intracellular carriers of fatty acids, delivering them to subcellular organelles, such as mitochondria, where they can be oxidised.

Before fatty acids can take part in metabolic reactions they are esterified to coenzyme A (CoA), forming the thiol ester acyl CoA. The formation of acyl CoAs is catalysed by several acyl CoA synthetases, which differ in their subcellular location and their specificity for fatty acids of different chain length (see further details in Section *evolve* 7.4 (a) 📖).

FATTY ACID SYNTHESIS

De novo fatty acid synthesis usually signifies an excess of energy-yielding substrates; carbon for fatty acid synthesis is supplied by carbohydrate or, in some cases, amino acids. As discussed in Section 6.5 under 'The oxidation of pyruvate to acetyl CoA', these precursors are metabolised to acetyl CoA in the mitochondria. There are three major steps in the pathway leading to the synthesis of fatty acids: (i) the transport of acetyl CoA to the cytoplasm, (ii) the formation of malonyl CoA and (iii) elongation of the fatty acid chain.

Under conditions which favour fatty acid synthesis, citrate that has been formed in the mitochondrion by condensation of acetyl CoA and oxaloacetate (see Fig. 6.2) is transported into the cytosol where it is cleaved by ATP citrate lyase to yield acetyl CoA and oxaloacetate. This compartmentalisation separates fatty acid synthesis, which occurs in the cytosol, from fatty acid oxidation, which occurs exclusively in mitochondria, and the transport step is therefore crucial in the control of fatty acid synthesis. The oxaloacetate re-enters the mitochondria as pyruvate (see Fig. *evolve* 7.7 🖁), yielding about half the NADPH required for fatty acid synthesis in the process; the other half comes from the pentose phosphate pathway (see Section 6.5, under 'The pentose phosphate pathway – an alternative to glycolysis').

Fatty acids are synthesised by the successive addition of two-carbon units from acetyl CoA, followed by reduction. Two key multi-enzyme complexes are responsible for the synthesis of fatty acids from acetyl CoA. The first is acetyl CoA carboxylase, which catalyses the carboxylation of acetyl CoA to malonyl CoA, a 3-carbon unit. Its activity is regulated in response to insulin and glucagon. Malonyl CoA is not only the substrate for fatty acid synthesis, but also a potent inhibitor of carnitine palmitoyl transferase (see Section 7.4 'Oxidation of fatty acids', below), so inhibiting the uptake of fatty acids into the mitochondria for β-oxidation. The second enzyme complex is fatty acid synthase (FAS), which catalyses a series of reactions involving the successive addition of 2-carbon units to a growing fatty acid chain, using malonyl CoA as the donor of each 2-carbon unit (see Fig. *evolve* 7.8 🖁). The enzymes required for fatty acid synthesis form a multi-enzyme complex, arranged in a series of concentric rings around a central acyl carrier protein (ACP), which carries the growing fatty acid chain from one enzyme to the next.

The malonyl group formed by acetyl CoA carboxylase is transferred onto an acyl carrier protein, and then reacts with the growing fatty acid chain, bound to the central acyl carrier protein of the fatty acid synthase complex. The carbon dioxide that was added to form malonyl CoA is lost in this reaction. For the first cycle of reactions, the central acyl carrier protein carries an acetyl group, and the product of reaction with malonyl CoA is acetoacetyl ACP; in subsequent reaction cycles, it is the growing fatty acid chain that occupies the central ACP, and the product of reaction with malonyl CoA is a keto-acyl ACP.

This intermediate is reduced then dehydrated to yield a carbon–carbon double bond, which is further reduced to yield a saturated fatty acid chain. Thus, the sequence of chemical reactions is the reverse of that in β-oxidation (see 'Oxidation of fatty acids', below). For both reduction reactions in fatty acid synthesis, NADPH is the hydrogen donor.

The normal end-product of FAS action is palmitic acid, a saturated, 16-carbon fatty acid, which is cleaved from the complex by an integral thioesterase. However, many membranes contain longer-chain fatty acids, which may be unsaturated. These are formed by elongation and/or desaturation of fatty acids after palmitic acid has been cleaved from the FAS complex.

ELONGATION AND DESATURATION OF FATTY ACIDS

Elongases are enzymes that add carbon atoms to preformed fatty acids that either have been synthesised de novo or originate from the diet. Two elongation systems exist in many tissues, one in the mitochondria and the other in the endoplasmic reticulum. The mitochondrial system involves the addition of 2-carbon units from acetyl CoA, whereas elongation in the endoplasmic reticulum employs malonyl CoA as the donor.

One of the most important roles of the elongases and desaturases is the conversion of the essential fatty acids, linoleic acid and α-linolenic acid, to their longer-chain derivatives. Thus, linoleoyl-CoA undergoes sequential desaturation and elongation to form intermediates of the n-6 family of polyunsaturated fatty acids, the key end-product of which is arachidonic acid. As a result of the sequential nature of these reactions, polyunsaturated fatty acids usually contain methylene-interrupted double bonds. A similar series of desaturations and elongations generates the n-3 family of polyunsaturated fatty acids. The derivatives of linoleic and α-linolenic acid are often termed 'conditionally essential', since their synthesis is determined by the presence of the essential fatty acid precursors. The extent and regulation of conversion of α-linolenic acid to EPA, docosapentaenoic acid (DPA) and DHA remains unclear. It appears that in human beings, α-linolenic acid can be converted to EPA and DPA, but only very low levels of DHA are synthesised. This needs to be borne in mind when considering the theoretical pathway for metabolism depicted in Figure *evolve* 7.9 . Importantly, the elongation and desaturation pathways for linoleic and α-linolenic acid share one set of desaturase and elongase enzymes, which means that there is competition between the n-6 and n-3 families of fatty acids. The elongation and desaturation of oleic acid does not occur to a significant degree in mammalian tissues, However, if essential fatty acid deficiency occurs, oleic acid is desaturated and elongated, usually to mead acid (C20:3 n-9). The presence of mead acid in biological samples is interpreted as a sign of essential fatty acid deficiency.

OXIDATION OF FATTY ACIDS

Fatty acids can undergo oxidation starting at the α-, β- or ω-carbon; β-oxidation is the most physiologically important pathway – see Figure *evolve* 7.10 and also Section *evolve* 7.4(b) .

In β-oxidation, fatty acids are degraded by the sequential liberation of acetyl CoA units. Although mitochondria are the major site for β-oxidation, the peroxisomes also contain the enzymes for this pathway. This additional site is particularly important in the liver, serving to oxidise very-long-chain fatty acids to medium-chain products, which are subsequently transported to the mitochondria for complete oxidation. In addition to partial oxidation of long-chain fatty acids, peroxisomes are also the site for the degradation of xenobiotics and eicosanoids.

Once it has entered the mitochondria, a fatty acyl CoA undergoes a repeating series of four reactions, as shown in Figure *evolve* 7.10 , which results in the cleavage of the fatty acid molecule to give acetyl CoA and a new fatty acyl CoA which is two carbons shorter than the initial substrate. This new, shorter, fatty acyl CoA is then a substrate for the same sequence of reactions, which is repeated until the final result is cleavage to yield two molecules of acetyl CoA. The reactions of β-oxidation are chemically the same as those in the conversion of succinate to oxaloacetate in the citric acid cycle, and the reverse of those in fatty acid synthesis (see 'Fatty acid synthesis', above):

1. Removal of two hydrogens from the fatty acid forms a carbon–carbon double bond – an oxidation reaction which yields a reduced flavin, so for each double bond formed in this way there is a yield of ~ 2 ATP.
2. The newly formed double bond in the fatty acyl CoA then reacts with water, yielding a hydroxyl group – a hydration reaction.
3. The hydroxylated fatty acyl CoA undergoes a second oxidation in which the hydroxyl group is oxidised to an oxo group, yielding NADH (equivalent to ~ 3 ATP).
4. The oxo-acyl CoA is then cleaved by reaction with CoA, to form acetyl CoA and the shorter fatty acyl CoA, which undergoes the same sequence of reactions.

Regulation of the rate of β-oxidation

See also Section *evolve* 7.4 (b) .

The rate of β-oxidation is regulated by two mechanisms, the availability of fatty acids and the rate of utilisation of β-oxidation products. The availability of fatty acids in turn is dictated by the insulin:glucagon ratio, which, when high, inhibits the breakdown of triacylglycerols from adipose tissue and therefore the release of NEFAs from adipose stores. The insulin:glucagon ratio will be high in the fed state, when there is adequate availability of fuel from the ingested food and the release of NEFAs from adipose tissue is therefore not required. In muscle, the rate of β-oxidation is dependent on the plasma NEFA concentration and the energy demand of the tissue. A reduction in energy demand (e.g. when physical activity is low) will lead to an accumulation of NADH (which will inhibit the citric acid cycle) and acetyl CoA.

The role of carnitine in fatty acid uptake for oxidation

Fatty acyl CoA cannot cross the mitochondrial membranes to enter the matrix. On the outer face of the outer mitochondrial membrane, the fatty acid is transferred from CoA onto carnitine, forming acylcarnitine, which enters the inter-membrane space through an acylcarnitine transporter.

Acylcarnitine can cross the inner mitochondrial membrane on a counter-transport system which takes in acylcarnitine in exchange for free carnitine being returned to the inter membrane space. Once inside the mitochondrial inner membrane, acylcarnitine transfers the acyl group onto CoA ready to undergo β-oxidation. This counter-transport system provides regulation of the uptake of fatty acids into the mitochondrion for oxidation. As long as there is free CoA available in the mitochondrial matrix, fatty acids can be taken up, and the carnitine returned to the outer membrane for uptake of more fatty acids. However, if most of the CoA in the mitochondria is acylated, then there is no need for further fatty acid uptake immediately, and indeed, it is not possible. Further control is exerted by malonyl CoA (the precursor for fatty acid synthesis; see 'Fatty acid synthesis', above) which is a potent inhibitor of carnitine palmitoyl transferase I in the outer mitochondrial membrane.

SYNTHESIS OF KETONE BODIES

In the liver, the acetyl CoA formed by β-oxidation is positioned at a crossroad for two important metabolic fates. It can react with either oxaloacetate to form citrate (and hence undergo complete oxidation) or with acetoacetyl CoA to form ketone bodies (ketogenesis). Its fate is determined chiefly by the rate of β-oxidation and the availability of oxaloacetate. If the rate of β-oxidation is high (as in fasting), then oxaloacetate will be diverted towards gluconeogenesis, so reducing the amount of acetyl CoA entering the citric acid cycle. In this situation, acetyl CoA will be directed towards ketogenesis.

Under conditions that favour ketone body synthesis (i.e. extended starvation), plasma insulin levels are low and fatty acid oxidation to acetyl CoA predominates in the liver and other tissues that are able to oxidise fatty acids. As the liver oxidises fatty acids to acetyl CoA, the citric acid cycle becomes progressively less able fully to oxidise the acetyl CoA formed, partly because high amounts of ATP begin to inhibit the activity of the cycle and partly because oxaloacetate is diverted towards gluconeogenesis (see Section 6.5) and so becomes limiting for citric acid cycle activity. This is a situation specific to the liver because of its important role in synthesising and secreting glucose during starvation. Acetyl CoA that does not undergo further oxidation is condensed to form the 4-carbon compound acetoacetyl CoA, which is further metabolised to form the ketone bodies acetoacetate and β-hydroxybutyrate (see Fig. *evolve* 7.11).

Most ketone bodies are converted back into acetyl CoA by muscle and other tissues that are able to use ketone bodies as a fuel (see Fig. *evolve* 7.12), and the acetyl CoA is oxidised in the citric acid cycle.

The formation of ketone bodies from fatty acids released by adipose tissue during starvation is extremely important because ketone bodies provide a water-soluble fuel to meet part of the energy requirements of the brain, which cannot oxidise fatty acids, so sparing glucose. Normal levels of circulating ketone bodies in the fed state are approximately 0.01 mmol/l, but they can rise to 0.1 mmol/l after an overnight fast and 6–8 mmol/l following several days of starvation. Excessively high concentrations of ketone bodies (which are acidic) can cause acidosis, inducing coma or death if untreated. This usually only occurs in uncontrolled type 1 diabetes mellitus, when it is termed diabetic ketoacidosis (see Ch. 21).

SYNTHESIS OF CHOLESTEROL

Cholesterol can be obtained through the diet, but all nucleated cells have the capacity to synthesise cholesterol, with the liver being quantitatively the most important site. An important function of cholesterol is its structural role in membranes, but it is also important as a precursor for the synthesis of bile acids and steroid hormones. The precursor for the synthesis of cholesterol is cytosolic acetyl CoA (see Section *evolve* 7.4(c)). Since high levels of unesterified cholesterol are likely to be undesirable for cells, and cells (other than the liver) are unable to oxidise cholesterol, excess cholesterol is converted into cholesteryl esters by the enzyme acyl CoA cholesterol acyltransferase, which is located on the endoplasmic reticulum. The cholesteryl esters can be stored in lipid droplets within the cytosol; these are commonly observed in steroidogenic tissues.

SYNTHESIS AND UTILISATION OF TRIACYLGLYCEROLS

See also Section *evolve* 7.4(d).

Triacylglycerols (TAGs) are both the chief form of dietary fat, and also the main form of fat stored in the body. Triacylglycerols provides a highly reduced, anhydrous form of metabolic fuel, which can be stored in very large amounts. Whenever energy supply from the diet exceeds the energy expenditure of the body, triacylglycerol is deposited in adipose tissue. In particular cases triacylglycerol may be stored in alternative sites such as muscle, liver or pancreas, referred to as ectopic fat storage. This generally occurs in obese individuals, with its occurrence leading to dysregulation of tissue metabolism. Ectopic fat storage is considered to be an underlying cause of insulin resistance.

As discussed in Section 4.2, white adipose tissue is distributed throughout the body, surrounding many internal organs, and provides a protective subcutaneous layer. The cells within adipose tissue are adipocytes, which are bound together by connective tissue and are supplied by an extensive network of blood vessels. When a fat-containing meal is consumed, adipocytes acquire fat from circulating lipoproteins by hydrolytic breakdown of triacylglycerol by LPL, releasing fatty acids (see 'Triacylglycerol', below). In the reverse situation, when there is a demand for fatty acids for metabolism, triacylglycerol is mobilised by the enzyme hormone-sensitive lipase (HSL). These phases are integrated and controlled by the nutritional status of the individual through a number of hormones, the most important of which is insulin (see 'Integration of fat metabolism from the fasted to the fed state at the whole body level', below).

Biosynthesis of triacylglycerol involves the esterification of three fatty acids (acyl groups) to a glycerol backbone. It can occur in a number of tissues, the most predominant of which are adipose tissue, liver, enterocytes and the mammary gland during lactation.

Under conditions where the demand for mobilisation of fuel reserves increases, usually signalled by low concentrations of insulin, biosynthetic pathways are inhibited and HSL is activated within adipocytes (for more detailed description of both TAG synthesis and breakdown, refer to Section *evolve* 7.4(d)). Once released, the NEFAs are bound to plasma albumin and may be taken up by tissues that are able to utilise fatty acids as a fuel source.

7.5 INTEGRATION, CONTROL AND DYNAMICS OF FAT METABOLISM

COORDINATED REGULATION OF FATTY ACID SYNTHESIS AND OXIDATION

In the fed state, when carbohydrate may be converted to fatty acids, the level of malonyl CoA is raised and this results in inhibition of carnitine palmitoyl transferase 1 (CPT1), which controls the uptake of acyl CoA into mitochondria for oxidation and hence inhibits β-oxidation of fatty acids (see 'Fatty acid synthesis', above). In the fasting state, the reverse situation occurs and CPT1 activity is high, stimulating β-oxidation and ketogenesis. Coinciding with this, in the fasting state, a low insulin:glucagon ratio and/or the release of adrenaline (epinephrine) inhibits acetyl CoA carboxylase activity, reducing the synthesis of malonyl CoA and relieving the inhibition of CPT (for details of this regulation, see Section *evolve* 7.5).

Tissues, such as muscle, that oxidise fatty acids but do not synthesise them also have acetyl CoA carboxylase, and produce malonyl CoA in order to control the activity of carnitine palmitoyl transferase I, and thus control the mitochondrial uptake and β-oxidation of fatty acids. Tissues also have malonyl CoA decarboxylase, which acts to remove malonyl CoA and so reduce the inhibition of carnitine palmitoyl transferase I. The two enzymes are regulated in opposite directions in response to insulin, which stimulates fatty acid synthesis and reduces β-oxidation, and glucagon, which reduces fatty acid synthesis and increases β-oxidation.

Fatty acids are the major fuel for red muscle fibres, which are the main type involved in moderate exercise. Children who lack one or other of the enzymes required for carnitine synthesis, and are therefore reliant on dietary intake, have poor exercise tolerance, because they have an impaired ability to transport fatty acids into the mitochondria for β-oxidation. Provision of supplements of carnitine to the affected children overcomes the problem.

INTEGRATION OF FAT METABOLISM WITH THE METABOLISM OF CARBOHYDRATE AND PROTEIN

As described above, fats can circulate in the blood in the form of NEFAs, as triacylglycerols in lipoproteins and as ketone bodies in prolonged starvation. In addition to these fat-derived fuels, carbohydrates circulate as glucose, lactate, pyruvate or glycerol and proteins as amino acids. What determines which of these fuels are oxidised by a tissue at any given time? This question is best answered by considering:

● The ability of tissue to oxidise the fuel; some tissues are anaerobic, or lack mitochondria, and therefore cannot oxidise fatty acids or ketone bodies

● The availability of fuel; this will be determined by the prevailing conditions. If an individual has been fasting for 18 hours, it is likely that the liver glycogen stores will be depleted and the circulating concentration of fatty acids will be high.

In summary, fatty acids are the preferred fuel for oxidation whenever their circulating concentrations are high and glucose is spared whenever necessary (see Fig. *evolve* 7.13 🖱). When the energy provided by the diet exceeds immediate requirements, excess carbohydrate is preferentially used to replenish liver glycogen stores (see Section 6.5). Excess amino acids will be oxidised only after satisfying the needs for protein synthesis (see Section 8.5). Any remaining excess of fuel will be used for fatty acid and triacylglycerol synthesis for storage in adipose tissue (see Fig. *evolve* 7.13 🖱). All of these processes will be coordinated by changes in the circulating levels of hormones, the most important of which are insulin and glucagon.

INTERCONVERSION OF FUELS AND THE ENERGY PARADOX

The following rules regarding interconversion of fuels are absolutely central to understanding the integration of metabolic pathways.

● Fatty acids can be made from carbohydrates and amino acids, but cannot be converted to either.

● Carbohydrates can be made from amino acids and can be used to make triacylglycerols.

The inability to convert fatty acids to glucose gives rise to what is known as the 'energy paradox'. The basis of this paradox is that the brain requires 500 kcal of water-soluble fuel (usually glucose) per day, yet the chief energy store in the body is fat, not glycogen, and fatty acids cannot be converted to glucose. The energy paradox is dealt with in four ways:

1. The oxidation of fatty acids (especially by muscle) spares glucose.
2. Lipolysis of triacylglycerol during starvation releases glycerol as well as fatty acids and the glycerol can be used as a substrate for gluconeogenesis. Thus glucose can be synthesised from the glycerol component of triacylglycerol.

3. Fatty acid oxidation in the liver provides the ATP required for gluconeogenesis.
4. Fatty acids can be converted to ketone bodies, a water-soluble fuel which can be used by the brain to meet perhaps one-fifth of its energy needs in starvation.

MECHANISMS FOR INTEGRATION OF FAT AND CARBOHYDRATE METABOLISM

Control of phosphofructokinase (PFK) activity

As discussed in Chapter 6, phosphofructokinase (PFK) catalyses a key irreversible and controlling step in glycolysis. Control of this enzyme is key to the integration of the metabolism of fat and carbohydrate. High levels of ATP inhibit PFK and therefore inhibit glycolysis. In tissues that are oxidising fatty acids (e.g. during starvation or exercise), large amounts of ATP are generated. As a result, the oxidation of fatty acids will prevent oxidation of glucose by inhibiting glycolysis and glucose will be spared for other tissues. This regulatory mechanism is termed the 'glucose–fatty acid cycle'.

Control of pyruvate dehydrogenase (PDH) activity

Pyruvate dehydrogenase (PDH) catalyses the irreversible oxidation of pyruvate to acetyl CoA. When glucose is freely available, PDH is active and acetyl CoA does not accumulate because it is rapidly used for synthesis of citrate and either complete oxidation in the citric acid cycle or fatty acid synthesis (if carbohydrate is in excess). However, when glucose supplies are diminished and plasma NEFA levels increase as a result of lipolysis in adipose tissue, the oxidation of fatty acids in tissues results in an increase in intracellular acetyl CoA, ATP and NADH. These inhibit PDH activity, reinforcing the glucose–fatty acid cycle. Thus, oxidising fatty acids will conserve glucose by inhibiting both PFK and PDH.

INTEGRATION OF FAT METABOLISM FROM THE FASTED TO THE FED STATE AT THE WHOLE BODY LEVEL

Non-esterified fatty acids

Following an overnight fast, the plasma NEFA concentration is normally about 0.5 mmol/l and the triacylglycerol concentration about 1 mmol/l (largely contributed by VLDL). The NEFAs are released by lipolysis of adipose tissue triacylglycerol by HSL and they are taken up by a number of tissues, including skeletal muscle and liver. The regulatory mechanisms which lead to the activation of hormone-sensitive lipase and of the reverse process, the esterification of fatty acids in adipose tissue, are key determinants of the plasma concentration of NEFAs. The rate of oxidation of NEFAs by tissues depends mainly on the plasma concentration, so that the higher the concentration, the greater the rate of utilisation. Hence, the plasma concentration of NEFAs is directly related to rate of release from adipose tissue (and therefore activation of HSL versus esterification). Since the key regulatory signal for activation of HSL is a fall in insulin concentration, the plasma NEFA concentration over the course of a day is normally an inverse reflection of the plasma concentrations of glucose and insulin. In the fasting state the concentrations of glucose and insulin are at their lowest and those of NEFAs highest. The plasma concentration of NEFAs has an upper limit of approximately 2 mmol/l, because above this concentration, the relative proportion of NEFAs which are not bound to albumin increases; NEFAs not bound to albumin will cause significant haemolysis and may also have adverse effects on other tissues, particularly the heart.

Following consumption of a meal (the absorptive phase), the rise in blood glucose concentration stimulates insulin secretion, which suppresses HSL activity, and the plasma concentration of NEFAs will subsequently fall to <0.1 mmol/l. The concentration at which insulin inhibits the activity of HSL is much lower than the concentration at which it stimulates glucose metabolism. This means that NEFAs fall very rapidly and dramatically very soon after food ingestion. The activity of this enzyme is never completely suppressed, even at very high concentrations of insulin. However, the increase in plasma glucose and insulin concentrations will also increase the uptake of glucose and of glycolysis within the adipocyte, and, as a result, glycerol-3-phosphate will become available for re-esterification of fatty acids, so any NEFAs released by the action of HSL will be re-esterified. After a meal, therefore, release of NEFAs from adipose tissue will be almost completely suppressed.

As a result of the fall in NEFA concentration, tissues that were oxidising fatty acids in the fasted state (and so sparing glucose) will reduce their uptake and oxidation of fatty acids and utilise glucose once more. The increased insulin: glucagon ratio on feeding also leads to a reduction in the synthesis of ketone bodies by the liver, so that plasma levels of ketone bodies fall from overnight fasted values of 0.1–0.2 mmol/l to levels that are almost undetectable. The absorptive phase finally begins to decline after about 5 hours, the exact time depending on the composition of the meal, allowing insulin concentrations to decline and relaxing the restraint on fat mobilisation. In general, a meal containing a significant amount of fat slows absorption.

Triacylglycerol

After an overnight fast, the plasma triacylglycerol concentration is normally about 1 mmol/l, almost all in the endogenous triacylglycerol-rich lipoprotein particles (VLDL). Consumption of a meal containing fat results in the formation of chylomicrons in the enterocyte and their entry into the bloodstream (as described in 'The exogenous lipoprotein pathway', above) approximately 3–5 hours after a meal. The postprandial plasma concentration of triacylglycerol can rise to between 1.5 mmol/l and 3.0 mmol/l, depending on the amount of fat in the meal and the metabolic capacity of the individual. The magnitude and duration of the postprandial lipaemic response will depend on the efficiency of the regulatory mechanisms for the disposal and storage of the triacylglycerol. Lipoprotein lipase is activated by insulin and will therefore be most active following a meal; in adipose tissue its activity reaches a peak approximately 3–4 hours after a meal, coinciding with the peak in postprandial plasma triacylglycerol. Insulin clearly plays a key role in the coordination of all aspects of fat metabolism, since both the hydrolysis of chylomicron-triacylglycerol by LPL and the subsequent uptake of the liberated fatty acids are facilitated by the fact that the activity of HSL is suppressed. Furthermore, insulin also promotes the re-esterification of fatty acids to form triacylglycerol for storage. However, adipose tissue is not the only tissue able to utilise the fatty acids released from chylomicron-triacylglycerol by the action of LPL. Skeletal muscle, for example, uses fatty acids from chylomicrons (or VLDL) as a source of energy.

During the postprandial period, chylomicron-triacylglycerol represents only a proportion of the total plasma triacylglycerol (perhaps 0.3–0.4 mmol/l after a very fatty meal). This is because the endogenous pathway (VLDL synthesis) is always active and after a meal the hydrolysis of VLDL is suppressed in favour of hydrolysis of chylomicrons. In addition, not all the NEFA released from chylomicrons is taken up and re-esterified in adipose tissue; much remains in the circulation and is taken up by liver, where it is used as substrate to drive synthesis of VLDL. Thus, a significant proportion of the postprandial lipaemic response is, in fact, contributed by VLDL. It should also be noted that the duration of elevation of triacylglycerols following a fat-containing meal is quite prolonged. It may be 6–8 hours before concentrations return towards the fasted values and because most people eat fat-containing meals throughout the day, postprandial lipaemia is the normal state. Once chylomicrons have been completely hydrolysed and their remnants removed by the liver, the exogenous pathway ceases and the endogenous pathway once again becomes the dominant route of triacylglycerol metabolism in the body.

KEY POINTS

- Fats perform a range of essential functions in the body; they can be stored for later release of energy, they are important structural components of cell membranes, they play roles in cell signalling, are essential for the absorption of fat-soluble vitamins and are precursors for the synthesis of hormones and other physiological mediators.
- Dietary fats are packaged into chylomicrons in enterocytes within the small intestine and enter the exogenous lipoprotein pathway via the lymph system. The triacylglycerol they carry is hydrolysed by the enzyme lipoprotein lipase, which is found on the surface of endothelial cells lining capillaries. The NEFAs released are taken up for use by the tissues.
- The endogenous pathway of lipoprotein metabolism involves the synthesis of VLDL by the liver and its subsequent metabolism to LDL. Chylomicrons and VLDL are carriers of triacylglycerol, while LDL and HDL transport cholesterol.
- Linoleic and α-linolenic acids are essential because they cannot be synthesised by animal cells. These essential fatty acids give rise to the n-6 and n-3 polyunsaturated fatty acids respectively through the action of desaturases and elongases. The metabolism of the essential fatty acids is competitive because the same set of enzymes is shared by the n-6 and n-3 pathways.
- The oxidation of fatty acids is regulated by their availability and their rate of utilisation. Fatty acids are stored as triacylglycerol in adipose tissue, which can be mobilised by the action of hormone-sensitive lipase during fasting. Fats can circulate as triacylglycerol in lipoproteins, NEFA or ketone bodies (in prolonged starvation). Fatty acids are the preferred fuel for oxidation whenever their circulating concentrations are high and glucose is spared whenever necessary.

References

Assmann G, Schulte H: Relation of high density lipoprotein cholesterol and triglycerides to incidence of atherosclerotic coronary artery disease (the PROCAM Experience), American Journal of Cardiology 70:733–737, 1992.

Austin MA, King M-C, Vranizan KM, Krauss RM: Atherogenic lipoprotein phenotype. A proposed genetic marker for coronary heart disease, Circulation 82:495–506, 1990.

Castelli WP: The triglyceride issue: a view from Framingham, Amerivcan Heart Journal 112:432–437, 1986.

Goldstein JL, Kita T, Brown MS: Defective lipoprotein receptors and atherosclerosis, New England Journal of Medicine 286:283–296 1983.

Havel R: McCollum Award Lecture 1993. Triglyceride-rich lipoproteins and atherosclerosis: new perspectives, American Journal of Clinical Nutrition 59:795–799, 1994.

Minihane AM, Khan S, Leigh-Firbank EC, Talmud P, Wright JW, Murphy MC, Griffin BA, Williams CM: ApoE polymorphism and fish oil supplementation in subjects with an atherogenic lipoprotein phenotype, Arteriosclerosis Thrombosis and Vascular Biology 20:1990–1997, 2000.

Ruotolo G, Howard BV: Dyslipidaemia of the metabolic syndrome, Current Cardiology Reports 4:494–500, 2002.

Sethi S, Gibney MJ, Williams CM: Postprandial lipoprotein metabolism, Nutrition Research 6:161–183, 1993.

Further reading

Key papers

Brown MS, Kovanen PT, Goldstein JL: Regulation of plasma cholesterol by lipoprotein receptors, *Science* 212:628–635, 1981.

Hussain MM, Strickland DK, Bakillah A: The mammalian low-density lipoprotein receptor family, *Annual Review of Nutrition* 19:141–172, 1999.

Mensink RP, Zock PL, Kester AD, Katan MB: Effects of dietary fatty acids and carbohydrates on the ratio of serum total to HDL cholesterol and on serum lipids and apolipoproteins: a meta-analysis of 60 controlled trials, *American Journal of Clinical Nutrition* 77:1146–1155, 2003.

Key textbooks

Assmann G, editor: *Lipoprotein metabolism disorders and coronary heart disease*, Munich, 1993, MMV Medizin Verlag.

Betteridge DJ, Illingworth DR, Shepherd J: *Lipoproteins in health and disease*, London, 1999, Arnold.

British Nutrition Foundation: *Unsaturated fatty acids: nutritional and physiological significance. Report of the British Nutrition Foundation's Task Force*, London, 1992, Chapman and Hall.

Frayn KN: *Metabolic regulation, a human perspective*, 2nd edn. Frontiers in Metabolism series, Oxford, 2003, Blackwell Science.

Gunstone FD, Harwood JL, Padley FB: *The lipid handbook*, 2nd edn. London, 1994, Chapman and Hall.

Gurr MI: *Role of fats in food and nutrition*, London, 1992, Elsevier Applied Science Publishers.

Gurr MI, Harwood JL, Frayn KN: *Lipid biochemistry – an introduction*, 5th edn. Oxford, 2002, Blackwell Science.

Vance DE, Vance JE: *Biochemistry of lipids, lipoproteins and membranes*, Amsterdam, 1996, Elsevier.

EVOLVE CONTENTS (available online at: evolve.elsevier.com/Geissler/nutrition)

Chapter 8

Protein metabolism and requirements

David A Bender and D Joe Millward

CHAPTER CONTENTS

© 2010 Elsevier Ltd/Inc/BV
DOI: 10.1016/B978-0-7020-3118-2.00008-5

OBJECTIVES

By the end of this chapter you should be able to:

- describe the key features of protein structure and the main functions of proteins
- explain what is meant by nitrogen balance and describe how it can be used to determine protein requirements
- explain what is meant by dynamic equilibrium
- describe in outline the mechanisms of protein synthesis and catabolism and explain the energy cost of protein turnover
- describe how protein synthesis is controlled by hormones and nutrients
- explain what is meant by dispensable and indispensable amino acids, the problem of unavailable amino acids
- describe the metabolism of amino acids
- explain the difficulty of determining amino acid and protein requirements
- describe the effects of physical activity and special needs on protein requirements
- explain what is meant by protein quality and describe the different ways of expressing it
- describe the stable isotope methods of determining protein and amino acid requirements, and explain the problems inherent in each.

8.1 INTRODUCTION

Protein is the most complex of the macronutrients. Indeed, dietary protein is not a single entity but rather a complex mixture of many different proteins, each with its own amino acid composition. Any individual protein may contain between 50 and 1000 amino acids; the sequence of these amino acids is specific for that protein.

The need for protein in the diet was demonstrated early in the nineteenth century, when it was shown that animals that were fed only on fats, carbohydrates and mineral salts were unable to maintain their body weight and showed severe wasting of muscle and other tissues. It was known that proteins contain nitrogen (mainly in the amino groups of their constituent amino acids), and methods of measuring total amounts of nitrogenous compounds in foods and excreta were soon developed.

The nutritional requirement is not only for total protein intake but for the various amino acids in the proportions that are required to maintain turnover of the complex mixture of body proteins. There are some 30000 to 50000 different proteins in the human body and they are broken down and replaced at different rates.

8.2 PROTEIN STRUCTURE AND FUNCTION

Proteins are composed of linear chains of amino acids joined by condensation of the carboxyl group of one with the amino group of another to form a peptide bond. Chains of amino acids linked in this way are known as polypeptides.

THE AMINO ACIDS

Twenty-one amino acids are involved in the synthesis of proteins, together with a number that occur in proteins as a result of chemical modification after the protein has been synthesised. In addition, a number of amino acids occur as metabolic intermediates but are not involved in proteins.

Chemically the amino acids all have the same basic structure – an amino group ($-NH_3^+$) and a carboxylic acid group ($-COO^-$) attached to the same carbon atom (the α-carbon). As shown in Figure 8.1, what differs between them is the nature of the other group that is attached to the α-carbon. In the

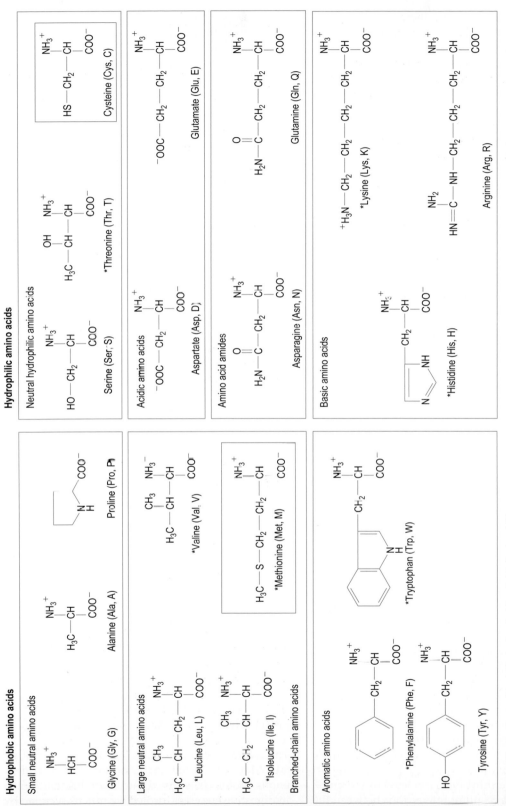

Fig. 8.1 The amino acids; left, hydrophobic; right, hydrophilic.

simplest amino acid, glycine, there are two hydrogen atoms, while in all other amino acids there is one hydrogen atom and a side-chain. Figure 8.1 does not show the structure of the 21st amino acid, the selenium analogue of cysteine, selenocysteine (see Ch. 12, Section 12.6).

The amino acids can be classified according to the chemical nature of the side-chain: whether it is hydrophobic (on the left of Fig. 8.1) or hydrophilic (on the right of Fig. 8.1); and the chemical nature of the group: hydrophobic, branched chain, aromatic, S-containing, neutral hydrophilic, acidic or basic.

The sequence of amino acids in a protein is its primary structure. It is different for each protein, although proteins that are closely related to each other often have similar primary structures. The primary structure of a protein is determined by the gene containing the information for that protein (see Section 8.3 under 'Protein synthesis').

FOLDING OF THE PROTEIN CHAIN

The linear chain of amino acids in a polypeptide folds in a variety of ways to form secondary and tertiary levels of structure. As a result of this, amino acids that may be far apart in the primary sequence come close together to form reactive regions that bind ligands (in receptor and transport proteins, and enzymes) and catalyse chemical reactions (in enzymes). Two main types of chemical interaction are responsible for the folding of the polypeptide chain: hydrogen bonds between the oxygen of one peptide bond and the nitrogen of another, and interactions between the side-chains of the amino acids.

The folding of the protein chain also provides proteins with physical properties: most soluble proteins have a relatively compact globular structure; structural proteins such as collagen (in bone and connective tissue) and keratin (in skin and hair) have a fibrous structure, with considerable cross-linkage between adjacent fibres, so that they are flexible but resist stretching. Elastin, the structural protein of elastic connective tissue, as in the arteries, has multiple cross-links between three or four adjacent chains, forming a three-dimensional network that is both flexible and elastic.

Having formed regions of secondary structure (regular helices and pleated sheets), the whole protein molecule then folds up into a compact shape. This is the third (tertiary) level of structure, and is largely the result of interactions between the side-chains of the amino acids, with each other and with the environment.

Two further interactions between amino acid side-chains may be involved in tertiary structure, forming covalent links between regions of the peptide chain:

● The ε-amino group on the side-chain of lysine can form a peptide bond with the carboxyl group on the side-chain of aspartate or glutamate. This is nutritionally important, since the side-chain peptide bond is not hydrolysed by digestive enzymes, and the lysine, which is an indispensable amino acid, is not available for absorption (see Section 8.4 under 'Unavailable amino acids').

● The sulphydryl (–SH) groups of two cysteine molecules may be oxidised to form a disulphide bridge between two parts of the protein chain.

Some proteins consist of more than one polypeptide chain; the way in which the chains interact with each other after they have separately formed their secondary and tertiary structures constitutes the quaternary structure of the protein. Interactions between the subunits of multi-subunit proteins, involving changes in quaternary structure and the conformation of the protein, affecting activity, are important in a number of regulatory enzymes.

DENATURATION OF PROTEINS

Because of their compact structures, most proteins are resistant to digestion; few bonds are accessible to proteolytic enzymes. However, the native structure of proteins is maintained by relatively weak non-covalent forces that are disrupted by heat and acid. When this happens, proteins become insoluble (the process of denaturation), and most of the peptide bonds are accessible to digestive enzymes. Gastric acid is also important, since relatively strong acid will disrupt hydrogen bonds and denature proteins.

8.3 NITROGEN BALANCE AND PROTEIN TURNOVER

The average dietary intake of protein is around 80 g/day, and about the same amount of endogenous protein is secreted into the intestinal lumen in digestive enzymes, protective mucus secreted by intestinal mucosal goblet cells and shed intestinal epithelial cells, so that the total flux of protein through the intestinal tract is about twice the dietary intake.

There is a small faecal loss equivalent to about 10 g of protein/day; the remainder is hydrolysed to free amino acids and small peptides, and absorbed. The faecal loss of nitrogen is partly composed of undigested dietary protein, but the main contributors are intestinal bacteria and shed mucosal cells that are only partially broken down, and mucus. Mucin, the main protein in mucus, is especially resistant to enzymic hydrolysis, and contributes a considerable proportion of obligatory nitrogen losses.

There is only a small pool of free amino acids in the body, in equilibrium with proteins that are being catabolised and synthesised. Part of this is used for synthesis of a variety of specialised metabolites (including hormones and neurotransmitters, purines and pyrimidines). An amount of amino acids equivalent to that absorbed from the diet is oxidised, with the carbon skeletons being used as metabolic fuels or for gluconeogenesis (see Section 6.3), and the nitrogen being excreted mainly as urea.

The state of protein nutrition, and the overall state of body protein metabolism, can be determined by measuring the dietary intake of nitrogenous compounds and the output of nitrogenous compounds from the body. Nitrogen constitutes 16% of most proteins, and the protein content of foods is calculated on the basis of mg N × 6.25, although for some foods with an unusual amino acid composition other factors are used.

The output of N from the body is largely in the urine and faeces, but significant amounts may also be lost in sweat and shed skin cells. Although the intake of nitrogenous compounds is mainly protein, the output is mainly urea, although small amounts of a number of other products of amino acid metabolism are also excreted.

The difference between intake and output of nitrogenous compounds is nitrogen balance. Three states can be defined:

- An adult in good health and with an adequate intake of protein excretes the same amount of nitrogen each day as is taken in from the diet. This is nitrogen balance or nitrogen equilibrium: intake = output, and there is no change in the total body content of protein.

- In a growing child, a pregnant woman or someone recovering from protein loss, the excretion of nitrogenous compounds is less than the dietary intake – there is a net retention of nitrogen in the body, and an increase in the body content of protein. This is positive nitrogen balance: intake > output, and there is a net gain in total body protein.

- In response to trauma or infection, or if the intake of protein is inadequate to meet requirements, there is net a loss of nitrogen from the body – the output is greater than the intake. This is negative nitrogen balance: intake < output, and there is a loss of body protein.

DYNAMIC EQUILIBRIUM

The proteins of the body are continually being broken down and replaced. Some proteins (especially enzymes that control metabolic pathways) may turn over within minutes or hours; others last for days or weeks before they are broken down. This is dynamic equilibrium. An adult catabolises and replaces some 3–6 g of protein/kg body weight/day, with no change in total body protein content. However, if an isotopically labelled amino acid is given, the process of turnover can be followed.

Protein breakdown occurs at a more or less constant rate throughout the day. Replacement synthesis is greater than breakdown after a meal, when there is an abundant supply of amino acids and metabolic fuels, and less than breakdown in the fasting state, when amino acids are being used as substrates for gluconeogenesis.

Protein turnover also occurs in growing children, who synthesise considerably more protein per day than their net increase in body protein. Even children recovering from severe protein energy malnutrition, who are increasing their body protein rapidly, still synthesise two to three times more protein each day than the net increase.

Although an adult may be in overall N balance, this is the average of periods of negative balance in the fasting state and positive balance in the fed state. As discussed below under 'The energy cost of protein synthesis', protein synthesis is energy expensive, and in the fasting state the rate of synthesis is lower than that of protein catabolism. There is a loss of tissue protein, which provides amino acids for gluconeogenesis. In the fed state, when there is an abundant supply of amino acids and metabolic fuel, the rate of protein synthesis increases, and exceeds that of break-down, so that what is observed is an increase in tissue protein, replacing that which was lost in the fasting state.

Even in severe undernutrition, the rate of protein breakdown remains more or less constant, while the rate of replacement synthesis falls, as a result of the low availability of metabolic fuels. It is only in cachexia that there is increased protein catabolism as well as reduced replacement synthesis.

TISSUE PROTEIN CATABOLISM

The catabolism of tissue proteins is a highly regulated process; different proteins are catabolised (and replaced) at very different rates. Three different mechanisms are involved in the process: lysosomal cathepsins, the cytosolic protease calpain and the ubiquitin-proteasome system. Ubiquitin is a small peptide that is attached to the ε-amino groups of lysine residues in target proteins in an ATP-dependent process. The proteasome is a multi-enzyme complex that utilises ATP to catalyse the unfolding of proteins that have been targeted with ubiquitin, then catalyses hydrolysis into small peptide fragments.

It is the continual catabolism of tissue proteins that creates the requirement for dietary protein. Although some of the amino acids released by breakdown of tissue proteins can be reused, most are metabolised to intermediates that can be used as metabolic fuels and for gluconeogenesis; the nitrogen is metabolised to urea, which is excreted.

PROTEIN SYNTHESIS

The information for the amino acid sequence of each of the 30 000–50 000 different proteins in the body is contained in the DNA in the nucleus of each cell. As required, a working copy of the information for an individual protein (the gene for that protein) is transcribed, as messenger RNA (mRNA), and this is then translated during protein synthesis on the ribosomes. Both DNA and RNA are linear polymers of nucleotides. In RNA the sugar is ribose, while in DNA it is deoxyribose.

The structure and information content of DNA

DNA is a linear polymer of nucleotides. It consists of a backbone of deoxyribose linked by phosphate

diester bonds from carbon-3 of one sugar to carbon-5 of the next (see Fig. *evolve* 8.1). The bases of the nucleotides project from this sugar phosphate backbone. There are two strands of deoxyribonucleotides, held together by hydrogen bonds between a purine (adenine or guanine) and a pyrimidine (thymine or cytosine): adenine forms two hydrogen bonds to thymine, and guanine forms three hydrogen bonds to cytosine. The DNA double strand coils into a helix, the double helix.

A group of three bases in DNA or mRNA is known as a codon, and may contain any one of the four bases in each position, so that there are 64 possible combinations. This gives a code consisting of 64 words, while there is a need for codons for only 21 for amino acids, plus a code for the end of the message. As can be seen from the genetic code (transcribed to RNA) in Table *evolve* 8.1 , most amino acids are coded for by more than one codon. This provides a measure of protection against mutations – in many cases a single base change in a codon will not affect the amino acid that is incorporated into the protein, and therefore will have no functional significance.

Ribonucleic acid (RNA)

In RNA the sugar is ribose, rather than deoxyribose as in DNA, and RNA contains the pyrimidine uracil where DNA contains thymine. There are three main types of RNA in the cell: messenger RNA (mRNA), synthesised in the nucleus, as an edited copy of one strand of DNA; ribosomal RNA (rRNA), which forms the ribosomes on which protein is synthesised; and transfer RNA (tRNA), which provides the link between mRNA and the amino acids for protein synthesis on the ribosome (see below).

In the transcription of DNA to form mRNA a part of the desired region of DNA is uncoiled, and the two strands of the double helix are separated. A copy of one DNA strand is then synthesised by binding the complementary nucleotide triphosphate to each base of DNA in turn, followed by condensation to form the phospho-diester link between ribose moieties.

Transcription control sites in DNA include start and stop messages, and promoter and enhancer sequences. The main promoter region for any gene is about 25 bases before (upstream of) the beginning of the gene to be transcribed. It acts as a signal that what follows is a gene to be transcribed. Enhancer and promoter regions may be found further upstream of the message, downstream or sometimes even in the middle of the message. The function of these regions, and of hormone response elements, is to increase the rate at which the gene is transcribed.

After transcription the RNA is edited to splice out non-coding regions (introns), and undergoes further modification before it is exported from the nucleus into the cytosol for translation.

Translation of mRNA – the process of protein synthesis

The process of protein synthesis consists of translating the message carried by the sequence of bases on mRNA into amino acids, and then forming peptide bonds between the amino acids to form a protein. This occurs on the ribosome, and requires a variety of enzymes, as well as specific transfer RNA (tRNA) molecules for each amino acid. Amino acids bind to activating enzymes (amino acyl-tRNA synthetases), which recognise both the amino acid and the appropriate tRNA species, forming amino acyl tRNA.

The subcellular organelle concerned with protein synthesis is the ribosome, which assembles on mRNA, permitting the binding of the anti-codon region of amino acyl tRNA to the codon on mRNA, and aligning the amino acids for formation of peptide bonds. The peptide chain grows as the ribosome moves along the mRNA – and each mRNA is being translated by a number of ribosomes at the same time.

The energy cost of protein synthesis

The minimum estimate of the energy cost of protein synthesis is 4 ATP equivalents per peptide bond formed, or 2.8 kJ/gram of protein synthesised; if allowance is made for the energy cost of active transport of amino acids into cells, the cost of protein synthesis is increased to 3.6 kJ/gram. Allowing for the nucleoside triphosphates required for mRNA synthesis gives a total cost of 4.2 kJ/gram of protein synthesised.

In the fasting state, when the rate of protein synthesis is relatively low, about 8% of total energy expenditure (i.e. about 12% of the basal metabolic rate) is accounted for by protein synthesis. After a meal, when the rate of protein synthesis increases, it may account for 12–20% of total energy expenditure.

Hormonal control of protein turnover

Hormonal (and other) control of protein synthesis may be at the level of changes in the rate of transcription, changes in the stability of mRNA or changes in the rate of translation.

Insulin, secreted in the fed state, increases the rate of protein synthesis, both by direct actions and also by stimulating the uptake of glucose and amino acids into cells. In addition, the amino acid leucine has a specific role in increasing the rate of overall protein synthesis. There is increased expression of the enzymes of urea synthesis in response to a high protein intake (mediated by insulin) and in response to tissue protein catabolism in fasting and cachexia (mediated by glucagon and glucocorticoid hormones).

Vitamins A and D and steroid hormones act to regulate the synthesis of specific proteins, by binding, via nuclear receptor proteins, to hormone response elements that regulate the expression of genes (see Ch. 11). In some cases there is increased synthesis of the proteins (induction); in others there is reduced synthesis (repression). The glucocorticoid hormone cortisol acts at a whole body level to increase the rate of muscle protein catabolism and gluconeogenesis in the liver. It achieves this by inducing key regulatory enzymes of gluconeogenesis, and two liver enzymes that initiate the catabolism of two essential amino acids: tryptophan dioxygenase and tyrosine transaminase. As a result of increased catabolism of tryptophan and tyrosine, there is a lack of these two amino acids, leading to reduced protein synthesis (see below under 'nutrient regulation of protein synthesis'), and a surplus of other amino acids that cannot be used for protein synthesis but are used as metabolic fuel or for gluconeogenesis.

Nutrient regulation of protein synthesis

It was noted above that vitamins A and D act like steroid hormones to regulate gene expression, so this can be considered to be nutrient control of gene expression. The receptors for vitamin D and thyroid hormone, and the PPAR receptors (which bind long-chain PUFA derivatives) and liver X receptor (which binds cholesterol metabolites) all form heterodimers with the retinoic acid (RXR) receptor, and both deficiency and excess of vitamin A may affect their actions. In vitamin A deficiency there will be insufficient retinoic acid to form occupied RXR receptors. This will decrease the responsiveness to vitamin D, thyroid hormone, long-chain PUFA derivatives and cholesterol metabolites. However, the unoccupied RXR can also form heterodimers with these receptors, and these dimers bind to response elements in the gene and inhibit transcription. Conversely, a high intake of vitamin A will lead to formation of occupied RXR–RXR homodimers, so depleting the pool of occupied RXR to form heterodimers. Again the result is decreased responsiveness to vitamin D, thyroid hormone, long-chain PUFA derivatives and cholesterol metabolites.

Vitamin B_6 modulates responsiveness to steroid hormones by releasing the hormone-receptor complex from DNA binding. The result of this is that in vitamin B_6 deficiency there is increased responsiveness to steroid hormone action, because the activated receptors remain bound to response elements on DNA for longer, and, conversely, high intracellular concentrations of pyridoxal phosphate result in reduced responsiveness to steroid hormones.

Long-chain polyunsaturated fatty acids or their derivatives regulate the expression of regulatory enzymes in fatty acid synthesis, β-oxidation, ketogenesis and fatty acid desaturation by two mechanisms:

1. The steroid response element binding protein (SREBP) induces desaturases and the enzymes of fatty acid synthesis; long-chain PUFA reduce the stability of SREBP mRNA, so reducing translation. They also increase the catabolism of SREBP by the ubiquitin-proteasome system.
2. Long-chain PUFA derivatives bind to and activate the peroxisome proliferation activation receptors (PPARs); the activated PPARs form heterodimers with (occupied) RXR and induce the enzymes of β-oxidation and ketogenesis.

Cholesterol and its metabolites bind to the so-called liver X receptor, which forms heterodimers with the retinoic acid receptor; the activated receptor induces fatty acid Δ^9 desaturase and represses the synthesis of other desaturases. It also induces the synthesis of cholesterol side-chain oxidase and the ABC (ATP-binding cassette) proteins that act to secrete cholesterol from hepatocytes into the bile.

Its deleterious effects are in the induction of steroid response element binding protein (SREBP) and hence the induction of fatty acid synthesis and increased synthesis of VLDL.

In response to increased availability of glucose there is an increase in glycolysis and lipolysis. Part of this is the result of induction of SREBP in response to insulin and repression in response to glucagon; as noted above, SREBP induces synthesis of lipogenic enzymes. However, SREBP accounts for only about half the lipogenic response to glucose. The promoter regions of both lipogenic and glycolytic enzymes also have carbohydrate response elements, which are activated by the carbohydrate response element binding protein (ChoREBP). Under basal conditions this protein is in the cytosol. However, in response to a high level of glucose 6-phosphate (in the liver this is the result of increased phosphorylation of glucose, see Section 6.4), the ChoREBP is translocated from the cytosol into the nucleus, where it binds to carbohydrate response elements and increases transcription.

Lack of any one amino acid leads to a decrease in protein synthesis. This is partly the result of slower translation because of lack of the appropriate charged tRNA to bind to the ribosome, but there is also inactivation of translation initiation factors by phosphorylation in response to the presence of uncharged tRNA, leading to a decrease in general protein synthesis.

The synthesis of transferrin, which is involved in cell uptake of iron, and of ferritin, which is involved in intracellular storage of iron, is regulated coordinately and in opposite directions by post-transcriptional control in response to the presence of free intracellular iron (see also Section 29.2):

- Transferrin mRNA has an iron response element in the 3′ untranslated region. In the absence of iron, regulatory proteins bind to the response element and protect the mRNA from degradation, so that more transferrin is synthesised, permitting increased uptake of iron. In the presence of free intracellular iron the regulatory proteins are displaced and the mRNA is now more susceptible to degradation, so reducing transferrin synthesis.
- Ferritin mRNA has an iron response element in the 5′ untranslated region, and in the absence of iron the iron regulatory proteins bind and inhibit translation, so supplying free iron for the cell. In the presence of free intracellular iron

the regulatory protein does not bind, and ferritin synthesis increases to permit intracellular storage of iron.

8.4 AMINO ACID METABOLISM

DISPENSABLE AND INDISPENSABLE AMINO ACIDS

Early studies of nitrogen balance showed that not all proteins are nutritionally equivalent. More of some is needed to maintain nitrogen balance than of others. This is because different proteins contain different amounts of the various amino acids. The body's requirement is not simply for protein, but for the amino acids that make up proteins, in the correct proportions to replace the body proteins.

As shown in Table 8.1, the amino acids can be divided into indispensable and dispensable groups:

- There are nine indispensable or essential amino acids, which cannot be synthesised in the body. If one of these is provided in inadequate amount, then regardless of the total intake of protein, it will not be possible to maintain nitrogen balance, since there will not be an adequate amount of the amino acid for protein synthesis.
  - Two amino acids, cysteine and tyrosine, can be synthesised in the body, but only from essential amino acid precursors – cysteine from methionine and tyrosine from phenylalanine.
  - For premature infants, and possibly also for full-term infants, a tenth amino acid is essential – arginine. The capacity for arginine

synthesis is low in infants, and may not be adequate to meet the requirements for growth.
- The non-essential or dispensable amino acids, which can be synthesised from metabolic intermediates, as long as there is enough total protein in the diet. If one of these amino acids is omitted from the diet, nitrogen balance can still be maintained.
  - Only three amino acids, alanine, aspartate and glutamate, can be considered to be truly dispensable; they are synthesised from common metabolic intermediates (pyruvate, oxaloacetate and α-ketoglutarate, respectively).
  - The remaining amino acids are generally considered as non-essential, but under some circumstances the requirement may outstrip the capacity for synthesis.

Unavailable amino acids

Chemical analysis of the amino acid content of dietary proteins does not reflect their nutritional value, since some of the essential amino acids in dietary proteins are not released by digestive enzymes, i.e. they are biologically unavailable. Nutritionally, it is unavailable lysine that is most important, since in many proteins lysine is the limiting amino acid – it is present in the lowest amount compared with requirements. Lysine may be unavailable because of inter-chain peptide bonds from the ε-amino group to the side-chain carboxyl group of glutamic or aspartic acid, or as a result of reaction of the ε-amino group with a reducing sugar – the Maillard or non-enzymic browning reaction that occurs during cooking and storage of foods. Not only is the lysine that has undergone reaction unavailable, since the ε-amino bonds are not

Table 8.1	Indispensable and dispensable – essential amino acids		
INDISPENSABLE	**INDISPENSABLE PRECURSOR**	**DISPENSABLE**	**PARTIALLY DISPENSABLE**
Histidine		Alanine	Arginine
Isoleucine		Aspartate	Asparagine
Leucine		Glutamate	Glutamine
Lysine			Glycine
Methionine	Cysteine		Proline
Phenylalanine	Tyrosine		Serine
Threonine			
Tryptophan			
Valine			

susceptible to digestive enzymes, but several amino acids either side of the reacted lysine will also be unavailable, because the side-chain links impair the activity of intestinal proteolytic enzymes.

UTILISATION OF AMINO ACIDS OTHER THAN FOR PROTEIN SYNTHESIS

An adult has a requirement for a dietary intake of protein because there is continual oxidation of amino acids as a source of metabolic fuel and for gluconeogenesis in the fasting state. In the fed state, amino acids in excess of immediate requirements for protein synthesis are oxidised. Overall, for an adult in nitrogen balance, the total amount of amino acids being metabolised will be equal to the total intake of amino acids in dietary proteins.

Amino acids are also required for the synthesis of a variety of metabolic products, including:

- purines and pyrimidines for nucleic acid synthesis
- haem, synthesised from glycine
- the catecholamine neurotransmitters, dopamine, noradrenaline (norepinephrine) and adrenaline (epinephrine), synthesised from tyrosine
- the thyroid hormones thyroxine and tri-iodothyronine, synthesised from tyrosine
- melanin, the pigment of skin and hair, synthesised from tyrosine
- the nicotinamide ring of the coenzymes NAD and NADP, synthesised from tryptophan (see also Ch. 10, Fig. *evolve* 10.3 🖱)
- the neurotransmitter serotonin (5-hydroxytryptamine), synthesised from tryptophan
- the neurotransmitter histamine, synthesised from histidine
- the neurotransmitter GABA (γ-aminobutyrate) synthesised from glutamate
- carnitine, synthesised from lysine and methionine
- creatine, synthesised from arginine, glycine and methionine
- the phospholipid bases ethanolamine and choline, synthesised from serine and methionine; acetyl choline functions as a neurotransmitter
- taurine, synthesised from cysteine.

In general, the amounts of amino acids required for synthesis of these products are small compared with the requirement for maintenance of nitrogen balance and protein turnover.

METABOLISM OF THE AMINO GROUP NITROGEN

The initial step in the metabolism of amino acids is the removal of the amino group ($-NH_2$), leaving the carbon skeleton of the amino acid. Chemically, these carbon skeletons are ketoacids (more correctly, they are oxoacids). A ketoacid has a $-C=O$ group in place of the $HC-NH_2$ group of an amino acid.

Some amino acids can be directly oxidised to their corresponding ketoacids, releasing ammonia: the process of deamination (see Fig. *evolve* 8.2 🖱). There is a general amino acid oxidase that catalyses this reaction, but it has a low activity. Four amino acids (glycine, glutamate, serine and threonine) are deaminated by specific enzymes.

Most amino acids are not deaminated, but undergo the process of transamination, in which the amino group is transferred onto the enzyme, leaving the ketoacid, then transferred onto an acceptor, which is a different ketoacid, so forming the amino acid corresponding to that ketoacid. The acceptor for the amino group at the active site of the enzyme is pyridoxal phosphate, the metabolically active coenzyme derived from vitamin B_6 (see Ch. 10, Fig. 10.4).

Transamination is a reversible reaction, so that if the ketoacid can be synthesised in the body, so can the amino acid. The essential amino acids are those for which the only source of the ketoacid is the amino acid itself. Three of the ketoacids are common metabolic intermediates; they are the precursors of the three amino acids that can be considered to be completely dispensable, in that there is no requirement for them in the diet: pyruvate (forming alanine), α-ketoglutarate (forming glutamate) and oxaloacetate (forming aspartate). See Figure *evolve* 8.3 🖱.

If the acceptor ketoacid in a transamination reaction is α-ketoglutarate, then glutamate is formed, and glutamate can readily be oxidised back to α-ketoglutarate, catalysed by glutamate dehydrogenase, with the release of ammonia. Similarly, if the acceptor ketoacid is glyoxylate, then the product is glycine, which can be oxidised back to glyoxylate and ammonia, catalysed by glycine oxidase. Thus, by means of a variety of transaminases, and using the reactions of glutamate dehydrogenase and glycine oxidase, all of the amino acids can, indirectly, be converted to their ketoacids and ammonia (see also Fig. *evolve* 8.4 🖰).

The metabolism of ammonia

The deamination of amino acids (and a number of other reactions in the body) results in the formation of ammonium ions. Ammonium is highly toxic, and is rapidly metabolised, by the formation of glutamate, then glutamine, from α-ketoglutarate (see Fig. *evolve* 8.5 🖰).

In the liver, ammonium arising from the hydrolysis of glutamine and other reactions is used to synthesise urea, the main nitrogenous excretion product (see Fig. *evolve* 8.6 🖰).

The total amount of urea synthesised each day is several-fold higher than the amount that is excreted. Urea diffuses readily from the bloodstream into the large intestine, where it is hydrolysed by bacterial urease to carbon dioxide and ammonium. Much of the ammonium is reabsorbed, and used in the liver for the synthesis of glutamate and glutamine, and then a variety of other nitrogenous compounds.

THE METABOLISM OF AMINO ACID CARBON SKELETONS

Acetyl CoA and acetoacetate arising from the carbon skeletons of amino acids may be used for fatty acid synthesis or be oxidised as metabolic fuel, but cannot be utilised for the synthesis of glucose (gluconeogenesis). Amino acids that yield acetyl CoA or acetoacetate are termed ketogenic.

By contrast, those amino acids that yield intermediates that can be used for gluconeogenesis are termed glucogenic. As shown in Table *evolve* 8.2, only two amino acids are purely ketogenic: leucine and lysine 🖰. Three others yield both glucogenic fragments and either acetyl CoA or acetoacetate: tryptophan, isoleucine and phenylalanine. Figure *evolve* 6.7 shows the ways in which amino acid carbon skeletons enter central metabolic pathways 🖰.

8.5 PROTEIN AND AMINO ACID REQUIREMENTS (*D JOE MILLWARD*)

AN INHERENTLY DIFFICULT PROBLEM

Defining minimum amino acid and protein requirements has always been inherently difficult and remains so today. Human adults are exposed to a very wide range of protein intakes, which enable full expression of their genotypical lean body mass throughout the range. The intractable problem is that of identifying the lower limits of this range. There are several major difficulties. Firstly, for protein there are no unequivocal biochemical or physiological deficiency symptoms, apart from growth failure and tissue wasting, which marks a severe deficiency. Thus protein or amino acid deficiency can only be identified as an intake that is below the requirement. This means that the extent of protein deficiency goes up or down as requirement values change. Secondly the process of adaptation makes for great difficulties in defining protein requirements, because our derivation of RNI values assumes that there is no relationship between intakes and requirements. With adaptation, where intakes can influence apparent requirements, a more complex model is required.

Another difficulty relates to the balance method for determining requirements. Without biochemical indicators, protein and amino acid requirements can only be defined in terms of maintenance of body protein, requiring balance methods of one sort or another. Such methods are inherently imprecise and logistically difficult, as discussed below in 'Nitrogen balance and factorial models'. Stable isotope techniques were expected to remedy such inadequacies, but in fact they bring their own problems. Indeed all current stable isotope methods based on amino acid oxidation are variants of the balance study, measuring the relationship between amino acid intake and some function of losses as amino acid oxidation rates, and, like the N balance method, they also suffer from the problem of a poorly defined end-point around equilibrium.

Protein requirements are best discussed in terms of *metabolic demand, dietary requirement* and *dietary allowances*.

Metabolic demand

This is determined by the nature and extent of those metabolic pathways which consume amino acids, and which vary with the phenotype and the developmental and physiological state of the individual. As shown in Figure 8.2, *demands* are conventionally identified as *maintenance* and *special needs* such as growth, rehabilitation, pregnancy and lactation.

Maintenance comprises all those processes that consume amino acids and give rise to urinary,

Protein: metabolic demands and utilisation

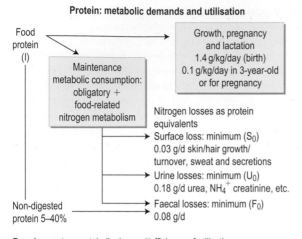

Food protein (I)

Maintenance metabolic consumption: obligatory + food-related nitrogen metabolism

Growth, pregnancy and lactation
1.4 g/kg/day (birth)
0.1 g/kg/day in 3-year-old or for pregnancy

Nitrogen losses as protein equivalents

→ Surface loss: minimum (S_0) 0.03 g/d skin/hair growth/turnover, sweat and secretions

→ Urine losses: minimum (U_0) 0.18 g/d urea, NH_4^+ creatinine, etc.

Non-digested protein 5–40%

→ Faecal losses: minimum (F_0) 0.08 g/d

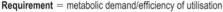

Requirement = metabolic demand/efficiency of utilisation

Metabolic demand:

minimum
= total obligatory N losses, ONL
= losses on protein-free diet
= $S_0 + U_0 + F_0$
= 46 mgN/kg ≡ 0.29 g body protein/kg/d

Utilisation = digestibility × biological value

Digestibility
(D, faecal losses) = $(I-F)/I$
true digestibility = $(I-(F-F_0))/I$

Biological value
(BV, urinary losses) = retained N/absorbed N
= $(I-F-U-S)/(I-F)$
true BV = $(I-(F-F_0)-(U-U_0)-(S-S_0))/(I-(F-F_0))$

Net protein utilisation
(NPU) = digestibility × biological value
= (intake−F−U−S)/intake
true NPU = $(I-(F-F_0)-(U-U_0)-(S-S_0))/I$

Fig. 8.2 Metabolic demands for protein and factors influencing utilisation.

faecal and other losses; net protein synthesis is only a very small part. Minimum metabolic demands, measured in subjects adapted to a protein-free diet when body protein provides for them, are quite low, amounting to about 46 mg N/kg/day, equivalent to 0.29 g/kg/day of body protein.

Dietary requirement

This is the amount of protein and/or its constituent amino acids that must be supplied in the diet in order to satisfy the metabolic demand and achieve nitrogen equilibrium. The requirement will in most cases be greater than the metabolic demand because of those factors which influence the efficiency of protein utilisation, i.e. *net protein utilisation*. These

are factors associated with digestion and absorption, which influence the digestibility and consequent amount of dietary nitrogen lost in the faeces, and the cellular bioavailability of the absorbed amino acids in relation to needs, which influences the *biological value*.

Dietary allowances

These are a range of intakes derived from estimates of individual requirements taking into account the variability between individuals.

8.6 METHODS OF DETERMINING PROTEIN REQUIREMENTS

The first estimates of protein requirements were made in the second part of the nineteenth century, with recommendations based on measurements of protein intakes of populations assumed to be healthy. The modern era began in 1957 with the first UN Food and Agriculture Organization (FAO) report, which derived estimates from nitrogen balance. These human studies have been supplemented with information about protein quality from animal studies. The most recent international report was published in 2007 (WHO 2007), and all requirement values below derive from this report.

NITROGEN BALANCE AND FACTORIAL MODELS

The metabolic demands can be estimated from measurement of all losses of nitrogen in subjects adapted to a protein-free diet. This is the obligatory nitrogen loss (ONL). When losses are measured over a range of intakes, balance is calculated at each intake as intake minus losses, and the equation of the balance curve calculated to predict the requirement. As shown in Figure *evolve* 8.7 🐭, which represents all published N balance studies up to 2001 (Rand et al 2003), a linear regression of balance against intake will allow prediction of the ONL as the zero intake intercept. The slope of the curve will indicate the efficiency of utilisation and the maintenance requirement, i.e. the amount that must be fed to balance losses and produce equilibrium, ONL/efficiency of utilisation. From these data the currently accepted maintenance requirement is 0.66 g/kg body weight/day.

Inherent difficulties with nitrogen balance studies

This apparently simple, but laborious, approach is beset with a large number of quite serious problems, as listed in Table 8.2.

Balance is the small difference between two large amounts and can seldom be precisely measured. Because of systematic errors (an overestimation of intake because subjects might eat less than the test meals, and an underestimation of the losses) balance is usually overestimated, with weight stable adults appearing to gain large amounts of body protein.

As might be expected, individual balance curves are not linear, so that curve fitting must be used to predict the intake for zero balance. Figure *evolve* 8.8 🖰 shows an important example from a study of the lysine requirement (Jones et al 1956). Subjects were fed amino acid mixtures containing varying amounts of lysine and the balance curve calculated from just urinary and faecal losses. The curve is very shallow at equilibrium so that the problem of accounting for all losses becomes critical, to the extent that the values for N equilibrium vary markedly according to the unmeasured integumental losses. At different points on the curve, the lysine requirements are 8, 17 or 36 mg/kg/day, at assumed integumental losses of zero, 5 or 8 mg N/kg/day. The currently accepted value is 5 mg N/kg/day; 8 mg N/kg/day was used in the past and is now known to be excessive for subjects in temperate climates.

Design problems: influence of energy and intakes of other nutrients on losses

Body protein equilibrium can be influenced by intakes of other nutrients or energy, and ensuring that energy intakes are sufficient is difficult. Excess energy intake leads to weight, and some lean tissue gain, whilst with too little energy intake, protein is oxidised as an energy source. This means that the protein requirement is a function of the state of energy balance. According to one analysis of N balance (NB) according to intakes of energy (EI) and N (NI), NB = 0.171 NI + 1.006 EI − 69.13. This means that the intake for N equilibrium (the requirement) will vary from 0.32 to 1.4 g/kg/day according to whether energy intakes are equal to or two times the resting metabolic rate. Two-thirds of the overall variability reported in the meta-analysis shown in Figure *evolve* 8.7 🖰 could be accounted for by an error of only about 0.2% of basal metabolic rate (BMR) in estimating the true energy needs of a subject.

Since N balance varies as a function of energy intake, it might be argued that protein requirements can only be defined in terms of a specified energy intake level, raising difficult and currently unanswered questions. Should populations with low protein staples consume more energy to achieve body protein equilibrium? Will this predispose to obesity?

N balance at varying levels of physical activity

Our understanding of the way physical activity influences N balance is limited. Assuming subjects maintain energy balance, there is evidence that physical activity influences protein utilisation, improving efficiency and increasing metabolic demands, depending on the type of activity, the degree of training and the habitual protein intake. Thus the intake to maintain N equilibrium may be higher, lower or unchanged and it is often quite difficult to predict. However, protein intakes with mixed diets that meet energy needs will usually exceed requirements.

Time dependency of adaptive mechanisms governing losses

Day-to-day variability

Although N balance is expressed in terms of daily amounts, measurements are usually made

---

Table 8.2	Potential problems relating to nitrogen balance methodology (see Millward 2001)

1. Imprecise
2. Systematic errors: intake overestimated, loss underestimated due to problem of accounting for all losses: e.g.
   (a) Skin surface and secretions
   (b) Loss of N_2 gas
   (c) Expired ammonia
   (d) Endogenous NO production gives urinary nitrate, faecal ammonia and nitrite
   (e) Changing size of the body urea pool
3. Non-linearity of the balance curve
4. Design
   (a) Dietary energy intake and physical activity influences balance
   (b) Accounting for adaptation

over at least 3–4 days at each intake level, to take into account daily variability, especially in faecal loss.

Long-term adaptation

A more serious problem is that when protein intake changes, the metabolic adjustment involved with matching amino acid oxidation to the new intake takes time to adapt. The actual time taken for complete adaptation is poorly understood and controversial. In practice, most balance studies are 'short term' with dietary periods of 2 weeks at each intake studied, and with diet periods randomised to minimise metabolic carryover of prior diets. Two weeks is the time to stabilise excretion in subjects fed a protein-free diet, which is an extreme metabolic change, and adaptation may occur more rapidly than adjustment from one intake to another. Other studies show that a new equilibrium takes much longer than 2 weeks to achieve.

Implications of adaptation for the interpretation of N balance data

The range of individual values from the reported N balance meta-analysis of Rand et al (2003) is shown in Figure *evolve* 8.9 . Analysis of individual risk of deficiency (intake < requirement) assumes that the requirement is not correlated with the intake so that for an individual with an intake equal to the mean requirement value, the risk of deficiency is 50%, falling to <2.5% at the higher intake equal to the RNI.

The serious implication of lack of complete adaptation in short-term balance studies is that, because of the very wide range of protein intakes in the human diet, the apparent requirement may still reflect the prior habitual diet because of an adaptive component of amino acid oxidation set to balance previous intakes. This may explain the very wide range of reported apparent requirements of 0.4 to >1.1 g protein/kg/day. If adaptation does account for the variability, the RNI would be much lower, and the risk of deficiency for fully adapted individuals would not increase until intakes fell to very low levels, close to the ONL. Such adaptive models as proposed by Millward (2003) pose difficult questions for public health nutrition (see Section 8.12).

8.7 PROTEIN REQUIREMENTS FOR GROWTH AND SPECIAL NEEDS

For infants, children and pregnant and lactating women, protein requirements are derived by a semi-factorial analysis of the components of the metabolic demands shown in Figure 8.2. The main components (WHO 2007) are shown in Figure *evolve* 8.10 . The maintenance value is assumed to be the same as that identified in adult N balance studies. The dietary requirements for growth derive from measured rates of protein accretion adjusted for an efficiency of utilisation of 58%. To account for inter-individual variability the RNI includes the addition of 2 × SD calculated from the weighted mean of the coefficient of variation values for maintenance (12%) and growth (43%).

Pregnancy requirements allow for protein retention in the products of conception and in the maternal tissues associated with a gestational weight gain of 13.8 kg. The factorial model calculates the additional dietary protein intake needed during pregnancy from the newly deposited protein and the maintenance costs associated with increased body weight assuming an efficiency of protein utilization of 42%. The safe level was derived from this average requirement, assuming a coefficient of variation of 12%. On this basis an additional 1, 9 and 31 g/day protein in the first, second and third trimesters, respectively, are required to support a 13.8 kg gestational weight gain. In view of the literature indicating a controversial increase in neonatal death with supplements that are very high in protein, it is recommended that the higher intake during pregnancy should consist of normal food, rather than commercially prepared high protein supplements.

Lactation requirements are calculated from rates of milk produced by well-nourished women exclusively breastfeeding their infants during the first 6 months postpartum and partially breastfeeding in the second 6 months postpartum. The mean concentrations of protein and non-protein nitrogen in human milk give average milk protein outputs. The additional dietary requirement to meet this is calculated, assuming an efficiency of 47% utilisation of dietary protein, at 19–20 g/day during the first 6 months and 12.5 g/d after that.

For the elderly, requirements are assumed to be the same as for younger adults although measurements of metabolic demand and efficiency of utilisation suggest if anything a lower requirement (see Table *evolve* 8.4).

8.8 EXPRESSION OF REQUIREMENTS: NUTRIENT BASED (G/KG/DAY) OR NUTRIENT DENSITY (PROTEIN : ENERGY RATIOS)?

In the past, protein requirements have been expressed as amounts per person or more precisely per kilogram body weight. Whilst this is adequate for calculating recommended intakes for an individual, it is less useful when advice is given about the types of diets and foods to be recommended and in assessing the adequacy of intakes. Energy expenditure determines overall energy and nutrient intakes, so that food-based guidelines, especially the use of nutrient density, can result in a better definition of nutritional priorities for specific populations. The calculation of the protein:energy (P:E) ratio of requirements is shown in Figure *evolve* 8.11 🖱. The changes with age in the RNI for protein and the energy requirements are shown at the top and the resultant safe P:E ratio in the bottom figure; i.e.:

$$\text{Safe PE\%} = 100 \times (\text{protein requirement} \\ (g/kg/day \times 16.7\ kJ/kg/day)/ \\ (\text{energy requirements } kJ/kg/day)$$

In fact calculation of a safe PE% value is complicated (WHO 2007) because account must be taken of the variability in the energy requirements. In practice the safe PE% value can be approximated to protein EAR + 3SDs/energy requirement and this value is shown in Figure *evolve* 8.11 🖱.

Because the very high energy requirements during infancy and childhood decrease with age at a greater rate than the fall in the protein requirement, the P:E ratio of the requirements for infants is low and increases with age. This means that a diet which can meet both energy and protein needs of the infant can satisfy energy needs of older children or adults while failing to meet their protein needs.

IMPORTANCE OF PHYSICAL ACTIVITY FOR NUTRIENT INTAKES AND RISK OF DEFICIENCY

Protein requirements are generally not considered to vary with energy expenditure (but see 'N balance at varying levels of physical activity', above) and protein requirements are usually provided by the increased food energy intakes. With energy requirements predicted from BMR × physical activity level,

energy requirements per kilogram will vary markedly with age (falling), with gender (women < men), with body weight (large < small) and with physical activity. The calculations in Figure *evolve* 8.11 🖱 are for mean values for males and females weighing 70 kg as adults, and with a moderate rate of energy expenditure (an energy requirement based on 1.75 × predicted BMR). Clearly as energy requirements increase, the P:E ratio of the protein requirements will fall, so that for adults and the elderly, increased physical activity reduces the P:E ratio of the protein requirement.

PROTEIN : ENERGY RATIOS: KEY IMPLICATIONS

- Protein dense foods are more important for adults, especially the elderly, than for infants and children.
- Energy dense foods are more important for children than for adults.
- Protein deficiency is more likely in the elderly than in children.
- Protein deficiency at any age is less likely as physical activity increases.

8.9 METHODS OF EVALUATING PROTEIN QUALITY AND ASSESSING AMINO ACID REQUIREMENTS

The nutritional importance of protein quality was established very early in the twentieth century, from N balance studies in human beings and growth studies in rats. The identification of separate metabolic demands for amino acids for maintenance and growth was an early discovery; as shown in Figure *evolve* 8.12 🖱, rats fed zein, the main protein in maize, were unable to maintain weight and died. Various amino acids were added but only tryptophan allowed weight maintenance; lysine did not. However, when lysine was added with tryptophan, normal growth occurred. This established not only that zein was deficient in both tryptophan and lysine, but that the metabolic demands for amino acids include growth (net protein synthesis) and maintenance, as indicated in Figure 8.2. Zein is inadequate for either maintenance, through tryptophan deficiency, or growth, through tryptophan plus lysine deficiency. W. C. Rose showed that rats could grow maximally on purified amino acid mixtures and then, with others, quantified the maintenance requirement of the essential amino acids with N balance studies in men and women. These data represent a major source of our understanding of amino acid requirements.

PROTEIN QUALITY EVALUATION IN ANIMALS

The rat growth assay for protein quality was developed from the early studies of Osborne and Mendel, and is still in use to day.

Protein efficiency ratio (PER) is the simplest measure: g weight gain/g protein intake from a diet containing 9–10% of protein. Very marked differences are apparent, with values of 3.8, 2.0 and 0.3 for whole egg, soya and wheat gluten. It does not reveal why differences in weight gain might occur in terms of digestibility, and biological value (see Fig. 8.2).

Digestibility can vary through restriction of digestion by plant cell walls and the presence in plant foods of anti-nutritional factors. Values range from 60–80% in legumes and cereals with tough cell walls such as millet and sorghum to 97% for egg (see Table *evolve* 8.3). Anti-nutritional factors in legumes and seeds include amylase and trypsin inhibitors, tannins in most legumes and cyanogens in lima beans. *Biological value (BV)* varies mainly through the composition of the absorbed amino acid mixture in relation to the pattern of the metabolic demand for maintenance and net protein deposition. Chemical modification of amino acids in food protein during processing can also reduce their bioavailability even though they are absorbed. The rat growth assay of BV shows marked differences between proteins when they are assessed individually in line with amounts of indispensable amino acids in the protein compared with tissue protein composition. In general, the overall amino acid composition is influenced by the number of different codons assigned to each amino acid in the genetic code (see Table *evolve* 8.1), with high levels of leucine and serine and low levels of methionine and tryptophan. However, since this is the same for both dietary and tissue proteins, it need not necessarily pose a nutritional problem. BV is low for cereal and legume proteins, because of low levels of lysine and tryptophan in cereals and of the sulphur-containing amino acids in legumes in relation to metabolic demands. However, because the limiting amino acids differ between types of

plant proteins, when they are combined they complement each other, so that mixed plant protein diets exhibit much higher BV values and may be similar to animal proteins.

Net protein utilisation (NPU, see Fig. 8.2) represents a specific measure of protein utilisation. It can be measured by means of N balance studies allowing separate evaluation of both digestibility and BV.

Because faecal and urinary losses include endogenous losses which occur on a protein-free diet (the ONL) the measurements need to differentiate between these and exogenous losses due to poor utilisation of food protein.

Endogenous losses $(S_0 + U_0 + F_0)$ (see Fig. 8.2) indicate metabolic demands and are measured in response to a protein-free diet.

Food-related losses $(S + U + F - (S_0 + U_0 + F_0))$ determine efficiency of utilisation.

DIRECT MEASUREMENTS OF NITROGEN RETENTION

In practice, N balance studies are very laborious and Bender & Miller devised a simplified, more accurate method based on direct measurement of N retention in the rat carcass, as shown in Figure *evolve* 8.13 . Food protein intake and total carcass N are measured after 10 days on either the test diet or a protein-free diet. NPU for both maintenance and growth is calculated from the difference in carcass N content between the two diets. With this approach, digestibility and BV are not separately indicated.

PROTEIN QUALITY EVALUATION IN HUMAN NUTRITION

Protein quality assessment in rat growth assays measures mainly the needs for rapid tissue growth. It is this work with animals that has resulted in the concept of first and second class proteins. However, this concept is much less relevant in human nutrition.

For human beings, as shown in Figure *evolve* 8.10 , metabolic demands for growth fall rapidly during the first year of life, so that amino acid needs are mainly for maintenance, and we know from extensive work in farm animals and rats that the amino acid pattern of these demands is quite different from the metabolic demands for growth. In particular, there is a much lower proportion of indispensable amino acids. Consistent with this is the difficulty of demonstrating differences in protein quality in human nutrition, especially with mixed plant food diets. N balance studies in adults indicate very small differences when comparisons are made between single proteins, and in the meta-analysis of all N balance studies in adults by Rand et al (2003), no differences in intakes to maintain N equilibrium were observed between diets based on plant protein and those based on animal protein sources. Several long-term balance studies with US college students fed largely bread showed maintenance of weight, N balance and fitness on these diets. Because of these difficulties in assessing protein quality in human nutrition current approaches attempt to predict quality from measured amino acid content; i.e. amino acid scoring.

AMINO ACID SCORING: THE PDCAAS METHOD

If the pattern of amino acid requirements is known, then in theory the measured BV of a dietary protein should be predictable from its amino acid pattern relative to that of the requirement pattern. Block and Mitchell introduced this concept using whole egg as the reference (the requirement pattern was unknown). The procedure involves two stages.

The single limiting amino acid is identified from the ratios of each individual amino acid in the protein with that in the reference pattern. Values <1 indicate potential deficiency but the limiting amino acid will have the lowest ratio.

The extent of the limitation is indicated by the value of the lowest ratio. In theory if the lysine content of wheat gluten is only 0.5 of the reference pattern, then the BV should be 0.5 and to achieve the required intake of lysine the intake of the gluten will have to be increased by 1/0.5 = 2 times the intake of the reference protein. At this level of intake sufficient of all amino acids are supplied.

The reference pattern is that of an ideal protein which would provide requirement levels of all amino acids when fed at the protein requirement level, so that:

$$\text{reference pattern} = \frac{\dfrac{\text{amino acid requirement/kg}}{\text{as mg/g}}}{\text{protein requirement/kg}}$$

This approach was first recommended in the 1985 FAO/WHO/UNU report on protein and energy requirements, and further endorsed in a 1991 FAO report on protein quality evaluation and in the most recent WHO/FAO/UNU report (WHO 2007). Quality is defined as digestibility × amino acid score. This is the PDCAAS method: Protein Digestibility Corrected Amino Acid Score. Digestibility values obtained in rat studies are reasonable predictors of digestibility in humans. However, the major problem focuses on identification of amino acid requirements from which a reference pattern for scoring can be calculated, a subject of considerable controversy.

DEFINING AMINO ACID REQUIREMENT LEVELS: N BALANCE STUDIES

The 1985 FAO/WHO/UNU report defined age-related changes in amino acid requirements and scoring patterns from data on protein and amino acid requirement values for infants, children and adults. In fact, the amino acid data, all from N balance studies, were very limited and are no longer believed to be credible in any way, apart from the adult values. However, the adult values are recognised as too low, because no allowances were made for surface N losses. Thus balance was overestimated and requirements underestimated. To correct for this error they can be adjusted, and Figure evolve 8.8 🖱 shows the effects of such an error for lysine. A reanalysis of all the data with the addition of 5 mg N for miscellaneous losses (Millward 1999) is shown in Table 8.3.

STABLE ISOTOPE STUDIES OF PROTEIN AND AMINO ACID REQUIREMENTS

Stable isotopes, being non-hazardous, allow tracer studies of amino acid metabolism in human beings; they were introduced to remedy the inadequacies of N balance studies, and to provide greater insight into amino acid homeostasis. Tracer studies of amino acid oxidation have proved to be most useful but are often quite difficult to interpret. Most of the N balance problems identified above are equally applicable to stable isotope studies, and like the N balance method, they also suffer from the problem of a poorly defined end-point around equilibrium in studies on adults. Other specific problems are listed in Table 8.4.

Table 8.3   Amino acid requirement values from FAO/WHO/UNU (1985) recalculated to allow for miscellaneous losses (Millward 1999) and as published in the recent WHO (2007) report

	FAO/WHO/UNU (1985) N BALANCE (mg/kg/day)	RECALCULATED N BALANCE (mg/kg/day)	WHO (2007) (STABLE ISOTOPES) (mg/kg/day)
Histidine	–	–	10
Isoleucine	10	18	20
Leucine	14	26	39
Lysine	12	19	30
Methionine + cysteine	13	16	15
Phenylalanine + tyrosine	14	20	25
Threonine	7	16	15
Tryptophan	3.5	3.7	4
Valine	10	14	26
Total	84	133	184

Table 8.4   Potential problems relating to stable isotope balance methodology (see Millward 2001)

1. Practical problems which are potentially soluble
   (a) Need for subject restriction and only short periods of study possible (24 hours current maximum)
   (b) The extent of ^{13}C retention as bicarbonate
   (c) Measurement of CO_2 production rates
   (d) Variation in background tracer enrichment
   (e) Quantitative excretion of ^{13}C as CO_2 and underestimation of losses due to non CO_2 routes
   (f) Oxidation rates as a tracer for overall N excretion influenced by mismatch of food and body tissue amino acid composition
   (g) Excessive positive balances in some studies
2. Model problems which are less tractable and possibly insoluble
   (h) Amount of 'tracer' excessive, invalidating 'tracer' kinetic assumption, precluding true study of responses to very low intakes of tracer or the post-absorptive/fasting state and requiring tracer to be incorporated into balance calculations and may influence balance
   (i) True precursor amino acid enrichment compared with measured value
   (j) Validity: no measure of the relationship between 'requirement' and true adequacy in terms of weight and lean body mass maintenance

[^{13}C-1]Leucine balance studies

Measurement of balance has been attempted for a number of ^{13}C-labelled amino acids in subjects fed diets based on amino acid mixtures with varying levels of the test amino acid, e.g. lysine, threonine, valine and leucine. [^{13}C-1] leucine is probably the most useful since its oxidation can be measured quite accurately. The first step in its catabolism after transamination to α-keto isocaproate, KIC, involves loss of carbon-1 as $^{13}CO_2$, so measurement of $^{13}CO_2$ production is a good measure of leucine oxidation.

Postprandial protein utilisation (PPU)

This approach is shown in Figure *evolve* 8.14 🐾, and is based on estimating acute changes in N balance from measurements of [^{13}C-1]leucine balance during a constant infusion of [^{13}C-1]leucine. The method assumes an adaptive metabolic demand model (Millward 2003), in which metabolic demands include both obligatory and adaptive components, the latter varying (very slowly) with habitual protein intake. Losses in the post-absorptive state (at least 12 hours after the last meal) are assumed to represent consumption of body protein to provide for metabolic demands, which occurs continuously throughout each 24-hour period.

The efficiency of protein utilisation is determined by the increases in losses in response to feeding. Since feeding improves balance by a combination of energy reducing post-absorptive loss, and protein mediating net protein gain (to replace post-absorptive losses), PPU is best measured as Δbalance/Δintake between feeding isoenergetic low and high protein meals. Leucine balance (from intake and oxidation) is assumed to represent changes in protein bound leucine balance (taking into account changes in the free leucine pool), which can be converted to N balance from the known composition of body protein. The derived

PPU value is a measure of biological value since the intake value is an estimate of digestible intake.

Examples of how this approach is used are shown in Table *evolve* 8.4 🖱. Compared with the near perfect efficiency of milk protein utilisation, that of wheat gluten was lower although not as low as predicted. Measurements of age-related changes in protein utilisation show no change in PPU in healthy elderly men or women compared with younger adults. However, the metabolic demands appear to fall with age, so that the apparent protein requirement is lower in the elderly. Adaptive changes in response to short-term (2 weeks) feeding of varying protein intakes have been measured. Thus, whilst PPU with egg and dairy protein meals remains high, metabolic demands and consequent apparent protein requirements (MD/PPU) vary with the level of intake, although it cannot be assumed that these adaptive changes are complete.

The PPU method of protein quality evaluation can help identify minimum amino acid requirements where specific amino acids are known to be limiting, as with lysine in wheat. Thus the amount of wheat protein which would provide the average protein requirement can be calculated from the PPU for wheat as $0.6/PPU_{wheat}$ where 0.6 g/kg/day is the estimated average requirement for protein, i.e. 0.99 g/kg/day for wheat gluten, and 0.88 g/kg/day for whole wheat. The amount of lysine in these amounts of wheat protein at 18.7 mg lysine/g gluten and 26 mg lysine/g whole wheat protein is 19 and 23 mg lysine/kg/day, respectively. Clearly this approach means that the derived lysine requirement will go up or down as the value for the estimated average requirement (EAR) for protein changes.

The weakness of this approach is (a) the dependency on leucine:N conversion factors for calculation of N retention, (b) the artificiality of the feeding regime, frequent small meals. However, a protocol based on a single large meal gives very similar results (see Table *evolve* 8.4 🖱). In fact the values obtained for the lysine requirement are not inconsistent with that from N balance methods shown in Table 8.3.

Indicator amino acid oxidation studies

This approach to estimating amino acid requirements is, in principle, free from some of the problems associated with tracer balance studies. It was developed to study rapidly growing animals and rather than estimate balance, the end-point in this case is a change, or breakpoint, in amino acid oxidation when the intake supports growth or net protein synthesis. A fixed amount of an amino acid mixture is fed with varying amounts of the amino acid under test (e.g. lysine), below and above the likely requirement. The oxidation of a second 'indicator' labelled amino acid is measured. When the intake of the test amino acid is too low to support net protein synthesis, the rest of the amino acid intake is oxidised, including the indicator amino acid. As the test requirement intake is approached or exceeded, all of the amino acid intake, including the indicator, will be utilized, so that indicator oxidation falls. Typical results are shown in Figure *evolve* 8.15 🖱. The indicator amino acid oxidation method works best with rapidly growing animals such as the piglet, where the method gives a clear breakpoint. However, in human studies, with net protein synthesis during feeding measured, as with the PPU method, this does not seem to result in such a clear end-point, and the exact intake for the breakpoint is model dependent.

In some studies an indirect measure of amino acid oxidation is reported, $^{13}CO_2$ production uncorrected for precursor enrichment. The main feature of these studies is the use of breakpoint analysis (two phase linear regression after assuming zero slope for the higher intakes). The value shown in Figure *evolve* 8.15 🖱 is obtained by this analysis but it is clear that a lower value between 20 and 30 could be identified by an alternative analysis, since none of the mean values above an intake of 20 mg/kg/day are different. This would fit with the changes in plasma lysine concentrations with intake, where increases occurred between 20 and 30 mg/kg/day. The fact that the breakpoint is so difficult to identify means that there is a great deal of variability in the results. In a study of tryptophan requirements with this approach values ranged from 1.7 to 5.4 mg/kg/day.

Twenty–four–hour [^{13}C] leucine oxidation studies

These represent the limits of development of tracer methodologies with a 24-hour infusion of tracer during periods of feeding and fasting, and continuous collection of expired $^{13}CO_2$. [^{13}C-1] leucine balance studies have been conducted in subjects fed amino acid mixtures with varying levels of leucine, lysine and threonine, with up to 2 weeks on the diets. Because the studies are so logistically difficult, the number of different intakes tested is limited, with those aimed at identifying lysine requirements testing four different levels of intake. These studies have proved difficult to interpret. As shown in Figure *evolve* 8.16 🖱, in subjects fed amino acid mixtures supplying about 1 g/kg/day with variable lysine, 24-hour leucine balances are dependent not only on the lysine intake, as expected, but also on the leucine intake, so that 24-hour leucine equilibrium has proved an inadequate criterion of adequacy. Thus rather than use leucine balance, breakpoint analysis has been adopted, identifying about 30 mg lysine/kg/day as the requirement in each study.

8.10 DEFINITION OF REFERENCE AMINO ACID PATTERNS

It is clear that there is much uncertainty about the actual values for amino acid requirements from which scoring patterns can be constructed but there is agreement on the principles. For infants prior to weaning the amino acid composition of breast milk is assumed to represent a reference pattern although it is recognised that such intakes may be generous compared with actual demands. From weaning at 6 months once an agreed maintenance pattern has been defined, a factorial calculation of amino acid requirements can be derived from maintenance and the composition and amount of tissue protein gain (corrected for 58% efficiency of utilisation of dietary protein). Since it is quite clear that after the first year of life, growth is relatively slow (see Fig. *evolve* 8.10 🖱), amino acid requirements will not vary much between the preschool child and the adult. For this reason the WHO has recommended that when judging protein quality for schoolchildren and adolescents, it is probably more practical to use just one pattern, i.e. that derived for the age group 3–10 years. The values for breast milk, the infant at weaning, the 3–10-year-old child and the adult are shown in Figure *evolve* 8.17 🖱, which derive from the 2007 WHO/FAO/UNU report.

QUALITY OF ANIMAL AND PLANT PROTEINS

Table *evolve* 8.5 🖱 shows PDCAAS values based on the adult scoring pattern shown in Figure *evolve* 8.17 🖱 and adjusted P:E ratios of dietary protein sources. The important measure is available protein in foods, the adjusted P:E ratio, which is determined by both protein content and quality.

Animal foods generally perform well on both counts. Lysine is the limiting amino acid for cereal proteins, yam and cassava. Maize also contains less than the reference tryptophan level, but at 83% of reference, compared with lysine at 64%, lysine is limiting, and adjusting intake to supply lysine needs will supply more than enough tryptophan. The improved maize variety opaque maize, with a higher ratio of cytoplasmic proteins to storage protein (zein), has adequate tryptophan and 89% of the reference lysine. Soya, in common with all legumes, has low levels of sulphur amino acids but, with this scoring pattern, is just sufficient.

Potatoes provide sufficient of all amino acids. It is interesting that even after correcting for digestibility the adjusted P:E ratio of potato at 8.2% is higher than that of breast milk. The idea that the potato is a high protein food compared with breast milk may seem incredible but it is the case as indicated by these figures. However even though the protein density of potato is adequate the growth of a newborn could not be supported on mashed potato because its energy density is insufficient: i.e. mashed potato would be too bulky to allow the new-born to eat enough to satisfy energy needs. Breast milk is high fat and therefore energy dense. In contrast, for a young adult, energy requirements are only half that of infants (per kg) so the potato could supply all of the energy needs. However the safe P:E ratio shown in Figure *evolve* 8.11 🖱 for a moderately active person is 9.0% energy. This means that the adjusted P:E ratio of potato (8.2%) is slightly less than the safe requirement and energy intakes would have to increase by about 10% to meet the protein needs.

The high protein level in wheat together with its high digestibility means that it provides a much higher level of utilisable protein (PDCAAS-adjusted P:E ratio) than yam or cassava, even though wheat has the lowest lysine level of any staple at 58% of the reference. Clearly cassava does badly mainly due to its low protein content so that only 1.9% of its energy is utilisable protein.

8.11 THE GREAT DEBATE: 1. ARE THE DEVELOPING COUNTRIES PROTEIN–DEFICIENT BECAUSE OF LYSINE DEFICIENCY?

Stable isotope studies have advanced our understanding of amino acid homeostasis but their initial promise of providing an alternative to nitrogen balance has yet to be fully realised. All methods published to date have serious methodological problems of one sort or another, and none can provide answers to the problem at the core of the protein quality debate: are minimally supplemented cereal-based diets as consumed in the developing world adequate?

It is the case that long-term studies (published in the 1960s–1970s) showed that wheat-based diets, providing 18–20 mg lysine/kg, enabled maintenance of body weight, N balance and fitness, but such studies tend to be ignored.

The US DRI report (Food and Nutrition Board 2002) has embraced the values from stable isotope studies to derive its age-related requirement values used to derive scoring patterns, arguing that the 1–3-year-old pattern be used for everyone. In Table *evolve* 8.6 , diets in the UK and India are scored with lysine values based on either recalculated N balance data for the lysine requirement (Millward 1999), the adult value shown in Figure *evolve* 8.17 (WHO 2007) or the DRI recommended value. It is clear that cereal-based diets in all parts of India would be judged markedly lysine deficient with the highest lysine reference value, with some regions approaching adequacy with the mid range value and with all regions adequate with the lower lysine value. In order for adequacy to be achieved 22–23% energy would need to be replaced from soya as shown. In the 1960s there was a UN call for 'international action to avert the impending protein crisis', which proved a false alarm. Some have repeated that call, but we need to be sure about our facts and some believe there is insufficient convincing evidence (Millward & Jackson 2004).Clearly this important debate needs to continue.

8.12 THE GREAT DEBATE: 2. IMPLICATIONS OF ADAPTATION FOR NUTRITION POLICY

The use of dietary guidelines in public health nutrition has recently been reviewed (Institute of Medicine 2000). In general, protein requirement figures serve two purposes.

One is as a basis for prescription, i.e. advice on safe diets through recommending appropriate dietary intakes. The adaptive model shown in Figure *evolve* 8.9b implies a much lower, but difficult to define, RNI. Formulation of policy will inevitably and correctly be most concerned with satisfying the upper range of demands for protein and, where there is uncertainty, including positive margins of error. In this case it may be unwise to adopt an adaptive model and reduce the RNI. Indeed an adaptive model does not mean that protein is an unimportant nutrient for the maintenance of human health and well-being, but that indicators other than balance need to be identified. There is growing experimental evidence for potential benefit of protein intakes considerably above the current RNI for bone health in the elderly, and epidemiological evidence for benefit with respect to hypertension and ischaemic heart disease (see WHO 2007). This results in a dilemma for those attempting to frame dietary guidelines. It is probably wise to retain current values until it becomes possible to quantify the benefits (and any risks) of protein intakes within the adaptive range.

The other purpose of requirement figures is as a diagnostic indicator of risk, in population groups rather than individuals. In this case indicators used to estimate prevalence of disease states, or deficit risk, are carefully chosen so as to strike an acceptable balance between false positives and false negatives. The main implication of adaptation for estimating risk of deficiency defined only as intake < requirements, is a dramatic reduction in the prevalence of risk for most populations compared with that assessed according to the current model. As in the prescriptive context, this low risk of deficiency applies only to that of being unable to maintain N balance after full adaptation with otherwise nutritionally adequate diets satisfying the energy demands. Whether such populations enjoy optimal protein-related health is a separate issue. It has been suggested that maintenance of N balance can no longer be used as a surrogate of adequate protein-related health and that current lack of quantifiable alternative indicators is no excuse for ignoring the issue of adaptation.

KEY POINTS

- Proteins are large polymers of 21 different amino acids; the amino acid sequence of each protein is different, and is determined by the gene for that protein.
- Folding of the protein chain produces proteins that act as receptors, transport proteins and enzymes, and serve structural functions
- An adult is overall in nitrogen equilibrium, with intake of nitrogenous compounds (mainly protein) matched by excretion of nitrogenous metabolites.
- In growth and recovery from loss there is positive nitrogen balance; in response to trauma, or an inadequate intake, there is negative nitrogen balance. There is continual catabolism of tissue proteins, and replacement synthesis, so there is a dynamic equilibrium – even in an adult who is not increasing the total body protein content.
- In the fasting state protein catabolism exceeds synthesis, and in the fed state synthesis exceeds catabolism.
- Both protein synthesis and catabolism are energy-requiring processes, and a significant proportion of total energy expenditure is accounted for by protein turnover.
- Protein synthesis is controlled both by hormones and also by nutrients. Fatty acids, iron and cholesterol regulate the synthesis of enzymes involved in their metabolism; carbohydrates regulate the synthesis of lipogenic and glycolytic enzymes; amino acid availability regulates overall protein synthesis.
- After synthesis on the ribosome, many proteins undergo post-synthetic modification, resulting in the formation of a number of amino acids that cannot be utilised for new protein synthesis, but are metabolised or excreted unchanged after protein catabolism.
- Nine amino acids cannot be synthesised in the body, but must be provided in the diet – these are the essential or indispensable amino acids.
- Although the remaining amino acids can be synthesised in the body, only three (alanine, aspartic and glutamic acids) can be considered to be wholly dispensable.
- In addition to the requirement for protein synthesis, a variety of other important compounds are synthesised from amino acids.
- The catabolism of amino acids leads to the formation of ammonium by transamination linked to deamination; this is transported in the body as glutamine, and metabolised in the liver to form urea, the main urinary nitrogenous compound.
- The carbon skeletons of amino acids may provide substrates for energy-yielding metabolism, fatty acid synthesis or gluconeogenesis.
- The determination of protein and amino acid requirements is inherently difficult, partly because of adaptation over a wide range of intakes.
- Protein requirements can be considered in terms of the metabolic demand for total protein and individual amino acids, and the dietary requirement, taking into account the digestibility and nutritional value of different proteins.
- Protein requirements can be determined by nitrogen balance studies and factorial calculation; there are inherent problems in this method.
- Protein requirements may be calculated on the basis of intake per kilogram body weight or on the basis of energy density.
- Various methods can be used to estimate protein quality, either in experimental animals or in human beings.
- Protein and amino acid requirements can be determined by a variety of stable isotope tracer studies; there are inherent problems in the various methods that have been used.

References

FAO/WHO/UNU: *Energy and protein requirements*. 15. Report of a joint FAO/WHO/UNU expert consultation. Technical report series 724, Geneva, 1985, WHO.

FAO/WHO: *Protein quality evaluation. Report of a joint FAO/WHO Expert Consultation*, Rome, 1991, FAO.

Food and Nutrition Board, Institute of Medicine: *Dietary reference intakes for energy, carbohydrate, fiber, fat, fatty acids, cholesterol, protein, and amino acids (macronutrients)*, Washington DC, 2002, National Academy Press.

Institute of Medicine: *Dietary reference intakes: application in dietary assessment*, Washington DC, 2000, National Academy Press.

Jones EM, Bauman CA, Reynolds MS: Nitrogen balances in women maintained on various levels of lysine, *Journal of Nutrition* 60:549–559, 1956.

Millward DJ: The nutritional value of plant based diets in relation to human amino acid and protein requirements, *Proceedings of the Nutrition Society* 58:249–260, 1999.

Millward DJ: Workshop on 'Protein and Amino Acid Requirements and Recommendations' methodological considerations, *Proceedings of the Nutrition Society* 60:1–4, 2001.

Millward DJ: An adaptive metabolic demand model for protein and amino acid requirements, *British Journal of Nutrition* 90:249–260, 2003.

Millward DJ, Jackson AA: Protein/energy ratios of current diets in developed and developing countries compared with a safe protein/energy ratio: implications for recommended protein and amino acid intakes, *Public Health Nutrition* 7(3):387–405, 2004.

Rand WM, Pellett PL, Young VR: Meta-analysis of nitrogen balance studies for estimating protein requirements in healthy adults, *American Journal of Clinical Nutrition* 77:109–127, 2003.

WHO: Protein and amino acid requirements in human nutrition. Report of a joint WHO/FAO/UNU expert consultation. WHO Tech Rep Ser 935, Geneva, 2007, WHO.

Further reading

Bolourchi S, Friedmann CM, Mickelsen O: Wheat flour as a source of protein for human subjects. *American Journal of Clinical Nutrition* 21:827–835, 1968.

Department of Health: *Dietary reference values for food energy and nutrients for the United Kingdom.* Report on Health and Social Subjects no. 41, London, 1991, HMSO.

Dewey K G, Beaton G, Fjeld C, Lonnerdal B, Reeds P: Protein requirements of infants and children. *European Journal of Clinical Nutrition* 50:S119–S150, 1996.

Edwards CH, Booker LK, Rumph CH, et al: Utilization of wheat by adult man: nitrogen metabolism, plasma amino acids and lipids. *American Journal of Clinical Nutrition* 24:181–193, 1971.

Institute of Medicine: *Dietary reference intakes: application in dietary assessment.* Washington DC, 2000, National Academy Press.

Millward DJ: Inherent difficulties in defining amino acid requirements. *In: The role of protein and amino acids in sustaining and enhancing performance.* Committee on Military Nutrition Research, Food and Nutrition Board, Institute of Medicine, Washington DC, 1999, National Academy Press, pp 169–208.

Millward DJ: Optimal intakes of dietary protein. *Proceedings of the Nutrition Society* 58:403–413, 1999.

Millward DJ, Pacy PJ: Postprandial protein utilisation and protein quality assessment in man. *Clinical Science* 88:597–606, 1995.

Millward DJ, Fereday A, Gibson NR, Pacy PJ: Efficiency of utilization and apparent requirements for wheat protein and lysine determined by a single meal [^{13}C-1] leucine balance comparison with milk protein in healthy adults. *American Journal of Clinical Nutrition* 76:1326–1334, 2002.

Pellett PL, Young VR: The effects of different levels of energy intake on protein metabolism and of different levels of protein intake on energy metabolism: a statistical evaluation from the published literature. In Scrimshaw NS, Schurch B, editors: *Protein Energy Interactions,* Waterville Valley, NH, 1992, IDECG, pp 81–136.

Young VR, Scrimshaw NS, Pellett PL: Significance of dietary protein source in human nutrition. Animal or plant protein? In Waterlow JC, Armstrong DG, Fouden L, Riley R, editors: *Feeding a world population of more than eight billion people. A challenge to science,* Oxford, 1998, Oxford University Press, in association with The Rank Prize Funds, pp 205–222.

Chapter 9

Alcohol metabolism: implications for nutrition and health

Ross Hunter, Timothy J Peters and Victor R Preedy

CHAPTER CONTENTS

OBJECTIVES

By the end of this chapter, you should be able to:
- appreciate the varying intake of alcohol by different population groups and the contribution that alcohol makes to energy intake
- understand the main features of alcohol metabolism
- explain the basis of nutritional deficiencies in alcoholism
- understand how alcohol damages virtually all organs in the body especially the liver.

DOI: 10.1016/B978-0-7020-3118-2.00009-7

9.1   INTRODUCTION

Alcohol is commonly used interchangeably with *ethanol* or ethyl alcohol. Ethanol, acetaldehyde and acetic acid/acetate (two metabolites of ethanol oxidation) are the current preferred names though there may be usage of systematic names, i.e. for acetaldehyde and acetic acid these would be ethanal and ethanoic acid, respectively. The term 'drinking' is often used to describe the consumption of beverages containing alcohol.

Individuals will consume wide-ranging quantities of alcohol but some countries or communities expressly forbid the consumption of alcohol on religious, cultural or moral grounds. Individuals may gain pleasure from the psycho-pharmacological effects of alcohol whereas others may react quite badly, with flushing, nausea and palpitations due to a genetic variation in alcohol- or acetaldehyde-metabolising enzymes. In excess, alcohol may cause malnutrition or act as a toxin and induce pathological changes in a variety of tissues. By contrast, a substantial proportion of individuals consume moderate amounts of alcohol, comprising up to 5% of total dietary energy, and some controversial data suggest that moderate alcohol consumption may be beneficial in reducing cardiovascular and other risk factors. Thus, it is important to take a balanced view of ethanol's effects.

Recent *Guidance on the consumption of alcohol by children and young people* from the Chief Medical Officers of England, Wales and Northern Ireland has suggested that children under 15 should not drink alcohol.

Apart from the impact on physical health, detrimental effects will arise due to lack of inhibitions and psychosocial factors such as increased risk taking. This leads to accidents and also inappropriate sexual activity. Furthermore it is advised that women who are pregnant or about to become pregnant should avoid drinking alcohol, particularly in the first 3 months post-conception. Certainly women who are pregnant should not consume more than one or two units once or twice a week. Nursing mothers should also be aware of the problems of drinking alcohol. Breast milk will contain traces of alcohol and smell differently, thus affecting the baby's nutritional intake and/or feeding patterns.

THE CHEMICAL NATURE OF ALCOHOL

Ethanol is produced from glucose via the fermentation of yeast to produce ethanol, carbon dioxide and ATP. As a consequence of its combined polar (OH group) and non-polar (C_2H_5 groups) properties, and because it is relatively uncharged, ethanol is miscible with water and can cross cell membranes by passive diffusion. It also has the ability to dissolve lipids, hence its disordering affects on biological membranes.

The immediate metabolite of ethanol oxidation, acetaldehyde (Fig. 9.1), is a highly toxic and chemically reactive molecule that can bind irreversibly with proteins and nucleic acids. The importance of acetaldehyde in the aetiology of disease was highlighted by the fact that it was the focus of a Novartis (formally CIBA) Foundation Symposium and readers are referred to this for additional reading (Novartis 2007) Acetate, the product of acetaldehyde metabolism, is either oxidised peripherally to CO_2 in the Krebs (citric acid) cycle or used for synthesis of fatty acids and triglycerides. Acetate *per se* also has some biological activity, e.g. it dilates resistance and capacitance blood vessels. However, in illicit or home brewed beverages and even in some commercially available beverages, there may be significant quantities of compounds that have putative toxic properties. These include ethylene glycol, diethylene glycol, acetaldehyde, acetone, methanol and butanol.

THE CONTRIBUTION TO THE ENERGY INTAKE OF DIFFERENT POPULATION GROUPS

Energy content of alcoholic beverages and the Unit system

The chemical energy content of ethanol is 29.7 kJ (7.1 kcal) per gram. In the UK, an alcoholic drink or 'Unit of alcohol' containing 10 ml of ethanol by volume will contain 8 g of ethanol (Table 9.1). However, there is a wide international variation in the amount of alcohol in a Unit: from 7 to 14 g ethanol (Table 9.1). The alcohol content of beverages can vary from 0.5% for low alcohol beers to 40–50% for distilled spirits such as vodka or whisky (Table 9.2).

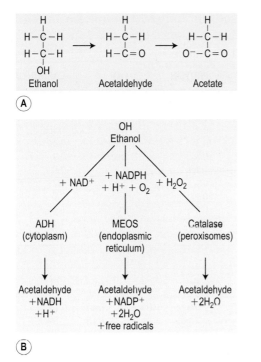

Fig. 9.1 **Metabolism of alcohol.** A. Simplistic representation of conversion of alcohol to acetaldehyde and then acetate. B. Three major route of ethanol oxidation.

Table 9.1	The Unit system

A.
The Unit system of alcohol consumption
One Unit
Half a pint of beer
One glass (125 ml) of wine
One measure (50 ml) of fortified wine (sherry, port)
One measure (25 ml) of spirits (whisky, gin, vodka etc)

B.
Ethanol comprising one Unit

UK	8 g
Australia and New Zealand	10 g
USA	12 g
Japan	14 g

The Unit system of alcohol ingestion is a convenient way of abstracting the amount of ethanol consumed by individuals and offers a suitable means to give practical guidance. The amount of alcohol in each Unit will vary, for example depending on geographical location. The unit system may also be misleading as the volume of drinks served and the percentage alcohol by volume are variable.

Recommended limits for alcohol consumption

The medical Royal Colleges have recommended that a consumption of either 21 Units (men) or 14 Units (women) per week are sensible limits and these are now generally accepted. The Department of Health (UK) also have guidelines based on daily amounts, namely 3–4 or 2–3 Units a day for men and women, respectively, and apply to whether consumption is daily, one or two times a week, or occasionally (Table 9.3). The original intention was to provide a user-friendly way people could keep track of what they drink, and curtail this if needed. However, changes in the volume and strength of alcohol sold to the consumer is making this increasingly misleading. A Unit of alcohol should contain 8 g of alcohol, which is equal to a 125 ml glass of wine containing 8% alcohol by volume or half a pint of 'ordinary' strength beer containing 3.5% by volume. If we then look at what is sold in pubs in the UK we see that most beers are around 5% (1.5 Units per half pint). Wine is often sold as medium (175 ml) or large (250 ml) servings, containing around 12% by volume (equating to around 2 and 3 Units respectively).

Public awareness of these guidelines is still lacking; despite much effort on publicity campaigns the 2008 statistics from the Institute of Alcohol Studies (IAS) report that although 69% of adults surveyed had heard of these guidelines, only 40% of these knew what the recommendations were. Taking the adult population as a whole, about 31% of males and 20% of females in the UK drink more than 21 or 14 Units per week, respectively (Table *evolve* 9.1). There is a staggering number of men and women in the UK who drink alcohol above either the daily (8.6 million) or weekly (9.1 million) guidelines. If one takes into account that previous figures were deficient in that they did not take into account the higher concentration of alcohol in beers and wines, or that wine serving sizes have increased, then there may be over 10 million people who exceed either weekly or daily guidelines. The estimates for alcohol dependence in the UK are high at 7% and 2% of the adult male and female population, respectively (Table *evolve* 9.2). There are an estimated 2.8 million individuals classified as alcohol-dependent. There has also been a worrying trend towards increased alcohol consumption in women and in the young.

Table 9.2   Composition of alcoholic beverages

	PER 100 ml (ALL AS g EXCEPT ENERGY)					
	kcal	kJ	ALCOHOL	PROTEIN	FAT	CARBOHYDRATE
Alcohol free lager	7	31	Trace	0.4	Trace	1.5
Low alcohol lager	10	41	0.5	0.2	0	1.5
Lager	29	131	4.0	0.3	Trace	Trace
Special strength lager	59	244	6.9	0.3	Trace	2.4
Bitter	30	124	2.9	0.3	Trace	2.2
Cider (dry)	36	152	3.8	Trace	0	2.6
Wine (red, dry)	68	283	9.6	0.1	0	0.2
Wine (white, dry)	66	275	9.1	0.1	0	0.6
Wine (white, sweet)	94	394	10.2	0.2	0	5.9
Sherry (dry)	116	481	15.7	0.2	0	1.4
Spirits (various; 40% proof)	222	919	31.7	Trace	0	Trace

	PER 100 ml (ALL AS g)									
	Na	K	Ca	Mg	P	Fe	Cu	Zn	Cl	Mn
Alcohol free lager	2	44	3	7	19	Trace	Trace	Trace	Trace	0.01
Low alcohol lager	12	56	8	12	10	Trace	Trace	Trace	Trace	0.01
Lager	7	39	5	7	19	Trace	Trace	Trace	20	0.01
Special strength lager	7	39	5	7	19	Trace	Trace	Trace	20	0.01
Bitter	6	32	8	7	14	0.1	0.001	0.1	24	0.03
Cider (dry)	7	72	8	3	3	0.5	0.04	Trace	6	Trace
Wine (red, dry)	7	110	7	11	13	0.9	0.06	0.1	11	0.10
Wine (white, dry)	4	61	9	8	6	0.5	0.01	Trace	10	0.10
Wine (white, sweet)	13	110	14	11	13	0.6	0.05	Trace	7	0.10
Sherry (dry)	10	57	7	13	11	0.4	0.03	N	14	Trace
Spirits (various; 40% proof)	Trace	Trace	Trace	Trace	Trace	Trace	Trace	Trace	Trace	Trace

	PER 100 ml							
	RIBOFLAVIN	NIACIN	TRYPT/60	B6	B12	FOLATE	PANTOTHENATE	BIOTIN
	(mg)	(mg)	(mg)	(mg)	(μg)	(μg)	(μg)	(μg)
Alcohol free lager	0.02	0.6	0.4	0.03	Trace	5	0.09	Trace
Low alcohol lager	0.02	0.5	0.3	0.03	Trace	6	0.07	Trace
Lager	0.04	0.7	0.3	0.06	Trace	12	0.03	1
Special strength lager	0.04	0.7	0.3	0.06	Trace	12	0.03	1
Bitter	0.03	0.2	0.2	0.07	Trace	5	0.05	1
Cider (dry)	Trace	0	Trace	0.01	Trace	N	0.04	1
Wine (red, dry)	0.02	0.1	Trace	0.03	Trace	1	0.04	2
Wine (white, dry)	0.01	0.1	Trace	0.02	Trace	Trace	0.03	N
Wine (white, sweet)	0.01	0.1	Trace	0.01	Trace	Trace	0.03	N
Sherry (dry)	0.01	0.1	Trace	0.01	Trace	Trace	Trace	N
Spirits (various; 40% proof)	0	0	0	0	0	0	0	0

This table only gives an estimate of some of the compounds that will be present in alcoholic beverages. In addition, there will also be other compounds, which are not tabulated, such as fluoride, polyphenols and other organic and non-organic compounds that impart characteristics of taste and smell. Data from Foods Standards Agency 2002.

Table 9.3	Categorisation of weekly alcohol consumption using Units	
	MEN	WOMEN
Low risk	0–21	0–14
Increasing risk	22–50	15–35
Harmful	>50	>35

Summary of Department of Health (UK) recommendations
Men:
- Protection: 1–2 Units per day, possibly protection against heart disease (over 40)
- Low risk: 3–4 Units a day (all ages).
- Not advised: consistently drinking 4 or more Units a day

Women:
- Protection: 1–2 Units day, possibly protection against heart disease (past menopause)
- Low risk: 2–3 Units a day (all ages).
- Not advised: consistently drinking 3 or more Units a day
- Harmful: more than 1 or 2 Units of alcohol, once or twice a week when pregnant or about to become pregnant

Guidelines are designed to limit harm (Department of Health 1995). Whilst the Royal Colleges' guidelines pertain to weekly consumption rates, the Department of Health's guidelines are more directed to daily rates.

Drinking in the young and gender susceptibility

The results of a UK survey showed that one fifth of children aged 11–15 had drunk alcohol in the past week. There have been recent increases in the quantity of alcohol consumed by children in this age category who drink, which presently averages 11 Units/week (Table *evolve* 9.3). Drinking by school children and adolescents has at least six serious consequences: (a) alcohol poisoning and fatalities; (b) drinking in formative years will predict the extent of alcohol misuse later on; (c) drinking may be compounded by polydrug and other substance misuse, including tobacco; (d) total lifetime intake of alcohol, rather than recent intakes, is a good predicator of alcohol-related harm (Saunders & Devereaux 2002); (e) tissues in the young are particularly sensitive to alcohol; (f) there is an association with antisocial behaviour, poor academic performance and crime, hence there is a wider social impact.

Boys and men are more avid consumers of alcohol than girls (Tables *evolve* 9.1, 9.2, 9.3) but women are more susceptible to alcohol-induced injury such as cardiomyopathy, skeletal muscle myopathy, brain damage and liver disease. This may be related to lower clearance rates of alcohol on 'first pass metabolism', as a consequence of smaller liver size, or gastric alcohol metabolising enzymes, endocrine factors, body fat composition or even psycho-social factors in reporting alcohol consumption. Compared with men, women also have higher blood acetaldehyde levels following the same amount of alcohol per unit body weight. It has been estimated that whilst men will show an increased chance of developing liver disease at an intake rate of 40–60 g ethanol/day, the threshold level for women is lower: 20 g/day. A comprehensive analysis of the vulnerability of women compared to men has been reviewed and readers are referred to this work (Fernandez-Sola et al 2005).

Energy and micronutrient content of alcoholic beverages

Ten ml of ethanol will yield approximately 234 kJ (56 kcal). This underestimates the true energy content of alcoholic beverages as they also contain other constituents, such as carbohydrates, amino acids and fatty acids (see Table 9.2; Food Standards Agency 2002). The energy composition of alcoholic beverages varies from about 125 to 920 kJ (30–220 kcal)/100 ml. Low or zero alcohol beverages will of course have a lower energy content although usually a higher carbohydrate content. Alcoholic beverages will also contain trace amounts of compounds that impart flavour or characteristics of taste and smell, e.g. aliphatic carbonyls, other alcohols, monocarboxylic acids, sulphur containing compounds, tannins, polyphenols, inorganic salts or metals (Aceto 2003). Some of these compounds, such as fluoride, vitamins or polyphenols, are reported to have beneficial properties (see Ch. 13).

Ethanol's contribution to energy in the diet

In the UK, the mean daily total energy intake excluding alcohol is 8834 and 6506 kJ (2110 and 1554 kcal) for men and women, respectively, and 9672 and 6824 kJ (2310 and 1630 kcal) including alcohol (Henderson et al 2003). The mean daily intake of alcohol in all men (consumers and non-consumers) is 22 g (27 g for just consumers) and 9 g for all women (13 g for just consumers) (Table 9.4). Other recent estimates have shown similar data for overall consumption by all men and women, i.e. 18 g and 9 g of ethanol per day (Lader & Meltzer 2002). Consideration must be taken of non-alcoholic

Table 9.4   Ethanol consumption as dietary energy in the UK

	MEN					WOMEN				
	19–24	25–34	35–49	50–64	ALL	19–24	25–34	35–49	50–64	ALL
All										
Mean daily intake										
g/day	20.4	22.2	23.1	21.1	21.9	11.4	9.1	9.2	8.6	9.3
kcal/d	143	158	164	150	155	81	65	65	61	66
% total										
energy	6	6.6	6.8	6.4	6.5	4.6	4.0	3.9	3.7	3.9
Consumers only										
Mean daily intake										
g/day	25.6	27.2	27.4	27.5	27.2	16.1	13.2	13.2	12.9	13.5
kcal/d	182	193	195	195	193	114	94	94	92	96
% total										
energy	7.6	8.1	8.1	8.3	8.1	6.4	5.8	5.6	5.4	5.7

In the above calculations, it was assumed that the energy value of alcohol was 7.1 kcal/g. It should be recognised that specific dietary questionnaires that include alcohol as a constituent may give different answers from questionnaires designed specifically to investigate the intake of alcohol per se, especially in alcohol misusers or alcohol-dependent subjects where the reliability of such questionnaires has been called into question. (Data adapted from Henderson et al 2003.)

energy contained within the beverages, for example carbohydrates or mixers that might accompany drinks.

Most of the consumption of alcohol in the UK is in the form of beer and wine (Table *evolve* 9.4). Overall (i.e. in alcohol consumers and non-consumers) the contribution of ethanol to total energy intake is 6.5% in men and 3.9% in women, respectively. In consumers, the contributions are 8.1% and 5.7%, respectively (Henderson et al 2003). However, the contribution of ethanol-derived calories increases significantly in dependent alcoholics. In one recent study, patients attending an inner city Alcohol Misuse clinic in the UK consumed on average 160 g ethanol/day; contributing to about 60% of dietary energy intake. However, alcohol consumption may be under-reported in women and over-reported in men and no food frequency questionnaires have been unequivocally validated in alcohol misusers. Typical patients with chronic liver disease may consume 160–250 g ethanol/day (1140–1770 kcal/day). This has nutritional consequences as ethanol may be perceived as being 'empty,' i.e. having negligible or minor quantities of micro- or macronutrients. High ethanol loads also impair the normal functions of the liver (see below).

THE SERIOUS NEGATIVE CONSEQUENCES OF CHRONIC ALCOHOL INGESTION ON HEALTH

There are at least 60–120 different alcohol-related pathologies (Table 9.5; Preedy & Watson 2005) and the myth that the most affected organs are the brain and liver should be dispelled. Many of the deleterious effects relate in some way to ethanol metabolism, altering cellular biochemistry either because of ethanol *per se*, or its immediate metabolite, acetaldehyde. Approximately 10–15% of chronic alcohol misusers will have cirrhosis and 30% will have gastrointestinal pathologies (Table 9.6). In terms of the gastrointestinal tract, all regions can be affected from the mouth to the rectum. For example oral mucosal lesions have be shown to occur in as many as 28% of chronic alcoholics. The relative risk of rectal cancers increases about fourfold in chronic alcohol misusers. Fatty liver will occur in 80% and 50% will have bone marrow changes (perturbing red blood cell morphology). Half of chronic alcoholics will have damaged skeletal tissue (osteoporosis, osteopenia, fractures, including post-fracture malunion) whereas between 20–30% will exhibit a spectrum of subclinical or clinical cardiac

Table 9.5   Systems and tissues affected by alcohol misuse

Hepato-pancreatobiliary	Genitourinary
Hepatomegaly – fatty liver, alcoholic hepatitis and fibrosis Cirrhosis and hepatocellular carcinoma Acute and chronic relapsing pancreatitis – malabsorptive syndrome	IgA nephropathy Renal tubular acidosis. Renal tract infections Female and male hypogonadism, subfertility Impotence Spontaneous abortion Fetal alcohol syndrome
Central, peripheral and autonomic nervous systems	**Cardiovascular**

Acute intoxication
Progressive euphoria, incoordination, ataxia, stupor, coma and
   death
Alcohol withdrawal symptoms including delirium tremens,
   morning nausea, retching and vomiting, nightmares and night
   terrors, blackouts and withdrawal seizures
	Cardiomyopathy, including dysrrhythmias
	Hypertension
	Binge strokes
	Cardiovascular disease (including stroke)
	Myocardial infarction

Nutritional deficiencies	**Dermatological**
Wernicke–Korsakoff syndrome. Pellagra Tobacco–alcohol amblyopia	Skin stigmata of liver disease – rosacea, spider naevi, palmar erythema, finger clubbing Skin infections – bacterial, fungal and viral Local cutaneous vascular effects Psoriasis Discoid eczema Nutritional deficiencies (including pellagra)
Others	

Cerebral dementia, cerebellar degeneration
Demyelinating syndromes – central pontine myelinolysis,
Marchiafava–Bignami syndrome, associated with electrolyte
   disturbances
Fetal alcohol syndrome – full-blown syndrome, mental
   impairment, attention deficit and hyperkinetic disorders, specific
   learning difficulties
	Respiratory

	Chronic bronchitis Respiratory tract malignancy Asthma Postoperative complications
Peripheral nervous system	**Oro-gastrointestinal**
Sensory, motor and mixed neuropathy	Periodontal disease and caries Oral infections, leukoplakia and malignancy
Autonomic neuropathy	Alcoholic gastritis and haemorrhage
Musculoskeletal	Alcoholic enteropathy and malabsorption Colonic malignancy

Proximal metabolic myopathy, principally affecting type II (white)
   fibres
Neuromyopathy secondary to motor nerve damage
Atrophy of smooth muscle of gastrointestinal tract, leading to
   motility disorders
Osteopenia – impaired bone formation, degradation, nutritional
   deficiencies (e.g. calcium, magnesium, phosphate, vitamin D)
Avascular necrosis (e.g. femoral head)
Fractures – malunion
	Haematological

	RBCs – macrocytosis, anaemia because of blood loss, folate deficiency and malabsorption, haemolysis (rarely) WBCs – neutropenia, lymphopenia Platelets – thrombocytopenia

This table is designed to show that diseases associated with alcohol misuse are not confined to the liver and brain. Virtually all tissues and organs systems can be affected adversely but only some are life threatening. However, not all individuals will get the diseases identified, perhaps because of inherent protective, dietary or genetic factors. (Compiled from Peters & Preedy 1998.)

abnormalities (i.e. alcoholic cardiomyopathy) or other cardiovascular diseases including hypertension. A staggering 80% of subjects will have skin lesions including those of vascular, fungal, bacterial or viral origin and 40–60% will have alcoholic myopathy. Abnormal gonadal function will occur in 50% of male alcoholics. As a rule of thumb, 50% of chronic alcohol misusers will have one or more organ or tissue abnormalities (Table 9.7).

Although many of these aforementioned diseases are considered to be 'organ specific' there may be secondary consequences. For example, the impact of liver disease on the body is well known and affects wide a range of tissues and organs, such as the skin, muscle, bone and brain. However, the effects of autonomic neuropathy in alcoholics are less well documented. Symptoms of autonomic neuropathy include dry eyes and/or mouth,

Table 9.6	Prevalence of alcohol–induced pathologies in chronic alcohol abusers	
		(%)
Skin disorders		80
Alcoholic myopathy		50
Bone disorders		50
Gonadal dysfunction		50
Gastroenterological disorders		30
Cirrhosis		15
Neuropathy		15
Cardiomyopathy		10
Brain disease (organic)		10

The prevalence of alcohol-related disorders relates to chronic alcohol-dependent subjects.

Table 9.7   Rule of thumb in alcohol misuse

The five 'rules of thumb' for alcohol induced pathologies
1. All tissues and organ systems have the potential to be affected by alcohol or its immediate metabolites.
2. Alcohol or its immediate metabolites has the potential to affect all biochemical pathways, subcellular organelles and other cellular systems and/or structures.
3. Not all individuals will suffer the consequences of alcohol ingestion because of cellular, nutritional or genetic protective systems.
4. 50% of alcoholics will have one or more organ or tissue pathologies.
5. 50% of alcoholics will have a deficiency of one or more micro- or macronutrient.

The above rules of thumb are gross generalisations and one should take into account differences due to gender, socio-ethnicity, and geographical and regional variations in alcohol ingestion.

---

sensory dysfunction (taste; vision), upper and lower gastrointestinal symptoms, genitourinary abnormalities including loss of bladder control and erectile problems, thermoregulatory dysfunction including sweating and cardiovascular dysfunction such as postural hypotension and arrhythmias. It is estimated that autonomic dysfunction will occur in between one-quarter and three-quarters of alcoholics. The definition of autonomic dysfunction usually depends on a number of tests but individual features may occur more frequently.

Very often dependent drinkers smoke cigarettes, i.e. they are addicted to nicotine and this has a greater effect on the development of disease than either addiction alone. This is particularly relevant with respect to cancers of the upper aerodigestive tract, and these synergistic effects of smoking and drinking have also been seen in the development of other diseases such as cirrhosis. It is important to remember that alcohol misuse not only has effects on body systems but also leads to perturbations in behaviours and life style activities, and quality of life measures.

In Europe and the Americas, between 15% and 55% of people attending hospital (as either inpatients or outpatients) or primary care centres are classified as dependent or hazardous alcohol abusers. However, fewer than 5% of adults have such misuse or dependency recorded in their medical records. Prevalence rates of alcohol misuse will depend on geographical and socio-economic factors. In London (UK), a third of all acute hospital admissions are alcohol related and the prevalence of alcohol misuse in inpatients in city hospitals may be as high as 50%. In fracture clinics, 40–70% of patients score positively for alcohol-related dependency or abuse syndromes.

There are numerous instruments designed to detect alcohol misuse; these include the CAGE (Cut down, Annoyed, Guilty, Eye-opener), AUDIT (Alcohol Use Disorders Identification Test), BMAST (Brief Michigan Alcoholism Screening Test), and PAT (Paddington Alcohol Test) questionnaires. In some circumstances these can be more useful than laboratory tests on serum, plasma, urine or saliva.

9.2 ALCOHOL METABOLISM

Many of the pathologies associated with drinking alcoholic beverages are due to the effects of acetaldehyde, or the ensuing metabolic changes (e.g. redox state, antioxidant or endocrine status) that accompany ethanol oxidation (see Fig. *evolve* 9.1 for a scheme of ethanol metabolism). All pathways and cell structures have the potential to be targeted by ethanol or its related metabolites. Central to these effects is the liver, where 60–90% of ethanol metabolism occurs. Up to 90% of the substrates utilised in conventional metabolic pathways in liver may be displaced by ethanol oxidation. Ethanol ingestion can inhibit protein and fat oxidation in the body by approximately 40 and 75% respectively. The 2.5-fold increase in oxidation of carbohydrate after a glucose load is also abolished by ethanol.

Oxidation of ethanol by gastric first pass metabolism will account for 5–25% of ethanol oxidation and 2–10% will appear in the breath, sweat or urine.

THE METABOLIC FATE OF ALCOHOL FOLLOWING DIGESTION AND ABSORPTION

Ethanol is rapidly absorbed, primarily in the upper gastrointestinal tract, and appears in the blood as quickly as 5 min after ingestion. Its distribution will approximate total body water. Its elimination thereafter will approximate to Michaelis–Menten kinetics though zero-order and elimination analyses have also been described. Blood alcohol levels depend on pathophysiological factors, such as absorption rate, first pass metabolism, the extent to which liver function has been altered and blood flow.

The rate at which alcohol is oxidised, or disappears from the blood, varies from 6 to10 g per hour. This is reflected in plasma levels, which fall by 9–20 mg/100 ml/hour. In response to a moderate dose of alcohol of 0.6–0.9 g/kg body weight, the elimination rate from the blood is approximately 15 mg/100 ml blood/hour on an empty stomach though there is considerable individual variation.

Food in the stomach will delay the absorption of alcohol and blunt the peak blood alcohol concentration. The peak blood level is the point at which the rate of elimination equals the rate of absorption. Using a standard dose of ethanol/kg body weight, it has been shown that the peak is lower after a meal compared with an empty stomach. The time to metabolise the alcohol was 2 hours shorter in the fed state than the fasted state, indicative of a postabsorptive enhancement of ethanol oxidation which can be as much as 35–50% (Jones 2000).

The type of food taken with alcoholic beverage will also alter the peak ethanol level: after a standard dose of ethanol of 0.3 g/kg, meals rich in fat, carbohydrate and protein result in peak ethanol levels of 16.6, 17.7 and 13.3 mg/100 ml, respectively (Jones 2000). Part of this variation may be due to increased portal blood flow in response to feeding, which will essentially deliver more ethanol to the liver for oxidation.

The concentrations of ethanol in beverages will also influence peak blood concentration. Thus, in the fed state for a given amount of ethanol, a lower peak level is obtained with high concentrations compared with the equivalent amount of ethanol in a more dilute beverage. In fasted subjects, high and low ethanol concentrations give similar blood alcohol concentrations and areas under the curve. For example, in the fed state, beer produces higher peak blood levels compared to whisky for a given alcohol load. In the fasted state, beer produces lower mean blood alcohol concentration and areas under the curve than whisky (Roine 2000). These differences are related to one of the primary determinants of alcohol metabolism: namely the rate of gastric emptying. In simple terms, the small intestine is the main site of ethanol absorption and food will have little effect on large volumes of ethanol-containing liquid (beer) compared to smaller volumes of high-ethanol-containing liquids (whisky) (Roine 2000).

First pass metabolism and the contribution of the stomach

First pass metabolism is principally due to the liver (*hepatic first pass metabolism*), but a small proportion of alcohol is also metabolised by the stomach (*gastric first pass metabolism*). Stomach ADH (sigma-ADH) is a different isoform from the enzyme in the liver (see Table *evolve* 9.5 🖰). Physiological factors that influence gastric emptying will also influence the contribution of this pathway to ethanol elimination. In one study, where ethanol (0.3 g/kg body weight) was administered by different routes, it was calculated that the amount of ethanol absorbed (0.224 g/kg body weight) was 75% of the administered dose: the difference being ascribed to first pass metabolism. The rate of gastric ethanol metabolism has been reported to be about 1.8 g of ethanol per hour (Haber 2000).

Reduced first pass metabolism and/or reduced gastric ADH will occur in *Helicobacter pylori* infection and during histamine H_2-receptor antagonist therapy. There are also ethnic differences: Orientals have a lower stomach ADH/first pass metabolism compared with Caucasians. Chronic alcoholism reduces the capacity of this route of ethanol oxidation due to the development of gastritis.

Gender differences in alcohol metabolism

There are gender differences in the rate of ethanol elimination rates that have also been partially ascribed to first-pass metabolism. The activity of gastric ADH in women is lower than in men, though this is less apparent in women over 50 years old. Compared with men, women will have higher blood ethanol levels after an equivalent load. The lower first-pass metabolism activities account for the higher ethanol levels in women, rather than differences in gastric emptying or rate of ethanol oxidation in the liver. It has however, been proposed that women and men have comparable peak blood alcohol concentrations when dosage is based on total body water.

THE SPEED WITH WHICH ALCOHOL IS DISTRIBUTED IN BODY WATER

Alcohol is rapidly distributed around the body. After ingestion, alcohol that is not immediately absorbed traverses the gastrointestinal tract. Very high ethanol levels occur in the small intestine compared with serum. Effectively, there is a gradient down the gastrointestinal tract. For example, a dose of 0.8 g ethanol/kg body weight (equivalent to 56 g ethanol = 7 Units = 3.5 pints of ordinary beer, consumed by a 70 kg male) will result in blood ethanol levels of 100–200 mg/100 ml between 15 and 120 min after dosage. Maximum blood concentrations occur after about 30–90 min. Gastric levels peak at 8 g/100 ml of luminal contents; jejunal levels are approximately 4 g/100 ml compared to approximately 0.15 g/100 ml in the ileum. Levels in the ileum reflect serum levels, i.e. from the vascular space. After about 2 hours, ethanol concentrations in the stomach and jejunum will approximate levels in serum (Mezey 1985). In the post-absorption phase, the distribution of alcohol in the body will reflect body water to the extent that, for a given dose of alcohol, blood levels will reflect lean body mass. The solubility of ethanol in bone and lipid is negligible. Whole blood levels (which includes plasma and cellular contents) of ethanol are about 10% lower than plasma levels because red blood cells have less water than plasma.

METABOLISM BY ALCOHOL AND ALDEHYDE DEHYDROGENASES AND OTHER ROUTES

Alcohol is oxidised to acetaldehyde by three routes (Fig. 9.1), namely: ADH (alcohol dehydrogenase; cystosolic); MEOS (microsomal ethanol oxidising system; in endoplasmic reticulum) and catalase (in peroxisomes). There are at least six classes of ADH

and oxidised substrates include steroids and some intermediates in the mevalonate pathway as well as fatty acid β-oxidation and retinoids (Table *evolve* 9.5 ; Lieber 2000).

There is an excess of reducing equivalents produced via ADH, so that the ratio of NADH:NAD$^+$ is increased, with a corresponding increase in the lactate:pyruvate ratio. The conversion of acetaldehyde to acetate via aldehyde dehydrogenase (ALDH; principally in the mitochondria), will also generate NADH, so compounding the elevated ratio. Changes in the cellular (via ADH) or mitochondrial (via ALDH) redox state may explain such metabolic abnormalities in alcoholism as hyperlactacidaemia, hyperuricaemia, increased lipogenesis, decreased β-oxidation of fatty acids in mitochondria, hypoglycaemia and disturbances in the tissue responsiveness to hormones.

The hypothesis that the altered NADH:NAD$^+$ ratio can explain most or all of the metabolic abnormalities in the liver is unproven, and many metabolic abnormalities are thought to be due to a number of processes, such as free radical damage, adduct formation, DNA damage and/or altered gene expression, apoptosis, perturbed proteolytic cascades, translational defects, membrane changes and alterations in cellular trafficking (Lieber 1996). Extrahepatic tissues, e.g. mouth, oesophagus, duodenum, jejunum, rectum and muscle, also contain ethanol metabolising enzyme leading to localised damage.

Peroxisomal catalase plays only a minor role in ethanol oxidation, and requires the concomitant presence of a hydrogen peroxide (H_2O_2) generating system (Figs 9.1 and *evolve* 9.1). When there is an increase in H_2O_2 generation, e.g. from the oxidation of long chain fatty acids in the peroxisomes, there may also be an increase in catalase-mediated ethanol oxidation.

In simple terms, acetaldehyde is toxic and any situation that results in exposure of cells to this agent is harmful. Once acetaldehyde is formed, it is further oxidised to acetate via NAD$^+$-dependent aldehyde dehydrogenase (ALDH). As with ADH, there are several classes of ALDH (Table *evolve* 9.6). The most important are ALDH2 and ALDH1, which are mitochondrial and cytosolic, respectively. The location of ALDHs in extrahepatic tissues such as heart may be protective whereas lower levels in brain may explain the vulnerability of CNS tissues in alcoholism (Kwo & Crabb 2002).

Some acetaldehyde becomes bound to cellular constituents such as proteins, lipids and nucleic acids generating harmful 'hybrid' molecules called adducts. Adduct formation not only changes the biochemical characteristic of the target molecule but the new structure may also be recognised as foreign (i.e. a neoantigen), thus initiating an immunological response (Freeman et al 2005).

Genetic or ethnic variations in ADH and ALDH may also explain some of the pathologies of alcoholism, and why some individuals will develop certain diseases when others do not. For example, many Orientals (about 40%) will have a deficiency of ALDH2 activity due to a gene modification and this results in an elevation in acetaldehyde with a visible flushing of the skin after alcohol ingestion. The modified allele is designated ALDH2*2 whilst the normal is ALDH2*1. There are also genetic differences in ADH between populations and these contribute to variation in ethanol oxidation. This has implications for addiction and target organ damage including those that have a role in nutritional metabolism. For example, a low ALDH activity will raise acetaldehyde, which will deter individuals from drinking alcohol. If those with low ALDH activity were to drink alcohol, then the high acetaldehyde levels will induce greater degrees or prevalence of harm and tissue damage. This has also been shown experimentally when agents such as cyanamide (an inhibitor of ALDH) can inhibit ALDH and cause greater metabolic perturbations in alcohol exposed tissues.

Formation of phosphatidylethanol and fatty acid ethyl esters (FAEE) are two other important routes of ethanol metabolism albeit by a non-oxidative pathway (Fig. 9.2; Laposata 1998). Phosphatidylethanol is formed when ethanol becomes the polar group of a phospholipid in a reaction catalysed by phospholipase D. It is found in the blood of alcoholics and organs exposed to ethanol, including liver, intestines, stomach, lung, spleen and muscle, in a dose- and time-dependent manner. FAEE are formed from fatty acids and ethanol in reactions catalysed by either cytosolic or microsomal FAEE synthase. In the former reaction, the immediate precursor is fatty acid, whereas the microsomal pathway utilises fatty acid CoA. The FAEE are broken down by a cytosolic hydrolase or may traverse the membrane into the intravascular space. Both phosphatidylethanol and FAEE are cytotoxic and may perturb cell-signalling and protein synthesis.

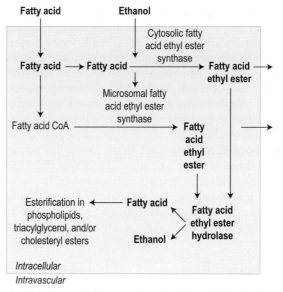

Fig. 9.2 Non-oxidative routes of ethanol metabolism. Illustration of the formation of fatty acid ethyl esters in tissues (Laposata 1998).

INDUCTION OF MICROSOMAL CYTOCHROMES FOLLOWING REPEATED INGESTION OF ALCOHOL

With the MEOS system, which utilises NADPH, there is free radical regeneration and induction of the cytochrome system (Figs 9.1 and *evolve* 9.1 ; Lieber 1996). The MEOS is especially important in chronic ethanol ingestion as it is an inducible pathway of ethanol metabolism and is thus of particular significance in chronic ethanol misusers where the existing enzymes are unable to cope with the high ethanol load. The MEOS has a higher K_m for ethanol (8–10 mmol/l) compared with ADH (0.2–2.0 mmol/l). The purified protein of MEOS is commonly referred to as CYP2EI or 2EI (formally IIEI) and its induction is due to increases in mRNA levels and its rate of translation.

UNCOUPLING OF METABOLISM FROM OXIDATIVE PHOSPHORYLATION

Some subjects on experimental alcohol feeding regimens have reduced weight, when compared with those on isocaloric diets without alcohol, suggesting inadequate utilisation of metabolic fuels. Contributory factors responsible for the weight loss or energy deficits in ethanol consumers pertain to the induction of the MEOS, which is energetically wasteful, leads to inadequate coupling of ATP production and may involve increased hydrolysis of ATP via Na⁺-ATPase activities. Additionally, maldigestion or malabsorption, poor dietary intakes and defects in tissue protein turnover may also contribute to such weight loss in alcohol misusers. Finally, alcohol intake will cause anorexia directly or indirectly via gastrointestinal damage such as gastritis.

Obesity is not apparent in all alcoholics but in some subjects who consume moderate to high amounts of alcohol, obesity may increase. The relationship between alcohol consumption and obesity is controversial and may relate to gender, genetic and dietary factors as well as the levels of alcohol consumed.

THE METABOLIC BASIS FOR 'FATTY LIVER' OF CHRONIC ALCOHOL INGESTION

Traditionally, alcohol-induced liver disease has been thought to have three stages, namely fatty liver (steatosis), alcoholic hepatitis with fibrosis, and cirrhosis, though fatty liver may progress directly to cirrhosis. The ability of the liver to develop steatosis in the presence of low fat diets has led to the hypothesis that the *de novo* synthesis of triacylglycerols may arise via increases in fatty acid synthesis in the liver. Fatty liver occurs in about 80–90% of chronic alcohol misusers and is usually asymptomatic. However, when it is combined with inflammatory reactions, i.e. steatohepatitis, the patients are at significant risk and may be hospitalised. Fatty liver, however, is not itself fatal and indeed may occur in a variety of other conditions such as diabetes mellitus or hyperlipidemia/obesity associated with insulin resistance, oxidative stress/imbalance. The changes in alcoholic fatty liver have some distinct biochemical differences from other non-alcohol fatty liver pathologies such as diabetes, reflecting their different aetiologies.

Increased fatty acids in the liver present a greater biochemical 'target' for the free radicals generated as a consequence of alcohol metabolism. This leads to peroxidation of fatty acids within the liver generating malondialdehyde, which in turn can form malondialdehyde–protein adducts. As with acetaldehyde–protein adducts, the malondialdehyde–protein adducts are immunogenic, increase inflammation and are cytotoxic. There are at least five different protein-adduct species formed in alcohol-exposed tissues.

The metabolic basis for fatty liver is still a matter of conjecture (Bathgate & Simpson 2002). The lipid in affected liver is largely triacyglycerol, which may increase between 10- and 50-fold; there is also a, less marked, increase in esterified cholesterol. Concomitant changes also include an increase in palmitic acid and a fall in arachidonic and linoleic acids in phospholipid. Contributing factors include some or all of the following (for a comprehensive review see Bathgate & Simpson 2002):

1. **Increased NADH/NAD⁺ ratio.** Some groups consider this the driving force for the defects in triacylglycerol synthesis and fatty acid oxidation. Alternatively, H⁺ derived from excess NADH may be transferred to NADPH, which provides reducing power for biosynthesis of fatty acids.

2. **Enhanced substrate supply, including glycerol-3-phosphate and fatty acyl CoA esters.** Glycerol-3-phosphate is formed by reduction of dihydroxyacetone phosphate, in a reaction catalysed by glycerate-3-phosphate reductase, which is dependent on NADH, and the increased NADH arising from alcohol or acetaldehyde oxidation may drive this reaction in favour of glyceraldehyde-3-phosphate.

3. **Increased fatty acid uptake.** Fatty acid uptake may increase in response to ethanol, possibly reflecting upregulation of intracellular fatty acid binding protein, or decreased peripheral clearance of chylomicrons. De novo synthesis of fatty acids may use ethanol-derived carbon, but acetate derived from ethanol is mainly metabolised in skeletal muscle.

Increased fatty acid synthesis (as a result of increased NADPH derived by transfer of H⁺ from NADH) has been a favoured hypothesis. However, in human percutaneous liver biopsy samples, reduced fatty acid synthesis occurs and correlates with lipid content in the specimens. Furthermore, the activities of key enzymes in the hepatic synthesis of fatty acids (e.g. acetyl CoA carboxylase) are reduced in the livers of subjects with alcohol-induced steatosis.

Impairment in the rate of mitochondrial β-oxidation of fatty acids may also be another route whereby fatty liver occurs in alcoholism possibly via effects on specific enzymes such as carnitine palmitoyl transferase I or acyl CoA dehydrogenase.

Esterification of free fatty acids may also be increased in alcoholic steatosis. Phosphatidate phosphohydrolase is a rate limiting enzyme in triacylglycerol synthesis and increases in both human and animal liver exposed chronically to ethanol, correlated with the degree of steatosis in clinical samples. Diacylglycerol transferase activity also increases.

4. **Export from the liver**. The impact of ethanol and/or acetaldehyde on the physiological export processes has been described previously with respect to albumin. The export of triacylglycerol-rich VLDL may also be impaired due to defects in the Golgi apparatus and/or microtubules via adduct formation with acetaldehyde (Bathgate & Simpson 2002).

LACTIC ACIDOSIS RESULTING FROM ALCOHOL INGESTION

The increased tissue NADH levels because of alcohol and acetaldehyde metabolism also increases the lactate/pyruvate ratio leading to lactic acidosis which may also be combined with a β-hydroxybutyrate predominant ketoacidosis under some conditions. Blood pH may fall to 7.1 and hypoglycaemia may occur. In severe situations of ketoacidosis and hypoglycaemia permanent brain damage may arise. Though in general the prognosis of alcoholic acidosis is good, it is dependent on liver function. These conditions may be exacerbated by thiamin deficiency and indeed thiamin deficiency per se may hasten acute episodes of lactic acidosis (see Chapter 10, Section 10.1). The high concentration of lactic acid also impairs the kidney's ability to excrete uric acid and consequently blood uric acid levels rise (hyperuricemia), causing gout.

9.3 TOXIC EFFECTS OF CHRONIC ALCOHOL INGESTION

ALCOHOL INGESTION LEADS TO THE RELEASE OF CATECHOLAMINES AND STEROID EXCESS

Alcohol causes increased activation of the sympathetic nervous system, with increased circulating catecholamines secreted by the adrenal medulla.

Increased circulating cortisol from the adrenal cortex can, very rarely, lead to a pseudo-Cushing's syndrome with typical symptoms of moon face, truncal obesity and muscle weakness, due to hypothalamic–pituitary stimulation. These changes in circulating catecholamines and cortisol have been considered to cause some of the pathology of alcoholism, but contribute little to the major complications such as myopathy, cardiomyopathy and alcoholic liver disease.

Alcoholism also affects the hypothalamo-pituitary–gonadal axis, and these effects are further exacerbated by alcoholic liver disease. There are conflicting data regarding the changes observed. Plasma testosterone is either normal or decreased in men, and increased in women, with oestradiol levels being increased in both men and women, and rising with worsening liver disease. The production of sex-hormone-binding globulin is also perturbed by alcohol, complicating the picture further. Feminisation of males, with gynaecomastia and testicular atrophy, tends to occur only after cirrhosis begins, and is more severe in alcoholic compared to non-alcoholic cirrhosis. In women, these changes can cause decreased libido, disturbances in menstruation and early onset of menopause. Sexual dysfunction is also common in men with reduced libido and impotence. Fertility may also be reduced, with decreased spermatozoon count and motility. It is worth remembering that alcohol misuse can affect virtually every endocrine axis (Gluud 2002).

SYMPTOMS OF EXCESS ALCOHOL INTAKE

Perhaps the most obvious effects of alcohol are on the central nervous system. These are dose dependent and begin with the so-called social modulating effects of alcohol, including increasing cheerfulness, loss of inhibitions and impaired judgement. Heavier consumption leads to agitation, slurred speech, loss of memory, with double vision and staggering. This may then progress to a depressed level of consciousness. This is of particular concern in emergency departments as, when people present drunk with a depressed level of consciousness and a head injury, it can be difficult to determine whether there is co-existent pathology such as an extradural haematoma. A good rule of thumb is not to assume that alcohol is solely responsible for any disturbance in consciousness. Ultimately loss of airway control may occur, with danger of suffocation or aspiration of vomitus and ultimately death. There is a great disparity in the effects of alcohol between individuals. This is due to varying effects of alcohol on the body, and differences in the metabolism of alcohol and waste products of its metabolism.

Acute effects of alcohol on the cardiovascular system involve both the heart and the peripheral vasculature. Peripheral vasodilation causes a sensation of warmth. Although this can be interpreted by the subject as being warmer, it can be dangerous, especially in cold weather or when swimming, as heat loss is rapid but lack of awareness leaves people vulnerable to hypothermia. Cardiac effects are usually in the form of arrhythmias, in particular atrial flutter and atrial fibrillation. These can occur whilst intoxicated or after drinking too much (i.e. the 'holiday heart' syndrome), although there is also an increase in the prevalence of these arrhythmias occurring chronically in those have a moderate to heavy alcohol intake.

EFFECTS OF ALCOHOL ON MUSCLE WEAKNESS

Alcoholic myopathy is common, affecting 40–60% all chronic alcohol abusers, and is a major cause of morbidity. It is characterised by muscle weakness, myalgia, muscle cramps and loss of lean tissue; up to 30% of muscle may be lost. Histological assessment correlates well with symptoms, and shows selective atrophy of Type II muscle fibres. Reductions in muscle protein and RNA, with reduced rate of protein synthesis, also occur. Rates of protein degradation appear either unaltered or reduced. Recently attention has focused on a role for free radicals in the pathogenesis of alcoholic myopathy. Cholesterol hydroperoxides are increased in alcohol-exposed muscle implying membrane damage.

EFFECTS OF ALCOHOL ON FACIAL FLUSHING

Facial flushing with patchy erythematous rash on the trunk and arms is seen in approximately 40% of Orientals and is thought to be due to a deficiency of ALDH2. This results in an accumulation of acetaldehyde, with plasma levels around 20 times higher in people with this deficiency. Acetaldehyde is thought to be chiefly responsible for many of the adverse effects of alcohol. Plasma and urinary catecholamine levels have been shown to be greatly increased in people with aldehyde dehydrogenase deficiency after alcohol consumption. Flushing in Europeans (5%) is due to other mechanisms of unknown aetiology.

Acetaldehyde acts partially through catecholamines, although other mechanisms have also been implicated, including histamine, bradykinin, prostaglandin and endogenous opioids (as well as adduct formation). Administration of aspirin (which irreversibly acetylates and inactivates cyclooxygenase, preventing prostaglandin production) has been shown to block the facial flushing response in some people, implicating a role for prostaglandins. Use of naloxone (an opioid antagonist) has also been shown to reduce flushing in people in whom cyclooxygenase inhibitors had an effect, implicating an interaction between endogenous opioids and prostaglandins.

EFFECTS OF ALCOHOL ON DEHYDRATION

Ethanol affects hypothalamic osmoreceptors, reducing antidiuretic hormone release, so causing reduced salt and water reabsorption in the distal tubule. This results in polyuria and may cause dehydration, especially in spirit drinkers who do not consume much water with their alcoholic drinks. A loss of hypothalamic neurons secreting antidiuretic hormone has also been described in chronic alcoholics, suggesting long term consequences for fluid balance. Increased plasma atrial natriuretic factor after alcohol consumption may also contribute to this diuresis and resultant dehydration.

EFFECTS OF ALCOHOL ON LIVER FUNCTION

The pathological mechanisms by which cirrhosis occurs are complex, and are still the subject of intensive research. Induction of the MEOS system and breakdown of ethanol by catalase results in free radical production. Glutathione (a free radical scavenger) is also reduced in alcoholics, decreasing the cell's ability dispose of free radicals. Mitochondrial damage occurs, limiting their ability to oxidise fatty acids, which are then oxidised in peroxisomes, further increasing free radical production. These changes eventually result in hepatocyte necrosis, and inflammation and fibrosis then ensue. Acetaldehyde also contributes at this stage by promoting collagen synthesis and fibrosis.

Fatty changes are usually asymptomatic, but can be detected on ultrasound or CT, and are associated with abnormal liver function tests (e.g. raised activities of aminotransferases in serum). Progression to alcoholic hepatitis involves invasion of the liver by neutrophils with hepatocyte necrosis. Giant mitochondria are visible and dense cytoplasmic lesions, known as Mallory bodies, are seen. Alcoholic hepatitis can be asymptomatic but usually presents with abdominal pain, fever and jaundice, or, depending on the severity of disease, patients may have encephalopathy, ascites and ankle oedema and mortality rates up to 50% have been reported. Continued alcohol consumption may lead to cirrhosis. There is increasing fibrocollagenous deposition, with scarring and disruption of surrounding hepatic architecture. There is ongoing necrosis with concurrent regeneration. This is classically said to be micronodular, but often a mixed pattern is present. Alcoholics usually present with one of the complications of cirrhosis such as gastrointestinal haemorrhage (often due to bleeding from oesophageal varices), ascites, encephalopathy or renal failure. It is uncertain why only a fraction of alcoholics go on to develop cirrhosis. It has been suggested that there may be genetic factors, and that differences in immune response may play a role. Dietary factors may also contribute. For example, with inadequate intake of cysteine and glycine, glutathione production may be impaired. Poor intake of vitamins A, C and E and β-carotene will also reduce the ability of the hepatocyte to cope with the oxidative stress imposed by alcoholism.

9.4 ALCOHOL AND NUTRITION

A variety of studies have shown that chronic ethanol misusers have impaired nutritional status due either to inadequate dietary intake, persistent damage to the hepatointestinal system or the redirection of funds that would otherwise be used to purchase food. Malnutrition frequently occurs in alcohol misuse and will further compromise alcohol-associated pathologies. However, it is worth distinguishing between hazardous, harmful drinkers and the addicted or dependent alcoholic. Such different categorisations of alcohol misuse will have different nutritional consequences. These terms have been defined by the WHO but in simple terms those described as 'hazardous' drinkers are at risk

of developing alcohol problems but have no overt alcohol-related pathologies. On the other hand those categorised as 'harmful' do indeed have a defined problem or problems without demonstrable dependence. Those who are 'addicted' or 'dependent' may have the same or worse pathologies as those described as harmful but at the same time exhibit a degree of psychological or physical symptoms upon withdrawal of alcohol. Dependence may be categorised as moderate or severe. Thus, in general the degree of nutritional impairment is: severe dependent > moderate dependent > harmful > hazardous drinker.

Chronic alcoholics frequently have deficient intakes of micronutrients (e.g. vitamins B_1, A, C, E and folate) and minerals (e.g. zinc and selenium). Ethanol-induced effects on digestion, absorption and storage will exaggerate these deficiencies. For example, hepatic stores of total retinoids (vitamin A) decrease in chronic ethanol misusers and correlate with the severity of liver disease. In contrast, iron status may be adequate in some alcohol misusers as a result of increased absorption. In very severe cases of alcoholism, classical symptoms of beri-beri and pellagra arise, although these are less common.

A recent study in UK alcoholics attending an inner city alcohol misuse clinic showed that 95–100% of patients had low (below UK RNIs) intakes of vitamin E, folate and selenium. Between 50 and 85% of all patients had low intakes of calcium, zinc and vitamins A, B_1, B_2, B_6 and C. Reduced intakes of magnesium and iron were reported in about 45% of subjects. Although the usage of RNIs in this study may be flawed (LNRI or EAR should have been used), it still illustrates the potential for malnutrition. However, studies on middle-class alcoholics, free from major organ disease, suggest that when malnutrition is present it is only mild to moderate.

Alcohol will also affect the metabolism of a number of nutrients including thiamin and it has been suggested that about half of alcoholics with liver disease will have thiamin deficiency (see Section 10.1). A recent UK study showed that 45% of alcohol misusers without liver disease had either reduced erythrocyte thiamin-dependent transketolase activity or a high activation ratio. This is of concern as Wernicke's encephalopathy/Wernicke–Korsakoff syndrome is a frequent manifestation of thiamin deficiency, particularly in alcohol misusers. Thiamin deficiency will arise from both inadequate intake and alcohol-induced interference with active transport of the vitamin in the gut. Formation of thiamin pyrophosphate may also be impaired by diseased hepatic tissue in alcoholism.

Acute or chronic alcohol impairs the absorption of galactose, glucose, other hexoses, amino acids, biotin, folate and vitamin C. There is no strong evidence that alcohol impairs the absorption of magnesium, riboflavin or pyridoxine so these deficiencies will arise as a result of poor intakes and/or excess loss. Hepato-gastrointestinal damage of course may have an important role in impairing the absorption of some nutrients such as the fat-soluble vitamins, due to villous injury, bacterial overgrowth of the intestine, pancreatic damage or cholestasis.

The muscle wastage that occurs in alcoholic myopathy arises directly as a consequence of alcohol or acetaldehyde on muscle, and is not associated with malnutrition *per se*. This implies that there is a fundamental problem in assessing malnutrition in chronic alcoholics using anthropometric measures such as muscle or limb circumference due to the presence of alcoholic myopathy.

A question arises as to whether the deleterious effects of alcohol on organs and tissues are the direct consequence of malnutrition. However, this belief is no longer held since the pioneering work of Charles Lieber in the 1960s showed that many pathologies, such as alcoholic hepatitis and cirrhosis, could be reproduced in laboratory animals fed an adequate diet. Nevertheless, the concomitant presence of alcoholism and malnutrition exacerbates organ damage and/or nutritional status.

9.5 LINKS BETWEEN ALCOHOL INTAKE AND RISK OF CARDIOVASCULAR DISEASE

A number of epidemiological studies have suggested that light–moderate amounts (1–6 Units per day) of alcohol are cardioprotective and reduce coronary heart disease, particularly in middle-aged men and post-menopausal women. This protective effect is not seen at higher levels of intake and indeed may increase incidence of cardiovascular disease including hypertension. In other words, there is a J- or U-shaped mortality curve. However, there is some uncertainty as to the exact shape of this curve and the point at which the putative protective effect of alcohol becomes harmful. Other studies have challenged any causal relationship between alcohol intake and the cardioprotective phenomena. In one study, a decreased risk of coronary heart disease was seen at 0–20 g/day and evident up to 72 g/day, whilst consumption of greater than 89 g/day was associated with an increased risk of coronary heart disease. Increases in alcohol consumption from one drink per week or less to one to six drinks per week over 7 years is associated with a 29% fall in the risk of cardiovascular disease.

This effect of alcohol on coronary disease and overall cardiovascular mortality is quite separate from the toxic effects on heart muscle. Chronic alcohol misuse can cause a progressive cardiac failure. This characteristic picture of a dilated impaired left ventricle without other cause has been termed alcoholic cardiomyopathy. This is thought to be due to a reduction in protein synthesis which causes reduced cardiac contractile protein content. Often this can normalise with medical management of heart failure and abstinence from alcohol.

Some studies have shown that in men there is a linear relationship between alcohol consumption and blood pressure, but a J-shaped relationship in women. Moderate to heavy drinking is associated with an increased risk of stroke. Consumption of up to 3 Units/day, however, reduces ischaemic strokes but binge drinking increases the risk of all types of stroke. There are several studies showing an association between long term alcohol use and atrial fibrillation. This association has been demonstrated only with prolonged heavy alcohol use in men, but there is evidence of an association with only moderate alcohol use in women (Conen et al 2008).

However, when considering the public health consequences of such data, one must also take into account the other effects of alcohol. Consuming only one Unit of alcohol a day may increase the risk of death from some cancers, accidents and violence. Furthermore, there is a substantial body of evidence to support the notion that the total cumulative intake of ethanol (i.e. over a lifetime) will predict disease severity, particularly of the heart, muscle and liver.

The reported cardioprotective effects of alcohol may be due to antioxidants or other substances in the beverages such as polyphenols in red wine (although it is now believed that all forms of alcohol can convey a cardioprotective effect). Protective effects may also occur via an antithrombotic effect, reducing circulating levels of fibrinogen, factor VII and plasminogen activator. Platelet aggregability may also be reduced by alcohol. An effect of alcohol in increasing serum HDL-cholesterol may be another mechanism.

9.6 LINKS BETWEEN ALCOHOL INTAKE AND RISK OF CANCERS

There has been increasing recognition over the last decade that there is an association between alcohol and various cancers, and this has been highlighted in a recent report by the World Cancer Research Fund. Alcohol consumption is associated with modest but significant increases in cancer of most of the gastrointestinal tract (the mouth, pharynx, larynx, oesophagus, colon and rectum) as well as that of the breast. The association with cancer of the liver is most marked but may be mediated by the development of cirrhosis rather than a direct toxic effect of alcohol per se. Otherwise, it appears that ethanol itself is the carcinogen, with the level of consumption being the main determinant of risk. The risk of these cancers appears linear, and there is no evidence of a 'safe threshold' or 'J-shaped curve'. The form in which the alcohol is consumed has only a small impact, with beer and spirit drinkers having more cancers of the upper gastrointestinal tract than wine drinkers. The mechanism for this is uncertain and several possibilities have been proposed. The toxic effects of acetaldehyde causing formation of protein adducts, reactive oxygen species causing membrane peroxidation, increased production of prostaglandins, and the solvent effect of alcohol causing increased membrane permeability to toxins have all been suggested as potential mediators.

KEY POINTS

Alcohol misuse is common: in the UK about 10 million people drink more than recommended guidelines.
- The young (school children and adolescents) and women are particularly vulnerable or susceptible to the deleterious effects of alcohol.
- In the UK, the overall contribution of ethanol to total energy intake is 6.5% in men and 3.9% in women.
- In alcohol misusers, the overall contribution of ethanol to total energy intake may rise to 60% or higher.
- Alcohol absorption and metabolism are affected by a number of variables, including gastric alcohol-metabolising enzymes, ethnicity, gender, presence of different foods and body size.
- It is a myth that the most affected organs are the brain and liver: organic brain disease and cirrhosis only occur in about 10–15% of chronic alcoholics.
- There are at least 60–120 different alcohol-related pathologies.
- 50% of chronic alcohol misusers will have one or more organ or tissue abnormalities
- Alcoholic myopathy is particularly prevalent, affecting 40–60% of chronic alcoholics.
- The immediate metabolite of ethanol oxidation, acetaldehyde, is highly toxic.

- The effects of alcohol or acetaldehyde on the body are due to many processes, such as adduct formation, changes in protein, carbohydrate and lipid metabolism, membrane dysfunction, altered cytokines and impaired immunological status, perturbations in gene expression, enhanced apoptosis, reactive oxygen species/oxidative stress and changes in intracellular signalling. Many of these will be exacerbated by malnutrition.
- All pathways and cell structures have the potential to be targeted by ethanol or its related metabolites.
- There are a number of routes of ethanol metabolism. The microsomal ethanol oxidising system (MEOS) is particularly important in chronic alcoholism.
- The metabolic basis for 'fatty liver' in chronic alcohol ingestion is still a matter of conjecture and may reflect the fact that a number of processes are affected.
- About 50% of alcoholics will have nutritional deficiencies and these can arise via a number of processes including poor dietary intakes, displacement of foods (empty calories theory), maldigestion and malabsorption.
- Low to moderate amounts of alcohol may reduce cardiovascular disease, particularly in middle aged men.

References

Aceto M: Metals in wine. In Preedy VR, Watson RR, editors: *Reviews in food and nutrition toxicity*, London, 2003, Taylor & Francis, pp 169–203.

Bathgate AJ, Simpson KJ: Alcoholic fatty liver. In Sherman DIN, Preedy VR, Watson RR, editors: *Ethanol and the Liver. Mechanisms and Management*, London, 2002, Taylor & Francis, pp 3–20.

Conen D, Tedrow UB, Cook NR: Alcohol consumption and risk of incident atrial fibrillation in women, *JAMA* 300:2489–2496, 2008.

Department of Health: *Sensible drinking: the report of an inter-departmental working group*, London, 1995, Department of Health.

Department of Health: *Statistical Bulletin. Statistics on alcohol: England, 1978 onwards*, London, 2001, Department of Health.

Fernandez–Sola J, Nicolas JM, Estruch RM, Urbano-Márquez A: Gender differences in alcohol pathology. In Preedy VR, Watson RR, editors: *Comprehensive Handbook of Alcohol Related Pathology, Vol. 1,* Amsterdam, 2005, Elsevier Academic Press, pp 261–278.

Food Standards Agency: *McCance and Widdowson's The Composition of Foods*, Cambridge, 2002, Royal Society of Chemistry.

Freeman TL, Tuma DJ, Thiele GM, et al: Recent advances in alcohol-induced adduct formation. *Alcoholism – Clinical and Experimental Research* 29:1310–1306, 2005.

Gluud C: Endocrine system. In Sherman DIN, Preedy VR, Watson RR, editors: *Ethanol and the Liver. Mechanisms and Management,* London, 2002, Taylor & Francis, pp 472–494.

Haber PS: Metabolism of alcohol by the human stomach. *Alcoholism: Clinical & Experimental Research* 24:407–408, 2000.

Henderson L, Gregory J: *J. National diet and nutrition survey: adults aged 19 to 64 years. Vol. 1. Types and quantities of foods consumed*, London, 2002, HMSO.

Henderson L, Gregory J, Irving K: *National diet and nutrition survey: adults aged 19 to 64 years. Vol. 2. Energy, protein, carbohydrate, fat and alcohol intakes*, London, 2003, HMSO.

Jones AW: Aspects of in-vivo pharmacokinetics of ethanol. [Review] [12 refs], *Alcoholism: Clinical & Experimental Research* 24:400–402, 2000.

Kwo PY, Crabb DW: Genetics of ethanol metabolism and alcoholic liver disease. In Sherman DIN, Preedy VR, Watson RR, editors: *Ethanol and the Liver. Mechanisms and Management,* London, 2002, Taylor & Francis, pp 95–129.

Lader D, Meltzer H: *Drinking: Adults' behaviour and knowledge in 2002.* London, 2002, Office for National Statistics.

Laposata M: Fatty acid ethyl esters: nonoxidative metabolites of ethanol. *Addiction Biology* 3:5–14, 1998.

Lieber CS: The metabolism of alcohol and its implications for the pathogenesis of disease. In Preedy VR, Watson RR, editors: *Alcohol and the gastrointestinal tract*, Boca Raton, 1996, CRC Press, pp 19–39.

Lieber CS: Alcohol: its metabolism and interaction with nutrients. *Annual Review of Nutrition* 20:395–430, 2000.

Mezey E: Effect of ethanol on intestinal morphology, metabolism and function. In Seitz HK, Kommerell B, editors: *Alcohol related diseases in gastroenterology*, Berlin, 1985, Springer-Verlag, pp. 342–360

NHS: *Pregnancy and alcohol*, London, 2008, Department of Health.

Novartis: *Acetaldehyde-Related Pathology: Bridging the Trans-Disciplinary Divide (Novartis Foundation Symposia) by Novartis Foundation*, Chichester, West Sussex, 2007, John Wiley & Sons Ltd.

Peters TJ, Preedy VR: Metabolic consequences of alcohol ingestion, *Novartis Foundation Symposium* 216:19–24, 1998.

Preedy VR, Watson RR: *Comprehensive handbook of alcohol related pathology.* San Diego, 2005, Academic Press.

Roine R: Interaction of prandial state and beverage concentration on alcohol absorption, *Alcoholism–Clinical and Experimental Research* 24:411–412, 2000.

Royal Colleges: Alcohol and the heart in perspective. Sensible limits reaffirmed. A Working Group of the Royal Colleges of Physicians, Psychiatrists and General Practitioners, *Journal of the Royal College of Physicians of London* 29:266–271, 1995.

Saunders JB, Devereaux BM: Epidemiology and comparative incidence of alcohol-induced liver disease. In Sherman DIN, Preedy VR, Watson RR, editors: *Ethanol and the Liver. Mechanisms and Management,* London, 2002, Taylor & Francis, pp 389–410.

Watson RR, Preedy VR: *Nutrition and Alcohol: Linking Nutrient Interactions and Dietary Intake,* London, 2003, CRC press.

Further reading

Institute of Alcohol Studies: *Statistics on Alcohol: England, available on line at:* http://www.ias.org.uk/, 2008.

World Cancer Research Fund and the American Institute for Cancer Research: *Food, nutrition, physical activity, and the prevention of cancer: a global perspective.* November 2007, available on line at: http://www.wcrf-uk.org.

EVOLVE CONTENTS (available online at: evolve.elsevier.com/Geissler/nutrition

PART 3

Micronutrient function

Chapter 10

Water–soluble vitamins

David A Bender

CHAPTER CONTENTS

© 2010 Elsevier Ltd/Inc/BV
DOI: 10.1016/B978-0-7020-3118-2.00010-3

OBJECTIVES

By the end of this chapter you should be able to:

- identify the compounds classified as water-soluble vitamins
- identify good sources of each
- summarise the absorption and transport of each
- summarise the main metabolic functions of each
- describe the main effects of deficiency and excess of each
- be aware of the methods of assessment of status
- discuss the basis for dietary requirements
- appreciate the metabolic interactions between water-soluble vitamins and other nutrients.

10.1 VITAMIN B$_1$ – THIAMIN

The peripheral nervous system disease beriberi, due to thiamin deficiency, became a major problem of public health in the Far East in the nineteenth century with the introduction of the steam-powered rice mill, which resulted in more widespread consumption of highly milled (polished) rice. While now largely eradicated, beriberi remains a problem in some parts of the world among people whose diet is especially high in carbohydrate. A different condition, affecting the central rather than peripheral nervous system, the Wernicke–Korsakoff syndrome, is also due to thiamin deficiency. It occurs in developed countries, especially among alcoholics and narcotic addicts.

FORMS OF THIAMIN IN FOODS AND GOOD FOOD SOURCES

In foods, most thiamin is present as the diphosphate (Fig. 10.1), also known as thiamin pyrophosphate; small amounts of mono- and triphosphate also occur. Pork is an especially rich source, but other meat and fish are good sources, as are potatoes, wheat, nuts and beans (see Table *evolve* 10.1). A number of biologically active allithiamins occur in plants.

Thiamin is labile to sulphite, and sulphite treatment of foods results in more or less complete loss of the vitamin.

ABSORPTION AND TRANSPORT OF THIAMIN

Dietary thiamin phosphates are hydrolysed by intestinal phosphatases, and thiamin is absorbed by active transport in the duodenum and proximal jejunum. The transport system is saturated at relatively low concentrations, so limiting the amount that can be absorbed. There is active transport from the intestinal cells into the bloodstream; this is inhibited by alcohol, leading to thiamin deficiency in alcoholics.

Much of the absorbed thiamin is phosphorylated in the liver, and both free thiamin and thiamin monophosphate circulate in plasma, bound to albumin. All tissues can take up both thiamin and thiamin monophosphate, and are able to phosphorylate them to the active di- and triphosphates.

A small amount of thiamin is excreted in the urine unchanged; the major excretory product is

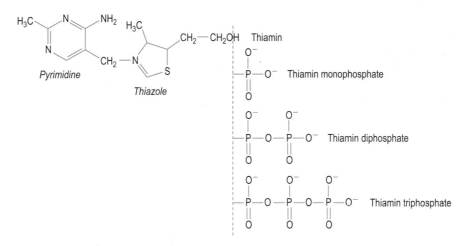

Fig. 10.1 Thiamin and the thiamin coenzymes.

thiochrome. Sweat may contain up to 30–56 nmol of thiamin/l, and in hot conditions this may represent a significant loss of the vitamin.

METABOLIC FUNCTIONS OF THIAMIN

Thiamin diphosphate is the coenzyme for three multi-enzyme complexes: pyruvate dehydrogenase (see Fig. *evolve* 10.1) and 2-oxoglutarate dehydrogenase in central energy-yielding metabolic pathways and the branched-chain oxo-acid dehydrogenase in the catabolism of leucine, isoleucine and valine. It is also the coenzyme for transketolase in the pentose phosphate pathway of carbohydrate metabolism (see Fig. *evolve* 10.2).

Thiamin also has a role in electrical conduction in nerve cells; thiamin triphosphate phosphorylates, and so activates, a chloride channel in nerve membranes.

THIAMIN DEFICIENCY

The biological half-life of thiamin is 10–20 days, and deficiency can develop rapidly during depletion. Diuresis increases the excretion of the vitamin, and patients who are treated with diuretics are potentially at risk of thiamin deficiency.

In deficiency there is impaired entry of pyruvate into the citric acid cycle. Especially on a relatively high carbohydrate diet, this results in increased plasma concentrations of lactate and pyruvate, which may lead to life-threatening acidosis.

Thiamin deficiency can result in three distinct syndromes: a chronic peripheral neuritis, beriberi, which may or may not be associated with heart failure and oedema; acute pernicious (fulminating) beriberi (shoshin beriberi), in which heart failure and metabolic abnormalities predominate, with little evidence of peripheral neuritis; and Wernicke's encephalopathy with Korsakoff's psychosis, associated especially with alcoholism, narcotic abuse and HIV-AIDS. Results from post mortem examination and brain imaging suggest that Wernicke's encephalopathy is significantly underdiagnosed.

In general, a relatively acute deficiency is involved in the central nervous system lesions of the Wernicke–Korsakoff syndrome. Dry beriberi is associated with a more prolonged, and presumably less severe, deficiency, with a generally low food intake, while higher carbohydrate intake and physical activity predispose to oedema and hence wet beriberi.

ASSESSMENT OF THIAMIN NUTRITIONAL STATUS

The activation of apo-transketolase in erythrocyte lysate by thiamin diphosphate added in vitro is the most widely used index of thiamin nutritional status. An activation coefficient >1.25 is indicative of deficiency, and <1.15 is considered to reflect adequate thiamin nutrition.

Urinary excretion of thiamin plus thiochrome reflects intake, and has also been used to assess status.

THE BASIS FOR SETTING DIETARY THIAMIN REQUIREMENTS

Thiamin requirements depend largely on carbohydrate intake. In practice, requirements are calculated on the basis of total energy intake, assuming that the average diet provides 40% of energy from fat. For diets that are lower in fat, and hence higher in carbohydrate and protein, thiamin requirements will be higher.

On the basis of depletion/repletion studies, an intake of 0.3 mg/1000 kcal is required for a normal transketolase activation coefficient. Reference intakes are based on 0.5 mg/1000 kcal (0.12 mg/MJ) for adults consuming more than 2000 kcal/day, with the proviso that even in fasting there is a requirement for 0.8 mg of thiamin/day to permit the metabolism of endogenous substrates.

There is no evidence of any toxic effect of high intakes of thiamin, although high parenteral doses have been reported to cause anaphylactic shock. The absorption of dietary thiamin is limited, and no more than about 2.5 mg (10 µmol) can be absorbed from a single dose; free thiamin is rapidly filtered by the kidneys and excreted.

CURRENT TOPICS

Studies in thiamin-deficient animals have revealed the presence of Alzheimer-like amyloid plaques in the brain, and although there is no evidence of similar plaque formation in the brains of patients with the Wernicke–Korsakoff syndrome, this has led to trials of thiamin for treatment of Alzheimer's disease. While some studies have shown beneficial effects, a systematic review has concluded that there is no evidence of beneficial effects of thiamin supplementation in Alzheimer's disease.

KEY POINTS

- Thiamin functions as a coenzyme in energy-yielding metabolism, and in nervous system electrical activity.
- The classical thiamin deficiency disease, beriberi, affecting the peripheral nervous system, is now rare, although it is still a problem in some areas of the world.
- Thiamin deficiency, leading to central nervous system damage, is a significant, and underdiagnosed, problem among alcoholics and people with HIV-AIDS.

- Thiamin requirements depend largely on carbohydrate intake, and are generally calculated on the basis of energy intake or expenditure.
- Thiamin status is assessed by erythrocyte transketolase activation coefficient.

10.2 RIBOFLAVIN – VITAMIN B$_2$

Riboflavin has a central role as a coenzyme in energy-yielding metabolism, and a more recently discovered role as the prosthetic group of the cryptochromes, the blue-sensitive pigments in the eye that are responsible for sensitivity to day length and setting circadian rhythms.

There is very efficient conservation and reutilisation of riboflavin in tissues in deficiency, so that while dietary deficiency is relatively widespread, it is rarely, if ever, fatal.

Reoxidation of reduced flavin coenzymes is the major source of oxygen radicals in the body, and riboflavin is also capable of generating reactive oxygen species non-enzymically. As protection against this there is very strict control over the body content of riboflavin; absorption is limited, and any in excess of requirements is rapidly excreted.

FORMS OF RIBOFLAVIN IN FOOD AND DIETARY SOURCES

The structure of riboflavin is shown in Figure 10.2. Apart from milk and eggs, which contain relatively large amounts of free riboflavin, most of the vitamin in foods is as flavin coenzymes (riboflavin phosphate and FAD, flavin adenine dinucleotide) bound to enzymes. Because of its intense yellow colour, riboflavin is used as a food colour (E-101). A small proportion of riboflavin in foods is covalently bound to enzymes and hence is not biologically available.

Liver, milk, meat and fish are good sources of riboflavin; some green leafy vegetables also provide significant amounts (see Table *evolve* 10.3). In average Western diets some 25–30% of riboflavin comes from milk.

ABSORPTION AND TRANSPORT OF RIBOFLAVIN

FAD and riboflavin phosphate in foods are hydrolysed in the intestinal lumen to yield free riboflavin, which is absorbed in the upper small intestine by a

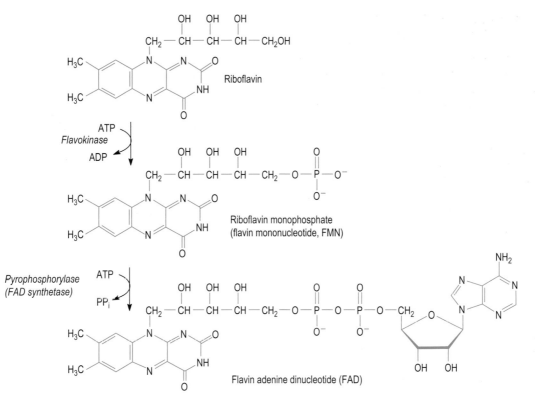

Fig. 10.2 Riboflavin and the flavin coenzymes.

sodium-dependent mechanism that is readily saturated. Intestinal bacteria synthesise riboflavin, which may be absorbed in the colon. Much of the absorbed riboflavin is phosphorylated in the intestinal mucosa, and enters the bloodstream as riboflavin phosphate. Free riboflavin and FAD are the main transport forms in plasma, with a small amount of riboflavin phosphate.

Most riboflavin in tissues is as coenzymes, bound to enzymes; unbound coenzymes are rapidly hydrolysed and free riboflavin leaves cells. There is no evidence of any significant storage of riboflavin; surplus intake is excreted rapidly. In animals, the maximum growth response is achieved with intakes that give about 75% saturation of tissues, and the intake to achieve tissue saturation is that at which there is quantitative urinary excretion of the vitamin. Equally, there is very efficient conservation of tissue riboflavin in deficiency, with only a four-fold difference between the minimum tissue concentration seen in deficiency and saturation.

METABOLIC FUNCTIONS OF RIBOFLAVIN

The metabolic function of the flavin coenzymes is as electron carriers in a wide variety of oxidation and reduction reactions central to all metabolic processes, including the mitochondrial electron transport chain.

Flavin oxidases make a significant contribution to the oxidant stress of the body, because the reoxidation of reduced flavins in oxidase reactions leads to the production of oxygen radicals. Overall, some 3–5% of the daily consumption of about 30 mol of oxygen by an adult human being is converted to reactive oxygen species daily, potentially capable of causing damage to membrane lipids, proteins and nucleic acids.

Cryptochromes are photosensitive proteins in the inner layer of the retina, behind the rods and cones involved in vision. They contain both methylene tetrahydrofolate and FAD, and act to set the circadian clock in response to day length.

RIBOFLAVIN DEFICIENCY

Riboflavin deficiency is relatively common, yet there is no clear deficiency disease and the condition seems never to be fatal. Almost all of the flavin coenzyme released by enzyme turnover is reutilised.

Clinically, deficiency is characterised by lesions of the margin of the lips (cheilosis) and corners of the mouth (angular stomatitis), a painful desquamation of the tongue, so that it is red, dry and atrophic (so-called 'magenta tongue') and a sebhorroeic dermatitis, with filiform excrescences. There may also be conjunctivitis with vascularisation of the cornea, and opacity of the lens.

The main metabolic effect of deficiency is decreased oxidation of fatty acids; deficient animals have a lower metabolic rate than controls, and require a 15–20% higher food intake to maintain body weight.

A number of studies have noted that, in areas where malaria is endemic, riboflavin-deficient people are relatively resistant and have a lower parasite burden than adequately nourished people. However, although parasitaemia is lower, the course of the disease may be more severe.

Secondary nutrient deficiencies in riboflavin deficiency

Riboflavin deficiency is associated with hypochromic anaemia as a result of secondary iron deficiency. Animal studies have shown that the absorption of iron is impaired and there is an increased rate of iron loss from the gastrointestinal tract. These effects appear to be modulated by changes in the morphology and cytokinetics of the small intestine including an increased rate of enterocyte transit along the villi and fewer, but longer, villi with deeper crypts. Additionally, riboflavin deficiency may impair the mobilisation of iron from intracellular stores, such as hepatic ferritin.

Riboflavin deficiency can also result in vitamin B_6 deficiency, because pyridoxine oxidase is a flavoprotein that is very sensitive to riboflavin depletion. Impaired tryptophan metabolism in riboflavin deficiency, due to impairment of kynurenine hydroxylase, can result in reduced synthesis of NAD, and may be a factor in the aetiology of pellagra.

Iatrogenic riboflavin deficiency

A variety of drugs, including phenothiazines, tricyclic antidepressants, antimalarials and Adriamycin, are structural analogues of riboflavin and inhibit flavokinase, leading to functional deficiency.

Neonatal hyperbilirubinaemia is normally treated by phototherapy. The peak wavelength for photolysis of bilirubin is the same as that for photolysis of riboflavin. Infants undergoing phototherapy show biochemical evidence of riboflavin depletion, but because photolysis products of riboflavin can cause damage to DNA, riboflavin supplements are not provided during phototherapy.

ASSESSMENT OF RIBOFLAVIN NUTRITIONAL STATUS

Two methods of assessing riboflavin status are generally used: urinary excretion of the vitamin and its metabolites and activation of erythrocyte glutathione reductase by FAD added in vitro. Criteria of riboflavin adequacy are shown in Table *evolve* 10.4 .

At intakes below about 1.1 mg/day there is very little urinary excretion; thereafter there is a sharp increase with increasing intake. Excretion is only correlated with intake in subjects who are maintaining nitrogen balance. In negative nitrogen balance there may be more urinary excretion than would be expected, as a result of net catabolism of tissue flavoproteins, and loss of their prosthetic groups. Higher intakes of protein than are required to maintain nitrogen balance do not affect indices of riboflavin nutritional status.

THE BASIS OF RIBOFLAVIN REQUIREMENTS

On the basis of depletion/repletion studies, the minimum adult requirement is 0.5–0.8 mg/day. In population studies, erythrocyte glutathione reductase activation coefficient <1.3 is seen in people whose habitual intake of riboflavin is 1.2–1.5 mg/day. At intakes between 1.1 and 1.6 mg/day urinary excretion rises sharply, suggesting that tissue reserves are saturated. On the basis of such studies, reference intakes are in the range of 1.2–1.8 mg/day.

Because of the central role of flavin coenzymes in energy-yielding metabolism, reference intakes are sometimes calculated on the basis of energy intake: 0.6–0.8 mg/1000 kcal (0.14–0.19 mg/MJ). However, in view of the wide range of riboflavin-dependent reactions, in addition to energy-yielding metabolism, it is difficult to justify this basis for the calculation of requirements.

CURRENT TOPICS: RIBOFLAVIN, MTHFR AND RIBOFLAVIN STATUS

Methylene tetrahydrofolate reductase is a key enzyme in folate metabolism (see 'Metabolic functions of folate', below), and is a flavoprotein. There is some evidence that marginal riboflavin status may be a factor in hyperhomocysteinaemia, and that riboflavin supplements may be beneficial in lowering plasma homocysteine.

Data from recent surveys in UK suggest that there has been a considerable increase in the prevalence of low riboflavin status over the last two decades. However, it is more likely that this is explained by subtle changes in the method used for determination of the erythrocyte glutathione reductase activation coefficient, rather than a significant reduction in riboflavin intake.

KEY POINTS

- Riboflavin functions as a coenzyme in a wide variety of reactions, including key reactions in energy-yielding metabolism. It is also the cofactor of the cryptochrome pigments in the eye that are responsible for setting circadian rhythms.
- Riboflavin deficiency is relatively common, but rarely (if ever) fatal, because there is efficient conservation of the vitamin in deficiency.
- Riboflavin deficiency is associated with resistance to malaria.
- Riboflavin deficiency can cause secondary deficiency of iron and functional deficiency of vitamin B_6 and impaired niacin synthesis, leading to development of pellagra.
- A number of drugs, and also phototherapy for neonatal hyperbilirubinaemia, can cause iatrogenic riboflavin deficiency.
- Riboflavin status is assessed by urinary excretion and erythrocyte glutathione reductase activation coefficient.
- Riboflavin metabolism is the main source of oxygen radicals in the body.

10.3 NIACIN

Niacin was discovered as a chemical compound, nicotinic acid produced by the oxidation of nicotine, in 1867 – long before there was any suspicion that it might have a role in nutrition.

The main metabolic role of niacin is as the precursor of the nicotinamide moiety of the coenzymes NAD and NADP, which can be synthesised in vivo from the essential amino acid tryptophan. In developed countries, average intakes of protein provide more than enough tryptophan to meet requirements for NAD synthesis without any need for preformed niacin; it is only when tryptophan metabolism is disturbed, or intake of the amino acid is inadequate, that niacin becomes a dietary essential. Thus, while it is usual to regard pellagra as a niacin deficiency disease, and tryptophan as a 'substitute' for niacin when the dietary intake of the vitamin is inadequate, pellagra should be regarded as being due to a deficiency of both tryptophan and niacin.

FORMS OF NIACIN IN FOODS AND GOOD FOOD SOURCES

The term niacin is the generic descriptor for the two compounds that have the biological action of the vitamin: nicotinic acid and nicotinamide (Fig. 10.3). Tryptophan is not considered to be a niacin vitamer.

Meat (especially liver and heart) and fish are good sources of preformed niacin; nuts and some fruits and vegetables provide significant amounts, as does coffee (see Table *evolve* 10.5).

Most of the niacin in cereals is biologically unavailable, since it is bound as niacytin – a variety of nicotinoyl esters to macromolecules. In calculation of niacin intakes, it is conventional to ignore the niacin content of cereals completely, although up to about 10% of niacytin may be labile to gastric acid and hence biologically available.

Quantitatively, synthesis from tryptophan is more important than dietary preformed niacin, and therefore foods that are good sources of protein are also good sources of niacin.

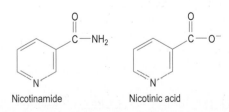

Fig. 10.3 The niacin vitamers, nicotinamide and nicotinic acid.

Total niacin intakes are calculated as mg niacin equivalents: the sum of preformed niacin plus 1/60 of tryptophan (the average equivalence of dietary tryptophan and niacin).

ABSORPTION AND TRANSPORT OF PREFORMED NIACIN

Niacin is present in tissues, and therefore in foods, largely as the nicotinamide coenzymes; post-mortem hydrolysis is extremely rapid, so that much of the niacin of meat is free nicotinamide. Any remaining coenzymes in the intestine are also hydrolysed to nicotinamide. A significant proportion of dietary nicotinamide may be deamidated to nicotinic acid by intestinal bacteria. Both vitamers are absorbed from the small intestine by a sodium-dependent saturable process.

In the liver, NAD is synthesised from tryptophan, and then hydrolysed to release nicotinamide, which is exported to other tissues, which can take up both nicotinamide and nicotinic acid to synthesise coenzymes.

There is little or no urinary excretion of either nicotinamide or nicotinic acid, until the plasma concentration is so high that the renal transport mechanism is saturated. The principal metabolites of nicotinamide are N^1-methyl nicotinamide and its oxidation products, methyl pyridone carboxamides.

METABOLIC FUNCTIONS OF NIACIN

Nicotinamide is the reactive moiety of the nicotinamide nucleotide coenzymes NAD (nicotinamide adenine dinucleotide) and NADP (nicotinamide adenine dinucleotide phosphate), which are coenzymes in a wide variety of oxidation and reduction reactions in energy-yielding metabolism.

In general, NAD is involved as an electron acceptor in energy-yielding metabolism, and the resultant NADH is oxidised by the mitochondrial electron transport chain. The major coenzyme for reductive synthetic reactions is NADPH.

NAD is the source of ADP-ribose for the reversible modification of proteins by mono-ADP-ribosylation, catalysed by ADP-ribosyltransferases, and poly(ADP-ribosylation), catalysed by poly(ADP-ribose) polymerase. A variety of guanine nucleotide-binding proteins (G-proteins) involved with the regulation of adenylate cyclase activity are regulated by ADP-ribosylation, and poly(ADP-ribosylation) of nuclear proteins is an important step in the DNA repair mechanism.

NAD is also the precursor of two second messengers that act to increase the release of calcium from intracellular stores in response to hormones: cyclic ADP-ribose and nicotinic acid adenine dinucleotide phosphate (NAADP).

EFFECTS OF NIACIN DEFICIENCY AND EXCESS

Pellagra is the disease due to deficiency of tryptophan and niacin. It is characterised by a photosensitive dermatitis, like severe sunburn, affecting regions of the skin that are exposed to sunlight. Advanced pellagra is also accompanied by a 'dementia' or depressive psychosis, and there may be diarrhoea. Untreated pellagra is fatal.

Pellagra was a major problem of public health in the early part of the twentieth century, and continued to be a problem until the 1980s in some parts of the world. It is now rare, although there have been reports of outbreaks among refugees in war zones, and occasional cases are reported in alcoholics, and among people being treated with isoniazid.

The synthesis of NAD from tryptophan requires both riboflavin and vitamin B_6, and deficiency of either may lead to the development of secondary pellagra when intakes of tryptophan and preformed niacin are marginal. Similarly, an excessive intake of leucine, as occurs in parts of India where the dietary staple is jowar (Sorghum vulgare), inhibits tryptophan metabolism and may be a factor in the development of pellagra.

ASSESSMENT OF NIACIN STATUS

The two methods of assessing niacin nutritional status are measurement of blood nicotinamide nucleotides and the urinary excretion of niacin metabolites, neither of which is wholly satisfactory. Criteria of adequacy are shown in Table evolve 10.6 🖱.

THE BASIS OF SETTING DIETARY REQUIREMENTS FOR NIACIN

Because of the central role of the nicotinamide nucleotides in energy-yielding metabolism, niacin requirements are conventionally expressed/unit of energy expenditure (i.e. /kcal or /MJ).

From depletion/repletion studies the average niacin requirement is 5.5 mg/1000 kcal (1.3 mg/MJ). Allowing for individual variation, reference intakes are set at 6.6 mg niacin equivalents (preformed niacin + 1/60 of the dietary tryptophan)/1000 kcal (1.6 mg/MJ). Even when energy intakes are very low, it must be assumed that energy expenditure will not fall below about 2000 kcal, and this is the basis for the calculation of reference intakes for subjects with very low energy intakes.

Upper levels of niacin intake

High intakes of niacin cause liver damage. Sustained release preparations are associated with more severe liver damage and clinical liver failure, because they permit more prolonged maintenance of high tissue concentrations of the vitamin. Nicotinic acid is used clinically to treat hyperlipidaemia. It causes a marked vasodilatation, with flushing, burning and itching of the skin and possibly also hypotension.

The tolerable upper limit of niacin intake is 35 mg/day for adults. The European Health Food Manufacturers' Federation restricts over-the-counter supplements to 500 mg/day. Where it is being used to treat hyperlipidaemia, and in trials for the prevention of type 1 diabetes mellitus, a tentative upper limit has been set at 3 g/day.

CURRENT TOPICS: NICOTINAMIDE FOR THE PREVENTION OF TYPE 1 DIABETES MELLITUS

In experimental animals, nicotinamide protects against the destruction of pancreatic β-islet cells by diabetogenic agents. Type 1 diabetes mellitus is caused by autoimmune destruction of β-cells, and autoantibodies against β-cell proteins can be detected in the circulation several years before the onset of disease. It has been suggested that nicotinamide may delay the development of diabetes in susceptible subjects, although it has no effect once diabetes has developed. However, two large intervention trials have shown no benefit of nicotinamide supplements.

KEY POINTS

- There are two niacin vitamers: nicotinic acid and nicotinamide.
- Niacin is not strictly a vitamin; endogenous synthesis from tryptophan is more important than dietary intake of preformed niacin.
- Niacin intake is calculated as mg niacin equivalents: preformed niacin + 1/60 tryptophan intake.
- Deficiency of riboflavin or vitamin B_6 impairs tryptophan metabolism and may lead to the development of pellagra, as may a number of drugs that react with vitamin B_6.
- Niacin functions as the nicotinamide ring of the coenzymes NAD and NADP in oxidation and reduction reactions.
- NAD is the source of ADP-ribose for ADP-ribosylation of G-proteins and poly(ADP-ribosylation) of nuclear proteins for DNA repair.
- NAD is the precursor for synthesis of second messengers that regulate intracellular calcium concentrations in response to hormones.
- Current methods of assessing niacin status are unsatisfactory.
- Niacin requirements are calculated on the basis of energy intake.
- High intakes of niacin cause liver damage, and high intakes of nicotinic acid cause vasodilatation.
- Nicotinic acid is used in pharmacological doses to treat hyperlipidaemia.

10.4 VITAMIN B_6

Vitamin B_6 has a central role in the metabolism of amino acids, is the cofactor for glycogen phosphorylase, and has a role in the modulation of steroid hormone action and regulation of gene expression.

The vitamin is widely distributed in foods, and clinical deficiency is virtually unknown. However, marginal status, affecting amino acid metabolism and steroid hormone responsiveness, is relatively common.

Oestrogens cause abnormalities of tryptophan B_6 metabolism that resemble those seen in vitamin deficiency, and the vitamin is widely used to treat the side-effects of the premenstrual syndrome, although there is little evidence of efficacy. High doses of the vitamin, of the order of 100 times reference intakes, cause peripheral sensory neuropathy.

FORMS OF VITAMIN B₆ IN FOODS AND GOOD FOOD SOURCES

The generic descriptor vitamin B_6 includes six vitamers: the alcohol pyridoxine, the aldehyde pyridoxal, the amine pyridoxamine and their 5'-phosphates (Fig. 10.4). The vitamers are metabolically interconvertible, and as far as is known, they have equal biological activity.

Meat, fish, potatoes and bananas are good sources of vitamin B_6; milk, nuts, beans and vegetables provide significant amounts (see Table *evolve* 10.7 🖱). Up to 75% of the vitamin B_6 in plant foods is present as glycosides, which have limited availability.

A proportion of the vitamin B_6 in foods may be biologically unavailable after heating, as a result of the formation of (phospho)pyridoxyllysine by reduction of the bond by which the vitamin is bound to the ε-amino groups of lysine in proteins. Pyridoxyllysine is a vitamin B_6 antimetabolite, and formation of pyridoxyllysine also reduces the nutritional value of proteins in which lysine is the limiting amino acid (see Ch. 8, Section 8.4).

ABSORPTION AND TRANSPORT OF VITAMIN B₆

The phosphorylated vitamers are hydrolysed by alkaline phosphatase in the intestinal mucosa; pyridoxal, pyridoxamine and pyridoxine are all absorbed by carrier-mediated diffusion, and there is net accumulation by metabolic trapping as pyridoxal phosphate.

Liver exports both pyridoxal phosphate, bound to albumin, and pyridoxal, which circulates bound to both albumin and haemoglobin. Extrahepatic tissues take up pyridoxal after hydrolysis of pyridoxal phosphate in plasma by extracellular alkaline phosphatase, followed by phosphorylation to trap the vitamin in cells. In the liver, vitamin B_6 in excess of requirements is oxidised to 4-pyridoxic acid, which is the main excretory product.

Some 80% of the body's total vitamin B_6 is pyridoxal phosphate in muscle, bound to glycogen phosphorylase. This is not released from muscle in deficiency, but rather in prolonged starvation, as muscle glycogen reserves are exhausted. Under these conditions it is available for redistribution to other tissues, and especially liver and kidney, to meet the requirement for gluconeogenesis from amino acids.

METABOLIC FUNCTIONS OF VITAMIN B₆

The metabolically active vitamer is pyridoxal phosphate, which is involved in many reactions of amino acid metabolism, in glycogen phosphorylase and in the recycling of steroid hormone receptors from tight nuclear binding.

Vitamin-B_6-dependent enzymes catalyse four main types of reaction involving amino acids: transamination (permitting both utilisation of amino acid carbon skeletons for gluconeogenesis or ketogenesis and also the synthesis of non-essential amino acids); decarboxylation to form a variety of biologically active amines; racemisation; and a variety of side-chain reactions.

Steroid hormones act by binding to nuclear receptors that then bind to hormone response elements on DNA, altering the transcription of specific genes. Pyridoxal phosphate acts to release the hormone-receptor complex from DNA binding, so terminating the nuclear action of the hormone. In experimental animals, vitamin B_6 deficiency results in increased and prolonged nuclear uptake and retention of steroid hormones in target tissues, and enhanced end-organ responsiveness to low doses of hormones.

EFFECTS OF VITAMIN B₆ DEFICIENCY AND EXCESS

Clinical deficiency of vitamin B_6 is extremely rare. The vitamin is widely distributed in foods and it is

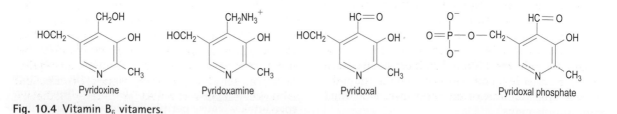

Fig. 10.4 Vitamin B₆ vitamers.

synthesised by intestinal flora. However, several studies have shown that 10–20% of the population of developed countries have marginal or inadequate status.

Much of our knowledge of human vitamin B_6 deficiency is derived from an 'outbreak' in the early 1950s, which resulted from an infant milk preparation that had undergone severe heating in manufacture. The result was the formation of the antimetabolite pyridoxyllysine by reaction between pyridoxal phosphate and the ε-amino groups of lysine in proteins. In addition to a number of metabolic abnormalities, many of the affected infants convulsed. They responded to the administration of vitamin B_6.

Vitamin B_6 deficiency may result from the prolonged administration of drugs that can form biologically inactive adducts with pyridoxal, such as penicillamine and isoniazid. Drug-induced vitamin B_6 deficiency frequently manifests as the tryptophan–niacin deficiency disease pellagra because synthesis of the nicotinamide nucleotide coenzymes from tryptophan is pyridoxal-phosphate-dependent.

Vitamin B_6 toxicity

Supplements of 50–200 mg vitamin B_6/day are widely prescribed and self-prescribed for a variety of conditions, including premenstrual syndrome, depression, morning sickness in pregnancy, hypertension and carpal tunnel syndrome, although the evidence of efficacy is slight. There are promising results from trials of pyridoxamine to prevent non-enzymic glycation of proteins in diabetic patients, and hence slow the development of the adverse effects of poor glycaemic control.

Animal studies have shown that vitamin B_6 in gross excess is neurotoxic, causing peripheral neuropathy. Sensory neuropathy has been reported in patients who had been taking 2000–7000 mg of pyridoxine/day for several months. On withdrawal of the supplements there was substantial recovery of nerve function, although there was residual damage in some patients.

There is little evidence that intakes up to 200 mg vitamin B_6/day are associated with adverse effects. The US Food and Nutrition Board set a tolerable upper level for adults of 100 mg/day; the EU Scientific Committee on Food level is 25 mg/day.

THE ASSESSMENT OF VITAMIN B_6 NUTRITIONAL STATUS

There are a number of indices of vitamin B_6 status available: plasma concentrations of the vitamin, urinary excretion of 4-pyridoxic acid, activation of erythrocyte aminotransferases by pyridoxal phosphate added in vitro, and the ability to metabolise test doses of tryptophan and methionine. None is wholly satisfactory, and where more than one index has been used in population studies there is poor agreement between different methods. Criteria of adequacy are shown in Table *evolve* 10.8 .

The oxidation of tryptophan (see Fig. *evolve* 10.3) includes the vitamin-B_6-dependent enzyme kynureninase and in deficiency, after a test dose of tryptophan, there is a considerable increase in the urinary excretion of xanthurenic and kynurenic acids. However, cortisol induces the first enzyme of the pathway, tryptophan dioxygenase, leading to a rate of metabolism that is greater than the capacity of kynureninase, so that people who are stressed will show results that falsely suggest vitamin B_6 deficiency. Similarly, oestrogen metabolites inhibit kynureninase and again give results that falsely suggest vitamin B_6 deficiency.

The conversion of homocysteine (arising from methionine) to cysteine (see Fig. *evolve* 10.4) includes two pyridoxal-phosphate-dependent steps. In vitamin B_6 deficiency there is an increase in the urinary excretion of homocysteine after a loading dose of methionine. However, the metabolic fate of homocysteine is determined mainly by the need for cysteine and the rate at which it is remethylated to methionine, so increased excretion of homocysteine following a test dose of methionine cannot necessarily be regarded as evidence of vitamin B_6 deficiency.

THE BASIS OF SETTING DIETARY VITAMIN B_6 REQUIREMENTS

Early studies of vitamin B_6 requirements used the development of abnormalities of tryptophan or methionine metabolism during depletion, and normalisation during repletion. Abnormalities develop faster during depletion in subjects maintained on a high protein diet, and during repletion normalisation occurs faster in subjects maintained on a low protein diet. From such studies the average requirement was set at 13 µg/gram dietary protein, and reference intakes were based on 15–16 µg/g dietary protein.

More recent studies, using more sensitive indices of status, have shown average requirements of 15–16 µg/g of dietary protein, suggesting a reference intake of 18–20 µg/g protein.

In 1998 the reference intake in the USA and Canada was reduced from the previous RDA of 2 mg/day for men and 1.6 mg/day for women to 1.3 mg/day for both. The report cites six studies that demonstrated that this level of intake would maintain a plasma concentration of pyridoxal phosphate of at least 20 nmol/l, although, as shown in Table *evolve* 10.8 🔋, the more generally accepted criterion of adequacy is 30 nmol/l.

CURRENT TOPICS: VITAMIN B_6 AND HYPERHOMOCYSTEINAEMIA, VITAMIN B_6 AND HORMONE–DEPENDENT CANCER

Epidemiological studies suggest that hyperhomocysteinaemia is most significantly correlated with low folate status, but there is also a significant association with low vitamin B_6 status. Supplementation trials have shown that while folate supplements lower fasting homocysteine in moderately hyperhomocysteinaemic subjects, supplements of 10 mg/day vitamin B_6 have no effect, although supplements do reduce the peak plasma concentration of homocysteine following a test dose of methionine. It thus seems unlikely that intakes of vitamin B_6 above amounts that are adequate to prevent metabolic signs of deficiency will be beneficial in lowering plasma concentrations of homocysteine.

The role of pyridoxal phosphate in attenuating the actions of steroid hormones suggests either that inadequate vitamin B_6 status may be a factor in the development of hormone-dependent cancer of the breast, uterus and prostate, or that supplements may be protective. There is no evidence as yet on which to base recommendations for higher intakes of the vitamin.

KEY POINTS

- Vitamin B_6 functions as a coenzyme in a wide variety of reactions of amino acids, in glycogen phosphorylase and to regulate the actions of steroid hormones.
- Clinical deficiency of vitamin B_6 is more or less unknown, but marginal status is widespread.
- Inadequate vitamin B_6 status may be a factor in hyperhomocysteinaemia, and hence cardiovascular disease, and in steroid-dependent cancer.

- A number of drugs react with vitamin B_6 and may cause deficiency that manifests as pellagra due to impaired synthesis of niacin from tryptophan.
- Vitamin B_6 status can be assessed by measuring blood levels, excretion of 4-pyridoxic acid, erythrocyte aminotransferase activation coefficient or the metabolism of test doses of tryptophan or methionine.
- Vitamin B_6 requirements are calculated per unit dietary protein intake.
- Vitamin B_6 supplements are used to treat premenstrual syndrome and some other conditions (with little evidence of efficacy).
- Very high doses of vitamin B_6 cause sensory nerve damage.

10.5 FOLATES

Folic acid derivatives function in the transfer of one-carbon fragments in a variety of reactions.

Although folate is widely distributed in foods, deficiency is not uncommon, and a number of commonly used drugs can cause folate depletion. Marginal folate status is a factor in the development of neural tube defects, and supplements of 400 µg/day periconceptionally reduce the incidence significantly. High intakes of folate lower the plasma concentration of homocysteine in people genetically at risk of hyperhomocysteinaemia, and may reduce the risk of cardiovascular disease. There is also evidence that low folate status is associated with increased risk of colorectal and other cancers. Mandatory enrichment of cereal products with folic acid has been introduced in the USA and elsewhere, and considered in other countries.

FORMS IN FOODS AND GOOD FOOD SOURCES

The structure of folic acid is shown in Figure 10.5. In the coenzymes the ring is fully reduced to tetrahydrofolate, and there are up to six additional glutamate residues, linked by γ-glutamyl peptide bonds. Although the terms 'folic acid' and 'folate' are often used interchangeably, correctly 'folic acid' refers to the oxidised compound, dihydrofolate monoglutamate, and the tetrahydrofolate derivatives are collectively known as 'folates'.

Tetrahydrofolate can carry one-carbon fragments attached to N-5 (formyl, formimino or methyl groups), N-10 (formyl) or bridging N-5-N-10

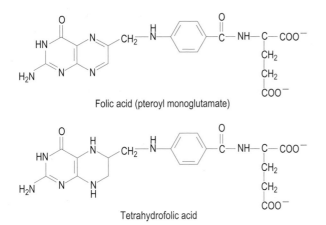

Folic acid (pteroyl monoglutamate)

Tetrahydrofolic acid

Fig. 10.5 Folic acid.

(methylene or methenyl groups) (see Fig. *evolve* 10.5 🐭).

5 Formyl-tetrahydrofolate is more stable to atmospheric oxidation than folic acid, and is commonly used in pharmaceutical preparations; it is also known as folinic acid, and the synthetic (racemic) compound as leucovorin.

The folate in foods consists of a mixture of different one-carbon substituted derivatives, with varying numbers of conjugated glutamyl residues; their biological availability differs, but is consistently lower than that of folic acid, which is the compound used in studies to determine requirements, and in food fortification. In order to permit calculation of folate intakes in terms of both naturally occurring mixed food folates and added folic acid, 1 μg dietary folate equivalent has been defined as the sum of μg food folate + 1.7 × μg folic acid.

Liver is an especially rich source of folate; green leafy vegetables, beans, nuts and milk are good sources, as are some fruits (see Table *evolve* 10.9 🐭).

ABSORPTION AND TRANSPORT OF FOLATE

In the intestinal lumen, folate conjugates are hydrolysed by conjugase, a zinc-dependent enzyme, and folate is absorbed in the jejunum. The biological availability of folate from milk is considerably greater than that of unbound folate, because it is bound to a binding protein and the protein–folate complex is absorbed intact, from the ileum, by a different mechanism. The availability of folate from cereal foods, or of free folic acid taken with cereal foods, is lower.

Most of the folate undergoes reduction and methylation in the intestinal mucosa, so that what enters the bloodstream is mainly methyltetrahydrofolate, which circulates bound to albumin, and is the main vitamer for uptake by tissues. Small amounts of other one-carbon substituted folates also circulate, and are also available for tissue uptake. In contrast, recent investigations show that the principal site of metabolic transformation of folic acid is the liver; most of a physiological dose of folic acid will be transferred to the liver from the gastrointestinal mucosa, for reduction and methylation.

Folate monoglutamates cross cell membranes readily, while polyglutamates do not, so formation of conjugates permits intracellular accumulation of folate. Rapid formation of at least a diglutamate is essential for tissue uptake and retention. Further conjugation to form the metabolically active coenzymes proceeds more slowly.

One-carbon substituted folates are poor substrates for conjugation; since the main form that is taken up into tissues is methyltetrahydrofolate, demethylation by the action of methionine synthetase is essential for tissue accumulation.

METABOLIC FUNCTIONS OF FOLATE

The metabolic role of folate is as a carrier of one-carbon fragments, both in catabolism and biosynthetic reactions. The major sources of the one-carbon fragments, their uses, and interconversion of substituted folates, are shown in Figure 10.6.

The major point of entry for one-carbon fragments into substituted folates is methylene-tetrahydrofolate, which is formed by the catabolism of glycine, serine and choline. Serine is the major source of one-carbon substituted folates for biosynthetic reactions. The other sources of one-carbon-substituted folate are important for catabolism of the substrates rather than provision of one-carbon units for biosynthetic reactions.

Methylene, methenyl and 10-formyl tetrahydrofolates are freely interconvertible. This means that single carbon fragments entering the folate pool in any form other than methyltetrahydrofolate are available for any of the biosynthetic reactions shown in Figure 10.6. When there is a greater entry of one-carbon units into the folate pool than is required for biosynthetic reactions, the surplus can be oxidised to CO_2 by way of 10-formyl-tetrahydrofolate, thus ensuring a continuing supply of free tetrahydrofolate for catabolic reactions.

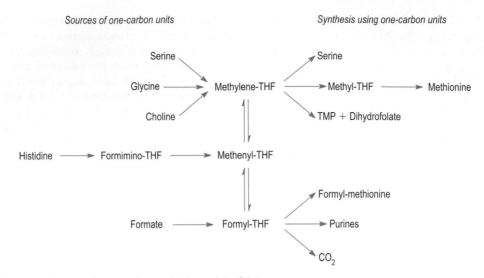

Fig. 10.6 Sources and uses of one-carbon units bound to folate.

The reduction of methylene tetrahydrofolate to methyltetrahydrofolate, catalysed by methylene tetrahydrofolate reductase, is irreversible and methyltetrahydrofolate, which is the main form of folate taken up into tissues, can only be utilised after demethylation, catalysed by methionine synthetase.

EFFECTS OF FOLATE DEFICIENCY AND EXCESS

Folate deficiency is relatively common; some 8–10% of the population of developed countries have low folate stores. Deficiency results in megaloblastic anaemia – the release into the circulation of immature red blood cell precursors due to a failure of the normal process of maturation in the bone marrow, because of impaired synthesis of purines and pyrimidines for DNA synthesis. There may also be a low white cell and platelet count, as well as hypersegmented neutrophils. Deficiency is frequently accompanied by depression, insomnia, forgetfulness and irritability, and sometimes cognitive impairment and dementia. Suboptimal folate status is also associated with increased incidence of neural tube defects, hyperhomocysteinaemia leading to increased risk of cardiovascular disease and altered methylation of DNA, which may increase cancer risk.

Folate deficiency and neural tube defects

The development of the brain and spinal cord begins around day 18 of gestation; closure begins about day 21 and is complete by day 24 – before the woman knows she is pregnant. The closed neural tube stimulates the development of the bony structures that will become the spinal cord and skull. Bone does not form over unclosed regions, leading to the congenital defects collectively known as neural tube defects, anencephaly and spina bifida, which affect between 0.5 and 8 per 1000 live births, depending on genetic and environmental factors.

A number of studies in the 1960s suggested that low folate status was a factor in neural tube defects, and in the 1990s intervention studies showed that supplements of 400 µg/day of folic acid, begun before conception, halved the incidence. It is unlikely that an increase in folate intake equivalent to 400 µg/day of folic acid could be achieved from unfortified foods, and where fortification of cereal products with folic acid is not mandatory, women who are planning a pregnancy are advised to take supplements.

Drug-induced folate deficiency

A number of folate antimetabolites are used clinically, as cancer chemotherapy, and as antibacterial and antimalarial agents, and their prolonged use can result in iatrogenic folate deficiency. The older antiepileptic drugs, such as diphenylhydantoin (phenytoin), phenobarbital and primidone, can also cause folate deficiency.

Upper levels of folate intake

Although folic acid has low toxicity, two groups of people are at risk of adverse effects of high intakes that might result from widespread enrichment of foods or indiscriminate use of supplements:

1. High intakes of folic acid mask the development of megaloblastic anaemia due to vitamin B_{12} deficiency, so that irreversible nerve damage is the presenting sign. The elderly are especially vulnerable, because of atrophic gastritis. An intake of 1000 µg/day is considered unlikely to mask the development of megaloblastic anaemia in elderly people, and this can be considered to be an upper level of habitual intake.

2. Intakes of folic acid in excess of about 5000 µg/ day antagonise the anticonvulsants used in treatment of epilepsy, leading to an increase in fit frequency.

In countries where there has been mandatory fortification of flour with folate for the last decade, there has been a considerable reduction in the incidence of neural tube defects, with no evidence of adverse effects on the population groups potentially at risk from high intakes of the vitamin. In 2006 the Scientific Advisory Committee on Nutrition of the UK Food Standards Agency recommended mandatory fortification of flour with 270 µg of folic acid/100 g flour, but stated that if this were enacted there should be an end to voluntary fortification of other foods with folic acid. This was based on consideration of the number of people aged over 50 who would be exposed to intakes greater than 1000 µg/day, and the number of neural tube defects that would be prevented, at various levels of enrichment of flour.

ASSESSMENT OF FOLATE STATUS

A number of methods have been developed to permit assessment of folate status and to differentiate between deficiency of folate and deficiency of vitamin B_{12} as the cause of megaloblastic anaemia. Criteria of folate status are shown in Table *evolve* 10.10 .

The serum or erythrocyte concentration of folate can be measured by radioligand binding and microbiological assays. Folate is incorporated into erythrocytes during erythropoiesis, and does not enter the cells in the circulation to any significant extent; erythrocyte folate is generally considered to give an indication of folate status over 1–3 months (the lifespan of erythrocytes in the circulation is 120 days), and not to be subject to variations in recent intake.

The ability to metabolise a test dose of histidine provides a sensitive functional test of folate status; formiminoglutamate (FIGLU) is an intermediate in histidine catabolism, and is metabolised by a folate-dependent enzyme. In deficiency the activity of this enzyme is impaired, and FIGLU accumulates and is excreted in the urine.

The ability of deoxyuridine to suppress the incorporation of [^{3}H]thymidine into DNA in rapidly dividing cells (bone marrow biopsy or transformed lymphocytes) also gives an index of folate status. Cells that have been pre-incubated with deoxyuridine then exposed to [^{3}H]thymidine incorporate little or none of the labelled material into DNA, because of dilution by the larger pool of newly synthesised thymidine monophosphate (TMP). In normal cells the incorporation of [^{3}H]thymidine into DNA after pre-incubation with dUMP is 1.4–1.8% of that without pre-incubation. By contrast, folate-deficient cells form little or no thymidine from dUMP, and hence incorporate as much of the [^{3}H]thymidine after incubation with dUMP as they do without pre-incubation.

THE BASIS OF SETTING DIETARY REQUIREMENTS

At the time that the UK and EU reference intakes of folate shown in Appendix Table A13 were being discussed, the results of intervention trials for the prevention of neural tube defects were only just becoming available, and there was no information concerning the effects of folate status on hyperhomocysteinaemia. The US/Canadian report noted specifically that protective effects with respect to neural tube defects were not considered relevant to the determination of the dietary reference intake of folate, and there was insufficient evidence to associate higher intakes of folate with reduced risk of cardiovascular disease.

The total body pool of folate in adults is some 17 µmol (7.5 mg), with a biological half-life of 101 days, suggesting a minimum requirement for replacement of 85 nmol (37 µg) per day. Studies of the urinary excretion of folate metabolites in subjects maintained on folate-free diets suggest that there is catabolism of some 170 nmol (80 µg) of folate/day.

Depletion/repletion studies to determine folate requirements suggest a requirement of the order of 170–220 nmol (80–100 µg)/day. However, because of the problems of determining the availability of the mixed folates in foods, reference intakes allow a wide margin of safety, and are generally based on an allowance of 3–6 µg (7–14 nmol)/kg body weight; 200–400 µg/day for adults.

CURRENT TOPICS: FOLIC ACID, HYPERHOMOCYSTEINAEMIA, CARDIOVASCULAR DISEASE AND COLORECTAL CANCER

A genetic polymorphism of methylene tetrahydrofolate reductase results in the enzyme being thermolabile (i.e. unstable to heating to about 40–45°C) (see Section 29.5). The variant enzyme is also unstable in vivo; people who are homozygous for the thermolabile enzyme have about 50% of normal enzyme activity in tissues. A number of studies have shown that the thermolabile variant is two- to three-fold more common among people with atherosclerosis and coronary heart disease than among disease-free people of the same ethnic origin.

Being homozygous for the variant of the enzyme is a necessary, but not sufficient, condition for the development of hyperhomocysteinaemia. Homozygotes with a high folate intake have plasma concentrations of homocysteine as low as heterozygotes or people who are homozygous for the stable enzyme. Two possible mechanisms have been proposed to explain how a high intake of folate can mask the effect of being homozygous for the enzyme.

Most dietary folate is methylated to methyltetrahydrofolate in the intestinal mucosa. Intestinal mucosal cells have a rapid turnover, typically 48 hours from proliferation in the crypt to shedding at the tip of the villus. An unstable enzyme, which loses activity over a shorter time than normal, is irrelevant in cells that have a rapid turnover. A high intake of folate will therefore result in a high rate of supply of methyltetrahydrofolate to tissues, arising from newly absorbed folate, so that impaired turnover of folate within tissues would be less important.

Methylene tetrahydrofolate reductase may be more stable in the presence of its substrate. Hence it is possible that high tissue levels of methylene tetrahydrofolate (resulting from a high folate status) may protect the enzyme and enhance its stability.

A number of epidemiological studies during the 1990s identified elevation of plasma homocysteine as an independent risk factor for cardiovascular disease, and supplements of folate lower plasma homocysteine in many hyperhomocysteinaemic subjects. Some intervention trials have shown improvement in some intermediate markers of cardiovascular disease, and reduced mortality from stroke, but no effect on death from ischaemic heart disease

Epidemiological studies also suggest that low folate status is associated with an increased risk of colorectal and other cancers. It is difficult to determine the importance of folate per se, since the vegetables that are major sources of folate are also sources of a variety of other compounds that have potentially protective effects. There is, however, evidence that folate deficiency leads to aberrant methylation of DNA. Methylation is important in the silencing of genes during development and tissue differentiation, and altered methylation may result in dedifferentiation and the development of cancer. However, there are also some reports of increased incidence of colorectal cancer associated with high intakes of folic acid, possibly as a result of excessive or inappropriate methylation of DNA.

KEY POINTS

- Folate functions as a coenzyme in one-carbon transfer reactions.
- The availability of mixed food folates is lower than that of free folic acid.
- Folate deficiency is not uncommon; deficiency results in megaloblastic anaemia.
- Low folate status is associated with neural tube defects, and periconceptional supplements, or enrichment of foods with folic acid, reduce the incidence.
- Low folate status is associated with hyperhomocysteinaemia and cardiovascular disease; high folate status overcomes the hyperhomocysteinaemia associated with the thermolabile variant of methylene tetrahydrofolate reductase.

- Low folate status is associated with altered methylation of DNA, and possibly cancer.
- Folate status can be assessed by measuring plasma or erythrocyte concentrations, metabolism of a test dose of histidine, or suppression of the incorporation in vitro of [^{3}H]thymidine into DNA by dUMP.
- Current estimates of folate requirements include a wide margin of safety because of the lack of information on the availability of mixed food folates. They do not take account of the higher intakes required to reduce neural tube defects or lower plasma homocysteine.
- High intakes of folate may mask the megaloblastic anaemia of vitamin B_{12} deficiency due to atrophic gastritis in the elderly, and may antagonise antiepileptic medication.

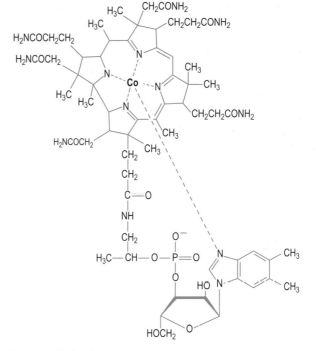

Fig. 10.7 Vitamin B_{12}.

10.6 VITAMIN B_{12}

Dietary deficiency of vitamin B_{12} only occurs among strict vegans, but deficiency as a result of impaired absorption is not uncommon, especially among elderly people with atrophic gastritis. Deficiency results in the development of pernicious anaemia – megaloblastic anaemia (as seen in folate deficiency) with degeneration of the spinal cord.

FORMS OF VITAMIN B_{12} IN FOODS AND GOOD FOOD SOURCES

The structure of vitamin B_{12} is shown in Figure 10.7; the various vitamers have different groups chelated to the central cobalt atom: CN^- (cyanocobalamin); OH^- (hydroxocobalamin); H_2O (aquocobalamin); $-CH_3$ (methylcobalamin); 5′-deoxy-5′adenosine (adenosylcobalamin).

Cyanocobalamin is not an important naturally occurring vitamer; because it is more stable to light than the other vitamers it is used in pharmaceutical preparations.

Vitamin B_{12} is found only in foods of animal origin; there are no plant sources. Rich sources include liver, fish and meat (see Table *evolve* 10.11). A number of reports have suggested that vitamin B_{12} occurs in some algae, but this is probably the result of bacterial contamination of the water in which they were grown.

A number of related compounds in plants do not have vitamin activity (and indeed are antimetabo-

lites of the vitamin), but are growth factors for B_{12}-dependent microorganisms, and hence give a misleading result when the vitamin is measured microbiologically.

ABSORPTION AND TRANSPORT OF VITAMIN B_{12}

Very small amounts of vitamin B_{12} can be absorbed by diffusion across the intestinal mucosa, but under normal conditions this is insignificant; the major route of vitamin B_{12} absorption is by way of binding to intrinsic factor, a glycoprotein secreted by the gastric parietal cells.

Both gastric acid and pepsin are important in vitamin B_{12} nutrition, serving to release the vitamin from protein binding. Between 10 and 15% of people over 60 show some degree of deficiency as a result of impaired absorption due to atrophic gastritis. In the early stages there is failure of acid secretion, resulting in failure to release the vitamin from dietary proteins, although the absorption of free crystalline vitamin is unaffected. As the condition progresses, so there is also failure of the secretion of intrinsic factor.

In the stomach, vitamin B_{12} binds to cobalophilin, a binding protein secreted in saliva. In the duodenum cobalophilin is hydrolysed, releasing the vitamin for binding to intrinsic factor. The vitamin B_{12}–intrinsic factor complex is absorbed from the distal third of the ileum by receptor-mediated endocytosis. Inside the mucosal cell, the vitamin is released by proteolysis and is bound to transcobalamin II for export from the enterocytes. Tissue uptake is by receptor-mediated endocytosis of holotranscobalamin II, followed by proteolysis to release hydroxocobalamin, which may either undergo methylation to methylcobalamin in the cytosol, or enter the mitochondria to form adenosylcobalamin.

Although transcobalamin II is the metabolically important pool of plasma vitamin B_{12}, it accounts for only 10–15% of the total circulating vitamin. The majority is bound to haptocorrin (also known as transcobalamin I). The function of haptocorrin is not well understood; it does not seem to be involved in tissue uptake or inter-tissue transport of the vitamin. A third plasma vitamin-B_{12}-binding protein, transcobalamin III, provides a mechanism for returning vitamin B_{12} and its metabolites from peripheral tissues to the liver.

There is considerable enterohepatic circulation of vitamin B_{12}; between 1 and 9 μg is secreted in the bile each day, and is mainly reabsorbed bound to intrinsic factor. This seems to be a mechanism for excretion of inactive metabolites of the vitamin; only active vitamin B_{12} binds to intrinsic factor, while transcobalamins and cobalophilins bind a variety of inactive analogues as well.

METABOLIC FUNCTIONS OF VITAMIN B_{12}

There are three vitamin-B_{12}-dependent mammalian enzymes:

1. Methionine synthetase, which catalyses the transfer of the methyl group from methyltetrahydrofolate to homocysteine.
2. Methylmalonyl CoA mutase, which catalyses the rearrangement of methylmalonyl CoA, an intermediate in the metabolism of valine, cholesterol and odd-carbon fatty acids, to succinyl CoA.
3. Leucine aminomutase, which catalyses the interconversion of leucine and β-leucine and acts mainly to metabolise β-leucine arising from intestinal bacteria.

EFFECTS OF DEFICIENCY AND EXCESS OF VITAMIN B_{12}

Pernicious anaemia is the megaloblastic anaemia due to vitamin B_{12} deficiency, commonly as a result of failure of intrinsic factor secretion, in which there is also spinal cord degeneration and peripheral neuropathy. High intakes of folate prevent the development of megaloblastic anaemia, and in up to one-third of patients the (irreversible) neurological signs develop without megaloblastosis.

Failure of intrinsic factor secretion is often due to autoimmune disease; 90% of patients with pernicious anaemia have antibodies against gastric parietal cells and 70% also have anti-intrinsic factor antibodies. Only about 10% of patients are aged under 40; by the age of 60 about 1% of the population are affected, rising to 2–5% of people aged over 65, as a result of atrophic gastritis.

The neurological damage is caused by demyelination due to failure of methylation of arginine-107 of myelin basic protein. The nervous system is especially vulnerable to lack of methionine for methylation reactions because, unlike other tissues, it contains only methionine synthetase, which is vitamin-B_{12}-dependent, and not the vitamin-B_{12}-independent homocysteine methyltransferase that uses betaine as the methyl donor.

It is difficult to account for megaloblastic anaemia in vitamin B_{12} deficiency; none of the B_{12}-dependent enzymes is associated with the synthesis of DNA or nucleotides. The most likely explanation is that vitamin B_{12} deficiency causes functional folate deficiency. Most folate is transported between tissues as methyltetrahydrofolate, and the only reaction that releases free folate is the vitamin-B_{12}-dependent reaction of methionine synthetase. Hence in vitamin B_{12} deficiency folate is trapped as (unusable) methyltetrahydrofolate.

There is no evidence of any adverse effects of high intakes of vitamin B_{12}.

Drug–induced vitamin B_{12} deficiency

Nitrous oxide inhibits methionine synthetase, by oxidising the cobalt of methylcobalamin. Patients with hitherto undiagnosed vitamin B_{12} deficiency can develop neurological signs after surgery when nitrous oxide is used as the anaesthetic agent, and there are a number of reports of neurological damage due to vitamin B_{12} depletion among dental surgeons and others occupationally exposed to nitrous oxide.

The histamine H_2 receptor antagonists and proton pump inhibitors used to treat gastric ulcers and gastro-oesophageal reflux act by reducing the secretion of gastric acid, and may result in impairment of the absorption of protein-bound vitamin B_{12}. However, a number of studies have shown that even prolonged use of these drugs does not lead to significant depletion of vitamin B_{12} reserves.

ASSESSMENT OF VITAMIN B_{12} STATUS

Serum vitamin B_{12} is measured by radioligand binding assay. A serum concentration below 110 pmol/l is associated with megaloblastic bone marrow, incipient anaemia and myelin damage. Below 150 pmol/l there are early bone marrow changes, abnormalities of the dUMP suppression test and methylmalonic aciduria after a valine load; this is considered to be the lower limit of adequacy. Criteria of adequacy are shown in Table *evolve* 10.12 🖱.

The Schilling test for vitamin B_{12} absorption

The absorption of vitamin B_{12} is determined by giving an oral dose of [^{57}Co] or [^{58}Co]vitamin B_{12} together with a parenteral dose of 1 mg of non-radioactive vitamin (the Schilling test); urinary excretion of radioactivity shows the absorption of the oral dose. Normal subjects excrete 16–45% of the radioactivity over 24 hours, while patients lacking intrinsic factor or with anti-intrinsic factor antibodies excrete less than 5%.

Atrophic gastritis causes decreased secretion of gastric acid before there is impairment of intrinsic factor secretion. This means that the absorption of crystalline vitamin B_{12}, as used in the Schilling test, is normal, but the absorption of protein-bound vitamin B_{12} from foods will be impaired and the test will give a false negative result.

Methylmalonic acid excretion

Moderate vitamin B_{12} deficiency impairs the activity of methylmalonyl CoA mutase, resulting in urinary excretion of methylmalonic acid, especially after a loading dose of valine. This can be used to detect subclinical deficiency. However, up to 25% of patients with confirmed pernicious anaemia excrete normal amounts of methylmalonic acid even after a dose of valine.

THE BASIS FOR SETTING DIETARY REQUIREMENTS OF VITAMIN B_{12}

The total body pool of vitamin B_{12} is of the order of 1.8 μmol (2.5 mg), with a minimum desirable body pool of about 0.3 μmol (1 mg). The daily loss is about 0.1% of the body pool in subjects with normal intrinsic factor secretion and enterohepatic circulation of the vitamin. On this basis the requirement is 0.3–1.8 nmol (1–2.5 μg)/day. This is probably a considerable overestimate of requirements, since parenteral administration of less than 0.3 nmol/day is adequate to maintain normal haematology in patients with pernicious anaemia, in whom the enterohepatic recycling of the vitamin is grossly impaired.

Requirements are probably between 0.1 and 1 μg/day; as shown in Appendix Table A14 reference intakes range between 1 and 2.4 μg/day, compared with an average intake of some 5 μg/day by non-vegetarians in most countries.

KEY POINTS

- Dietary deficiency of vitamin B_{12} occurs only in strict vegans; there are no plant sources of the vitamin.
- Functional deficiency, due to failure of absorption, is relatively common among elderly people, as a result of atrophic gastritis.
- Deficiency causes pernicious anaemia – megaloblastic anaemia with spinal cord degeneration. The nerve damage is the result of failure of methylation of myelin basic protein.
- The anaemia is due to functional folate deficiency, as a result of the failure to demethylate methyltetrahydrofolate because of the impaired activity of vitamin-B_{12}-dependent methionine synthetase. High intakes of folate can prevent the development of anaemia.
- Vitamin B_{12} status can be assessed by measurement of the serum concentration, the excretion of methylmalonic acid after a test dose of valine, or suppression of the incorporation in vitro of [^{3}H]thymidine into DNA by dUMP.
- The absorption of vitamin B_{12} can be assessed by the Schilling test, using an oral dose of radioactive vitamin and a large parenteral dose of non-radioactive vitamin.
- Current estimates of requirements are almost certainly an overestimate of true requirements, but considerably lower than average intakes by omnivores.

10.7 VITAMIN C (ASCORBIC ACID)

Vitamin C is a vitamin for only a limited number of vertebrate species: humans and the other primates, the guinea pig, bats, some birds and fishes. It is synthesised as an intermediate in the gulonolactone pathway of glucose metabolism; in those species for which it is a vitamin, one enzyme of the pathway, gulonolactone oxidase, is absent.

Vitamin C is the cofactor for some hydroxylation reactions, and also functions as a non-specific reducing agent and antioxidant.

FORMS IN FOODS AND GOOD FOOD SOURCES

The physiologically important compound is L-ascorbic acid (Fig. 10.8). It can undergo oxidation to the monodehydroascorbate radical and dehydroascorbate, both of which have vitamin activity because they can be reduced to ascorbate. D-Isoascorbic acid (erythorbic acid) has some vitamin activity; it is not a naturally occurring compound, but is widely used, interchangeably with ascorbic acid, in cured meats and as an antioxidant in a variety of foods.

Fruits and vegetables are rich sources; blackcurrants and guava provide about five times the reference intake in a single serving, and potatoes are an important source in many countries (see Table *evolve* 10.13).

ABSORPTION AND TRANSPORT OF VITAMIN C

Some 80–95% of dietary ascorbate is absorbed at intakes up to about 100 mg/day; the absorption of larger amounts of the vitamin is lower – about 50% of a 1.5 g dose is absorbed. Unabsorbed ascorbate is a substrate for intestinal bacterial metabolism.

Ascorbate is absorbed by active transport; dehydroascorbate by a carrier-mediated (equilibrium) transport, followed by reduction to ascorbate inside the intestinal epithelial cell.

Ascorbate enters tissues by way of sodium-dependent transporters, while dehydroascorbate enters by way of the (insulin-dependent) glucose transporter, and is reduced to ascorbate intracellularly. Tissue uptake of dehydroascorbate is impaired in poorly controlled diabetes mellitus, and functional signs of deficiency may develop despite an adequate intake of vitamin C.

About 70% of ascorbate in the blood circulation is in plasma and erythrocytes (which do not concentrate the vitamin). The remainder is in white cells, which have a marked ability to concentrate ascorbate; mononuclear leukocytes achieve 80-fold, platelets 40-fold and granulocytes 25-fold concentration compared with plasma.

There is no specific storage organ for ascorbate; apart from leukocytes (which account for only 10% of total blood ascorbate), the only tissues showing a significant concentration of the vitamin are the adrenal and pituitary glands. Although the concentration of ascorbate in muscle is relatively low, skeletal muscle contains much of the body's pool of 5–8.5 mmol (900–1500 mg) of ascorbate.

The major fate of ascorbic acid is urinary excretion, either unchanged or as dehydroascorbate and diketogulonate. At plasma concentrations above about 85 μmol/l the renal transport system is saturated, and ascorbate is excreted quantitatively with increasing intake.

METABOLIC FUNCTIONS OF VITAMIN C

Ascorbic acid has specific and well-defined roles in two classes of enzymes:

1. Copper-containing hydroxylases, such as dopamine β-hydroxylase and peptidyl glycine

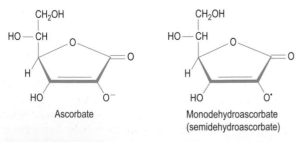

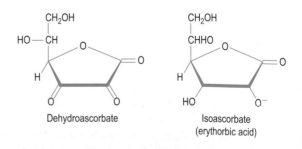

Ascorbate

Monodehydroascorbate
(semidehydroascorbate)

Dehydroascorbate

Isoascorbate
(erythorbic acid)

Fig. 10.8 Vitamin C.

hydroxylase. The enzymes contain Cu^+, which is oxidised to Cu^{2+} during the reaction; reduction back to Cu^+ requires ascorbate, which is oxidised to monodehydroascorbate.

2. The 2-oxoglutarate-linked iron-containing hydroxylases, of which the best studied are the proline and lysine hydroxylases involved in synthesis of collagen and other connective tissue proteins. Although ascorbate is consumed in these reactions, it is not stoichiometric with the formation of product. The enzymes contain Fe^{2+}, and the iron is not oxidised during the reaction. However, it is occasionally (accidentally) oxidised to Fe^{3+}, inactivating the enzyme. Ascorbate is required to reduce the enzyme-bound iron back to the active form.

Ascorbate can act as a radical-trapping antioxidant, reacting with superoxide and a proton to yield hydrogen peroxide, or with the hydroxyl radical to yield water. In each case the product is monodehydroascorbate. It also reduces the α-tocopheroxyl radical formed in cell membranes and plasma lipoproteins during the oxidation of vitamin E, so sparing vitamin E.

VITAMIN C DEFICIENCY AND EXCESS

Although there is no specific site of vitamin C storage in the body, signs of deficiency do not develop until previously adequately nourished subjects have been deprived of the vitamin for 4–6 months, by which time plasma and tissue concentrations have fallen considerably.

The name scurvy for the vitamin C deficiency disease is derived from the Italian *scorbutico*, meaning an irritable person; deficiency is associated with listlessness and general malaise, and sometimes changes in personality and psychomotor performance. The behavioural effects are due to impaired synthesis of catecholamines as a result of reduced activity of dopamine β-hydroxylase.

Most of the other signs of scurvy are due to impaired collagen synthesis. The earliest signs are skin changes, beginning with plugging of hair follicles by horny material, followed by petechial haemorrhage and increased fragility of blood capillaries leading to extravasation of red cells. Later there is haemorrhage of the gums and loss of dental cement. Wounds show only superficial healing in scurvy, with little or no formation of (collagen-rich) scar tissue, so that healing is delayed and wounds can readily be reopened.

Anaemia is common in scurvy, and may be either macrocytic, indicative of folate deficiency, or hypochromic, indicative of iron deficiency. Folate deficiency may be epiphenomenal, since the major sources of folate are the same as those of ascorbate. Iron deficiency in scurvy may well be secondary to reduced absorption of inorganic iron, and impaired mobilisation of tissue iron reserves.

A significant number of people consume gram amounts of vitamin C supplements. There is no evidence that this either confers any benefit or presents any significant hazard. The US/Canadian tolerable upper level of intake is 2 g/day. High intakes of ascorbate lead to acidification of the urine, which will increase the risk of forming oxalate and urate renal stones, but reduce the risk of forming phosphate stones. Ascorbate can also react non-enzymically with amino groups in proteins, glycating them in the same way as occurs with glucose in poorly controlled diabetes mellitus, and there is some evidence of increased cardiovascular disease in diabetics who take high supplements of the vitamin.

Unabsorbed ascorbate in the intestinal lumen is a substrate for bacterial fermentation, which may explain the diarrhoea and intestinal discomfort reported in some studies with high doses of the vitamin.

ASSESSMENT OF VITAMIN C STATUS

Vitamin C status is generally assessed measuring plasma and leukocyte concentrations of the vitamin – criteria of adequacy are shown in Table *evolve* 10.14 . At intakes above about 100 mg/day the plasma concentration of ascorbate reaches a plateau around 70–85 µmol/l, because of quantitative excretion of the vitamin as the renal threshold is exceeded.

Different types of leukocyte have different capacities to accumulate ascorbate, so that a change in the proportion of granulocytes, platelets and mononuclear leukocytes will result in a change in the total concentration of ascorbate/10^6 cells, although there may well be no change in status. Stress, myocardial infarction, infection, burns and surgical trauma all result in an increase in the proportion of granulocytes, which achieve saturation at a lower concentration of ascorbate than other leukocytes, and hence an apparent change in leukocyte ascorbate. This has been misinterpreted to indicate an increased requirement for vitamin C in these conditions. Without a differential white cell count, leukocyte ascorbate concentration cannot be considered to give a meaningful reflection of vitamin C status.

Urinary excretion of hydroxyproline-containing peptides is reduced in people with inadequate vitamin C status, but a number of other factors that affect bone and connective tissue turnover confound interpretation of the results. Excretion of compounds derived from collagen cross-links provides a more useful index, but is affected by copper status.

There is increased formation of 8-hydroxyguanine (a marker of oxidative radical damage) in DNA during vitamin C depletion, suggesting that measurement of 8-hydroxyguanine excretion may provide a way of estimating requirements to meet a biomarker of optimum status.

THE BASIS OF SETTING DIETARY VITAMIN C REQUIREMENTS

The minimum requirement for vitamin C was established in a depletion/repletion study in Sheffield in the 1940s; 7–10 mg/day will prevent or cure scurvy; but wound healing requires 20 mg/day. From these data 30 mg/day was established as a reference intake.

As intake rises above 30 mg/day, the plasma concentration increases, reaching a plateau of 70–85 μmol/l at intakes between 70 and 100 mg, when the renal threshold is reached and the vitamin is excreted quantitatively with increasing intake. The midpoint of the curve, where the plasma concentration increases more or less linearly with intake, represents a state where tissue reserves are adequate. This corresponds to an intake of 40 mg/day and is the basis of the UK and EU reference intakes shown in Appendix Table A8. At this level of intake the total body pool is about 900 mg (5.1 mmol).

The US/Canadian reference intakes of 75 mg for women and 90 mg for men are based on studies of leukocyte saturation.

Clinical signs of scurvy are seen when the total body pool of ascorbate is below 1.7 mmol (300 mg). The pool increases with intake, reaching a maximum of about 8.5 mmol (1500 mg). The fractional turnover rate of ascorbate is 3–4% daily, suggesting a need for 45–60 mg/day for maintenance of this maximum pool. If a total body pool of 900 mg (5.1 mmol) is considered adequate (it is three-fold higher than the minimum required to prevent scurvy) then 40 mg/day is adequate.

PHARMACOLOGICAL USES OF VITAMIN C

Ascorbate enhances the intestinal absorption of inorganic iron, and therefore it is frequently prescribed with iron supplements. Iron is absorbed as Fe^{2+}, and not as Fe^{3+}; ascorbic acid in the intestinal lumen will both maintain iron in the reduced state and also chelate it; a dose of 25 mg of vitamin C taken together with a semi-synthetic meal increases the absorption of iron some 65%, while a 1 g dose gives a nine-fold increase.

Vitamin C is also used when it is desired to acidify the urine, for example in conjunction with some antibiotics. Supplements of vitamin C are widely consumed to protect against cancer, cardiovascular disease and viral infections, although there is little evidence of efficacy. Results from the Physicians' Health Study in USA show no benefits of vitamin C supplements.

High doses of vitamin C are popularly recommended for the prevention and treatment of the common cold. The evidence from controlled trials is unconvincing, and a recent Cochrane review of the literature reported that high-dose supplementation of vitamin C does not reduce the incidence of the common cold in the normal population.

KEY POINTS

- Vitamin C acts as a coenzyme for two classes of hydroxylase, and has a non-specific antioxidant activity; it is especially important in reducing the tocopheroxyl radical formed by oxidation of vitamin E in membranes and plasma lipoproteins.
- Deficiency (scurvy) results in mood and behavioural changes, skin lesions and impaired wound healing (due to impaired synthesis of collagen).
- Vitamin C status is assessed by plasma and leukocyte concentrations. Different types of leukocyte have different ability to concentrate the vitamin, and without a differential white cell count, total leukocyte vitamin C does not give useful information.
- Current estimates of vitamin C requirements differ from one country to another, depending on the criteria selected: plasma concentration of the vitamin, metabolic turnover during depletion/repletion studies or leukocyte saturation.

- Vitamin C enhances the absorption of inorganic iron very considerably, and may also reduce the formation of carcinogenic nitrosamines from dietary amines and nitrite.
- At intakes above about 100 mg/day the vitamin is excreted quantitatively with intake in the urine.
- There is little evidence that high intakes have any beneficial effects, but equally there is little evidence of any significant hazard from high intakes.

10.8 PANTOTHENIC ACID

Pantothenic acid has a central role in energy-yielding metabolism as the functional moiety of coenzyme A, in the biosynthesis of fatty acids as the prosthetic group of acyl carrier protein, and through its role in CoA in a wide variety of other reactions.

Pantothenic acid is widely distributed in all foodstuffs (see Table *evolve* 10.15) and it is absorbed throughout the small intestine, so intestinal bacterial synthesis contributes to intake. As a result, deficiency has not been unequivocally reported except in depletion studies, which have frequently also used the antagonist ω-methyl pantothenic acid.

Prisoners of war in the Far East in the 1940s, who were severely malnourished, showed a new condition of paraesthesia and severe pain in the feet and toes, which was called the 'burning foot' syndrome or nutritional melalgia. Although it was tentatively attributed to pantothenic acid deficiency, no specific trials of pantothenic acid were performed; rather they were given rich sources of all vitamins as part of an urgent programme of nutritional rehabilitation. There seem to be no reports of neurological damage in deficient animals that would explain the 'burning foot' syndrome.

The naturally occurring vitamer is D-pantothenic acid, shown in Figure 10.9. Free pantothenic acid and its sodium salt are chemically unstable, and the usual pharmacological preparation is the calcium salt (calcium dipantothenate). The alcohol pantothenol is a synthetic compound that has biological activity because it is oxidised to pantothenic acid in vivo.

There are no functional tests of pantothenic acid nutritional status that are generally applicable. From the limited studies that have been performed it is not

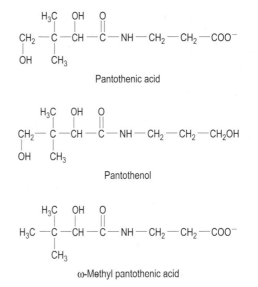

Fig. 10.9 Pantothenic acid.

possible to establish requirements for pantothenic acid. Average intakes are around 27 mg/day; this is obviously adequate, since deficiency is unknown under normal conditions. The US/Canadian adequate intake for adults is 5 mg/day.

KEY POINTS

- Pantothenic acid is required for synthesis of coenzyme A and the acyl carrier protein for fatty acid synthesis.
- Pantothenic acid deficiency is unknown except in depletion studies; the vitamin is widely distributed in foods and is synthesised by intestinal bacteria.
- There is no evidence on which to base estimates of requirements.

10.9 BIOTIN (VITAMIN H)

Biotin was discovered as the protective or curative factor in 'egg white injury' – the disease caused in experimental animals by feeding diets containing large amounts of uncooked egg white. The glycoprotein avidin in egg white binds biotin, rendering it unavailable.

Dietary deficiency of biotin sufficient to cause clinical signs is extremely rare. The vitamin is widely distributed in many foods (see Table *evolve* 10.16) and is synthesised by intestinal flora.

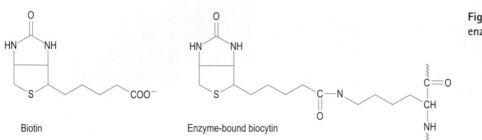

Fig. 10.10 Biotin and enzyme–bound biocytin.

However, there is increasing evidence that suboptimal biotin status may be relatively common.

The few early reports of biotin deficiency all concerned people who consumed abnormally large amounts of uncooked eggs. More recently, signs of biotin deficiency (hair loss and a scaly erythematous dermatitis) have been observed in patients receiving total parenteral nutrition for prolonged periods.

The structure of biotin is shown in Figure 10.10; it occurs in foods covalently bound to proteins by the formation of a peptide bond between the carboxyl group of the side-chain and the ε-amino group of a lysine residue, forming biocytin (biotinyl-lysine). Biocytin is hydrolysed by biotinidase in the pancreatic juice and intestinal mucosal secretions.

Metabolically, biotin is of central importance in lipogenesis and gluconeogenesis, acting as the coenzyme for carboxylation reactions. In addition, it induces the synthesis of a number of key enzymes of glycolysis and gluconeogenesis. It is essential for cell proliferation, acting to biotinylate histones and so regulate the cell cycle.

Biotin deficiency in experimental animals is teratogenic, and a number of the resultant defects resemble human birth defects. Up to half of women in the first trimester of pregnancy show metabolic abnormalities that respond to supplements of biotin, suggesting that marginal status may be widespread, and a possible factor in the aetiology of some birth defects.

There is little information concerning biotin requirements, and no evidence on which to base recommendations. Average intakes range between 15 and 70 μg/day. The safe and adequate range of intakes is set at 10–200 μg/day; the US/Canadian adequate intake for adults is 30 μg/day.

KEY POINTS

- Biotin functions as a coenzyme in carboxylation reactions, and has a role in regulating the cell cycle.
- Clinical deficiency of biotin occurs only in people consuming large amounts of uncooked egg white or receiving long-term total parenteral nutrition.
- Marginal biotin status is common in women in the first trimester of pregnancy, and may be associated with birth defects.
- There is no evidence on which to base estimates of requirements.

Further reading

Section 10.1 – Thiamin

Bender DA: Chapter 6, Thiamin. *In: Nutritional biochemistry of the vitamins*, ed 2, New York, 2003, Cambridge University Press.

Butterworth RF: Thiamin deficiency and brain disorders, *Nutrition Research Reviews* 16(2):277–283, 2003.

Section 10.2 – Riboflavin

Bates CJ: Human requirements for riboflavin, *American Journal of Clinical Nutrition* 46:122–123, 1987.

Bender DA: Chapter 7, Riboflavin. *In: Nutritional biochemistry of the vitamins*, ed 2, New York, 2003, Cambridge University Press.

McNulty H, McKinley MC, Wilson B, et al: Impaired functioning of thermolabile methylenetetrahydrofolate reductase is dependent on riboflavin status: implications for riboflavin requirements, *American Journal of Clinical Nutrition* 76:436–441, 2002.

Powers HJ: Riboflavin (vitamin B2) and health, *American Journal of*

Clinical Nutrition 77(6):1352–1360 Review, 2003.

Section 10.3 – Niacin
Bender DA: Chapter 8, Niacin. In: Nutritional biochemistry of the vitamins, ed 2, New York, 2003, Cambridge University Press.

Bender DA, Bender AE: Niacin and tryptophan metabolism: the biochemical basis of niacin requirements and recommendations, Nutrition Abstracts and Reviews (Series A) 56:695–719, 1986.

Takasawa S: Recent advances in physiological and pathological significance of NAD$^+$ metabolites: Roles of poly(ADP-ribose) and cyclic ADP-ribose in insulin secretion and diabetogenesis, Nutrition Research Reviews 16(2): 253–266, 2003.

Young GS, Kirkland JB: The role of dietary niacin intake and the adenosine-5'-diphosphate-ribosyl cyclase enzyme CD38 in spatial learning ability: is cyclic adenosine diphosphate ribose the link between diet and behaviour? Nutrition Research Reviews 21:42–55, 2008.

Section 10.4 – Vitamin B$_6$
Bender DA: Oestrogens and vitamin B$_6$ – actions and interactions, World Review of Nutrition and Dietetics 51:140–188, 1987.

Bender DA: Non-nutritional uses of vitamin B$_6$, British Journal of Nutrition 81:7–20, 1999.

Bender DA: Chapter 9, Vitamin B$_6$. In: Nutritional biochemistry of the vitamins, ed 2, New York, 2003, Cambridge University Press.

Oka T: Modulation of gene expression by vitamin B$_6$, Nutrition Research Reviews 14:257–265, 2001.

Ubbink JB: The role of vitamins in the pathogenesis and treatment of hyperhomocyst(e)inaemia, Journal of Inherited Metabolic Disease 20:316–325, 1997.

Section 10.5 – Folates
Bailey LB, Gregory JF, 3rd: Folate metabolism and requirements, Journal of Nutrition 129:779–782, 1999.

Bender DA: Chapter 10, Folic acid and vitamin B$_{12}$. In: Nutritional biochemistry of the vitamins, ed 2, New York, 2003, Cambridge University Press.

Brouwer IA, van Dusseldorp, M, West CE, Steegers-Theunissen RPM: Bioavailability and bioefficacy of folate and folic acid in man, Nutrition Research Reviews 14:267–293, 2001.

Choi SW, Mason JB: Folate and carcinogenesis: an integrated scheme, Journal of Nutrition 130:129–132, 2000.

Scientific Advisory Committee on Nutrition: Folate and disease prevention, The Stationery Office (available from http://www.sacn.gov.uk/pdfs/folate_and_disease_prevention_report.pdf), 2006.

Section 10.6 – Vitamin B$_{12}$
Bender DA: Chapter 10, Folic acid and vitamin B$_{12}$. In: Nutritional biochemistry of the vitamins, ed 2, New York, 2003, Cambridge University Press.

Carmel R: Current concepts in cobalamin deficiency, Annual Review of Medicine 51:357–375, 2000.

Section 10.7 – Vitamin C
Bender DA: Chapter 13, Vitamin C. In: Nutritional biochemistry of the vitamins, ed 2, New York, 2003, Cambridge University Press.

Benzie IF: Vitamin C: prospective functional markers for defining optimal nutritional status, Proceedings of the Nutrition Society 58:469–476, 1999.

Halliwell B: Vitamin C and genomic stability, Mutation Research 475:29–35, 2001.

Wilson JX: Regulation of vitamin C transport, Annual Review of Nutrition 25:105–125, 2005.

Section 10.8 – Pantothenic acid
Bender DA: Chapter 12, Pantothenic acid. In: Nutritional biochemistry of the vitamins, ed 2, New York, 2003, Cambridge University Press.

Tahiliani AG, Beinlich CJ: Pantothenic acid in health and disease, Vitamins and Hormones 46:165–228, 1991.

Section 10.9 – Biotin
Bender DA: Chapter 11, Biotin. In: Nutritional biochemistry of the vitamins, ed 2, New York, 2003, Cambridge University Press.

McMahon RJ: Biotin in metabolism and molecular biology, Annual Review of Nutrition 22:221–239, 2002.

Zempleni J, Mock DM: Biotin homeostasis during the cell cycle, Nutrition Research Reviews 14:45–64, 2001.

Zempleni J: Uptake, localisation, and noncarboxylase roles of biotin, Annual Review of Nutrition 25:175–196, 2005.

Chapter 11

Fat-soluble vitamins

David A Bender

CHAPTER CONTENTS

OBJECTIVES

By the end of this chapter you should be able to:
- identify the compounds classified as fat-soluble vitamins
- identify good food sources of each
- summarise the absorption and transport of each
- summarise the main metabolic functions of each

© 2010 Elsevier Ltd/Inc/BV
DOI: 10.1016/B978-0-7020-3118-2.00011-5

- describe the main effects of deficiency and excess of each
- be aware of the methods of assessment of status
- discuss the basis for dietary requirements
- appreciate the metabolic interactions between fat-soluble vitamins and other nutrients.

11.1 VITAMIN A: RETINOIDS AND CAROTENOIDS

Vitamin A deficiency is a serious problem of public health nutrition, second only to protein-energy malnutrition worldwide, and is probably the most important cause of preventable blindness among children in developing countries. Marginal deficiency is a factor in childhood susceptibility to infection, and hence morbidity and mortality, in developing countries. Even in developed countries

vitamin A (along with iron) is the nutrient most likely to be supplied in marginal amounts.

Preformed vitamin A (retinol) is found only in animals and a small number of bacteria. β-Carotene and some of the other carotenes in plants can be oxidised to retinol. The main physiologically active forms of vitamin A are retinaldehyde (in the visual system) and retinoic acid, which modulates gene expression and tissue differentiation.

FORMS IN FOODS AND GOOD FOOD SOURCES

The term vitamin A includes both provitamin A carotenoids, and retinol and its active metabolites. The term retinoid is used to include retinol and its derivatives and analogues, either naturally occurring or synthetic, with or without the biological activity of the vitamin. The main biologically active retinoids are shown in Figure 11.1; until the late

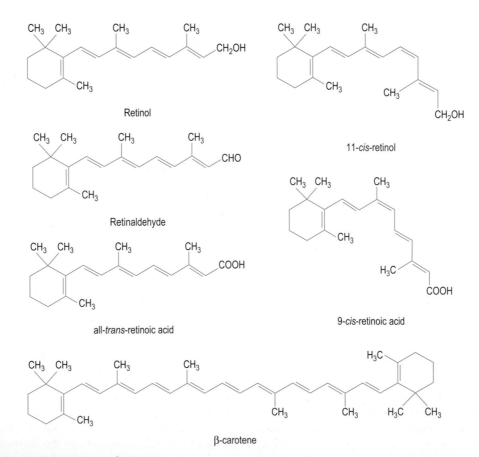

Fig. 11.1 Vitamin A vitamers and β-carotene.

1990s only retinol, retinaldehyde, all-*trans*- and 9-*cis*-retinoic acid were known to be biologically active, but a number of other retinoids are now known to have important functions (see Fig. *evolve* 11.1 🖰).

Free retinol is chemically unstable, and the main form in foods is the palmitate. Retinoic acid occurs in foods in only small amounts. Liver, full-fat dairy produce, fortified margarine, oily fish and kidneys are good sources of retinol (see Table *evolve* 11.1 🖰).

Carotenes that can be oxidised to retinaldehyde are known as provitamin A carotenoids. Relatively few foods are rich sources of retinol, so that carotenes are nutritionally important. In developed countries, with a relatively high intake of animal foods, some 25–30% of vitamin A is derived from carotenoids; in developing countries 80% or more of vitamin A is from carotenoids. The major dietary carotenoids are shown in Figure *evolve* 11.2 🖰. Good dietary sources of carotenes are dark green, yellow, red and orange fruits and vegetables (see Table *evolve* 11.2 🖰 for information about carotenoid-rich foods and Table *evolve* 11.3 🖰 for foods rich in total vitamin A).

International units and retinol equivalents

The international unit of vitamin A activity (now obsolete), was based on biological assay of the ability of the test compound to support growth in animals; 1 iu = 10.47 nmol of retinol = 0.3 μg free retinol or 0.344 μg retinyl acetate.

The total vitamin A content of foods is expressed as μg retinol equivalents – the sum of that provided by retinoids and that from carotenoids; 6 μg β-carotene is 1 μg retinol equivalent. β-Carotene is absorbed very much better from milk than from other foods, and in milk 2 μg β-carotene is 1 μg retinol equivalent. Other provitamin A carotenoids yield a maximum of half the retinol of β-carotene, and 12 μg of these compounds = 1 μg retinol equivalent. On this basis, 1 iu of vitamin A activity = 1.8 μg β-carotene or 3.6 μg of other provitamin A carotenoids.

In 2001 the USA/Canadian Dietary Reference Values report introduced the term *retinol activity equivalent* (RAE) to take account of the incomplete absorption and metabolism of carotenoids; 1 RAE = 1 μg all-*trans*-retinol, 12 μg β-carotene, 24 μg α-carotene or β-cryptoxanthin. On this basis, 1 iu of vitamin A activity = 3.6 μg β-carotene or 7.2 μg of other provitamin A carotenoids.

ABSORPTION AND TRANSPORT OF VITAMIN A

Dietary retinyl esters are hydrolysed by intestinal lipases, and 70–90% of dietary retinol is absorbed. Uptake into enterocytes is by facilitated diffusion from lipid micelles, followed by esterification to retinyl palmitate, with small amounts of other esters. Retinyl esters enter the lymphatic circulation, and then the bloodstream, in chylomicrons, together with dietary lipid and carotenoids.

Carotenoids are absorbed dissolved in lipid micelles. The absorption of carotene is between 5 and 60%, depending on the nature of the food, whether it is cooked or raw, and the amount of fat in the meal. Provitamin A carotenoids undergo oxidative cleavage to retinaldehyde in the intestinal mucosa, catalysed by carotene dioxygenase. Retinaldehyde is reduced to retinol, then esterified and secreted in chylomicrons.

Only a relatively small proportion of carotene is oxidised in the intestinal mucosa, and a significant amount of carotene enters the circulation in chylomicrons. There is some hepatic cleavage of carotene taken up from chylomicron remnants, again giving rise to retinaldehyde and retinyl esters; the remainder is secreted in very low density lipoproteins, and may be taken up and cleaved by carotene dioxygenase in extrahepatic tissues.

Central oxidative cleavage of β-carotene gives rise to two molecules of retinaldehyde, which can be reduced to retinol. However, the biological activity of β-carotene on a molar basis is considerably lower than that of retinol, not two-fold higher as might be expected. Three factors may account for this: limited absorption of carotenoids from the intestinal lumen, limited activity of carotene dioxygenase and excentric (asymmetric) cleavage. In addition, other carotenoids in the diet, which are not substrates, such as canthaxanthin and zeaxanthin, may inhibit carotene dioxygenase.

Tissues can take up retinyl esters from chylomicrons, but most is left in the chylomicron remnants that are cleared by the liver. Retinyl esters are hydrolysed and free retinol is transferred to the rough endoplasmic reticulum, where it binds to apo-retinol binding protein (RBP). Holo-RBP is secreted as a 1 : 1 complex with the thyroid hormone binding protein, transthyretin. Impaired synthesis of RBP in protein-energy malnutrition can result in failure of retinol release from the liver, and hence functional vitamin A deficiency, even if liver reserves are adequate.

Binding to RBP serves to maintain the vitamin in aqueous solution, protects it against oxidation, and also delivers the vitamin to target tissues. RBP is a small molecule, which would be filtered by the kidney; formation of the complex between RBP and transthyretin prevents urinary loss of retinol. Moderate renal damage, or the increased permeability of the glomerulus in infection, may result in considerable loss of vitamin A bound to RBP–transthyretin.

Cell surface receptors in target tissues take up retinol from the RBP–transthyretin complex. The receptors also remove the carboxy terminal arginine residue from RBP, so inactivating it, and apo-RBP is catabolised in the kidney, not recycled.

Retinoic acid is the main metabolite of retinol. It is not a catabolic product, but the ligand for nuclear receptors involved in modulation of gene expression. It may be formed in liver, although there is no hepatic storage, and is then transported bound to serum albumin rather than retinol binding protein. Other tissues are also able to form retinoic acid from retinol, but retinoic acid cannot be reduced back to retinol or retinaldehyde.

The main excretory product of both retinol and retinoic acid is retinoyl glucuronide, which is secreted in the bile. At high levels of intake the capacity to metabolise retinol is saturated; excess retinol is toxic.

METABOLIC FUNCTIONS OF VITAMIN A

Vitamin A has four metabolic roles: as the prosthetic group of the visual pigments; as a nuclear modulator of gene expression; as a carrier of mannosyl units in the synthesis of hydrophobic glycoproteins; and in the retinoylation of proteins. The major targets for retinoylation are the regulatory subunits of cAMP-dependent protein kinases, suggesting a role for retinoic acid in modulation of the actions of cell-surface-acting hormones and neurotransmitters.

Retinol and retinaldehyde in the visual cycle

The light-sensitive pigment in the photoreceptor cells of the retina is retinaldehyde bound to the protein opsin; excitation by a single photon results in the propagation of a nerve impulse.

The pigment epithelium of the retina isomerises all-*trans*-retinol to 11-*cis*-retinol, which may either be stored as esters or be oxidised to 11-*cis*-retinaldehyde and transported to the photoreceptor cells bound to the inter-photoreceptor retinoid binding protein.

11-*cis*-Retinaldehyde binds to a lysine residue in opsin, forming rhodopsin. Opsins are cell-type specific; they serve to shift the absorption of 11-*cis*-retinaldehyde from the ultraviolet into what we call, in consequence, the visible range – either a relatively broad spectrum of sensitivity for vision in dim light (in the rods, with an absorbance peak at 500 nm) or more defined spectral peaks for differentiation of colours in stronger light (in the cones), with absorption maxima at 425 (blue), 530 (green) or 560 nm (red), depending on the cell type.

The absorption of light by rhodopsin results in a change in the configuration of the retinaldehyde from the 11-*cis* to the all-*trans* isomer, together with a conformational change in opsin. This results in both the release of retinaldehyde from the protein and the initiation of a nerve impulse. The overall process is known as bleaching, since it results in the loss of the colour of rhodopsin.

Under conditions of low light intensity, the all-*trans*-retinaldehyde released from rhodopsin is reduced to all-*trans*-retinol, which is then transported to the pigment epithelium bound to the inter-photoreceptor retinoid binding protein. Under conditions of high light intensity, all-*trans*-retinaldehyde undergoes photoisomerisation to 11-*cis*-retinaldehyde and reduction to 11-*cis*-retinol in the photoreceptor cell.

The rate-limiting step in initiation of the visual cycle is the regeneration of 11-*cis*-retinaldehyde. In vitamin A deficiency, when there is little stored 11-*cis*-retinyl ester in the pigment epithelium, both the time taken to adapt to darkness and the ability to see in poor light are impaired.

Genomic actions of retinoic acid

Retinoic acid has both a general role in growth and a specific morphogenic role in development and tissue differentiation. These functions are the result of nuclear actions, modulating gene expression by activation of nuclear receptors. Both deficiency and excess of retinoic acid cause severe developmental abnormalities.

There are two families of nuclear retinoid receptors: the retinoic acid receptors (RAR), which bind all-*trans*-retinoic acid, and the retinoid X receptors (RXR), so called because their physiological ligand was unknown when they were first discovered. It is now known to be 9-*cis*-retinoic acid, which also binds to, and activates, the retinoic acid receptors. A number of other retinoids also bind to, and activate, the RAR family of receptors, at physiological concentrations, but do not bind to the RXR family.

RXR forms active homodimers, and also forms heterodimers with the calcitriol (vitamin D) receptor, the thyroid hormone receptor, the peroxisome proliferation activated receptor (PPAR, whose physiological ligand is a long-chain polyunsaturated fatty acid derivative), and the chicken ovalbumin upstream promoter (COUP) receptor, an orphan receptor whose physiological ligand is unknown.

In the presence of all-*trans*- or 9-*cis*-retinoic acid the receptor heterodimers are transcriptional activators. However, the heterodimers will also bind to DNA in the absence of retinoic acid, in which case they act as repressors of gene expression.

EFFECTS OF VITAMIN A DEFICIENCY AND EXCESS

Vitamin A deficiency (xerophthalmia) is a major problem of children under 5 in developing countries, being the single most common preventable cause of blindness. The increased susceptibility to infection and impairment of immune responses in vitamin A deficiency cause significant childhood mortality, and a number of trials of vitamin A supplementation in areas of endemic deficiency show a 20–35% reduction in child mortality.

A mild infection such as measles commonly triggers the development of xerophthalmia in children whose vitamin A status is marginal. In addition to functional deficiency as a result of impaired synthesis of retinol binding protein and transthyretin in response to infection, there may be considerable urinary loss of vitamin A due to increased renal epithelial permeability and proteinuria, permitting loss of retinol bound to RBP–transthyretin. Vitamin A supplements are generally recommended for children who have been hospitalised with measles.

In adults, excessive alcohol consumption reduces liver reserves of vitamin A, both as a result of alcoholic liver damage and also by induction of cytochrome P450 enzymes that catalyse the oxidation of retinol to retinoic acid (as also occurs with chronic use of barbiturates).

Mild deficiency results in impaired dark adaptation; as the deficiency progresses there is inability to see in dim light (night blindness). More prolonged and severe deficiency leads to conjunctival xerosis – squamous metaplasia and keratinisation of the epithelial cells of the conjunctiva with loss of goblet cells in the conjunctival mucosa, leading to dryness, wrinkling and thickening of the cornea (xerophthalmia). As the deficiency progresses, so there is keratinisation of the cornea. At this stage the condition is still reversible, although there may be residual scarring of the cornea. In advanced xerosis, yellow-grey foamy patches of keratinised cells and bacteria (Bitot's spots) may accumulate on the surface of the conjunctiva. Finally there is ulceration of the cornea due to increased proteolytic action, causing irreversible blindness. Table *evolve* 11.4 🕮 shows the WHO classification of xerophthalmia.

Other epithelia are affected by vitamin A deficiency, earlier than the more readily observed diagnostic changes in the eye. There is increased intestinal permeability to disaccharides, and later a reduction in the number of goblet cells and mucus secretion. There is also atrophy of respiratory epithelium, with loss of goblet cells, and keratinisation.

Toxicity of vitamin A

Vitamin A is both acutely and chronically toxic. Acutely, large doses of vitamin A (in excess of 300 mg in a single dose to adults) cause nausea, vomiting and headache, which disappear within a few days. After a very large dose there may also be itching and exfoliation of the skin, and extremely high doses can prove fatal. Single doses of 60 mg of retinol are given to children in developing countries as a prophylactic against vitamin A deficiency – an amount adequate to meet the child's needs for 4–6 months. About 1% of children so treated show transient signs of toxicity, but this is considered to be acceptable in view of the considerable benefit of preventing xerophthalmia.

The chronic toxicity of vitamin A is a more general cause for concern; prolonged and regular intake of more than about 7500–9000 µg/day by adults (and significantly less for children) causes signs and symptoms of toxicity affecting the skin, central nervous system, liver and bones.

Carotenoids do not cause hypervitaminosis A, because of the limited oxidation to retinol. Accumulation of even abnormally large amounts of carotene seems to have no short-term adverse effects, although plasma, body fat and skin can have a strong orange-yellow colour (hypercarotinaemia) following prolonged high intakes. However, two large-scale intervention trials have shown an increased incidence of cancers in people receiving high dose supplements of β-carotene. The adverse effect of β-carotene supplementation was largely confined to heavy smokers.

Synthetic retinoids used to treat dermatological conditions are highly teratogenic. By extrapolation, it has been assumed that retinol is also teratogenic, although there is little evidence, and it has been suggested that the plasma concentration associated with teratogenic effects is unlikely to be reached with intakes below 7500 µg/day. Nevertheless, as a precaution, pregnant women are advised not to consume more than 3000–3300 µg/day.

ASSESSMENT OF VITAMIN A STATUS

An early sign of vitamin A deficiency is impaired dark adaptation – an increase in the time taken to adapt to seeing in dim light. The apparatus required is not suitable for use in field studies, or for use with children (the group most at risk from deficiency), and the dark adaptation test is largely of historical interest.

Criteria of vitamin A status are shown in Table *evolve* 11.5 🖰. Because retinol binding protein is released from liver only as the holo-protein, and apo-RBP is cleared from the circulation rapidly after tissue uptake of retinol, the fasting plasma concentration of retinol remains constant over a wide range of intakes. It is only when liver reserves are nearly depleted that plasma retinol falls significantly, and it only rises significantly at the onset of toxic signs.

Interpretation of plasma concentrations of retinol is confounded by the fact that both RBP and transthyretin are negative acute phase proteins, and their synthesis falls, and hence the plasma concentration of retinol falls, in response to infection. Similarly, both protein-energy malnutrition and zinc deficiency result in a low plasma concentration, despite possibly adequate liver reserves, as a result of impaired synthesis of RBP.

The most sensitive assessment of vitamin A status is the relative dose response test – a test of the ability of a dose of vitamin A to raise the plasma concentration of retinol several hours later, after chylomicrons have been cleared from the circulation. In subjects who are retinol deficient, a test dose will produce a large increase in plasma retinol, because of the accumulation of apo-retinol binding protein in the liver; in those whose problem is due to lack of retinol binding protein then little of the dose will be released into the circulation. A relative dose response greater than 20% indicates depletion of liver reserves of retinol to less than 70 µmol/kg.

Early changes in vitamin A deficiency include loss of the mucus secreting goblet cells from the conjunctival epithelium, and the appearance of enlarged, flattened and partially keratinised epithelial cells. An impression of the conjunctiva is taken by blotting onto cellulose acetate, then fixing and staining prior to histological examination. The technique identifies children who do not yet show any clinical signs, and whose serum retinol is within the normal range.

THE BASIS OF DIETARY REQUIREMENTS

On the basis of depletion/repletion studies in a very small number of people, the reference intake for adult men was set at 1000 µg retinol equivalent, with a minimum physiological requirement of 600 µg/day. Requirements have been estimated by measuring turnover of the vitamin using a radioactive tracer. The fractional catabolic rate is 0.5%/day; assuming 50% 'efficiency' of storage of dietary retinol, this gives a mean requirement of 6.7 µg/kg body weight, and a reference intake of 650–700 µg for adult men.

Although there is some evidence that carotenoids may have actions in their own right, apart from provitamin A activity, there is no evidence on which to base any recommendations or suggestions of requirements other than as a precursor of retinol.

Vitamin A and carotene in cancer prevention

Since the discovery of vitamin A, the observation of hyperplasia and loss of differentiation of squamous epithelium in deficiency has raised speculation that the vitamin may be associated with carcinogenesis – either that deficiency may be a risk factor for cancer, or that increased intake may be protective.

Deficient animals develop more spontaneous tumours, and are more sensitive to chemical carcinogens.

The doses of retinol that are protective in animals are in the toxic range and therefore unlikely to be useful in cancer therapy or prevention. A number of synthetic retinoids have been developed, in a search for compounds that show anti-cancer activity, but are metabolised, stored and transported differently, or bind to different subtypes of retinoid receptor, and so are less toxic.

In addition to their importance as precursors of vitamin A, carotenes can also act, at least in vitro (and under conditions of low oxygen tension), as antioxidants, trapping singlet oxygen generated by photochemical reactions or lipid peroxidation of membranes. Epidemiological and case-control studies show a negative association between β-carotene intake and a number of cancers, suggesting that β-carotene may have a protective effect against some forms of cancer, and hence a function in its own right, not simply as a precursor of retinol. In an intervention trial in China, supplements of β-carotene, vitamin E and selenium to a malnourished population led to a reduction in mortality from a variety of cancers. However, intervention trials in Finland (in which heavy smokers were given supplements of β-carotene and/or vitamin E) and USA (involving smokers and people who had been exposed to asbestos dust, who received β-carotene and retinyl palmitate) both showed increased lung cancer mortality among those receiving carotene supplements. The UK Food Standards Agency has advised that smokers should not take β-carotene supplements.

KEY POINTS

■ Vitamin A deficiency is a major public health problem worldwide, and the commonest preventable cause of blindness among children in developing countries.

■ Vitamin A may be provided as preformed retinol, or it may be synthesised from dietary carotenoids. The absorption and oxidation of carotene is poor, and the yield of retinol is significantly less than would be predicted.

■ Vitamin A has two main functions: as the prosthetic group of the visual pigments, and as the ligand for a variety of nuclear receptors that regulate gene expression and tissue differentiation.

■ In addition to their role as precursors of retinol, carotenoids may act as antioxidants.

■ Vitamin A deficiency causes corneal damage and blindness; even mild deficiency severely impairs immune responses.

■ Functional vitamin A deficiency can occur despite adequate liver stores in protein-energy malnutrition and zinc deficiency, because of failure of synthesis of the retinol binding protein that is required for plasma transport.

■ Vitamin A is both acutely and chronically toxic in excess, and is also teratogenic.

■ Vitamin A status is assessed by measurement of the plasma concentration of the vitamin or retinol binding protein, by measurement of the increase in plasma concentration several hours after a test dose (the relative dose response) or by conjunctival impression cytology.

■ Vitamin A requirements have been estimated by measuring the fractional rate of turnover during depletion/repletion studies. There is no evidence on which to base estimates of requirements for carotene except as a precursor of retinol.

11.2 VITAMIN D

Vitamin D is not strictly a vitamin, rather it is the precursor of one of the hormones involved in calcium homeostasis and the regulation of cell proliferation and differentiation, where it has both endocrine and paracrine actions. Dietary sources are relatively unimportant compared with endogenous synthesis in the skin; problems of deficiency arise when there is inadequate exposure to sunlight. The deficiency diseases (rickets in children and osteomalacia in adults) are therefore largely problems of temperate and sub-arctic regions, although cultural factors that result in little exposure to sunlight may also cause problems in subtropical and tropical areas. Few foods are rich sources of vitamin D, and it is generally accepted that supplements are necessary for young children and the house-bound elderly. Excessively high intakes of vitamin D are associated with hypercalcaemia and calcinosis.

The active metabolite of vitamin D, calcitriol, acts like a steroid hormone, binding to a nuclear receptor protein in target tissues and regulating gene expression. As a result of studies of the distribution of calcitriol receptors and the induced proteins, a number of functions have been discovered for the vitamin other than in the maintenance of calcium balance, including roles in cell proliferation and differentiation, in the modulation of immune system responses and in the secretion of insulin, and thyroid and parathyroid hormones. Calcitriol also has rapid actions, acting via cell surface receptors.

FORMS IN FOODS AND GOOD FOOD SOURCES

Two compounds have the biological activity of vitamin D, cholecalciferol (vitamin D_3), which is the compound formed in the skin, and ergocalciferol (vitamin D_2), which is synthesised by ultraviolet irradiation of ergosterol (Fig. 11.2).

The (obsolete) international unit of vitamin D activity is equivalent to 25 ng (65 pmol) cholecalciferol. 1 μg cholecalciferol is equivalent to 40 iu; 1 nmol is 104 iu. Cholecalciferol and ergocalciferol are not equipotent, because there is faster metabolic clearance of ergocalciferol and hence less formation of active metabolites. The active metabolites, calcitriol and ercalcitriol, are equipotent.

There are few dietary sources of cholecalciferol; the richest sources are oily fish, and especially fish liver oils, although eggs also contain a relatively large amount, and there is a modest amount in full fat milk products and liver (see Table evolve 11.6). In many countries margarine, and sometimes also milk, is fortified with ergocalciferol. No common plant foods contain vitamin D.

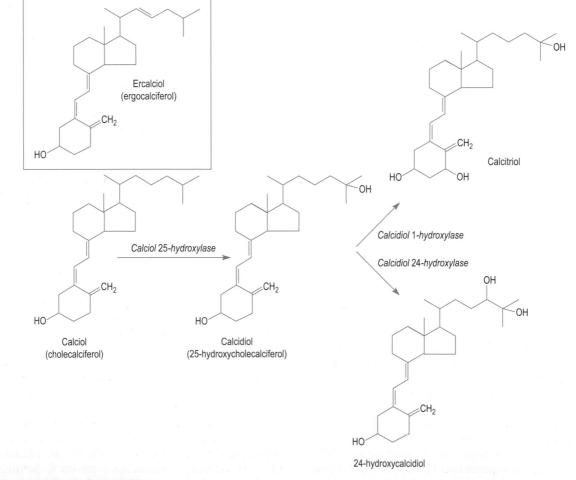

Fig. 11.2 Vitamin D metabolism.

ABSORPTION, TRANSPORT AND METABOLISM OF VITAMIN D

Dietary vitamin D is absorbed in chylomicrons and taken up rapidly by the liver as chylomicron remnants are cleared from the circulation. Vitamin D synthesised in the skin is bound to a plasma binding protein and is metabolised more gradually.

Cholecalciferol and its active metabolites (calcidiol, calcitriol and 24-hydroxycalcidiol) are all transported bound to the same plasma binding protein – Gc-globulin, also known as the 'group-specific component' or transcalciferin. Cholecalciferol is also transported in plasma lipoproteins, so that about 60% is normally bound to Gc-globulin and 40% is in lipoproteins. In addition to its role in the plasma transport of vitamin D, Gc-globulin represents the major storage site for the vitamin, mainly as calcidiol.

Both dietary and endogenously synthesised vitamin D undergo 25-hydroxylation in the liver to yield calcidiol (25-hydroxycholecalciferol), which is the main circulating form of the vitamin. This undergoes 1-hydroxylation in the kidney to produce the active hormone calcitriol (1,25-dihydroxycholecalciferol), or 24-hydroxylation in the kidney and other tissues, to yield 24-hydroxycalcidiol (24,25-dihydroxycholecalciferol). Calcitriol also undergoes 24-hydroxylation, followed by oxidation to calcitroic acid, which is the main excretory product of the vitamin (see Fig. *evolve* 11.3 and Table *evolve* 11.7).

There is little storage of vitamin D in the liver, except in oily fish. In human liver, concentrations of vitamin D do not exceed about 25 nmol/kg, and the main storage of the vitamin is as plasma calcidiol.

Photosynthesis of cholecalciferol in the skin

Cholecalciferol is formed non-enzymically in the skin by ultraviolet (UV) irradiation of 7-dehydrocholesterol, an intermediate in the synthesis of cholesterol that accumulates in skin, but not other tissues. In addition to low exposure to sunlight, the elderly are at risk of vitamin D deficiency because of decreased formation of 7-dehydrocholesterol in the epidermis.

The peak wavelength for the reaction of 7-dehydrocholesterol to precalciferol is 296.5 nm; for practical purposes the useful range of solar radiation is the UV-B range, between 290 and 320 nm, although at 310 nm the yield is only 1% of that at 296.5 nm. Precalciferol undergoes slow isomerisation to cholecalciferol. Excessive sunlight exposure does not cause hypervitaminosis, because the photolysis of 7-dehydrocholesterol is reversible, yielding either 7-dehydrocholesterol or lumisterol, which does not undergo reaction to yield precalciferol. In addition, precalciferol undergoes photo-isomerisation to tachysterol, which is biologically inactive (see Fig. *evolve* 11.4).

Sunshine is not strictly essential for synthesis of cholecalciferol, since UV-B penetrates cloud reasonably well; it also penetrates light clothing. However, low intensity irradiation does not result in significant formation of previtamin D. In temperate regions (beyond about 40°N or S), the intensity of UV-B is below the threshold in winter, so there is unlikely to be any significant cutaneous synthesis of the vitamin, and plasma concentrations of calcidiol show a marked seasonal variation in temperate regions. There is no evidence that skin pigmentation has any significant effect on the synthesis of cholecalciferol.

REGULATION OF VITAMIN D METABOLISM

The main physiological function of vitamin D is in the control of calcium homeostasis, and in turn vitamin D metabolism is regulated largely by the state of calcium balance. The activities of the kidney calcidiol 1- and 24-hydroxylases are regulated in opposite directions and early studies suggested that 24-hydroxylation was a pathway for inactivation of vitamin D, although there is some evidence that 24-hydroxycalcidiol has biological actions. The major determinant of the relative activities of calcidiol 1- and 24-hydroxylases is the availability of calcitriol. It is likely that the high prevalence of vitamin D deficiency among people from the Indian subcontinent is due to genetically determined high activity of calcidiol 24-hydroxylase rather than cultural and dietary factors.

Parathyroid hormone acts to raise plasma calcium by effects on bone resorption and renal reabsorption of calcium, and by regulating the metabolism of vitamin D. It increases the activity of 1-hydroxylase and decreases that of 24-hydroxylase. In turn, calcitriol represses expression of the parathyroid hormone gene. In chronic renal failure there is reduced synthesis of calcitriol, leading to the development of secondary hyperparathyroidism, with excessive mobilisation of bone mineral, hypercalcaemia, hypercalciuria, hyper-phosphaturia and the development of calcium phosphate renal stones.

Calcitonin is secreted by the C-cells of the thyroid gland in response to hypercalcaemia. Its primary action is to oppose the actions of parathyroid hormone by suppressing osteoclast actions. It also stimulates calcidiol 1-hydroxylation in the kidney.

METABOLIC FUNCTIONS OF VITAMIN D

Calcitriol maintains the plasma concentration of calcium by increasing intestinal absorption of calcium, reducing excretion by increasing reabsorption in the distal renal tubule, and mobilising the mineral from bone.

Calcitriol binds to, and activates, nuclear receptors that modulate gene expression. More than 50 genes are known to be regulated by calcitriol, including: calcidiol 1- and 24-hydroxylases; calbindin, a calcium binding protein in the intestinal mucosa and other tissues; the vitamin-K-dependent protein osteocalcin in bone; osteopontin, which permits the attachment of osteoclasts to bone surfaces; and the osteoclast cell membrane protein integrin. In addition, calcitriol affects the secretion of insulin and the synthesis and secretion of parathyroid and thyroid hormones – these actions may be secondary to changes in intracellular calcium concentrations resulting from induction of calbindin. Calcitriol also has a role in the regulation of cell proliferation and differentiation.

The vitamin D receptor acts as a heterodimer with the RXR retinoid receptor. Binding of calcitriol permits dimerisation with occupied or unoccupied RXR, leading to activation. Abnormally high concentrations of 9-*cis*-retinoic acid result in sequestration of RXR as the homodimers, meaning that it is unavailable to form heterodimers with the vitamin D receptor; excessive vitamin A can therefore antagonise the nuclear actions of vitamin D.

In addition to its nuclear actions, calcitriol has two non-genomic actions:

1. In intestinal mucosal cells it acts to recruit membrane calcium transport proteins from intracellular vesicles to the cell surface, resulting in a rapid increase in calcium absorption, before there has been induction of calbindin.

2. In a variety of cells it acts via cell-surface receptors, leading to opening of intracellular calcium channels and activation of protein kinase C and mitogen-activated protein kinases (MAP kinases). The effect of this is inhibition of cell proliferation, and induction of differentiation.

Calcitriol affects the proliferation, differentiation and immune function of lymphocytes and mono-cytes. Activated macrophages have calcidiol 1-hydroxylase, and can synthesise calcitriol from calcidiol, suggesting that in addition to its endocrine role calcitriol may have a paracrine or autocrine role in the immune system.

Calcitriol receptors have been identified in a variety of tumour cells. At low concentrations it is a growth promoter, while at higher concentrations it has both antiproliferative and pro-apoptotic actions in cancer cells in culture. There is an epidemiological association between low vitamin D status and prostate and colorectal cancer.

Adipocytes have vitamin D receptors, and there is evidence that vitamin D suppresses adipocyte development. It has been suggested that vitamin D inadequacy may be a factor in the development of the metabolic syndrome ('syndrome X', the combination of insulin resistance, hyperlipidaemia and atherosclerosis associated with abdominal obesity). Sunlight exposure, and hence vitamin D status, may be a factor in the difference in incidence of atherosclerosis between northern and southern European countries.

EFFECTS OF VITAMIN D DEFICIENCY AND EXCESS

Rickets is a disease of young children and adolescents, resulting from a failure of the mineralisation of newly formed bone. In infants, epiphyseal cartilage continues to grow, but is not replaced by bone matrix and mineral. The earliest sign of this is craniotabes – the occurrence of unossified areas in the skull. At a later stage there is enlargement of the epiphyses. When the child begins to walk, the weight of the body deforms the undermineralised long bones, leading to bow legs or knock knees, as well as deformity of the pelvis. Similar problems may develop during the adolescent growth spurt.

Osteomalacia is the defective remineralisation of bone during normal bone turnover in adults, so that there is a progressive demineralisation, but with adequate bone matrix, leading to bone pain and skeletal deformities, with muscle weakness. Women with inadequate vitamin D status are especially at risk of osteomalacia after repeated pregnancies, because of the drain on calcium reserves for fetal bone mineralisation and lactation. The elderly are at risk of osteomalacia, because of both decreased synthesis of 7-dehydrocholesterol in the skin with increasing age and low exposure to sunlight.

Osteoporosis, the loss of bone mineral and matrix that may affect 40% of women and 12% of men as they age, is not due to vitamin D deficiency, but an intake of 10–15 µg/day, together with 1200–1500 mg calcium, is recommended for treatment of osteoporosis, together with hormone replacement therapy or treatment with antiresorptive agents such as bisphosphonates.

Vitamin D toxicity

Intoxication with vitamin D causes weakness, nausea, loss of appetite, headache, abdominal pains, cramp and diarrhoea. More seriously, it also causes hypercalcaemia, with plasma concentrations of calcium between 2.75 and 4.5 mmol/l, compared with the normal range of 2.2–2.5 mmol/l. Above 3.75 mmol/l, vascular smooth muscle may contract abnormally, leading to hypertension. Hypercalciuria may also result in the precipitation of calcium phosphate in the renal tubules and the development of urinary calculi. Hypervitaminosis also results in increased uptake of calcium into tissues, leading to calcinosis – the calcification of soft tissues, including kidney, heart, lungs and blood vessels.

Rickets was more or less eradicated as a nutritional deficiency disease during the 1950s, by widespread enrichment of infant foods with vitamin D. However, some children are sensitive to hypercalcaemia and calcinosis with vitamin D intakes as low as 45 µg/day, and the level of enrichment was reduced because of the development of hypercalcaemia in a small number of susceptible infants. As a result, rickets has re-emerged, especially in northern cities in temperate countries.

The tolerable upper level of intake is 50 µg/day for adults and 25 µg/day for infants. Reports of hypercalcaemia in adults have involved intakes in excess of 1000 µg/day.

ASSESSMENT OF VITAMIN D STATUS

Before anatomical deformities are apparent in vitamin-D-deficient children, bone density is lower than normal – radiological rickets. At an earlier stage of deficiency there is a marked elevation of plasma alkaline phosphatase released by osteoblast activity – biochemical rickets.

The plasma concentration of calcidiol is the most sensitive index of vitamin D status, and is correlated with elevated plasma parathyroid hormone and alkaline phosphatase activity. The reference range of plasma calcidiol is between 20 and 150 nmol/l, with a two-fold seasonal variation in temperate regions. Concentrations below 20 nmol/l are considered to indicate impending deficiency, and osteomalacia is seen in adults when plasma calcidiol falls below 10 nmol/l. In children, clinical signs of rickets are seen when plasma calcidiol falls below 20 nmol/l (see Table *evolve* 11.8).

THE BASIS FOR SETTING DIETARY REQUIREMENTS

Dietary vitamin D makes little contribution to status, and the major factor is exposure to sunlight. There are no reference intakes for young adults in UK and Europe; for the house-bound elderly, the reference intake is 10 µg/day, based on the intake required to maintain a plasma concentration of calcidiol of 20 nmol/l. This will almost certainly require supplements of the vitamin, since average intakes are less than half this amount. The US/Canadian adequate intake is 5 µg/day up to age 50, increasing to 10 µg between 51 and 70, and to 15 µg over 70 years of age. However, intakes above 5 µg/day are required to prevent osteoporosis and secondary hyperparathyroidism, and normal sunlight exposure may provide the equivalent of 20–50 µg/day.

There is growing evidence that higher vitamin D status might be protective against various cancers, including prostate and colorectal cancer, and also against prediabetes and the metabolic syndrome. Desirable levels of intake may be considerably higher than the reference intakes discussed above, and could certainly not be met from unfortified foods. While increased sunlight exposure would meet the need, it carries the risk of developing skin cancer.

The vitamin D content of human milk is probably inadequate to meet the requirements of breast-fed infants without exposure to sunlight, especially during the winter, when the mother's reserves of the vitamin are low. Infant formulae normally provide 10 µg of cholecalciferol/day, and a similar amount is recommended for breastfed infants and children aged under 3 years – this maintains the plasma concentration of calcidiol above 20 nmol/l.

KEY POINTS

- Vitamin D is really a steroid hormone, and dietary intake is relatively unimportant compared with sunlight exposure for endogenous synthesis, except for infants and the elderly.
- The main body reserve of vitamin D is circulating calcidiol.
- The main function of vitamin D is in maintenance of calcium homeostasis; it has both nuclear actions to induce synthesis of calcium binding proteins and also rapid actions to enhance calcium uptake into cells and movement of calcium within cells.
- Vitamin D also acts to regulate cell proliferation in a variety of tissues, and is involved in the secretion of a number of hormones.
- Vitamin D deficiency leads to rickets in children and adolescents, and osteomalacia in adults, both of which are due to undermineralisation of bone.
- Osteoporosis in not due to vitamin D deficiency, but vitamin D may be beneficial in treatment.
- There are few rich sources of vitamin D and it is unlikely that requirements of infants and the elderly can be met without the use of supplements or food fortification.
- Intakes of vitamin D considerably higher than are required to prevent deficiency may provide protection against various cancers and the metabolic syndrome.
- Some infants are especially sensitive to hypercalcaemia due to vitamin D toxicity; fortification of infant foods has to avoid endangering these vulnerable people, resulting in a proportion of the population being at risk of developing rickets.

11.3 VITAMIN E

For a long time it was considered that, unlike the other vitamins, vitamin E had no specific functions; rather it was the major lipid-soluble radical trapping antioxidant in membranes. Many of its functions can be met by synthetic antioxidants; however, some of the effects of vitamin E deficiency in experimental animals do not respond to synthetic antioxidants. More recent studies have shown that vitamin E also has roles in cell signalling, by inhibition or inactivation of protein kinase C, and in modulation of gene expression, inhibition of cell proliferation and platelet aggregation. These effects are specific for α-tocopherol, and are independent of the antioxidant properties of the vitamin.

FORMS IN FOOD AND RICH FOOD SOURCES

As shown in Figure 11.3 and Figure *evolve* 11.5, there are eight vitamers of vitamin E; the tocopherols have a saturated side-chain and the tocotrienols an unsaturated. The four forms of each (α, β, γ and δ) differ in the methylation of the ring. Tocotrienols occur in foods as both the free alcohols and as esters; tocopherols occur naturally as the free alcohols, but acetate and succinate esters are used in pharmaceutical preparations because of their greater stability.

The different vitamers have different biological activity (see Table *evolve* 11.9). The (obsolete) international unit of vitamin E potency was equated with the activity of 1 mg of (synthetic) DL-α-tocopherol acetate; on this basis D-α-tocopherol (*RRR*-α-tocopherol, the most potent vitamer) is 1.49 iu/mg. It is now usual to express the vitamin E content of foods in terms of mg equivalents of (*RRR*)-α-tocopherol, based on their biological activities. For the major vitamers present in foods, total α-tocopherol equivalent is calculated as the sum of mg α-tocopherol + 0.4 × mg β-tocopherol + 0.3 × mg γ-tocopherol + 0.01 × mg δ-tocopherol + 0.3 × mg α-tocotrienol + 0.05 × mg β-tocotrienol + 0.01 × mg γ-tocotrienol.

The naturally occurring compound is D-α-tocopherol, in which all three asymmetric centres have the *R*-configuration (2*R*, 4′*R*, 8′*R*, or all-*R* (*RRR*)-α-tocopherol). Chemical synthesis yields a mixture of eight possible stereo-isomers which have different biological activity (all-*rac*-α-tocopherol). The synthetic all-*rac* mixture has 0.74 × the activity of *RRR*-α-tocopherol. In the USA and Canada only the 2*R* isomers are considered to contribute to vitamin E intake, giving an equivalence of 0.45 iu/mg for synthetic all-*rac*-α-tocopherol.

Oily fish, nuts and seeds (and hence vegetable oils), beans and green leafy vegetables are rich sources of vitamin E (see Table *evolve* 11.10).

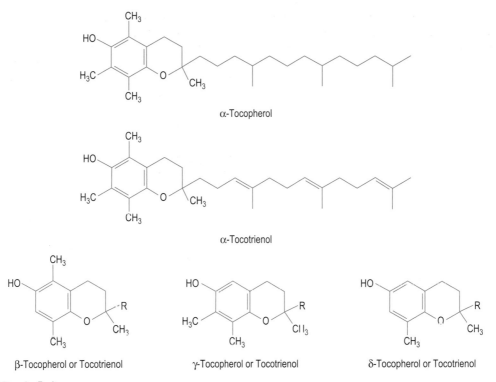

Fig. 11.3 Vitamin E vitamers.

ABSORPTION AND TRANSPORT OF VITAMIN E

Vitamin E is absorbed in micelles with other dietary lipids, but only 20–40% of a test dose is absorbed from the small intestine. Esters are hydrolysed in the intestinal lumen by pancreatic esterase, and also by intracellular esterases in the mucosal cells.

In intestinal mucosal cells, all vitamers of vitamin E are incorporated into chylomicrons, and tissues take up some vitamin E from chylomicrons. Most, however, goes to the liver in chylomicron remnants. α-Tocopherol, which binds to the liver α-tocopherol transfer protein, is then exported in very low density lipoprotein, and is available for tissue uptake. The other vitamers, which do not bind well to the α-tocopherol transfer protein, are not incorporated into VLDL, but are metabolised in the liver and excreted.

Tocopherol can undergo reversible oxidation to an epoxide, followed by ring cleavage to yield a quinone, which is reduced to the hydroquinone and conjugated with glucuronic acid, then excreted in the bile. There may also be significant excretion of the vitamin by the skin.

METABOLIC FUNCTIONS OF VITAMIN E

The best established function of vitamin E is as a lipid-soluble antioxidant in plasma lipoproteins and cell membranes. Many of the antioxidant actions are unspecific, and both selenium and synthetic antioxidants have a vitamin E sparing effect. α-Tocopherol, but not the other vitamers, has a role in modulation of gene expression and regulation of cell proliferation. Dietary tocotrienols, but not tocopherols, have a cholesterol-lowering effect by reducing the activity of HMG CoA reductase.

Antioxidant functions of vitamin E

Vitamin E is the major lipid-soluble antioxidant in tissues. The tocopheroxyl radical formed by reaction of α-tocopherol with a lipid peroxide radical can be reduced back to tocopherol by reaction with:

- ascorbate to yield monodehydroascorbate, which can be reduced back to ascorbate (see Section 10.7, under 'Metabolic functions of vitamin C')

- glutathione, catalysed by a membrane-specific isoenzyme of glutathione peroxidase, which is a seleno-enzyme
- other lipid-soluble antioxidants in the membrane or lipoprotein, including ubiquinone.

Most of the studies of the antioxidant activity of vitamin E have used relatively strong oxidants as the source of oxygen radicals. Studies of lipoproteins treated in vitro with low concentrations of sources of radicals suggest that vitamin E may also have a pro-oxidant action. This is perhaps unsurprising; radical trapping antioxidants are effective because they form stable radicals that persist long enough to undergo reaction to non-radical products. It is therefore to be expected that they are also capable of perpetuating the radical chain reaction deeper into lipoproteins or membranes, and therefore causing increased damage in the absence of co-antioxidants such as ascorbate or ubiquinone.

Non-antioxidant actions of vitamin E

α-Tocopherol (but not other vitamers) inhibits platelet aggregation and vascular smooth muscle proliferation. In monocytes it reduces formation of reactive oxygen species, cell adhesion to the endothelium and release of interleukins and tumour necrosis factor.

α-Tocopherol modulates transcription of a number of genes, including the scavenger receptor for oxidised LDL in macrophages and smooth muscle. As yet no response element for intracellular vitamin E binding protein has been identified on any of the proposed target genes.

In experimental animals, vitamin E deficiency depresses immune system function, with reduced mitogenesis of B- and T-lymphocytes, reduced phagocytosis and chemotaxis and reduced production of antibodies and interleukin-2, suggesting a signalling role in the immune system.

Vitamin E deficiency and excess

Vitamin E deficiency in experimental animals was first described in 1922, when vitamin E was discovered to be essential for fertility. It was not until 1983 that vitamin E was demonstrated to be a dietary essential for human beings, when the devastating neurological damage due to lack of vitamin E in patients with hereditary abetalipoproteinaemia was first described.

Vitamin E deficiency in experimental animals results in a number of different conditions, with considerable differences between species. Some of the lesions can be prevented or cured by synthetic antioxidants, and others respond to selenium. Most of these effects of vitamin E deficiency can be attributed to oxidative damage to membranes.

Dietary vitamin E deficiency is not a problem even among people living on relatively poor diets. In depletion studies, very low intakes of vitamin E must be maintained for many months before there is any significant fall in circulating α-tocopherol, because there are relatively large tissue reserves of the vitamin.

Deficiency develops in patients with severe fat malabsorption, cystic fibrosis, chronic cholestatic hepatobiliary disease and in two rare groups of patients with genetic diseases:

- Patients with congenital abetalipoproteinaemia, who are unable to synthesise VLDL. They have undetectably low plasma levels of α-tocopherol and develop 'devastating' ataxic neuropathy and pigmentary retinopathy.
- Patients who lack the hepatic tocopherol transfer protein and suffer from what has been called AVED (ataxia with vitamin E deficiency) are unable to export α-tocopherol from the liver in VLDL.

In both groups of patients the only source of vitamin E for peripheral tissues will be recently ingested vitamin E in chylomicrons. Without supplements they develop cerebellar ataxia, axonal degeneration of sensory neurons, skeletal myopathy and pigmented retinopathy similar to those seen in experimental animals.

In premature infants, whose reserves of the vitamin are inadequate, vitamin E deficiency causes haemolytic anaemia. When premature infants are treated with hyperbaric oxygen, there is a risk of damage to the retina (retrolental fibroplasia), and vitamin E supplements may be protective, although this is not firmly established.

Vitamin E has low toxicity, and many people take relatively large supplements for protection against atherosclerosis and coronary heart disease. There is little evidence from intervention trials that this is effective, and meta-analysis of intervention trials shows that there is increased all-cause mortality among people taking vitamin E supplements. The Physicians' Health Study in the USA has shown no benefit of modest vitamin E supplements taken over many years.

Very high intakes may antagonise vitamin K and potentiate anticoagulant therapy. On the basis of prolonged prothrombin time in people receiving anticoagulants and consuming vitamin E supplements, the tolerable upper level is set at 1000 mg vitamin E per day.

ASSESSMENT OF VITAMIN E STATUS

The most commonly used index of vitamin E nutritional status is the plasma concentration of α-tocopherol; because it is transported in plasma lipoproteins, it is best expressed /mol cholesterol or /mg total plasma lipids. The reference range is 12–37 μmol/l; ranges associated with inadequate and desirable status are shown in Table *evolve* 11.11; epidemiological studies suggest that an optimum concentration for protection against cardiovascular disease and cancer is >30 μmol/l.

Erythrocytes are incapable of de novo lipid synthesis, so oxidative damage has a serious effect, shortening red cell life and possibly precipitating haemolytic anaemia in vitamin E deficiency. The haemolysis induced in vitro by hydrogen peroxide or dialuric acid provides a means of assessing functional status, albeit one that will be masked by adequate selenium intake and may be affected by other, unrelated, factors.

Overall antioxidant status, rather than specifically vitamin E status, can be assessed by a variety of measures of lipid peroxidation.

THE BASIS FOR SETTING DIETARY REQUIREMENTS

Early reports suggested that vitamin E requirements increase with intake of polyunsaturated fatty acids. Neither the UK nor the EU set reference intakes for vitamin E, but both suggested that an acceptable intake was 0.4 mg α-tocopherol equivalent/g dietary polyunsaturated fatty acid. This should be readily achievable from PUFA-rich oils, which are also rich sources of vitamin E. There is little evidence to support the figure of 0.4 mg α-tocopherol equivalent/g dietary PUFA, and indeed the need for vitamin E (and other antioxidants) depends more on the degree of unsaturation of fatty acids than the total amount.

From the plasma concentration of α-tocopherol required to prevent haemolysis in vitro, the average requirement is 12 mg/day, which was the basis of the 2000 US/Canadian RDA of 15 mg/day. This was a 50% increase on the previous (1989) RDA, partly as a result of considering only the $2R$ isomers in dietary intake.

Pharmacological uses of vitamin E

Although vitamin E deficiency causes infertility in experimental animals, there is no evidence that deficiency has any similar effects on human fertility, and it is a considerable leap of logic from the effects of gross depletion in experimental animals to the popular, and unfounded, claims for vitamin E in enhancing human fertility and virility.

Animal studies show some protective effects of tocopherol supplements against a variety of radical generating chemical toxicants, and it has been assumed that vitamin E may similarly be protective against degenerative diseases that are associated with radical damage. However, there is little evidence from intervention trials that vitamin E reduces cancer risk, cardiovascular disease, cataract or neurodegenerative diseases, and supplements may increase mortality.

KEY POINTS

- Vitamin E is the major lipid-soluble antioxidant in cell membranes and plasma lipoproteins.
- There are eight vitamers, with differing biological activity and antioxidant action.
- α-Tocopherol has actions in regulating platelet coagulability and vascular smooth muscle proliferation, and gene expression.
- The tocotrienols downregulate cholesterol synthesis.
- Vitamin E deficiency only occurs in people with severe fat malabsorption, and rare patients with a genetic lack of β-lipoprotein or hepatic tocopherol transfer protein, who suffer devastating nerve damage.
- Premature infants have inadequate vitamin E status and are susceptible to haemolytic anaemia.
- There is little evidence on which to estimate requirements for vitamin E.

11.4 VITAMIN K

Vitamin K was discovered in 1935 as a result of studies of a haemorrhagic disease of chickens fed on solvent-extracted fat-free diets and cattle fed on silage made from spoiled sweet clover. The problem in the chickens was a lack of the vitamin in the diet, while in the cattle it was due to the presence of dicoumarol, an antimetabolite of the vitamin. It soon became apparent that vitamin K was required for the synthesis of several of the proteins required for blood clotting, but it was not until 1974 that the mechanism of action of the vitamin was elucidated. A new amino acid, γ-carboxyglutamate (Gla), was found to be present in the vitamin K dependent proteins, but absent from the abnormal precursors that circulate in deficiency.

A number of other proteins undergo the same vitamin K-dependent carboxylation of glutamate to γ-carboxyglutamate, including osteocalcin and the matrix Gla protein in bone, nephrocalcin in kidney and the product of the growth arrest specific gene Gas6, which is involved in both the regulation of differentiation and development in the nervous system, and control of apoptosis in other tissues. All of these γ-carboxyglutamate containing proteins bind calcium, which causes a conformational change so that they interact with membrane phospholipids.

FORMS IN FOODS AND GOOD FOOD SOURCES

As shown in Figure 11.4, there are two naturally occurring vitamers: phylloquinone from plants (vitamin K_1) has a phytyl side-chain, while the bacterial menaquinones (vitamin K_2) have a polyisoprenyl side-chain, with up to 15 isoprenyl units (most commonly 6–10), shown by menaquinone-n. The synthetic compounds menadione and menadiol are vitamin K_3. Menadiol diacetate (acetomenaphthone) is used in pharmaceutical preparations, and two water-soluble derivatives, menadione sodium bisulphite and menadiol sodium phosphate, have been used for administration of the vitamin by injection and in patients with malabsorption syndromes which would impair the absorption of menadione, phylloquinone and menaquinones, which are lipid-soluble.

Menaquinones are synthesised by intestinal bacteria, but it is unclear how much they contribute to vitamin K nutrition, since they are extremely hydrophobic, and will only be absorbed from regions of the gastrointestinal tract where bile salts are present – mainly the terminal ileum. However, prolonged use of antibiotics can lead to vitamin K deficiency and the development of vitamin-K-responsive hypoprothrominaemia, as can dietary deprivation of phylloquinone.

The main dietary sources of vitamin K are nuts and seeds, and the oils prepared from them.

ABSORPTION AND TRANSPORT OF VITAMIN K

Phylloquinone is absorbed in the proximal small intestine, and is incorporated into chylomicrons. Extrahepatic tissues take up phylloquinone from chylomicrons and very low density lipoprotein, and synthesise menaquinone-4, which is the principal vitamer in most tissues.

THE METABOLIC FUNCTIONS OF VITAMIN K

The main metabolic function of vitamin K is as the coenzyme in the carboxylation of protein-incorporated glutamate residues to yield γ-carboxyglutamate. Four vitamin-K-dependent proteins involved in blood coagulation, prothrombin and factors VII, IX and X, were discovered early in the investigations of the vitamin, as a result of the haemorrhagic disease caused by deficiency. The function of γ-carboxyglutamate in these

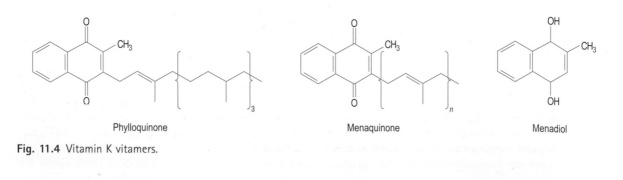

Phylloquinone   Menaquinone   Menadiol

Fig. 11.4 Vitamin K vitamers.

proteins is to chelate calcium, and induce a conformational change that permits binding of the proteins to membrane phospholipids. In addition to blood clotting, γ-carboxyglutamate-containing proteins are found in: bone (osteocalcin and bone matrix Gla protein), the kidney cortex (nephrocalcin), hydroxyapatite and calcium oxalate containing urinary stones, atherosclerotic plaque (atherocalcin), the intermembrane space of mitochondria, the central nervous system and other tissues (Gas6), and a number of proteins involved in cell signalling and as cell surface receptors.

A specific vitamin-K-binding protein has been identified in the nucleus in osteoblasts, suggesting that the vitamin may also have direct nuclear actions. Phylloquinone, but not menaquinones, downregulates osteoclastic bone resorption by inducing apoptosis in osteoclasts.

The vitamin–K-dependent carboxylase

The vitamin-K-dependent carboxylase is a membrane protein. The initial reaction is oxidation of vitamin K hydroquinone to the epoxide, linked to activation of the glutamate residue that is to be carboxylated, catalysed by vitamin K epoxidase (see Fig. *evolve* 11.6 🔋). Vitamin K epoxide is reduced to the quinone in a reaction involving oxidation of a dithiol to the disulphide, catalysed by epoxide reductase, a reaction that is inhibited by the anticoagulant warfarin.

Vitamin K quinone is reduced to the active hydroquinone substrate for the epoxidase reaction by either the same enzyme or a warfarin-insensitive quinone reductase. In the presence of adequate amounts of vitamin K, the carboxylation of glutamate residues can proceed normally, despite the presence of warfarin, with the stoichiometric formation of vitamin K epoxide, which cannot be re-utilised. Small amounts of vitamin K epoxide are normally found in plasma; in warfarin-treated patients there is a significant increase in the plasma concentration and urinary excretion of metabolites of the epoxide.

Vitamin–K-dependent proteins in cell signalling – Gas6

The product of the growth arrest specific gene 6 (Gas6) is a γ-carboxyglutamate containing protein that is important in the regulation of growth and development. The γ-carboxyglutamate region of Gas6 is required for binding to phosphatidylserine in cell membranes before interacting with a receptor tyrosine kinase, leading to the induction of mitogen-activated protein kinase (MAP kinase). Phosphatidylserine is normally deep in the membrane phospholipid bilayer, but it is exposed at the cell surface in senescent red blood cells and apoptotic cells, suggesting that Gas6 has a role in the recognition of cells that are to undergo phagocytosis, and hence regulation of apoptosis and cell survival.

VITAMIN K DEFICIENCY

Vitamin K deficiency results in prolonged prothrombin time, and haemorrhagic disease, because of impaired synthesis of the vitamin-K-dependent blood clotting proteins. Osteocalcin synthesis is similarly impaired, and there is evidence that undercarboxylated osteocalcin is formed in people with marginal intakes of vitamin K who show no impairment of blood clotting.

Treatment with warfarin or other anticoagulants during pregnancy can lead to bone abnormalities in the fetus, the so-called fetal warfarin syndrome, which is due to impaired synthesis of osteocalcin.

Newborn infants have low plasma levels of prothrombin and the other vitamin-K-dependent clotting factors (about 30–60% of the adult concentrations, depending on gestational age). To a great extent this is the result of the relatively late development of liver glutamate carboxylase, but they are also short of vitamin K, as a result of the placental barrier that limits fetal uptake of the vitamin. This is probably a way of regulating the activity of Gas6 and other vitamin-K-dependent proteins in development and differentiation.

Over the first 6 weeks of postnatal life the plasma concentrations of clotting factors gradually rise to the adult level; in the meantime infants are at risk of potentially fatal haemorrhage which was formerly called 'haemorrhagic disease of the newborn', and is now known as vitamin K deficiency bleeding in infancy. It is usual to give all newborn infants prophylactic vitamin K, either orally or by intramuscular injection. At one time menadione was used, but because of a possible association between menadione and childhood leukaemia, phylloquinone is preferred.

ASSESSMENT OF VITAMIN K STATUS

The usual method of assessing vitamin K status, or monitoring the efficacy of anticoagulant therapy, is to measure the time taken for the formation of a fibrin clot in citrated plasma after the addition of calcium ions and thromboplastin to activate the extrinsic clotting system – the prothrombin time. The normal prothrombin time is 11–13 seconds; greater than 25 seconds is associated with severe bleeding.

Measurement of plasma preprothrombin also provides an index of status, but measurement of undercarboxylated osteocalcin in plasma is more sensitive; it is detectable, and responds to supplements of vitamin K in people with normal clotting time and no detectable preprothrombin.

The urinary excretion of γ-carboxyglutamate, as both the free amino acid and in small peptides, also reflects functional vitamin K status, since γ-carboxyglutamate released by the catabolism of proteins is neither reutilised nor metabolised.

THE BASIS FOR SETTING DIETARY REQUIREMENTS

The total body pool of vitamin K is 150–200 nmol (70–100 mg), with a half-life of 17 hours, suggesting a requirement for replacement of 50–70 mg/day. Preprothrombin is elevated at intakes between 40–60 mg/day, but not at intakes above 80 mg/day.

The US/Canadian Adequate Intake is 120 µg for men and 90 µg for women. This is based on observed intakes, but there is some evidence that average intakes may be inadequate to permit full carboxylation of osteocalcin.

KEY POINTS

- Although intestinal bacteria synthesise vitamin K, it is not known to what extent this contributes to intake and status.
- The metabolic function of vitamin K is as cofactor for carboxylation of glutamate in precursors of proteins involved in blood clotting and a range of other functions, including the product of the growth arrest specific gene Gas6 that is involved in regulation of growth and development, and osteocalcin in bone.
- Clinically used anticoagulants for treatment of people at risk of thrombosis act as antimetabolites of vitamin K.
- Dietary deficiency of vitamin K is rare, and there is little evidence on which to base estimates of requirements.
- Newborn infants have low vitamin K status and are at risk of severe bleeding unless given prophylactic vitamin K.
- Vitamin K status is assessed by blood clotting (the prothrombin time) and sometimes measurement of undercarboxylated prothrombin and osteocalcin.

Further reading

Section 11.1 – Vitamin A

Bender DA: Chapter 2, Vitamin A. *In: Nutritional biochemistry of the vitamins*, ed 2, New York, 2003, Cambridge University Press.

Blomhoff R, Green MH, Green JB, et al: Vitamin A metabolism: new perspectives on absorption, transport, and storage, *Physiological Reviews* 71:951–990, 1991.

Clagett-Dame M, DeLuca HF: The role of vitamin A in mammalian reproduction and embryonic development, *Annual Review of Nutrition* 22:347–381, 2002.

Harrison EH: Mechanisms of digestion and absorption of dietary vitamin A, *Annual Review of Nutrition* 25:87–103, 2005.

Yeum K-J, Russell RM: Carotenoid bioavailability and bioconversion, *Annual Review of Nutrition* 22:483–504, 2002.

Section 11.2 – Vitamin D

Baeke F, van Etten E, Overbergh L, Mathieu C: Vitamin D3 and the immune system: maintaining the balance in health and disease, *Nutrition Research Reviews* 20:106–118, 2007.

Bender DA: Chapter 3, Vitamin D. *In: Nutritional biochemistry of the vitamins*, ed 2, New York, 2003, Cambridge University Press.

Chatterjee M: Vitamin D and genomic stability, *Mutation Research* 475:69–87, 2001.

Fleet JC, Hong J, Zhang Z: Reshaping the way we view vitamin D signalling and the role of vitamin D in health, *Nutrition Research Reviews* 17:241–248, 2004.

Flores M: A role of vitamin D in low-intensity chronic inflammation and insulin resistance in type 2 diabetes mellitus? *Nutrition Research Reviews* 18:175–182, 2005.

Griffin MD, Xing N, Kumar R: Vitamin D and its analogs as regulators of immune activation and antigen presentation, *Annual Review of Nutrition* 23:117–145, 2003.

Haussler MR, Haussler CA, Jurutka PW, et al: The vitamin D hormone and its nuclear receptor: molecular actions and disease states, *Journal of Endocrinology* 154(suppl):S57–S73, 1997.

Omdahl JL, Morris HA, May BK: Hydroxylase enzymes of the vitamin D pathway: expression, function, and regulation, *Annual Review of Nutrition* 22:139–166, 2002.

Section 11.3 – Vitamin E

Azzi A, Breyer I, Feher M, et al: Nonantioxidant functions of alpha-tocopherol in smooth muscle cells, *Journal of Nutrition* 131:378S–381S 2001.

Azzi A, Ricciarelli R, Zingg JM: Non-antioxidant molecular functions of alpha-tocopherol (vitamin E), *FEBS Letters* 519:8–10, 2002.

Azzi A, Gysin R, et al: Vitamin E mediates cell signaling and regulation of gene expression, *Annals of the New York Academy of Science* 1031:86–95, 2004.

Bender DA: Chapter 4, Vitamin E. *In: Nutritional biochemistry of the vitamins*, ed 2, New York, 2003, Cambridge University Press.

Brigelius-Flohé R: Bioactivity of vitamin E, *Nutrition Research Reviews* 19:174–186, 2006.

Miller ER, Pastor-Barriuso R, et al: Meta-analysis: high-dosage vitamin E supplementation may increase all-cause mortality, *Annals of Internal Medicine* 142:37–46, 2005.

Packer L, Weber SU, Rimbach G: Molecular aspects of alpha-tocotrienol antioxidant action and cell signalling, *Journal of Nutrition* 131:369S–373S, 2001.

Singh U, Devaraj S, Jialal I: Vitamin E, oxidative stress, and inflammation, *Annual Review of Nutrition* 25:151–174, 2005.

Traber MG: Vitamin E regulatory mechanisms, *Annual Review of Nutrition* 27:347–362, 2007.

Section 11.4 – Vitamin K

Bender DA: Chapter 5, Vitamin K. *In: Nutritional biochemistry of the vitamins*, ed 2, New York, 2003, Cambridge University Press.

Berkner KL: The vitamin K-dependent carboxylase, *Annual Review of Nutrition* 25:127–149, 2005.

Bolton-Smith CPR, Fenton ST, Harrington DJ, Shearer MJ: Compilation of a provisional UK database for the phylloquinone (vitamin K1) content of foods, *British Journal of Nutrition* 83:389–399, 2000.

Weber P: Vitamin K and bone health, *Nutrition* 17:880–887, 2001.

Chapter **12**

Minerals and trace elements

Paul Sharp

CHAPTER CONTENTS

© 2010 Elsevier Ltd/Inc/BV
DOI: 10.1016/B978-0-7020-3118-2.00012-7

OBJECTIVES

By the end of this chapter you should be able to:
- identify the most important food sources of minerals and trace elements
- understand the main features of their absorption, metabolism and tissue distribution
- describe their important functions in the body
- appreciate the effects of deficiency and excess, and their importance in the UK and elsewhere
- discuss the basis for dietary recommendations.

12.1 INTRODUCTION

This chapter deals with the key minerals and trace elements essential to a number of important biochemical and physiological functions in the body. The focus is placed on dietary sources of the various minerals and their homeostatic regulation in the body (i.e. the balance between bioavailability and absorption versus regulation and excretion). This is followed by discussion of the major metabolic functions of the minerals and trace elements and the consequences of deficiency and excess of individual elements. Each section closes by discussing the current methodologies used to assess the body status of these minerals and trace elements and the basis of the current dietary recommendations for intakes of these micronutrients. Five minerals are dealt with in detail. Calcium and phosphorus are discussed together because of their close interrelationship in maintaining bone health. This is followed by a discussion of the essential roles of iron, zinc and iodine in human metabolism. Further information on the essential nature of these micronutrients as well as their interactions with other nutrients will be provided elsewhere in this book: Section 11.2, under 'Regulation if vitamin D metabolism' Chapter 13; Chapter 24; Chapter 25; Chapter 28. Additional information is provided on the accompanying *evolve* website .

12.2 CALCIUM AND PHOSPHORUS

Calcium is the most abundant mineral in the body, the majority of which is contained within the adult skeleton in the form of hydroxyapatite, a complex crystalline form of calcium phosphate, $Ca_{10}(PO_4)_6(OH)_2$. Accordingly, phosphorus is also abundant in bone (approximately 85% of total body phosphorus). More details of the roles of calcium and phosphorus in maintaining bone health are provided in Chapter 24.

FOOD SOURCES

The most important dietary sources of calcium in the Western world are milk and other dairy products including yoghurt, cheese and ice cream (see Table *evolve* 12.1). Phosphorus is also abundant in these products and its concentration is approximately equimolar with calcium. However, while the calcium content of these foods can contribute 50–75% of the daily dietary intake, dairy products only contribute 20–30% of daily phosphorus intake. Many cereal products in the UK are fortified with calcium (added as calcium carbonate). The Bread & Flour Regulations 1998 stipulate that the calcium content of all flours derived from wheat (with the exception of wholemeal flour) must be between 235 and 390mg/100g. Cereal and vegetable sources of calcium contribute less to total intake in Western countries (approximately 25%) than in developing countries where grains and cereals are staple foods. The phosphate content of cereals and vegetables is relatively high because of the presence of phytic acid (inositol hexaphosphate) and these foods contribute a further 25–35% of daily phosphorus intake. In addition, carbonated soft drinks, which are often rich in phosphates, contribute significantly to phosphorus intakes in some diets. The calcium content of meat and fish is low in comparison to dairy products and cereals but sardines are a rich source of both calcium and phosphorus. In addition to its abundance in bone, phosphate is also present at high levels in soft tissues such as muscle and therefore levels of phosphorus in meat and fish are much higher than those of calcium, and contribute a further 25–35% to daily phosphorus intake.

Whilst in most foods calcium is largely present as simple organic and inorganic salts (some of which form larger complexes with other dietary components), dietary phosphorus occurs in several forms including inorganic phosphate, organic phosphoproteins, phosphorylated sugars, sugar alcohols (e.g. phytate) and phospholipids. The relative amounts of organic versus inorganic phosphate vary depending on the food source; for example, organic complexes prevail in meat, whereas 80% of phosphorus in cereals and grains is phytic acid and 33% of phosphorus in milk is present as inorganic salts.

ABSORPTION AND METABOLISM

Bioavailability

Absorption of calcium from a mixed diet is fairly constant (25–35%). Bioavailability of calcium in milk and dairy products is improved by the presence of sugars (lactose) and casein phosphopeptides (Allen & Wood 1994). The absorption from calcium salts used as supplements (such as lactate, carbonate, gluconate and citrate) is similar to that from dairy products (30–40%). However, other dietary acids, especially oxalate and phytate, inhibit calcium uptake. Oxalate is the most potent inhibitor of calcium absorption and forms a highly insoluble complex, whereas phytate is less potent but is present at a much higher concentration in the intestinal lumen and is likely to be the major dietary inhibitor of calcium absorption – a dietary phytate to calcium molar ratio of 0.2 can increase the risk of calcium deficiency.

Phosphorus is absorbed very efficiently from the small intestine (approximately 60–70% of dietary intake) and is always absorbed as inorganic phosphate – phosphate groups are liberated from organic compounds prior to absorption by alkaline phosphatase on the luminal membrane of intestinal enterocytes. This enzyme has little activity towards phytate, which is largely non-bioavailable in its natural form. However, yeast added to leavened bread contains significant levels of the enzyme phytase, which is lacking from human intestinal secretions. Phytase readily releases phosphate from phytate and about 50% of phytate-derived phosphate in bread is thought to be absorbed.

Absorption

Intestinal calcium absorption occurs via both active transcellular and passive paracellular pathways (see Fig. *evolve* 12.1). The transcellular route is subject to tight homeostatic control by the calcium content of the diet and 1,25-dihydroxycholecalciferol (1,25-$(OH)_2D_3$; vitamin D_3), whereas the passive paracellular route is not regulated and is non-saturable. The trigger for vitamin D_3 synthesis is the release of parathyroid hormone (PTH) in response to decreased plasma calcium. Elevated PTH levels do not regulate intestinal calcium absorption directly, but act indirectly by increasing the production of active vitamin D_3 in the kidney.

The mechanisms involved in phosphate absorption are less well defined (see Fig. *evolve* 12.2). Phosphate absorption is regulated by long-term changes in dietary phosphorus content and body phosphorus status. In addition, there may be a regulatory role for vitamin D_3 in controlling dietary phosphate absorption.

Tissue distribution

The human body contains approximately 1.2 kg (30 mol) of calcium, 99% of which resides in mineralised tissues such as the bones and teeth. The majority of calcium in these tissues is present as hydroxyapatite; the remainder is found in blood (where plasma calcium is tightly regulated at 2.5 mmol/l), and extracellular fluid. Intracellular free calcium concentration is extremely low (approximately 100 nmol/l) but can rise dramatically following hormone- or neurotransmitter-induced release of calcium from the intracellular stores in the endoplasmic/sarcoplasmic reticulum, and influx from the extracellular fluid through plasma membrane calcium channels.

Body phosphorus is also largely associated with the bone; approximately 85% of the 600 g in the body is found in the skeleton. The remaining 15% is found in the soft tissues and blood largely as phospholipids, phosphoproteins and nucleic acids as well as inorganic phosphate.

Renal excretion and regulation

Approximately 50% of plasma calcium is present in the ionised form (Ca^{2+}) and is freely filtered by the renal glomerulus. Most of this calcium is reabsorbed as the tubular fluid passes through the nephron and this process is tightly regulated by the action of PTH and vitamin D_3, which increase calcium reabsorption (Fig. 12.1), and calcitonin, produced in the C-cells of the thyroid gland, which

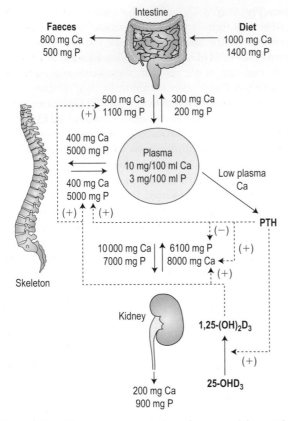

Figure 12.1 Homeostatic regulation of serum calcium and phosphorus. PTH, parathyroid hormone; 1, 25-(OH) 2D3, 1, 25-dihydroxycholecalciferol (vitamin D3).

promotes calcium excretion. PTH is released in response to a decrease in plasma calcium levels and has several actions, including promoting the synthesis of 1,25-$(OH)_2D_3$ (the active form of vitamin D_3), which in turn stimulates intestinal calcium absorption. In addition, PTH (and vitamin D_3) promotes bone resorption and increases renal calcium reabsorption. Together, these coordinated actions serve to raise plasma calcium back to normal levels within minutes to hours. Thyroid synthesis of calcitonin is promoted in response to elevated plasma calcium levels and release of this hormone acts to antagonise the effects of PTH, inhibiting bone resorption and renal calcium reabsorption, to lower plasma calcium.

As a consequence of bone resorption induced by PTH and vitamin D_3, plasma phosphate levels also rise. The excess phosphate, which could decrease ionised Ca^{2+} in the plasma, is eliminated via the kidney under the action of PTH, which inhibits its reabsorption in the renal tubules.

FUNCTIONS

Bone mineralisation

The major function of both calcium and phosphorus is in the formation of hydroxyapatite (see also Ch. 24). Calcium is deposited in bone at a rate of 150 mg/day during adolescence as the skeleton develops. In the adult, there is a dynamic equilibrium between calcium and phosphate deposition and resorption (400 mg Ca and 500 mg P are exchanged between the bone and plasma every day) due to the constant remodelling associated with the maintenance of the healthy skeleton.

Blood clotting

Integral to the formation of a blood clot is the presence of a series of irregular fibrils of the protein fibrin, formed by polymerisation of a soluble precursor, fibrinogen. Deposition of fibrin is the endpoint of a complicated cascade of enzyme reactions involving at least 10 other factors. This sequence of events can be initiated by blood coming into contact with a foreign surface such as collagen (the intrinsic clotting system) or following tissue damage (the extrinsic clotting system). Ca^{2+} (also known as factor IV) is a key component for the activation of both the intrinsic and extrinsic factor X activator complexes, the point at which the intrinsic and extrinsic coagulations systems converge. Calcium ions are further required at several subsequent stages of this cascade and a decrease in plasma calcium (below 2.5 mmol/l) is associated with a reduced ability to form blood clots (see also Section 11.4, under 'The metabolic functions of vitamin K').

Calcium and cell signalling

Intracellular free calcium concentrations are low (less than 100 nmol/l). Low cytosolic calcium is maintained because cell membranes are relatively impermeable to calcium. Any calcium that does enter the cell is rapidly removed from the cytosol through the action of a number of calcium transporters and channels present in the plasma membrane and in the membranes of intracellular organelles, in particular, the smooth endoplasmic/sarcoplasmic reticulum, which sequesters calcium and acts as an intracellular store. However, cytosolic calcium levels can increase dramatically following agonist-induced generation of the second messenger inositol-1,4,5-trisphosphate (IP_3), which binds to specific receptors on the smooth endoplasmic reticulum and leads to an increase in intracellular Ca^{2+} concentration by as much as 10-fold. The release of Ca^{2+} initiates further second messenger activity by binding to various target molecules, for example protein kinase C and calmodulin, which in turn trigger a number of diverse cellular responses including cell division, cell motility, contraction, secretion, endocytosis and fertility.

Phosphorus and energy metabolism

Phosphorus not incorporated into bone mineral is generally found in the soft tissues. Intracellular phosphorus (as the phosphate ion) participates in a number of processes associated with energy metabolism. Ultimately, energy produced from metabolism during oxidative phosphorylation in the mitochondria is stored as high-energy phosphate bonds in ATP (plus phosphocreatine in skeletal muscle).

A number of second messenger signalling cascades rely on phosphorylation or dephosphorylation as a mechanism for either activating or deactivating crucial enzymes. One of these second messengers is cyclic AMP, which is generated from ATP by the enzyme adenyl cyclase. Formation of cyclic AMP activates a specific protein kinase that modulates the activity of a number of proteins by adding phosphate groups. An example of one such target protein is glycogen phosphorylase.

EFFECT OF DEFICIENCY AND EXCESS

Every day there are obligatory losses of calcium in the urine and the faeces. If this calcium is not replaced by the dietary supply, plasma calcium is maintained by resorption of bone under the action of PTH. If a low intake of calcium persists, or if intestinal absorption is impaired over a prolonged period, bone resorption will cause a severe decrease in bone mass and this dietary imbalance, together with a number of other factors, contributes to an increased risk of osteoporosis (see Ch. 24). It is estimated that more than one-third of women and one-sixth of men will sustain an osteoporotic fracture during their lifetime.

Evidence for calcium toxicity is rare and adverse effects are limited to people taking high-level calcium supplements. However, the US Food and Nutrition Board has set a tolerable upper intake level of 2500 mg/day, which appears to be safe for most people. There have been some concerns that high intakes of calcium might reduce the absorption of other essential trace elements, especially iron, but there is no evidence to suggest that chronic calcium supplementation alters body iron status in the long term.

Since almost all food contains phosphorus, deficiency syndromes associated with inadequate phosphorus intake are extremely rare. When phosphorus intakes are low the body can adapt accordingly, increasing intestinal absorption and decreasing renal excretion. However, in some circumstances, for example in people with chronic gastrointestinal malabsorption syndromes or uncontrolled diabetes, there can be an imbalance in phosphorus homeostasis, which is regulated by demineralisation of the bone to maintain plasma phosphate levels. In severe situations, this can result in rickets in children or osteomalacia in adults. Similarly, rare genetic defects in the renal reabsorption of phosphate can cause rickets.

Toxicity associated with high phosphorus intakes is rare and is only likely to be a problem when calcium intakes are low. Elevated phosphorus intakes may lead to an increase in plasma phosphate concentration, which is thought to be a risk factor for a reduced bone mass. When plasma phosphate increases it results in a decrease in the plasma ionised calcium concentration that in turn leads to elevated serum PTH, which promotes bone resorption to re-establish plasma calcium levels. To this end there has been some concern in recent years that increasing dietary phosphorus intakes due to the large consumption of processed foods, which are often rich in phosphates, could have a detrimental effect on bone health.

STATUS ASSESSMENT

Currently there are no reliable biochemical indicators to accurately assess calcium status. As we have seen above, plasma calcium is so tightly regulated that it bears little relationship to body calcium status. However, since 99% of body calcium is retained within the skeleton, measures of bone mass such as the bone mineral content (of a specific region such as the femoral neck) and bone mineral density have proved to be useful indicators of body calcium status. The most common measure of phosphorus status is serum phosphate concentration.

THE BASIS OF DIETARY RECOMMENDATIONS

The dietary reference values (see Table *evolve* 12.2 🖱)) for the UK for calcium were determined by factorial analysis of the basal amounts of calcium required for bone growth and the maintenance of bone mineralisation (Department of Health 1991). In breastfed infants, calcium requirements (reference nutrient intake (RNI): 525 mg/day) are high and are met by the increased bioavailability of calcium from breast milk. Calcium retention in children increases significantly between the ages of 1 and 10 years as the skeleton develops. Absorption efficiency of calcium from a mixed diet in childhood is around 35%, less than from breast milk, and accordingly, the RNI has been calculated at 350 mg/day at age 2 rising to 550 mg/day at age 10. Assuming retention increases in adolescence to 250 mg/day for girls and 300 mg/day for boys the RNIs increase accordingly to 800 mg/day and 1000 mg/day, respectively. In adults following cessation of growth, there is still a significant calcium requirement based on calcium losses of 150 mg/day in the urine and 10 mg/day in sweat, skin and hair loss. Calcium absorption from an adult mixed diet is assumed to be 30%, giving an RNI of 700 mg/day.

No recommendation has been made for increasing calcium intakes during pregnancy because of higher rates of absorption compared with non-pregnant women. However, in adolescent pregnancies where females are still growing it may be advisable to increase calcium intakes. During lactation, the mother requires increased calcium for milk production, most (if not all) of which is derived from the diet. Initial estimates suggested that an extra 550 mg calcium/day was required for this purpose although this has recently been questioned because of potential adaptations in maternal calcium metabolism during lactation (Department of Health 1998).

In the UK and EU, phosphorus requirements are based on an equimolar intake with calcium and current recommendation is that the RNI for phosphorus should be equal to the calcium intake in mmol/day. Recently, the US Food and Nutrition Board set separate RDAs for phosphorus; for infants (0–6 months) 100 mg/day rising to 275 mg/day by 12 months of age; for children (1–3 years) 460 mg/day rising to 500 mg/day by age 8 years; for adolescents 1250 mg/day; for adults 700 mg/day. No further recommendations were made for pregnant or lactating adult women.

12.3 IRON

Iron is an essential trace metal and plays numerous biochemical roles in the body, including oxygen binding in haemoglobin and acting as an important catalytic centre in many enzymes, for example the cytochromes. However, in excess, iron is extremely toxic to cells and tissues because of its ability to rapidly alter its oxidation state and generate oxygen radicals. Consequently, body iron levels must be tightly regulated to avoid pathologies associated with both iron deficiency and overload. More than 2 billion people worldwide suffer from iron deficiency anaemia, making this the most common nutritional deficiency syndrome. At the same time 1 person in 200 of northern European descent is genetically predisposed to the iron loading disease haemochromatosis. The prevalence of these disorders highlights the importance of maintaining homeostatic control over iron nutriture.

FOOD SOURCES

Dietary iron is found in two basic forms, either as haem or non-haem iron. Haem is found in meat and meat products that are rich in two major haem-containing proteins, haemoglobin and myoglobin. The most important dietary sources of haem iron are those that are eaten in significant quantities, though these are not necessarily the richest sources of haem. Between 25% and 50% of the total iron content of meat is haem; the remainder is non-haem iron largely present in iron storage proteins such as ferritin. Therefore haem iron accounts for approximately 5–10% of the daily iron intake in industrialised countries, whereas in vegetarian diets and in developing countries the haem iron intake is negligible. The main form of iron in all diets is non-haem iron, found in cereals, vegetables, pulses, beans, fruits, etc. (see Table *evolve* 12.3 🖱)), present in these foods in a number of compounds ranging from simple iron oxides and salts to more complex organic chelates. Exogenous iron from the soil can be present in significant quantities on the surface of food. Average iron intakes in the UK have decreased significantly over the last 20 years, because of the amount of food consumed together with a reduction in the intake of meat.

Cereals contribute approximately half of our daily iron intake, yet most of the naturally occurring iron in cereals is in the seed coat. However, since the 1950s in the UK, all wheat flours (other than wholemeal) have been fortified with iron by law so that they contain at least 1.65 mg iron/100 g flour. In addition to flour, breakfast cereals and many infant foods are also fortified with iron. The iron source used to fortify foods is usually small particles of reduced elemental iron, which are partially soluble at gastric pH and therefore readily contribute to the non-haem dietary iron pool.

ABSORPTION AND METABOLISM

The absorption of iron by duodenal enterocytes is influenced by a number of variables, especially dietary factors (e.g. the iron content of foods, the type of iron present, bioavailability, other dietary constituents). Absorption is also regulated in line with metabolic demands that reflect the amount of iron stored in the body, and the requirements for red blood cell production (Fig. 12.2).

Bioavailability

Haem iron is the most bioavailable form of iron (see Table *evolve* 12.4). Although it only accounts for 5–10% of dietary iron in Western countries, absorption of iron from haem-containing foods is some 20–30%. Compared with non-haem iron, haem

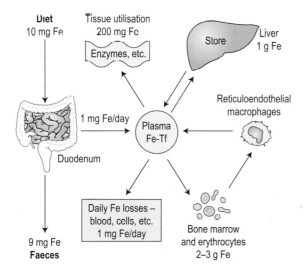

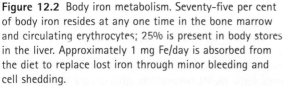

Figure 12.2 Body iron metabolism. Seventy-five per cent of body iron resides at any one time in the bone marrow and circulating erythrocytes; 25% is present in body stores in the liver. Approximately 1 mg Fe/day is absorbed from the diet to replace lost iron through minor bleeding and cell shedding.

absorption is less influenced by the iron status of individuals. The calcium content of the diet is thought to be the only other dietary factor to influence haem iron absorption, though the mechanism for this action is unknown. Food preparation alters haem iron bioavailability; prolonged cooking of meat at high temperatures is thought to degrade the porphyrin ring allowing the iron centre to be removed and join the non-haem iron pool.

Although non-haem iron is the most prevalent form of dietary iron only 1–10% is absorbed, because of the profound influence of other dietary components (see Table *evolve* 12.5). The most potent enhancer is ascorbic acid (vitamin C), which acts by reducing ferric iron to the more soluble and absorbable ferrous form. Other small organic acids, such as citric acid, and alcohol also promote the absorption of non-haem iron, possibly by forming stable soluble complexes with iron, thereby avoiding precipitation in the gut lumen. Meat and fish, as well as being abundant sources of haem and non-haem iron, also significantly promote the absorption of non-haem iron. The nature of the so-called 'meat factor' is still unclear; protein (high levels of cysteine- and histidine-containing peptides that could reduce ferric iron to ferrous); carbohydrate (glycosaminoglycans) and phospholipid (L-α-glycerophosphocholine) have all been shown to increase non-haem iron bioavailability.

The best-known dietary inhibitors of non-haem iron absorption are phytates, which are salts of inositol hexaphosphates found especially in cereal products. Phenolic compounds found in all plant food sources are also potent inhibitors of non-haem iron absorption. Perhaps the best-known group of compounds are the tannins found in abundance in tea and red wine. Both the phytates and phenolic compounds are thought to form insoluble ferric iron chelates in the intestinal lumen rendering the iron in a non-absorbable form.

In animals and plants, iron is stored intracellularly in ferritin. Surprisingly little attention is given to the possibility that ferritin may be an important dietary source of iron although a number of recent studies have shown that humans absorb plant and animal ferritins.

Intestinal absorption

Both haem and non-haem iron are absorbed in the duodenum, through completely independent mechanisms (see Fig. *evolve* 12.3). Haem is absorbed intact and inside the enterocyte the iron is removed by the action of haem oxygenase. Non-haem iron is largely present in the less soluble and non-absorbable ferric form and must first be reduced to ferrous iron before it becomes bioavailable. This is achieved by a combination of dietary reducing agents and enzymic activity of the enterocyte. The fate of the absorbed iron is determined largely by body iron requirements being stored in the enterocyte as ferritin when the body stores are replete, or leaving the cell and transported to other tissues on transferrin.

Transport and tissue distribution

Transferrin can bind two ferric iron molecules, delivering the iron to the sites of storage (mainly in the liver) or utilisation (e.g. the bone marrow) (Fig. 12.2). Body iron content is some 3–5 g (approximately 50 mg/kg body weight). Of this, approximately 70% is present in the circulating red blood cells, 20% is stored as ferritin and haemosiderin in the liver, 5% is incorporated into myoglobin in muscle and 5% is bound or utilised by various enzymes. Clearly erythrocyte production and destruction accounts for the majority of metabolic iron turnover in the body (some 20–30 mg/day). The typical lifespan of a red blood cell is 120 days and after this time senescent erythrocytes are engulfed by cells of the reticuloendothelial system (a combination of splenic macrophages and the Kupffer cells in the liver) and the iron recovered from haemoglobin by the action of haem oxygenase. This liberated iron is transported in the blood bound to transferrin back to the bone marrow for new red blood cell production or to the liver for storage.

Iron homeostasis

There are no defined excretory pathways for excess iron from the body. Iron losses are therefore restricted to that stored in cells shed from the lining of the gastrointestinal and urinary tracts, skin and hair, and losses through bleeding. Basal losses of iron amount to approximately 1.0 mg/day in men and 1.3–1.4 mg/day in premenopausal women (due to menstrual blood loss). These losses must be replaced by dietary intake to maintain body iron levels. The body has three basic mechanisms for maintaining iron homeostasis: (1) continuous re-utilisation of iron recovered from senescent red blood cells; (2) regulation of intestinal iron absorption; and (3) exploitation of an intracellular store (ferritin).

The main regulator of body iron homeostasis is hepcidin, a peptide synthesised in the liver. Hepcidin production is increased in response to elevated iron status and inflammatory stimuli (e.g. cytokines such as interleukin-6) and decreased when iron requirements are high. Hepcidin functions by inhibiting iron release from recycling macrophages, intestinal enterocytes and the hepatic iron stores. This mechanism serves to control the flow of iron between the absorptive, storage and recycling compartments and the bone marrow. In pathological situations, high levels of hepcidin lead iron to become trapped within the recycling macrophages resulting in inadequate erythropoiesis and ultimately the anaemia of chronic disease.

FUNCTIONS

Iron–containing enzymes

Iron plays a major role in regulating energy production via oxidative phosphorylation. The cytochromes are haem-containing enzymes consisting of a globin chain plus a haem group containing one iron atom.

The cytochromes function as efficient electron carriers and play a crucial role in the mitochondrial oxidation of fuels and formation of ATP. Iron is also an important component of other enzymes involved in energy metabolism, e.g. aconitase, succinate dehydrogenase and NADH-dehydrogenase, in which iron is present as non-haem iron. Haem iron is an important component of the antioxidant enzymes catalase and peroxidase.

Pro-oxidant activity

Despite its essential role in metabolism, iron is also a prospective pro-oxidant and is therefore potentially harmful (see also Section 13.5). Excess iron promotes lipid peroxidation and tissue damage, raising the possibility that, via these pro-oxidant effects, disturbances in iron metabolism play a pathogenic role in a number of diseases.

Immune function

Iron contributes to the regulation of immune function. Iron is an important growth promoter for a number of crucial immune responses including lymphocyte proliferation, and hence cell-mediated immunity may be compromised by iron deficiency.

However, iron is also a growth factor for microorganisms. Most iron in the body is either sequestered in ferritin or protein-bound and therefore unavailable as a nutrient for microbial growth but when there is a failure in body iron homeostasis, as in iron overload, an individual may be more at risk of infection.

EFFECTS OF IRON DEFICIENCY AND OVERLOAD

Anaemia

The most common cause of anaemia is nutritional iron deficiency (see Ch. 28). It is estimated that 2 billion of the world's population (largely in developing countries) have marked iron-deficiency anaemia (WHO 1997). Recent national dietary data show that, on average, 25% of British women have iron intakes below the lower RNI (8.0mg/day).

Whilst mild anaemia in many individuals is of little health consequence (because of a number of compensatory mechanisms such as increased cardiac output, diversion of blood flow to vital organs and increased release of oxygen from haemoglobin), severe anaemia exceeds the body's ability to adapt, resulting in impaired oxygen delivery to the tissues. This in turn has deleterious effects on a number of important body functions.

Work performance

Work performance, particularly physical work capacity, is severely limited in anaemia. In female tea pickers in Sri Lanka and in male Indonesian rubber plantation workers who had hookworm infection, reduced productivity was directly related to the severity of anaemia. Following supplementation therapy, iron-deficient subjects showed improved performance, with the greatest progress seen in those who had the most severe anaemia.

Cognitive function

The relationship between iron deficiency and impaired performance in mental and motor tests in children is well established (Lozoff et al 2000). Brain iron content increases throughout childhood and reaches its maximal levels in young adulthood between the ages of 20 and 30 years. Iron accumulation during infancy is especially important in determining both total brain iron content and brain development; an early deficit in brain iron is not compensated for in later years. Infants with iron deficiency anaemia fare less well in an array of psychomotor tests than non-anaemic age-matched counterparts. Even though measurable indices of body iron status can be normalised in these children by giving iron supplements, cognitive function is still impaired some 10 years later in those individuals who were severely iron-deficient in childhood.

Haemochromatosis

The majority of cases of primary iron overload are accounted for by the genetic disease haemochromatosis, an autosomal recessive disorder affecting mainly populations of European descent. The disease has a carrier frequency of approximately 1 in 10 and a homozygous frequency for the mutated gene of 1 in 200. Two mutations resulting in the disease have been mapped to the *HLA-H* (now called *HFE*) gene region of chromosome 6 and these account for more than 80% of the cases of haemochromatosis in northern Europeans.

Most cases of hereditary haemochromatosis are not diagnosed until patients present with clinical problems associated with organ failure (typically around 40–50 years of age). Simple and effective treatment of these patients can be achieved through the regular removal of excess body iron by phlebotomy. While it is not possible to treat haemochromatosis by dietary means, the Haemochromatosis Society have published dietary recommendations which include; avoiding iron supplements and breakfast cereals that are heavily fortified with iron, and high doses of vitamin C that would enhance uptake from the diet; restricting the consumption of red meat and offal, which are rich in haem iron; consuming tea with meals to limit iron bioavailability.

STATUS ASSESSMENT

Currently, there is no single test available to determine with complete accuracy perturbations in body iron status. Therefore, a wide variety of biochemical methods are employed to assess a number of key indices of iron metabolism (Table 12.1).

Table 12.1   Common methods for assessing body iron status

STATUS INDICATOR	NORMAL RANGE	ADDITIONAL INFORMATION
Serum ferritin	30–300 µg/l	1 µg/l serum ferritin = 10 mg tissue stored ferritin 12–15 µg/l indicates empty stores Acute phase protein – false high levels seen in infection and inflammation
Transferrin saturation	25–30%	Values below 16% are indicative of inadequate supply for erythropoiesis Values above 50–60% are generally indicative of haemochromatosis
Erythrocyte protoporphyrin	<80 µmol/mol haem	Protoporphyrin is the final intermediate in haem synthesis – levels rise when iron supply is limited Values >80 µmol/mol haem indicate iron-deficiency anaemia Also increased by other diseases, resulting in increased erythroid turnover
Serum transferrin receptor	2.8–8.5 mg/l	A measure of reticulocyte differentiation – shedding of TfR into serum Detectable receptor levels increase in iron deficiency Also increased in all diseases, increasing erythrocyte turnover Not affected by iron overload
Haemoglobin	120–180 g/l	Values below 110 g/l indicative of anaemia Not altered by iron overload Not altered in intermediate phases leading to anaemia
Mean cell volume	80–94 fl	Smaller erythrocyte volume in anaemia Cannot distinguish between iron deficiency anaemia and other anaemias

THE BASIS OF DIETARY RECOMMENDATIONS

Daily basal iron losses occur as a consequence of desquamation of cells lining the gastrointestinal tract (0.14 mg/day) and urinary tract (0.1 mg/day); blood loss accounts for a further 0.38 mg/day and bile losses amount to 0.24 mg/day (see Table *evolve* 12.6). Minor amounts are lost due to shedding of skin and hair. Thus basal iron losses are estimated at 14 mg/kg body weight/day. In infants, children and adolescents, in addition to basal losses, iron is also required for growth of the tissues and organs and for the expanding red blood cell mass. Within the first year of life the infant doubles its iron content and triples its body weight. Body iron content is again doubled between 1 and 6 years old. The growth spurt in adolescence also increases iron demand, as does the dramatic increase in haemoglobin concentration seen in males during puberty and at the onset of menarche in females. It is estimated that women also lose an average of 0.7 mg/day through menstrual blood loss. However, menstrual blood loss is not normally distributed within the population but is skewed to the right, and consequently the estimated average requirement for females for iron is set at the 75th percentile.

Dietary intakes to satisfy the metabolic requirements and iron losses depend largely on the bioavailability of iron in the diet. In most industrialised countries typical diets will be rich in meat, poultry and fish plus food containing high levels of ascorbic acid. Current UK guidelines assume that iron absorption from typical diets will be 15% and this has been used to calculate the current dietary reference values for iron (Department of Health 1991). Assuming average endogenous iron losses in adults are 1.0 mg/day in men and 1.7 mg/day in women, the estimated average requirement (EAR) for iron is 6.7 and 11.4 mg/day in men and women, respectively; with the RNI set at 8.7 mg/day for men and 14.8 mg/day for women.

The EAR for breast- or formula-fed infants aged 0–3 months is 1.3 mg/day, which trebles (in line with increased growth) over the next 6 months to 3.3 mg/day. There are no recommendations for increasing iron intake during pregnancy as the extra demand should be met by a combination of pre-existing body stores, lack of menstrual blood loss and the increased intestinal absorptive capacity during the second and third trimesters. Likewise, there are no recommendations for increasing iron intake during lactation, where iron losses (i.e. secreted in breast milk) are compensated for by the amenorrhoea associated with lactation.

12.4 ZINC

Human zinc deficiency was first noted in the 1960s in adolescents living in the Nile delta of Egypt and in rural Iran. Since these observations there has been a very significant increase in the understanding of human zinc metabolism. However, there are still significant nutritional questions to be addressed, including the assessment of marginal zinc status.

FOOD SOURCES

Daily zinc intake from an omnivorous diet is typically 10–12 mg/day (see Table *evolve* 12.7). The zinc content of foods varies greatly (see Table *evolve* 12.8), with the highest levels found in meat, whole grains and shellfish (particularly oysters). Animal sources provide the majority of dietary zinc in omnivorous diets (up to 70% of daily intake), mainly due to the high levels of zinc present in muscle (up to 50 mg/kg). In contrast, fat has a very low zinc content (5 mg/kg). In many cultures, cereal products are the major dietary energy sources but the zinc content decreases with an increase in the level of refinement of flour.

ABSORPTION AND METABOLISM

Bioavailability and absorption

Zinc is variably absorbed from different food groups (see Table *evolve* 12.9), with fractional absorption of around 30% being typical of solid diets (compared with 60–70% from aqueous solutions). The major inhibitor of absorption is phytate, which is negatively charged at food pH and readily forms insoluble complexes with positively charged ions such as zinc, thereby limiting bioavailability. This inhibitory effect on absorption can be partly overcome by food preparation techniques; for example, addition of yeast during bread-making increases phytase activity, reducing phytate levels. On the other hand, diets containing large quantities of unleavened bread are poor providers of zinc and are thought to be associated with the growth defects observed in adolescents living in the Nile delta of Egypt and rural Iran. There is also evidence that competition between zinc and other metals (e.g. copper, cadmium and possibly iron) at the level of intestinal absorption may limit zinc bioavailability.

Animal protein is thought to act as an 'antiphytic' agent and enhances the bioavailability of zinc. It is thought that small peptides and amino acids released during digestion improve the solubility of zinc and protect against the formation of insoluble phytate complexes. A typical omnivorous diet should provide adequate zinc to maintain body homeostasis, since animal protein intake would be sufficient to outweigh the inhibitory effects of the phytate.

Endogenous zinc is also present in the small intestine as a consequence of pancreatic and biliary secretions (zinc is an essential co-factor for the carboxypeptidases involved in protein digestion). This source of zinc is also available for absorption and is taken up by the intestinal epithelial cells by the same route as dietary zinc. Zinc absorption takes place in the small intestine, with the highest absorption rate in the jejunum. Uptake is transporter-mediated (an additional passive component may be evident at high luminal zinc concentrations) though the precise cellular mechanisms involved are still unclear (see Fig. *evolve* 12.4).

Transport and tissue distribution

Zinc entering the blood from the intestinal enterocytes is transported in the portal circulation to the liver bound mainly to albumin (70%) and α_2 macroglobulin (20–30%). Total body zinc amounts to some 2–3 g in a typical adult and is primarily localised intracellularly. Only 0.1% of total body zinc is found in the plasma whereas 60% is found in skeletal muscle and a further 30% is contained within bone (Fig. 12.3).

Homeostatic regulation of body zinc content

There is no recognised storage pool of zinc in the body but a number of tissues, especially the liver, are highly active in redistributing zinc between body organs. A key feature of this regulation appears to be the intracellular zinc binding protein metallothionein, a cysteine-rich protein that is induced by high dietary zinc levels and is thought to act as an intracellular zinc buffer.

The small intestine ultimately controls body zinc content by regulating both the amount of dietary zinc absorbed and the quantity of endogenous zinc, supplied by the intestinal, biliary and pancreatic secretions, lost in the faeces. Absorption (or reabsorption) of zinc is directly related to body zinc

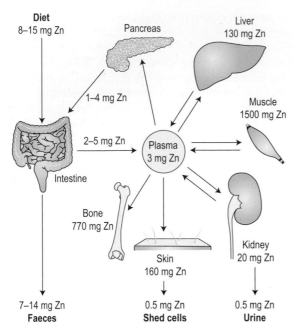

Figure 12.3 Body zinc distribution. Dietary intake (8–15 mg/day) matches endogenous losses in the faeces, urine and shed skin cells. Zinc is mainly an intracellular ion – hence low plasma but high tissue concentrations.

status. Zinc losses via the intestinal route include not only exogenous and endogenous zinc but also that lost as a consequence of shedding of cells lining the gastrointestinal tract. Total losses via this route normally range from 0.5 to 3 mg/day but can be greater in gastrointestinal disease.

In addition to intestinal losses, excretion of zinc via the kidney usually amounts to 0.5 mg/day in healthy adults. Most of the zinc filtered through the glomerulus is reabsorbed from the renal tubular fluid as it passes along the nephron. Urinary zinc excretion can be altered significantly in renal disease, insulin-dependent diabetes mellitus, alcoholism and starvation.

Further zinc can be lost from the body via skin, hair and sweat (about 0.5 mg/day). Also zinc accumulates in the prostatic fluids and an ejaculation of semen contains up to 1 mg of zinc.

FUNCTIONS

The major function of zinc in human metabolism is as a cofactor for over 100 known metalloproteins and enzymes; however, this may be an underestimate as recent genome analysis suggests that

3–10% of the human genome may encode zinc metalloproteins.

Several key enzymes involved in the synthesis of RNA and DNA are zinc-dependent, including the DNA and RNA polymerases. In addition, zinc plays a key role in gene transcription as an essential structural component of the zinc finger motifs found in several nuclear hormone receptors (e.g. those for vitamin D, testosterone and oestrogen) and transcription factors. The ability of zinc-finger-containing transcription factors to bind DNA is highly zinc-dependent and may be lost in zinc deficiency.

In addition to zinc fingers, structural zinc centres are essential for several enzymes, including the antioxidant enzyme superoxide dismutase (SOD), which contains zinc and copper. Zinc exhibits further antioxidant actions, including induction of metallothionein synthesis, and the ability to bind to sulphydryl groups on various proteins, protecting them from oxidation.

Zinc has profound effects on carbohydrate metabolism. Zinc-deficient animals have significantly impaired glucose tolerance, due to a reduced ability to secrete insulin from the pancreas in response to an oral glucose load. In addition to corelease with insulin from the beta cell, zinc is thought to increase and stabilise insulin binding to its receptors on target tissues, prolonging its biological actions. Intriguingly, recent genome-wide analyses have linked a beta cell zinc transporter polymorphism with an increased risk of developing type 2 diabetes, further establishing the close relationship between zinc and insulin activity.

ZINC DEFICIENCY AND EXCESS

Zinc deficiency

A number of zinc deficiency states of varying severity occur, especially in low-income countries. Zinc deficiency, along with deficiency of vitamin A, is responsible for the largest disease burden attributable to micronutrient deficiencies globally in children under 5 years of age and is particularly prevalent in south Asia, sub-Saharan Africa and regions of Central and South America. In the UK, zinc intakes are sufficient to replace endogenous daily losses and therefore severe zinc deficiency does not occur.

The first observations of human zinc deficiency were made in the 1960s in Iran and Egypt (Prasad et al 1961, 1963). It was suggested that zinc deficiency was the major contributing factor to a syndrome in which adolescents presented with dwarfism and hypogonadism. A number of similar cases were subsequently identified, mainly in Middle Eastern countries. The primary causes of zinc deficiency in these patients were two-fold: nutritional deficiency due to poor zinc bioavailability from a diet rich in unleavened bread; and geophagia (the practice of eating clay), which would further reduce zinc absorption.

Cases of severe zinc deficiency have been reported in industrialised countries and are characterised by dermatitis, diarrhoea and impaired immunity leading to greater susceptibility to infections. This syndrome, called acrodermatitis enteropathica, does not have its origins in nutritional deficiency but rather develops due to an autosomal recessive inborn error of zinc metabolism leading to a decrease in the absorption of dietary zinc. Recently, an intestinal zinc transport protein (ZIP4) has been shown to be mutated and functionally impaired in a number of families affected with acrodermatitis enteropathica, demonstrating that this defective protein contributes to the aetiology of the disease.

Zinc deficiency inhibits growth and zinc supplementation studies have shown improved growth in infants and children (Gibson 1994).

Zinc is found associated with the skeleton where it is thought to play a central role in the turnover and metabolism of the connective tissues. Zinc deficiency has a negative influence on bone formation, which might result from imbalances in DNA synthesis and protein metabolism. Zinc is also an essential cofactor for a number of crucial enzymes including alkaline phosphatase, which plays a major role in bone mineralisation, and collagenase, which is fundamental to the development and remodelling of bone structure.

Zinc excess

Whilst on the whole zinc is considered to have low toxicity, acute excessive intake (of the order of 2 g zinc) can cause symptoms such as nausea, abdominal pain, vomiting, diarrhoea and fever. In addition, there are some concerns that high doses of zinc (75–300 mg/day) over a prolonged period of time might adversely influence the metabolism of other important trace elements, in particular copper and iron.

STATUS ASSESSMENT

The intracellular nature of zinc, its tissue distribution (and homeostatic redistribution) and the absence of a defined storage pool make the assessment of zinc status difficult. Several indices of zinc status are in use including zinc levels in plasma, erythrocytes, leukocytes, neutrophils and hair as well as various physiological measurements, including the activity of a number of metalloenzymes, dark adaptation and taste acuity, but all have limitations. However, recent studies suggest that plasma or serum zinc may still be a useful biomarker of zinc deficiency and response to supplementation at the population level but further research is required.

THE BASIS OF DIETARY RECOMMENDATIONS

Endogenous losses of zinc are dependent on zinc intake and the homeostatic mechanisms controlling faecal loss. Zinc requirements are based on replenishing basal losses. A number of methods have been used to determine these, including metabolic balance studies, turnover time of radiolabelled endogenous zinc pools and measurement of total endogenous zinc loss. In people eating a typical Western diet providing 10–12 mg zinc/day, endogenous losses amount to 2–3 mg/day and this amount needs to be replaced. The dietary reference values for the UK are based on these figures and assume that 30% of dietary zinc is bioavailable for absorption. This translates into RNIs of 9.5 and 7.0 mg/day for men and women, respectively (Department of Health 1991). For infants and children, factorial analysis has suggested that zinc losses are related to body size and that the zinc requirements for growth increase incrementally with age. Consequently, the RNI for infants is 4.0 mg/day, rising to 9.0 mg/day in prepubescent children. Currently, the estimates for dietary zinc requirements for the elderly are the same as for the general adult population. However, there is evidence that zinc status is reduced in the elderly, possibly as a consequence of reduced absorptive efficiency and this requires further research.

In the UK there is no recommendation for additional zinc in pregnancy as the additional requirements seem to be offset by adaptive responses. In lactation, additional zinc requirements have been calculated on the basis of a zinc secretion in milk of

2.13 mg/day, giving an increase in the RNI of 6.0 mg/day. Requirements fall after 4 months of lactation, as milk secretion decreases, to an additional 2.5 mg/day over the RNI.

12.5 IODINE

Iodine is an essential micronutrient that forms a vital component of the thyroid hormones thyroxine (T_4) and triiodothyronine (T_3), which are crucial regulators of the metabolic rate and physical and mental development in humans. Iodine deficiency is relatively rare in the UK but is still prevalent in many areas in the world, where it constitutes a major problem of public health nutrition.

DIETARY SOURCES

Iodine is usually found in food as inorganic iodide or iodate. The iodine content of plants and cereals varies dramatically (from 10 µg/kg to 1 mg/kg) depending on the iodine content of the soil. Similarly the iodine concentration in drinking water lies in the range 0.01–70 µg/l, depending on geographical location and therefore for many population groups does not constitute a major dietary source (see Table *evolve* 12.7 📖). In the UK, cow's milk has become the major iodine-containing food in the diet because of the use of supplemented feeds and the provision of iodinated casein as a lactation promoter (Wenlock 1987). The richest sources of iodine in the diet are marine fish, shellfish and sea salt. Significant amounts of iodine are also provided by multivitamin and mineral supplements and by seaweed. In some regions of the world where iodine deficiency is a significant problem, extra iodine is provided in the diet in the form of iodide- or iodate-supplemented salt or bread (see Table *evolve* 12.8 📖).

ABSORPTION AND METABOLISM

Bioavailability

Iodine is rapidly and efficiently absorbed in the proximal small intestine as iodide. In addition, some organic iodine complexes, such as thyroid hormones added to animal feeds, can be absorbed intact. The remaining larger organic complexes are lost in the faeces. Other iodine-containing foods and iodates, which are often used for example as salt fortificants or as food additives, are readily broken down and reduced to iodide in the intestinal lumen.

Iodine content of foods can be significantly affected by the way that foods are cooked. For example, boiling foods reduces their iodine content by approximately half whereas frying decreases iodine by less than 20%. Bioavailability and absorption is also influenced by other dietary components, especially by brassicas (e.g. cabbage, broccoli, etc.) that are rich in sulphur-containing glucosides, which can liberate the 'goitrogens' thiocyanates and isothiocyanates that compete with iodide for absorption and tissue uptake.

Transport and tissue distribution

The mechanisms involved in iodide absorption in the intestine are still unclear; however, following absorption free iodide appears rapidly in the blood. Unlike the majority of trace elements, iodide in the blood does not appear to be bound to plasma proteins and is available for uptake by all the tissues of the body. The majority of the circulating iodide (approximately 80%) is rapidly taken up by the thyroid gland, but significant amounts are also accumulated by the salivary glands, choroid plexus (the area on the ventricles of the brain where cerebrospinal fluid is produced) and the lactating mammary gland. Uptake of iodide by all of these tissues employs a similar mechanism utilising a sodium/iodide symporter, which is stimulated by the thyroid-stimulating hormone (TSH) released from the pituitary gland. Total body iodine levels are 15–20 mg in healthy adults. Once the iodine requirements for thyroid hormone production have been met, excess circulating iodide is removed from the blood by the kidney and excreted in the urine. Urinary iodide is a good indicator of body iodine status.

FUNCTION – THE THYROID HORMONES

Iodide is taken up from the circulation by the follicle cells of the thyroid and passes into the inner colloidal space where it is rapidly oxidised to iodine (I_2), by thyroid peroxidase, and reacts with the tyrosine residues on thyroglobulin, a large glycoprotein, to produce monoiodotyrosine (MIT) and diiodotyrosine (DIT). These two precursors can condense to form the thyroid hormones T_3 and T_4.

These remain bound to thyroglobulin and are stored within the colloid until the thyroid is stimulated by TSH, whereupon thyroglobulin is taken up by the follicle cells and acted on by lysosomal enzymes to liberate active T_3 and T_4, which are subsequently released into the circulation. T_4 has a relatively low biological activity and serves as a reservoir for the production of the more active T_3 following removal of a 5' iodine by selenium-dependent deiodinases present in the liver, kidney, muscle and pituitary.

The major functions of the thyroid hormones are the maintenance of the metabolic rate, cellular metabolism and growth. Their function is elicited by binding to nuclear receptors that in turn bind to DNA and regulate the transcription of several genes in target tissues, in particular the brain, heart, liver and kidneys.

EFFECTS OF IODINE DEFICIENCY AND EXCESS

Iodine deficiency causes a wide range of disorders collectively known as iodine-deficiency disorders in which symptoms range from mild, such as goitre, to severe, including mental retardation or cretinism (see also Ch. 28). The fetal brain is particularly susceptible to iodine deficiency if the mother is iodine-deficient. The neurological damage caused by iodine deficiency in these children is irreversible and devastating, resulting in mental retardation, and hearing and speech defects.

Goitres are formed by enlargement of the thyroid gland. Iodine deficiency leads to a decrease in T_4 production, which in turn stimulates the pituitary gland to produce TSH. This increase in TSH production stimulates the thyroid follicles to enlarge and multiply, giving the characteristic goitre appearance. With very large goitres there can be additional problems such as blockage of the oesophagus and trachea as well as damage to the laryngeal nerves.

Most people are very tolerant to a wide range of iodine intakes, and no adverse effects of up to 2 mg iodine/day have been reported. These levels are unlikely to be achieved in the normal diet and are more likely to result from iodine contamination of food or water supply. Some individuals are sensitive to iodine and may experience mild skin irritations following higher than normal iodine intakes.

STATUS ASSESSMENT

Assessment of iodine status in populations living in areas at risk of iodine deficiency is based on a number of methods. The size of the thyroid is measured by palpation or ultrasound, giving a measure of the number of goitres that can be classified in accordance with WHO/UNICEF/ICCIDD guidelines. Urinary iodine can be measured by a simple colorimetric assay (values under 50 µg iodine/g creatinine are considered to indicate deficiency). Neonatal levels of TSH in the serum (normal range 0.5–5.5 mU/l) are used routinely in most developed countries to give an indication of congenital hypothyroidism.

DIETARY RECOMMENDATIONS

In adults, an iodine intake of 70 µg/day appears to be the minimum necessary to avoid the appearance of goitre and has therefore been set as the LRNI for the UK (Department of Health 1991). The RNI has been set at 140 µg/day to allow for different dietary patterns. Recent estimates for iodine intake in the UK suggest means of 215 and 159 µg/day for men and women, respectively (Food Standards Agency 2003) compared with 200 and 140 µg/day in the USA. Because of the possible risk of iodine toxicity, current dietary recommendations in the UK are that iodine intake should not exceed 1 mg/day.

12.6 SELENIUM

Selenium is a metalloid mineral that exists in a number of oxidation states. It is found in all soils and rocks at varying concentrations, depending on geological factors. Plant selenium content is determined by the concentration in soils and this consequently enters the animal and human food chain. Hence the geographical variation in soil selenium content has a dramatic impact on dietary selenium intake in different populations. Until the mid-1980s most wheat entering the UK food chain was imported from Canada. However, as a result of changes in the economic and political climate together with the advent of modern food manufacturing technologies, lower-selenium UK wheat now predominates. Consequently there has been a considerable reduction in selenium intakes and status in the UK over the last two decades (see Table *evolve* 12.7). To circumvent similar problems with falling selenium intakes, Finland has since 1984 been adding selenium to its food chain by including selenate in fertilisers used to treat arable crops. This has been associated with a consequent rise in plasma selenium levels, close to values at which glutathione peroxidase is optimally active.

DIETARY SOURCES

Selenium is found in a variety of foods, with cereals, meat, Brazil nuts and fish providing particularly rich sources (see Table *evolve* 12.8). Despite the decrease in selenium-rich North American wheat imports, bread and cereal products still contribute approximately 20% to daily UK selenium intakes. Meat (30%), fish (13%) and dairy products (15%) are the other major contributors. There are negligible amounts of selenium in drinking water.

ABSORPTION AND METABOLISM

Selenium is present in foods mainly in organic forms such as the amino acids selenocysteine (from animal products) and selenomethionine (mainly in cereals), but also exists in the environment as inorganic selenide, selenite and selenate compounds. Interestingly, in a number of plants (e.g. garlic) up to 50% of the selenium content is present as selenate. Selenite is usually only found in supplements and food fortificants.

The mechanisms involved in intestinal selenium absorption have not been fully elucidated; however there is good evidence that selenomethionine and selenocysteine share common transport pathways with methionine and cysteine, respectively. Unlike many micronutrients, the absorption of selenium does not appear to be regulated by metabolic demand. The average absorption of selenium from food is approximately 80% and there is evidence that organic forms (i.e. seleno-amino acids) are taken up more efficiently than inorganic compounds. In addition, there is evidence that the bioavailability of inorganic selenium compounds is decreased by heavy metals and by a high-sulphur diet. In humans, all absorbed forms of selenium are metabolised to hydrogen selenide. This in turn is converted to selenophosphate, which is used to synthesise selenocysteine. Selenium in the form of selenocysteine is incorporated into a number of selenoproteins and enzymes. Selenocysteine is the '21st amino acid' and has its own codon (UGA). In most translation events UGA acts as a stop codon

for protein synthesis; however in selenoproteins it permits the insertion of selenocysteine due to the presence of so-called SECIS (selenocysteine insertion sequence) elements in the 3′ untranslated region of target mRNAs.

FUNCTION

To date 25 human selenoproteins have been identified (see Table *evolve* 12.10), which include iodothyronine deiodinase, responsible for the conversion of T_4 to T_3, thioredoxin reductase, which reduces nucleotides in DNA synthesis, and members of the glutathione peroxidase (GSHPx) family, which are important antioxidant enzymes. One of the GSHPx isoforms is found in abundance in the sperm capsule, where it plays an essential function in maturation and motility of spermatozoa.

Epidemiological evidence as well as data from animal studies point to a role for selenium in reducing cancer incidence. The Nutritional Prevention of Cancer trial in 1996, carried out in the USA, was the first human study to test the hypothesis that selenium supplementation could reduce cancer risk. Subjects with a history of non-melanoma skin cancer were given either selenium supplements (200 μg/day selenium-enriched yeast containing predominantly selenomethionine) or a placebo. Interestingly, while there was no direct effect of selenium supplementation on non-melanoma skin cancer there was a significant reduction in both total cancer incidence and cancer mortality in the supplemented group. In particular, cancers of the prostate, colon and lung were greatly reduced in those in the supplemented group who had relatively low baseline selenium status, suggesting that the effects of selenium were tissue-specific and related to selenium status. The effect on prostate cancer incidence led to the Selenium and Vitamin E Cancer Prevention Trial (SELECT) in 2001. However, in summer 2008 the trial was stopped, as there was no evidence of a beneficial effect on prostate cancer incidence.

EFFECTS OF SELENIUM DEFICIENCY AND EXCESS

The best characterised selenium deficiency syndrome is Keshan disease, a cardiomyopathy that affects children and women of child-bearing years in rural China where soils are selenium-deficient.

Symptoms are further exacerbated by viral infection. Kashin–Beck disease, a form of osteoarthropathy observed in rural China, is also associated with severe selenium deficiency but other factors including low iodine status and food mycotoxins are also important in the aetiology of this disease. Low selenium status has also been associated with a number of other health problems including a decrease in immune function and increased susceptibility to viral infection, lower reproductive capacity, decreased thyroid function and reduced antioxidant status. Pathologies associated with selenium deficiency are linked to decreased activity of a number of selenoenzymes.

While selenium is an essential micronutrient and supplementation or fortification of foods may in many cases be advantageous, selenium is exceedingly toxic in excess. While selenosis is less common than selenium deficiency, a three- to four-fold change in selenium intake can be the difference between beneficial and harmful intakes. Symptoms of selenium excess (consumption of >800μg/day) include brittle hair and nails, skin lesions and garlic odour on the breath due to expiration of the metabolite dimethyl selenide.

STATUS ASSESSMENT

Selenium status can be assessed by measuring selenium levels in a number of tissues including plasma or serum. A serum selenium level of 100 ng/ml is generally seen as a measure of nutritional adequacy. Selenium levels in red blood cells, hair and toenails are seen as good indicators of long-term selenium intakes. The antioxidant activity of plasma glutathione peroxidase (GSHPx3) has emerged as a functional biomarker of selenium status but it is a poor indicator of status in individuals with moderate or high intakes. Current UK dietary recommendations are based on the calculated intake of selenium required to optimise the activity of the plasma GSHPx3.

DIETARY RECOMMENDATIONS

Keshan disease is not seen in populations where selenium intake is >20 μg/day. On this basis the World Health Organization has set the basal requirements (i.e. the amount required to prevent pathology) at 21 μg/day for males and 16 μg/day for females and its recommended intakes at 40 μg/day for males and 30 μg/day for females. The

current UK RNI for selenium is 75 μg/day for men and 60 μg/day for women. UK selenium intakes, however, are falling and are currently estimated to be below the LRNI (40 μg/day). In contrast, selenium intakes in New Zealand have increased in recent years due to the import of selenium-rich wheat from Australia. Nutrient reference values in New Zealand were set in 2005 at 75 μg/day for men and 60 μg/day for women. In the USA, where median intakes are substantially higher than in the UK (154 μg/day for men and 98 μg/day for women), RDA for selenium is set at 55 μg/day with no gender difference.

12.7 OTHER IMPORTANT TRACE ELEMENTS

COPPER

Copper is the third most abundant dietary trace metal (see Table *evolve* 12.7) and is found at high levels in shellfish, liver, kidney, nuts and whole-grain cereals (see Table *evolve* 12.8). The absorption efficiency ranges from 10 to 50% and is variable depending on both requirements and the bioavailability of the diet. The majority of absorption occurs in the duodenum and jejunum via a carrier-mediated mechanism (see Fig. *evolve* 12.5); a limited amount is also absorbed in the stomach. Copper homeostasis is tightly maintained by regulating absorptive efficiency and biliary excretion. The major function of copper is as a catalytic centre in numerous enzymes involved in redox reactions (see Table *evolve* 12.11).

Dietary induced copper deficiency is relatively rare in human beings due to the plentiful and varied supply in the diet and the high efficiency of absorption (see Table *evolve* 12.12). However, the assessment of marginal copper deficiency is problematic because of the lack of a sensitive and specific biomarker of copper status. Most reported incidences of deficiency are in association with prolonged diarrhoea and/or malnutrition, particularly in infants. Nutrient–nutrient interactions have also been linked with deficiency, with over-the-counter zinc supplements suppressing dietary copper absorption and ultimately resulting in deficiency.

Menke's disease, a rare congenital condition, involves failure of copper absorption and leads to severely impaired mental development, inability to keratinise hair, and skeletal and vascular problems. These symptoms are associated with impairment of a number of copper-dependent enzymes. Dietary copper overloading is also rare because of the body's ability to excrete excess copper in the bile. These mechanisms fail in a second congenital disease, Wilson's disease, which leads to copper accumulation in the body, particularly in the liver and the basal nuclei of the brain, with consequent pathological damage.

CHROMIUM

The main chromium-rich foods are meat, nuts, cereal grains, brewer's yeast and molasses. Absorption from these foods is extremely low (0.5–2%). Consequently, total body chromium content is less than 6 mg. Chromium (III) is the active form of this nutrient and its main functions appear to be associated with carbohydrate and lipid metabolism. Cr (III) enhances the actions of insulin, either by optimising the number of receptors on target tissues, acting as a cofactor to improve insulin binding or contributing to the phosphorylation and dephosphorylation events in the downstream insulin signalling pathway. Subjects receiving adequate dietary chromium have better control over blood glucose and an improved lipid profile, linked to good regulation of plasma insulin. Indeed one major characteristic of marginal chromium deficiency is impaired glucose tolerance, which can be improved by chromium supplementation, although chromium supplements do not enhance insulin action further in people who were not initially deficient.

FLUORIDE

Fluoride is present in most foods at varying levels and also in drinking water, either naturally occurring or added deliberately. The main function of fluoride in the body is in the mineralisation of bones and teeth (as calcium fluoroapatite). Fluoride content of teeth and bones is directly proportional to the amount ingested and absorbed from the diet. In addition, some fluoride from drinking water can be directly incorporated into dental enamel forming fluorohydroxyapatite, which is less soluble than hydroxyapatite itself. This function plus the bacteriostatic action of fluoride on the bacteria in dental plaque protects teeth from dental caries. Adding fluoride to drinking water is a controversial issue because, while low supplementary levels (1 mg/l) may be beneficial, higher intakes (10 mg/l) of fluoride are toxic, leading to fluorosis. Symptoms of fluorosis may be mild (mottled tooth enamel) or severe (skeletal fluorosis). Skeletal changes include calcification of ligaments and tendons leading to stiffness, joint pain and spinal defects due to hypercalcification of the vertebrae. The most severe symptoms develop only with chronic excess intakes of fluoride (over at least 10 years) and are extremely rare in the Western world, with only 5–10 recorded cases. However, fluorosis is common in parts of southern Africa, the Indian subcontinent and China where there is a high fluoride content in the subsoil water, which enters the food chain either directly or via plants.

KEY POINTS

■ Calcium and phosphorus are the major bone minerals; 99% of total body calcium and 85% of total body phosphorus are present in the bone and are in a dynamic equilibrium with the plasma that is controlled by the hormones PTH, 1,25-$(OH)_2D_3$ and calcitonin.

■ Non-haem iron absorption from the diet is strongly influenced by other dietary components that may act to promote (e.g. ascorbic acid) or inhibit (e.g. phytic acid) bioavailability. The amount of iron absorbed is usually sufficient to replace basal losses, and satisfy metabolic demand for growth and red blood cell formation. However, if intake drops then there is a risk of developing iron-deficiency anaemia, the most common nutritional deficiency disease in the world.

■ Zinc is essential for a wide array of biochemical processes that play a central role in growth and development. Its major function is as a structural and/or catalytic centre in a number of metalloenzymes and proteins that rely on the presence of zinc for their activity.

■ Iodine is an essential nutrient because it is a constituent of the thyroid hormones thyroxine and tri-iodothyronine. These hormones are required for normal growth and maintenance of the metabolic rate. If iodine intake is low, iodine deficiency diseases can become prevalent and symptoms can range from mild (e.g. goitre) to severe (e.g. cretinism).

■ For these and many other key minerals and trace elements there is a requirement for better functional markers of body nutritional status. In particular, these markers where possible should relate to physiological or biochemical factors connected to the known essential function of these micronutrients and should be able to identify changes in body stores as well as dietary intakes.

- Furthermore, there is a requirement to fully evaluate specific health risks associated with marginal deficiencies of specific minerals and trace elements that have not developed into a full deficiency syndrome. Similarly, more information is required regarding the effects of excess intakes of many of these elements.

ACKNOWLEDGEMENTS

The author would like to thank Susan Fairweather-Tait, Diane Ford, Linda Harvey, Rachel Hurst and Victor Preedy for their helpful comments.

References

Allen LH, Wood RJ: Calcium and phosphorus. In Shils ME, Olson JA, Shike M, editors: *Modern nutrition in health and disease*, ed 8. Philadelphia, 1994, Lea & Febiger, pp 144–163.

Department of Health: *Dietary reference values for food energy and nutrients for the United Kingdom*. Report on Health and Social Subjects 41. London, 1991, HMSO.

Department of Health: *Nutrition and bone health: with particular reference to Vitamin D and calcium*. Report on Health and Social Subjects 49. London, 1998, The Stationery Office.

Food Standards Agency: *The National Diet & Nutrition Survey: adults aged 19 to 64 years*, London, 2003, The Stationery Office.

Garrow JS, James WPT, Ralph A: *Human Nutrition and Dietetics*, 10th edn, Edinburgh, 2000, Churchill Livingstone.

Gibson RS: Zinc nutrition in developing countries, *Nutrition Research Reviews* 7:151–173, 1994.

Lozoff B, Jimenez E, Hagen J, et al: Poorer behavioral and developmental outcome more than 10 years after treatment for iron deficiency in infancy, *Pediatrics* 105:E51, 2000.

Prasad AS, Halstead JA, Nadimi M: Syndrome of iron deficiency anaemia hepatosplenomegaly, hypogonadism, dwarfism and geophagia, *American Journal of Medicine* 31:532–546, 1961.

Prasad AS, Mial A, Farid Z, et al: Zinc metabolism in patients with the syndrome of iron deficiency anaemia, hypogonadism and dwarfism, *Journal of Laboratory and Clinical Medicine* 61:537–549, 1963.

The Bread and Flour Regulations 1998, London, 1998, The Stationery Office.

Wenlock RW: Changing patterns of dietary iodine intake in Britain. In *Dietary iodine and other aetiological factors in hyperthyroidism*. Conference Report, Southampton, 1987, MRC Environmental Epidemiology Unit (MRC Scientific Report No. 9), pp 1–6.

WHO: The World Health Report. Conquering suffering, enriching humanity. Geneva, 1997, World Health Organization.

Further reading

Bowman B, Russel R, editors: *Present knowledge in nutrition*, ed 8. Washington DC, 2001, ILIS Press.

British Nutrition Foundation: *Iron nutrition and physiological significance*. London, 1995, Chapman & Hall.

British Nutrition Foundation: Selenium and Health. BNF Briefing Paper. 2001. http://www.nutrition.org.uk/upload/Selenium%20and%20Health.pdf

Centers for Disease Control and Prevention: Recommendations to prevent and control iron deficiency in the United States. *Morbidity and Mortality Weekly Report* 47(RR-3):1–29, 1998.

Journal of Nutrition 2000 vol. 130: part 5, supplement 'Zinc and health: current status and future directions'. Several papers.

Lozoff B: Behavioural alterations in iron deficiency, *Advances in Paediatrics* 35:331–359, 1988.

Nemeth E, Ganz T: Regulation of iron metabolism by hepcidin, *Annual Review of Nutrition* 26:323–342, 2006.

Sharp P, Srai SK: Molecular mechanisms involved in intestinal iron absorption, *World Journal of Gastroenterology* 13:4716–4724, 2007.

Theobald HE: Dietary calcium and health, *BNF Briefing Paper Nutrition Bulletin* 30:237–277, 2005.

EVOLVE CONTENTS (available online at: evolve.elsevier.com/Geissler/nutrition)

Chapter 13

Inter-micronutrient topics

David Thurnham

CHAPTER CONTENTS

OBJECTIVES

By the end of this chapter you should be able to:
- summarise drug–micronutrient interactions
- describe the role of micronutrients in the immune response
- understand which micronutrients play a role in gene expression
- discuss the roles of micronutrients as pro- or antioxidants
- describe the potential protective effects of polyphenols and phytoestrogens.

13.1 INTRODUCTION

Poor diets are rarely just deficient in only one nutrient. The nutrient that is least adequate in the diet may cause the main clinical or subclinical effects

© 2010 Elsevier Ltd/Inc/BV
DOI: 10.1016/B978-0-7020-3118-2.00013-9

but if only that nutrient is replaced, other nutrients may then become limiting, preventing any response to treatment. There is considerable potential for adverse consequences from both single and multi-nutrient supplements through interaction with dietary components. Supplements usually contain a disproportionately large amount of nutrient relative to normal dietary intakes as the objective is to improve nutritional status rapidly (Beaton et al 1993). Giving large amounts of supplements can have surprisingly adverse effects. Nutrients may have toxic effects themselves on the body as in the case of vitamin A. Even non-toxic β-carotene increased mortality from lung cancer in smokers in two large intervention studies. Nutrients can interact with one another and block absorption, as happens with iron and zinc. Supplementary nutrients may exacerbate inflammation and thus worsen the effects of disease on the body. Iron is a good example of this, but there are also reports that supplements of vitamin A can adversely affect respiratory disease and there is one report that vitamin A supplements increased transmission of HIV to infants from the mother.

We adapt to handle nutrients and other substances at the concentrations in our diet and environment. We have in-built safety mechanisms to handle large amounts of nutrients as well as the many thousands of xenobiotics in our diet (Guengerich 1995, Kane & Lipsky 2000). The biotransformation of such compounds is handled by what are known as phase I and II reactions. Most end-products of such bio-transformations can be safely excreted but there are some well-known exceptions. Intermediate compounds formed from dietary nitrosamines and aflatoxins are more active than the original and, in these cases, are carcinogenic. The activity of phase I enzymes can be both depressed and stimulated by substances in our diet and the actual activity of these enzymes may be a product of the habitual dietary environment in which we live. Hence persons regularly consuming diets high in fruit and vegetables may metabolise potential carcinogens differently from those whose diet is low in these foods, and thereby will have a lower risk of developing cancers. A well-balanced diet should contain adequate amounts of nutrients to maintain normal metabolism but also a wide range of non-nutrients to optimise phase I and II metabolic processes.

This chapter examines a selection of issues relating to micronutrient interactions. Section 13.2 addresses drug–nutrient interactions and this includes lifestyle factors like smoking and alcohol use. Section 13.3 looks at issues relating to the immune response and micronutrients whilst section 13.4 addresses some issues relating to gene–nutrient interactions. Section 13.5 considers inter-relationships between the antioxidant nutrients and their significance in maintaining health. Finally Sections 13.6 and 13.7 deal with two specific groups of antioxidants, namely (1) phenols and polyphenols and (2) phytoestrogens and the possible importance of their antioxidant properties in determining biological activity.

13.2 DRUG–NUTRIENT INTERACTIONS

A drug–nutrient interaction refers to the effect of a medication on nutrients in the food we eat or those already in our bodies or the converse, where food or dietary treatments may have an influence on the effectiveness of a drug. Food ingestion can profoundly affect a drug's pharmacodynamics and can either accelerate or retard drug absorption. Where prolonged medication is prescribed, the potential interaction between food and drugs may be increased and this becomes of greater importance in older people (Thomas & Burns 1998). Risk factors that increase the potential for drug–nutrient interactions are multiple medications, reduced intakes, nutrient loss from poor cooking habits, restrictive diets, anorexia, eating disorders, alcoholism, drug dependency or addiction, and renal and hepatic dysfunction.

Drug–nutrient interaction can be categorised as physicochemical, physiological or pathophysiological. An example of a physicochemical interaction is chelation of a nutrient by a drug, causing loss of a nutrient and lower activity of a drug. Physiological interactions include drug-induced changes in appetite, digestion, gastric emptying, metabolism and excretion. Pathophysiological interactions occur when a drug impairs nutrient absorption or metabolism, or a drug causes an inhibition of metabolic processes. For example, female sex hormones alter the metabolism of vitamins A and D, producing higher plasma concentrations of retinol and 25-hydroxycholecalciferol.

Frequently, drug–nutrient interactions are bi-directional. For example, while the bioavailability of minerals is reduced by co-administration with some drugs, drug absorption is also reduced by nutrients, especially minerals. Iron–drug interactions of clinical significance may involve tetracycline derivatives, penicillamine, methyldopa, thyroxine and other drugs. Furthermore, disease itself depresses circulating concentrations of some nutrients and may increase requirements (Thurnham & Northrop-Clewes 2004). Plasma concentrations of iron, retinol, ascorbate and zinc are rapidly and almost universally depressed by the inflammatory response and recent evidence suggests that carotenoids, selenium and pyridoxal phosphate are similarly affected.

COMMON DRUGS THAT INFLUENCE THE HANDLING OR TURNOVER OF NUTRIENTS

Medications may decrease appetite but usually the effects of the drugs are to alter nutrient absorption, metabolism or excretion (Table 13.1). The interactions described in this section are those that may lead to impaired nutritional status.

The short-term use of drugs is less likely to have adverse effects on nutritional status than long-term treatments. The problem is that the long-term use of many drugs is escalating. Over the last forty years, life expectancy has increased by almost 10 years in industrialised countries and by 20 years in parts of the developing world. As people live longer, the incidence of chronic diseases rises and the use of long-term drug therapy for chronic diseases such as arthritis, hypertension, coronary artery disease and adult onset diabetes will continue to increase. Many classes of drugs including antimicrobials, hypoglycaemic and hypocholesterolaemic agents can be affected by the presence of food, with the elderly patient being particularly at risk.

Aspirin and other non-steroidal anti-inflammatory drugs commonly cause gastric irritation and should be consumed with food. Aspirin is also reported to lower plasma vitamin C concentrations, but the mechanism is not known. Severe irritation to the stomach lining can cause bleeding leading to the loss of blood and the risk of anaemia through iron deficiency. In addition, it is suggested that aspirin alters the transport of folate by competition for binding sites on serum proteins; 70% of patients with rheumatoid arthritis have low plasma folate concentrations.

Antacids neutralise stomach acid and acid blockers reduce its secretion. Antacids may alter a substance's solubility both by modifying gastric pH and by chelation. Aluminium, a constituent of many antacids, can produce a relaxing effect on gastric smooth muscle that leads to a delay in gastric emptying time. Increased gastric pH leads to a reduced absorption of calcium, iron, magnesium and zinc. Long-term use of antacids such as H_2-receptor antagonists, proton-pump inhibitors and biguanides lowers the absorption of vitamin B_{12} in about 20% of elderly people (Dali-Youcef & Andrès 2009) since an acid environment is needed for its release from dietary proteins. As discussed in Section 10.6, the elderly are already at risk of vitamin B_{12} deficiency as a result of atrophic gastritis.

Antibiotics are used to treat bacterial infections. When they are taken by mouth they will reduce the number and range of bacteria found in the large intestine. Although the relative importance of dietary vitamin K (phylloquinone) and intestinal bacterial menaquinones is unclear (see Section 11.4), antibiotics can cause vitamin K deficiency and impair blood clotting. Cephalosporins containing the N-methyl-thiotetrazole side-chain are inhibitors of hepatic vitamin K epoxide reductase.

Tetracycline antibiotics bind to calcium in dairy products, which is a major food source of calcium in most industrialised countries (Thomas & Burns 1998). The interaction prevents the absorption of both calcium and the antibiotic. Calcium deficiency leads to mobilisation of bone calcium and subsequently to osteoporosis, a common feature of ageing. The elderly are also at risk from increasing gastric pH which retards the absorption of calcium and increased use of loop diuretics which enhance urinary loss of calcium.

Anticoagulants such as warfarin slow the process of blood clotting and this can decrease the risk of strokes in persons whose blood shows tendency to clot too easily. Such drugs function by interfering in the metabolism of vitamin K. Effective therapy is achieved by balancing the amount of anticoagulant against the usual intake of vitamin K. Hence physicians warn against the consumption of foods high in vitamin K in case an elevated dietary intake of the vitamin impairs the effectiveness of the treatment. In addition, haemorrhage caused by the anti-vitamin K action of such drugs can be exaggerated in the elderly by taking antioxidants such as tocopherol or very large doses of vitamin C ($\geq$10 g).

Anticonvulsant drugs used to control epilepsy, such as phenytoin, phenobarbital and primidone,

Table 13.1   Examples of some drug–nutrient interactions

ALTERING ABSORPTION		ALTERING NUTRIENT METABOLISM		ALTERING NUTRIENT EXCRETION	
DRUG	NUTRIENT MALABSORBED	DRUG	NUTRIENT	DRUG	NUTRIENT WITH INCREASED EXCRETION
Bisacodyl (laxative)	Potassium	Hydralazine (antihypertensive)	Vitamin B_6 antagonism	Aspirin (anti-inflammatory)	Vitamin C, potassium
Cholestyramine (anti-hyperlipaemic)	Iron, carotene, vitamins A, D and K, folate	Isoniazid (antitubercular)	Vitamin B_6 antagonism	Furosemide (diuretic)	Vitamin B_1, potassium, calcium, magnesium, sodium, chloride
Aluminium hydroxide (antacid)	Phosphate, vitamins A and B_1	Methotrexate (antineoplastic, antipsoriatic)	Folate antagonist, malabsorption of vitamin B_{12} and fat	Spironolactone (diuretic)	Sodium, chloride
Colchicine (anti-gout)	Sodium, potassium, carotene, vitamin B_{12}	Penicillamine (chelating agent)	Inhibits vitamin-B_6-dependent enzymes, chelates copper, iron and zinc	Thiazide (diuretic)	Potassium, magnesium and sodium but decrease urinary calcium
Mineral oil (laxative)	Carotene, vitamins A, D, E and K, calcium and phosphorus	Phenobarbital (anticonvulsant)	Increased turnover of vitamin D due to hepatic enzyme induction	Tetracycline (antibiotic)	Vitamin C
Phenolphthalein (laxative)	Vitamin D, calcium and other minerals	Phenytoin (anticonvulsant)	As above and also decreased folic acid levels		
Sulfasalazine (anti-inflammatory)	Folate	Pyrimethamine (antimalarial)	Inhibits dihydrofolate reductase and lowers folic acid levels		
Captopril (antihypertensive)	Iron and other minerals	Triamterene (diuretic)	Weak folic acid antagonist		
Olestra (anti-obesity)	Small decreases in carotene and vitamins D and E	Aspirin (anti-inflammatory)	Gastric irritation can cause iron deficiency		
Stanols and sterols (anti-obesity)	Small decreases in carotene	Corticosteroids	Anti-vitamin-D activity can reduce calcium absorption and cause osteoporosis		
		Oestrogen-containing oral contraceptive	Increase turnover of vitamin C and B_6 Elevate serum retinol concentrations		

Modified from Smith C H, Bidlack W R 1984 Dietary concerns associated with the use of medications. Journal of the American Dietetics Association 84: 901–914.

can cause diarrhoea and decrease appetite, so reducing the availability of many nutrients. They also increase vitamin D turnover and catabolism by inducing the hepatic microsomal drug metabolising system, so that vitamin D supplements may be needed.

Anticonvulsants also interact with folate; blood levels fall shortly after the onset of therapy. Folic acid supplements will counter the adverse effects on folate status but they also adversely affect the efficacy of anticonvulsant treatment, so folic acid supplementation has to be monitored carefully (as discussed in Section 10.5, under 'Upper levels of folate intake', this is one of the problems in considering widespread enrichment of foods with folic acid). The anti-epilepsy drug valproic acid is associated with folate deficiency and birth defects; in experimental animals it alters embryonic folate distribution, producing elevated concentrations of tetrahydrofolate and lower concentrations of formylated forms of folate. Such alterations are partially prevented by co-administration of folinic acid (5-formyl tetrahydrofolate) and S-adenosylmethionine but could cause hypomethylation of DNA and induce teratogenesis.

Antihyperlipaemic drugs are used to reduce blood cholesterol levels. Such drugs work by reducing fat absorption, the side effect of which is a reduction in absorption of the fat-soluble vitamins A, D, E and K and carotenoids. It is also reported that the absorption of vitamin B_{12}, folate and calcium may be affected.

The unabsorbed fat replacer Olestra (a sucrose polyester) and the plant sterols and stanols used to reduce cholesterol absorption cause small variable decreases in plasma carotenoid concentrations but minimal detectable effects on serum concentrations of vitamins A, D, E and K.

Antihypertensive drugs used to control blood pressure can affect body levels of potassium, calcium and zinc. Captopril, a hypotensive drug and an inhibitor of angiotensin-converting enzyme, can bind to iron in the gut if jointly administered with iron-containing mineral preparations, thus reducing absorption of the drug. Food also interferes with the absorption of captopril since food retards gastric emptying and elevates gastric pH.

Antineoplastic drugs used in cancer chemotherapy frequently irritate the lining of the mouth, stomach and intestines and can damage mucosal cells, thus altering digestion. Many cause nausea, vomiting and/or diarrhoea. All of these effects can potentially influence nutrient status.

The antineoplastic drug methotrexate is a folate antagonist that competitively inhibits key enzymes of intracellular folate metabolism and reduces the availability of methyl groups derived from single carbon compounds. Supplies of both folate coenzymes and the tetrahydropteroyl glutamate substrate for the conversion to polyglutamate derivatives (and liver storage) are impaired. Methotrexate also inhibits folate transport across the intestine and into hepatocytes.

The anti-tuberculosis drug isoniazid (isonicotinic acid hydrazide) reacts with pyridoxal phosphate and increases the risk of vitamin B_6 deficiency. Although older treatment regimens using high doses of isoniazid frequently included vitamin B_6, more modern low-dose regimens do not; however, a significant proportion of the population are genetically slow metabolisers of isoniazid, and hence are at risk of vitamin B_6 deficiency even at low doses. Isoniazid-induced vitamin B_6 deficiency frequently presents as the niacin deficiency disease pellagra, as a result of impaired synthesis of niacin from tryptophan (see Section 10.3), although it may also present as seizures due to changes in brain neurotransmitter synthesis. Isoniazid can also inhibit hepatic vitamin D 25-hydroxylation and possibly affect metabolism of the vitamin.

Diuretics stimulate increased excretion of urine and with it the risk of increased excretion of potassium, magnesium and calcium and the water-soluble vitamins. Thiamin status in the elderly is of particular concern in relation to the use of diuretics. Total thiamin body stores are small and thiamin has a high turnover rate with a half-life of 10–18 days, so a regular intake is required in conjunction with diuretics. Furosemide, in particular, has been associated with thiamin deficiency in elderly patients; in addition to increased urinary loss, it has been shown to impair the uptake of thiamin by cardiac cells in vitro. Thiamin supplements should be considered in patients undergoing sustained diuresis, especially if there is a risk of dietary deficiency.

Laxatives speed up the movement of material through the digestive tract, so reducing the time for nutrient absorption. They may therefore deplete vitamins and minerals, and there may also be increased fluid losses leading to dehydration.

INFLUENCE OF NUTRIENTS OR NUTRITIONAL STATUS ON DRUG HANDLING

The processing or detoxication of drugs and the many foreign compounds that enter our bodies daily occurs through phase I and phase II reactions. Phase I reactions include oxidation, hydroxylation, reduction or hydrolysis, introducing reactive groups on molecules. They occur predominantly in the liver and comprise the microsomal or mixed function oxidase systems (MFOS), NADPH-dependent enzymes and cytochrome P450, the latter in liver, lung and small intestine (Guengerich 1995). The second phase of the transformation involves conjugation with glucuronate, sulphate or glycine to render the metabolites water-soluble and permit excretion in the urine or bile. In general the intermediate compounds formed by these reactions are safe but there are exceptions, and a number of otherwise inert compounds are rendered carcinogenic by phase I metabolism.

Many nutrients and micronutrients may affect phase I activity; niacin and riboflavin are needed for oxidation, iron and glycine for haem synthesis for cytochrome P450 and minerals like calcium, zinc and magnesium to maintain membranes (Hoyumpa & Schenker 1982). It is difficult to establish to what extent low nutritional status influences MFOS activity but considerable experimental work suggests that the cytochrome P450 system is sensitive to deficiency of vitamins A, B-group, C and E. The pentobarbital sleeping time is prolonged in scorbutic guinea pigs, reflecting slower metabolism of the drug. However, it is uncertain whether human cytochrome P450 enzymes are also sensitive to vitamin C deficiency since the rate of metabolism of ^{13}C-labelled methacetin was not sensitive to vitamin C supplementation. Deficiencies of both protein and carbohydrate, on the other hand, clearly do reduce P450-catalysed oxidations in humans. For example, children with kwashiorkor have lower rates of drug metabolism.

Some food constituents can reduce human cytochrome P450 activity in amounts that are within the normal dietary intake, including flavonoids, the sulphur compounds in onions and garlic, the isothiocyanates and indoles in cruciferous plants, and capsaicin in capsicum fruits. Experimental studies with compounds that inhibit phase I or activate phase II metabolism show they reduce tumour formation in animals and there is growing evidence of their effectiveness in human beings.

The role of dietary inadequacies and excesses in influencing P450 activity in humans is also of fundamental importance in obtaining a better understanding of the aetiology of several diet-related cancers. For example, alcohol consumption is associated with head and neck cancers, smoking with lung cancers and a diet high in salt is associated with gastric cancers. By contrast, diets high in fruit and vegetables are associated with a general protection against many cancers and, as indicated above, there are several classes of compounds now known to inhibit or induce different P450 enzymes with potential anti-cancer properties.

EFFECTS OF LIFESTYLE HABITS ON NUTRIENT STATUS

Polyphenol-containing beverages, such as tea, reduce the bioavailability of non-haem iron, raising the possibility that tea consumption might cause anaemia. A review of published studies concluded that tea consumption does not influence iron status in Western populations where most people have adequate iron stores Temme & van Hoydonck 2002). Among people with marginal iron status there was a weak negative association between ferritin or haemoglobin and tea consumption. Recent experimental work suggests that flesh foods (beef, poultry and seafood), phytic acid and vitamin C are probably the most important dietary factors determining iron bioavailability.

Smoking is associated with lower consumption of many foods including fruit and vegetables and dairy products. Furthermore, smokers frequently have lower plasma concentrations of nutrients (especially vitamin C and carotenoids) than non-smokers even when dietary intake is taken into account. There is some evidence that smoking increases the rate of vitamin C metabolism.

There is an increased risk of bone demineralisation, fractures and osteoporosis in women who smoke and there is some evidence that smokers consume significantly less calcium and vitamin D than non-smokers, never smokers or ex-smokers. Although dietary vitamin D is usually a poor predictor of vitamin D status, since sunlight provides our main supply, one study in two groups of elderly women reported that plasma 25-hydroxycholecalciferol concentrations were significantly lower in heavy smokers than in non-smokers and this was accompanied by lower calcium absorption, but there was no difference in bone density at any site. In a recent review of the evidence for the effects of smoking and alcohol use on micronutrient requirements in pregnancy, it was suggested that vitamin C requirements increase for pregnant smokers and that plasma β-carotene, vitamin B_{12}, vitamin B_6 and folate concentrations were lower in pregnant than non-pregnant smokers. It is not clear whether the lower concentrations were due to increased requirements, lower dietary or supplement intakes or other factors. There is some evidence that iron supplementation partially ameliorates impaired fetal growth caused by cadmium intake from cigarette smoke.

The consumption of alcohol impairs the absorption of thiamin by inhibiting the active but not the passive process of thiamin absorption and, as discussed in Section 10.1, thiamin deficiency is a significant problem among alcoholics. Reduced absorptive capacity for thiamin persists despite supplementation with thiamin, but the effects of the alcohol are reversible since thiamin absorption, general nutritional status and hepatic morphology return to normal after a 2–3-month period of adequate nutrition and abstinence from alcohol.

Animal studies suggest that chronic alcohol consumption (at levels of 20–50% of energy intake) during pregnancy may mobilise fetal vitamin A from the liver, resulting in increases in vitamin A in various organs and birth defects. These results are of questionable relevance to human beings as the human infant has very little hepatic vitamin A at birth. However, chronic alcohol abuse is known to interfere with the storage of liver vitamin A in adults, and poor control of plasma retinol concentrations could have adverse effects; excess vitamin A is known to be teratogenic (see Section 11.1, under 'Toxicity of vitamin A').

Ethanol is oxidised to acetaldehyde in the liver by two enzyme systems, alcohol dehydrogenase and the microsomal ethanol oxidising system. The predominant enzyme in the latter system is cytochrome P4502E1 (CYP2E1). Isozymes of alcohol and other dehydrogenases convert ethanol and retinol to their corresponding aldehydes in vitro. In addition, new pathways of retinol metabolism have been described in hepatic microsomes that involve, in part, cytochrome P450s, which can metabolise various drugs. In view of these overlapping metabolic pathways, it is not surprising that multiple interactions between retinol, ethanol and other drugs occur. Accordingly prolonged use of alcohol, drugs or both not only results in decreased dietary intake of retinoids and carotenoids but also accelerates the breakdown of retinol through cross-induction of degradative enzymes. In addition, acetaldehyde interacts with liver stellate cells, the main storage sites of retinol in the body, stimulating their capacity to produce fibrous tissue and impairing the ability to store retinol.

13.3 MICRONUTRIENTS AND THE IMMUNE RESPONSE

As discussed in Chapter 26, the immune response is part of an orchestrated series of responses by the body known as the acute phase response (APR) that follows infection or trauma. The APR is essentially a protective response of the body against the danger posed by disease and is designed to facilitate both the inflammatory and repair processes, and to protect the organism against the potentially destructive action of inflammatory products. For example, tissue damage can be controlled or reduced by limiting cytokine production, neutralising reactive oxygen intermediates, inhibiting proteinases, etc. A reduction occurs in the concentration of several plasma nutrients with the onset of the immune response and these are frequently misinterpreted as nutrient deficiencies (Thurnham & Northrop-Clewes 2004). However, as circulating nutrient concentrations can fall very rapidly, they may be a part of the APR. If such 'apparent-deficient states' are protective, then administering large quantities of micronutrients at such times may upset this homeostasis and be counterproductive. This section will attempt to examine some of these issues and suggest explanations for the changes seen. Low plasma nutrient concentrations also occur in nutrient-deficient states when the body maximises mechanisms for nutrient economy and possibly the same mechanisms operate in disease states.

VITAMIN A

Low plasma retinol is an early feature of many infections, predominantly due to reduced hepatic synthesis of retinol binding protein (RBP; see Section 11.1, under 'Absorption and transport of vitamin A'). RBP, like transthyretin (TTR), albumin and transferrin, is a negative acute phase protein (APP) that responds rapidly following infection, suggesting that the changes in RBP synthesis accompany those of the other APPs initiated by cytokines IL-1 and IL-6. The rapid fall in plasma retinol associated with infection may initially be due to increased capillary permeability facilitating quicker distribution of retinol to tissues where it is needed to counter the infection. Labelling studies suggest that vitamin A in the extravascular pool is returned only slowly (37 days) to the plasma, hence the recovery of plasma retinol concentrations following infection is dependent on a resumption of RBP synthesis and mobilisation from the liver (Blomhoff 1994).

Vitamin A has been known as the anti-infection vitamin for more than half a century. Meta-analysis of eight major community vitamin A supplementation studies has shown an overall reduction in mortality of 23% (Beaton et al 1993) and vitamin A supplements have also been shown to reduce severity of severe diarrhoea and to be vitally important for the treatment of measles. Vitamin A enhances T-cell maturation, differentiation and proliferation. In animal models, vitamin A deficiency is associated with a shift from type 2 to type 1 cytokine responses. Type 2 responses include generating humoral immunity, antibody production and immunoglobulin maturation, hence the beneficial effect of vitamin A supplements on measles (Jason et al 2002). In contrast, type 1 cytokine responses are associated with low plasma retinol concentrations, with a raised proportion of natural killer cells and a higher proportion of lymphocytes producing both pro-inflammatory cytokines TNF-α and IFN-γ. IFN-γ plays a central role in activating macrophages.

The active form of vitamin A is retinoic acid and this acts at the nuclear level by binding to two types of response elements. One of these response elements can form heterodimers with the vitamin D response element. Where the heterodimer controls immune activity a relative deficiency of vitamin A may allow the inhibitory effects of calcitriol on T cell function to be expressed more strongly and influence T cell activity. Recent evidence also suggests that interplay between retinoic acid and calcitriol influences lymphocyte migratory capacity or 'homing'. Calcitriol blocks retinoic acid-induced upregulation of gut-homing receptors on human T-cells (Mora et al 2008). See also 'Vitamin D' and 'Vitamins A and D and gene regulation', below, and Section 11.2, under 'Metabolic functions of vitamin D'.

VITAMIN C

Evidence for changes in blood vitamin C concentrations associated with infection was first reported in the early 1970s when a rapid fall in leukocyte ascorbate concentration was documented within 24 hours of the onset of the common cold or following surgery. Leukocyte ascorbate concentration normalised over the next 3–6 days and the changes were shown to be due to the rapid influx into the circulation of newly synthesised white cells, most of which were neutrophils and contained very little vitamin C. Normalisation in leukocyte ascorbate concentration can be accompanied by a lower plasma concentration. The leukocytosis is of course a feature of the APR, and the dilution of the resident polymorphonuclear (PMN) leukocytes by the newly synthesised, vitamin-C-depleted PMN leukocytes accounts for the observed fall in leukocyte ascorbate concentration associated with stress conditions.

The accumulation of ascorbate by neutrophils in response to stress is a necessary part of neutrophil function and the production of superoxide when stimulated. However, large supplements of vitamin C (≥600 mg/day) can inhibit superoxide production while smaller amounts (200 mg/day) enhance it. Thus large vitamin C supplements may be counterproductive to neutrophil free radical generation and cytotoxic action.

Large doses of vitamin C can potentially aggravate oxidant damage within tissues and the uptake of ascorbate by neutrophils may provide a safe store for an important antioxidant and reduce the risk of increasing inflammation at the site of trauma. However, in convalescent states, there are suggestions that vitamin C supplements may have beneficial effects. Evidence suggests that vitamin C alters the redox state of arterial smooth muscle guanyl cyclase, altering arterial sensitivity to nitric oxide; measurement of flow-mediated dilation of the brachial artery shows a significant improvement following treatment with vitamin C.

A progressive neutrophil leukocyte infiltration of damaged myocardium has been observed during the first 24 hours after infarction. This is initially a beneficial process designed to remove damaged tissue. However, if the process continues it may exacerbate myocardial injury due to overproduction of reactive oxygen intermediates (ROI), and endothelial cells can be the primary target of immunological injury resulting in vasculopathy and organ dysfunction. Supplements of vitamins C and E increase neutrophil adherence, chemotactic and phagocytic capacity, coupled with a reduction in superoxide production, and 250 mg vitamin C daily for 6 weeks was found to significantly reduce monocyte adhesion to endothelial cells in subjects with low compared with high concentrations of plasma ascorbate (mean 32 and 67 µmol/l respectively). Thus vitamin C (± vitamin E) supplements in convalescent states such as coronary artery disease appear to improve blood flow through damaged tissues, reduce infiltration by monocytes and possibly reduce the net superoxide production from infiltrating neutrophils. Vitamin C supplements in the post-traumatic stage may assist the healing process, by promoting endothelial function.

VITAMIN D

As discussed in Section 11.2 under 'Metabolic functions of vitamin D', in addition to its role in calcium homeostasis, the active metabolite of vitamin D, calcitriol, has profound antiproliferative, pro-differentiating and immunosuppressive effects on the immune system. This has led to clinical applications of calcitriol or its analogues for its anti-inflammatory properties, e.g. in the treatment of psoriasis. In addition, calcitriol and analogues of vitamin D have been shown to have immunosuppressive properties in autoimmune disease and organ transplantation.

Although the primary source of calcitriol is the proximal convoluted tubular (PCT) cells in the kidney and the main function is to regulate calcium status (see Section 11.2), calcitriol synthesis is possible in many cells of the haematolymphopoietic system. 1α-hydroxylase activity has also been demonstrated in mature monocytes and macrophages, and activated T- and B-lymphocytes and the enzyme is induced by bacterial lipopolysaccharide (LPS). In addition, relatively high concentrations of extracellular calcium at sites of injury and infection may modify immune responses and enhance monocyte chemotaxis by increased synthesis of calcitriol.

Thus the production of calcitriol at sites other than the PCT cells appears to be responsive to infection and to promote maturation and differentiation of the monocyte/macrophage. Overall, calcitriol depresses cell-mediated immunity by blocking the induction of T-helper-1-cells (T_H1) and the production of their cytokines, particularly IFN-γ, while promoting T_H2 cell responses. Likewise, cells of the innate immune system are inhibited by calcitriol except for monocytes. Calcitriol also increased production of IL-1 and the bactericidal peptide cathelicidin by monocytes and macrophages (Mora et al 2008) confirming other reports that calcitriol promoted phagocytosis and intracellular killing by macrophages (Lemire 1995). In addition, evidence suggests that calcitriol inhibits the expression of B7.2 molecules, expressed on antigen-presenting cells to engage with the counter-receptor, CD28, on T-cells. Thus although calcitriol stimulated macrophage activation it blocked stimulation of T-cells by antigen.

IRON

Nutritional deficiency of iron results in anaemia; growth may also be impaired. Both anaemia and poor growth are common in many developing countries where exposure to and rates of infection are particularly high. There are rapid falls in the plasma concentrations of iron and zinc following the onset of infection, even before the onset of any fever (Thurnham & Northrop-Clewes 2004) and the greatest falls occur in those who subsequently develop fever. Recently the hypoferraemia of infection has been attributed to the actions of hepcidin, a peptide hormone (Collins et al 2008). The induction of hepcidin expression is brought about by the action of IL-6 on hepatocytes and causes inhibition of intestinal iron absorption, iron recycling from macrophages and iron mobilisation from hepatic stores (Ganz 2007). The hypoferraemia of infection is accompanied by changes in plasma concentrations of several iron-binding proteins that facilitate the uptake of iron from effete erythrocytes by the reticuloendothelial system and prevent its reutilisation for the synthesis of haemoglobin. To understand the potential role of infection in contributing to iron and zinc deficiencies it is important to understand the purpose and possible functions of those pathological responses to infection that affect these minerals. See also 'Inflammation and vitamin C' below for discussion on pro-oxidant properties of iron and the potentially protective role of hypoferraemia.

Iron affects both lymphocyte activation and proliferation and how macrophages handle iron. The proliferative phase of lymphocyte activation is an iron-requiring step as iron is essential for enzymes such as ribonucleotide reductase, which is involved in DNA synthesis. Hence a large number of clinical studies have found reduced T-cell function in vivo as manifest by impaired skin-test reactions and reduced in vitro proliferation of T-cells in iron-deficient individuals. The extent to which mild anaemia, the major problem in developing countries, impairs lymphocyte proliferation and immune responses is more difficult to evaluate.

ZINC

As discussed in Section 12.4, zinc is an essential component of a large number of enzymes, and the highly proliferative immune system is reliant on zinc-dependent proteins involved in cellular functions such as replication, transcription and signal transduction. Experimental data suggest that zinc deficiency depresses recruitment and chemotaxis of neutrophils, impairs natural killer cell activity, impairs phagocytosis by macrophages and neutrophils, and impairs the generation of the oxidative burst. Homeostatic regulation of zinc concentrations appears to be in the hands of a group of zinc transporter proteins, the so-called ZIP and ZnT families regulating both absorption and excretion. ZIP-4 is associated with the intestinal absorption of zinc and a recessive mutation of the gene that codes for the ZIP-4 transporter is associated with the severe zinc deficiency in the disease acrodermatitis enterohepatica, which is accompanied by thymic atrophy and a high frequency of bacterial, viral and fungal infections if not treated.

Zinc influences all immune cell subsets but is especially important in the maturation and function of T-lymphocytes because it is the cofactor for the thymus hormone thymulin. The control of T-lymphocyte activation is delicately regulated by zinc, and the physiological plasma zinc concentration 12–16 μmol/l is optimally balanced for T-cell function. Th1 lymphocytes are important in cell-mediated immunity and are responsible for interleukin-2 (IL-2) and interferon-γ release, while Th2 cells are linked to antibody-mediated immunity and the production of IL-4, IL-6, IL-10 and IL-13. It is suggested that zinc influences Th1 more than Th2 cells.

With the onset of infection, plasma zinc concentrations fall rapidly and in febrile illness the fall can be as much as 70%. It was recently shown that ZIP-14 concentration rises in response to IL-6 during inflammation and may be responsible for the hypozincaemia. During this acute phase response, zinc is redistributed from the plasma to the liver and lymphocytes. The advantage to the host of this response may be deprivation of zinc from invading pathogens. It is also important to note that while 12–16 μmol/l is the optimal plasma zinc concentration for T-cell function in healthy subjects, higher concentrations can be inhibitory; thus a reduction in plasma zinc may be anti-inflammatory. The mitogenic properties of zinc, i.e. the direct induction by zinc of cytokine production in polymorphonuclear leukocytes, is enhanced by bacterial LPS and phytohaemagglutinin at concentrations that would not normally be mitogenic. Hence apparent immunological disadvantages of low plasma zinc concentrations at the start of infection may be overcome by synergisms with bacterial antigens.

Low plasma zinc concentrations (<10.7 μmol/l) have been associated with not only reduced growth and development but also impaired immunity and increased morbidity from infectious diseases. The response to zinc supplements, however, is variable and may be dependent on whether plasma zinc concentrations reflect a true zinc deficiency or an infection-associated depression of plasma zinc. A meta-analysis of supplementation studies in children aged under 13 years showed that overall there was a highly significant positive impact of zinc on change in weight, although a review of eight randomised controlled intervention trials in pregnant women performed in less developed countries found no evidence that maternal zinc supplementation promotes intrauterine growth. There was evidence to suggest beneficial effects on neonatal immune status, early neonatal morbidity and infant infections but evidence was conflicting with respect to labour and delivery complications, gestational age at birth, maternal zinc status and health and fetal neuro-behavioural development.

Zinc supplements have been shown to be beneficial against diarrhoea and this is possibly the best evidence of the widespread nature of zinc deficiency in developing countries, since in experimental zinc deficiency, inducible nitric oxide synthase is more readily upregulated in intestinal cells by exposure to infection, with the production of diarrhoea.

Adverse effects of zinc supplementation have also been reported. Fever was greater in patients on home parenteral nutrition with catheter sepsis who were given zinc supplements (30 mg/day) compared with those given 0 or 23 mg/day. Depressed immune responses were observed in another study where patients were given 100–300 mg/day. One study is particularly revealing. Zinc supplements were given to children (6 months to 3 years) 3 days after admission with severe protein–energy malnutrition (PEM) and there was higher morbidity in those who received 6 mg/kg elemental zinc compared with 2 mg/kg. Most of the infants died of sepsis-related conditions and the authors suggested that the higher mortality may have been because many of the children would not have recovered from intercurrent infections present on admission. The study serves to illustrate the importance of the hypozincaemia in the infective process. Hypozincaemia may be important to deprive bacteria of an essential nutrient or reduce the potential pro-oxidant effects of zinc. This is similar to the situation with iron, where early iron supplementation of children with severe PEM also caused high mortality (see 'Transition metals' below).

SELENIUM

As discussed in Section 12.6, selenium, as seleno-cysteine, provides the active site of glutathione peroxidase, one of whose main functions is to convert lipid peroxides to hydroxy acids and hydrogen peroxide to water. Thyrodoxin is a specific seleno-peroxidase in the thyroid, and selenium deficiency partially blunts the thyroid response to iodine supplements. In addition to this, selenium is required in the deiodinases that form active tri-iodothyronine from thyroxine (see Section 12.5). Selenium deficiency exacerbates the effects of iodine deficiency. When selenium is deficient, a high iodine intake may cause thyroid damage due to a lack of selenium-dependent glutathione peroxidase activity during thyroid stimulation.

It is also apparent that serum selenium concentrations are lower in the presence of inflammation and selenium has been described as a negative acute phase reactant (Galloway et al 2000). It is not transported on carrier proteins and main plasma selenoproteins are selenoprotein-P and glutathione peroxidase. The reduction in selenium concentrations in inflammation appears to be associated with decreases in both selenoproteins. The reason for the decrease in serum selenium concentrations in the presence of inflammation is not clear but the fact that it occurs needs to be considered when interpreting epidemiological data on selenium concentrations and disease risks.

Disease and trauma are linked with increases in redox stress within tissues and experimental studies indicate that certain viruses may take advantage of compromised antioxidant status. Keshan disease in China is geographically associated with selenium deficiency but temporal fluctuations in incidence suggested that other factors were involved in its aetiology. Enteroviruses, and particularly coxsackieviruses, are believed to be responsible for the cardiomyopathy of Keshan disease, and experimental studies showed that Se-deficient mice were more susceptible than Se-supplemented mice to the cardiotoxic effects of coxsackievirus B4, which had been isolated from the blood of a patient with Keshan disease. Susceptibility to these viruses was not specifically associated with Se deficiency but could also be increased by vitamin E deficiency or a combination of vitamin E deficiency and polyunsaturated fatty acid (PUFA) excess. A previously avirulent strain of coxsackievirus CVB3/0 was changed to a virulent phenotype when passaged through vitamin-E-deficient animals. Similar effects have been observed in mice given excess iron and in glutathione-peroxidase-'knock-out' mice. Analysis of the genomic structure of the newly developing viruses suggests that increased oxidative stress in disease facilitates the enhanced growth rate of the invading virus, increasing the likelihood of development of more virulent mutations. That is, it was not selenium deficiency specifically that promoted development of more virulent viruses, but impaired antioxidant status in appropriate tissues and cells.

13.4 MICRONUTRIENTS IN GENE EXPRESSION

VITAMINS A AND D AND GENE REGULATION

The process of cell differentiation takes place in all tissues throughout the body. It has been known for a long time that epithelial tissue differentiation is sensitive to vitamin A deficiency as the normal mucus-secreting cells are replaced by keratin-producing cells. This is the basis of the pathological process termed xerosis that leads to drying of the conjunctiva and cornea of the eye in vitamin A deficiency (see Section 11.1, under 'Effects of vitamin A deficiency and excess'). As discussed in Section 11.1, under 'Genomic actions of retinoic acid', it has become clear that vitamin A plays a hormone-like role in controlling differentiation of cells in tissues and organs throughout the body.

As discussed in Section 11.2, under 'Metabolic functions of vitamin D', calcitriol, the active form of vitamin D, also exerts its effects on gene transcription through vitamin D receptors (VDR), and the vitamin D receptor forms a heterodimer with the retinoid X receptor, so that both vitamins A and D are required for many, if not all, of the genomic functions of vitamin D.

It is interesting to speculate whether the possible need for vitamin A to permit vitamin-D-induced calcium absorption can explain the effect of oestrogen therapy in the prevention of bone loss in postmenopausal women, apart from the direct effects of oestrogens on bone metabolism (see Ch. 24). Oestradiol has no direct effect on calcium transport, and does not directly increase the effect of calcitriol. However, hormone replacement therapy significantly increases plasma retinol and this might increase tissue retinoic acid concentrations, and so enhance calcitriol actions.

CONTROL OF IRON METABOLISM

The regulation of iron metabolism has recently been shown to be under the control of hepcidin produced primarily by the liver and secreted into the circulation. Its synthesis is increased in response to iron and inflammation and reduced in response to erythropoiesis, anaemia and hypoxia. IL-6 is the most important cytokine regulating hepcidin. Hepcidin regulates systemic iron metabolism by interacting with its receptor ferroportin, a transmembrane iron-exporter protein. Ferroportin is abundantly expressed on the cell surface membrane of reticuloendothelial (RE) macrophages, i.e. resident macrophages in the liver, spleen and bone marrow, and on the basolateral membrane of the duodenal enterocytes. Hepcidin inhibits iron release at these sites by binding to ferroportin and the complex is internalized and degraded. RE macrophages are especially important for the re-use of 20–25 mg iron daily from senescent red cells, and duodenal enterocytes release 1–2 mg dietary iron into the circulation each day. RE iron normally undergoes rapid turnover; thus iron retention in this cell population acutely lowers circulating iron concentrations (Collins et al 2008, Fleming 2008).

In addition to hepcidin, iron metabolism is under the control of iron-regulatory proteins (IRP). These are cytoplasmic proteins that coordinate cellular iron traffic by binding to iron-responsive elements on mRNA for a number of proteins responsible for iron uptake, storage and utilisation, protecting them from degradation. In iron deficiency IRP binds to mRNA and promotes the synthesis of transferrin receptor protein while ferritin synthesis is repressed. Hence the utilisation and absorption of iron is increased. When iron is adequate, ferritin synthesis is promoted, iron storage occurs and serum ferritin concentrations also increase. The presence of ferritin in the serum, however, is not sufficient by itself to indicate iron storage since ferritin mRNA is increased by both iron and the inflammatory cytokines. Thus infection and inflammation exert powerful control over iron metabolism.

Nitric oxide (NO) is produced both by macrophages in vivo as a physiological response to infection and by a variety of cell types as an intracellular messenger. It is central to macrophage-mediated cytotoxicity. It is increased in infection and may have a direct role in the post-transcriptional gene regulation mediated by IPR. In a low-iron environment, IFN-γ, TNF-α, IL-1 or LPS induces macrophage nitric oxide synthase (NOS). NO activates the mRNA-binding activity of IRP and so mimics iron deficiency. However, NO-induced binding of IRP to iron responsive elements specifically represses the synthesis of the cellular iron-storage protein, ferritin.

Hereditary haemochromatosis is a disease characterised by progressive iron overload which if undetected can lead to cirrhosis, diabetes mellitus, cardiac disease, arthritis or hepatocellular carcinoma or a combination of these. Recent evidence suggests that the disease is the result of perturbed hepcidin expression in the liver (Collins et al 2008). A two-point mutation in a high-iron gene (HFE) that regulates hepcidin production results in inappropriately low hepcidin expression and iron overload as a result. The lack of hepcidin increases iron absorption, decreases in iron excretion and production of preferential deposits of iron in hepatic parenchymal cells rather than Kupffer cells.

POLYMORPHISM IN THE HAPTOGLOBIN GENE, VITAMIN C AND IRON

Serum haptoglobin (Hp) comprises two protein chains and there are two forms of the α chain, giving rise to three variants of Hp in serum. It seems that Hp 1-1 has the best haemoglobin-binding capacity, while Hp 2-2 is the best at promoting immune function. Caucasians tend to have approximately 10–20% Hp 1-1, blacks 30–50% and Asians 10%. The Hp 2-2 is commonest in Asians (50%), lowest in blacks and middling in Caucasians.

One phenotype of the haptoglobin gene has been reported to influence vitamin C metabolism. The results indicate a lower stability of vitamin C (a higher rate of oxidation) in haptoglobin Hp 2-2 carriers than in those with Hp 1-1 and Hp 2-1. There is potentially less haptoglobin in the blood of Hp 2-2 individuals, so there will be more haemoglobin iron present in serum, causing the oxidation of ascorbate.

Likewise the Hp 2-2 phenotype has also been reported to influence iron metabolism. People with this phenotype accumulate more iron and have higher serum ferritin concentrations than those of the haptoglobin 1-1 or 2-1 phenotypes. Thus possession of the Hp 2-2 phenotype may make individuals more susceptible to disease by lowering plasma vitamin C concentrations (although this might be viewed as protective – see 'Inflammation and vitamin C' below) and increasing potential inflammatory damage as a result of increased tissue iron concentrations.

CONTROL OF PLASMA HOMOCYSTEINE CONCENTRATIONS

As discussed in Section 10.5, homocysteine is an intermediate in one-carbon metabolism. Intracellular homocysteine is either converted to cysteine via the vitamin-B_6-dependent *trans*-sulphuration pathway or is re-methylated to methionine by the vitamin-B_{12}-dependent methionine synthase which requires 5-methyl-tetrahydrofolate as methyl donor. This means that vitamin B_{12} and folic acid are major determinants of plasma homocysteine.

The synthesis of 5-methyl-tetrahydrofolate is catalysed by methylene tetrahydrofolate reductase (MTHFR). A commonly occurring polymorphism of the MTHFR gene reduces the stability and activity of the enzyme and is associated with moderate increases in homocysteine, particularly in subjects with low folate status. Supplementation with folate in doses from 0.2 to 10 mg/day has been shown to reduce both normal and elevated plasma homocysteine concentrations.

As discussed in Section 10.2 under 'Metabolic functions of riboflavin', riboflavin is a precursor of the flavin coenzymes which are cofactors for enzymes involved in the metabolism of folate and vitamins B_6 and B_{12}. FAD is the cofactor for MTHFR, which catalyses the formation of 5-methyl-

tetrahydrofolate, the methyl donor for methionine synthase.

The possibility that riboflavin status might influence homocysteine concentrations was initially demonstrated in blood donors, where plasma homocysteine concentrations were 1.4 µmol/l higher in the quartile with the lowest riboflavin concentrations. This compared with a 2.8 µmol/l difference between the quartiles for folate and 1.0 µmol/l in the case of vitamin B_{12}. The riboflavin–homocysteine relationship was mainly confined to subjects with the unstable variant of the MTHFR gene. Further studies confirm that riboflavin status can be an independent determinant of plasma homocysteine but the modulating effect of genotype is less clear.

Elevated total homocysteine (tHcy) concentrations have been associated with cognitive impairment but it was unclear whether it was low vitamin B_{12} or folate status that was responsible. A prospective cohort study in Oxford found that serum holotranscobalamin (a marker of reduced vitamin B_{12} status), tHcy and methylmalonic acid concentrations predicted cognitive decline, but folate did not. After adjustment for all vitamin markers simultaneously, the associations of cognitive decline with biomarkers of low vitamin B_{12} status remained significant. It needs to be tested whether randomized supplementation trials with vitamin B_{12} will prevent dementia (Clarke et al 2007).

13.5 MICRONUTRIENTS AS PRO- AND ANTIOXIDANTS

ANTIOXIDANT NUTRIENTS

Cellular integrity

Disruption of cellular integrity leads to the rapid release of cytokines by non-specific immune cells of the innate or natural immune system distributed through the body. The cytokines help to mount an inflammatory response and to recruit specialised cells such as mononuclear phagocytes, natural killer cells and neutrophils to the site of damage or infection. It is now known that the rapid induction of the synthesis of these cytokines is coordinated by a common cellular element, a transcription factor known as nuclear factor kappa-B (NF-κB) (Kopp & Ghosh 1995).

NF-κB is critical for the inducible expression of many genes involved in the immune and inflammatory responses including IL-1, -2, -6, -8, TNF-α, TNF-β and serum amyloid A protein. It is reported that NF-κB exists in almost all cells but that it remains in the cytoplasm bound to an inhibitory protein, inhibitory of kappa-B (IκB). Exposure of cells to various inducers such as TNF-α leads to the dissociation of the cytoplasmic complex and the translocation of the free NF-κB to the nucleus. Significant activation of NF-κB occurs within minutes, allowing NF-κB to function as an effective signal transducer and rapidly connect events in the cytoplasm to response genes in the nucleus. One such response is the rapid upregulation of IκB-α synthesis, which then helps to shut down the NF-κB response and provide a feedback loop to control a transient inducer of responsive genes. However, a unique feature of signalling through NF-κB is the diversity of both signalling molecules, including viruses, ROIs, mitogens and cytokines and situations that activate NF-κB, and the types of genes responsive to NF-κB. Nevertheless the common feature of the inducers is that they all signal situations of stress, infection or injury to the organism.

NF-κB can be activated by ROI and common inducers can be inhibited by antioxidants. Thus the NF-κB mechanism is of particular interest to those wishing to account for the health advantages associated with antioxidant-rich fruit and vegetable diets. N-acetyl-L-cysteine is a precursor of the antioxidant reduced glutathione, and a scavenger of ROI, and suppresses the activation of NF-κB by many agents. This supports the idea that the redox state of the cell plays a general role in the activity of NF-κB. However, in vitro studies with micronutrients which influence the redox state have to be interpreted with caution. In neutrophils, deficiency of iron can reduce myeloperoxidase activity and supplements of vitamins C and E suppress production of oxygen free radicals, so potentially both dietary deficiency and dietary excess could impair the killing of bacteria and/or reduce tissue damage. Among the questions that need to be answered are: is there an optimal redox state in vivo to enable efficient bacterial killing with minimal damage to surrounding tissues and are certain antioxidant nutrients more important than others in regulating this state?

Vitamin E

As discussed in Section 11.3 under 'Antioxidant functions of vitamin E', vitamin E is a conventional phenolic antioxidant. The amount of vitamin E in membranes is several thousand-fold less than the amount of potentially oxidisable lipid. Under oxidative stress, vitamin E undergoes a very rapid transfer of phenolic hydrogen to the recipient free radical with the formation of a resonance-stabilised phenoxyl radical from the vitamin E. The phenoxyl radical is relatively unreactive towards lipid or oxygen and therefore does not propagate the chain reaction; however, it is not an antioxidant and to maintain the antioxidant properties of membranes the vitamin E must be regenerated. Water-soluble vitamin C is believed to be the main reductant of the phenoxyl radical, but thiols and particularly glutathione can also function in vitro.

Vitamin C

As discussed in Section 10.7 under 'Metabolic functions of vitamin C', ascorbic acid is a powerful reducing agent and many if not all of the biological properties of vitamin C are linked to its redox properties. In the eye, vitamin C concentrations are 50 times higher than those in the plasma and may protect against oxidative damage initiated by light. Spermatogenesis may need ascorbate to protect DNA from oxidative damage. Spermatogenesis needs many more cell divisions than oogenesis, and reports suggest that DNA damage at this site varies inversely with the intake of vitamin C between 5 and 250 mg/day. Vitamin C is superior to other biological antioxidants in protecting plasma lipids exposed ex vivo to a variety of sources of oxidant stress. Lastly, folate, homocysteine and probably many other plasma components require vitamin C for stability and when blood plasma is separated from erythrocytes, vitamin C is one of the first antioxidants to disappear.

Carotenoids

As discussed in Section 11.1 under 'Vitamin A and carotene in cancer prevention', carotenoids can act as antioxidants because of their extended system of conjugated double bonds and the various functional groups on the terminal ring structures. Although there are many hundreds of carotenoids found in nature, there are relatively few found in human tissues, the five main ones being β-carotene, α-carotene, lycopene, β-cryptoxanthin and lutein. The ROIs scavenged by carotenoids are peroxyl radicals, and carotenoids in general, and especially lycopene, are very efficient at quenching singlet oxygen. Singlet oxygen is generated during photosynthesis; therefore carotenoids are important in protecting plant tissues but there is limited evidence for this role in human beings. However, β-carotene has been used in the treatment of erythropoietic protoporphyria, a light-sensitive condition where singlet oxygen might be involved in pathogenesis, with some success. Otherwise results from studies suggesting that β-carotene provides protection against solar radiation are somewhat equivocal. There was no benefit reported when large amounts of β-carotene were used to treat persons with a high risk of non-melanomatous skin cancer. However, lutein and zeaxanthin, which occur in the retinal epithelium, may be particularly important antioxidants. These hydroxyl-carotenoids together with meso-zeaxanthin are the major ones in the eye. Concentrations of zeaxanthin and meso-zeaxanthin are highest in the macula of the eye and evidence suggests they may protect against age-related macular degeneration (ARMD). Meso-zeaxanthin is probably synthesized from lutein since there is little to none in the diet (Thurnham 2007, Johnson et al 2005).

The antioxidant properties of carotenoids may depend on oxygen tension in the surrounding tissue. For example, at low oxygen tension, β-carotene acts as a chain-breaking antioxidant whereas at high oxygen tension it readily autoxidises and exhibits pro-oxidant behaviour. As discussed in Section 11.1 under 'Vitamin A and carotene in cancer prevention', the widespread distribution of carotenoids in plants and the considerable epidemiological evidence that consumption of fruit and vegetables was protective against heart disease led to three major β-carotene intervention studies. In two of these the subjects were smokers or people who had previously been exposed to asbestos. In both there was excessive mortality from lung cancer in the β-carotene-treated groups. In the third study, the subjects were not primarily smokers and the overall conclusion was that β-carotene caused neither benefit nor harm. β-Carotene is essentially non-toxic but one possible explanation is that the large amount of β-carotene induced one or more of the cytochromes that increase carcinogenicity of smoking-associated toxins, such as nitroso compounds, and increase the risk of cancer (Paolini et al 1999).

Flavonoids and polyphenols

Polyphenols are compounds which by definition are made up from multiple phenol rings. They can be classified into two groups, flavonoids and non-flavonoids. Flavonoids are the most common and widely distributed group of phenolics; over 4000 individual flavonoids occur in nature. They can be free, polymerised or linked to sugars or other non-flavonoid phenols. Dietary sources of flavonoids are predominantly fruits and vegetables, or products derived from these foods, such as wines and fruit juices. The simpler flavonoids tend to be water-soluble and are usually conjugated with various sugars in the form of glycosides. Cooking usually has little effect on the glycosides but colonic bacterial β-glycosidases will hydrolyse the glycosidic link, releasing the aglycone (Day et al 2000). The aglycones tend to be insoluble and, to be absorbed, must be conjugated to glucuronide or sulphate groups by phase II enzymes (see 'Influence of nutrients or nutritional status on drug handling', above).

Quercetin is a major flavonol (a subclass of the flavonoids) which is found ubiquitously in the diet. There is much evidence to suggest that it is a bioactive constituent of the human diet with powerful antioxidant activity and free-radical scavenging properties. However, most of the experimental work with quercetin has used the aglycone. After feeding sources of quercetin (such as 200 g of onion), only a very small amount is present in plasma as the aglycone; most is present as a variety of metabolites. While some of the metabolites will retain the biological properties of the aglycone, others will not and much work is being done to re-evaluate the earlier experimental work with flavonoid aglycones to characterise the important metabolites and their biological activity.

PRO-OXIDANT NUTRIENTS

Most biological antioxidants are potentially pro-oxidants. When an antioxidant molecule accepts an unpaired electron from a free radical, the intermediate formed by the antioxidant becomes itself a free radical. Fortunately, this is mainly a problem of food chemistry rather than physiology. However, in the case of vitamin C, changes in plasma concentrations occur which may be linked to its potential to be a pro-oxidant in inflammatory conditions. Likewise, although iron in healthy subjects is carefully controlled and unlikely to have pro-oxidant effects, in inflammation and disease there is indirect evidence that iron may become pro-oxidant since changes occur in the handling of iron to minimise potential pro-oxidant effects.

Inflammation and vitamin C

Several metabolic changes occur during inflammation which depress the concentration of vitamin C. Within 24 hours of surgery or following an attack of influenza, leukocyte vitamin C concentrations are depressed, due to the mobilisation of new neutrophils from bone marrow, which enter the circulation with low concentrations of ascorbate. The depression continues for 3 to 5 days while the cells gradually acquire vitamin C, probably from the plasma. Granulocytes actively take up ascorbate in vitro and where residual inflammation remains, plasma ascorbate concentration tends also to be low. It has been suggested that granulocytes require the ascorbate to protect them from free radical products that they produce during phagocytosis.

An alternative reason why plasma ascorbate concentrations fall in inflammation may be to prevent oxidation of transition metals. Inflammation is associated with tissue damage which increases the concentration of transition metals in the circulation. Interaction with vitamin C increases the risk of formation of ferrous and cuprous ions from iron and copper. Ferrous iron in particular is a powerful catalyst of the non-enzymic reactions that form hydroxyl radicals, with potentially damaging consequences for any molecule in the vicinity. In the stomach, vitamin C is secreted into the gastric juice where its ability to convert ferric to ferrous iron probably assists in the absorption of iron. However the presence of ferrous iron in intestinal lumen is a potential source of proxidant damage and the unpleasant side effects associated with taking iron tablets may be an illustration of this.

Ascorbate frequently catalyses damage in tissues in vitro probably because any tissue preparation is likely to be contaminated with unbound iron. This may be the explanation for the suggestion that ascorbate and many of its derivatives have anti-cancer properties. In vitro experiments with a malignant leukaemia cell line (P388D1) suggested that the concentration of ascorbate that inhibited cell growth by 50% (ED50) was approximately 17 µmol/l, within the range of plasma ascorbate of 11–20 µmol/l seen in populations where there is a risk of chronic disease (e.g. the elderly) or there is increased exposure to disease. Although plasma ascorbate is strongly correlated with dietary intake of vitamin C, healthy populations tend to have higher plasma concentrations than those exposed to sickness/trauma or who are sick.

Other workers have suggested that the cytotoxic properties of the ascorbate derivatives against human tumour cell lines are due to their ability to generate hydrogen peroxide and showed that cytotoxic activity of sodium ascorbate was almost completely inhibited by the addition of catalase to the assay. The generation of hydrogen peroxide by sodium ascorbate is probably an artefact of the experimental conditions, due to reaction of ascorbate with transition metals in the medium. Nevertheless, the treatment of cancer is often aggressive and likely to cause inflammation as indicated by the usefulness of iron chelators to lessen side effects of chemotherapy. However, the use of large amounts (up to 45 g) of vitamin C to treat cancer was not successful, and it was later pointed out that the four patient deaths from haemorrhagic tumour necrosis soon after treatment was started could have been due to the pro-oxidant effects of vitamin C.

Transition metals

In the absence of inflammation, zinc, copper, magnesium and selenium are involved in protecting the body against oxidative stress. Superoxide dismutase (SOD) is found in all aerobic cells and is responsible for the dismutation of the free radical superoxide (to hydrogen peroxide and oxygen). The cytoplasmic enzyme uses zinc and copper as cofactors, while mitochondrial enzyme uses zinc and magnesium. The hydrogen peroxide produced by the reaction is reduced to water by glutathione peroxidase (GPx), a selenium-dependent enzyme, using reduced glutathione as the reductant. Cellular concentrations of glutathione are maintained by the enzyme glutathione reductase, which is a riboflavin-dependent enzyme.

SOD and GPx are widely distributed in aerobic tissues and if no catalytic metal ions are around, endogenously produced superoxide and hydrogen peroxide at physiological concentrations have little, if any, damaging effect. However, during inflammation and disease, tissue structures break down, and in these conditions transition metals which are normally tightly bound to proteins are freed and potentially able to generate the highly reactive hydroxyl radical (OH) by non-enzymic reactions. In addition, pathological conditions greatly increase the concentrations of both superoxide and nitric oxide, and the formation of the toxic intermediate peroxynitrite (ONOO) with the reactivity of the hydroxyl radical has also been demonstrated in macrophages, neutrophils and cultured endothelium. Thus with the onset of disease, the potential for highly damaging reactions in tissues increases considerably.

Serum iron concentrations fall abruptly during the incubation period of most generalised infectious processes. (See also section on zinc in Section 13.3 for similarities with iron.) This can be viewed as a measure by the body to counter potential pro-oxidant damage. The body alters the transport and distribution of iron by blocking iron mobilisation and stimulating iron uptake from plasma into liver, spleen and RE-macrophages. In addition, as noted in 'Control of iron metabolism' above, nitric oxide mimics the consequences of iron starvation, leading to cellular uptake of iron. These changes in the control of iron traffic are part of a generalised response known as the acute phase response which in the short term is considered protective. It is widely accepted that the hypoferraemia of infection protected the host by reducing the iron available for bacterial growth. This is undoubtedly true for some bacteria but other pathogenic bacteria have powerful siderophores enabling them to compete successfully against the iron-binding proteins in the plasma. However, whether the role the hypoferraemia is to prevent or reduce the severity of infection, or to directly influence the redox status in the tissues, ultimately the body is protected. The pro-oxidant properties of iron potentially exacerbate tissue damage at sites of inflammation. In this connection it is interesting to point out that lactoferrin is secreted by neutrophils at sites of inflammation. Lactoferrin has a higher affinity for iron than transferrin and can also bind iron under acid conditions such as those found at sites of inflammation. Thus a reduction in plasma ascorbate and iron can be viewed as a physiopathological response to the potential pro-oxidant conditions that can arise as a result of inflammation and disease.

13.6 PHENOLS AND POLYPHENOLS

OCCURRENCE, STRUCTURES AND ABSORPTION

Phenols (derived from hydroxybenzene) and polyphenols (compounds containing two or more phenolic groups) are widely distributed in the plant kingdom and there are more than 8000 known compounds. There is a range of biological structures from the very simple, such as phenol itself, to highly complex and diverse forms, such as the tannins. The best-characterised group of polyphenols is the flavonoids of which there are over 5000 known compounds. Some of the major subgroups within the flavonoids are the flavones (e.g. rutin, luteolin), flavonols (e.g. quercetin, kaempferol), flavanols (e.g. catechin, epicatechin), flavonones (naringin, hesperidin), stilbenes (e.g. resveratrol), isoflavonoids (genistein, daidzein) and proanthocyanidins (e.g. cyanidin, malvidin: condensed tannins). The structures of the major classes of flavonoids are shown in Figure 13.1.

Most dietary flavonoids occur in food as 3-*O*-glycosides, most commonly of glucose, and some are glycosylated at carbon-7 in the A ring or carbons-39 and -49 in the B ring. Two β-endoglucosidases capable of hydrolysing the glycosides have been identified in human small intestine and studies with everted gut sacs have shown that several glucosides can cross the intestine, undergoing complete hydrolysis to the aglycone. Subsequent work has shown that the aglycone undergoes sulphation and/or methylation prior to appearing in the plasma. In a study in which four people consumed 200 g cooked onion containing ~79 mg quercetin glycosides, a fifth of the absorbed quercetin was methylated and a third was present as the sulphate conjugate. The average concentration in the plasma was ~0.6 μmol (~160 mg). Others have also reported identical metabolic profiles after consumption of quercetin-glucuronide from onion, buckwheat tea, quercetin-49-glucoside and quercetin-3-rhamnoglucoside supplements. In contrast to glucosides, however, hydrolysis by intestinal bacteria is essential for the absorption of other flavonoids. Where hydrolysis occurs, it will influence when and how much flavonoid appears in plasma and may also influence the extent of liver involvement in the production of secondary metabolites.

ANTIOXIDANT PROPERTIES

Most of the beneficial health effects of flavonoids are attributed to their antioxidant and chelating abilities. In vitro data consistently demonstrate the antioxidant efficacy of structurally diverse flavonoids under many circumstances of oxidative stress. For a flavonoid to be an effective antioxidant, it requires:

- a hydroxyl group on the unsaturated C ring at position 3 (to facilitate delocalisation of electrons)

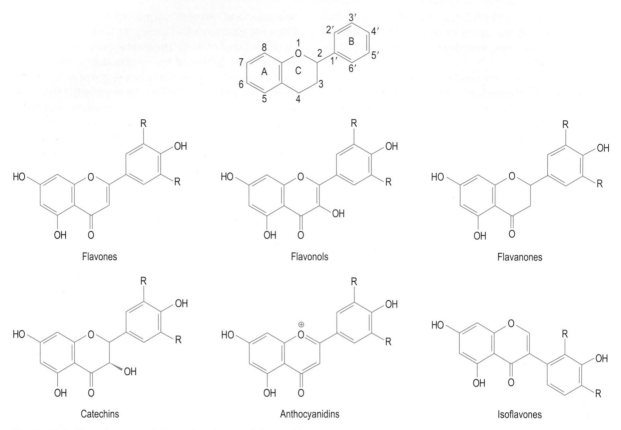

Figure 13.1 The structures of the major classes of flavonoids.

- a 2,3-double bond in conjugation with an oxo group at position 4 in the C ring and –OH groups at positions 3 and 5 in the A and C rings
- an *o*-dihydroxy structure in the B ring.

The B ring configuration is the most significant determinant of scavenging capacity for reactive oxygen species (ROS), reactive nitrogen species, peroxyl radicals and superoxide, and for inhibition of lipid peroxidation. Quercetin is a flavonol that has all three of the above characteristics and is one of the most powerful flavonoid antioxidants. If a hydroxyl group is linked to a sugar moiety then the potential antioxidant capacity is reduced, so the aglycones show higher scavenging ability than the parent glycosides.

Mineral chelating activity of polyphenols has both good and bad aspects. In vivo, polyphenols will potentially assist mineral-binding proteins and other mechanisms to scavenge body fluids for divalent cations and reduce the risk of Fenton-type reactions and free radical formation. Chelating complexes with divalent cations may form between the 5-OH and 4-oxo group on the C ring and between the 3'- and 4'-OH groups on the B ring. However, the mineral-binding properties of polyphenols compete in the absorption of important elements like iron and zinc. Phytic acid is a major dietary component in cereal flours. It is a phenyl ring with six phosphorylated hydroxyl groups and renders iron and zinc unavailable for absorption unless destroyed by the leavening process. Likewise, tannic acid in tea has been implicated in interfering with iron absorption, although a recent review of published studies suggested that tea consumption has no significant influence on haemoglobin concentrations in industrialised countries (see 'Effects of lifestyle habits on nutrient status', above).

Much of the work on the assessment of antioxidant properties of polyphenols has used the naturally occurring glycosides or the aglycones. For example, one study compared the effects of feeding red wine extract (equivalent to 375 ml red wine and comprising a mixture of flavonoid glycosides and aglycones) and quercetin aglycone (30 mg) on lipoprotein oxidisability. Following 2 weeks' supplementation to male volunteers, resistance to oxidation was increased by 18% and 16% for the wine extract and quercetin groups, respectively. However, there is no way of comparing the efficiency of absorption of the respective components in these two treatments, since the wine extract contained a mixture of flavonoid glycosides and aglycones while the quercetin was the pure aglycone. Not only do absorption characteristics vary between foods and also between individuals but the type of sugar glycosylating the flavonoid and the position of conjugation will also influence absorption. Furthermore, new metabolites are formed during absorption and structure–activity relationships suggest that they will have different antioxidant properties from those of the pure compounds tested in vitro, with potentially different biological activities. An aspect that should be considered is that the new metabolites may well have less pro-oxidant activity than native flavonoids (see 'Adverse effects of polyphenols', below). Consequently, it is important to determine the exact nature of the metabolites in plasma.

ANTI-CARCINOGENIC PROPERTIES

Quercetin has been shown to be chemopreventative in several animal models and in vitro it inhibits the proliferation of colorectal, breast, gastric, ovarian and lymphoid cancer cell lines. The protective effects of quercetin and other flavonoids have been attributed to inhibition of key signalling enzymes, e.g. protein kinase C, tyrosine kinase and phosphoinositide 3-kinase involved in the regulation of cell proliferation, angiogenesis and apoptosis, as well as antioxidant effects such as radical scavenging.

There is also evidence that polyphenols may inhibit cancer cell growth by effects on P450 enzymes 1A and 2B1 (see 'Influence of nutrients or nutritional status on drug handling', above). Repression of phase I enzymes involved in cancer initiation will guard against cancer development. A number of in vitro and trial cancer models have shown that green tea polyphenols appear to inhibit cancer development by blocking nitrosamine activation. In addition, green tea and citrus fruit polyphenols have been shown to increase the activity of the detoxifying phase II enzymes. However, a review of studies of green tea consumption in relation to various cancers reported mixed results. Only for gastric cancer did most of the evidence suggest that tea consumption might be beneficial, since 6 out of 10 studies found an inverse association. For colon, rectum and bladder cancers, no conclusion could be drawn as tea consumption was associated with both increased and decreased risks. Thus although green tea contains polyphenols with powerful antioxidant effects and one cup of tea usually contains ~400 mg polyphenols, the evidence for a protective effect against cancer in human studies is weak.

CARDIOVASCULAR PROPERTIES

Red wine is an especially rich source of phenolic compounds and the protective effects of moderate wine consumption against heart disease, and in providing a possible explanation for the 'French paradox', are well known. Tea is also a rich source of flavonoids and it has recently been shown that tea consumption can reverse endothelial dysfunction in patients with proven coronary artery disease; both short-term and long-term consumption of tea improved flow-mediated dilatation of the brachial artery.

High flavonoid intake mainly from black tea (61%), onions (13%) and apples (10%) was first associated with a lower mortality from cardiovascular disease and a lower incidence of myocardial infarction in the Zutphen study of older men. Catechin is the main flavonoid in tea but it is also present in wine, fruit juices and chocolate, and later studies suggested that sources of catechin intake from foods other than tea might explain 20% of the reduction in ischaemic heart disease mortality risk. Although not all studies have found similar effects, a recent meta-analysis on 10 cohort and 7 case-control studies suggested that the incidence rate for myocardial infarction in those consuming three cups of tea per day was 11% lower than that in those consuming no tea (Peters et al 2001). Reasons for inconsistencies in the epidemiological data are not clear. The antioxidant properties of black and green teas are similar and although milk is usually added to black tea, the flavonoid–protein complex formed does not appear to inhibit the absorption of flavonoids. For black tea, a cup (235 ml) contains 172 mg flavonoids and dose–response evidence suggests that 150 mg is needed to trigger an antioxidant effect and increase the anti-thrombotic lipid prostacyclin. However, the strength of tea as drunk varies enormously not only between populations but also within households and this may be the most important factor responsible for inconsistencies in the epidemiological findings.

ADVERSE EFFECTS OF POLYPHENOLS

In spite of the many potentially health-benefiting effects of polyphenols, adverse effects are known. Many polyphenols are synthesised by plants to protect themselves from predators. For example, resveratrol and catechins are antifungal agents produced by plants grown in conditions that encourage mould growth. Thus possible toxic properties in many of these compounds should be expected.

There are reports that mutagenicity is related to flavonoid-mediated oxidative damage and it appears that some of the same structural attributes that optimise antioxidant capacity may also exacerbate oxidative stress and tissue damage. Prooxidant activity is thought to be directly proportional to the total number of hydroxyl groups and in vitro studies show that flavonoids with multiple hydroxyl groups, especially in the B ring, increased the production of hydroxyl radicals in vitro. Various studies have reported cytotoxic and pro-apoptotic effects, induction of DNA strand breakage and even that the unsaturated 2,3-bond and 4-oxo arrangement may promote the induction of ROS in the presence of copper ions and oxygen. However, glycosylation and methylation attenuate the prooxidant behaviour of flavonoids, so the production of secondary metabolites of flavonoids following absorption may well be protective.

There are suggestions that hot tea consumption might be one of the factors responsible for the high risk of oesophageal cancer in China, but opinions seem to indicate that it is the hotness rather than the components that is responsible for the risk. Although a cup of green tea may provide 300–400 mg flavonoids, in the author's experience the tea consumed in some parts of China is very weak indeed and little more than ~400 ml scalding hot water containing one or two small leaves. In these circumstances, the hot water hypothesis seems more tenable.

13.7 PHYTOESTROGENS

A number of polyphenols that occur in plant foods as glycosides and other conjugates have weak oestrogenic/anti-oestrogenic actions, and are collectively known as phytoestrogens. As shown in Figure 13.2, they have two hydroxyl groups that are the same distance apart as the hydroxyl groups of oestradiol, and hence can bind to oestrogen receptors. They produce typical oestrogenic responses in animals, with a biological activity 1/500–1/1000 of that of oestradiol.

High consumption of legumes, and especially soya beans, which are particularly rich sources of phytoestrogens, is associated with lower incidence of breast and uterine cancer, as well as lower incidence of osteoporosis. The oestrogenic action is probably responsible for the effects on the development of osteoporosis, while three factors may be involved in the effect on hormone-dependent cancer:

1. The isoflavones are mainly anti-oestrogenic, since they compete with oestradiol for receptor binding, but the phytoestrogen-receptor complex does not undergo normal activation, so has only a weak effect on hormone response elements on DNA. Even those phytoestrogens that have a mainly oestrogenic action will reduce responsiveness to oestradiol because they compete for receptor binding but have lower biological activity.

2. The phytoestrogens increase the synthesis of sex hormone binding globulin in the liver by stabilising mRNA, leading to a lower circulating concentration of free oestradiol.

3. Some of the phytoestrogens inhibit aromatase and therefore reduce the endogenous synthesis of oestradiol, especially the unregulated synthesis that occurs in adipose tissue.

Recent concern that the increasing consumption of soy foods in the American population might interfere with the effectiveness of the anti-oestrogenic drug tamoxifen in the treatment of breast cancer was found in one study to be unjustified (Lannersfeld et al 2009).

Figure 13.2 The structures of oestradiol and the major phytoestrogens.

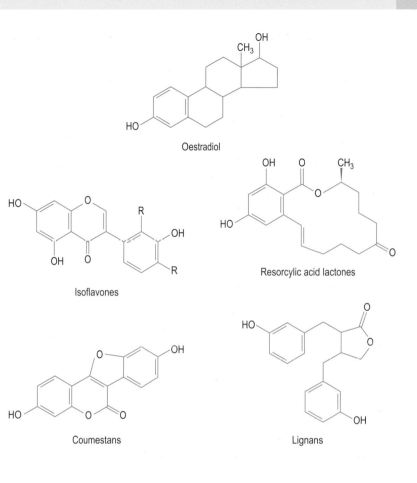

Oestradiol

Isoflavones

Resorcylic acid lactones

Coumestans

Lignans

KEY POINTS

- A large number of prescribed drugs can interfere with micronutrient metabolism, mainly by reducing absorption. The people who are most vulnerable to malnutrition from drug–nutrient interactions are those regularly consuming drugs, such as individuals with chronic diseases and the elderly.
- Lifestyle factors are well known for their sometimes debilitating effects on nutritional status and for having specific effects on vitamin C and carotenoids (smoking) and thiamin (alcohol). Tea consumption, although suspected of impairing iron absorption, would appear to have little effect on iron status in industrialised countries.
- The immune response has a major impact on several nutrients. Plasma retinol, ascorbate, iron and zinc concentrations are depressed as part of the acute phase response, and make important contributions to the body in infection.

- Vitamins A and D are important in regulating gene expression.
- Hepcidin is the single most important factor controlling iron metabolism. It is highly sensitive to both iron status and infection but the latter appears to be the dominant controlling factor.
- Haptoglobin polymorphisms also influence plasma vitamin C concentrations and plasma homocysteine concentrations are influenced by folate, riboflavin and vitamin B_{12} status.
- Several micronutrients exhibit antioxidant properties and interact in the maintenance of cellular integrity but recent evidence suggests the hydroxyl carotenoids may play a particularly important role in eye health and vision.
- Antioxidant nutrients can potentially become pro-oxidants and depression of plasma vitamin C, iron and zinc at the onset of infection may protect

the tissues against excessive free-radical-initiated oxidative damage.

- Polyphenols from a variety of foods act as radical scavenging antioxidants, and may also be protective against cancer and cardiovascular disease for other reasons as well. Some may also have pro-oxidant actions and may be mutagenic or carcinogenic.

- Some polyphenols (phytoestrogens) have both weak oestrogenic and anti-oestrogenic activity, and may provide protection against hormone-dependent cancer of the breast, uterus and prostate, as well as protection against postmenopausal development of osteoporosis.

References

Beaton GH, Martorell R, Aronson KJ, et al: *Effectiveness of vitamin A supplementation in the control of young child morbidity and mortality in developing countries,* Geneva, 1993, World Health Organization.

Blomhoff R: *Vitamin A in health and disease,* New York, 1994, Marcel Dekker.

Clarke R, Birks J, Nexo E, et al: Low vitamin B-12 status and risk of cognitive decline in older adults, *American Journal of Clinical Nutrition* 86:1384–1391, 2007.

Collins JF, Wessling-Resnick M, Knutson MD: Hepcidin regulation of iron transport, *Journal of Nutrition* 138:2284–2288, 2008.

Dali-Youcef M, Andrès E: An update on cobalamin deficiency in adults, *Quarterly Journal of Medicine* 102:17–28, 2009.

Day AJ, Canada FJ, Diaz JC, et al: Dietary flavonoid and isoflavone glycosides are hydrolysed by the lactase site of lactase phlorizin hydrolase, *FEBS Letters* 468:166–170, 2000.

Fleming R: Iron and inflammation: cross-talk between pathways regulating hepcidin, *Journal of Molecular Medicine* 86:491–494, 2008.

Galloway P, McMillan DC, Sattar N: Effect of the inflammatory response on trace element and vitamin status, *Annals of Clinical Biochemistry* 37:289–297, 2000.

Ganz T: Molecular control of iron transport, *Journal of the American*

Society of Nephrology 18:394–400, 2007.

Guengerich FP: Influence of nutrients and other dietary materials on cytochrome P450 enzymes. *American Journal of Clinical Nutrition* 61:651S–658S, 1995.

Hoyumpa AM, Schenker S: Major drug interactions: effect of liver disease, alcohol and malnutrition, *Annual Review of Medicine* 33:113–149, 1982.

Jason J, Archibald LK, Nwanyawu OC, et al: Vitamin A levels and immunity in humans, *Clinical Diagnosis and Laboratory Immunology* 9:616–621, 2002.

Johnson EJ, Neuringer M, Russell RM, Schalch W, Snodderly DM: Nutritional manipulation of primate retinas, III: Effects of lutein or zeaxanthin supplementation on adipose tissue and retina of xanthophyll-free monkeys, *Investigations in Ophthalmology and Vision Science* 46:692–702, 2005.

Kane GC, Lipsky JJ: Drug-grapefruit juice interactions, *Mayo Clinical Proceedings* 75:933–942, 2000.

Kopp EB, Ghosh S: NF-kB and rel proteins in innate immunity, *Advances in Immunology* 58:1–27, 1995.

Lannersfeld CA, King J, Walker S, et al: Prevalence, sources, and predictors of soy consumption in breast cancer, *Nutrition Journal* 8, 2009.

Lemire JM: Immunomodulatory actions of 1,25-dihydroxyvitamin

D3, *Journal of Steroid Biochemistry and Molecular Biology* 53:599–602, 1995.

Mora JR, Iwata M, von Andriano UH: Vitamin effects on the immune system: vitamins A and D take centre stage, *Nature Reviews in Immunology* 8:685–698, 2008.

Paolini M, Cantelli-Forti G, Perocco P, Pedulli GF, Abdel-Rahman SZ: Co-carcinogenic effect of β-carotene, *Nature* 398:760–761, 1999.

Peters U, Poole C, Arab L: Does tea affect cardiovascular disease? A meta-analysis, *American Journal of Epidemiology* 154:495–503, 2001.

Temme EHM, van Hoydonck PGA: Tea consumption and iron status, *European Journal of Clinical Nutrition* 56:379–386, 2002.

Thomas JA, Burns RA: Important drug-nutrient interactions in the elderly, *Drugs and Aging* 13:199–209, 1998.

Thurnham DI: Macular zeaxanthins and lutein – a review of dietary sources and bioavailability and some relationships with macular pigment optical density and age-related macular disease, *Nutrition Research Reviews* 20:163–179, 2007.

Thurnham DI, Northrop-Clewes CA: Effects of infection on nutritional and immune status. In Hughes DA, Darlington LG, Bendich A, editors: *Diet and human immune function,* Totowa, NJ, 2004, Humana Press, pp 35–64.

Further reading

Blumberg J, Couris R: Pharmacology, nutrition and the elderly: interactions and implications. In Chernoff R, editor: *Geriatric nutrition: the health professionals handbook,* Gaithersberg, MD, 1999, Aspen Publishers, pp 342–365.

Brown KH, Hess SY, editors: Systematic reviews of zinc intervention strategies. International Zinc Consultative Group Technical Document #2. *Food & Nutrition Bulletin,* Boston, 2009, UNU University 30 supplement 1.

Cooper KA, Chopra M, Thurnham DI: Wine polyphenols and promotion of cardiac health: A review, *Nutrition Research Reviews* 17:111–129, 2004.

Dali-Youcef N, Andrès E: An update on cobalamin deficiency in adults, *Quarterly Journal of Medicine* 102:17–28, 2009.

Goldman P: Olestra: assessing its potential to interact with drugs in the gastrointestinal tract, *Journal of Clinical Pharmacology and Therapeutics* 61:613–618, 1997.

Harbourne JB, editor: *The flavonoids: advances in research since 1986,* London, 1994, Chapman & Hall.

Kraemer K, Zimmermann MB, editors: *Nutritional Anemia,* Basel, 2007, Sight & Life Press.

Mangelsdorf DJ: Vitamin A receptors, *Nutrition Reviews* 52:S32–S44, 1994.

Thomas JA: Drug-nutrient interactions, *Nutrition Reviews* 53:271–282, 1995.

Thurnham DI: Iron as a pro-oxidant. In Wharton BA, Ashwell M, editors: *Iron, nutritional and physiological significance,* London, 1995, Chapman & Hall, pp 31–41.

Thurnham DI: An overview of interactions between micronutrients and of micronutrients with drugs, genes and immune mechanisms *Nutrition Research Reviews* 17:211–240, 2004.

PART 4

Dietary requirements for specific groups

Chapter 14

Infancy, childhood and adolescence

Elizabeth M E Poskitt and Jane B Morgan

CHAPTER CONTENTS

OBJECTIVES

By the end of this chapter you should be able to:
- describe the changing characteristics of growth and maturation from birth to adult that alter nutrient requirements
- understand the degree of immaturity of the digestive tract and organs during infancy, including pre-term infants, and the implications for diet
- discuss the composition of maternal milk and compare with alternatives
- explain the weaning process and associated risks
- have an informed opinion about the application of 'healthy eating' beliefs to children, e.g. high fibre, vegetarian/veganism
- be aware of the social and psychological factors that affect food intake during adolescence
- explain the basis of calculation of dietary requirements for infants, children and adolescents.

© 2010 Elsevier Ltd/Inc/BV
DOI: 10.1016/B978-0-7020-3118-2.00014-0

14.1 INTRODUCTION

Nutrition in childhood must be considered in conjunction with children's age, growth and development. Interactions between individuals' genetic endowments for growth and their nurturing environments determine body size and composition. Growth has specific nutritional needs but is not a steady process, proceeding rapidly in early life, slowing in middle childhood and accelerating at puberty before linear growth ceases. With increasing age also come physical and psychomotor maturation, which influence activity and body composition and, through feeding skills and food choices, dietary intakes.

14.2 BODY COMPOSITION IN CHILDHOOD

Table 14.1 shows age- and sex-related changes in body composition. After birth total body water falls and the proportion of extracellular fluid also declines. Percentage body weight that is fat (% BF) increases rapidly to a peak around 6 months old. Early infancy is followed by a period of natural 'slimming' until around 5 years. Typically this is followed by a second phase of relatively rapid fat deposition, the adiposity rebound, which continues almost unabated in girls until growth ceases. In boys the adiposity rebound reverses with the rapid lean tissue deposition of late puberty.

Each organ has a unique pattern of growth and maturation. At birth, brain weight is 25%, and at 5 years 90%, of expected adult brain weight.

Seventy-five per cent of postnatal brain growth takes place in the first 2 years of life. By contrast, about 30% of male adult body mass is acquired during adolescence.

14.3 NUTRITIONAL ASSESSMENT IN CHILDHOOD

(For further information see Section *evolve* 14.3 📑, and Chapters 28 and 31.4.)

Body weight for age is frequently used as an indicator of nutritional status but weight-for-age (WFA) is heavily influenced by height-for-age (HFA). Childhood nutritional assessment commonly uses either weight-for-height (WFH) independent of age, or WFA in relation to HFA.

Normally growing individuals follow growth trajectories which usually have similar relationships to population means throughout childhood, although deviating from these temporarily in adolescence. Reference standards for growth and development (Freeman et al 1995) do not distinguish the abnormal from the extremes of normal. If only anthropometric criteria are used for assessment, cut off points will inevitably include overlap between normally and abnormally growing children. Further, tall parents tend to have tall-for-age children and short parents tend to have relatively short-for-age children.

In 2006 WHO produced new growth standards for children from birth to 5 years (www.who.int/childgrowth/standards/en) based on infants who were exclusively or predominantly breast fed for at least 4 months after birth, regarded as close to ideal.

Table 14.1   Variation in body composition with age in childhood

AGE	MEAN WEIGHT (kg)	WHOLE BODY: WATER % BODY WEIGHT	WHOLE BODY: FAT % BODY WEIGHT	FFM: WATER % LBM	FFM: PROTEIN % LBM
Birth	3.5	72	14	84	14
4 months	7	60	26	82	15
12 months	10	59	24	78	19
2 years	12	60	21	78	18
5 years	18	60	16	74	20
10 years	32	60	17	72	20
25-year-old men	70	60	12	72	21
25-year-old women	60	55	25	72	21

FFM, fat-free mass; LBM, lean body mass.
From Poskitt 2003 © John Wiley & Sons Ltd. Reproduced with permission.

The growth of these infants was considered more or less optimal. The WHO 2006 charts are therefore seen as representing growth standards to emulate rather than simply reference charts (WHO Multicentre Growth Reference Study Group 2006).

Birth weights in UK are, on average, higher than those from the WHO data and, using the WHO 2006 data, fewer infants are defined as underweight and more classified as overweight than with previous UK reference charts (Wright et al 2008). UK 2009 growth charts combine UK 1990 growth references (Freeman et al 1995) and WHO 2006.

UNDERNUTRITION

For definitions of underweight, wasting and stunting see Chapter 28. Stunting, as growth retardation associated with socioeconomic deprivation, is a significant problem in westernised as well as in less affluent societies and usually responds better with changes in psychosocial and/or economic environments than with specifically nutritional interventions.

OVERNUTRITION

In adults, body mass index (BMI: weight in kg/(height in m)^2) is used to define overweight and obesity. In children mean BMI varies non-linearly with age. The International Obesity Task Force (IOTF) defines childhood overweight and obesity as the BMI SD score (or Z score) which, if maintained throughout childhood, would achieve the adult overweight and obesity BMI cut-off points of 25 and 30 kg/m^2 at 18 years. The 85th and 95th centiles are usually considered the cutoff points for overweight and obesity in epidemiological studies (NICE 2006).These definitions need to be used widely to evaluate their specificity and sensitivity.

14.4 DEVELOPMENT AND MATURATION

PHYSICAL MATURATION

The age at onset of puberty and the pubertal growth spurt vary widely between individuals. Secular trends towards increased HFA and WFA and earlier age at puberty, judged from age at menarche or age at cessation of linear growth, have slowed or ceased in recent years in much of Europe and North America but continue elsewhere, most notably in the Far East. These secular trends are attributed to positive changes in health and nutrition.

The age for 'normal' onset of the secondary sexual development characteristic of puberty is considered as between 8 and 13 years in girls and 9 and 13.5 years in boys, with similar mean age (11.5 years) in both sexes. In girls the first manifestations of puberty vary but the growth spurt always occurs early in the progression of puberty with peak height velocity (PHV – the point of most rapid growth in height) on average 0.7 years after the onset of puberty and before menarche. In boys testicular enlargement is the first observable sign of the onset of puberty. Growth acceleration in boys occurs relatively late in the pubertal process, with PHV occurring on average 1.5 years after the first signs of puberty, and continuing longer than in girls. Peak rates of deposition of bone mineral occur 0.7 years after PHV in both sexes and peak bone mass (PBM) is achieved 2 years after cessation of growth (mean: girls 16 years; boys 18 years). Pubertal changes in body size and composition (Table 14.1) lead to greater differences in nutrient requirements between males and females than were present in earlier childhood. In adolescent girls the nutritional needs of pregnancy and lactation may have to be added to those of growth and menstruation. In adolescent boys increased LBM leads to greater nutritional demands/kg body weight.

PSYCHOMOTOR MATURATION RELEVANT TO FEEDING

Table 14.2 outlines some of the important developmental 'milestones' that occur with age and which impact on children's independence and ability to feed themselves. The period of infancy (birth to 12 months) is one of almost total dependency on others for the provision of warmth, food, shelter and emotional needs. As children grow and become more independent, they begin to understand the implications of choice, make their wishes understood and learn to use food to manipulate those around them.

Once at school and mixing with their peers, children take their cues for food preferences from their friends as well as from their families. They may be heavily influenced by the portrayal of foods on television and by other advertising pressures. Then, in adolescence, peer approved fashions for certain foods and eating styles can lead to haphazard eating and bizarre diets with risk of compromising the good quality diets needed to meet the demands

Table 14.2	Age at average development of feeding/nutrition skills
AGE OF CHILD	**FEEDING SKILLS ACQUIRED**
36 weeks gestation to birth	Integrated sucking and swallowing reflexes
Three months	Conveys bolus of food from front of mouth to back of mouth
Five months	Conveys objects placed in hand to mouth Drinks from hand-held cup with biting movements
Five and a half months	Reaches out for objects and conveys them to mouth
Six and a half months	Begins to make chewing movements Feeds self with biscuit, rusk or other small item Transfers objects from one hand to the other
Seven months	Learns to shut mouth, shake head and indicate 'No'
Nine months	Picks up raisin-sized object with thumb and forefinger Throws food to ground with great enthusiasm – and expects someone else to pick it up
Ten months	Holds beaker of liquid but drops it when finished
Twelve months	Tries to spoon feed but unable to stop rotation of spoon (and loss of food) before it reaches mouth
Fifteen months	Manipulates spoon and food on spoon to mouth
Eighteen months	Determined to be independent at mealtimes
Two years	Expresses own self and independence in – often irrational – food refusal. This spell may last some years
Five years	Eating in company with peers may lead to eating a greater variety of foods than previously accepted May also lead to strong preferences for 'popular' foods

From Poskitt 2003 © John Wiley & Sons Ltd. Reproduced with permission.

of growth and maturation. At home the deliberate choice of unconventional foods and meal patterns may be used to express independence of the family. Those living away from home for the first time may have difficulty accessing foods and may lack the cooking skills required for a good diet. Habits such as drug addiction and smoking may also conflict with the needs for good nutrition. Lifestyles adopted in the adolescent years can continue into adult life.

Many adolescents feel very strongly about 'issues'. Anxieties about the environment, food additives, killing animals for food, becoming overweight, or even achieving 'healthy diets', may result in vegetarianism, unusual mixtures of foods, enthusiasm for 'quack' foods and supplements, or, more worryingly, macrobiotic and other extreme diets. In the 1997 National Diet and Nutrition Survey (Gregory & Lowe 2000) of children and adolescents, 2% of boys and 7% of girls aged 11–14 years stated they were vegetarian or vegan. Although only 1% of boys aged 15–18 were making the same statement, 10% of 15–18-year-old girls claimed to be following vegetarian or vegan diets at the time of the survey.

Adolescents and, increasingly, younger children, may demonstrate psychiatric instability through anorexia nervosa or bulimia. These two conditions have profound, even fatal, effects. Management should be approached through psychiatric methodologies rather than solely nutritional rehabilitation.

NUTRITION, GROWTH AND LATER DISEASE

The work of Barker (1998) and colleagues in the 1980s and 1990s has led to a worldwide explosion of research into the relation of fetal and early infant growth and nutrition with health and disease in adulthood. Low birthweight (LBW), particularly when there is rapid catch-up growth postnatally, is associated with increased prevalence of coronary heart disease and type 2 diabetes mellitus in adult life. The pathophysiological mechanisms for these and other fetal and infant programming events are currently subject to intense study. Causal explanations for associations between the diets of pregnant women, their offspring and later health, have still to be established. However, parental attitudes and family circumstances influence infant feeding practices and diet later in childhood, making it often unclear whether associations, such as between infant feeding practices and later obesity, are true programming or the consequences of common environment and related lifestyle choices. It does appear however that the later expression of genes may be influenced by the events and environment in utero and early postnatal life.

IMMUNOLOGICAL DEVELOPMENT

Food allergy and intolerance and the maturation of the immune system in relation to dietary components are discussed in detail in Chapter 26. Infants are born with essentially untried and immature immune systems. Gastrointestinal resistance to invasion by foreign proteins relies in part on the mucus secretions which contain protective substances such as secretory immunoglobulin A (sIgA) and IgM. The epithelial cells contain enzymes which destroy histamine and active substances in the gut. The immune barrier produced by IgG in blood and tissues under the epithelium also helps protect against sensitisation to foreign substances. Low levels of sIgA and lack of specifically sensitised IgM and IgG probably make young infants more at risk of sensitisation to foreign proteins which cross the mucosal barrier.

The relationship between infant feeding and infantile and later atopic conditions is not clear cut (for further information see Section *evolve* 14.4(a)). Exclusive breast feeding for the first 4 months of life is associated with prevention, or at least delay in onset, of early childhood atopic dermatitis, cow's milk protein allergy and wheezing. Thus the recommendations for infants with a strong family history of atopic disease would be the same as those for other infants: exclusive breast feeding for 6 months. If an infant formula is needed after 6 months of breast feeding and the infant has developed evidence of cow's milk protein allergy, a hydrolysed cow's milk protein formula should be suitable. The early addition of prebiotics, non-digestible food components which may facilitate growth and effect of beneficial bacteria in the colon, to infant formula might have some value in reducing infantile eczema although this is an area which needs much more research.

In the past, soy protein formulas were sometimes recommended for infants with evidence or risk of atopic conditions but the risk of allergy to soy protein is similar to that for cow's milk protein.

DEVELOPMENT OF GASTROINTESTINAL FUNCTION

Digestion and absorption in breastfed infants are promoted by many specific components in breast milk (Table 14.3). Immaturity of gastrointestinal enzymatic function makes digestion and absorption less efficient with infant formula than with breast

Table 14.3   Some specific components of breast milk which facilitate nutrient absorption

TYPE OF NUTRIENT	SPECIFIC COMPONENT OF MILK	EFFECTS ON GASTROINTESTINAL ABSORPTION
Carbohydrates	Lactose	Digested to glucose and galactose which are readily absorbed Fermentation of any lactose in colon produces lactic acid and low pH which encourage growth of non-pathogenic colonic bacteria Facilitates absorption of calcium as soluble calcium lactate
Fats	Presence of bile-salt-stimulated lipase in breast milk	Helps digestion of fat in milk in young infants in whom pancreatic lipase activity is low
	Relatively small fat droplet size	Small droplets offer larger surface area for volume, encouraging enzymatic digestion
	Saturated fatty acids – palmitic acid	Position of palmitic and other saturated fatty acids in middle of triglyceride molecule facilitates fatty acid absorption as monoacylglycerol which is more readily absorbed than free palmitic acid. Good absorption of palmitic acid discourages precipitation of calcium as calcium palmitate
Nitrogen-containing compounds	Casein: whey ratio	More soluble whey proteins predominate
	Casein composition	Human milk casein micellar structure creates small, easily digested flocculates in stomach
	Urea	May be used as nitrogen source by colonic bacteria to combine with organic acids and form amino acids which can be absorbed
Micronutrients	Lactoferrin and other micronutrient binding compounds	Many specific binding compounds in breast milk facilitate absorption of iron, folic acid, vitamin B_{12}, zinc and other micronutrients

milk in the first months of life. Fat absorption is particularly likely to be less in formula-fed infants than in breastfed infants. Pancreatic lipase, amylase and bile salt pool size are low in the newborn compared with older infants. Lactase levels in the newborn are quite low, increase as milk feeding begins and may decline later as milk ceases to be the predominant feed. Low lactase levels and lactose intolerance are common in older African and Asian children and adults but less common in Caucasian children and adults.

DEVELOPMENT OF RENAL FUNCTION

Young infants cannot dilute or concentrate their urine as much as older children and adults. This makes them particularly susceptible to fluid overload or to overload from food-derived non-metabolisable substances which have to be excreted via the kidney (the potential renal solute load: PRSL). The PRSL is expressed as milliosmoles per litre (mOsm/l) and indicates the total number of ionic or molecular particles in the fluid. For infant feeds it is calculated as: PRSL (mOsm/l) = Na + K + P + Cl + protein (mg)/175 when the dietary intakes of sodium (Na), potassium (K), phosphorus (P) and chloride (Cl) are expressed in mmol/l.

The PRSL for breast milk is ≈ 93 mOsm/l; for infant formula ≈ 135 mOsm/l; and for cow's milk ≈ 308 mOsm/l. The unmodified cow's milk formulas used before 1972, sometimes with complementary foods, gave young infants difficulty excreting sufficiently concentrated urine to expel the necessary solutes. Blood osmolality, plasma sodium and urea were at the upper limits of normal and even mild fluid deficiency precipitated hypernatraemia, uraemia and extracellular hyperosmolality. The ensuing intracellular hyperosmolality, especially in the brain, had disastrous, often fatal, consequences. UK legislation in the early 1970s which lowered the acceptable levels of sodium, phosphate and protein in infant formulas was followed later by similar EC Directives.

The high phosphate content of unmodified cow's milk based formulas also caused problems in young infants who were feeding well. The phosphate ions ingested in large quantities by term infants feeding well on infant formula were not readily excreted. Levels of plasma phosphate rose, precipitating falls in plasma calcium, hypocalcaemic tetany and convulsions in otherwise healthy infants around 7–10 days old. The condition resolved readily with intra-venous calcium and change to lower-phosphate formula. Changes to low-phosphate infant formula have virtually eliminated the problem (Poskitt 1994).

UK government recommendations on infant feeding have changed in recent years from the recommendation that infants be exclusively breast fed until 4–6 months old to following the WHO recommendation that infants be exclusively breast fed until 6 months of age. Current UK Department of Health guidelines on infant feeding are:

- Breastmilk is the best form of nutrition for infants; it provides all the nutrients a baby needs.
- Exclusive breastfeeding is recommended for the first 6 months of an infant's life.
- Six months is the recommended age for the introduction of solid foods for both breast- and formula-fed infants.
- Breastfeeding (and/or breastmilk substitutes, if used) should continue beyond the first 6 months along with appropriate types and amounts of solid foods.
- Mothers who are unable to, or choose not to, follow these recommendations should be supported to optimise their infants' nutrition (Department of Health 2003).

BREASTFEEDING PREVALENCE AND PROMOTION

Despite the almost universal consensus that breast milk is the best food (Table 14.4) for normal infants with healthy mothers and despite widespread publicity and promotion for breastfeeding, it has proved extremely difficult to improve 'breastfeeding statistics' in the UK. In 2005 only 63% of infants received breast milk at 1 week and only 25% at 6 months. Although breastfeeding exclusively to six months is the ideal, it is little practised in the UK. Fewer than 1% of infants still received only breast milk at 6 months in 2005. Breastfeeding rates are higher for more educated women, older women and black and minority ethnic women, which highlights continuing problems in getting young and disadvantaged mothers to breastfeed in the first place and then to continue exclusive breastfeeding for at least 4 months let alone the ideal of 6 months (for further details see Section *evolve* 14.4(b), Tables *evolve* 14.1 and 14.2 , and Ch. 15).

Table 14.4	Advantages of human milk for young infants
FACTOR	**ADVANTAGE**
Colostrum	High in vitamin A, zinc, sIgA
Convenience	Ready to feed but convenience dependent on local acceptability of breastfeeding
Low cost	Mother may have stores of fat laid down in pregnancy to mobilise for provision of fat in breast milk. Mother does not have to eat expensive food to produce milk
Clean	Breast milk is not sterile but bacteria present are usually non-pathogenic and milk contains antibodies to bacteria in maternal gastrointestinal system
Composition	Appropriate amino acid profile; contains long-chain PUFA; high organic acid residues in infant large bowel may be converted to amino acids by colonic flora
Facilitated absorption of micronutrients	Binding proteins, such as lactoferrin, facilitate absorption of many micronutrients
Enzymes	Breast milk contains enzymes the role of which is not understood in all cases. However, bile-salt-stimulated lipase may improve the efficiency of fat absorption in early infancy
Other non-nutritional factors in breast milk	Breast milk contains hormones, growth-promoting factors, cytokines and prostaglandins. The role of many of these is not clear but they may be relevant to the protective effects of breastfeeding against infection and possibly against non-communicable disease of later life
Anti-infective properties	These are varied: see Table 14.6

HUMAN BREAST MILK COMPOSITION

Human milk does not have constant composition (DHSS 1977). The first milk, colostrum, is low in volume and high in proteins, especially secretory immunoglobulin A (sIgA), as well as vitamin A and zinc. Over the first few days of lactation as the volumes of milk secreted increase, milk composition modifies to 'transitional' and then 'mature' milk. Table 14.5 outlines the biochemical composition of colostrum and human milk, together with indications of the range of nutrients in modern infant formulas – and neat cow's milk for comparison. Volumes of milk produced and precise composition of breast milk vary between individual women. The fat content of human milk falls in concentration with duration of lactation. Secretory IgA levels decline gradually with time although lactoferrin levels remain high beyond 6 months' lactation. Milk composition also varies according to the time of day and the stage of feed, with fat levels being higher in the morning and towards the end of a feed. The fatty acid composition of human milk fat partly reflects the fatty acid composition of the mother's diet.

Anti-infective properties

Human milk contains cells (macrophages, lymphocytes, neutrophils) and humoral components which protect infants against infection in the first months of life (Table 14.6). Secretory IgA resists digestion, adheres to the intestinal mucosa, and can be detected in infants' stools. It prevents adherence of viruses and bacteria to mucosal cells (often a preliminary to pathogenic invasion), allowing destruction of pathogens by the phagocytic components of milk. Secretory IgA specific to organisms affecting the mother–infant dyad appears rapidly in milk. Lymphocytes in the Peyer's patches are sensitised to organisms present in the maternal gastrointestinal tract and to those transferred from the infant during maternal contact. These lymphocytes, sensitised to produce relevant sIgA, seem specifically directed to the mammary glands and from there migrate into the milk. Nutrient binding proteins in milk such as lactoferrin, which binds iron, facilitate absorption of some nutrients essential for microorganism growth, thus inhibiting pathogen multiplication in the gastrointestinal tract.

There are other factors in milk which discourage pathogen growth in the infant intestine. Colonisation of the colon by *Lactobacillus bifidus* and *Bifidobacterium* spp. is promoted by the glycoprotein components of whey proteins and by N-acetyl-D-glucosamine-containing oligosaccharides ('bifidus factor') in human milk but not present in cow's milk. *Lactobacillus* and *Bifidobacterium* spp. promote lactic and acetic acid production from metabolism of lactose reaching the large bowel, creating an

Table 14.5 Comparative outline of energy, macronutrient and selected micronutrients/100 ml of colostrum, mature human milk, infant formula, preterm formula and cow's milk (information derived from various sources)

NUTRIENT	COLOSTRUM	MATURE HUMAN MILK	INFANT FORMULA (WHEY DOMINATED)	PRETERM FORMULA	COW'S MILK
Energy (kcal) (kJ)	69 (290)	70 (295)	67 (280)	80 (335)	67 (280)
Protein (g)	2.0[a]	1.3	1.5	2.4	3.3
Fat (g)	2.6	4.2	3.6	4.4	3.8
Carbohydrate (g)	6.6	7.0	7.2	7.8	4.8
Calcium (mg)	28	35	46	100	115
Sodium (mg)	47	15	16	41	55
Zinc (mg)	0.6	0.3	0.6	0.7	0.4
Iron (mg)	0.1	0.1	0.8	0.9	0.05
Retinol (µg)	155	60	75	75	52
Vitamin D (µg)	N	0.04	1.0	5.0	0.03
Vitamin C (mg)	7	4	9	16	1

N: significant quantities but no reliable information.
[a] Since much of this protein is sIgA it is not clear how much is digested and absorbed and how much remains in the gastrointestinal tract.

Table 14.6 Anti-infective properties in human milk

TYPE OF FACTOR	SPECIFIC FACTORS	METHOD OF PROTECTING AGAINST INFECTION
Cellular	Macrophages and neutrophils	Act as scavengers in infant gastrointestinal tract
	Lymphocytes	Synthesise sIgA. May be sensitised to organisms in maternal gastrointestinal tract
Humoral	sIgA	Adheres to intestinal mucosa preventing adherence of pathogenic microorganisms
	Lactoferrin and other nutrient binding compounds	Facilitate absorption of micronutrients, making them unavailable for microorganism growth and multiplication
	Bifidus factor, low buffering capacity, high lactose content	All facilitate maintenance of low colonic pH, encouraging growth of lactobacilli and bifidobacteria and discouraging growth of pathogenic organisms
	Interferon, complement, lysozymes	Facilitate immunological destruction of microorganisms
	Hormones, enzymes and other humoral factors	May have a significant role but this not yet clarified

environment of pH < 5 which discourages growth of potential pathogens such as *E. coli* and *Shigella* spp. Other active protective compounds in human milk include anti-staphylococcal and anti-*Giardia* factors.

Carbohydrates

Lactose, the main carbohydrate (80%) in milk, accounts for approximately 40% of total milk energy. Its particular suitability as the carbohydrate in milk lies in its high solubility, promotion (already discussed) of protective intestinal flora, and facilita-tion of calcium absorption through the relative solubility of calcium lactate. Other carbohydrates in milk include monosaccharides, oligosaccharides and protein-bound carbohydrates.

Proteins

Human milk protein is 30–40% casein to 70–60% whey. Whey proteins include lactalbumin, sIgA, lactoferrin and lysozymes. Casein is a mixture of proteins associated with magnesium, phosphate and citrate ions, bound with calcium as 'calcium caseinate complex'. Human milk casein forms smaller micelles with looser structure than the casein of cow's milk. The structure facilitates enzymic action. Precipitation of tough, undigested casein curds in the stomach is less likely than with cow's milk or unmodified cow's milk formula. Heat treatment of cow's milk protein in the manufacture of infant formulas affects casein micellar structure and enhances digestibility (Poskitt 1994).

The newborn liver has little cystathionine β-synthase, an enzyme involved in the synthesis of cysteine from methionine. Deficiency is greater in immature infants. However, provided there is sufficient methionine in the diet, cysteine deficiency does not seem to arise. There is cystathionine synthase activity in organs other than the liver which may account for this paradox.

About 25% of total nitrogen in human milk is non-protein nitrogen, of which 50% is urea, with small amounts of glucosamines, nucleotides, free amino acids, polyamines and biologically active peptides. Taurine is present in unusually high amounts amongst the free amino acids (DHSS 1977). Levels of taurine are lower in cow's milk and some infant formulas are supplemented with taurine. Infants fed low-taurine diets conjugate bile acids with glycine rather than taurine and these conjugated bile acids are less stable than taurine-containing bile acids, although evidence of disadvantage for normal full-term infants does not exist. All amino acids are potentially essential in infancy if rapid protein synthesis (e.g. in catch-up growth) outstrips the synthesis of amino acids from precursors.

Fat

Although the quantities of fat in human and cow's milk are not very different, the component fatty acids are very different. Human milk fat is higher in unsaturated fat, particularly the essential fatty acids linoleic (18:2ω6) and α-linolenic (18:3ω3) acid and also contains the long-chain polyunsaturated fatty acids (LCPUFA) arachidonic (20:4ω6), eicosapentaenoic (20:5ω3) and docosahexaenoic (22:6ω3) acid. Interest in the role of these LCPUFAs in neurological development particularly has been huge since it was shown that the levels of LCPUFAs in the brains of infants who were breastfed were higher than in those fed unsupplemented cow's milk formula. LCPUFAs are seen as conditionally essential for fast growing premature infants who may have difficulty synthesising LCPUFAs from precursors sufficiently rapidly to meet the needs of

the rapidly growing premature brain. The real importance of these fatty acids in full-term infants has yet to be determined but LCPUFAs are seen as justifiable fortifying compounds for modern term infant formulas.

The fats in human milk are more readily digested and absorbed than those of cow's milk since saturated fatty acids, especially palmitic, tend to be attached to the middle carbon of the glycerol molecule, encouraging absorption bound to micelles as monoglycerides rather than free fatty acids. Fat absorption from breast milk is also facilitated by the presence of bile-salt-stimulated breast milk lipase, although this is probably not of great significance except in immature infants. Most infant formulas now contain fats derived predominantly from vegetable oils with rather different proportions of fatty acids from those found in human milk fat. The relative proportions of fatty acids in plant fats are largely determined by plant genetics. The relative proportions of fatty acids in the milk of mammals, human and otherwise, reflect in part dietary fatty acid content.

Human milk has a surprisingly high level of cholesterol. The explanation for this is not obvious. Human milk also contains relatively high levels of carnitine – an amino acid like substance which is involved in mitochondrial oxidation of fatty acids. Infants can sythesise carnitine, but premature infants and those undergoing very rapid catch-up growth may be unable to synthesise carnitine at a sufficiently rapid rate to meet demand. This may limit the rate of fatty acid oxidation.

Enzymes and hormones

The roles of the many enzymes, other than breast milk lipase, and of the hormones in human milk remain largely undetermined. One enzyme – glucuronidase – can cause minor problems in early infancy. Newborn infants are prone to jaundice due to poor hepatic capacity to form bilirubin glucuronide which is excreted via the bile. Jaundice may have pathological significance since it is more likely not only with prematurity but with infection, dehydration and undernutrition. High levels of glucuronidase in the milk of some mothers deconjugate bilirubin glucuronide excreted in the bile, allowing resorption of bilirubin, increased bilirubin load on the liver, and 'breast milk jaundice'. The jaundice, usually developing at 7–10 days, is mild and occurring in otherwise healthy infants who are feeding and gaining weight well. It resolves gradually as liver function matures.

PROBLEMS WHICH MAY ARISE FROM COMPOSITION OF BREAST MILK

Breastfeeding is not without problems (see Table *evolve* 14.4). Rarely infants present with failure to thrive in association with inappropriate breast-feeding technique or, even more rarely, failure of breast milk production. When this happens the infants present with gross weight loss and sometimes hypernatraemia. Jaundice, mother–child transmission of infection and vitamin K deficiency bleeding (VKDB) are other medical concerns.

Transmission of infection via breast milk

Breast milk may transfer viral infection, most notably hepatitis B, cytomegalovirus (CMV) and human immunodeficiency virus (HIV), from mothers to infants. The risk from CMV in maternal milk is low since antibodies are also transferred unless mothers are acutely infected with CMV during lactation. Infants of mothers positive for hepatitis B surface antigen are at risk irrespective of the feeding method and should be actively immunised at birth. HIV risk of infection increases with duration of breastfeeding such that 5% infants are infected by 6 months and 15–20% by 24 months of lactation. The risk is greatest when breastfeeding is not exclusive. Current UK advice for HIV-positive and high-risk, but not serologically tested, women is to avoid breastfeeding. Where mothers are determined to breastfeed or where the risks of infection and undernutrition make formula feeding undesirable, breastfeeding should be exclusive for 6 months and then infants should be moved on to complementary feeding and breastfeeding stopped as quickly as practical.

VITAMIN SUPPLEMENTATION IN INFANCY AND EARLY CHILDHOOD

Rapid growth rates in young infants demand relatively high levels of micronutrients. Infants formulas contain sufficient supplementary vitamins and iron for normal term infants until weaning around 6 months old. The vitamin content of breast milk is affected by maternal nutritional status. Breastfed infants under 6 months do not need vitamin supplementation provided their mothers have ade-

quate vitamin status during pregnancy and lactation. Low maternal levels of vitamins and/or low levels of maternal intake may be reflected in low levels of these nutrients in breast milk (Table *evolve* 14.4). The vitamin probably most likely to be present in inadequate amounts in breast milk, other than vitamin K discussed below, is vitamin D, particularly for infants with mothers of Asian, African and Afro-Caribbean or Middle Eastern origin. Northern climes also make children more at risk of vitamin D deficiency since the period of the year when sunlight of wavelength around 300 nm, suitable for synthesis of vitamin D in the skin, penetrates the atmosphere is less.

The UK health departments recommend a daily dose of vitamins A, C and D for:

- breastfed infants from 6 months (or from 1 month if there is any doubt about the mother's vitamin status during pregnancy)
- formula-fed infants who are over 6 months and taking less than 500 ml infant formula per day
- children under 5 years of age (Department of Health 1994).

'Healthy Start', the UK government scheme with a focus on the nutrient intakes of pregnant women, nursing mothers and their children, endorses the UK recommendations for supplementary vitamins A, C and D for infants and children (Department of Health 2008). Daily supplements contain 7.5 µg of vitamin D, 233 µg of vitamin A and 20 mg of vitamin C.

Vitamin K and haemorrhagic disease of the newborn (VKDB)

Plasma vitamin K levels are low in the newborn. At birth infants lack the colonic flora that synthesise vitamin K. The ability to absorb vitamin K from milk or formula varies, as does breast milk vitamin K (mean = 15 µg/l). Levels of vitamin K in cow's milk are higher than in human milk and modern infant formulas are supplemented with vitamin K. Thus breastfed infants are at most risk of VKDB, which can cause minor bruising, blood loss from (for example) the umbilical stump, or major haemorrhage in the brain in later stages (> 7 days after birth). Prophylaxis and treatment are vitamin K as phytomenadione (Busfield et al 2007, Clarke & Shearer 2007). All term newborn infants in UK should receive prophylactic oral, or parenteral if oral is not practical, vitamin K at birth to prevent early (first 24 hours) or classical (1–7 days age) VKDB. Oral prophylaxis is by two doses of 2 mg of a colloidal preparation of phytomenadione in the first week of life with the first dose given as soon as possible after birth. Parenteral dose is 1 mg menadione intramuscularly at birth. If the oral dose is vomited, it should be repeated. Breast fed infants should be given a further dose of 2 mg oral colloidal phytomenadione at one month of age. Infants who are formula fed should have sufficient vitamin K from formula and do not need the third dose. Premature infants, infants thought to be at high risk of bleeding postnatally, and infants with perinatal trauma, should receive 400 µg/kg, to a maximum of 1 mg, vitamin K parenterally as soon as possible after birth. Refusal by parents to allow vitamin K supplementation, more likely when it is given parenterally, is associated with some cases of VKDB.

FORMULA FEEDING

The energy and nutrient content of breast milk provides the basis for developing infant dietary reference values (DRVs) (see Tables *evolve* 14.5 and *evolve* 14.6). However, questions raised by generally slower growth rates of breastfed than formula-fed infants, doubly labelled water estimations of breast milk energy content as closer to 600 than 700 kcal (2.5 rather than 2.9 MJ)/l, the relevance of Atwater factors, which estimate metabolisable energy of foods from constituent proteins, fats and carbohydrates extrapolated from adult values, in assessing energy content of breast milk, suggest the nutritional requirements of non-breastfed infants cannot be directly extrapolated from breast milk composition. Safety factors, developed with educated guesswork, are incorporated in energy and nutrient recommendations and formula composition.

All infant formulas are now highly modified from their base of cow's milk or, rarely (see below), soya protein (Table 14.5). Many formulas are available and differ according to content, whether they contain LCPUFAs, taurine, carnitine and even nucleotides, and to presentation such as traditional powder in tins with a measuring scoop, powder and scoop sachets, 1 litre ready to feed (RTF) versions and smaller 'one feed' RTF. Infant formulas are designed to provide appropriate nutrition for babies whose mothers are unable to, or chose not to, breastfeed, or who breastfeed in combination

with formula. Essential nutrient components are in line with the compositional standards set out in the UK/EU legislation. Infant formula is suitable from birth until neat cow's milk is introduced which should not be before 12 months.

Legal controls on the composition and use of formulas

Since the 1970s a series of UK government and international agency reports have made recommendations on the composition and promotion of infant formula. In 1981, the WHO adopted the International Code of Marketing of Breast Milk Substitutes promoting breastfeeding and the correct use of infant formulas. The implementation of this Code is closely watched by UNICEF and other international non-governmental organisations. In 2006 the EU published a directive on the composition, labelling and marketing of infant and follow-on formulas. The Directive was incorporated into UK law in 2007 (Statutory Instrument No. 3521, 2007). The legislation provides compositional standards for infant and follow-on formula together with detail on the labelling and marketing of the products.

SPECIALISED INFANT FORMULAS

Follow–on formulas

Follow-on formulas are designed to provide appropriate nutrition for infants over 6 months of age who are receiving complementary foods and probably taking less formula/kg weight than fully formula-fed infants. They provide more protein, micronutrients and energy per unit volume than term formula. They are a particularly useful source of iron during the weaning stage and research has shown that infants at risk of iron deficiency can benefit from the use of a follow-on formula. Since the introduction of follow-on formulas, the use of cow's milk as the main drink before the recommended age of 12 months has declined.

Formulas for LBW infants

These are developed to meet the enhanced nutrient needs of LBW and premature infants and include formulas for LBW infants in neonatal units and formulas for non-breastfed infants after hospital discharge.

Hypoallergenic formulas

These are based on partially or fully hydrolysed cow's milk. Fully hydrolysed milk formula is used as a feed for infants with diagnosed cow milk protein allergy. Partially hydrolysed formulas are used in cases where there is a strong family history of atopy to reduce the risk of development of allergies. Soy-protein-based formula is no longer recommended as a feed for infants, even those with suspected atopy.

Vegan formulas

Vegans do not consume milk products. Rearing infants on vegan diets can be problematic and is best avoided. If mothers insist on following a vegan regimen for their infants but fail to breastfeed, soya-protein-based formulas with vegetable fats are suitable for infants and compatible with the regimen. They should be used for vegan infants who are not breastfed as the alternative to cow's-milk-based formula but should be continued as part of the vegan diet in the post-infancy (toddler) period as they provide useful contributions to protein and micronutrient intakes.

Other formulas

There are many very specific formulas developed to meet the needs of infants with inborn errors of metabolism and other specific illnesses. Textbooks of paediatrics should be consulted for further information. Children fed these very highly modified formulas need supplements of micronutrients and conditionally essential substances such as carnitine and biotin.

14.5 NUTRITION OF LBW INFANTS

Low birthweight infants (<2500 g birthweight) may be preterm (born before the completion of 37 weeks' gestation) and/or small for gestational age (SGA), usually considered to be <2SD or below tenth centile weight for gestational age. Nourishing LBW infants is more difficult when the problems of immaturity are added to those of small size. They have less fat and higher total body water and extracellular fluid than more mature infants, and are at above average risk of hypothermia, hypoglycaemia and infection

(for management of feeding and care see Section *evolve* 14.5 and Table *evolve* 14.7 ⬛).

14.6 THE TRANSITION TO MIXED FEEDING: WEANING OR COMPLEMENTARY FEEDING

DEFINITIONS AND THE AGE OF INTRODUCTION OF FOODS OTHER THAN BREAST MILK

(For further information see Section *evolve* 14.6 ⬛.)

Weaning, also known as complementary feeding, has been defined as 'the process of expanding the diet to include foods and drinks other than breast milk or infant formula' (Department of Health 1994). Since the term 'weaning' is also used to indicate complete cessation of breastfeeding, WHO has recommended that the terms 'weaning' and 'weaning foods' are avoided and the terms 'complementary feeding' and 'complementary foods' used instead. However there is still some confusion in terminology since infant formulas, sometimes counted as complementary feeds, may be fed from birth. We use the term complementary feeding to embrace the use of all foods and liquids other than breast milk or infant formula. WHO and more recently the UK Department of Health formally adopted the policy that:

> Breast feeding is the best form of nutrition for infants. Exclusive breast feeding is recommended for the first six months (26 weeks) of an infant's life as it provides all the nutrients a baby needs.
>
> (Department of Health 2003)

An ESPGHAN (2008) review has challenged this recommendation as it is based on breastfed infants. The need for complementary foods may be different for formula-fed infants, individual mothers may be unable or unwilling to follow the recommendation and yet need support, and it is unrealistic to expect all infants to change from no complementary feeding to complementary feeding at the same time of 6 months (Ward Platt 2009). They conclude that exclusive breastfeeding for around 6 months is a desirable goal and that 'the introduction of complementary feeds should not be before 17 weeks but should not be delayed beyond 26 weeks'. Their recommendations for complementary feeding are summarised in Table 14.7.

Table 14.7	Recommendations for complementary feeding*

1. Exclusive or full breastfeeding for about 6 months is a desirable goal
2. The term 'complementary feeding' should include all solid foods and liquids other than breast milk, infant and follow-on formulas
3. Recommendations for complementary feeding should embrace both breastfed and formula-fed infants
4. Avoidance or delayed introduction of potentially allergenic foods is unnecessary since this has not been convincingly shown to reduce allergies
5. During complementary feeding, bioavailable iron sufficient to provide more than 90% of the infant's requirements should come from the complementary foods.
6. Cow's milk should not be used as the main drink before 12 months. Small volumes may be added to complementary foods
7. Prudent avoidance of early (<4 months) and late (>7 months) introduction of gluten. Introducing gluten while the infant is still breastfeeding may reduce the risk of coeliac disease, type 1 diabetes mellitus and wheat allergy.
8. Infants and young children receiving vegetarian diets should receive ≈ 500 ml breast milk or formula and dairy products daily.
9. Infants and young children should not receive a vegan diet.

*Abbreviated from ESPGHAN Committee on Nutrition 2008

MATERNAL CHOICE IN COMPLEMENTARY FEEDING

Early introduction of complementary feeds is associated with low maternal age, formula feeding and maternal smoking. Maternal practices seem influenced by infant growth since infant weight at 6 weeks predicts age at introduction of complementary foods better than birthweight or early weight gain, with heavy infants introduced earlier than light infants. Breastfed infants are often switched to infant formula with the introduction of complementary foods.

Digestion is not a problem for full-term infants introduced prematurely to complementary foods. For example, starchy foods (e.g. cereal) fed before pancreatic enzymes reach mature levels, around 4 months of age, can be digested fully. Increased salivary amylase and intestinal glycoamylase activities compensate for low pancreatic amylase. Table 14.8 outlines some advantages and disadvantages of introducing complementary feeds.

What foods

Complementary foods may be home prepared or commercially produced. Initially one small feed is introduced per day but feed frequency may increase quite quickly. Some recommendations suggest foods are introduced one at a time so as to recognise intolerance to specific foods but this seems an unnecessarily cautious approach which could threaten mothers' confidence over introducing new foods. Offering a variety of foods from the onset of complementary feeding should be perfectly satisfactory but later dietary preferences do seem to relate to early dietary experience so feeding very sweet foods could have disadvantages for later 'healthy' food choices.

Energy

Whilst breast milk (or formula) remains the main source of energy early in complementary feeding, cereal-based complementary foods, with energy density enhanced by additional fat source, should be introduced early. Rice preparations are usually recommended since rice is gluten-free. With wheat-based foods there is slight risk of malabsorption from either temporary gluten intolerance following gastrointestinal infection, or permanent gluten intolerance in coeliac syndrome. There is some evidence that delaying introduction to gluten-containing foods until after 7 months of age may increase the risk of coeliac disease. Introducing gluten when the infant is still breastfed may reduce the risk of developing intolerance (ESPGHAN 2008).

Fat

Fat in the diet can increase the energy density of foods, thus facilitating energy sufficiency and optimum infant growth with the relatively small volumes of food tolerated by infants' small gastric capacities. Fats also act as sources of fat-soluble vitamins, essential fatty acids and exogenous cholesterol and enhance taste and food texture and thus palatability.

Protein

Dietary surveys consistently show mean protein intakes well above DRVs in infancy. Provided breast milk, formula or, later, cow's milk intakes are

Table 14.8   Advantages and disadvantages for infant nutrition of introduction of complementary foods around 6 months of age

ADVANTAGE	DISADVANTAGE
Possible introduction of high energy and micronutrient (e.g. iron) sources to meet restricted provision of these in breast milk may prevent growth faltering in second 6 months of life	Complementary diet, particularly if vegetables and 'puddings', may be lower in energy and micronutrients than breast milk
Encouraging hand–mouth skills through feeding process	Failure to provide foods that require feeding techniques other than suckling may lead to delay in learning appropriate feeding skills
Maintenance of good nutrition through effective complementary feeding can help relatively non-immune young infant fight infections likely to develop in second 6 months of life	Anti-infective effects of breast milk coupled with its relative sterility may be more beneficial than nutrient gains if poor hygiene during complementary diet preparation. Anti-infective effect of breast milk reduced by mixed feeding Increased respiratory tract infection in infants introduced to complementary feeding early
Ability to eat with family and develop social skills	Eating along with the family may give less attention to the infant's diet and may disadvantage the infant by hurrying meal process. Rest of family may consume food infant needs
Permeability of infant gastrointestinal mucosa to foreign proteins greatly reduced after 4 months age so introduction of non-breastmilk foods after this probably does not affect level of foreign protein absorption	Early introduction of complementary foods may lead to increased problems with allergic reactions to foods
Breastfeeding can continue to provide a significant contribution to diet	Breast milk output tends to fall as complementary feeding is introduced and suckling frequency may reduce. Mixed breast and complementary feeding more likely to lead to HIV transmission to infant if mother seropositive

around 500 ml/day, protein intakes are likely to be adequate even if complementary feeds are low in protein and amino acid variety (as may happen in diets with a single plant staple).

HOME-PREPARED VERSUS COMMERCIAL COMPLEMENTARY FOODS

UK legislation specifies a range of nutritional contents for commercially produced infant foods. Thus infants receiving commercial complementary foods may have more balanced nutrient intakes than those fed home-prepared foods. Stordy and colleagues (1995) reported, in their study involving chemical analysis of foods, that 40% of home-prepared complementary/weaning foods had an energy content lower than breast milk and were lower in fat, iron and vitamin D and higher in sodium than commercially prepared infant foods. The 2005 Infant Feeding Survey (Bolling et al 2007) showed that mothers feeding complementary foods before 6 months were likely to feed commercial preparations but after 6 months infants' diets were more likely to be home-prepared foods.

Cultural and personal dietary choices mean that some mothers are uncertain about the acceptability of some commercial savoury dishes. (Which animal source? Is the meat 'halal'?) As a consequence, they may feed their infants commercial fruit, vegetable and pudding products only. If only these are offered as complementary foods, energy needs are unlikely to be met as the foods displace breast milk and formula in the diet but are usually less energy-dense. Minority groups, particularly if hampered by language as well as cultural problems, may benefit from complementary feeding advice from suitably trained health visitors or paediatric dieticians.

Food consistency

Complementary feeding is a progressive process. Early foods offered are semisolid. Infants quickly learn to cope with solid and lumpy foods and ultimately foods which require chewing prior to swallowing. This progression is important. Prolonged partial breastfeeding without adequate addition of weaning foods, excessive juice intake, the offering of inadequate foods because of perceived food 'allergens', the inappropriate provision of a milk-free diet that is low in protein can all lead to undernutrition. Prolonged bottle feeding, beyond 1 year, can lead to failure to thrive (FTT) due to the 'comfort' aspect of sucking and the low energy density of fluids proffered. Infants should be moved from fluids fed by bottle to predominantly fluids fed by cup over the second 6 months of life.

High solute load and low iron content make unmodified cow's milk unsuitable for early complementary feeding. Cow's milk protein intolerance (CMPI) can cause incipient or overt gastrointestinal blood loss. Current UK recommendations are that cow's milk should not be given as a drink to infants under 1 year. When it forms part of family recipes, small amounts may be safe before this age.

Vegan infants and other at-risk groups

Vegan mothers have higher levels of unsaturated fatty acids in their milk than omnivore mothers. This may be advantageous to the infants. Even so, feeding infants according to a vegan regimen is nutritionally hazardous. If mothers are determined to feed their infants from a vegan regimen, soya-based infant formulas, supplemented with micronutrients and appropriately balanced energy and protein, should be used as alternatives to breast milk as breast milk output declines, and continued beyond infancy. Vitamin deficiencies in infants born to deficient mothers, particularly for B_1 and B_{12}, may be exacerbated by low breast milk vitamin content. In vegans low levels of breast milk vitamin B_{12} reflect maternal intakes during lactation rather than maternal stores, so deficiency in infants may be exacerbated by breastfeeding even without evidence of maternal deficiency. ESPGHAN (2008) state very definitely that 'infants and young children should not receive a vegan diet'.

COMPLEMENTARY FEEDING FOR PRETERM INFANTS

After discharge from neonatal units, preterm (PT) infants still have higher than normal requirements for energy, protein, LCPUFA, zinc, iron, calcium and selenium. Current recommendations for age of introduction to complementary foods, when the infant 'weighs at least 5 kg, has lost the extrusion reflex and is able to eat from a spoon' (Department of Health 1994), fail to take account of differences in nutritional requirements between PT and normal birthweight term infants. Complementary feeding tends to begin earlier in PT infants who had little exposure to human milk in the neonatal period and whose mothers smoke.

14.7 NUTRITION IN CHILDREN AND ADOLESCENTS

Digestion and absorption in preschool children enable them to consume the same foods as adults but nutrient needs and feeding skills are different. Table 14.9 lists some of the issues to consider in child and adolescent nutrition. Children's small stomachs limit the amounts of food taken at any one meal. They do not consume food overnight. Young children should therefore be fed three meals a day and perhaps two between-meal snacks, the timing of which depends on mealtimes. One snack or meal should be close to bedtime. Small eaters and 'fussy' eaters may have difficulty consuming sufficient energy to meet needs so recommendations for adults to consume <35% dietary energy from fat do not apply to young children. The transition from >50% dietary energy derived from fat provided by exclusive breastfeeding to <35% energy derived from fat should be spread over the first 5 years of life. Similarly, adult recommendations for fibre intake should not apply in early childhood since high fibre content lowers food energy density and phytates reduce absorption of micronutrients. Diets with <30% energy derived from fat are quite common amongst preschool children who consume large quantities of 'juice' and sweets instead of meals of varied content. These are likely to lead to FTT if prolonged.

Persuading children to eat family meals is not always easy. All over the world children seem reluctant to eat green leafy vegetables. Inexperience with chewing may be a contributing factor. UK government recommendations for supplementary vitamins A and D and more recently vitamin C in Healthy Start vitamins to children under 5 years, recognise the difficulties of achieving varied diets in young children. Nevertheless, relatively few children receive supplementary vitamins after infancy.

Table 14.9   Modifications to quality of diet needed for child to progress from infant diet to that of adult

AGE	DIET	NUTRITIONAL ISSUES
Young infant	Wholly breastfed	Entirely liquid diet Quite low-energy food, ~0.7 kcal/ml All essential nutrients in one food No fibre in diet >50% total energy from fat
Weaning diet	Milk: formula or breast plus some 'solid' foods as purees and porridges	Diet low energy density, ~1 kcal/g Very little or no fibre May be low in fat – some weaning diets even in developed countries may have fat content <30% total energy Often high refined sugar content to diet
Young child	Mixed diet. May be quite limited in variety Little unprocessed meat Children often not keen to chew and whole fruit largely absent Vegetables usually eaten only with reluctance	Varies according to food offered and children's pickiness Fat content may range from 25% to >40% total energy Iron content may be very low Fibre intake largely from breakfast cereals
Schoolchild	Diet may be influenced by school meal. School dinners whether provided from home or canteen often high in total energy, energy from fat and refined sugar and low in vegetable fibre. Micronutrient intake in school dinners commonly low	School dinners may achieve >45% energy from fat Saturated fat may be majority of fat Sugar and sweetened drinks very popular May be high salt intake Fibre predominantly from breakfast cereals
Adolescent	May be a balanced adult diet or a thoroughly irregular diet Diet eaten away from home without supervision. May be excessive soft drink consumption	Important that diet is encouraged to follow recommendations for adults whenever possible Other aspects of 'healthy living' important as well as diet

From Poskitt 2003 © John Wiley & Sons Ltd. Reproduced with permission.

As children grow up they become more independent in their eating habits. Meals should be spread over the day and snacks regulated to facilitate recognition of hunger and satiety.

NUTRITIONAL PROBLEMS IN CHILDREN AND ADOLESCENTS

Failure to thrive (FTT)

Failure to thrive (FTT) is failure to gain in weight and height at the expected rate, the expected rate being that indicated by the child's weight and/or height velocity compared with reference standards for age (see Table *evolve* 14.8 for further details 🐭). Resolution of FTT through catch-up growth (CUG) can be very rapid with treatable cause and the provision of extra nutrients to support catch-up. Where resolution of the precipitating cause is impossible, as with cystic fibrosis and with some congenital heart disease with high cardiac output,

increasing the energy and nutrient density of the diet so children ingest more energy and nutrients without increasing food volume can lead to improved growth rates.

FTT: psychosocial deprivation syndrome

Psychosocial deprivation (PSD) may be the commonest form of FTT in the UK today although often unrecognised. Overt cases come from homes where the nurturing environment is in some way deficient in the love, warmth, enjoyment and stimulus which enable normal growth. The explanation for the poor growth must be multifactorial with inadequate food offered or ingested as the most reasonable explanation for some cases. Some children steal food, eat food off others' plates at school, and show other attention-seeking behaviours. Children with PSD may have low levels of growth hormone and ACTH secretion when in their deprived environments. Changing the adverse environments so as to provide more positive nurture rapidly normalises hormone levels and results in catch-up growth.

Obesity

(See also Ch. 20.)

Childhood obesity has increased dramatically in UK over the past 20 years. The situation is often described as an obesity 'epidemic'. The UK National Child Measurement Programme (Information Centre 2008) has measured weights and heights in reception (4–5 years) and year 6 (10–11 years) school classes for the past few years. In 2007/8 13.0% of 4–5-year-olds were considered overweight and a further 9.6% obese. For 10–11-year-olds figures were 14.3% overweight and 18.3% obese. Differences between the sexes were small and figures were very similar to those of the previous year although considerably greater than data for the year 2000. The UK government obesity prevention and reduction programme hopes to bring the prevalence of overweight/obesity back to 2000 levels. Levels of obesity at school entry are particularly disturbing since in the past the prevalence of overweight/obesity in the toddler age group was low and most children showed declining %BF between 1 and 5 years.

Most westernised countries show a dramatic rise in the prevalence of childhood obesity. In many transitional and developing countries childhood obesity is also extremely common amongst the affluent urban elite (Poskitt 2009). Highest prevalence amongst the elite is in contrast to well established western economies where overweight/obesity is more common amongst socioeconomically deprived urban children.

Obesity is a matter of major public health concern. Psychological distress and the physical handicap of gross size contribute to underachievement at school. More childhood overweight/obesity and more prevalent adult obesity inevitably mean more overweight/obese children continue into adult overweight and associated complications. More concerning is the appearance of some of the complications previously associated with adult obesity not only amongst adolescents but in prepubertal children. Type 2 diabetes mellitus in an obese child under 10 years is no longer a rarity.

Causes of childhood obesity

The vast majority of obese children have no recognisable underlying medical cause for their obesity.

Around 80% of obese children have one obese parent and 20–40% have both parents obese. Presumably a genetic predisposition and an obesogenic environment combine in many children to produce obesity. Very rare, single gene defect, obesity syndromes associated with abnormalities of leptin metabolism are described. Such children usually show unrelenting increase in fatness from birth but dramatic and sustained fat loss with leptin therapy.

A few uncommon medical conditions are also associated with increased risk of obesity in children (see Table *evolve* 14.9). Most childhood obesity 'secondary' to other recognised conditions includes short stature as a feature, often with other clinical findings and/or psycho-developmental problems. Prader–Willi syndrome is the most likely condition to present with obesity as the prime concern, although short stature and low IQ usually alert clinicians to the possibility of 'secondary' obesity.

Explanations for the rise in childhood obesity must be multifactorial (see Table *evolve* 14.10). Contrary to what might be expected, recorded energy intakes in the UK fell for several decades during which time the prevalence of overweight/obesity increased. The National Diet and Nutrition Survey (Gregory & Lowe 2000) showed that total energy intakes for 10–11-year-old UK children decreased on average by 1.6 MJ/day between 1983 and 1997. For the same period and age group, the percentage of energy derived from fat decreased from a mean of 37.4% energy from fat in 1983 to 35.7% in 1997. These dietary patterns were replicated in all age groups in the National Diet and Nutrition Survey (NDNS) studies and in other countries as well. Some of this decline may reflect failure of previous studies to account adequately for food eaten outside the home. Unfortunately there have been no recent national surveys of UK children's dietary intakes with which to compare these data but it is now widely acknowledged that food intake is only one of the many lifestyle changes that contribute to childhood, and adult, obesity prevalence.

Energy expenditures must have declined more than energy intakes to explain the increased prevalence of obesity. For the same movement the obese expend more energy than their lean lighter peers, making it difficult to judge energy needs but studies suggest UK children today spend little time in moderate to vigorous physical activity and have long periods of sedentary behaviour. In one study of children of 5–8 years old, only 42% of boys and 11%

of girls met the government recommendations of at least 60 minutes a day of moderately intense activity.

Studies from a number of countries have associated obesity in individuals with the hours spent watching television. Whilst most of these studies focus on teenage boys, the concerning prevalence of overweight/obesity in young children could relate to the widespread use of television as entertainment and often almost a 'baby sitter' for young children. Television viewing is associated with very low levels of energy expenditure. The role of computers in contributing to the obesity epidemic is less studied but it would seem likely that all forms of modern sedentary entertainment play a part in facilitating energy intake exceeding energy expenditure. Increased sedentary behaviour could be the most significant societal change leading to increased prevalence of childhood overweight/obesity.

Children in Copenhagen brought up in disadvantaged areas showed increased risk of obesity in later life irrespective of their families' income. This suggests that an environment of deprivation which includes, for example, lack of shops selling fresh fruit, vegetables and wholemeal breads and lack of places to play or walk, and which leads to parental depression, may have a role in driving the obesity epidemic. Another interesting sociological factor which may be contributing to the obesity epidemic is sleep duration. There is some evidence to suggest that the more hours children sleep, the less the prevalence of overweight/obesity. This may simply be that it is not possible to be sleeping and eating at the same time. However both leptin and ghrelin, hormones associated with appetite suppression and appetite stimulus respectively, are affected by sleep, with lack of sleep tending to raise circulating ghrelin and lower leptin levels so there could be physiological reasons for this finding. Whilst there are few if any studies of changing patterns of sleeping in children, it would seem likely that the availability of 24-hour television, computers and televisions commonly in bedrooms, working parents who want their children's company in the evenings and less disciplined bedtimes than common in the past could be contributing to less sleep for many children.

Treatment and prevention

Programmes to treat already existing obesity have not produced impressive results even when they have been invasive. Rebound after a period of treatment is almost expected. Children are normally acquiring both fat and lean tissue as they grow. Drastically energy-reduced diets can lead to impaired linear growth although modest 'slimming' programmes usually allow continuation of normal linear growth. Interventions to reduce childhood obesity include: individual and family actions to attain sustainable dietary and lifestyle practices; community actions including public policies to facilitate weight control; commercial actions to remove promotion to children of energy-dense, micronutrient-poor, tasty foods requiring little effort to eat; and food labelling to provide higher-quality, more readily understandable, labelling of manufactured and packaged foods.

Policies for the prevention of childhood obesity differ little from those we recommend for treatment except they are less intense, aimed at families and communities and promoting lifestyle changes compatible with balanced nutrition and with recommendations for the reduction of heart disease and cancer. Indeed efforts to reduce overweight, to reduce cancer and heart disease and to save the environment have very similar lifestyle goals (for further detail see Section *evolve* 14.7 🔒 and Ch. 33).

Anorexia nervosa

Increasing prevalence of anorexia in children and adolescents is sometimes seen as a consequence of excessive dieting in overweight children. Anorexic children sometimes describe themselves as previously obese but impaired body image is a feature of anorexia and most such individuals have only *perceived* themselves as obese. Nevertheless, there is some risk that *non-obese* adolescents who are psychologically susceptible may develop anorexia following publicity promoting slimming diets and lean physique. Public health policies aiming to reduce childhood obesity should emphasise the benefits of healthy lifestyles rather than the attractions of a slim figure.

Anaemia

The definition of anaemia in childhood is not straightforward because of physiological variations in haemoglobin levels with age (Table 14.10). In utero haemoglobin levels are high in order to maximise oxygen uptake from the low oxygen tension of the environment. At birth oxygen tension increases, high haemoglobin levels are no longer

Table 14.10	Minimum acceptable levels of haemoglobin according to age
AGE (YEARS)	**HAEMOGLOBIN LEVEL (G/L)**
0.5–6.0	110
>6.0–14	120
>14 boys	130
>14 girls	120
Adult men	130
Adult women	120
Pregnant women	110

Adapted from WHO 1972.

necessary, and the bone marrow becomes relatively quiescent. Haemoglobin levels fall as ageing red cells (red cells have shorter lifespan in the first months of life) are broken down and iron is stored in the bone marrow. After 4–8 weeks, bone marrow activity increases but haemoglobin levels remain low because red blood cell production only just keeps up with the increasing body size and blood volume.

Anaemia is not uncommon in UK children. In the Gregory & Lowe (2000) study of children aged 4–18 years, 9% of boys aged 4–6 years and 11–14 years and 9% of girls aged 4–6 years and 15–18 years had low haemoglobin levels. Other groups were less affected. Deficiencies of iron (by far the commonest deficient micronutrient), folic acid, vitamins A, B_{12}, C, E, riboflavin, copper and probably other micronutrients may contribute to anaemia. Childhood DRVs for iron are shown in Table *evolve* 14.12 🖰.

Iron deficiency

In the most recent NDNS of children, the level of consumption of breakfast cereals (mostly fortified with iron in the UK) was directly associated with dietary iron intakes in children over 11 years. Non-meat-eaters and non-Caucasian adolescent girls had greatest risk of poor iron status. Table *evolve* 14.13 outlines some of the clinical and dietary factors contributing to iron deficiency 🖰.

Most iron is transferred across the placenta in the last trimester so PT neonates have less iron/kg body weight than term infants. In all infants, iron stores are consumed in early growth as the blood volume increases with the increase in body size. By 6 months, and often earlier in PT infants, iron stores

are minimal. Complementary foods providing good sources of iron are necessary. Iron stores build up only after growth has slowed considerably around 5 years of age. Iron requirements increase in adolescence with increase in body size and the needs for growth and, in girls, the onset of menstruation. The NDNS of children 4–18 years (Gregory & Lowe 2000) found most children's iron intakes were adequate but 44% of girls aged 11–18 years had intakes below the lower reference nutrient intake for iron.

Depletion of iron stores even in the absence of anaemia may lead to psychological changes. Depression, irritability, loss of appetite, apathy, and evidence of impaired learning and cognition and slowed growth rates have all been associated with iron-deficiency anaemia (IDA). The extent to which these symptoms occur with iron deficiency in the absence of anaemia is not clear.

Children with IDA are often tired and anorexic, look pale and may be breathless. As IDA usually develops over months, physiological adaptations to falling haemoglobin may obscure symptoms until there is severe anaemia (e.g. Hb <40 g/l). Blood transfusion to raise haemoglobin levels risks upsetting the physiological adaptation and precipitating cardiac failure. Oral iron – provided it is taken – is effective, safe treatment. Additional vitamin C will help to sustain iron in the more absorbable ferrous form.

Bone mineralisation: calcium and vitamin D

Although the total daily calcium increment is highest in adolescence, the proportion of calcium taken up compared with total body, or total bone mineral, weight is highest immediately after birth and in PT infants. In the term fetus, 300 mg of calcium is transferred across the placenta to the fetus each day. Calcium needs in adolescence are less clear but recommendations range from 600 to 1000 mg calcium daily (see Table *evolve* 14.14 🖰). Dietary phytates and substances competing with calcium binding sites may affect calcium requirements significantly in childhood (see Ch. 24).

Calcium and vitamin D nutrition are inescapably linked. The active form of vitamin D, 1,25-(OH)$_2$D, is necessary for absorption of calcium, maintenance of circulating calcium levels and bone mineralisation (see Ch. 24). Children at most risk of deficiency are those growing most rapidly – infants, especially LBW, and adolescents. The main source of vitamin

D both during and after infancy is from conversion of 7–dehydrocalciferol to cholecalciferol by ultraviolet light radiation of approximately 300 nm to the skin. This accounts for the seasonal changes in plasma 25-(OH)D levels with peaks in August/September and troughs in February in the UK. Most children with adequate summer sunshine exposure should have no need for dietary vitamin D (see Table *evolve* 14.15 💊) but those with heavily pigmented skin and/or little exposure to summer sunlight in Britain are at risk of low levels of circulating vitamin D metabolites. Drugs such as anticonvulsants and cortisol, which stimulate metabolism of cholecalciferol to inactive metabolites excreted via the bile duct, increase susceptibility to vitamin D deficiency. Table *evolve* 14.16 outlines some causes of vitamin D deficiency 💊.

The cardinal clinical signs of vitamin D deficiency in childhood are those of rickets (see Ch. 24) which remains a common problem in children and adolescents in the UK (Bishop 2006). Other congenital or acquired paediatric conditions can mimic nutritional rickets and may need to be distinguished. Calcification of cartilage at the growing end of the shaft of long bones fails and uncalcified cartilage and osteoid accumulate, causing swelling at the epiphyseal plate. Overall bone mineralisation is poor. In membranous bones of the skull, the growing brain encourages bossing of the soft skull bones. Soft long bones bend with weight bearing, leading to bowed arm bones in crawling children and bowed leg bones in those who are walking. Because of poor calcification of cartilage and bone, there is delay in development of the epiphyseal centres in bones. Growth rates are reduced. Vitamin D has effects on many tissues other than bone. Muscle tone is reduced leading to hypotonia and weakness with distended abdomen due to lax abdominal musculature. Weak respiratory muscles lead to ineffective coughing and thus a tendency for lower respiratory tract infections. The soft lower rib cage is pulled in by diaphragmatic contraction during respiration causing the typical indrawing of the lower chest or 'Harrison's sulcus'. This, with the swelling at the costochondral junctions which cause the 'rickety rosary', gives the characteristic appearances of the chest.

Secondary hyperparathyroidism in response to the fall in plasma calcium with vitamin D deficiency leads to bone demineralisation and loss of phosphate through the kidney. Thus the biochemical findings in rickets are usually those of borderline low plasma calcium, low plasma phosphate and very high alkaline phosphatase. Alkaline phosphatase, a manifestation of osteoclastic activity, may remain high throughout the healing period. Oral vitamin D (cholecalciferol) is very effective in restoring bone architecture to normal after time. However, with adolescent girls there may be insufficient growth time left for resolution of pelvic deformity and the risk of cephalopelvic disproportion during childbirth. Subclinical hypovitaminosis D in adolescence, probably related to inadequate sunlight exposure, is not uncommon and could contribute to suboptimal PBM.

Metabolic bone disease, or 'rickets of prematurity', is common in PT infants but is more complex in aetiology than simple vitamin D deficiency. Mineral needs are high in rapidly growing PT infants and bone disease can result from calcium or phosphate deficiency. Use of the diuretic furosemide for fluid overload can worsen the situation by increasing urinary excretion of phosphate. Modern PT infant formulas and intravenous nutrition solutions aim to meet PT infants' needs for bone growth and mineralisation. However, nutritional requirements cannot always be met when infants are sick and not tolerating large fluid volumes either enterally or parenterally. Vitamin D supplementation of all LBW infants is advisable to maximise calcium absorption. The parathyroid hormone response to low plasma calcium is poorly developed in PT and newborn infants. Symptomatic hypocalcaemia, including tetany and convulsions, in neonatal vitamin D deficiency is common whilst plasma phosphate levels are often more or less normal.

Bone health and later life

The likelihood of the loss of bone mineral in middle and old age leading to clinical osteoporosis is partly determined by peak bone mass (PBM). Weight-bearing activity in adult life and old age appears to reduce the loss of bone mineral with age but in childhood weight-bearing activity contributes positively to developing PBM. Although calcium intakes should have some influence on bone mineralisation, work from The Gambia suggests that normal bone mineralisation can take place on diets that are very low in calcium compared with recommended requirements. Calcium supplementation (1000 g/day) to pre-adolescent children on very low calcium traditional diets improves bone mineralisation but has no effect on growth.

Macronutrient undernutrition may also have negative impact on bone mineralisation. Anorexic individuals, as well as ballet dancers and gymnasts who deliberately undereat so as to remain light and small, have low PBM. The importance of energy and protein for developing the collagen matrix on which bone mineral is deposited may explain the apparently better response to calcium supplementation in trials where calcium is supplied as extra milk, with all its extra nutrients, rather than as calcium salts.

14.8 CONCLUSIONS

Growth, dependency and development make infants and children susceptible to nutritional imbalance and deficiencies. It may seem that broad knowledge of nutrition is necessary in order to feed children appropriately. Clearly this is not so since the nutritional knowledge of most families is slight yet the majority of children survive with good nutrition even in environments less advantageous than in western Europe. Nevertheless, it is wise to promote meals varied in content, texture and taste for children. Variety leads, almost certainly, to nutritionally adequate combinations of macro- and micronutrients, even when there is no specific nutritional knowledge. Meals should be made enjoyable social affairs offered without excessive pressure to eat. Snacks should be planned rather than opportunistic or continuous. Wholemeal cereals, fruits and vegetables should be seen as enjoyable components of the diet. In this way children can eat to requirement whilst allowing opportunity to develop and recognise satiety and hunger. Linking family nutrition with a caring, stimulating environment encourages both normal growth and development, and the prospect of sustainable healthy lifestyles continuing into adulthood. Table *evolve* 14.17 suggests how this may be achieved 🖱.

KEY POINTS

- There are sound and varied physiological reasons why breast milk is most suitable for the young infant.
- The adaptations in modified formula milks accommodate the needs of young infants, even those with very low birthweight or with inborn errors of metabolism, where breast milk may have limitations.
- The transition from breast milk/formula milk to a solid diet is a time when young children are vulnerable to nutritional problems.
- Vitamin and mineral deficiencies present problems in child nutrition even in affluent developed countries.

- Overnutrition as overweight and obesity is a problem of increasing concern to public health and child nutrition. It presents challenges which involve not only diet but lifestyle change for prevention or cure.
- Adolescence is an age of both nutritional vulnerability and opportunity for nutritional education for a healthy adult lifestyle.
- Healthy nutrition encompasses not only what is eaten but when and how it is consumed and includes many aspects of lifestyle such as activity.

References

Barker DJP: *Mothers, babies and health in later life*, 2nd edn. Edinburgh, 1998, Churchill Livingstone.

Bishop N: Don't ignore vitamin D. *Archives of Disease in Childhood* 91:549–550, 2006.

Bolling K, Grant C, Hamlyn B, Thornton A: Infant feeding 2005. The Information Centre. Available on line at: http://www.ic.nhs.uk 2007.

Busfield A, McNinch A, Tripp J: Neonatal vitamin K prophylaxis in Great Britain and Ireland: the impact of perceived risk and product licensing on effectiveness, *Archives of Disease in Childhood* 92:754–758, 2007.

Clarke P, Shearer MJ: Vitamin K deficiency bleeding: the readiness is all, *Archives of Disease in Childhood* 92:741–743, 2007.

Department of Health: Breast feeding, http://www.dh.gov.uk. reference number: 2003/0185 (12 May 2003), 2003.

Department of Health: *Weaning and the weaning diet. Report on health and social subjects no 45,* London, 1994, HMSO.

Department of Health: Healthy Start, http://www.healthystart.nhs.uk. Web page access on 30 October 2008, 2008.

Department of Health and Social Security (DHSS): *Composition of human milk. Report on health and social subjects no 12,* London, 1977, HMSO.

ESPGHAN Committee on Nutrition: Complementary feeding: a commentary by the ESPGHAN Committee on Nutrition, *Journal Pediatric Gastroenterology & Nutrition* 46:99–110, 2008.

Freeman JV, Cole TJ, Chinn S, et al: Cross sectional stature and weight reference curves for the UK 1990, *Archives of Disease in Childhood* 73:17–24, 1995.

Gregory JR, Lowe S: *National diet and nutrition survey – young people aged 4 to 18 years, Volume 1: Report of the diet and nutrition survey,* London, 2000, The Stationery Office.

Information Centre: National child measurement programme: results from the 2006/7 school year, http://www.ic.mhs.uk/statistics-and-data-collections/health-and-lifestyles/obesity, 2008.

NICE (National Institute for Health and Clinical Excellence): Obesity: the prevention, identification, assessment, and management of overweight and obesity in adults and children, London The Stationery Office, www.nice.org.uk/guidance/CG43, 2006.

Poskitt EME: Use of cows' milk in infant feeding with emphasis on the compositional differences between human and cows' milk. In: Walker AF, Rolls BA, editors: *Infant nutrition: issues in nutrition and toxicology 2,* London, 1994, Chapman & Hall, p 162–185.

Poskitt EME: Nutrition in Childhood. In: Morgan JB, Dickerson JWT, editors: *Nutrition in early life,* Chichester, 2003, John Wiley, p 291–323.

Poskitt EME: Countries in transition: underweight to obesity non stop? *Annals of Tropical Paediatrics and International Child Health,* 29:1–11, 2009.

Statutory Instruments 3521: Infant formula and follow- on formula regulation, http://www.opsi.gov.uk/si/si2007/uksi_20073521_en_1, 2007.

Stordy BJ, Redfern AM, Morgan JB: Healthy eating for infants – mothers' actions, *Acta Paediatrica* 84:733–741, 1995.

Ward Platt, MP: Demand weaning: infants' answer to professionals' dilemmas, *Archives of Disease in Childhood* 94:79–80, 2009.

WHO: *Nutritional anemia,* WHO Technical Report Series number 3, Geneva, 1972, WHO.

WHO Multicentre Growth Reference Study Group: WHO child growth standards based on length/height, weight and age, *Acta Paediatrica* Suppl 450:76–85, 2006.

Wright C, Lakshman R, Emmett P, Ong KK: Implications of adopting the WHO 2006 Child Growth Standard in the UK: two prospective cohort studies, *Archives of Disease in Childhood* 93:566–569, 2008.

Further reading

Burniat W, Cole TJ, Lissau I, Poskitt EME: *Child and adolescent obesity,* Cambridge, 2002, Cambridge University Press.

De Onis M, Garza C, Onyango A, Martorell R: WHO child growth standards, *Acta Paediatrica* Suppl 450:1–104, 2006.

Fomon SJ: *Nutrition of normal infants,* St Louis, 1993, Mosby.

Lobstein T, Baur L, Uauy R: Obesity in children and young people – a crisis in public health. Report to WHO, *Obesity Reviews* 5(Suppl 1), 2004.

Morgan JB, Dickerson JWT: *Nutrition in early life,* Chichester, 2003, Wiley.

Royal College of Physicians, Royal College of Paediatrics and Child Health and the Faculty of Public Health: *Storing up problems: the medical case for a slimmer nation,* London, 2004, Royal College of Physicians.

SACN: Update on vitamin D, http://www.sacn.gov.uk/pdfs/sacn_position_vitamin_d_2007_05_07.pdf, 2007.

Websites

World Health Organization
http://www.who.dk/nutrition/Infant/20020808
http://www.who.dk/nutrition/Infant/20020730

(Both refer to baby-friendly hospital initiatives.)
SACN (Standing Advisory Committee on Nutrition)
http://sacn.gov.uk

Chapter 15

Prepregnancy, pregnancy and lactation

Robert Fraser and Fiona Ford

CHAPTER CONTENTS

OBJECTIVES

By the end of this chapter you should be able to:
- discuss the role of nutrition in healthy conception
- describe the changes in body composition during pregnancy and lactation and determining factors such as metabolic changes, activity, control of intake
- explain the impact of nutrition in pregnancy on birthweight and long-term health
- discuss the effects of lactation on birth spacing and mother's nutritional status
- describe the effects of inadequate nutrition on milk volume and composition
- explain the basis of calculating requirements for pregnancy and lactation.

15.1 INTRODUCTION

It is self-evident from worldwide demographic change that human reproduction is a highly successful process. High rates of infant survival to adulthood have enabled humans to populate many parts of the world. Optimal nutrition prior to pregnancy, during pregnancy and in lactation will make a significant contribution to that success. A continuum of reproductive casualty has been suggested (Table 15.1). Of couples across the globe attempting to achieve a pregnancy 90% will have been successful after approximately 18 months of regular sexual intercourse. The remaining 10% are subfertile but many of these couples can now be helped to have a successful pregnancy as a result of medical management, such as in vitro fertilisation (IVF). Once pregnancy has been achieved and in the absence of any medical interference the maternal death rate is

DOI: 10.1016/B978-0-7020-3118-2.00015-2

Table 15.1   Continuum of reproductive casualty

- Fecundability/fertility
- Maternal morbidity
- Maternal mortality
- Miscarriage
- Late fetal death
- Aneuploidy
- Structural congenital anomaly
- Neonatal death
- Cerebral palsy/psychomotor impairment
- Susceptibility to disease in adult life

approximately 1 in 200 pregnancies and 1 in 20 babies will die before birth, or in the first week of life. With intervention by health professionals, including nutritional advice, 1/10 000 pregnancies result in a maternal death and 1 in 200 pregnancies result in the loss of the infant. Both these figures may be higher than this in the developing world where deficiency of specific nutrients, poor provision of medical services and/or intercurrent infectious disease may each play a part (Rush 2000).

The concept of the continuum of reproductive casualty is quite useful because when recommending an intervention such as a nutritional supplement perhaps to achieve a beneficial outcome in one aspect of the continuum, e.g. to reduce miscarriage, one must be careful that the result of the intervention does not lead to an increase in unwanted effects elsewhere in the continuum such as the birth of more infants with congenital malformations. A recent suggestion, for instance, has been that the periconceptional supplementation with folic acid of a woman planning a pregnancy, which will reduce her risk of producing an infant with a neural tube defect (spina bifida), may have the unwanted effect of increasing the spontaneous twinning rate. As twinning increases infant deaths and handicaps, principally because of an excess of premature births, the overall burden of disease and disability may be greater than before. This important concept must be understood by all those who would wish to advise or prescribe for the would-be pregnant or pregnant woman. It is also prominent in the minds of such women – the constant query to the health professional offering advice on nutrition or pharmaceutical drug use in pregnancy is – 'will it harm my baby?'

15.2 PREPREGNANCY

NUTRITIONAL REQUIREMENTS FOR HEALTHY CONCEPTION

The opinions of Frisch and her colleagues regarding the relevance of body composition, particularly the percentage of fat, in achieving pregnancy are now generally accepted (Frisch 1994). Her principal observation was that an improved plane of nutrition in adolescent girls was associated with an increasingly early date of menarche signalling the onset of fertility. The mean body weight at which menarche occurred in US girls was 48 kg with a mean height of 1.59 m at 12.9 years. Of the mean body weight at the completion of growth (16–18 years) 16 kg was fat, representing an energy reserve for reproduction of 602 MJ (144 000 kcal). Such an energy reserve would provide the theoretical energy requirement of both pregnancy and 3 months of lactation. Of course in athletes in training or those involved in hard physical work this body weight can be achieved with a relatively low proportion of fat. Frisch's observation was that body fat proportion of less than 22% of body weight was associated with the absence of ovulation and that healthy fertile women who were ovulating on a monthly basis had an average body fat proportion of 28%. Menarche and the onset of fertility can be delayed by athletic training or eating disorders and accelerated by excess nutrient consumption. Early menarche may be a particular problem in girls exposed to famine in childhood who are then re-fed with a high energy diet. If they live in a society where the onset of menarche is a trigger for marriage and reproduction they may get into serious difficulties in trying to give birth before they have achieved full adult stature and their bony birth canal has reached full adult dimensions. Natural labour may become obstructed if the baby's head is too large to pass easily through the mother's pelvis.

The basic mechanism involved in body fat as a determinant of a healthy conception appears to be a requirement for a certain energy store to permit reproduction to take place. In natural experiments when severe famine has affected populations of women who are *already* established in pregnancy there is no significant change in mean birthweight if this occurs during the first 6 months of pregnancy. There is a modest reduction in birthweight of approximately 5–10% if famine affects women during the last 3 months of pregnancy. Most surprisingly perhaps, successful lactation can continue for up to 3 months in the face of severe energy deprivation of the mother. These physiological adaptations in extreme conditions are clearly factors in successful human reproduction. What is seen in the non-pregnant female population exposed to acute famine is a failure of ovulation in at least 50% of females even before the fat store has been catabolised.

In summary, a population exposed to a low plane of nutrition during childhood will have a relative delay in reaching full adult stature and reproductive maturity. Refeeding of the chronically undernourished child may lead to accelerated development and onset of puberty, which may lead to pregnancy before full adult stature has been obtained. In the absence of adequate medical and midwifery resources such pregnant young women may die as the result of neglected obstructed labour. When energy deficits affect women after the achievement of natural puberty and full adult stature there is an acute reduction in fertility and with chronic undernutrition ovulation will cease. In acute undernutrition during an established pregnancy utilisation of stored energy from the maternal adipose tissue is capable of protecting the baby's nutrient supply to a large extent during pregnancy and indeed through the early months of lactation.

INFLUENCE OF OBESITY ON CONCEPTION

Obesity with or without the problem of the polycystic ovarian syndrome (PCOS) is associated with a doubling in the rate of ovulatory infertility (Rich-Edwards et al 1994) (see Fig. *evolve* 15.1 🔳). In both polycystic ovarian syndrome and simple obesity weight reduction is associated with a return of ovulation, menstruation and fertility, in many cases.

It is therefore appropriate to assess body mass index (BMI) and general nutritional status in women who wish to get pregnant but are anovulatory. Therapies designed to raise or lower the BMI into the normal weight range represent a simple non-pharmacological and often successful approach to anovular infertility. Anti-obesity drugs such as orlistat (Xenical) and sibutramine may be prescribed to achieve weight targets that will return a woman to normal fertility, but because of unknown effects on embryo development, these should be discontinued before the woman stops using contraceptive methods.

PERICONCEPTIONAL NUTRITION AND FETAL MALFORMATIONS

Periconceptional nutrition may be a factor in structural congenital malformations. In human populations major handicapping or lethal malformations complicate 1 in 80 pregnancies. The major nutritional influence on malformation which has been scientifically tested is the benefit of folic acid supplementation in the prevention of neural tube defects (NTD). The neural tube, which runs from the brain to the lower end of the spinal cord, normally closes in embryonic development in the third and fourth post-fertilisation weeks. Periconceptional supplementation with a dose of 400 µg of folic acid per day or a diet rich in folates can reduce the incidence of these major handicapping conditions from affecting 3–4/1000 pregnancies to less than 1/1000 pregnancies. In some countries such as the USA and Canada folic acid fortification has been made universal through flour, and these countries are reporting reductions in the rate of NTD of up to 40% for their populations since the change of policy in 1998. In the landmark study from Hungary by Czeizel and colleagues (1992) a multivitamin supplement which included 800 µg per day of folic acid was associated not only with the prevention of NTD in the treated group of women and a statistically significant reduction in structural congenital malformations overall.

Other specific micronutrient deficiencies operating during embryonic development that may lead to avoidable congenital malformations deserve further exploration but appropriate experiments in the human are expensive and difficult to mount. In the meantime the advice about periconceptional folic acid should be made available to all, particularly in countries where mandatory folic acid fortification of flour is not government policy, as is the case for the UK. It is recommended that for that small group of women who have had a previous pregnancy affected by NTDs the periconceptional supplement should be 5 mg of folic acid not 400 µg. In the UK, surveys show that major efforts to disseminate the public health message have resulted in take-up of voluntary supplementation of only between 35% and 50% of eligible women.

NUTRITION IN PLANNED AND UNPLANNED PREGNANCIES

Half of women who plan their pregnancies are not taking periconceptional folic acid supplements. A large proportion of pregnancies are unplanned and obviously in these circumstances the majority of women are not taking periconceptional supplements. Surveys suggest that the groups who are either planning a pregnancy but not taking supplements or who are more likely to have unplanned pregnancies include teenagers, women who smoke and those on low incomes. This group is particularly at risk of low intakes of folates and other micronutrients, which may partly explain the social class gradient in the incidence of NTDs, which are more common in low income women.

In those women who are planning a pregnancy there is an opportunity to give lifestyle advice over and above folic acid and/or multivitamin supplementation which may improve their fitness for pregnancy. As suggested above, normalisation of BMI either up or down will improve their ability to become pregnant. The reduction or elimination of alcohol consumption and cigarette smoking might also be considered to be important lifestyle measures to be taken in preparation for pregnancy.

15.3 PREGNANCY

PHYSIOLOGICAL CHANGES IN PREGNANCY

The nutritional background to pregnancy can only be understood with a knowledge of the physiological changes which the mother experiences. These were characterised by Hytten as follows:

- the changes precede fetal demands and are therefore anticipatory
- the changes are in excess of possible fetal requirements
- the maternal internal milieu is altered to favour placental exchange of nutrient substrates and fetal metabolic processes (Campbell-Brown & Hytten 1998).

The genital organs

The uterine weight rises from a non-pregnant mean of 46 g to 1000 g at the end of pregnancy. This is achieved by hyperplasia and hypertrophy of the smooth muscle and an increase in vascularity, particularly in the region of the placental bed. In preparation for lactation there is hyperplasia of the mammary tissue and an increase in breast volume of about 50% by the end of pregnancy.

Blood volume and haemodynamics

There is an increase in the circulating blood volume of approximately 1600 ml by the end of the pregnancy. Eighty per cent of this increase is required to perfuse the placental bed in the last few weeks of pregnancy. The increased blood volume consists of a rise in the plasma volume from 2500 ml in the non-pregnant state to 3800 ml at term and an increase in the red cell volume of 1400 ml to 1640 ml at term. Thus although the red cell mass is increasing and oxygen-carrying capacity is enhanced, there is a dilution of the red cells because of the relatively greater increase in plasma volume. This leads to a fall in the haemoglobin concentration from a non-pregnant average of 13–14 g/dl to levels of 10–11 g/dl in late pregnancy. Because the haemoglobin concentration will rise in response to oral iron therapy some have described this change as 'dilutional anaemia'. This a physiological change, not a pathological one, designed to reduce blood viscosity to improve placental perfusion, and therefore oxygen and nutrient exchange at the placental bed. Blood pressure tends to fall slightly in the middle of pregnancy with a rise towards full term. The heart rate increases from an average non-pregnant rate of 70 beats per minute to a rate of 80 to 85 beats per minute at full term. This is accompanied by an increase in the stroke volume, the amount of blood pumped by one cardiac cycle, from 65 ml in the non-pregnant state to 70 ml at term. The effect of this combination is to increase the cardiac output, the amount of blood pumped per minute from a non-pregnant average of 5000 ml to 6500 ml at term.

Respiratory system

The pregnant woman has an increasing metabolising mass and an increasing requirement for oxygen as the pregnancy develops. The tidal volume, the amount of air inspired per breath, increases from a non-pregnant mean of 400 ml to 550 ml at term. This is achieved by a physiological change in the relationships of the rib cage to the diaphragm. The subcostal angle increases, widening the area through which the diaphragm oscillates. Oxygen consumption is increased by about 15% from a non-pregnant average of about 250 ml/min. Chemoreceptors are reset to allow the mother to tolerate her PCO_2 at 4 kPa rather than the non-pregnant average of 4.7 kPa. Carbon dioxide is excreted through the lungs, but fetal production of CO_2 must be excreted to the mother via the placenta before reaching *her* lungs. The physiological lowering of the homeostatic level of CO_2 (PCO_2) by about 15–20% facilitates diffusion of CO_2 from fetus to mother, and is a vital physiological shift in maternal homeostasis. For the mother the deeper breathing required to lower the PCO_2 produces the common symptom of breathlessness but her fetus benefits from an increased concentration gradient of CO_2 across the placenta and facilitated excretion of CO_2.

Renal system

Renal plasma flow increases by about 30% with the corresponding increase in glomerular filtration rate. Serum albumin falls, unrelated to diet but as a physiological change designed to reduce the plasma oncotic pressure, allowing increased renal glomerular filtration. An unwanted effect of the increased glomerular filtration is that significant glycosuria and aminoaciduria are common in normal pregnancy and can occasionally contribute to generalised nutrient depletion.

Gastrointestinal system

There is a generalised relaxation of smooth muscle in the gastrointestinal tract present from about 10 weeks of gestation and persisting through to term. Women commonly report altered appetite, often with dulled sensation leading to craving, particularly for highly flavoured or spiced foods or for sweets, chocolate, milk and dairy foods. They may also develop aversions to common dietary items such as tea, coffee or meat and some women thereby experience a major alteration in their pattern of nutrient intake from early pregnancy onwards. Pica is a rare condition when non-food items are eaten, such as coal, clay, toothpaste, chalk etc. This habit is potentially harmful and, when recognised, demands medical referral. Endocrine changes are probably responsible for the symptoms of anorexia, nausea and vomiting, which are particularly common problems from about 10–16 weeks of gestation, possibly related to the high levels of human chorionic gonadotrophin (HCG) when levels of this hormone peak. Observational studies have, however, found no association between absolute HCG levels in serum and symptoms in the individual woman. In about 1% of cases the vomiting is severe enough to require hospital admission and parenteral nutritional support (hyperemesis gravidarum). Although it is a major concern for many women that their nutrient intake is severely compromised by the duration of nausea and vomiting there is no evidence, except in the most severe cases, of fetal harm resulting from a temporary acute fall in nutrient intakes. In fact the evidence is that those women who suffer more from nausea and vomiting have relatively higher birthweight infants.

A further common symptom is ptyalism, the sensation of producing excessive saliva, which may be spat out rather than swallowed when the woman is nauseated. Objective testing has not shown any measured increase in saliva production.

Relaxation of the cardiac sphincter in the stomach is thought to be at the root of the common symptom of acid reflux which results in heartburn. Delayed gastric emptying can lead to a feeling of fullness after meals. Motor sluggishness in the small intestine increases transit time from stomach to caecum from a mean of 52 hours in the non-pregnant, to 58 hours in pregnant subjects. Animal studies report an increase in villous density and absorptive area in the small bowel in pregnancy. Assuming such changes appear in the human the combined effect would be to increase nutrient uptakes. Evidence for this is scanty but calcium absorption is greater in early pregnancy up to 24 weeks, with no subsequent increase. Iron absorption in contrast increases throughout pregnancy and may be 40% higher towards the later stages. In contrast again experiments with oral folate uptake demonstrated no increased absorption in pregnancy.

The reduced peristalsis in the large bowel is associated with increased water reabsorption and production of hard stools leading to the common symptom of constipation.

PLACENTAL TRANSFER

The placenta is responsible for maternal fetal exchange and grows with the fetus. It is perfused on the fetal side by fetal blood and on the maternal side by maternal blood, exchange taking place across the cellular interface which is the syncytiotrophoblast. Major physiological changes take place in the terminal branches of the uterine artery at the placental site to allow expansion of the placental blood flow with advancing pregnancy. At term the placental blood flow reaches 800 ml/min.

The structural modifications of these terminal arteries follow invasion of the trophoblast into the uterine wall and the arterial walls in the first half of pregnancy. A failure of adequate trophoblast invasion is a feature of disorders such as pre-eclampsia. Despite this abnormal vascularisation placental perfusion is adequate in early pregnancy whilst the demands are small but fails to increase progressively in later gestation leading to retardation of fetal growth. Other barriers to adequate placental perfusion and therefore normal late fetal growth include factors such as maternal cigarette smoking. Placental transfer of nutrients takes place through four mechanisms: simple diffusion, facilitated diffusion, active transport and pinocytosis. The placenta is also the source of several placental proteins with endocrine functions including HCG (the hormone detected in the maternal blood or urine in pregnancy testing), human placental lactogen and human placental growth hormone. The latter two have insulin counter-regulatory effects and therefore may modify the nutrient substrate mixture presented to the placenta by the mother. A number of other pregnancy-specific placental proteins have been identified, most of which appear to have a role in early pregnancy to facilitate uterine implantation.

Transfer of the principal fetal substrates is discussed below.

Maternal homeostasis of fetal nutrient substrates

Plasma levels of water-soluble and fat-soluble nutrients adopt different homeostatic relationships in the maternal plasma in pregnancy, characterised as a fall in maternal plasma levels of the water-soluble nutrients and a relative rise in the plasma levels of lipid-soluble nutrients. These are established at two stages in pregnancy, the majority having taken place by about 10–12 weeks following fertilisation, long before fetal demands could cause maternal depletion. These are homeostatic resettings which are potentially beneficial to the fetus but the relationships have not as yet been well characterised. A second wave of changes in substrate availability occurs at the end of the mid trimester, approximately 24–28 weeks into the pregnancy, when women in the developed world almost universally show relative insulin resistance. Insulin resistance is associated with an increased availability of all potential fetal substrates, particularly in the postprandial period when glucose, amino acid and lipid levels are raised. Insulin resistance is also

a factor in enhanced lipolysis which is seen during overnight fasting in pregnancy and generates glycerol and free fatty acids as potential fetal or maternal energetic substrates.

Women on typical diets of the developing world, particularly those that are rich in unrefined carbohydrate sources, do not show the picture of insulin resistance in the second half of pregnancy and therefore are presenting a different substrate mix to the placental circulation. The implication of these observations for normal fetal growth and proportions of fetal body composition remains the subject of continuing research.

Carbohydrates

Glucose provides at least 75% of fetal energy requirements. Glucose homeostasis is reset, resulting in approximately 15–20% lower plasma levels during overnight fasting and during the postabsorptive phase throughout gestation. Postprandially, however, the glucose peaks are relatively higher and there is increased glucose flux across the placenta during the postprandial period, particularly in the second half of pregnancy when insulin resistance has been established.

Glucose transport is by transcellular carrier-mediated facilitated diffusion up to a saturable maximum of 17 mmol/l. Experiments with large animals suggest an eight-fold rise in fetal glucose requirements between mid and late gestation, facilitated by increased amounts of the GLUT1 transporter in syncytiotrophoblast and endothelial cells and an increase in the density of GLUT1 in fetal endothelial cells.

The human fetoplacental unit appears to have no mechanism to prevent excess glucose transfer across the placenta below the saturable maximum, and in the pathological model of pregnancy complicated by maternal diabetes the excess glucose transfer has serious harmful effects on fetal growth and development (see Section *evolve* 15.3(a) 🖰).

Protein and amino acids

Although small IgG class immunoglobulins may cross the placenta by the process of pinocytosis the placenta is effectively a barrier to the transport of larger protein molecules. Amino acids are actively transported across the placenta by both sodium-dependent and sodium-independent mechanisms. Amino acids appear in higher concentrations in the fetal than maternal circulation. In the studies of Phelps and colleagues (1981) measurements of eight neutral amino acids (leucine, isoleucine, valine, tyrosine, phenylalanine, serine and proline) showed a similar profile to that of glucose in that fasting and preprandial levels were lower in pregnancy but post-meal increments were greater and more sustained than in non-pregnant women. Throughout the diurnal cycle these amino acids appear in higher concentrations in the fetal circulation than the maternal circulation as a result of active transport across the placenta. There are at least 15 transport systems in the placenta for amino acids, some of which are sodium-dependent, others not. Transferred amino acids are required for new tissue formation in the fetus, placental metabolism and consumption and placental interconversion. Basic amino acids are transferred to the fetus in adequate amounts for new tissue formation. Neutral amino acids are transferred in excess of requirement for new tissue formation and may be utilised as an energy source.

Lipids

Fat accumulates rapidly in the fetus in the last third of pregnancy when fetal synthesis makes a significant contribution. Triglycerides do not appear to cross the placenta but fatty acids will cross the placenta by concentration-dependent diffusion. The pattern of fatty acids seen in fetal triglycerides after re-esterification mimics the triglyceride pattern in the mother's adipose tissue.

Placental transfer of lipoprotein complexes is slow but significant in that up to half of fetal cholesterol is of maternal origin. This transfer follows proteolysis in placental lysosomes. Phospholipids are hydrolysed by the placenta and resynthesised by the fetus. Selective transport mechanisms for n-3 and n-6 essential fatty acids (EFAs) are present for the requirements of placental metabolism and fetal central nervous system (CNS) development during the second half of pregnancy. Maternal diets deficient in EFAs may fail to provide adequate fetal substrate for normal brain development, but there is insufficient evidence for this to be certain (see below under 'Nutrient requirements of pregnancy').

Ketone bodies resulting from maternal lipolysis cross the placenta freely by diffusion. As well as representing an oxidative substrate there is evidence that structural carbon atoms derived from maternal ketones can be incorporated into fetal tissue. Excessive ketone transfer across the placenta in late pregnancy may be associated with impaired IQ in the offspring. Plausible mechanisms for this observation have not yet been identified but it is of potential concern because of the very common finding of relatively enhanced lipolysis during overnight fasting as an apparent physiological shift in late pregnancy. This has been interpreted as sparing glucose for fetal transfer by encouraging oxidation of ketone bodies to maintain maternal oxidative processes.

Micronutrients

Vitamin A

The placenta transfers maternal retinol, bound to retinol binding protein, through the putative RBP receptor on the syncytiotrophoblast (the epithelium separating maternal from fetal circulation). Retinol passes into the fetal circulation. The placenta is able to metabolise retinol, specifically to esterify retinol, and to store retinyl esters. The placenta may thereby play an important role in protecting the fetus from the risks of excess vitamin A. The concentration of retinol is lower in the fetus than in the maternal circulation.

Vitamin D and calcium

Both 25-hydroxycholecalciferol (25-(OH)D$_3$) and 1,25-dihydroxycholecalciferol (1,25-(OH)$_2$D$_3$) cross the human placenta in perfusion experiments. The latter is transferred at 10 times the rate of the former, which is probably because of tight binding to a specific globulin. Whilst a mechanism for interconversion exists it is considered doubtful whether this process in the placenta contributes to fetal levels of 1,25-(OH)$_2$D$_3$.

The fetal plasma concentration of calcium is higher than the maternal concentration, and this is maintained through active placental transfer, regulated by fetal parathyroid hormone receptor protein (PTHrP), thereby contributing to fetal calcium homeostasis.

Vitamin E and vitamin K

Placental transfer of vitamins E and K occurs slowly, and the process seems relatively unresponsive to maternal supplementation. Similarly to vitamin A the concentrations of vitamins E and K in the fetus and the newborn are lower than in the mother.

Vitamin C

Vitamin C is transported across the placenta in its oxidised form, dehydroascorbic acid (DHA), which usually constitutes <5% of plasma concentration. DHA is transported across the placenta by facilitated diffusion and this maintains a higher plasma concentration in the fetal circulation than in the mother. The transfer is regulated at least in part by the D-glucose transporter. There has therefore been some interest in the possibility that maternal hyperglycaemia might influence placental transport of this vitamin, but studies so far suggest that moderate maternal hyperglycaemia does not alter placental transfer of DHA.

B vitamins

The human placenta contains high affinity folate-binding receptors which maintain a high fetal–maternal concentration gradient that is only moderately sensitive to changing maternal folate status. The process may occur in two stages, with the final transfer from the placenta to the fetal circulation taking place down a concentration gradient. The placenta also carries specific receptors for vitamin B_{12}.

Vitamin B_6 is probably transported across the placenta by passive transport (mainly as pyridoxal and pyridoxine), with substantive binding in the placenta, phosphorylation, and final release into the fetal circulation as pyridoxal 5-phosphate. The placental transfer of thiamin has been studied in in vitro placental perfusion systems. Results indicate an active transport mechanism, which maintains a higher concentration in the fetal plasma than in the mother. Riboflavin in the fetal circulation is at a higher concentration than in the mother, mainly as the mononucleotide (FMN). Studies suggest an efficient, saturable active transport system from mother to fetus.

Minerals and trace elements

Most of the work in this area has used in vitro perfusion of human placental lobules.

Magnesium

Magnesium is thought to cross the placenta by an active transport mechanism but there is no clear relationship between maternal and fetal plasma concentrations.

Zinc

Zinc is probably actively transported in its albumin bound form and fetal cord blood levels are about 50% higher than maternal plasma levels.

Iron

In late pregnancy a large proportion of available iron from the mother is transferred to the fetus. Placental transferrin receptors are present to facilitate transfer of transferrin-bound iron by endocytosis.

Other trace elements

Copper and selenium appear to be transported by passive diffusion.

GROWTH AND DEVELOPMENT OF THE CONCEPTUS

Following fertilisation, human gestation goes through three phases: blastocyst formation, embryogenesis and fetal growth. Blastocyst formation lasts for 2 weeks after fertilisation and then embryogenesis for 6 weeks. During embryogenesis all the tissues and organs are defined anatomically, and any teratogens are likely to have their greatest impact. Therefore when a pregnant woman is 10 weeks post her last menstrual period the structure and anatomical relationships of her infant's tissues and organs have been established. The remaining 30 weeks of gestation comprise the fetal period of life when the fetus grows from a weight of about 10–30 g to its birthweight, which on average in white women is 3.3 kg with an additional 0.7 kg represented by the placenta (see Fig. *evolve* 15.2). In pregnancy about 800—1000 ml of amniotic fluid accumulates and therefore the average total weight of the products of conception at full term is about 4.8 kg.

ENERGY COSTS OF PREGNANCY

The nutritional costs of pregnancy comprise the energetic value of new tissue laid down both by the mother and in the products of conception and the additional energetic costs associated with the increasing metabolising mass of the pregnant woman as her pregnancy advances. The classic studies of Hytten and Leitch on the accumulation of new tissue in relation to advancing pregnancy are summarised in Table 15.2. In addition to the new tissue laid down as products of conception

Table 15.2   Mean daily increments of protein and fat in the fetus and maternal body

| | WEEKS OF PREGNANCY | | | | CUMULATIVE TOTAL |
	0–10	10–20	20–30	30–40	
Protein (g)	0.64	1.84	4.76	6.1	925.0
Fat (g)	5.85	24.80	21.85	3.3	3825.0

detailed above, Hytten calculated the tissue accretion in maternal anabolism as follows: uterus 0.9 kg; breasts 0.4 kg; blood 1.2 kg; extracellular fluid 1.2 kg; fat 3.5 kg. This gives a total average maternal weight gain of 7.2 kg, which combined with the weight of the products of conception produces an average weight gain for human pregnancy of 13 kg, but with a very wide range. 'Normal weight gain for pregnancy' is difficult to define and hence advice on energy intakes during pregnancy to optimise fetal growth has no physiological basis.

Hytten calculated the theoretical energy requirements for pregnancy on the basis of weight gain, using the mother's pre-pregnancy physiological status as a baseline. In an average pregnancy the energy requirement for the stored fetal and placental tissue is 177 MJ (42 500 kcal), the maintenance energy an additional 146 MJ (35 000 kcal), and the conversion energy for creating new tissue approximately 33 MJ (8000 kcal). This represents a cumulative increased energy requirement over the whole of pregnancy of 334–356 MJ (80 000–85 000 kcal), or a daily energy increase of approximately 1.3 MJ (310 kcal). This gave rise to the widespread advice that women, in order to have a successful pregnancy, must increase their energy intakes by 1–1.5 MJ (250–350 calories) per day– the widespread layperson's idea that the mother should 'eat for two'.

However dietary surveys by and large do not match these theoretical calculations. For example the longitudinal study of energy balance in healthy pregnant women in Glasgow by Durnin et al (1987) showed a gradual rise in intakes during the duration of pregnancy, but the calculated total extra energy intake in pregnancy was less than 84 MJ (20 000 kcal). Basal metabolic rate (BMR) fell in early pregnancy, followed by a rise in the last 10 weeks. There was no extra requirement in the first 30 weeks and the increase in the last trimester could have been met by a small increase

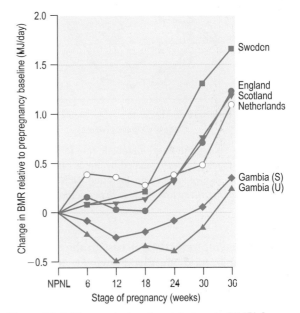

Figure 15.1 Changes in basal metabolic rate (BMR) from the non-pregnant state and at 6-weekly intervals in pregnancy in women studied by indirect calorimetry in four European countries and one African country. Gambian women were on their normal diet (U) or randomised to receive a high calorie supplement (S). *(Adapted from Prentice et al 1989, with permission.)*

in energy intake or a reduction in physical activity.

Durnin's study was expanded into a collaborative international project in selected developing and developed countries. The increase in basal metabolic rates (BMR) in pregnancy show very wide geographical variations, with women in the developed world having increases compatible with increased total energy expenditure (TEE) similar to the hypothetical calculation (Fig. 15.1), while women in the developing world may go through pregnancy with an apparent reduction in energy expenditure, indicating a very powerful adaptation

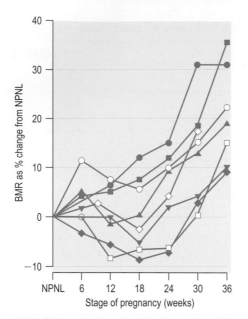

Figure 15.2 Changes in basal metabolic rate in eight individual European subjects studied by direct calorimetry. Baseline is the non-pregnant non-lactating (NPNL) state. *(Adapted from Prentice et al 1989, with permission.)*

Table 15.3	EAR energy for women in the UK
	ENERGY MJ/DAY (KCAL/DAY)
Women (19–50)	8.1 (1940)
Pregnancy	10.8 (200)[a]
Lactation (1 month)	11.9 (450)
Lactation (2 months)	12.2 (530)
Lactation (3 months)	12.4 (570)
Lactation (4–6 months)[b]	12.0 (480)
Lactation (4–6 months)[c]	12.4 (570)
Lactation (>6 months)[b]	11.0 (240)
Lactation (>6 months)[c]	12.3 (550)

[a]Third trimester only.
[b]Non-exclusive breastfeeding – weaning commenced.
[c]Exclusive breastfeeding – weaning not commenced.

to guarantee reproductive success in the context of an unreliable food supply. However, individual studies on eight healthy Cambridge women (Prentice et al 1989), using whole body calorimetry, show a very variable individual pattern in total energy expenditure, with half being energy-profligate during pregnancy whilst the other half were energy-sparing (Fig. 15.2). It is therefore impossible to recommend an ideal energy intake. Current estimated average requirements (EARs) for energy intake in pregnancy and lactation are shown in Table 15.3.

EFFECTS OF ACTIVITY ON PREGNANCY AND OF PREGNANCY ON ACTIVITY

Whilst there is now much interest in the developed world in the relationship of activity and exercise to pregnancy outcomes it must be borne in mind that for many women in the developing world manual labour throughout pregnancy is not something they have a choice about. In addition, both in the developed and developing world the mother who has the day-to-day care of younger children at the time of the pregnancy may find that she does not have the opportunity to significantly reduce her physical activity.

For those who are able to reduce activity or give up demanding physical work during the last few weeks of pregnancy, the altered pattern of energy expenditure is bound to have an effect on substrate availability to the fetus. Studies such as that of Clapp & Dickstein (1984) suggested that women who maintained a high level of recreational exercise throughout pregnancy gained less weight, delivered their children earlier, and produced infants of lower birthweight. A study from the developing world, of women who were involved in hard physical work despite lower than recommended calorie intakes, found similar effects on birthweight.

Overall, studies suggest that women who exercise before pregnancy and continue to do so during pregnancy tend to weigh less initially, to gain less weight, and to deliver smaller babies than (non-randomised) control subjects. There is insufficient evidence in the literature to make a judgement whether active women have better pregnancy outcomes than women who are predominantly sedentary in the second half of pregnancy, although one observational study from France reported that premature delivery rates more than doubled in women working more than 40 hours a week during pregnancy compared to those working for less than 40 hours per week. Apart from this there is little information from good quality studies to indicate whether active women have better pregnancy outcomes than less active women. The Royal College of Obstetricians and Gynaecologists has issued some guidance to women about exercise patterns during pregnancy. Whilst these are empirical they may be useful as a practical guide (see Section *evolve* 15.3(b) for details 🖱)).

An important consideration when advising women about exercise in pregnancy is to consider diet as well. Diets high in carbohydrate, particularly from low glycaemic index sources, will alter the availability of fetal substrates, and thus a relatively unrefined diet associated with hard physical work or programmed exercise in pregnancy can lead to a reduction in birthweight. It is an interesting argument as to whether the non-exercising woman on the usual Western diet or her exercising sister on a high carbohydrate traditional type of diet should be recognised as the physiological norm in studies of pregnancy outcome.

NUTRIENT REQUIREMENTS OF PREGNANCY

The current UK recommendations for nutrient intakes in pregnancy (and lactation) are summarised in Table 15.4. The reference nutrient intake (RNI) represents a nutritional intake at which about 97% of the population will obtain their daily requirements. Increased intakes are recommended during pregnancy for a small number of nutrients discussed below.

Protein

The recommendation for increased dietary protein content is based on the protein requirement of the new tissue formation outlined above. It is likely, however, that maternal resources would be made available to the fetus on a short-term basis in the face of any acute deficiency of protein intake. Pregnant women are advised to consume protein-rich foods such as lean meat and chicken, two servings of fish per week, including one of oily fish, eggs and pulses.

Non-starch polysaccharides

Requirements for non-starch polysaccharides (NSP) during pregnancy are not increased. Evidence

Table 15.4	RNI for women in the UK			
	WOMEN	LACTATION	LACTATION	
	NUTRIENT/DAY	(19–50 YEARS) PREGNANCY	(0–4 MONTHS)	(4+ MONTHS)
Protein (q)	45	16	111	18
Thiamin (mg)	0.8	10.1[a]	10.2	10.2
Riboflavin (mg)	1.1	10.3	10.5	10.5
Niacin (mg)	13	[b]	10.2	10.2
Vitamin B$_6$ (mg)	1.2	[b]	[b]	[b]
Vitamin B$_{12}$ (μg)	1.5	[b]	10.5	10.5
Folate (μg)	200	1100	160	160
Vitamin C (mg)	40	110	130	130
Vitamin A (μg)	600	1100	1350	1350
Vitamin D (μg)	–	10	10	10
Calcium (mg)	700	[b]	1550	1550
Phosphorus (mg)	550	[b]	1440	1440
Magnesium (mg)	270	[b]	150	150
Sodium (mg)	1600	[b]	[b]	[b]
Potassium (mg)	3500	[b]	[b]	[b]
Chloride (mg)	2500	[b]	[b]	[b]
Iron (mg)	14.8	[b]	[b]	[b]
Zinc (mg)	7.0	[b]	16	12.5
Copper (mg)	1.2	[b]	10.3	10.3
Selenium (μg)	60	[b]	115	115
Iodine (μg)	140	[b]	[b]	[b]

[a] Third trimester only.
[b] No increment.

suggests that NSPs are an integral part of a healthy and balanced diet which appear to have both direct and indirect positive effects on health. The COMA Panel recommends that the diet of the adult population should contain on average 18 g per day nonstarch polysaccharides (individual range of 12–24 g per day). The latest National Diet and Nutrition Survey (NDNS) of British adults aged indicates that a significant proportion of women of childbearing age have intakes of NSP below these recommendations. Pregnant women are advised to increase their intake of NSP which, as a side affect, might help alleviate constipation, a common symptom during pregnancy.

A low GI diet with a high NSP content has been shown to enhance insulin sensitivity in pregnancy and may therefore prevent progression to gestational diabetes (GDM) in susceptible individuals.

Vitamins

Thiamin and riboflavin

The third trimester increase in thiamin intake is recommended to accompany the suggested increase in carbohydrate intake but there is no evidence of thiamin depletion arising as a result of pregnancy or indeed in lactation. Similarly an increase in riboflavin in pregnancy and lactation is recommended over the third trimester but there is little evidence to suggest that riboflavin depletion is a particular problem of pregnancy in the developed world.

Folate

The potentially beneficial effects of folic acid supplementation in the periconceptional period are discussed above in 'Periconceptional nutrition and fetal malformations'. On theoretical grounds, with so much new tissue formation, an increased folate intake is recommended for pregnancy, and indeed folate prophylaxis against megaloblastic anaemia is a widespread prescription for healthy pregnant women. The evidence of benefit is limited and the recommendation is simply based on observations that in pregnancy an extra 100 μg per day intake of folic acid is required to maintain plasma and red cell folate levels at or above those of non-pregnant women. Folate depletion may arise in association with poor general nutrition in women on low incomes where fresh fruit and vegetables do not comprise a significant or regular component of the habitual diet. Doyle and colleagues (2001) in deprived areas of London found a mean daily folate intake of 162 μg/day in women judged to have inadequate diets compared with 331 μg/day in those with adequate diets.

Despite public health campaigns to increase awareness of the importance of folic acid supplementation when planning a pregnancy in the UK, compliance remains patchy; also, many pregnancies are unplanned. In the USA and Canada where the mandatory folic acid fortification of flour was implemented in 1998, NTD prevalence has been reduced by 20–50%. Mandatory fortification of flour with folic acid has been debated in the UK but implementation has been delayed pending the results of studies on related health concerns (see also Section 10.5 and Ch. 33).

Ascorbic acid

Vitamin C depletion is rare in pregnancy but again may be a feature of a generally poor quality diet. The vitamin is actively transported across the placenta to the fetus and the COMA panel recommended an increased intake of 10 mg daily in pregnancy and 30 mg daily in lactation. Pregnant women are encourages to consume foods or drinks containing vitamin C, together with iron-rich meals, in order to help with iron absorption (see Sections 10.7 and 12.3).

Vitamin A

Vitamin A occupies a confusing role in relation to pregnancy. Both low levels and high levels periconceptionally may be associated with teratogenesis. The problem with overdosage seems to relate to preformed vitamin A (retinol) of animal origin. The UK Scientific Advisory Committee on Nutrition (SACN) concluded that there was insufficient evidence to establish a safe upper level for vitamin A intake. Current recommendations in the UK advise against the consumption of supplements containing vitamin A and of liver or liver products by pregnant women or women who might become pregnant. Dietary deficiency of vitamin A is rare in the developed world and although the recommendation is for an extra 100 mg per day, supplementation is rarely indicated. In contrast there are geographical areas in the developing world where vitamin A deficiency is widespread and in these areas appropriate levels of supplementation are associated with reduced maternal mortality and improved vitamin A status of the infant and in some studies improved fetal growth, and reduced xerophthalmia (see also Sections 11.1 and 28.3).

Vitamin D

Vitamin D deficiency in pregnancy is rare. Low Vitamin D status (25-OH D concentration below 25 nmol/L) is seen in 10% of 15–18-year-old, 28% of 19–24-year-old, and 13% of 25–34-year-old females in the UK, therefore peaking in the reproductive years. This may represent widespread deficiency, although as a similar pattern is seen in males it may represent a physiological change associated with a maturing skeleton. Those at high risk of deficiency in pregnancy are dark-skinned women living in northern climates with limited skin exposure to summer sunlight, women who consume a diet low in vitamin D and women with a pre-pregnancy BMI above 30.

Their infants may have deficient calcification of the skeleton and suffer from neonatal tetany without prescription of maternal supplements. In one double-blind placebo-controlled study of vitamin D supplements in pregnancy, tetany was not seen in the infants of 59 supplemented women but five cases occurred in 67 control women. Also in the follow-up of this study infant growth was better and dental enamel dysplasia reduced in the infants of the supplemented women.

The report *Update on vitamin D* (SACN 2007) recommends that all pregnant and breastfeeding women should consider taking a daily supplement of vitamin D (10 µg–400 iu) to ensure their own requirement for vitamin D and to generate adequate fetal stores for the demands of early infancy.

Essential fatty acids

Transplacental transfer of essential fatty acids (EFAs) is obviously of crucial importance for fetal development, particularly membrane formation and cellular development in the brain. Modern diets have lower n-3 EFA intakes in particular, mainly due to a decline in oily fish consumption, and there is considerable scientific interest in the reproductive outcomes of women with high and low n-3 intakes from fish or fish oil supplements.

A Cochrane review (2006) of supplementation studies reported a mean prolongation of pregnancy of 2.6 days with fish oil compared to placebo, with a possible particular benefit in preterm delivery below 34 weeks of gestation (relative risk 0.69 (95% CI 0.49–0.99)) There was a mean increase in birthweight of 47 g but no reductions in low birthweight or pre-eclampsia. However, a multicentre European study of supplementation of pregnant women with docosahexaenoic acid (DHA), eicosapentaenoic acid (EPA) and/or folic acid or placebo, administered from 22 weeks gestation revealed no differences in pregnancy outcomes or fetal development between the groups. (Krauss-Etschmann et al 2007. Essential fatty acid deficiency is rare, however, and the combination of considerable body reserves in the adipose tissue with efficient placental transfer suggests that maternal supplementation has little to offer. Studies of cord, blood and maternal plasma at the time of birth confirm the concentrating power of the placenta for EFA Table 15.5.) The possibility of EFA deficiency being related to fetal or infant brain and retinal development means that considerable research activity continues in this area (see also Section 7.2).

Minerals

Calcium

Additional calcium intakes are not recommended in pregnancy although there are major physiological changes in calcium metabolism, presumably designed to meet the fetal requirements. In early pregnancy there is an increase in bone turnover with increased bone resorption liberating calcium to the plasma pool. There is also increased gut absorption of calcium and an increase of urinary calcium excretion in healthy pregnant women of about 100%, which would suggest that the combination of the above factors is more than adequate to provide the calcium required for fetal skeleton and membranes. There is considerable remodelling of bone with an increase in bone mineral density in the long bones of the arms and legs and a reduction in bone mineral density in the pelvis and spine being a feature of late pregnancy (Naylor

Table 15.5	Fatty acids in maternal and cord plasma phospholipids at the time of birth (median and interquartile range)	
	MATERNAL PLASMA	PHOSPHOLIPIDS CORD PLASMA
C20: 4n-6	7.68(1.90)	16.14(2.49)
C22: 6n-3	2.89(0.99)	4.76(1.70)
Modified from Berghaus et al 1998.		

et al 2000). No increase in calcium intake is recommended although problems may arise with exclusion diets in those who do not consume milk or milk products or who exclude cheese from their diet in pregnancy because of concerns about the risk of transmission of *Listeria*, for instance (see also Section 12.2).

Iron

The combination of new tissue formation, haematopoiesis in the fetus and the mother, and typical blood losses at delivery, suggest an additional iron requirement of approximately 900 mg in pregnancy. This would justify iron supplementation in many women, particularly those with low iron intakes on their habitual diet, were it not for evidence that small bowel absorption of iron, along with other divalent cations, is enhanced in pregnancy. Whilst iron-deficiency anaemia is a feature of pregnancy in many parts of the developing world where poor iron intakes are combined with other causes of anaemia, such as malaria or hookworm, in the developed world confusion continues to arise from the observation that, even in those women who appear to be iron-sufficient based on measurements of iron stores, supplementation with oral iron leads to a rise in the haemoglobin concentration. A response of this nature would normally be interpreted as confirming the presence of anaemia but careful studies of red cell indices in relation to iron suggest a different phenomenon. What in fact is seen with supplementation is an increase in the haemoglobin content of the individual red cell leading to a rise in the mean corpuscular volume. This is a change associated with alteration of the shape of the usual biconcave disc, a shape associated with maximum oxygen transfer, to a rounder cell with a reduction in surface area. Although there is no experimental evidence of harm, the altered shape of these red cells increases the blood viscosity and may impair placental perfusion. The National Institute of Clinical Excellence (NICE) recommends against routine iron supplementation of pregnant women as it does not benefit the health of either mother or baby and may have unpleasant maternal side effects (NICE 2008) (see also Sections 12.3 and 28.5).

Zinc

There is a theoretical increased zinc requirement in late pregnancy but zinc deficiency is rare on usual diets, and experiments with zinc supplementation have failed to demonstrate any beneficial outcome for either mother or infant in pregnancy (see also Section 12.4).

Iodine

For most women recommended intakes (see Appendix Table A27) are achieved from dietary sources such as cow's milk or fish, but principally from iodised table salt. Plasma levels of 150–249 µg represent adequate iodine intakes. Iodine deficiency remains a major problem, however, on a geographical basis in some areas of the developing world. It is particularly important in relation to pregnancy because of the risk of cretinism and lesser degrees of mental impairment in the offspring of iodine-deficient mothers. These are handicapping conditions which are almost entirely preventable by manipulation of the pregnancy diet. Where iodine deficiency is known to exist, iodised table salt or iodised cooking oil should be available to all the population and pregnant women in particular (see also Sections 12.5 and 28.4).

NUTRITION AND ADVERSE PREGNANCY OUTCOMES

Foodborne disease in pregnancy

Listeriosis is a disease more common in the immunocompromised. Pregnancy represents a state of relative immune compromise and in the rare case of primary infection during pregnancy transplacental infection of the fetus has been responsible for fetal death. Because of the behaviour of the organism and its proliferation in common foodstuffs such as mould-ripened cheese, liver pate and cook–chill foods, major anxiety has been provoked amongst pregnant women in recent years. Sensible advice is that women should avoid mould-ripened cheese whilst pregnant and only eat pate from manufacturing processes where pasteurisation has taken place. As far as cook–chill food is concerned it should be consumed within the recommended shelf life and properly heated through before serving. Current awareness in the UK has resulted in the reduced incidence of pregnancy-associated listeriosis from a peak of 114 cases per year in 1988 and 1989 to 28 cases in 2007.

Toxoplasma gondii is a parasitic protozoal infection which non-immune women may be at increased risk of during pregnancy. It is caught from the ingestion of parasites from undercooked meat or from contact with cat faeces as a result of gardening or cleaning cat litter trays. In the fetus it can be responsible for brain infection and particularly defects of vision. Sensible advice to women in pregnancy who may be at risk is to cook all meat thoroughly before consumption and to either avoid gardening and cat litter trays or only to undertake these tasks with strong rubber gloves.

Maternal mortality

Maternal mortality rates are extremely low in the developed world, in the order of 1 in 10 000 births, but in the developing world rates may be as high as 6 per 1000 pregnancies. Nutrition may contribute to this increased mortality in two respects. Firstly protein calorie malnutrition or rickets in childhood may lead to a failure to reach full genetic potential of adult height. This in turn may be associated with inadequate pelvic dimensions and obstructed labour in adulthood. Obstructed labour is a major cause of maternal death where facilities for safe caesarean section are not available.

Severe anaemia is also a contributor to maternal death, often in association with intercurrent illness such as malaria and the absence of safe blood transfusion to deal with antepartum or postpartum haemorrhage. Evidence, reviewed by Rush (2000), would suggest that moderate anaemia is not a major risk factor but severe anaemia (Hb 8.0 g/dl) has been associated with a doubling of death rates in urban-dwelling women and a quadrupling of death rates in rural-dwelling women. For example, when the relationship between haematocrit and maternal death in northern Nigeria was examined there were 36 maternal deaths amongst 760 anaemic women (4.7%) but only 142 deaths in 11 699 non-anaemic women (1.2%), a relative risk of death of 3.9.

Low birthweight

Poor weight gain in pregnancy has been associated with poor fetal growth but of course to some extent this is self-fulfilling as the normal growth of the products of conception must be a factor in the maternal weight gain. Although advice to increase energy intakes will result in enhanced maternal weight gain there is no published evidence that this enhanced weight gain acts in the fetal interest.

In any obstetric population the prevalence of low birthweight is a good surrogate marker for risk of perinatal death (this is a combination of deaths before birth plus those in the first week of life). There are two principal causes of low birthweight – preterm delivery, in which the infant may be normally grown but born in an immature state, and intrauterine growth retardation (IUGR), where inefficient placental transfer of oxygen and/or nutrients has led to a reduced rate of growth. The WHO definition simply is 'birthweight of less than 2.5 kg'. This must include a mixture of the two diagnostic groups, although the proportions may vary depending on factors such as maternal stature, smoking and alcohol consumption, altitude above sea level, etc. Evidence is that low calorie intakes do not significantly contribute to low birthweight above a threshold value of an average energy intake somewhere between 5.8 and 7.0 MJ (1400 and 1700 kcal). Below this threshold there is good evidence that carbohydrate supplementation can significantly reduce the number of low birthweight babies. Above the threshold there is no clear evidence of such a benefit from supplementation.

Energy supplementation experiments both in the developed and developing world in women with calorie intakes above the threshold have negligible effects on birthweight and indeed experiments with protein-dense supplements have been associated with a relative *reduction* in birthweight. Rush reviewed the published studies in 1989 and reported a reduction in birthweight when the percentage of calories as protein in supplements exceeded 20% (Rush 1989). Nutrient supplementation of healthy pregnant women at a time of enhanced energetic efficiency may simply result in increased rates of maternal obesity postpartum.

Concerns about inadequate nutrient intakes in low-income pregnant women encouraged the UK government to reform the long-standing Welfare Food Scheme (WFS), with the Healthy Start (HS) Scheme in 2006. This provides vouchers that can be exchanged for fresh fruit and vegetables, liquid cow's milk and infant formula and the opportunity to access good quality health advice, including diet in pregnancy, breastfeeding, stopping smoking, and the roles of milk, fresh fruit, vegetables and vitamins in the diet (Ford et al 2008). It is too early to say whether the effects of this scheme on dietary quantity and quality will be followed by a reduction in low birthweight and influence early-years nutrition (see also Ch. 33 and Section *evolve* 15.3(c) 🔧 for a summary of NICE guidance on maternal and child nutrition in low-income families).

The effect of individual nutrient supplements in the prevention of low birthweight has been studied. Calcium supplementation appears be effective in the reduction of both preterm birth and the incidence of low birthweight (Atallah et al 2001). It may be that calcium supplementation has a role in the prevention of pregnancy-induced hypertension (see below) and that the increased mean birthweight is simply a reflection of prolongation of pregnancy. Although several experiments have been performed there is no evidence to support the use of magnesium supplementation during pregnancy to prevent low birthweight. There is similarly no evidence that routine iron supplementation prevents low birthweight. There is some suggestion from trials that folate supplementation may be effective in reducing the incidence of low birthweight in infants born at full term but folate supplementation has no preventative effect on preterm labour. In contrast, trials of zinc supplementation have suggested that lower rates of preterm delivery may be seen, although this evidence is not considered strong enough to influence practice at present. Meta-analyses of zinc supplementation studies suggest a non-significant reduction in low birthweight at term which again does not justify zinc supplementation in practice. Some studies suggest that vitamin D supplementation in pregnancy may have a beneficial effect on fetal growth but these are not of sufficient quality to influence practice and further research is in progress in this particular area.

No other specific nutrient supplement has been shown to be beneficial in properly designed trials in either reducing preterm birth rates or reducing term intrauterine growth retardation.

Obesity and pregnancy outcome

Obesity creates problems throughout the continuum of reproductive casualty. A BMI above 30 is associated with a doubling of the rate of ovulatory infertility and an even greater increase when the obesity is associated with the polycystic ovarian syndrome (see Fig. *evolve* 15.1). During pregnancy obese women are at increased risk of developing gestational diabetes, venous thromboembolism and pregnancy-induced hypertension. There is also evidence that labour in the obese is more likely to be prolonged and unsuccessful, and should delivery by caesarean section be necessary,

the procedure can be technically fraught because of difficulties with surgical access to the uterus through the obese abdomen. Offspring of obese mothers are heavier than those of height- and age-matched non-obese women when obese diabetic women are excluded from the analysis.

Nutrition and the hypertensive disorders of pregnancy

Pregnancy is complicated by the development of hypertension in about 8% of cases worldwide, with a predominance of first pregnancies. When hypertension is established and accompanied by proteinuria the condition is referred to as pre-eclampsia and is associated with increased maternal and perinatal mortality and morbidity. There have been many attempts to identify the causes of pre-eclampsia and several nutritional hypotheses have been tested. Early observational studies for instance suggested that the conditions were more common in omnivores than in strict vegetarians. Generalised nutritional deprivation in wartime has also been associated with a reduction in the frequency of pregnancy-associated hypertension. More recently attempts to prevent the condition have been made by dietary interventions including high protein diets, or establishing a high plane of general nutrition by eating a well-balanced diet. In contrast, some workers have suggested that voluntary dieting leading to weight gain restriction in pregnancy was beneficial in preventing hypertensive disease.

The evidence for dietary prevention of hypertension in pregnancy is of limited quality – and there is no suggestion that manipulating the diet can alter the incidence of these conditions. It may be able to prevent or moderate the secondary effects of disease in some circumstances.

As stated earlier, maternal obesity is associated with increased rates of pregnancy-associated hypertension and high weight gains during pregnancy have been reported in association with this disease. Once again this is probably self-fulfilling as these hypertensive conditions are often accompanied by fluid retention in the form of oedema.

In the past women have been recommended to reduce their salt intake but the only comparative study of low versus normal salt intakes showed lower rates of hypertensive disease in the higher salt intake group.

A number of experiments using calcium supplements have secured a lowering of mean blood pressure compared to placebo and in one study the calcium-supplemented subjects had one-third of the incidence of pregnancy-associated hypertension compared to the placebo group. Meta-analysis has confirmed this apparent benefit. It is not clear whether the benefit is in reducing the incidence of hypocalcaemia where the women's diet is low in calcium, or whether similar benefits are seen in calcium-sufficient women. In the meta-analysis pre-eclampsia incidence was reduced by calcium supplementation (RR 0.48; 95%CI 0.33–0.69), but the reduction appeared greatest in those judged to have pre-existing risk factors for pre-eclampsia and where low baseline calcium intakes were recorded. In studies of women with adequate calcium intakes the effect on pre-eclampsia incidence was not significantly reduced (RR 0.62; CI 0.32–1.20) (Hofmeyr et al 2007). Studies on the role of zinc supplementation in the prevention of pre-eclampsia have been conflicting, as have some experiments in which multivitamin and mineral preparations have been offered to pregnant women. There are good theoretical reasons to suggest that intakes of essential fatty acids may have a part to play in vascular sensitivity in women at risk of pregnancy-associated hypertension. Dietary surveys show no difference in essential fatty acid intakes between women with and without pregnancy-associated hypertension, and a recent Cochrane review found no clear difference between fish-oil-supplemented and placebo groups in the relative risk of pre-eclampsia (Makrides et al 2006).

A further therapeutic intervention which has been the subject of recent randomised controlled trials in the modification of preeclampsia is a possible role for antioxidant vitamins. Markers of oxidative stress are present in the placenta and maternal circulation and early small-scale studies had suggested a role for a supplement containing 1000 mg vitamin C and 400 iu vitamin E in prevention of progress of the disorder. Large-scale RCTs, however, have failed to confirm any benefit in women studied in the developed world (Poston et al 2006) or in the developing world (Villar et al 2009). In the former study there was a small unexpected increase in low birthweight in the treated group, but this finding was not replicated in the second study. At present there is no case to recommend antioxidant supplements for women at increased risk of pre-eclampsia.

15.4 LACTATION

CHANGES IN BODY COMPOSITION DURING LACTATION

Studies have been performed in the developing and developed world addressed to the possible effects of lactation on maternal body composition. These studies are generally difficult to interpret because of variations in nutrient availability, physiological changes in maternal energy consumption (see below), and differences in the average age of the child at weaning.

Studies performed on 22 healthy Swedish women who all commenced breastfeeding and 12 of whom were still at least partially breastfeeding when the infant was 6 months of age were reported in 1988. Prepregnancy mean body weight was 61.0 kg (69.9) compared to 61.9 kg (610.9) 6 months postpartum. When body composition was compared, the most striking difference was that total body fat was 17.2 kg (66.9) prepregnancy but 20.4 kg (67.9) 6 months post-delivery. This raised the important question as to whether pregnancy and subsequent lactation were associated with major changes of body composition. Our own studies addressing this question reached similar conclusions but reported that in women with pre-existing obesity there was persistence of increased suprailiac skinfold thickness at 6 months postpartum with a corresponding increase in the waist:hip ratio.

In contrast, undernourished women studied in the developing world (Taiwan) revealed increases of weight and upper arm skinfold thicknesses during prolonged lactation in approximately a third of women whilst the remaining two-thirds demonstrated a pattern of weight gain similar to that seen in the studies reported above (Adair et al 1984).

ENERGY REQUIREMENT OF LACTATION

Studies of lactation are bedevilled by differences in practice. In many societies 99% of women lactate and produce enough milk to represent their infant's sole nutritional requirement for at least the first 6 months of its life and a significant component for up to 2 years. In other societies, particularly in the developed world, lactation rates may be as low as 30% or 40% and artificial formula feeding is more common. Again the timing and extent of introduction of weaning foods will affect both the infant's energy intake and growth rate and indeed postpartum changes in maternal body composition. Although it has been suggested that the net gain of fat seen in women in the developed world is a reserve against lactation there seems to be no evidence that these fat deposits are mobilised during lactation.

To understand the energy requirement of lactation, which is after all the physiological situation, it is necessary to calculate the milk volume and nutrient density along with changes which occur over time. Unfortunately much of the published literature on human milk contents may be biased by natural variations such as the composition of milk early in the feed compared to late in the feed and the timing of the sample throughout the day, with nitrogen and lactose being lower and fat higher during the night, and according to the gestational age at birth, with nitrogen higher when birth is premature, and the pattern of suckling, either on demand or controlled.

For the first postpartum week milk produced is colostrum, a relatively thick yellow fluid with a mean energy value of 67 kcal (0.3 MJ) per 100 ml with a volume of only 2–20 ml per feed during the first 3 days. From 7 days postpartum to 14 days postpartum the milk produced is called transitional and has a lower protein content and increased content of lactose, but a lower fat content than mature milk (Table 14.5). Milk volumes per 24 hours rise from about 700 ml in the first month to 900 ml in the fifth to sixth months. Thereafter with prolonged lactation milk volumes reduce slightly to about 750 ml by 12 months of lactation. During this time most women have introduced supplementary feeding for the infant and this alternative source of energy results in reduced milk demand by the infant and a reduction in the volume of milk being produced.

Accepting the provisos above as a guideline, the gross energy content of milk is approximately 0.67 kcal/ml (2.8 kJ), with a daily energy content of 500 kcal (2.09 MJ). Efficiency of milk production is thought to be between 80 and 95%; therefore the energy cost of milk synthesis to the mother during full lactation in the early months of the infant's life is between 25 and 125 kcal per day (100–525 kJ). The average fat gain in the developed world is 3.3 kg, and in the developing world 0.9 kg. It is assumed that this is a reserve for lactation but the outcome of the deposited fat is not shown to be closely related to lactational behaviour. In the developed world women have usually recovered

their prepregnancy body weight but body composition is altered with the retention of body fat at the expense of lean body mass.

There are conflicting studies about the possible role of suppression of diet-induced thermogenesis in the lactating mother. Illingworth and colleagues (1986; Fig. 15.3) suggest a 30% reduction in diet-induced thermogenesis, which would be an important adaptation to energy conservation and successful lactation as a physiological change. Other studies are conflicting, some suggesting that there is no alteration in diet-induced thermogenesis in lactation but some confirming the observation of Illingworth and colleagues (see 'Undernutrition in lactation', below). A review by Prentice et al (1996) showed a remarkable similarity in breast milk output of women from different nutritional cultural settings both in the developed world and in developing countries. Daily volumes of breast milk in women fully breastfeeding were 830 ml/day in months 3–6, 650 ml/day in months 6–12, and 600 ml/day in months 12–24. The energy content of average samples of milk was found to be 0.73 kcal/g (3.06 kJ/g), and energetic efficiency in the order of 94%, suggesting an energy requirement of about 557 kcal (2.3 MJ) per day. If the mother met the full cost of energy requirement for breast milk from her daily diet this would require 690 kcal (2.87 MJ) per day but this figure might reasonably be reduced to 540 kcal (2.2 MJ/day) on the assumption that maternal fat stores would be consumed at the rate of 500 g/month during the first 6

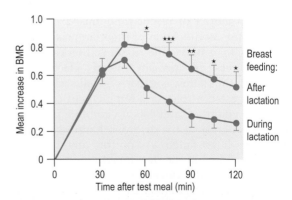

Figure 15.3 Mean increase (±SEM) in metabolic rate (kJ/min) in response to test meal in breastfeeding women during and after lactation; represents significant differences. *(Adapted from Illingworth et al 1986, with permission.)*

months of lactation. There is some evidence that lactation is associated with physiological shifts towards energy conservation and most women are probably in an energy-efficient mode during lactation (Fig. 15.3).

NUTRIENT REQUIREMENTS OF LACTATION

Although essential fatty acid concentrations are low in human milk and low in breast milk substitutes, there is no evidence that maternal supplementation with essential fatty acids is beneficial. In lactation there is a recommendation for increased calcium intake to match losses in the milk. In prolonged lactation bone mineral density reduces in relation to the volume of breast milk produced. The bone mineral density is restored rapidly on cessation of lactation and there is no evidence that lactation contributes to an increased risk of osteoporosis in post-menopausal life. Phosphorus requirements are judged to be equimolar to calcium requirements and phosphate deficiency is unrecognised in normal diets.

The recommended increases in nutrients for lactation are calculated based on the assumption that the energy costs of lactation are added to the typical energy expenditure of the non-pregnant, non-lactating state. The comments above with regard to alterations in diet-induced thermogenesis and possible metabolism of maternal stored fat obviously influence the validity of these calculations in the individual.

Essential fatty acid contents of breast milk range from 0.1 g/100 g total fat to 1.4 g/100 g total fat in different population groups. The predominant n-6 long-chain polyunsaturated fatty acid (LCPUFA) is arachidonic acid and docosahexaenoic acid (DHA) is the most common and most important n-3 LCPUFA in breast milk. The ratio of n-6 to n-3 fatty acids depends almost entirely on the intakes in the maternal habitual diet.

DIETARY REFERENCE VALUES

See Table 15.4.

UNWANTED COMPONENTS OF MATERNAL DIET WHICH PASS INTO MILK

General concerns about the effect of components of the maternal diet on infants' tolerance of breast milk are probably overstated. Essential oils in foods such as garlic and some spices produce characteristic odours in milk which the infant may object to, although in one study maternal garlic consumption was associated with increased length of suckling and the rate of suckling at subsequent feeds. Foods which can produce problems of tolerance for the infant are cabbage, turnips, broccoli and beans, which seem capable of producing colic in some infants. The same effect has been ascribed to rhubarb, apricots and prunes. It might be sensible to exclude such food items when a breastfed infant appears to be distressed by colic after feeds.

UNDERNUTRITION IN LACTATION

There are significant adaptive mechanisms to protect the newborn baby despite acute or chronic maternal undernutrition. The classic Bacon Chow studies performed in Taiwanese women who were given a nutrient-dense supplement or placebo during pregnancy and lactation revealed marginally improved weight maintenance through lactation in the supplemented women (Adair et al 1984). Some placebo-treated women, however, maintained their weight or even increased it during a period of 12 months of lactation following birth. Skinfold thicknesses in undernourished women were greater at the end of lactation after the second studied pregnancy whether given supplements or not. The conclusion drawn was that most mothers maintain an appropriate energy balance, compromising neither their own health status nor that of their developing infants despite the apparent marginal nutritional status of the whole population. Mothers on low energy intakes in lactation maintain their weight well and lactate successfully, suggesting that important adaptive mechanisms are operating.

LACTATIONAL AMENORRHOEA, BIRTH SPACING AND EFFECTS OF MATERNAL NUTRITIONAL STATUS

Fertile couples reproducing in the developing world without access to contraception typically show birth intervals of 3–4 years. This includes the duration of the pregnancy and approximately 18–24 months of lactational amenorrhoea during which there is no ovulation. In the developed world, freely available high-calorie intakes are associated with periods of lactational amenorrhoea which may be as short as 6–8 weeks after the delivery. Thus paradoxically a high nutritional plane may be associated with a shorter inter-pregnancy interval and possibly physiological derangements associated with frequent childbearing in the developed world, compared with the developing world. Studies performed in Bangladesh in poorly nourished women reported average durations of amenorrhoea of 17.9 months compared to 16.8 months in well-nourished women from the same population. Similar studies performed in Guatemala found periods of amenorrhoea of 14.8 months in the undernourished compared to 13.2 months in the better nourished. This is a different pattern of response in developed compared to developing countries and once again there may be a trigger related to body mass index for the resumption of ovulation and menstruation.

KEY POINTS

■ Nutritional status throughout the human reproductive cycle can affect outcomes.

■ Anovulatory infertility is seen in undernourished and overnourished women.

■ Periconceptional nutritional deficiencies may be associated with congenital malformations.

■ There is extensive maternal homeostatic change to produce a milieu favouring fetal growth and development.

■ Energy costs of pregnancy are variable and unpredictable.

■ Foodborne diseases such as listeriosis may be fatal for the fetus.

■ Maternal nutrient deficiencies such as iron predict increased maternal mortality in the developing world.

■ Reduced diet-induced thermogenesis is an energy-sparing mechanism in lactation.

References

Adair LS, Pollitt E, Mueller WH: The Bacon Chow study: effect of nutritional supplementation on maternal weight and skinfold thicknesses during pregnancy and lactation, *British Journal of Nutrition* 51:357–369, 1984.

Atallah AN, Hofmeyr GJ, Duley L: Calcium supplementation during pregnancy for preventing hypertensive disorders and related problems (Cochrane Review). In: The Cochrane Library, Issue 3, Oxford, 2001, Update Software.

Berghaus TM, Demmelmair H, Koletzko B: Fatty acid composition of lipid classes in maternal and cord plasma at birth, *European Journal of Paediatrics* 157:763–768, 1998.

Campbell-Brown M, Hytten F: Nutrition. In: Chamberlain G, Broughton-Pipkin F, editors: *Clinical physiology in obstetrics*, ed 3, Oxford, 1998, Blackwell Science, p 165–191.

Clapp JF, Dickstein S: Endurance exercise and pregnancy outcome, *Medicine and Science in Sports and Exercise* 16:556–562, 1984.

Czeizel AE, Dudas I: Prevention of the first occurrence of neural-tube defects by periconceptional vitamin supplementation, *New England Journal of Medicine* 327:1832–1835, 1992.

Doyle W, Srivostova A, Crawford MA, et al: Interpregnancy folate and iron status of women in an inner city population, *British Journal of Nutrition* 86:81–87, 2001.

Durnin JV, McKillop FM, Grant S, Fitzgerald G: *Energy requirements of pregnancy in Scotland*, Lancet ii:897–900, 1987.

Ford FA, Mouratidou T, Wademan SE, Fraser RB: Effect of the introduction of 'Healthy Start' on dietary behaviour during and after pregnancy: early results from the 'before and after' Sheffield study, *British Journal of Nutrition* 19:1–9, 2008.

Frisch R: The right weight: body fat, menarche and fertility, *Proceedings of the Nutrition Society* 53:113–129, 1994.

Hofmeyr GJ, Duley L, Atallah A: Dietary calcium supplementation for prevention of preeclampsia and related problems: a systematic review and commentary, *British Journal of Obstetrics and Gynaecology* 114:933–943, 2007.

Illingworth PJ, Jung RT, Howie PW, et al: Diminution in energy expenditure during lactation, *British Medical Journal* 292:437–441, 1986.

Krauss-Etschmann S, Shadid R, Campoy C, et al: Effects of fish-oil and folate supplementation of pregnant women on maternal and fetal plasma concentrations of docosahexaenoic acid and eicosapentaenoic acid: a European randomised multicentre trial, *American Journal of Clinical Nutrition* 85:1392–1400, 2007.

Makrides M, Duley L, Olsen SF: Marine oil, and other prostaglandin precursor, supplementation for pregnancy uncomplicated by pre-eclampsia or intrauterine growth restriction, *Cochrane Database of Systematic Reviews*, Issue 3:CD003402, 2006.

Naylor KE, Iqbal P, Fledelius C, et al: The effect of pregnancy on bone density and bone turnover, *Journal of Bone and Mineral Research* 15:129–137, 2000.

NICE (National Institute for Clinical Excellence): *Antenatal care: routine care for the healthy pregnant woman* (Clinical Guideline 62), London, 2008, RCOG Press.

Phelps RL, Metzger BE, Freinkel N: Carbohydrate metabolism in pregnancy. XVII Diurnal profiles of plasma glucose insulin free fatty acids, triglycerides, cholesterol and individual amino acids in late normal pregnancy, *American Journal of Obstetrics and Gynecology* 140: 730–736, 1981.

Poston L, Briley AL, Seed PT, et al: Vitamin C and Vitamin E in pregnant women at risk for pre-eclampsia (VIP Trial): randomised placebo controlled trial, *Lancet* 367:1145–1154, 2006.

Prentice AM, Goldberg GR, Davies HL et al: Energy sparing adaptations in human pregnancy assessed by whole body calorimetry, *British Journal of Nutrition* 62:5–22, 1989.

Prentice AM, Spaaij CJ, Goldberg GR, et al: Energy requirements of pregnant and lactating women, *European Journal of Clinical Nutrition* 50(suppl 1):S82–S118, 1996.

Rich-Edwards JW, Goldman MB, Willet WC, et al: Adolescent body mass index and infertility caused by ovulatory disorder, *American Journal of Obstetrics and Gynecology* 171:171–177, 1994.

Rush D: Effects of changes in maternal energy and protein intake during pregnancy, with special reference to fetal growth. In: Sharp F, Milner RDG, Fraser RB, editors: *Fetal growth*, London, 1989, RCOG Publications, p 203–229.

Rush D: Nutrition and maternal mortality in the developing world, *American Journal of Clinical Nutrition* 72(suppl):2125–2405, 2000.

Scientific Advisory Committee on Nutrition (SACN): *Update on vitamin D* (Position Statement), London, 2007, The Stationery Office.

Villar J, Purwar M, Merialdi M, et al: World Health Organisation multicentre randomised trial of supplementation with Vitamins C and E among pregnant women at high risk for pre-eclampsia in populations of low nutritional status from developing countries, *British Journal of Obstetrics and Gynecology* 116:780–788, 2009.

Further Reading

Frisch RL: *Female fertility and the body fat connection*, Chicago, 2002, University of Chicago Press

Lawrence RA: *Breast feeding, a guide for the medical profession*, ed 4, St Louis, 1994, Mosby-Year Book.

Mittlemark RA, Wiswell RA, Drinkwater BL: *Exercise in pregnancy*, ed 2, Baltimore, 1991, Williams & Wilkins.

Chapter 16

Ageing and the elderly

Salah Gariballa*

CHAPTER CONTENTS

OBJECTIVES

By the end of this chapter you should be able to:
- describe the physiological and pathological changes during ageing relevant to nutrition
- debate the adequacy of macro- and micronutrient changes in older people
- understand the interactions of current measures of nutritional status with ageing, disability and disease, and the consequent limitations for use in elderly people
- discuss the role of nutrition in the development, susceptibility to and outcome of common chronic disabling diseases in the elderly
- understand current important public health messages to maintain and improve nutritional status in elderly people.

*Updated and modified from the previous edition chapter written by Salah Gariballa and Alan Sinclair

16.1 INTRODUCTION

Globally, there has been, over the last century, a clear shift in population demographics, associated with an increase in life expectancy and a decline in fertility. This has created a need for a more complete understanding of age-related changes relevant to nutrition, and the role of nutrition in the prevention and treatment of chronic disabling diseases in the elderly. It is well recognised that with advancing age there is an increasing incidence of chronic diseases, and evidence points to the importance of nutrition in the development, susceptibility to, and outcome of these diseases. Undernutrition is recognized as a potential problem in the elderly, especially among the oldest age groups. There are, however, problems in diagnosing undernutrition in the elderly because of physical and biochemical changes which may take place as part of normal ageing. In addition, the neglect of nutritional assessment in the setting of acute clinical medicine is well known. For example, in the UK undernutrition is prevalent and largely unrecognised in hospital inpatients on admission and tends to deteriorate further during their hospital stay. There is no doubt that good nutrition contributes to the health and well-being of elderly people and to their ability to recover from illness (Fig. 16.1).

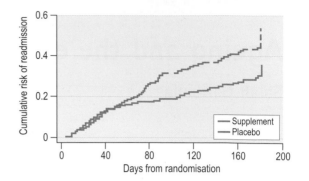

Fig. 16.1 Risk of hospital readmission in a 6-month follow-up is significantly lower in patients who received nutritional supplements (p = 0.018).

16.2 DEMOGRAPHIC TRENDS

Since the early 1930s the number of people aged over 65 in England has more than doubled and today a fifth of the population is over 60. Between 1995 and 2025 the number of people over the age of 80 is set to increase by almost a half and the number of people over 90 will double. It is predicted that by 2025 over 20% of the population in developed regions of the world will be aged 65 years and older and Asia will see the proportion of its elderly population almost double, from about 6% in 2000 to 10% in 2025. In absolute terms, this represents a stark increase in just 25 years from about 216 million to about 480 million older people worldwide (United Nations 2005).

The 2000 national statistics on the health of older people in England revealed that, of all those aged 65 years and over, 4% were resident in care homes and just over three-quarters of those were women, compared with 57% of those aged 65 years and over in private households. Women were more likely than men to have been living alone before admission.

As well as chronic illness, older people are also more likely to have a disability. Although no national register of disability or disabled older persons in Britain exists nearly two-thirds of disabled people are aged 65 years or older. The NHS for example spent around 40% of its budget – £10 billion – on people over the age of 65 in1998/99. In the same year social services spent nearly 50% of their budget on the over-65s, some £5.2 billion.

16.3 AGE-RELATED PHYSIOLOGICAL AND PATHOLOGICAL CHANGES RELEVANT TO NUTRITION

Ageing in humans may be accompanied by changes that impair access to food and its subsequent intake, but such changes are complex and difficult to document. Anorexia and weight loss are common and important clinical problems in the oldest age groups, and the causes are multifactorial. There is a growing recognition that age-related physiological anorexia may predispose to protein-energy undernutrition (PEU) in the elderly, particularly in the presence of other 'pathological' factors associated with aging, such as social, psychological, physical and medical factors, the majority of which are responsive to treatment. Additionally, overweight and obesity in older people carries associated health risks.

PHYSIOLOGICAL CHANGES

Hormonal changes

Compared with younger adults, older people have a reduced feeding drive and a higher degree of satiety whilst fasting (Sturm et al 2003), contributing to the 'anorexia of ageing'. Current evidence suggests that a combination of reduced sensory perception within the gastrointestinal tract, a decline in opioid modulation of feeding, particularly in older women, and an increase in the satiating effects of cholecystokinin (CCK) contribute to this anorexia. CCK, the best characterised of the gastrointestinal hormones, is known to play a role in the control of food intake (see Section 5.6). There is evidence that sensitivity to the satiating effects of CCK increases with age. The combination of increased circulating CCK concentrations and enhanced sensitivity to the satiating effects of CCK in older people suggests that CCK may be a significant contributor to the anorexia of ageing.

With increasing age, the time taken for the emptying of the stomach after a large volume of food is increased and this affects satiation. This may explain why older adults feel a greater satiating effect after an average meal compared with younger adults. Other hormones (e.g. leptin), neurotransmitters (e.g. opioids and nitric oxide) and cell signalling molecules (e.g. cytokines) may also have a role to play in anorexia and weight loss of ageing (MacIntosh et al 2000).

Other hormonal changes are also important during ageing. The increased prevalence of type 2 diabetes in older people may be partly associated with a decline in pancreatic beta cell function and a dysregulation of the normal profile of insulin secretion. It has even been suggested that changes in endocrine signalling pathways are key determinants of longevity (Russell & Kahn 2007).

Gastrointestinal tract

Objective changes in smell and taste have been observed in older adults, which may directly decrease food intake or alter the type of foods which are selected. In addition, the ability to identify foods while blindfolded decreases with advancing age. This is a common perceived problem among elderly individuals who complain of loss of both taste and smell (Exton-Smith 1980). Impaired appetite is often associated with reduction in taste and smell, which may occur in up to 50% of elderly people. Taste thresholds are higher among institutionalised than in healthy elderly men and the use of drugs, particularly antihypertensive medication, appears to be a contributing factor. Dental health is important in old age and 45% of the free-living elderly in the most recent National Diet and Nutrition Survey in the UK were edentulous (Finch et al 1998). Although there is evidence linking nutritional status to dentition a causal relationship is yet to be established in randomised controlled intervention trials (see Section 25.2, under 'Geographic and social class differences' and Section *evolve* 16.3).

Other gastrointestinal changes in the elderly have been documented which could affect their food intake. For example, changes in peristaltic activity of the oesophagus occur, which may result in delay of oesophageal emptying. Absorption of some nutrients, in particular vitamin B_{12}, may be impaired because of mild ageing-related achlorhydria. Some researchers have reported widespread nutritional deficiencies associated with bacterial contamination of the small bowel, whilst others found no association between bacterial contamination of the small bowel and nutritional status. The most likely interpretation of these apparently conflicting reports is that bacterial contamination of an anatomically normal small bowel in the elderly is the result rather than the cause of undernutrition. The mechanisms through which undernutrition might cause bacterial growth are not fully understood but there is evidence that the activity of several enzyme systems involved in bactericidal processes may be reduced in undernutrition.

Body composition

Changes in body composition seen with ageing include a decrease in lean body mass, which occurs faster after the eighth decade, and an increase in body fat. The decline in lean body mass is predominantly that of muscle, and the loss of muscle mass with ageing contributes to the loss of mobility and an increased frequency of falls in elderly people. A decrease in lean body mass is associated with a reduction in energy expenditure and this will lead to a reduction in energy intake. However, studies have shown that exercise can halt the decline in lean body mass with ageing, and limit the usual fall in energy intake with increasing age. (To read more on this topic see Section 4.3.) BMI has been proposed as a valuable indicator of nutritional status appropriate as a screening tool in the elderly. Data from the UK show that the prevalence of a lower BMI is much higher in institutionalised elderly people (about 15% BMI <20) than free-living elderly people (about 5% BMI < 20) (Finch et al 1998). A prospective study conducted among nearly 2000 elderly people in residential care in Australia showed that low BMI (<22kg/m^2) at baseline was a strong predictor of fracture and all-cause mortality 2 years later (Miller et al 2009). However, overweight is also a problem among older adults, and current UK estimates suggest that about 65% of free-living elderly people and 45% of institutionalised elderly are overweight (Finch et al 1998).

Many body composition assessment methods have limited application to the elderly. For example, underwater weighing may be unsuitable for disabled individuals, isotope dilution techniques are not universally accessible and other models face similar limitations because they require combinations of such measurements obtained in the same individual. Many studies have been undertaken using a variety of simple bedside measurement techniques from which body composition can be predicted, but these techniques have not been validated specifically for use in elderly people. A recent study has been carried out to evaluate a range of body composition prediction techniques and equations against total body water (TBW), measured using isotope dilution, which is considered to be a suitable method for elderly people. Body composition predictors including weight, height, skinfold thickness, bioelectrical impedance and near-infrared interactance were evaluated against TBW in 23 randomly selected men over 75 years old, and dual-energy X-ray absorptiometry (DXA) in 15 volunteers from this group. Comparisons were made between anthropometric and impedance methods for estimating limb muscle mass. The researchers found that some body composition predictions are unacceptable (at least for TBW) in older men, and care is recommended when selecting from these methods or equations. The authors also reported that DXA is not the most appropriate reference method for assessing muscle mass; further studies using scanning techniques, such as magnetic resonance imaging (MRI) and computer-aided tomography (CAT) scans, as the preferred reference methods, are recommended (Fuller et al 1996).

Bone mass

Peak bone mass is achieved at around 30 years of age and the actual peak bone mass, which is higher in men than women, is a determinant of bone mass in old age. The amount of bone falls from this point in time and the rate of decline after achieving this appears to have some common determinants including exercise, and calcium, energy and protein intake. The loss of bone associated with ageing may lead to a condition known as osteoporosis, particularly common in post-menopausal women. Severe osteoporosis may cause the bones in the legs to bow under the weight of the body. This bowing, together with changes in the spine, makes measurement of height unreliable in some elderly subjects even in those elderly who are able to stand unaided (see Ch. 24).

PATHOLOGICAL CHANGES

Medical and social factors

There are physical changes such as decreased visual acuity, joint problems, hand tremors and hearing problems, which in combination may make the task of food preparation and eating more difficult for the elderly. Other factors which may affect nutritional status in the elderly include loss of spouse, depression and bereavement, decreased mobility, dementia, anorexia due to disease especially cancer, medications, poor dentition, alcoholism and most important of all acute illness. In institutions, lack of supervision and assistance at mealtimes may be an important factor resulting in poor food intake. Because a disproportionate number of older people are isolated, on low income or disabled, socio-economic factors and disease are likely to have more influence on their nutritional status than age alone. There is evidence from across the globe that disability in the elderly can lead to difficulty in preparing food. The Nottingham Longitudinal Survey of Activity and Ageing (Morgan 1998) studied a sample of 1042 old people thought to be representative of the elderly population in the UK in terms of social class, age, sex and the number living alone. Subjects were asked whether they cooked or shopped: 6% of women aged 65–74 years said they did not do their own cooking, rising to 12% of women aged over 74 years; 11% of women aged 65–74 years did not do their shopping, rising to 30% for those over 74 years. Identification of those ambulatory elderly people at risk of undernutrition requires understanding of their social, cultural and economic environment.

Other studies from Europe (Bartali et al 2003) and the USA (Sharkey et al 2004) show a clear link between disability and diet quality.

Immune function

Aspects of the immune response are known to deteriorate with ageing and to be influenced by poor nutritional status (Lesourd 1997). However, studies in healthy elderly people have shown that many modifications in immune responses previously considered to be due to ageing per se may in fact be associated with pathological conditions. While ageing may induce dysregulation of the immune system on its own, undernutrition seems to be one of the main factors, leading to poor immune responses. Undernutrition, common in aged populations, induces lower immune responses, particularly in cell-mediated immunity. Protein–energy undernutrition is associated with decreased lymphocyte proliferation, reduced cytokine release and lower antibody response to vaccines. Micronutrient deficiencies, such as zinc, selenium, iron, copper, vitamins A, C, E, B_6 and folate, all of which are reported in elderly people, have important influences on immune responses. Because ageing and undernutrition appear to exert cumulative influences on immune responses, many elderly people have poor cell-mediated immune responses and are therefore at a high risk of infection.

Several groups have explored effects of improving nutritional status in the elderly on immune responses. Some groups reported a beneficial effect of energy or micronutrient supplements but results are not consistent. In a few studies, this was associated with reduced infections. However, more work is needed in this area of considerable public health importance to clarify the causal link between undernutrition and impaired immunity in the elderly.

Cognitive function

Cognitive decline and dementia are common in old age. For example, 1 in 5 of hospitalised older people have cognitive impairment at any one time, whereas dementia affects 1 in 20 people over the age of 65 and 1 in 5 over the age of 80.

The role of diet in determining cognitive function is not well understood; many studies have demonstrated associations between dietary intake or biomarkers of nutrient status and measures of cognitive function, but it is more difficult to demonstrate that such relationships are causal. Various epidemiological studies have shown associations between loss of cognitive function or dementia and biomarkers of inadequate B-group vitamin status in older people, including elevated plasma homocysteine. A recent Cochrane Review examined the effects of folic acid supplementation, with or without vitamin B_{12}, on elderly healthy or demented people, in preventing cognitive impairment or retarding its progress. The small number of studies available for review provided no consistent evidence to support a beneficial role for folic acid or vitamin B_{12} supplements in cognitive function in unselected healthy or cognitively impaired older people.

Some evidence supports the notion that oxidative damage and inflammation might contribute to cognitive decline and progression to dementia in older people. Other research suggests that the use of vitamin E supplements may have modest cognitive benefits in older women. Supplementation with vitamin E has also been found to lead to significant delay in the progression of dementia.

There is also interest in the potential importance of fish in the diet in protecting the elderly against decline in cognitive function and several studies have been carried out to examine this. A recent cross-sectional study conducted in >2000 elderly people in Hordaland, Norway, showed a dose-response relationship between fish intake and measures of cognitive function (Nurk et al 2007). It remains to be determined what the active components of the high fish diet are, but ω-fatty acids are currently a focus of interest.

The strength and causative nature of the relationship between inadequate nutrient status and loss of cognitive function in older people remains unclear. Advances in the understanding of this relationship may depend on the outcome of randomised controlled trials initiated in subjects prior to the onset of neurocognitive decline.

Depression and well-being

The relationship between diet and psychiatric disorders in the elderly has received little attention although several dietary components have been ascribed a role in the prevention or the exacerbation of depressive symptoms in the adult population, including folate, vitamin B_{12}, and ω-3 polyunsaturated fatty acids. A recent prospective cohort study of >3000 adults has reported an inverse association between intake of fish and long chain ω-fatty acids and depressive symptoms (Colangelo et al 2009), and this is an area in which more research is needed in the elderly. Quality of life is now recognised as a clinically relevant outcome measure when evaluating new treatment strategies in older patient populations. Studies have shown a close relationship between undernutrition and poor quality of life in institutionalised older people. Two related studies published recently have shown that oral nutritional supplementation of hospitalised acutely ill older patients can have a significant benefit on depressive symptoms and quality of life scores (Gariballa & Forster 2007a, b).

Obesity

The prevalence of obesity (defined as body mass index (BMI) greater than $30 \, kg/m^2$) has now reached 21% in both males and females in England, and has almost trebled since 1980. It is associated with a range of health problems and affects an increasing number of people across all ages. Ageing is associated with a high incidence of diseases such as hypertension, diabetes, atherosclerosis, arthritis and disability, most of which are associated with obesity. Access to obesity management services in the UK is currently variable and there is a need for the development of specialist services, involving primary and secondary care sectors, especially for those with severe morbid obesity.

16.4 AGE-RELATED CHANGES IN ENERGY REQUIREMENTS AND EXPENDITURE

ENERGY REQUIREMENTS

To date, the scientific evidence regarding energy requirements in the elderly has been incomplete and highly variable. The reasons for this include paucity and variability of data on energy intake and requirements; and most important of all, diversity of physical activity patterns in the elderly population. The Department of Health and Social Security (DHSS) longitudinal study in the UK, which examined energy intake in 365 elderly people in 1967/8 and 5 years later, found that the average energy intake had fallen from 2235 to 2151 kcal per day for men and from 1711 to 1636 kcal per day for women

(DHSS 1979). The most recent Diet and Nutrition Survey of British people aged 65 years and over (Finch et al 1998) reported lower mean energy intakes for free-living men and women (see Section 17.7). A similar trend for energy intakes to fall with age over 5 years was observed in a study of 269 elderly people in Sweden.

ENERGY EXPENDITURE

Basal metabolic rate (BMR)

BMR reflects the energy requirements for maintenance of the intracellular environment and the mechanical processes, such as respiration and cardiac function, which sustain the body at rest. It usually accounts for between 60 and 75% of total energy expenditure.

The FAO reported a decrease in BMR of about 2.9% (men) and 2.0% (women) for each decade increase in age in older adults (FAO/WHO/UNU 2005). The increase in fat mass and the decline in lean mass that occur with ageing will be a major component of this fall in BMR.

Physical activity

In most working populations physical activity accounts for 10–35% of total energy expenditure. The energy expenditure of different activities depends on the amount of work being carried out, the weight of the individual and the efficiency with which that work is carried out. In general ageing is associated with a reduction in efficiency, which may make standard tasks like walking up to 20% more energy-expensive in older people. This reduced efficiency may be one reason why older individuals slow down. For example, the energy cost of normal activities has been reported to increase with age for men. In Nottingham, healthy women aged 70 years had a 20% higher energy cost for walking at a standard speed than either men of the same age or younger women.

In a questionnaire survey based on a sample of the general population resident in private (non-institutional) households in the UK, information was collected from 3691 people aged 65 or over about participation in physical activities in the previous 4 weeks. In the 60–69-year age group about 70% recorded no outdoor activity in the previous 4 weeks and this proportion was even higher in the over-70-year age group. A survey in Nottingham of customary activity of elderly people found that the average reported daily time in active pursuits was less than one hour and lower still in those aged 75 years or more. Four years later a significant decline in activity levels was found in the 620 survivors. Another feature of ageing which may restrict physical activity is the liability to a variety of degenerative and chronic diseases such as chronic obstructive airway disease, angina and arthritis.

Thermogenesis

The term thermogenesis includes energy expenditure and heat generation associated with feeding, body temperature maintenance and thermogenic response to various specific stimuli such as smoking, caffeine and drugs. Thermogenesis has also been postulated to play a part in the regulation of body weight (see Ch. 5). This field of research is complex in humans, and the underlying theory is derived mainly from animal models. In the elderly, resting circulating catecholamine concentrations are elevated, and the responsiveness to catecholamines may decline with age, as is the case in experimental animals. The thermic response to meal ingestion (diet-induced thermogenesis, DIT), appears to be influenced by age, physical activity and body composition. However, results of human studies are inconsistent, with some showing a decrease and others showing an increase in DIT with ageing.

PROTEIN REQUIREMENTS

Determination of protein requirements in humans is a complex subject, posing difficult questions for nutritionists. (For a detailed discussion see Ch. 8, Section 8.5.) Total protein contained in lean body mass falls with age, and protein synthesis, turnover and breakdown all decrease with advancing age. The progressive loss of protein seems to be a feature of ageing throughout adult life. This appears to affect some tissues, notably skeletal muscle, more than others. There is no direct evidence to suggest that this erosion of tissue protein is due to lack of adequate amounts of protein in the average diet.

Ill health, trauma, sepsis and immobilisation may upset the equilibrium between protein synthesis and degradation. A group of researchers studied the dietary protein requirements of 12 elderly men and women aged 56–80 years using short-term nitrogen balance techniques and calculations recommended by the 1985 Joint FAO/WHO/UNU expert consultation. They also recalculated nitrogen-balance data from three previous protein requirement studies in elderly people. From the current and retrospective data they reported that a safe protein intake for elderly adults would be 1.0–1.25 g/kg/day.

16.5 AGE-RELATED CHANGES IN MICRONUTRIENT REQUIREMENTS

VITAMINS

Because of a reduced energy requirement and the associated lower food intake and the increased incidence of physical diseases, which may interfere with intake, absorption, metabolism and utilisation, vitamin deficiency is more likely in the elderly than in younger adults. The most recent National Diet and Nutrition Survey of the elderly in the UK revealed average intakes of most vitamins to be above current RNIs. However, older people comprise a very heterogeneous group within which there are subgroups at more risk of vitamin inadequacies than others. Vitamin D status is more likely to be poor in the institutionalised elderly, especially during the winter months. Lower vitamin intakes in lower socioeconomic groups, reported in young people, tracks into old age, and this is true for folate and vitamin C. Poor folate or vitamin B_{12} status has been associated with poor cognitive function and poor vitamin C status has been associated with evidence of impaired collagen metabolism, likely to contribute to poor wound healing in the elderly. The Euronut SENECA study of nutrition in the elderly in Europe was carried out among more than 2500 people between 70 and 75 years of age across Europe. A great deal of variation in dietary habits and nutritional status was evident between and within countries. Contributory factors included differences in meal frequency, regularity of cooked meals and whether individuals lived at home or not. There was little evidence of poor vitamin status, with the exception of vitamin B_6, vitamin B_{12} and vitamin E, for which evidence of biochemical deficiency was evident among a significant proportion of the study populations (Haller et al 1991).

B-group vitamins

Evidence for low intakes of riboflavin in institutionalised elderly people has been a consistent feature of national diet and nutrition surveys of the elderly in the UK, with biochemical deficiency in a modest proportion of the elderly. Red blood cell folate concentrations indicative of deficiency are reported in 8% of free-living elderly and 16% of institutionalised elderly people in the UK although estimates of the prevalence of folate deficiency vary greatly across Europe and the USA. There is some uncertainty regarding the true prevalence of vitamin B_{12} deficiency in the elderly, because of difficulties in interpreting plasma concentrations of vitamin B_{12}. Data from the National Health and Nutrition Examination Survey (1991–1994) in the USA revealed a high prevalence of elevated serum methylmalonic acid (MMA), considered to indicate a functional deficiency of vitamin B_{12}, with an inverse association with serum B_{12}. However, in about 15% of cases, elevated MMA was not associated with lower serum B_{12}, suggesting that other factors might be involved, perhaps impaired renal function. This observation has been made by several groups and it is clear that estimates of vitamin B_{12} deficiency in the elderly need to be examined carefully.

Several studies have demonstrated an association between neurocognitive function and B vitamin status in the elderly but data are not consistent (Balk et al 2006). This is an area of current research activity.

Homocysteine

Although several case-control and prospective cohort studies have shown associations between modest elevation of plasma total homocysteine and cardiovascular disease, including stroke, there is still disagreement as to whether the association suggests causation. Experimental studies have provided plausible explanations for a role for homocysteine in the development of vascular diseases, for example, the oxidation of low-density lipoprotein cholesterol, vascular smooth muscle cell proliferation, platelet and coagulation factors activation and endothelial dysfunction.

The prevalence of hyperhomocysteinaemia in the general population is between 5% and 10% but rates may be as high as 30–40% in the elderly population. Hyperhomocysteinaemia can occur because of dietary inadequacies, polymorphisms in genes expressing enzymes relevant to homocysteine metabolism, and renal dysfunction. Folate, vitamin B_{12}, B_2 and B_6 are all cofactors for enzymes involved in homocysteine metabolism, but epidemiological studies show that poor folate status is the most important dietary cause of elevated serum homocysteine. Nutritional deficiencies of folate, vitamin B_{12} and riboflavin all occur in elderly populations, and are more prevalent among elderly living in institutions. Additionally, some medications may impair homocysteine metabolism and increase the risk of hyperhomocysteinaemia, including folate antagonists such as methotrexate, and vitamin B_6 antagonists such as theophylline and azarabine. Renal impairment is also more common in the elderly than in younger adults.

In a prospective study of 2127 men and 2639 women aged 65–67 years in 1992/3 from Norway, 162 men and 97 women died during a median 4.1 years of follow-up. Subjects with an elevated plasma tHcy at baseline compared with the lowest quintile (<9 μmol/l) had a significantly increased risk of death from vascular and non-vascular causes. An increase in plasma tHcy of 5 μmol/l was associated with a 49% increase in all-cause mortality, a 50% increase in cardiovascular mortality, a 26% increase in cancer mortality, and a 104% increase in non-cancer, non-cardiovascular mortality. However, results of randomised controlled trials to examine effects of homocysteine-lowering treatments on measures of cardiovascular risk have generally failed to demonstrate a beneficial effect (Clarke et al 2007). Results of ongoing trials will help to clarify the potential benefits of homocysteine-lowering strategies on risk of cardiovascular events.

Evidence is accumulating from case-control, cross-sectional and prospective cohort studies that plasma tHcy is a risk factor for Alzheimer's disease (Kado et al 2005), although not all data are consistent. Results of Hcy-lowering trials that include measures of cognitive function will make an important contribution to our understanding of dietary determinants of cognitive function. A new hypothesis linking elevated plasma tHcy and depressed mood has emerged. A plausible explanation for the association relates to the neurotoxic effects of elevated homocysteine, resulting in neurotransmitter deficiency, which causes depression of mood. Intervention studies are needed to test this hypothesis.

Antioxidants

Epidemiological associations have been made between some antioxidant vitamins and cardiovascular disease and some cancers, although results of randomised controlled trials have been inconsistent and interest in the possible protective value of antioxidant supplements against disease of public health relevance has waned. Furthermore, whilst fruit and vegetable intervention trials have been shown to increase circulating concentrations of antioxidant vitamins, they have generally proved ineffective at changing biomarkers of oxidant status. Low intakes of vitamin C and associated biochemical deficiency have been reported in many studies of the elderly. Those living in institutions appear to be most at risk. A 20-year follow-up of 730 elderly people who had participated in a nutritional survey in the UK reported a strong inverse inverse relationship between risk of mortality from stroke and plasma ascorbic acid. Plasma concentrations of alpha tocopherol and ascorbic acid have been associated with markers of oxidative damage after acute ischaemic stroke, and plasma concentrations of β-carotene and ascorbic acid have been shown to predict carotid intima media thickness in an elderly population. In this context it can be argued that a diet rich in fruits and vegetables might be protective against some of the diseases of ageing. Indeed, the recent WCRF/AICR report on food, nutrition, physical activity and the prevention of cancer concluded that foods rich in folates, carotenoids and vitamin C may be protective against certain cancers, including oesophageal and lung. A study of elderly Italians (the InCHIANTI study) showed moderately strong correlations between plasma concentrations of antioxidants and measures of physical performance and muscle strength, but there is little information from prospective studies to support these observations (Cesari et al 2004).There is some evidence to suggest that free radical damage may be important in other diseases of ageing, such Parkinson's disease and Alzheimer's disease, but the evidence lacks consistency. A recent Cochrane review found no evidence to support the use of antioxidants in primary or secondary prevention of disease (Bjelakovic et al 2008).

MINERALS

Sodium and potassium

Hypertension and stroke are both more common in older people than younger adults. Studies in hypertensive rats have found that high potassium intake protects against death from stroke independent of effects on blood pressure. An inverse association of potassium intake with stroke mortality has been

reported in humans, irrespective of hypertensive status. Clinical, experimental and epidemiological evidence all suggest that a high dietary intake of potassium is associated with lower blood pressure. Excess salt intake causes hypertension not only through simple volume expansion but also through sodium-accelerated vascular smooth muscle cell proliferation and it enhances thrombosis by the acceleration of platelet aggregation. Moreover, there is some evidence that protective nutritional factors such as potassium, calcium, magnesium, dietary fibre, protein, some amino acids and some fatty acids may counteract the adverse effect of sodium or cholesterol intake on hypertension, atherosclerosis and thrombosis.

Calcium and vitamin D

Age-related renal impairment is reported to decrease renal hydroxylation of vitamin D, thereby decreasing the amount of active vitamin D available for regulating calcium absorption. Many institutionalised and free-living elderly (up to 50% in some studies) have poor vitamin D status; although sunlight deprivation, decreased intake of dairy products, lactose intolerance and malabsorption of fat-soluble vitamins have all been implicated in the aetiology, insufficient exposure to UV light is considered to be particularly relevant to the elderly. The UK Government's Scientific Advisory Committee on Nutrition advises that institutionalised elderly take supplements of vitamin D.

Bone mass declines with age, especially in white women. This is associated with osteoporosis and an increased fracture risk. Calcium alone (without oestrogens) cannot fully ameliorate post-menopausal bone loss, but calcium supplementation of 1000 mg daily with exercise does retard the rate of bone loss. Although calcium supplementation may be necessary for certain groups of elderly people it may be harmful in patients with a history of calcium stones, primary hyperparathyroidism, sarcoidosis or renal hypercalcuria. Randomised placebo-controlled trials in the elderly have demonstrated beneficial effects of calcium and vitamin D supplements in preventing bone loss at certain sites and the incidence of non-verterbral fractures. Institutionalised elderly people especially are likely to benefit from vitamin D supplements. Low dietary intakes of dairy products, calcium and vitamin D have been associated with increased risk of hypertension in middle-aged and older women, suggesting a possible role in the primary prevention of hypertension and cardiovascular complications.

Magnesium (Mg)

Plasma levels of magnesium are controlled by the kidneys and gastrointestinal tract and appear closely linked to calcium, potassium and sodium metabolism. In patients with chest pain admitted to hospital the frequency of hypokalaemia was found to be greater among hypomagnesaemic patients than normomagnesaemic patients. Stroke patients have been reported to exhibit deficits in serum and CSF magnesium. Acute magnesium or potassium deficiency can produce cerebrovascular spasm, and the lower the extracellular concentration of either magnesium or potassium the greater the magnitude of cerebral arterial contraction. Potential causes of magnesium deficiency such as low dietary intake and the use of diuretic therapy are more likely to occur in elderly people, especially those who are ill.

Iron (Fe)

Whilst iron-deficiency anaemia is more prevalent among elderly than in young adults, the prevalence is considerably higher among institutionalised elderly people. This partly reflects inadequate dietary intake of haem iron or of dietary factors that enhance the bioavailability of non-haem iron, but is also a result of a higher prevalence of disorders which interfere with iron absorption, such as atrophic gastritis and post-gastrectomy syndromes. Blood loss associated with hiatus hernia, peptic ulcer, haemorrhoids and cancer, as well as with non-steroidal anti-inflammatory drug use, is more likely in elderly people. Studies of house-bound and hospitalised elderly patients suggest that low iron intakes in these groups may often be a result of low energy intakes, indicating the importance of maintaining an adequate food intake in the elderly if micro nutrients needs are to be met from the diet.

Zinc (Zn)

In the UK, healthy elderly people living at home and eating a self-selected diet were in metabolic balance for zinc on a mean daily intake of 137 μmol (9 mg) with leukocyte zinc levels comparable to healthy young people. Institutionalised elderly subjects are at increased risk of zinc deficiency. Zinc has been found to promote healing of damaged tissues, especially skin, but only in those who are zinc-deficient. Zinc is also important in cell mediated immunity. In an open and uncontrolled study a group of zinc-deficient elderly who were anergic developed positive skin tests after zinc supplementation. Zinc deficiency adversely affects cellular immunity at all ages. A recent small observational study conducted in nursing home elderly residents in Boston, USA found that serum zinc concentrations in the normal range were associated with a decreased incidence and duration of pneumonia, a decreased number of antibiotic prescriptions and a decrease in the days of antibiotics used, compared with subjects with lower serum zinc.

Selenium (Se)

Selenium is an active component in various enzymes involved in immune function, oxidative stress and muscle function. Selenium deficiency is associated with skeletal myopathy and cardiomyopathy and low plasma selenium is reported to be independently associated with poor skeletal muscle strength in community-dwelling older adults. Further studies may clarify whether selenium supplementation can slow down the age-associated decline in muscle strength. Importantly for the elderly, in whom immunocompetence can be depressed, selenium supplementation of subjects with marginal selenium status has been shown to improve immune function.

OTHER TRACE ELEMENTS

Understanding of the exact role and dietary requirements for trace elements such as cobalt, copper, chromium, fluoride, iodine, manganese, molybdenum and selenium is incomplete. Deficiencies in humans are thought to be rare, although there may be problems of absorption associated with diseases of the gastrointestinal tract, and there is the potential for drug–trace-element interactions. For some trace elements there is still uncertainty with respect to dietary reference values, partly because of uncertainty with respect to the capacity for adaptation to low intakes.

16.6 ASSESSMENT OF NUTRITIONAL STATUS IN OLDER PEOPLE

The combination of advanced age, multiple chronic diseases and use of drugs leads to an increased risk of protein–energy undernutrition (PEU). The difficulties in detecting early signs of undernutrition are similar to those encountered in the early recognition of many diseases in old age. However, in the case of nutritional deficiency there are two further difficulties: for many nutrients there is a long latent period before a low intake leads to overt clinical manifestations, and early diagnosis must depend upon the findings of abnormalities of special tests, including biochemical and haematological investigations; secondly, in the elderly the true significance of abnormal results of these tests is not fully understood. Many abnormalities can be related to low intake of certain nutrients, but in old age there is considerable variation between individuals. In general in younger persons the margin of safety is wide, but in old age homeostatic mechanisms are often impaired and physical illness or environmental hazards to which the elderly are particularly prone may upset this precarious physiological balance.

At present, nutritional assessment in the elderly has three main goals. The first is to define the type and severity of undernutrition; the second is the identification of high-risk patients; and the third is to monitor the efficacy of nutritional support. Various anthropometric, haematological, biochemical and immunological variables have been used to assess nutritional status but the sensitivity and specificity and the relative contribution of each individual variable to the diagnostic accuracy of undernutrition have not been clearly defined. Table 16.1 shows some of these measurements, their role in identifying patients at risk of PEU and their limitations in relation to elderly people.

In summary, problems in diagnosing undernutrition in the elderly are common because of physical and biochemical changes which may take place as part of normal ageing processes; in addition, overt clinical signs of undernutrition may be late to appear, by which time much subclinical damage may have gone uncorrected. All of the clinically available nutrition screening instruments lack sensitivity and specificity and cannot be relied on individually as definitive diagnostic tests for PEU. However, in combination these screening instruments, including clinical assessment, food frequency questionnaires and selected anthropometric, haematological and biochemical variables, are accepted measurements of nutritional status. Of particular importance are involuntary body weight changes or values below an established population standard, arm muscle circumference, skinfold measurement and depressed secretory proteins.

16.7 NUTRITIONAL STATUS OF OLDER PEOPLE IN THE COMMUNITY

Risk factors for undernutrition in older people in the community include isolation, loss of spouse, depression and bereavement, decreased mobility, dementia, anorexia due to disease, especially cancer, medications, poor dentition, alcoholism and most important of all acute illness. In institutions, lack of supervision and assistance at mealtimes may be an important factor resulting in low food intake (Table 16.2). However, the National Diet and Nutrition Surveys of the UK population reveal that, although dietary inadequacies occur in older people this group consumes diets that are generally closer to recommendations than younger adults do.

Conducting surveys of nutritional status, and interpreting results, can be more difficult in elderly populations than in younger adults. As discussed in the previous section, ageing per se can impose practical obstacles to assessing nutritional status, and it is not always easy to disentangle effects of healthy ageing from effects of inadequate dietary intake.

Cohort studies in the elderly suffer from a reduction in numbers over time. Also, dietary intakes of elderly people are likely to show more profound changes over time than in younger adults, in association with changes in social factors as well as health status. It is generally assumed that those individuals who are better nourished at the start of a study outlive those who are initially less well-nourished (selective survival).

A detailed diet and nutrition survey was conducted in six towns in England and Scotland in 1967/8, which used dietary recall and diary methods to assess the energy and nutrient intakes. Full information was obtained in 764 people. A further study was carried out in 1972/3 of 365 surviving elderly people who had participated in the 1967/8 survey and who could be traced. These surveys excluded people in institutional care. In 1972/3 7% of the group surveyed were considered to be undernourished and this condition was more prevalent in those over 80 years of age. In the 1967/8 survey 3% were diagnosed as having undernutrition and three-quarters of these cases were in association with clinical disease. Several risk factors

Table 16.1   Assessment of nutritional status in elderly people

MEASURES OF NUTRITIONAL STATUS	COMMENTS	LIMITATION IN ELDERLY PEOPLE
Dietary surveys, types: 1. Dietary history by interview 2. Recall interviews (previous 24 h) 3. Weighted dietary intakes 4. Chemical analysis	More useful when used with social, economic, environmental, clinical and laboratory data. Dietary history or recalls give only crude information. Weighted records most appropriate when dietary intakes are to be related to clinical findings. Biochemical analysis most accurate, but expensive and time-consuming. Evidence suggests that unbiased retrospective estimates of diet are unobtainable	Increased age found to be associated with decreased recall ability in some studies Diet stability in the elderly may improve recall
Anthropometric measurements: 1. Skeletal size (height, demispan, arm span, weight and body mass index 2. Skinfold thickness (triceps (TSF), biceps, subscapular, dorsum of the hand, suprailiac, thigh skinfold thicknesses, arm fat area and waist:hip ratio) 3. Mid-arm circumference (MAC) and arm muscle circumference (AMC)	Total arm length and total span are reported to change with age less than height. Measurement does not need a trained observer and the subject can remain seated. Arm span approximates to height at maturity and is another alternative to measurement of height in the elderly The measurement of skinfold thickness using constant pressure calipers provides a cheap and non-invasive assessment of subcutaneous fat. The technique is reliable in practised hands	Changes in the spine as a result of ageing and inability of some of the elderly to stand makes height measurements alone unsatisfactory Although standards for the elderly exist for MAC and skin fold thickness the major difficulty is the definition of normality and referral values, and also lack of good correlation with biochemical measures
Biochemical measures: Serum albumin, transferrin, prealbumin, retinol binding protein, caeruloplasmin plasma fibronectin and urinary creatinine excretion (CHI)	CHI may be used as an estimate of skeletal muscle mass provided renal function is stable and there is no significant element of rhabdomyolysis present, such as in septic conditions	Values affected by presence of coexisting diseases and multiple drugs. Problems in collecting accurately timed urine samples, forgetfulness, dementia, incontinence make CHI measurement difficult
Immunological measures Lymphocytopenia and anergy to skin tests	There is some evidence to support a causal relationship between malnutrition, impaired cell-mediated response and infections	The similarity of the effects of ageing and malnutrition on immune function places the usefulness of routine immunological testing in this population in question
Clinical assessment scales 1. History and physical examinations 2. Mini Nutritional Assessment (MNA) 3. SCALES	MNA is said to be simple and a quick screening tool. It includes: anthropometric measurement, dietary questionnaire, global and subjective assessment SCALES (S = sadness; C = cholesterol; A = albumin; E = eat; S = shopping) reported to have high sensitivity to detect people potentially at risk of malnutrition	History and examination may be as effective as other objective measurements MNA and SCALES have not been tested on a wider scale

for undernutrition were identified of which the most important was being house-bound. A major conclusion of this survey was that, provided individual elderly people were in good health, their dietary patterns and the foods eaten were no different from those of younger people.

The most recent National Diet and Nutrition Survey, of British people aged 65 years and over found that the mean energy intake for free living men was 8.02MJ (1909 kcal) and for women was 5.98MJ (1422 kcal). Seven percent of men and 11% of women in the free-living group and 13% of men and 12% of women in institutions reported that they had been unwell during the dietary recording period and their eating has been affected. In the free-living group, these participants were found to have on

Table 16.2	Factors associated with poor nutritional status in older people in community and home care settings

Poor eyesight and hearing problems
Joint problems and hand tremors
Isolation
Inability to go out shopping and poor income
Depression and bereavement
Poor cognitive function
Nausea and vomiting
Poor appetite
Anorexia due to disease, especially cancer
Medications
Lack of assistance at mealtimes
Poor dentition and chewing problems
Acute illness

average lower intakes of protein, total carbohydrates and starch although there was no significant difference in energy intake. Free-living men who were unwell and whose eating was affected had lower intakes of vitamin A, D, pantothenic acid and riboflavin and lower intakes per unit of energy of retinol, vitamin B_{12} and vitamin D. These differences in vitamin intake were not seen in free-living women and there were few differences among institutionalised individuals (Finch et al 1998).

In the Euronut-Seneca Study (referred to in Section 16.5 under 'Vitamins'), data regarding nutrient and food intakes, dietary habits, diet awareness, nutritional status, health and lifestyle factors were collected. The authors reported considerable variability from site to site even within countries, in dietary intake, in both quantity and composition; blood biochemistry; lifestyle factors; health; and performance. Considerable diversity and variability in serum lipid profile and dietary intakes of all components were observed. However living conditions and social activities reflected a high quality of life and most of the elderly were still engaged in physical activities.

16.8 NUTRITIONAL STATUS OF OLDER PEOPLE IN ACUTE AND NON-ACUTE CARE SETTINGS

Studies of elderly people in hospitals and residential/nursing homes generally agree that food intakes are less than those reported for free-living elderly people and that undernutrition is prevalent and often unrecognised in patients admitted to hospitals and institutions.

The prevalence of undernutrition among patients admitted to hospitals reported in different studies has not changed over two decades. This does not necessarily imply failure of physicians to prevent or treat undernutrition, but may simply reflect interaction between disease and undernutrition. It could also be due to an increase in the number of elderly patients. The effect of ill health on the nutritional status of hospitalised patients can be limited to the time of acute illness. Once the patient recovers the nutritional disadvantage should be overcome, but elderly people are particularly at risk because of decreased nutritional reserves and the effect of repeated ill health. Researchers from Sweden studied the nutritional status by measuring weight, triceps skinfold, serum albumin and delayed cutaneous hypersensitivity reaction of 96 consecutive hospital admission over the age of 70 years and a 100 randomly selected age- and sex-matched free-living controls. Patients classified as undernourished were required to display at least two variables below the cut-off limits chosen according to national reference data and one of the variables had to be anthropometric. Thirty nine per cent of the patients were undernourished compared with the controls and undernutrition was related to the nature of the disease rather than age. There was a marked difference in undernutrition between free-living and hospitalised people, suggesting that disease played a major role in the development of a negative energy balance. Also, the highest prevalence and the most advanced forms of undernutrition were observed in patients with multiple organ disease and malignancy. The 1967/8 DHSS survey showed that elderly people who believed that they had poorer health than average tended to have lower energy intakes and lower body weight. Body weight, body composition and dietary intakes are reported to be markedly different in elderly people who are day patients or inpatients compared with free-living elderly. A house-bound group of people in Southampton, UK, aged from 69 to 85 years, suffering from various chronic disorders (although known hepatic, renal, gastrointestinal diseases, malignancies and acute illnesses were excluded) consumed diets that were more likely to be deficient in protein, zinc, copper, iron, selenium, calcium and phosphorus when compared with those of apparently healthy people of similar ages. A non-randomly selected group of institutionalised elderly from

Boston, USA had a dietary and nutritional assessment. Subjects were free of clinically apparent terminal or wasting illness and people who were mentally incompetent were excluded. Compared to a free-living elderly group the institutionalised group had lower values for circulating concentrations of vitamin A, retinol-binding protein, zinc, albumin, pre-albumin and transferrin but no specific nutrient deficiency was identified. Elderly long-stay hospital patients are reported to have lower values for triceps skinfold thickness, mid-arm circumference and arm fat area than fit elderly people living in the community, and a dietary energy intake that does not satisfy basal metabolic demands.

Several studies of acute care hospital and institutionalised patients have demonstrated a strong correlation between PEU and an increased risk for subsequent in-hospital morbid events. A large observational multi-centre study of the relationship between baseline nutritional status and 6 months clinical outcome in hospitalised stroke patients reported that baseline nutritional status, assessed by a simple bedside method, was independently associated with morbidity and mortality. Recently a graded and independent relationship was reported between nutritional status measured by mid-upper arm circumference and serum albumin and 1-year mortality in older patients (Figs 16.2 and 16.3).

As well as the possible effects of illness on nutritional status, many drugs that are commonly used in the elderly may have specific interaction with nutrition factors such as energy and nutrients intake, appetite, minerals and electrolyte homeostasis.

16.9 NUTRITIONAL SUPPORT IN ELDERLY PEOPLE

WHY DO ELDERLY PATIENTS NEED NUTRITIONAL SUPPORT, AND WHEN?

Prior to coming into hospital elderly people in the community are more likely to have premorbid decreases in energy intake, less lean body mass and impaired immune response, all of which may be associated with poor nutritional status. Their nutritional status is likely to deteriorate further as the result of the catabolism associated with the acute illness. This is compounded further by the demands of the sometimes-prolonged period of rehabilitation. Nutritional depletion during rehabilitation, however, may be more serious than during acute illness, since rehabilitation periods may extend over weeks and months, and weight loss, although less marked than in the early catabolic phase, may be greater overall.

Research has shown that baseline nutritional status of elderly stroke patients was worse among those who later died or remained in hospital than those discharged and most patients who remained in hospital showed marked and significant deterioration in all measures of nutritional status during the hospital stay (Gariballa et al 1998). Nutritional status was a strong and independent predictor of morbidity and mortality at 3 months following

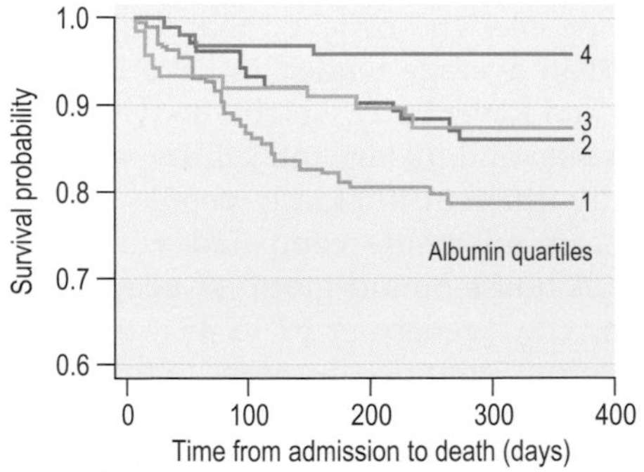

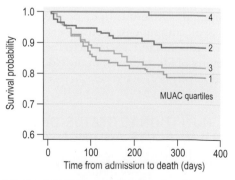

Fig. 16.2 Survival at 1 year according to serum albumin quartiles (1,2,3,4) on admission. The relationship between serum albumin on admission and 1-year survival is significant ($p < 0.01$).

Fig. 16.3 Survival at 1 year according to mid-upper arm circumference (MUAC) quartiles (1,2,3,4) on admission and 1-year survival is significant ($p < 0.001$).

acute stroke (FOOD trial collaboration 2003). Studies of the nutritional status and energy intake of 350 randomly selected admissions to a geriatric rehabilitation unit found that protein–energy malnutrition was a strong predictor of in-hospital and post-discharge mortality. Individuals with any amount of weight loss and no improvement in albumin concentrations in the early stages of hospitalisation are reportedly at a much higher risk of readmission than those who maintain or increase their post-discharge weight and increase their serum albumin concentrations.

A recent meta-analysis reported that aggressive nutritional support in surgical and critically ill patients who are known to be hypermetabolic (with a loss of 20–40g of nitrogen/day) and have increased nutrient requirements did not influence the overall mortality. However, it may reduce complication rates in already malnourished patients. A larger, systematic Cochrane Library review on protein and energy supplementation in elderly people at risk of malnutrition concluded that protein and energy supplements produce a small but consistent weight gain in this group of patients. Additional data from large multi-centre trials are required to provide clear evidence of benefit from protein and energy supplements on mortality and length of hospital stay.

Based on present evidence it is possible that the poor outcome in elderly patients following acute illness may at least be partly due to undernutrition and that aggressive nutritional support during the convalescent period is likely to improve nutritional status and lead to better rehabilitation outcome, decreased readmission rate and improved quality of life, and contribute to reducing Health Service cost.

See Section *evolve* 16.3 for a summary of the latest UK National Diet and Nutrition Survey of people aged 65 years and over (1998) and Section *evolve* 16.9 for a discussion of nutritional support studies in elderly patients. Consult Appendix Tables A1–A27 for recommended energy and nutrient intakes, including those for older people, and the *evolve* website Additional references and Further reading sections for additional reading.

KEY POINTS

- Dietary intakes of healthy elderly people are similar those of younger age.
- Older people are at risk of malnutrition due to body composition changes, physical and mental illness, disability and lack of mobility, resulting in reduced activity and food intake.
- The majority of 'pathological' factors associated with ageing such as social, psychological, physical and medical factors, which may predispose to malnutrition, are responsive to treatment.
- Older people should be advised to eat a balanced diet containing a variety of nutrient-dense foods; more fruits, vegetables and grains; foods containing adequate amounts of calcium and vitamin D; and this may need to be monitored in certain individuals.
- Elderly people should be encouraged to lead an active life, especially after episodes of intercurrent illness.
- All older people accessing the health services should be nutritionally screened using the MUST tool.
- Oral nutritional supplementation of acutely ill patients improves nutritional status and leads to clinical benefit.
- Dietetic advice is an integral part of the management of older people in hospital. It should be sought early to assess the most appropriate method of meeting individual nutritional requirements in those patients at risk, and provide advice for nursing and medical staff, catering and other health professionals involved.
- Dietary treatment strategies should be tailored to meet individual patients' needs and preferences. They should also be flexible, responsive and reviewed on a regular basis to maintain individual patients' enthusiasm and commitment.
- New evidence is emerging of the link between nutritional status and cognitive function in older people.
- Future research should focus on understanding the factors determining dietary intake and the role of adequate nutrition in prevention of disease in the ageing population.

References

Balk E, Chung M, Raman G, Tatsioni A, Ip S, DeVine D, Lau J: B vitamins and berries and age-related neurodegenerative disorders, *Evidence Report/Technology Assessment (Full Report)* 134:1–161, 2006.

Bartali B, Salvini S, Turrini A, et al: Age and disability affect dietary intake, *Journal of Nutrition* 133:2868–2873, 2003.

Bjelakovic G, Nikolova D, Gluud LL, Simonetti RG, Gluud C: Antioxidant supplements for prevention of mortality in healthy participants and patients with various diseases, *Cochrane Database of Systematic Reviews* 2008 Apr 16;(2): CD007176), 2008.

Cesari M, Pahor M, Bartali B, et al: Antioxidants and physical performance in elderly persons: the INvecchiare in Chianti (InCHIANTI) study, *American Journal of Clinical Nutrition* 79(2):289–294, 2004.

Clarke R, Armitage J, Lewington S, Collins R: B Vitamin Treatment Trialists' Collaboration: Homocysteine-lowering trials for prevention of cardiovascular disease: protocol for a collaborative meta-analysis, *Clinical Chemistry and Laboratory Medicine* 45(12):1575–1581, 2007, Review.

Colangelo LA, He K, Whooley MA, Daviglus ML, Liu K: Higher intake of long-chain ω-3 polyunsaturated fatty acids is inversely associated with depressive symptoms in women, *Nutrition* 25:1011–1019, 2009.

Department of Health and Social Security (DHSS): *Nutrition and health in old age*, London, 1979, HMSO, Report on health and social subjects 16.

Department of Health and Social Security (DHSS): *Nutrition in the elderly*, London, 1992, HMSO, Report on health and social subjects 43.

Exton-Smith AN: Nutritional status: diagnosis and prevention of malnutrition. In Exton-Smith AN, Caird FI, editors: *Metabolic and nutritional disorders in the elderly*, Bristol, 1980, John Wright & Sons.

FAO/WHO/UNU: Energy and protein requirements, *Report of a joint FAO/WHO/UNU Expert Consultation World Health Organisation Technical Report Series* 724:1–206, 1985.

FAO/WHO/UNU: Human energy requirements, *Report of a joint FAO/WHO/UNU Expert Consultation Food and Nutrition Bulletin* 26(1):166, 2005.

Finch S, Doyle W, Lowe C, Bates C, et al: National Diet and Nutrition Survey: people aged 65 years and over. *Volume I: Report of the Diet and Nutrition Survey*, London, 1998, The Stationery Office.

FOOD Trial Collaboration: Poor nutritional status on admission predicts poor outcome after stroke: observational data from the FOOD Trial, *Stroke* 34(6):1450–1456, 2003.

Fuller NJ, Sawyer MB, Laskey MA, Paxton P, Elia M: Prediction of body composition in elderly men over 75 years of age, *Annals of Human Biology* 23(2):127–147, 1996.

Gariballa S, Forster S: Effects of Dietary supplements on depressive symptoms in older patients: a randomised double-blind placebo-controlled trial, *Clinical Nutrition* 26:545–551, 2007a.

Gariballa S, Forster S: Dietary supplementation and quality of life in older patients: a randomised double-blind placebo-controlled trial, *Journal of American Geriatrics Society* 55:2030–2034, 2007b.

Gariballa SE, Taub N, Parker SG, Castledon CM: The influence of nutritional status on clinical outcome after acute stroke, *American Journal of Clinical Nutrition* 68:275–281, 1998.

Haller J, Lowik MR, Ferry M, Ferro-Luzzi A: Nutritional status: blood vitamins B6, B12, folic acid and carotene. Euronut SENECA investigators, *European Journal of Clinical Nutrition* 45(Suppl 3):63–82, 1991.

Kado D, Karlamangla A, Huang M, et al: Homocysteine versus the vitamin folate, B6 and B12 as predictors of cognitive function and decline in older high-functioning adults: MacArthur Studies of successful ageing, *American Journal of Medicine* 118:161–167, 2005.

Lesourd BM: Nutrition and immunity in the elderly, *American Journal of Clinical Nutrition* 66:478s–484s, 1997.

MacIntosh CG, Morley JE, Horowitz M, Chapman IM: Anorexia of ageing, *Nutrition* 16:983–995, 2000.

Miller MD, Thomas JM, Cameron ID, Chen JS, et al: BMI: a simple, rapid and clinically meaningful index of undernutrition in the oldest old? *British Journal of Nutrition* 101(90):1300–1305, 2009.

Morgan K: the Nottingham Longitudinal Study of Activity and Ageing: a methodological overview, *Age and Ageing* 27: Supplement 3, 5–11, 1998.

Nurk E, Drevon CA, Refsum H, Solvoll K, et al: Cognitive performance among the elderly and dietary fish intake: the Hordaland Health Study, *American Journal of Clinical Nutrition* 86(5):1470–1478, 2007.

ONS: *Population: by gender and age 1901–2026, Social Trends 31(ST 31103)*, London, 2001, Office for National Statistics.

Russell SJ, Kahn CR: Endocrine regulation of ageing, *Nature Reviews Molecular Cell Biology* 8:681–689, 2007.

Sharkey J, Branch L, Guiliani C, et al: Nutrient intake and BMI as predictors of severity of ADL disability over 1 year in housebound elders, *Journal of*

Nutrition and Healthy Ageing 8:131–139, 2004.

Sturm K, MacIntosh CG, Parker BA, et al: Appetite, food intake and plasma concentrations of cholecytokinin, ghrelin and other gastrointestinal hormones in undernourished older women and well-nourished young and old women, *Journal of Clinical Endocrinology and Metabolism* 88:3747–3755, 2003.

United Nations: World Population Prospects: the 2004 Revision (medium scenario), available on line at http://www.prb.org)/ presentations/j_trends-aging), 2005.

Weinsier RL, Heimburger DC: Distinguishing malnutrition from disease: the search goes on, *American Journal of Clinical Nutrition* 66:1063–1064, 1997.

Further reading

Guigoz, Vellas BJ, Garry PJ: Mini nutritional assessment. In Vellas BJ, Guigoz Y, Garry PJ, Albarede JL, editors: *Nutrition in the elderly:* Paris, 1994, Serdi Publishing, Suppl 2, pp 15–32.

Milne AC, Potter J, Avenell A: *Protein and energy supplementation in elderly people at risk of malnutrition,* Cochrane Library issue 3, Oxford, 2002.

Stanner S, Thompson R, Buttriss JL, editors: *Healthy ageing: the role of nutrition and lifestyle: the report of a British Nutrition Foundation task force,* Oxford, Wiley-Blackwell, 2009.

EVOLVE CONTENTS (available online at: evolve.elsevier.com/Geissler/nutrition)

Chapter **17**

Vegetarian diets

Tom A B Sanders

CHAPTER CONTENTS

OBJECTIVES

By the end of this chapter you should be able to:
- describe the different types of vegetarian diets
- understand the reasons why people follow vegetarian diets
- identify the nutrients most likely to be lacking from a vegetarian diet
- understand how the health of vegetarians/vegans differs from that of omnivores.

17.1 INTRODUCTION

Vegetarianism can be defined as avoiding the consumption of meat or flesh food. The commonplace use of the term vegetarian is to describe someone who does not eat animal flesh (meat, poultry, fish) but who includes eggs and dairy products in their diet. The terms *ovo-vegetarian, lacto-vegetarian* and *ovo-lacto-vegetarian* describe people who consume eggs, milk or both, respectively. The term *vegan* is used to describe people who consume no food of animal origin. Usually the first stage in becoming a vegetarian is to give up consuming red meat; this is followed by the exclusion of poultry and fish. Many vegetarians aspire to becoming vegans. Veganism is a way of life that avoids the exploitation of animals. Besides avoiding food of animal origin, vegans will not use products that have been derived from animals, such as leather, wool and vaccines. Fruitarianism is an extreme form of veganism where dietary intake is restricted to raw fruits, nuts and berries, which has resulted in severe malnutrition in children. Macrobiotic diets, which orig-

© 2010 Elsevier Ltd/Inc/BV
DOI: 10.1016/B978-0-7020-3118-2.00017-6

inate from the teachings of George Ohsawa, of the George Ohsawa Macrobiotic Foundation, consist of relatively large amounts of brown rice, accompanied by smaller amounts of fruits, vegetables and pulses; processed foods and Solanaceae species (tomatoes, aubergines and potatoes) are avoided; meat and fish are permitted if they are hunted or wild. In practice, however, most macrobiotic diets are vegetarian and contain only small amounts, if any, of milk products. It can be seen that these various definitions all depend upon the exclusion of certain foods from the diet, whereas the nutritional quality of diet is dependent on foods consumed.

The risk of nutrient deficiency is greatest in childhood as requirements relative to body weight are greater and children are unable to exert the same degree of control over what they eat as adults can. Indeed, there have been several reports of severe protein–energy malnutrition as well as deficiencies of iron, vitamins B_{12} and D in infants and toddlers fed inappropriate vegetarian diets. Older children are less susceptible to the dietary strictures imposed by their parents as they are able to forage for food at home independently. However, providing sufficient care is taken, children can be brought up healthily on both vegan and vegetarian diets. Many patients with eating disorders report following a vegetarian diet. Although the relationship is not necessarily causative, vegetarianism may be used as a device to restrict food intake. The health and diet of adult Western vegetarian groups has been extensively studied and generally appears to be good, and certain aspects of a vegan diet, notably the low saturated fat and high dietary fibre content, may offer certain advantages to the health of adults.

17.2 REASONS FOR FOLLOWING VEGETARIAN DIETS

Pythagoras was one of the earliest advocates of a vegetarian diet for its putative health benefits. Abstinence from 'flesh' has been associated with asceticism throughout history. Several religions refer to unclean meats (e.g. Judaism, Islam and Sikhism) and specify methods for the slaughter of animals, perhaps indicating early recognition that diseases could be transmitted from animals to humans. Some religions were more explicit and advocated avoiding meat. Vegetarianism is widely practised by believers of the Hindu and Buddhist faiths and is prescribed by the Seventh Day Adventist Church on health grounds. More extreme forms of vegetarianism are practised by the Jain sect, who will only eat food that grows above the ground, and Rastafarians advocate a restricted vegan diet based mainly on fruit.

The current popular belief that vegetarian diets are healthier than the typical Western diet has been reinforced by a series of food scares that involve the intensive production of poultry, meat and fish (e.g. salmonellosis in poultry, bovine spongiform encephalopathy in cattle and polychlorinated biphenyls in farmed salmon). The UK Vegetarian Society was founded in 1842 and was associated with the 'Mechanics Institutes', which represented a group of the emerging middle class who sought to improve themselves through education and temperance. Many of the leading characters in the Food Reform Movement in the nineteenth century, such as Kellogg, Graham, Cadbury and Elizabeth Fry, also espoused a vegetarian diet. More recently, vegetarianism has also been intertwined with the 'Green Movement', which is concerned with environmental issues, animal rights, opposition to genetically modified foods and the anti-globalisation movement – which amongst other things is opposed to the influence that multinational food companies have on the food chain. It is perhaps not surprising that vegetarianism appeals to the younger age groups and is associated with 'alternative' lifestyles. Some individuals style themselves as 'ethical vegetarians' to indicate that they regard meat eating as unethical. However, this term is rather unsatisfactory as it implies that all other vegetarians are unethical, and it also can be argued that individuals whose religion advocates a vegetarian diet follow their diet for ethical reasons.

The leading reason currently given in the UK for following a vegetarian diet is the belief that the diet is healthier. Other reasons are that it is wrong and cruel to eat animals. Some also argue that it is better for the environment to depend upon plant foods for our nutritional needs because it takes less land to feed a family on food of plant origin. In a survey commissioned by the UK Vegetarian Society in 2003 it was claimed that 8% of university and college students were following a vegetarian diet. A UK Food Standards Agency UK survey found that 5% of households followed a vegetarian diet. There is little doubt that the popularity of vegetarian diets has increased and most international airlines and restaurants now offer vegetarian options.

Most of the dietary and nutritional studies of vegans and vegetarians have been carried out on members of the Vegan and Vegetarian Societies or religious groups such as members of the Seventh Day Adventists Church. These subjects are generally keen to volunteer for studies in order to demonstrate their health and the adequacy of their diets. Consequently, they may not be truly representative of all vegetarians.

17.3 DIETARY ADEQUACY

Dietary diversity is important in maintaining the adequacy of a vegetarian diet as the nutrient density of plant foods is often lower than those of meat, fish, eggs and milk. In developing countries, economic factors are far more important in restricting food because this can result in a limited choice of foods. Overdependence on a nutritionally inadequate dietary staple such as polished rice is a well-known cause of malnutrition. However, there is also plenty of evidence to show that growth rates of infants reared on vegetarian diets are retarded, and in India, where poverty and intestinal infestation are common, they are at increased risk of anaemia compared with children eating mixed diets. On the other hand, when people of Indian origin migrate to developed countries and still maintain their vegetarian dietary practices but consume more dairy products, the impact of the vegetarian diet on growth is more limited.

In practice, there are surprisingly few qualitative differences in the intake of proximate nutrients between vegetarians/vegans compared with omnivores in developed countries (Table 17.1). Energy intakes appear to be similar to non-vegetarians although some reports, which have estimated energy intake by food frequency questionnaire, suggest that energy intakes are lower among vegans and vegetarians. However, this is not the case for weighed food intake surveys. The likely reason for the discrepancy between the two methods is that the portion sizes of plant foods consumed by vegetarians and vegans are often larger than those consumed by omnivores, particularly in the case of cereals.

Because the energy density of some plant foods is very low, some vegetarian diets may be so bulky that they restrict the energy intake of young children. For example, several studies have reported impaired growth in children under the age of 5 years fed vegan and macrobiotic diets associated with low energy intakes. Indeed, a fruitarian diet, which has the lowest energy density, resulted in the death of an infant in the UK.

PROTEIN

Protein intakes are slightly lower in vegetarians than in omnivores, typically supplying about 12% of the energy intake as opposed to 15% in omnivores (Table 17.1). However, these intakes support nitrogen balance. Although plant proteins have a

	ENERGY (MJ/DAY)	% ENERGY				FIBRE (G/DAY)
		PROTEIN	CARBOHYDRATE	SUGAR	FAT	
European men (UK)						
Omnivores	10.3	14.4	42	19	38	26
Vegetarians	9.4	12	48	21	37	34
Vegans	9.2	11.7	50	21	34	44
European women (UK)						
Omnivores	7.28	15.5	43	20	38	20
Vegetarians	7.67	12.6	46	20	37	33
Vegans	7.35	10.8	53	21	34	36
South Asian (UK)						
Men	9.3	12.6	47	–	38	23
Women	6.1	11.7	54	15	37	16

Table 17.1   Proximate nutrient intakes in vegetarians, vegans and omnivores

Data derived from: Draper et al 1993; Miller et al 1988; Reddy & Sanders 1992.

lower biological value than meat, the protein quality of vegetarian diets differs little from that of diets containing meat, as the constituent amino acids in the different plant proteins mutually complement each other. Many legumes contain protease inhibitors that can decrease the digestibility of protein. However, these are inactivated by heat treatment. Meat and fish, especially shellfish, are also rich sources of taurine. Taurine is thought to be an essential nutrient in the newborn where the capacity to synthesise it from cysteine is limited. Lower rates of urinary excretion of taurine have been found in vegan women compared with meat-eaters and markedly lower concentrations of taurine in breast milk of vegans. However, the concentration of taurine was still considerably greater than in unsupplemented breast milk substitutes.

CARBOHYDRATES

The intake of complex carbohydrates is generally high in vegan/vegetarian diets owing to their higher consumption of cereals compared with omnivores. Sugar intakes, on the other hand, are relatively similar. Intakes of dietary fibre (non-starch polysaccharide) are between 50% and 100% higher than in subjects on an omnivorous diet, depending on the source of dietary carbohydrate (i.e. wholegrain/wholemeal versus refined cereal): typical intakes are in the order of 30 g dietary fibre in vegetarians and 40 g in vegans. The higher fibre intake is associated with a faster faecal transit time and a larger faecal bulk (faecal weight is typically about 160 g/day in female vegetarians compared with 117 g in omnivores). Higher faecal bulk (186 g/day) has been reported in South Asian vegetarian women living in the UK, which does not appear to be related to the total fibre intake. It has been suggested that their diets contain more fermentable carbohydrate and this would also explain the reported lower faecal pH, presumably as it can be fermented within the colon to short-chain fatty acids (see Section 6.4 under 'Fermentation in the large intestine').

FATS

The proportion of energy derived from fat is only slightly lower in vegetarians/vegans than in omnivores and is typically in the region of 30–37% of the dietary energy. Saturated fatty acid intakes are slightly lower in vegetarians, being derived mainly from dairy fats, but markedly lower in vegans (around 6% energy) in comparison with omnivores. Cholesterol is virtually absent from plant foods but instead they provide small amounts of phytosterols (~0.5 g/day) which inhibit the reabsorption of cholesterol from the intestinal tract. The intake of polyunsaturated fatty acids is usually greater in vegetarian and vegan diets because of their preference for nuts, oilseeds and vegetable oils. Intakes of linoleic acid (18:2 n-6) are considerably greater in vegans and vegetarians than in omnivores. Intakes of linolenic acid (18:3 n-3) are more dependent on the types of oils used in food preparation. Intakes of linoleic acid may be as high as 12% of the energy in vegans. The long-chain n-3 fatty acids are lacking from vegan diets and in vegetarian diets depend upon intakes from eggs and dairy foods. Differences in the composition of dietary fat are well illustrated by the composition of breast milk in vegans, vegetarians and omnivores (Table 17.2).

NUTRIENTS USUALLY PROVIDED BY FOOD OF ANIMAL ORIGIN

Meat and fish provide several nutrients that are scarce or absent from common foods of plant origin and these include iodine, taurine, vitamin B_{12}, vitamin D and long-chain polyunsaturated fatty acids such as eicosapentaenoic (20:5 n-3) and docosahexaenoic (22:6 n-3). Meat and fish also make a significant contribution to protein intake but recommended intakes are easily met by vegetarian diets, especially if the proteins are derived from a variety of dietary sources. The forms of iron and zinc in meat and fish are also more bioavailable.

Table 17.2	Polyunsaturated fatty acids (wt %) in the breast milk of vegans, vegetarians and omnivores		
FATTY ACIDS	VEGANS	VEGETARIANS	OMNIVORES
18: 2 n-6	23.8	19.5	10.9
18: 3 n-3	1.36	1.25	0.49
20: 3 n-6	0.44	0.42	0.4
20: 4 n-6	0.32	0.38	0.35
22: 6 n-3	0.14	0.3	0.37

Source: Sanders & Reddy 1992.

Iron

Iron is found in a very wide variety of foods but in common with zinc its availability from foods of plant origin is low compared with that from meat. Eggs, dairy food and rice are poor sources of iron. Good sources of iron for vegetarians include wheat, pulses, dark green vegetables (especially low oxalate varieties), fortified cereals, dried fruit and iron cooking equipment. Vegetarians are more prone to iron deficiency than meat-eaters. The South Asian vegetarian population in the UK and North America has a higher incidence of iron-deficiency anaemia, particularly among women and infants, compared with the general population. The risk of anaemia is greatest among those who rely on rice rather than wheat. An increased prevalence of iron-deficiency anaemia has also been reported in macrobiotic vegetarians. However, iron intakes appear to be relatively high in vegetarians and vegans whose staple food is wholemeal bread, although bioavailability is low. Haemoglobin concentrations are generally normal in both Seventh-Day Adventist and ethical vegans and vegetarians. However, serum ferritin concentrations are low (below 12 mg/l) in both ethical white and Asian vegetarian women of childbearing age compared with women who eat meat. Meat is an important source of iron in the diet and the haem form is particularly well absorbed. Serum ferritin levels have been found in several studies to be strongly correlated with the intake of haem iron. While vegetarians are more prone to developing iron-deficiency anaemia than meat-eaters, those who carry the gene predisposing to haemochromatosis (HFE) are less likely to develop haemochromatosis.

Vitamin B$_{12}$

Cases of dietary vitamin B$_{12}$ deficiency, sometimes fatal, have been reported in both vegans and vegetarians. White vegans and vegetarians tend to present with neurological signs of deficiency (paraesthesia and subacute combined degeneration of the spinal cord and even optic nerve neuropathy) because of their high intake of folate which masks the megaloblastic anaemia of vitamin B$_{12}$ deficiency. Although dietary supplements and foods fortified with the vitamin are readily available, Lloyd-Wright et al (2003) found that 27% of vegan men and 2% of vegetarian men recruited into the European Prospective Investigation in Cancer had plasma B$_{12}$ concentrations consistent with deficiency (<130 ng/l). In a follow-up study 32% of the same men were found to have definite metabolic vitamin B$_{12}$ deficiency (increased plasma methylmalonic acid, severely increased plasma homocysteine and low serum vitamin B$_{12}$ concentrations) without megaloblastic anaemia (Fig. 17.1).

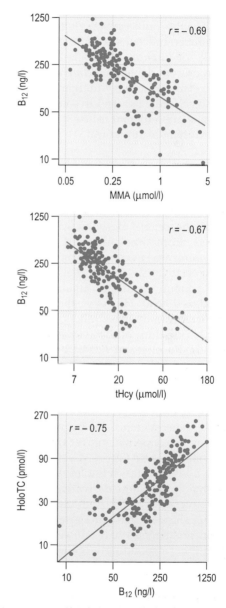

Fig. 17.1 Indices of vitamin B$_{12}$ deficiency in British vegan men. Plasma concentrations of methylmalonic acid (MMA) >0.75 mmol/l, homocysteine (tHcy) >15 mmol/l and holotranscobalamin (HoloTC) <25 pmol/l indicate vitamin B$_{12}$ deficiency. *Source: Lloyd-Wright et al (2003)*

Megaloblastic anaemia appears to be uncommon among vegetarians because their intakes of folate are generally high. The significance of the elevated plasma homocysteine in B_{12} deficiency is uncertain but it may increase the risk of neurological disorders and cardiovascular disease. Dietary vitamin B_{12} deficiency in an unsymptomatic mother can also result in severe neurological signs of deficiency in the offspring. There clearly is a need for vegans and vegetarians who only consume small amounts of dairy products and eggs to be vigilant regarding their intake of vitamin B_{12}. There are a variety of fortified foods available including soya milks, textured vegetable protein, margarine and yeast extracts which can be useful sources. However, some vegans are reluctant to use these products as they regard them as unnatural.

ω–3 Fatty acids

Docosahexaenoic acid (22:6n-3; DHA) is believed to play an important role in the development of the retina and the central nervous system. It can be synthesised from linolenic acid (18:3 n-3) or obtained preformed in the diet from food of animal origin, especially fish. Vegan diets are devoid of DHA but contain significant amounts of linolenic acid (Sanders 1999a). However, the levels of DHA in blood, arterial and breast milk lipids are approximately only one-third of those found in omnivores (Table 17.2). Rosell et al (2005) in a large cross-sectional study failed to show that the proportion of DHA falls according to the duration on a vegan or vegetarian diet. This would suggest that there is a basal rate of conversion of linolenicacid to DHA. There was some evidence to suggest that the proportions of eicosapentaenoic acid (20:5n-3) and docosapentaenoic acid (22:5n-3) were higher in subjects with a lower ratio of linoleic:linolenic acid in their plasma lipids. These derivatives may undergo further conversion to DHA in the brain. Reddy et al (1992) showed that cord arterial lipids from vegetarian pregnancies had a lower proportion of DHA and a correspondingly higher proportion of docosapentaenoic acid (22:5n-6, DPA) compared with omnivores. This would imply that the ability to convert linolenic acid to DHA is not limited in vegetarians but is more influenced by substrate availability. Short-term supplementation with linolenic acid does not lead to an increase in DHA in these lipids but relatively small amounts (~200 mg) of preformed DHA lead to a substantial increase.

Products acceptable to vegans, fortified with an algal source of DHA, are now available. Geppert et al (2006) in a high quality placebo controlled randomised controlled trial compared the effect of 0.94 g DHA in vegetarians versus placebo. This resulted in an increase in the proportion of DHA in plasma phospholipids from 2.8% to 7.3% and a 6.9% rise in LDL cholesterol. While there are cogent reasons for believing that a supply of DHA is important for normal visual and neurological development in the neonate, as yet there is no clear indication that the consumption of DHA by vegans has any clear health benefits.

Vitamin D and calcium

Vegetarians who consume milk and cheese regularly have relatively high intakes of calcium but vegans tend to have low intakes of calcium, usually well below the reference nutrient intake. Vegetarian diets may contain significant quantities of modifiers of the absorption of calcium such as phytic acid contributed by legumes and unrefined cereals (especially unleavened breads and brown rice). A high prevalence of rickets has been noted in children reared on macrobiotic diets who are predominantly vegetarians. However, rickets and osteomalacia do not appear to be significant problems among the white vegetarian population. To be acceptable to vegetarians, vitamin D needs to be provided as ergocalciferol in fortified foods and supplements. Rickets among vegans and vegetarians appears to be more related to the bioavailability of calcium from the diet than any other factor. High intakes of phytate from cereals such as brown rice or unleavened bread appear to be the main precipitating factor even in climates where exposure to sunlight may be high.

17.4 PREGNANCY

The duration of pregnancy was found to be approximately 4–5 days shorter in Hindu vegetarians and earlier onset of labour and caesarean section are more common than in the white population in the UK. Babies born to Hindus are lighter than those born to Muslims or white omnivores even when adjustments are made for gestational age and maternal frame size. Birthweights appear normal in white vegetarian women but a shorter duration of pregnancy has been observed in vegans. The pathophysiological significance of a slightly lower birthweight is uncertain. However, according to Barker's nutritional programming hypothesis, a lower birthweight and smaller head circumference may increase the risk of developing diabetes and cardiovascular disease in later life.

17.5 CHILD GROWTH AND DEVELOPMENT

Widdowson and McCance (1954) in their classic experiment carried out at the end of World War II clearly demonstrated that children will grow and develop quite normally on a diet consisting of plenty of bread and vegetables with minimal amounts of milk and meat. The growth rate of the white Seventh-Day Adventists vegetarian population appears to be virtually indistinguishable from that of white omnivores except for a later age of menarche. Lower rates of growth, particularly in the first 5 years of life, have been reported in children reared on vegan and macrobiotic diets. Despite these lower rates of growth in the first few years of life, catch-up growth occurs by the age of about 10 years. Height is normal but there is still a tendency for these children to be lighter in weight for height than children on mixed diets. The slower rates of growth observed in some of these children under the age of 5 can be attributed to low energy intakes. The significance of slightly slower rates of growth is debatable, but a small fraction of vegan children do show evidence of impaired growth.

It needs to be more widely recognised that severe nutritional deficiencies do occur in children reared on inappropriate vegetarian and vegan diets. With the increasing popularity of vegetarian diets and the trend for a small majority to ignore conventional nutritional wisdom, it seems inevitable that more children will fall victims to their parental folly.

17.6 THE HEALTH OF VEGETARIANS AND VEGANS

The health of Western vegetarian groups has been extensively studied and generally appears to be good, providing the known dietary pitfalls – low energy density, inadequate intakes of iron, vitamin B_{12} and D – are avoided. Assessing the health impact of vegetarianism is often compounded by other lifestyle factors such as socioeconomic status, non-smoking status and health consciousness. One approach has been to compare biomarkers of disease (such as plasma cholesterol and blood pressure) in vegan, vegetarian and omnivore groups. These studies show that on average serum cholesterol is 20% (~1 mmol/l) lower in vegans than in omnivores with intermediate values in vegetarians. Blood pressure has also been found to be lower in vegetarians and this appears to be an effect independent of salt intake or body mass index and appears to be due to a higher consumption of potassium from fruit and vegetables. Recent research has reported elevated homocysteine in vegetarians and vegans. This was particularly marked in subjects recruited in the report by Lloyd-Wright et al (2003) and was attributable to a low vitamin B_{12} intake rather than a low folate intake. This would be regarded as an adverse finding as elevated plasma homocysteine is associated with endothelial dysfunction and increased risk of cardiovascular disease (ischaemic heart disease, stroke and deep-vein thrombosis). Epidemiological studies suggest that a 3 mmol/l increase in plasma homocysteine is associated with a 15% increase in risk of cardiovascular disease (Wald et al 2002). The mean plasma homocysteine concentration in B_{12}-deficient vegans was 22 mmol/l compared with 10 mmol/l in healthy controls. Despite the findings of Lloyd-Wright et al (2003) elevated plasma homocysteine is often indicative of poor folate status, which is thought to have implications for risk of cancers at various sites.

An almost universal finding has been that vegetarians and vegans are lighter in weight than their meat-eating counterparts. The Oxford cohort of the EPIC Study found a difference of 1 unit of BMI (Spencer et al 2003). The lower BMI would be expected to be associated with a decreased risk of type 2 diabetes and gallstones. However, BMI tends to fall abruptly over the age of 60 in vegetarians and especially vegans compared with meat-eaters, which suggests that elderly vegans may have difficulty maintaining muscle mass in old age. This is of concern as a low body mass is associated with increased mortality particularly from respiratory disorders. As vegans have a low proportion of body fat, the decrease in BMI with age is likely to be due to a decrease in muscle mass. This finding would be consistent with the lower reported concentrations of insulin-like growth factor 1 (IGF-1) in vegans compared with omnivores (Allen et al 2000).

There was a suggestion that IGF-1 concentrations are related to protein intake and it is known IGF-1 plays an important role in maintaining muscle mass. As a group, vegetarians have been found to have lower age-standardised mortality rates compared with the general population (Table 17.3). However, a large proportion of this variability can be accounted for by lifestyle factors other than diet. For example, a comparison of members of the Seventh Day Adventists Church, the majority of whom are vegetarians, shows about half the rate of cancer compared with the average Californian population. However, similar observations have been made among other religious denominations that also proscribe smoking and alcohol use but who do not follow vegetarian diets, e.g. Mormons. A meta-analysis of prospective cohort studies suggests that vegetarians and vegans differ little from meat-eaters in terms of survival (Key et al 2003). However, compared with the general population the death rate ratios (the expected number of deaths compared with general population adjusted for age) were half the level expected. When comparisons were made with the meat-eating control populations in these studies, the death rate was significantly lower in the vegetarians only for ischaemic heart disease, which is consistent with their lower plasma cholesterol and blood pressure. However, cancer incidence was remarkably similar between vegetarians and omnivores when other lifestyle factors such as smoking and alcohol intake were taken into account. UK vegetarians and vegans have substantially greater intakes of soy phyto-estrogens than the general population but Travis et al (2008) were unable to find any protective effect on risk of breast cancer in the UK. The failure of a vegetarian diet to provide protection against colorectal cancer was surprising as it had been widely believed that a diet high in fibre and vegetables would offer some protection.

Table 17.3	Death rate ratios with 95% confidence intervals for vegetarians versus non–vegetarians	
DEATH RATE	**RATIOS**	
Ischaemic heart disease	0.76	(0.62–0.94)
Cerebrovascular disease	0.93	(0.74–1.17)
Stomach cancer	1.02	(0.64–1.62)
Colorectal cancer	0.99	(0.77–1.27)
Lung cancer	0.84	(0.59–1.18)
Breast cancer	0.95	(0.55–1.63)
Prostate cancer	0.91	(0.60–1.39)
All causes	0.95	(0.82–1.11)

Source: Key et al 1998.

17.7 CONCLUSION

Vegetarian diets as consumed in developed countries differ little in terms of nutrient composition from those containing meat in developed countries. However, in developing countries, where the choice of foods is more restricted, nutritional deficiencies are more likely, particularly those of iron and vitamin B_{12}. In isolated areas where soil levels of selenium and iodine are low, selenium deficiency and goitre are also more likely to occur on plant-based diets. Thus plant-based diets are nutritionally adequate providing they are not restricted in variety or quality. Particular care needs to be taken to ensure that plant foods are adequately processed to inactivate anti-nutritive substances such as phytates, trypsin inhibitors and cyanogenic glycosides. The lower intake of saturated fatty acids and cholesterol and the higher intake of fruit and vegetables probably explains much of the lower risk of ischaemic heart disease in vegetarians.

KEY POINTS

- Vegetarian diets are defined on the basis of the foods excluded whereas nutritional value depends on what constitutes the diet.
- People follow vegetarian diets for religious, ethical and health reasons.
- Diets high in fruit and vegetables can be bulky and low in energy.

- Vitamin B_{12} is the nutrient most likely to be lacking in vegan and to a lesser extent in vegetarian diets. Deficiency results in elevated plasma homocysteine concentrations and increased risk of neurological disorders.
- Vegetarians are at increased risk of iron-deficiency anaemia owing to the low bioavailability of iron from plant foods.

- Long-chain n-3 fatty acids are absent from vegan diets and their intakes of linoleic acid are high and this may be one explanation of the shorter duration of pregnancy in some vegetarian groups.
- Vegetarians tend to be lighter in weight than omnivores. Vegans may have difficulty maintaining weight in old age.
- Intakes of saturated fatty acids are much lower in vegans and coupled with the lack of cholesterol in the diet results in plasma cholesterol concentrations that are 20% lower than those of meat-eaters.
- The incidence of ischaemic heart disease is lower in vegetarians but that of cancer does not differ.

References

Allen NE, Appleby PN, Davey GK, Key TJ: Hormones and diet: low insulin-like growth factor-I but normal bioavailable androgens in vegan men, *British Journal of Cancer* 83:95–97, 2000.

Draper A, Lewis J, Malhotra N, Wheeler E: The energy and nutrient intakes of different types of vegetarian: a case for supplements? *British Journal of Nutrition* 70(3):812, 1993.

Geppert J, Kraft V, Demmelmair H, Koletzko B: Microalgal docosahexaenoic acid decreases plasma triacylglycerol in normolipidaemic vegetarians: a randomised trial, *British Journal of Nutrition* 95:779–786, 2006.

Key TJ, Fraser GE, Thorogood M, et al: Mortality in vegetarians and non-vegetarians: a collaborative analysis of 8300 deaths among 76000 men and women in five prospective studies, *Public Health Nutrition* 1:33–41, 1998.

Key TJ, Appleby PN, Davey GK, Allen NE, Spencer EA, Travis RC: Mortality in British vegetarians: review and preliminary results from EPIC-Oxford, *American Journal of Clinical Nutrition* 78(3 Suppl): 533S–538S, 2003.

Lloyd-Wright Z, Hvas AM, Moller J, Sanders TA, et al: Holotranscobalamin as an indicator of dietary vitamin B_{12} deficiency, *Clinical Chemistry* 49:2076–2078, 2003.

Miller GJ, Kotecha S, Wilkinson WH, et al: Dietary and other characteristics relevant for coronary heart disease in men of Indian, West Indian and European descent in London, *Atherosclerosis* 70(1–2):63–72, 1988.

Reddy S, Sanders TA: Lipoprotein risk factors in vegetarian women of Indian descent are unrelated to dietary intake, *Atherosclerosis* 95(2–3):223–229, 1992.

Rosell MS, Lloyd-Wright Z, Appleby PN, Sanders TA, Allen NE, Key TJ: Long-chain n-3 polyunsaturated fatty acids in plasma in British meat-eating, vegetarian, and vegan men, *American Journal of Clinical Nutrition* 82:327–334, 2005.

Sanders TA: Essential fatty acid requirements of vegetarians in pregnancy, lactation, and infancy, *American Journal of Clinical Nutrition* 70:555S–559S, 1999.

Sanders TA, Reddy S: The influence of a vegetarian diet on the fatty acid composition of human milk and the essential fatty acid status of the infant, *Journal of Pediatrics* 120:S71–S77, 1992.

Spencer EA, Appleby PN, Davey GK, Key TJ: Diet and body mass index in 38000 EPIC-Oxford meat-eaters, fish-eaters, vegetarians and vegans, *International Journal of Obesity and Related Metabolic Disorders* 27:728–734, 2003.

Travis RC, Allen NE, Appleby PN, Spencer EA, Roddam AW, Key TJ: A prospective study of vegetarianism and isoflavone intake in relation to breast cancer risk in British women, *International Journal of Cancer* 122(3):705–710, 2008.

Wald DS, Law M, Morris JK: Homocysteine and cardiovascular disease: evidence on causality from a meta-analysis, *British Medical Journal* 325:1202–1209, 2002.

Widdowson EM, McCance RA: *Studies on the nutritive value of bread and the effect of variations in the extraction rate of flour on the growth of undernourished children*, Medical Research Council Special Report Series No. 287, London, 1954, HMSO.

Further reading

Key TJ, Appleby PN, Rosell MS: Health effects of vegetarian and vegan diets, *Proceedings of the Nutrition Society 2006 Feb* 65(1):35–41, 2006.

EVOLVE CONTENT (available online at: evolve.elsevier.com/Geissler/nutrition)

Further reading from the book

Useful web links

Chapter 18

Dietary considerations for sport and exercise

Luc J C van Loon and Wim H M Saris

CHAPTER CONTENTS

OBJECTIVES

By the end of this chapter you should be able to:
- understand the basic physiology of muscle contraction
- appreciate the importance of usage of different fuels at different intensity exercise
- understand factors influencing fuel utilisation in individuals under different circumstances
- understand the feeding strategies for optimum physical performance for different situations
- be aware of the evidence for the use of different ergogenic aids

18.1 INTRODUCTION

Next to a certain genetic predisposition and participation in a regular and effective training regime, nutrition is a key factor in determining physical well-being and exercise performance capacity. Nutrition has become even more important for performance now that athletes have reached limits in training volume and intensity. This has led to a renewed interest among athletes, coaches and exercise physiologists regarding the role of nutrition and the influence of gastrointestinal problems on physical performance and well-being. Clear-cut nutritional counselling, however, is often difficult for a number of reasons. First of all, there is no generally accepted nutritional recommendation for the recreational and/or elite athlete involved in heavy physical training. In contrast, most countries have recommended nutrient intakes (RNIs) or recommended daily allowances (RDAs) for nutrients for different age groups and genders. The RDAs for people involved in heavy physical work are generally derived from studies of people performing strenuous manual labour for their profession. Information about the daily requirements of the elite and/or recreational athlete, who will differ with respect to the relative work intensities, is lacking. Secondly the elite athlete's diet is often obscured by secrecy. Following the efforts to ban the use of performance-enhancing drugs, there has been an increasing interest in the potential for the use of specific food products and/or food ingredients to optimise exercise performance. The use of food in this respect is not new and dates back to the days when sports were first practised, around 500 BC in Greece.

Examination of the literature suggests that a well-balanced, healthy diet, compensating for the metabolic demands imposed by intense exercise training and competition, is all that athletes require to optimise their performance. However, the question remains as to what extent a well-balanced diet for the elite and/or recreational athlete differs from a balanced diet for the normal population. Based on an increasing number of scientific studies, certain dietary manipulations have been shown to improve physical performance, in particular endurance performance. Consequently, the development of specific sports supplements, and carbohydrate-rich sports drinks in particular, has shown a rapid increase over the last 20 years. More recently, there has been an increasing interest in functional food ingredients, an area in which sports nutrition has led in developing concepts and products. Unfortunately, in such a booming market the number of 'exotic' (sports) drinks and supplements, claiming to improve health and/or exercise performance without any reasonable scientific justification, is growing fast. In this chapter a general overview is given on the most important aspects of the athlete's nutrition, the practical use of nutritional supplements and facts and fiction relating to the use of nutraceuticals as ergogenic aids.

18.2 MUSCLE STRUCTURE AND FUNCTION

To perform physical exercise our bone structure needs to be moved by muscle force. To generate such force chemical energy has to be transformed to mechanical energy within the muscle. The basic structure of a muscle consists of an outer layer of connective tissue, which covers a number of small bundles each containing up to 150 individual muscle fibres. A muscle fibre represents the individual muscle cell and usually extends the entire length of a muscle. At both ends the muscle fibre fuses with a tendon, which is attached to the bone. The contents of a muscle fibre are enclosed within its plasma membrane (sarcolemma). Within the sarcolemma there are three main structures that play an important role in enabling muscle contraction. First of all, the muscle fibre contains numerous myofibrils, which represent the contractile elements of the muscle. These myofibrils are long strands of smaller subunits, the sarcomeres. Secondly, an extensive network of transverse tubules (T tubules) passes laterally among the myofibrils through the muscle fibre. This network allows nerve impulses to the sarcolemma to reach all myofibrils. In addition, another network of tubules, the sarcoplasmic reticulum (SR complex), runs in parallel with the myofibrils and serves as a storage site for calcium ions, which are essential to enable muscle contraction (see next section). The subunits of the myofibril, the sarcomeres, are the basic functional units of the muscle. The latter contain two types of small protein filaments, the actin and the myosin filaments, which are responsible for the shortening and lengthening of the muscle.

For further information on muscle structure and function see Sections *evolve* 18.2(a), *evolve* 18.2(b) and *evolve* 18.2(c) 🖱.

MUSCLE CONTRACTION

A single motor nerve innervates several muscle fibres, and together they are referred to as a single motor unit. Muscle contraction is preceded by a series of events. First, a motor nerve impulse is generated and conducted through the motor neuron towards its nerve endings. There, an electrical charge can be generated and conducted throughout the entire muscle fibre. The T tubules system allows the electrical charge to reach all myofibrils in the muscle fibre. This so-called action potential triggers the SR complex to release its stored calcium ions. The calcium ions subsequently bind to the actin filaments, which allows the myosin filaments to attach. When these actin–myosin cross-bridges are repeatedly formed and released, these filaments can slide past each other, causing the sarcomere to shorten/lengthen. As such, this sliding filament principle explains the shortening of the muscle during contraction. This process of muscle contraction requires energy, which is provided by adenosine triphosphate (ATP), the universal energy donor in the living cell. When the muscle is no longer stimulated, the flow of calcium ions is halted and the actin–myosin interaction inhibited. To enable muscle relaxation calcium ions need to be pumped back into the SR complex, which also requires ATP. Though this describes the process of a single contraction in an individual muscle fibre, it should be clear that an extremely complex, well-orchestrated series of muscle contractions within numerous muscle fibres from various muscle groups is needed to enable even the simplest of movements.

MUSCLE FIBRE TYPES

Though all muscle fibres are generally of the same structure and function, certain differences between muscle fibres allow a classification into two main types. Skeletal muscle contains both type I and type II muscle fibres, also referred to as slow-twitch and fast-twitch fibres, respectively. This classification is based on the contractile and metabolic characteristics of the fibres. Type II fibre can be further classified into type IIa and IIb fibres. On average, most skeletal muscle contains about 50% type I, 25% type IIa and 25% type IIb fibres. However, there can be substantial differences in fibre type distribution between various muscle groups as well as between individuals. The main difference between the type I (slow-twitch) and type II (fast-twitch) muscle fibres is their contractile speed. The tension that can be generated is not much different between the individual type I and II muscle fibre. However, a type II motor unit can develop much greater strength than a type I motor unit. The latter is explained by the fact that a type II motor unit (recall that a motor unit is a motor nerve with the muscle fibres it innervates) contains a type II motor neuron which innervates between 300 and 800 different type II muscle fibres, whereas a type I motor neuron innervates only about 10 to 180 type I fibres. Besides these specific contractile differences, these muscle fibre types also show concomitant differences in their metabolic adaptation. The type I muscle fibres are relatively slow, more resistant to fatigue and have a high aerobic capacity. The latter means that they are optimised to generate ATP by oxidative metabolic pathways (see Section 18.3). In contrast, the type II muscle fibres are fast, fatigue easily

and therefore need a metabolic system optimised to provide energy fast. This implies that they need to derive most of their ATP through non-oxidative (or anaerobic) metabolic pathways (see Section 18.3). An overview of the main differences between the type I, IIa and IIb fibres is provided in Table 18.1.

Clearly, type I muscle fibres are well suited for prolonged endurance exercise, like marathon running, cycling, etc. In contrast, the type II muscle fibres are predominantly activated during short-term high intensity activities and resistance exercise, such as sprinting, weight-lifting, etc. Clearly, though the extent of type I and II motor unit recruitment depends on the physical activity, a combination of both is always apparent. Besides the sort (and intensity) of exercise, the duration of exercise can also result in changes in muscle fibre type recruitment. During prolonged endurance exercise the predominant use of type I motor units leads to the depletion of type I muscle fibre energy stores and subsequent fatigue. Consequently, in time more type II motor units need to be recruited to maintain exercise performance.

Fibre type composition has been reported to vary considerably between individuals, and is largely determined by genetic background. Elite athletes often have a muscle fibre type composition which more or less conforms to fibre type recruitment in their sport. For example, elite endurance runners and cross-country skiers often have a relatively high percentage of type I muscle fibres (up to 80%) in their muscle tissue, whereas athletes such as world-class weight-lifters, body-builders or sprinters tend to have relatively more type II muscle fibres. Clearly, genetic predisposition to develop a certain muscle fibre type composition (before birth

Table 18.1	Skeletal muscle fibre types		
MUSCLE FIBRE	**TYPE I**	**TYPE IIA**	**TYPE IIB**
Contractile properties			
Contractile speed	Slow	Fast	Fast
Fatigue resistance	High	Moderate	Low
Motor unit strength	Low	High	High
Metabolic properties			
Oxidative capacity	High	Moderate	Low
Non-oxidative	Low	High	Highest capacity
Adapted from Wilmore & Costill 1994.			

and/or during the early years of childhood) can provide an (dis-) advantage to excel in a certain sport. However, it should not be used as a predictive measure of athletic performance capacity, as muscle fibre type composition is merely one of the numerous factors that attribute to performance capacity. There are some suggestions that prolonged exercise training can also modify muscle fibre type distribution. Whether this is true or not, all muscle fibres show a tremendous capacity to adapt to the demands imposed upon them by regular exercise training. As such, endurance training can substantially increase the aerobic capacity of any muscle fibre, whereas regular sprint and/or resistance training increases their anaerobic capacity.

18.3 SKELETAL MUSCLE SUBSTRATE UTILISATION

The immediate source of chemical energy required for skeletal muscle to contract is provided by the hydrolysis of ATP. Intracellular ATP stores are small (5.0–5.5 mmol/g wet muscle) and would be depleted within seconds of maximal contraction if not adequately replenished. In addition, close to maximal ATP levels are essential for normal (muscle) cell function. Hence, metabolic pathways for ATP resynthesis need to be activated directly in response to an increase in ATP demand. To maintain ATP levels and enable ongoing contractile activity, ATP synthesis rate needs to be tightly coupled to the rate of hydrolysis. This requires a highly efficient and responsive interaction between the various metabolic pathways responsible for ATP generation, especially during the transition from rest to exercise when the demand for ATP synthesis, at the muscular level, can increase more than 100-fold. Depending on the ATP demands, both substrate level phosphorylation and oxidative phosphorylation contribute to ATP synthesis. ATP synthesis from substrate level phosphorylation is required to sustain high intensity, dynamic exercise when the high ATP demands cannot be matched (entirely) by oxidative phosphorylation. These ATP synthesis pathways include the phosphagen system and (anaerobic) glycolysis. The phosphagen system includes the breakdown of creatine phosphate, a high-energy compound stored in the muscle (25 mmol/g wet muscle), by creatine kinase, thereby providing energy for ATP synthesis. In

addition, some ATP can be generated by the adenylate kinase reaction ($2 ADP \rightarrow ATP + AMP$). For the cell to generate ATP by glycolysis, intracellular glucose or glycogen is converted to glucose-6-phosphate. Thereafter, in a series of enzymatic reactions, called glycolysis, glucose-6-phosphate is broken down to pyruvate, which under these conditions, is converted to lactate (see Section 6.5). Substrate level phosphorylation of ADP in these so-called anaerobic pathways, allows high rates of ATP synthesis (5–6 times higher than the rate of ATP synthesis provided by oxidative phosphorylation) but can only be maintained for a relatively short period due to the depletion of creatine phosphate and the accumulation of by-products of the adenylate kinase reaction and anaerobic glycolysis, including adenosine diphosphate (ADP), adenosine monophosphate (AMP), inosine monophosphate (IMP), ammonia (NH_3), hydrogen ions (H^+) and inorganic phosphate (P). At rest and during exercise (lasting more than 10 minutes) the vast majority of ATP required for muscle contraction is generated through oxidative phosphorylation. The principal substrates that fuel this aerobic ATP synthesis are fat and carbohydrate. As the ability of skeletal muscle to synthesise ATP at rest and during continuous exercise depends on the availability of both fat and carbohydrate, these substrates ultimately need to be provided by dietary intake. Because ATP has to be generated continuously, a readily available pool of metabolic fuels is essential. Therefore, the human body contains a variety of storage sites for carbohydrate and fat.

FUEL STORAGE

Carbohydrates are mainly stored as glycogen in skeletal muscle and in the liver. Carbohydrate stores are relatively small and normally range between 0.46 and 0.52 kg, corresponding to a total energy storage of 7.5–8.4 MJ (1785–2000 kcal). Fat is mainly stored as triacylglycerol (TAG) in subcutaneous and deep visceral adipose tissue. However, smaller quantities of TAG are present as lipid droplets inside muscle fibres (intramyocellular triacylglycerol or IMTG) (Hoppeler et al 1985). In addition, some fat is present in the circulation as non-esterified or free fatty acids (FFA) bound to albumin, or as TAG incorporated in circulating lipoprotein particles (chylomicrons and very-low, low-, intermediate- and high-density lipoproteins or VLDL, LDL, IDL and HDL, respectively). In contrast to carbohydrate, fat stores are quite large and range between 9 and 15 kg in the average, non-obese male (body mass ~70 kg), corresponding to a total energy storage of 350–586 MJ (80 000–140 000 kcal). An overview of the energy stores is provided in Table 18.2. As such, more than 97% of our entire energy storage is covered by endogenous fat sources. This apparent preference for the storage of fat as a fuel source is quite practical as fat contains more than twice the amount of energy per unit of weight compared to carbohydrate. However, an important advantage of carbohydrate as a fuel source is that more ATP can be generated per unit of time compared to the oxidation of fat.

The rate at which ATP can be generated depends on the biochemical pathways that are followed as well as on the substrate (source) from which ATP is derived. As mentioned, anaerobic ATP synthesis allows considerably higher rates of high-energy phosphate formation compared with the complete, oxygen-dependent, oxidation of carbohydrate and fat. In short, the maximal rate of ATP synthesis from fat can provide only enough energy to sustain exercise at 55–70% of maximal oxygen uptake (VO_2max), depending on the training status. However, the rate of energy generated from carbohydrate (aerobic and anaerobic) can provide enough energy to sustain exercise up to 100% of VO_2max. Consequently, during moderate-intensity endurance-type exercise, like a marathon, ATP demands can be provided entirely by oxidative phosphorylation of both intra- and extracellular carbohydrate and fat. The relative contribution of fat and carbohydrate oxidation to total energy expenditure during exercise can vary enormously and strongly depends on exercise intensity, training status and diet.

For further information on fuel storage see Section *evolve* 18.3 .

EXERCISE INTENSITY AND DURATION

Fat and carbohydrate are the main substrates that fuel aerobic ATP synthesis during prolonged exercise. Though both substrates will always contribute to total energy provision, their relative utilisation has been shown to vary with the intensity and duration of exercise. Most conclusions about substrate utilisation rates in relation to exercise intensity on a whole body level have been derived from stable isotope studies (van Loon et al 2001). Generally, the oxidation of blood-plasma-derived FFA provides the majority of energy during low intensity exercise (~30% of maximal oxygen uptake, or VO_2max), with little (or no) net utilisation of intramuscular or lipoprotein-derived TG and muscle glycogen and a relatively small amount of plasma glucose. During moderate intensity exercise (40–65% VO_2max) fat oxidation, from an absolute point of view, reaches maximal rates, with the fat stores contributing about 50% (40–60%) of total energy expenditure (Fig. 18.1). As plasma FFAs provide only about half

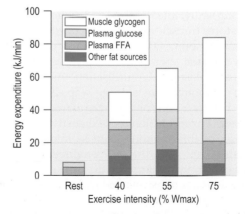

Fig. 18.1 Substrate utilisation during exercise of various intensities. Energy expenditure (expressed as kJ per minute) as a function of exercise intensity (expressed as percentage of maximal workload). The relative contributions of plasma glucose, muscle glycogen, plasma FFA and other fat sources (sum of intramuscular plus lipoprotein-derived TG) to energy expenditure are illustrated as described in the key. *Adapted from van Loon et al 2001.*

Table 18.2	Fuel stores in an average person	
FUEL SOURCE	**IN WEIGHT (G)**	**IN ENERGY (KJ)**
Fat		
Plasma FFA	0.4	16
Plasma TG	4.0	156
IMTG	300	11 700
Adipose tissue	12 000	468 000
Carbohydrate		
Plasma glucose	20	360
Liver glycogen	100	1 800
Muscle glycogen	350	6 300

Based on estimates for a normal, non-obese person with a body mass of ~70 kg. Fat provides 39 kJ/g and carbohydrate 18 kJ/g.

of the energy derived from fat oxidation, intramuscular TAGs (IMTGs) are likely to form an important substrate source. However, the latter estimate also includes the use of lipoprotein-derived TAG, as the applied stable isotope techniques do not enable the distinction between TAG derived from the IMTG stores and TAG from circulating lipoproteins.

The majority of the carbohydrates oxidised during moderate intensity exercise are derived from muscle glycogen stores, with an estimated use of plasma glucose ranging between 15% and 35% of total endogenous carbohydrate utilisation. As exercise intensity is further increased (up to 70–90% VO_2max) fat oxidation decreases substantially, from both a relative as well as a quantitative point of view, accounted for by a decrease in the use of plasma FFA as well as intramuscular and/or lipoprotein-derived TAG sources. At the same time, endogenous carbohydrate oxidation rates increase exponentially (Fig. 18.1), which is necessary to account for the high energy demands. Consequently, muscle glycogen becomes the most important substrate source during moderate-to-high intensity exercise.

Besides exercise intensity, exercise duration also plays an important role in substrate source utilisation. As moderate intensity exercise is prolonged and muscle glycogen stores gradually decline, plasma FFA levels continue to increase with a concomitant increase in plasma FFA oxidation rates. Concomitantly, the use of endogenous carbohydrate stores (muscle and liver glycogen) and the use of other fat sources (IMTG and lipoprotein-derived TAG) decrease over time, compensated for by the increased plasma FFA utilisation. As the endogenous carbohydrate storage capacity is quite limited, muscle and/or glycogen stores will become depleted during prolonged exhaustive endurance exercise. In this situation exercise intensity cannot be maintained since the ATP production will slow down due to the reliance on fat as a substrate. This phenomenon is often referred to as 'hitting the wall' and can occur as soon as 45 minutes after onset of intense exercise. The symptoms of fatigue during prolonged endurance exercise are strongly related to glycogen depletion in the exercising muscle, as shown in the early muscle biopsy studies by Bergström & Hultman (1966). Based on these physiological observations, it has become clear that the level of pre-exercise muscle glycogen concentration as well as carbohydrate ingestion during exercise

is important to delay the onset of fatigue (see Section 18.4).

TRAINING STATUS

The relative contribution of fat and carbohydrate oxidation to total energy expenditure during exercise is also determined by training status. In their classic studies, Christensen & Hansen (1939) already observed that endurance training leads to an increased capacity to utilise fat as a substrate source and reduces the reliance on the limited endogenous carbohydrate stores during exercise. This training-induced change in substrate utilisation has since been confirmed in numerous studies (Fig. 18.2).

The contribution of fat as a fuel source during exercise has been shown to be increased in an endurance-trained state, compared at the same absolute as well as the same relative (and therefore higher absolute) workload. The main metabolic adaptations to endurance training that are believed to be responsible for the increase in fat oxidative capacity include an increase in both the size and number of mitochondria and a concomitant upregulation of enzymes involved in the activation, mitochondrial transport and oxidation of FA as well as enzymes involved in the TCA cycle and respiratory chain. In addition, endurance training has been

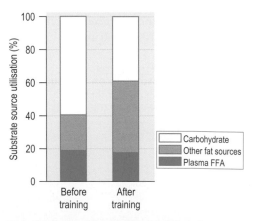

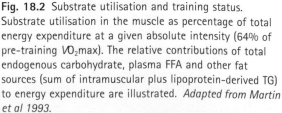

Fig. 18.2 Substrate utilisation and training status. Substrate utilisation in the muscle as percentage of total energy expenditure at a given absolute intensity (64% of pre-training VO_2max). The relative contributions of total endogenous carbohydrate, plasma FFA and other fat sources (sum of intramuscular plus lipoprotein-derived TG) to energy expenditure are illustrated. *Adapted from Martin et al 1993.*

shown to result in an increased capillary density of muscle tissue and increased FABP (FA-binding protein) and GLUT-4 (glucose transporter protein) content, suggesting an increased capacity to take up FFA and glucose from the circulation. However, the actual mechanisms responsible for the increased fat oxidative capacity, and reduced reliance on endogenous carbohydrate, following endurance training have not yet been fully elucidated.

Though the relative contribution of fat oxidation to energy expenditure increases substantially following endurance training, it is not quite clear which fat sources are utilised to a larger extent. Most studies do not report large differences in plasma FFA uptake in an endurance trained state. As such, it has been suggested that the increase in fat oxidation observed in an endurance-trained state is entirely accounted for by an increased contribution of IMTG utilisation (Fig. 18.2). In accordance with the increased reliance on IMTG as a substrate source in endurance athletes, studies have reported an increase in IMTG storage following endurance training. The regulation of IMTG metabolism has recently received much interest as excessive IMTG accumulation in obese and/or type 2 diabetes patients has been linked to the development of defects in the insulin signalling cascade, causing skeletal muscle insulin resistance (Shulman 2000). Obviously, there are important differences between the increased IMTG accumulation in the obese and/or type 2 diabetes patient compared to the endurance athlete, as athletes generally show an improved insulin sensitivity compared to untrained individuals. Clearly, regular exercise seems to play an important regulatory factor in the aetiology of obesity and insulin resistance. More research is warranted to evaluate the importance of regular exercise training in the obese and/or type 2 diabetes patient.

The observed decrease in the reliance on endogenous carbohydrate utilisation in an endurance-trained state has been shown to be accounted for by a decrease in both plasma glucose and muscle glycogen use during exercise (van Loon et al 1999). The effects of endurance training on carbohydrate metabolism are not limited to changes in the reliance on the use of endogenous carbohydrate during exercise but also affect carbohydrate storage. Trained individuals have an increased capacity to store glycogen, which is attributed to an increase in insulin sensitivity, GLUT-4 content and/or glycogen synthase activity. Clearly, endurance training

increases performance capacity by reducing the reliance on the limited endogenous carbohydrate stores as a substrate, as well as by increasing the storage capacity of muscle glycogen.

18.4 NUTRITIONAL INTERVENTIONS TO OPTIMISE PERFORMANCE

The first and clearest difference in nutritional needs between athletes and non-athletes is energy. The energy expenditure of a sedentary adult female/male amounts to approximately 8.5–12.0 MJ per day. Physical activity by means of training or competition will increase the daily energy expenditure by 2–4 MJ per hour of exercise, depending on physical fitness, duration, type and intensity of sport. For this reason, athletes must increase food consumption to meet their energy needs, according to the level of daily energy expenditure. This increased food intake should be well balanced with respect to an adequate macronutrient and micronutrient ingestion. The latter, however, is not always easy. Many athletic events are characterised by high exercise intensities. As a result, energy expenditure over a short period of time may be extremely high. For example, to run a marathon will take about 10–12 MJ. Depending on the time to finish, this may induce an energy expenditure of approximately 3.2 MJ/hour in a recreational athlete and 6.3 MJ/hour in an elite athlete who finishes in approximately 2–2.5 hours. A professional cycling race like the Tour de France will cost an athlete about 27 MJ/day, a figure that will increase to approximately 40 MJ/day when cycling over mountain passes (Saris et al 1989). Compensating for such high energy expenditure by ingesting normal solid meals will pose a problem to any athlete involved in such competition, since the digestion and absorption processes will be impaired during intensive physical activity. These problems are not only restricted to competition days. During intensive training days, energy expenditure is also high. In such circumstances, athletes tend to ingest a large number of 'in between meals' providing up to 40% of the total energy intake. These 'in between meals' are often energy-rich snacks, which are often low in protein and/or micronutrient content. As such, the diet becomes unbalanced. Specially adapted nutritious foods/fluids which are easily digestible and rapidly absorbable may solve this problem. In addition to the energy needs and the limited capacity and time to digest and metabolise, there is the importance of muscle fuel selection. Metabolic capacity and power output depend on this selection. During prolonged moderate-to-high intensity exercise, the muscle cell depends mainly on carbohydrate as a substrate (see Section 18.3). Therefore, diet selection is not only a matter of energy but also a selection of the right substrate source.

In contrast to the efforts to ingest ample energy to account for the high energy expenditure, some athletes (e.g. female runners, gymnasts and ballet dancers) are known to reduce their energy intake, whereas their energy expenditure is high. Energy expenditure in the average sedentary subject ranges between 1.4 and 1.6 times basal metabolic rate (BMR), while reported energy intake in elite (female) gymnasts is usually below this level, despite the fact that they work out between 3 and 4 hours a day. This can probably be explained by two factors: underreporting and the urge to limit energy intake, the first being a result of the latter. Whether the intake data are reliable or not, some of these athletes limit their energy intake to reduce body mass and fat mass with major consequences for energy turnover and performance.

CARBOHYDRATE

In Section 18.3, under 'Exercise intensity and duration', it was shown that the muscle glycogen stores, from a quantitative point of view, form the most important substrate source during prolonged moderate-to-high intensity exercise. Combined with the fact that endogenous substrate stores are relatively small, it is not surprising that endurance performance capacity is often limited by the availability of endogenous carbohydrate. Therefore, athletes involved in moderate-to-high intensity exercise lasting more than 45–60 minutes should ensure that their muscle glycogen stores are optimised before the start of an important event. Much research has been performed to develop nutritional regimes to maximise pre-competition muscle glycogen stores. Bergström & Hultman (1966) introduced a dietary intervention which increased muscle glycogen concentration more than two-fold. This regime included an exhaustive cycling test followed by 3 days of a low carbohydrate diet, after which a second exhaustive exercise test was performed followed by 3 days of a high carbohydrate diet. Though muscle glycogen stores increased more than two-fold following this classic glycogen loading regime, major disadvantages were reported when applied in practice. Side effects such as weight gain, gastrointestinal complaints, fatigue, irritability and nervousness were reported. To reduce these side effects a modified glycogen supercompensation regime was introduced. This 6-day glycogen loading regime included the tapering of training (reducing training volume, while maintaining training intensity) with an increase in the relative contribution of carbohydrate in the diet (from ~50% up to 70% of total energy intake). This modified regime results in slightly lower but comparable increases in muscle glycogen content without the apparent disadvantages of the classical regime.

Carbohydrate loading and the tapering of training before competition as a means to maximise precompetition muscle glycogen storage is nowadays widely practised by endurance athletes throughout the world.

Besides optimising pre-competition muscle glycogen content, carbohydrates can be ingested during exercise to provide an additional exogenous carbohydrate source (Wagenmakers et al 1993). Numerous studies have demonstrated that carbohydrate supplementation during prolonged endurance exercise increases exercise performance. The latter has been attributed to the maintenance of normal blood glucose concentrations and high carbohydrate oxidation rates throughout the latter stages of prolonged exercise. As an increase in plasma glucose availability leads to an increase in plasma glucose uptake and oxidation, it has often been suggested that carbohydrate supplementation also reduces the reliance on muscle glycogen. Though most research has been unable to demonstrate such a glycogen-sparing effect, a reduction in muscle glycogen use specific for type I muscle fibres has been observed during running. It has also been suggested that carbohydrate supplementation can be beneficial to performance in non-endurance sports (such as soccer, tennis and weight-lifting).

Carbohydrates are best provided during exercise in combination with water. A wide variety of studies have been performed to maximise exogenous glucose absorption and/or oxidation rates by varying the type, amount and feeding schedule of carbohydrate-containing solutions. Almost all carbohydrates are absorbed and oxidised at similar rates. This category includes glucose, maltose, sucrose and maltodextrins. Fructose and galactose are oxidised at considerably slower rates (50%) when ingested individually. However, the oxidation rate of carbohydrates ingested during exercise is limited. Even when extremely high amounts of carbohydrates are ingested during exercise, oxidation rates will not exceed 1.0–1.1 g/min. This shows that during exercise not more than ~60–70 g of carbohydrate should be ingested per hour. The ideal sports drink should, therefore, contain such a carbohydrate content that a total intake rate of 60 g carbohydrate per hour is practically achievable. On average the carbohydrate content in a good sports drink should be around 6–10% (certainly not exceeding 15%) and osmolality should not be too high (~350 mosmol/kg), as this would result in impaired gastric emptying followed by gastrointestinal complaints. It is advisable to ingest 6–8 ml per kg body mass of such a sports drink during the warm-up period immediately before the start of training or competition to fill the stomach, which stimulates gastric emptying. Thereafter, during exercise, smaller amounts should be ingested (2–3 ml/kg) at 15–20 min intervals. The oxidation of exogenous carbohydrate can provide a substantial contribution to total energy expenditure (~20%). There are no differences in the oxidation rate of ingested carbohydrates (provided by a sports drink) during moderate intensity exercise between untrained men and trained endurance athletes, implying that the recreational athlete as well as the elite athlete can profit from the use of carbohydrate-rich sports drinks during prolonged endurance exercise (van Loon et al 1999).

Following prolonged endurance exercise, muscle glycogen stores are substantially decreased. As such, post-exercise restoration of muscle glycogen stores is considered an important factor in determining the time needed to recover. Under normal conditions, muscle glycogen is restored at a rate of only 3–7% per hour, provided that an adequate amount of carbohydrate is ingested. Therefore, approximately 24 hours are required for the muscle glycogen stores to be fully restored. However, in multi-day sports events (such as the Tour de France) available recovery time is far less than 24 hours. Muscle glycogen resynthesis rates are highest during the first 2 hours after exercise. Therefore, one should start to consume ample carbohydrate immediately after cessation of exercise. As solid food is often not too well tolerated immediately post-exercise, carbohydrate-rich (recovery) sports drinks are an effective alternative. Thereafter, moderate-to-high glycaemic index foods (bread, pasta, potatoes etc.) should be consumed rather than low

glycaemic index foods. Though carbohydrate intake rates of 0.8 g/kg/hour have been advised to optimise muscle glycogen synthesis rates, recent studies suggest that about 1.2–1.5 g/kg/hour should be ingested, provided at short (30 min) intervals. The addition of an insulinotropic free amino acid/protein mixture to the carbohydrate-containing beverages has been suggested to be beneficial as a means of accelerating glycogen resynthesis.

FAT

The importance of optimising muscle and liver glycogen storage and the use of carbohydrate supplementation during exercise to reduce fatigue and improve athletic performance has led to a quite extensive understanding of carbohydrate metabolism during exercise. Far less information is available on the role of fat as an endogenous and/or exogenous substrate during exercise. As discussed above in 'Training status', endurance training increases fat oxidative capacity, which reduces the reliance on the limited endogenous carbohydrate stores and subsequently improves endurance performance capacity. As such, there is considerable interest in potential (nutritional) interventions to increase fat oxidative capacity.

Therefore, the effects of fat supplements and high fat diets on performance capacity have been the subject of concentrated research, particularly with respect to the use of medium-chain triacylglycerols (MCT). These C8 to C10 carbon triglycerides are more soluble in water and less likely to inhibit gastric emptying than long chain triglycerides (LC-TG). Furthermore, medium-chain fatty acid oxidation is not as limited by transport into the mitochondria as long-chain fatty acids are. Exercise studies with MCT supplementation have revealed that MCT is oxidised almost as rapidly as glucose and even better in combination with glucose. However, since MCT intake is limited due to gastrointestinal distress when ingesting larger amounts, their contribution to total energy expenditure is restricted to about 7%. Also, most performance studies have not yet shown an additional effect to carbohydrate feeding alone.

As well as the use of such fat supplements during exercise, research has also focused on the effect of using long-term high fat diets on performance. The use of such diets provokes adaptive responses, leading to an increase in the capacity to oxidise fat as a fuel and to the sparing of endogenous carbohydrate stores during exercise. Though a few studies have reported an increase in time to exhaustion following the use of a high fat diet followed by a short-term carbohydrate-rich diet, most studies investigating the effects of high fat diets on exercise performance do not report an increase in exercise performance. In addition, from a health perspective, long-term high fat diets are not generally recommended.

The recognition of the importance of carbohydrate has resulted in the recommendation of high carbohydrate diets in endurance athletes, and has led to a reduction in fat intake. In some cases this has been exaggerated, with fat intake being reduced to less than 20–25% of total energy intake. Recent findings suggest that this should not be recommended for athletes during recovery. Studies in trained athletes have shown that prolonged endurance exercise leads to a substantial net depletion of IMTG stores. Following post-exercise recovery the use of extremely low fat diets prevents the restoration of IMTG stores for up to 48 hours or more. In contrast, low and moderate fat-containing diets resulted in IMTG stores that did not return to pre-exercise levels until 24 hours of recovery. Clearly, more research needs to be performed to determine the importance of IMTG stores as a substrate source during exercise and its role in athletic performance.

PROTEIN

For many years the effects of exercise on dietary protein requirements has been a controversial topic. Most RDA committees have not provided an additional allowance for protein for physically active individuals. However, a considerable amount of experimental evidence indicates that regular exercise increases dietary protein needs. The latter is explained by the need for protein to repair exercise-induced muscle damage, as an additional substrate source during prolonged exercise, and to support training-induced muscle reconditioning with a concomitant increase in lean tissue mass. Clearly, the protein requirement of the individual athlete is likely to depend on the type (endurance or resistance), intensity and duration of the exercise training regime. Current evidence suggests that endurance-trained athletes should consume approximately 1.1 g/kg body weight per day (Phillips 2007). This is somewhat higher than normal

protein requirements in compensation for an enhanced utilisation of amino acids in oxidative energy production during regular exercise training. This process is known to be intensified at higher work levels and in a state of glycogen depletion. In general, the increased protein needs are covered by the concomitant increase in overall food intake in the athlete. For example, in a nationwide study in elite athletes, a close relation was found between protein and energy intake. In the extreme case of cyclists in the Tour de France, this resulted in an absolute protein intake of more than 3 g protein/kg/day, despite the fact that food selection was completely focused on carbohydrate-rich products.

Intense endurance training is likely to lead to a higher daily energy expenditure when compared to intense resistance training. However, the energy needs of experienced strength athletes and bodybuilders may be just as high as endurance athletes because of their much higher body weight and elevated fat-free mass. Resistance training is thought to increase protein requirements more than endurance exercise, and it is recommended that experienced male body-builders and strength athletes consume up to 1.4 g/kg body weight per day to allow for the maintenance and further increase of their already increased body weight and fat-free mass. Where energy expenditure is matched by energy intake the suggested protein requirements are easily met through normal dietary intake in both strength as well as endurance athletes. However, restricted food intake, as reported in athletes trying to reduce body weight (especially female endurance runners, gymnasts and weight-class athletes), is likely to result in inadequate protein intake.

A single bout of exercise can accelerate muscle protein synthesis for up to 24 h. However, exercise also stimulates muscle protein breakdown, albeit to a lesser extent than protein synthesis. Nonetheless, net muscle protein balance will remain negative in the absence of nutrient intake. Ingestion of protein and/or essential amino acids during post-exercise recovery inhibits protein breakdown and stimulates muscle protein synthesis, leading to net muscle protein accretion (Tipton et al 1999). Consequently, post-exercise protein ingestion has been suggested as an effective strategy to optimise post-exercise recovery and, as such, to facilitate skeletal muscle reconditioning. This has resulted in the widespread use of protein and/or amino acid supplements by strength and endurance athletes. Though carbohydrate co-ingestion does not seem to be required to maximise post-exercise muscle protein synthesis, it is likely that carbohydrate co-ingestion further inhibits the post-exercise increase in muscle protein breakdown, thereby improving net protein balance (Koopman et al 2007).

Branched-chain amino acids (BCAA; leucine, isoleucine, valine) and tryptophan have also been advocated as supplements for endurance athletes as a means to reduce central fatigue by serotonergic mechanisms. However, well-controlled studies investigating the effects of BCAA supplementation in athletes have failed to show any effect on fatigue and/or endurance exercise performance. Based on the experience in clinical nutrition and the observed reduction in plasma glutamine levels in overtrained athletes, it has also been proposed that oral glutamine supplementation could support the immune competence of athletes involved in intense daily training. However, no evidence has been provided that supports the hypothesis that glutamine supplementation is beneficial for athletes.

FLUIDS AND ELECTROLYTES

Most of the energy required for intensive endurance exercise is produced by oxidative metabolism. As such, each litre of oxygen consumed will contribute to an energy production of approximately 20 kJ. However, 75% of this energy is released as heat and only 25% is used for mechanical work. In order to avoid hyperthermia, the produced heat must be transferred from the working muscles to the periphery, primarily by circulating blood. This heat is eliminated at the surface of the body by radiation, convection and evaporation. Radiation and convection are the means by which dry heat is transferred to the immediate surroundings. Heat loss by convection can be increased substantially by wind or water. Evaporation of sweat is the most important way to eliminate heat when working in a warm environment because convection and radiation will be minimal under these circumstances. With intense physical activity sweat rates will then be maximised. At maximal sweat rates, a 70 kg male athlete may lose >30 ml/min or >1800 ml sweat/hour. Body size, training status, exercise intensity and weather conditions all influence the sweating rate. One of the highest sweat rates ever reported amounted to 3.7 l/hour in a 67 kg marathon runner. Without appropriate rehydration blood flow through the extremities and the skin will decrease. In addition, sweat response and heat flux will be diminished. This may cause hyperthermia with associated severe health risks when exercising in the heat. In any situation, dehydration substantially impairs exercise performance, with a ~10–15% decrease in performance capacity with each degree increase in body temperature.

With sweat loss, electrolytes are also excreted. Because sweat contains fewer minerals than plasma and water intake is inadequate to fully compensate the losses, the electrolyte concentration in blood normally increases as a result of intense endurance exercise. When water intake is equal to water loss by sweating, theoretically the plasma electrolyte levels, especially the major electrolytes sodium and chloride, should fall. However, due to the high plasma sodium content and the large extracellular space, this is not apparent until late in exercise, after significant amounts of water have been ingested. For example, if a 70 kg athlete (14 litres extracellular fluid) loses 6 litres of sweat (Na^+ concentration 30 mEq/l or 600 mg/l), then 180 mEq Na^+ would be lost. If the water loss occurs equally from extracellular fluid (containing 20–30 mEq Na^+) and intracellular fluid, then the extracellular Na^+ concentration would still be above 130 mEq/l. This may explain why drinking large amounts of plain water when competing in the heat has only been shown to result in significant hyponatraemia in about 10–20% of ultra-endurance runners and triathletes. Therefore, in most exercise events lasting less than 3 or 4 hours, the major concern is that fluid and glucose be available to prevent exhaustion and heat stroke. In the case of maximal performance, the availability of carbohydrate together with fluid may limit performance. In this respect both carbohydrate and sodium have beneficial characteristics stimulating water absorption. On the other hand, from a number of observational as well as experimental studies, it has become clear that there is a higher frequency of gastrointestinal distress symptoms when athletes are dehydrated, especially when fluid loss exceeds 4% of body weight.

Restoration of fluid balance after exercise is an important part of recovery. Rehydration after exercise can be achieved effectively only if both electrolyte and water losses are replaced. The sodium content of most sports drinks lies within a range of

200 to 600 mg/l. These values are already at the lower level for an effective rehydration solution. An ideal post-exercise rehydration drink should contain around 1100 mg/l sodium to optimise water retention. In comparison, regular soft drinks contain virtually no sodium and are therefore less suitable as a rapid rehydration solution.

MICRONUTRIENTS

Vitamins have attracted much attention in the world of sport because of their supposed capacity to enhance performance. Vitamin supplements are widely used by both professional and recreational athletes, often with extreme levels of intake exceeding 10 to 100 times the RDA. It is fair to assume that vitamin requirements are increased in the athlete involved in rigorous exercise training, due to the increased energy expenditure, sweat loss, core temperature, etc. However, as the increased energy expenditure in the athlete is compensated for by an increase in energy intake and assuming a healthy diet, increased vitamin intake fully compensates for any increase in vitamin requirements. As such, there are no indications that long-term vitamin intake among athletes is in any way insufficient. The only exception may be athletes involved in regular intense exercise training who consume either a (very) extreme low (<4.2 MJ/day) or high (>21 MJ/day) energetic diet for a prolonged period. The latter is explained by the fact that athletes requiring such an extreme high energy intake tend to consume energy-dense food and beverages (often during prolonged endurance exercise trials) which from a dietary viewpoint often tend to be of a lesser quality. These athletes (such as cyclists during the Tour de France) as well as those consuming extremely low energy diets (such as female endurance runners, gymnasts and ballet dancers) are prone to a marginal vitamin intake and can be at risk of developing vitamin deficiencies. Therefore, vitamin supplementation at moderate levels can contribute to adequate daily intake in these athletes. A vitamin deficiency may result in decreased performance and/or increased susceptibility to illness. However, vitamin supplementation at pharmacological levels has not been shown to improve performance.

In addition, vitamin E, C and β-carotene are important antioxidants. The interest in the health-related potential of antioxidants has also raised the interest of sport nutritionists. Exercise has been associated with increases in free radical production in skeletal muscle, with potential for tissue damage. It is suggested that especially in a state of overtraining the balance between oxidative stress and repair has been interrupted, leading to dysfunction of membranes and increased lipid peroxidation. However, it has also been shown that athletes have increased levels of cellular antioxidant enzymes, such as superoxide dismutase (SOD), catalase and glutathione peroxidase compared with untrained individuals. Most probably this is the result of a physiological adaptation to the higher oxidative stress and therefore it is questionable whether supplementation with antioxidants above the recommended intakes are of any benefit. So far, in this respect the available literature does not allow any claims.

With respect to the minerals, iron has probably attracted most attention regarding the advice on supplementation in athletes. Although other minerals, such as calcium, chromium, magnesium, zinc, copper and selenium, are just as important, the status of these minerals is generally adequate in most athletes. Iron loss is increased in athletes, partly due to some iron loss in sweat, increased gastrointestinal and/or urinary blood loss and foot strike haemolysis, as a consequence of the intensity and duration of the exercise. However, as mentioned before regarding other (micro) nutrients, increased iron loss is usually well compensated for by the increased dietary intake associated with the higher energy expenditure. Though many athletes, in particular females, tend to be iron-depleted, true iron deficiencies are rarely seen. Iron deficiency may be suspected in athletes who have a slightly lower than average haemoglobin (Hb), the so-called athletes' anaemia (Hb <14% in male and <12% in female endurance athletes). This is usually a training-induced physiological condition, caused by an increase in plasma volume. Despite a slightly reduced haemoglobin, the total red cell mass is normal or greater than usual. Although athletes' anaemia may be associated with low serum ferritin, this physiological condition does not respond to iron supplementation. Therefore, iron supplement use is generally considered unnecessary and supplementation without medical indication is not advised. The latter is because excessive iron supplementation can cause gastrointestinal disturbances and/or even haemosiderosis. Iron supplements have not been shown to enhance performance capacity, except where iron-deficiency anaemia exists.

18.5 ERGOGENIC AIDS

Following the recognition of glycogen loading and carbohydrate supplementation as means to improve exercise performance, much attention has been directed towards the use of nutritional supplements to optimise sports performance. In response, various nutrition companies started to develop specific sports nutrition products. Since then, sports nutrition has become a thriving branch of the food industry, and a wide variety of (sports) supplements is now available. These supplements range from the well-known sports drinks, high-energy bars and protein-shakes to a multitude of supplements containing vitamins, minerals, free amino acids, etc. These supplements are, in some cases, useful to compensate (temporarily) for a less than adequate diet, to meet the special nutrient demands induced by intense exercise training and/or to optimise exercise performance. An increasing interest has been directed towards novel ergogenic supplements, often referred to as functional foods or nutraceuticals. From the term nutraceuticals it is already clear that these supplements should be categorised somewhere between nutritional supplements and pharmaceuticals. In most cases these nutraceuticals contain compounds that do occur in a normal diet but are present in amounts far above recommended levels, or the amounts typically provided by food. Most of these supplements are proposed to increase performance capacity, often through a more pharmacological rather than a physiological effect. However, most of these claims rely on theoretical or anecdotal support rather than on documented results from scientific trials. It must be noted that such products are not registered like regular pharmaceuticals and, as such, are not under appropriate legislation or obligatory safety requirements. At present no clinical trials need to be carried out before these products are allowed to be advertised and marketed. Although the majority of the advertised nutraceuticals have not been clinically tested for their ergogenic potential nor for their safety, some nutraceuticals (e.g. caffeine, creatine, carnitine and sodium bicarbonate) have received much attention from scientists because of their proposed potential to affect muscle metabolism. Here, we will discuss the efficacy of a few currently popular ergogenic aids.

CAFFEINE

Caffeine is a well-known ergogenic aid, and was until January 2004 included on the banned substances list used by the IOC (International Olympic Committee), with an acceptance limit of 12 mg/ml in the urine. Several studies have provided evidence for the ergogenic properties of caffeine ingestion during prolonged endurance exercise tasks. These ergogenic effects have been observed even when caffeine was ingested in doses leading to urine concentrations well below IOC limits. An effective ingestion dose lies between 2 and 5 mg/kg body weight, comparable to the amount of caffeine in 2–6 cups of coffee. The performance-enhancing effect of caffeine is often attributed to its proposed stimulating effect on adipose tissue lipolysis and subsequent increase in fat oxidation rate. However, no direct in vivo evidence for this mechanism has yet been provided. A more plausible explanation would be the stimulating effect of caffeine on the central nervous system, the release and/or activity of adrenaline (epinephrine). Through this mechanism caffeine stimulates motivational aspects of behaviour, which probably explains the improved performance observed mainly during long-term endurance exercise tasks. Caffeine supplementation could be detrimental to performance capacity when an athlete is particularly sensitive to its diuretic effect. Other negative side effects associated with caffeine use include gastrointestinal distress, decreased motor control, shivering, headache, dizziness, and minor elevations in blood pressure and resting heart rate.

CREATINE

As the amount of ATP in the muscle is limited, ATP stores can only provide enough energy to perform maximum exercise for several seconds. Some of the energy necessary to rephosphorylate ADP to ATP can be derived rapidly and without oxygen by the transfer of chemical energy from creatine phosphate. Creatine phosphate levels in the cell are more than three to five times greater than ATP, and creatine phosphate serves an important function as a high-energy phosphate buffer (see Section 18.3). In healthy individuals, the total endogenous creatine pool is approximately 120 g, of which 95% is located in skeletal muscle. Each day 2 g is replenished by endogenous synthesis and dietary intake (meat and fish). Several studies have shown that oral creatine (monohydrate) supplementation increases total creatine and creatine phosphate concentrations in human skeletal muscle. Ingestion of 20 g creatine per day for a period of 2–6 days can lead to a ~20% increase in muscle creatine phosphate concentration. As an elevation in muscle creatine phosphate concentration increases the availability of energy for ATP rephosphorylation, it is not surprising that creatine supplementation has been shown to enhance performance in (repeated) high intensity, short-term exercise tasks, during which energy transfer is primarily derived from the ATP-creatine phosphate system. Consequently, creatine supplementation has become a common practice in both professional and amateur athletes (Terjung et al 2000). Most research has focused on the ergogenic effects of (short-term) creatine supplementation on (repeated) high intensity exercise performance (such as sprinting, jumping, weightlifting, volleyball, tennis, soccer, etc.). Several important possibilities concerning the long-term effects of creatine supplementation remain to be elucidated. Prolonged creatine use has been suggested to stimulate protein synthesis, especially when combined with exercise strength training. Others have speculated on the ergogenic possibilities of prolonged creatine use in endurance athletes as a means to increase oxidative capacity and increase fat oxidation. However, in vivo research has not shown any evidence for such an effect. In sports practice where body weight is an important factor in determining performance capacity of an athlete, it should be questioned whether the ergogenic metabolic effect of creatine use outweighs the concomitant increase in body weight secondary to water retention (1–2 kg) during the creatine loading phase. Though several concerns have been raised about possible side effects of creatine use, no evidence about associated health risks has been reported following short-term creatine use.

CARNITINE

Besides creatine, there is also a considerable amount of carnitine present in our skeletal muscle mass. Carnitine plays an important role in the transport of long-chain fatty acids over the mitochondrial membrane, after which they can be oxidised in the β-oxidation pathway. It has been suggested that increasing the intramuscular carnitine pool by using carnitine supplements could improve fatty acid import into the mitochondria and increase fat oxidative capacity. Consequently, claims were made suggesting that carnitine supplementation could stimulate weight loss and improve endurance performance, the latter because an increase in fat oxidative capacity would spare the limited endogenous glycogen stores. The use of carnitine became especially popular after reports in the media that the victory of the Italian football team in the 1982 World Cup could partly be attributed to the use of carnitine supplements. Carnitine, like creatine, is present in the diet (red meat and dairy products) as well as synthesised endogenously. Small amounts of carnitine are excreted in the urine and faeces. The daily excretion of carnitine (~60 mg per day) declines significantly (60–70%) when a carnitine-free diet is used. Even in such a situation endogenous synthesis rates are able to supply sufficient carnitine to maintain normal bodily functions in healthy subjects. Conversely, numerous studies have shown no change in muscle carnitine content after supplementation with substantial amounts of carnitine, leaving no room for further speculations about any ergogenic properties of carnitine supplementation in healthy subjects.

SODIUM BICARBONATE

Sodium bicarbonate ($NaHCO_3$), also known as 'baking soda', can also be regarded as an ergogenic aid. Anaerobic glycolysis is the major source of energy supply during exercise of near maximal intensity lasting longer than 20–30 seconds (see Section 18.3). The total capacity of this energy system is limited by the progressive increase in the acidity of the intracellular environment by the accumulation of hydrogen ions. The latter inhibits muscle contraction by impairing the role of calcium in this process and by reducing the activity of several glycolytic key enzymes. This leads to muscular pain and fatigue and the inability to maintain exercise intensity for a more prolonged period. As bicarbonate represents the most important extracellular buffer for the accumulation of hydrogen ions, it has been suggested that an increase in plasma bicarbonate levels might delay the onset of muscular fatigue during prolonged anaerobic metabolism. Studies have indeed shown that bicarbonate loading in athletes (0.3 g $NaHCO_3$ per kg body weight taken 1–2 hours before exercise with 1 litre water) can improve performance in exercise tasks lasting between 0.5 and 6.0 minutes of near maximal performance. The use of bicarbonate does not seem to pose any major health risks, but gastrointestinal distress as well as hyperosmotic diarrhoea have often been reported following bicarbonate loading.

ERGOGENIC AIDS IN SPORTS PRACTICE

Though nutraceuticals such as caffeine, creatine, carnitine and sodium bicarbonate have received much attention, scientific data on most ergogenic substances such as bee-pollen, royal jelly, hydroxycitrate, guarana, taurine, ginseng, yohimbe, colostrum and various other exotic ingredients are either scarce or not available at all. Therefore, one should be aware of the nutritional quackery which offers athletes a wide variety of products and misleading information about preferred dosages and applications. Only a few nutraceuticals, under specific circumstances and proper guidance, have been shown to improve performance capacity. Whether the use of such ergogenic aids should be encouraged in recreational and/or professional sports practice is highly questionable. More important is to realise that a healthy diet, compensating for the metabolic demands imposed by intense exercise training and competition, forms the basis of good nutritional practice and should be a first priority in any effort to optimise performance capacity.

KEY POINTS

- The main nutritional need of an athlete is to consume sufficient food to compensate for the increased energy expenditure.
- Daily energy needs may double for a marathon, and increase up to three- to four-fold during cycling events like the Tour de France.
- In athletes, between-meal snacks can supply up to 30% of daily energy intake, and therefore should be of good nutritional quality (containing not only carbohydrates but also fat, protein and micronutrients).
- Dietary intake in female endurance runners, ballet dancers and gymnasts has often been reported to be insufficient for the supply of adequate energy as well as micronutrients.
- From a quantitative point of view, muscle glycogen stores form the most important energy source during moderate-to-high intensity exercise.
- Endogenous carbohydrate stores are relatively small and therefore often play a key role in limiting endurance performance capacity.
- Carbohydrate loading in the days preceding endurance competition represents an effective means to optimise pre-exercise glycogen content.
- During prolonged endurance exercise (>45 minutes) carbohydrate ingestion (up to 1.1 g/min) can significantly improve performance capacity.
- Ingestion of low-protein, carbohydrate-rich drinks and food soon after cessation of exercise accelerates recovery.
- Endurance training increases fat oxidative capacity, thereby reducing reliance on the limited endogenous carbohydrate stores.
- Protein requirements of athletes range between 1.1 and 1.4 g/kg bodyweight/day. These requirements are easily met by the increased food intake of athletes.
- Fluids and electrolytes need to be supplied during prolonged exercise to compensate for sweat loss.
- In general, vitamin and mineral needs in the athlete are fully compensated for by the increased dietary intake. Therefore when a basic healthy diet is used, vitamin and mineral supplements are unnecessary. Vitamin and/or mineral supplementation does not improve performance capacity when no deficiencies are present.
- Only a few nutraceuticals (e.g. caffeine and creatine), under specific circumstances and proper guidance, have been shown to improve performance capacity. Caution is needed to assess the dubious nutritional merits of the wide range of sports supplements/nutraceuticals available to professional as well as recreational athletes.

References

Bergström J, Hultman E: Muscle glycogen synthesis after exercise: an enhancing factor localised in the muscle cells in man, *Nature* 210:309–312, 1966.

Christensen EH, Hansen O: Respiratorischer Quotient und O₂-Aufnahme, *Scandinavian Archives of Physiology* 81:180–189, 1939.

Hoppeler H, Howald H, Conley K, et al: Endurance training in humans: aerobic capacity and structure of skeletal muscle, *Journal of Applied Physiology* 59:320–327, 1985.

Koopman R, Beelen M, Stellingwerff T, et al: Coingestion of carbohydrate with protein does not further augment postexercise muscle protein synthesis, *American Journal of Physiology* 293:E833–E842, 2007.

Martin WH, Dalsky GP, Hurley BF, et al: Effect of endurance training on plasma FFA turnover and oxidation during exercise, *American Journal of Physiology* 256:E708–E714, 1993.

Phillips SM: Dietary protein for athletes: from requirements to metabolic advantage, *Applied Physiology, Nutrition, and Metabolism* 31:647–654, 2007.

Saris WHM, Van Erp-Baart AMJ, Brouns F: Study on food intake and energy expenditure during extreme sustained exercise: the Tour de France, *International Journal of Sports Medicine* 10(1):S26–S31, 1989.

Shulman GI: Cellular mechanisms of insulin resistance, *Journal of Clinical Investigation* 106:171–176, 2000.

Terjung RL, Clarkson P, Eichner ER, et al: American College of Sports Medicine roundtable. The physiological and health effects of oral creatine supplementation, *Medicine and Science in Sports and Exercise* 32(3):706–717, 2000.

Tipton KD, Ferrando AA, Phillips SM, et al: Postexercise net protein synthesis in human muscle from orally administered amino acids, *American Journal of Physiology* 276:E28–E634, 1999.

Van Loon LJC, Jeukendrup AE, Saris WHM, Wagenmakers AJM: Effect of training status on fuel selection during submaximal exercise with glucose ingestion, *Journal of Applied Physiology* 87(4):1413–1420, 1999.

Van Loon LJC, Greenhaff PL, Constantin-Teodosiu D, et al: The effects of increasing exercise intensity on muscle fuel utilisation in humans, *Journal of Physiology* 536:295–304, 2001.

Wagenmakers AJM, Brouns F, Saris WHM, Halliday D: Oxidation rates of orally ingested carbohydrates during prolonged exercise in men, *Journal of Applied Physiology* 77:2774–2780, 1993.

Wilmore JH, Costill DL: *Physiology of sport and exercise,* Champaign, 1994, Human Kinetics.

Further reading

Hultman E, Harris RC: Carbohydrate metabolism. In Poortmans JR, editor: *Principles of exercise biochemistry,* Basel, 1988, Karger, pp 78–119.

Jeukendrup AE, Raben A, Gijsen A: Glucose kinetics during prolonged exercise in highly trained human subjects: effect of glucose ingestion, *Journal of Physiology* 515:579–589, 1999.

Rehrer NJ, Wagenmakers AJM, Beckers EJ: Gastric emptying, absorption and carbohydrate oxidation during prolonged exercise, *Journal of Applied Physiology* 72:468–474, 1992.

Van Loon LJC, Saris WHM, Kruijshoop M, Wagenmakers AJM: Maximizing postexercise muscle glycogen synthesis: carbohydrate supplementation and the application of amino acid/protein hydrolyzate mixtures, *American Journal of Clinical Nutrition* 72:106–111, 2000.

Williams C, Devlin JT, editors: *Foods, nutrition and sports performance,* London, 1992, E & FN Spon.

Williams MH, Kreider RB, Branch JD: *Creatine; the power supplement,* Champaign, 1999, Human Kinetics.

PART 5

Clinical nutrition

Chapter 19

Cardiovascular disease

Jim Mann

CHAPTER CONTENTS

OBJECTIVES

At the end of this chapter you should:
- know the prevalence of cardiovascular disease in different parts of the world and be aware of the changing mortality rates in different countries
- know the risk factors for cardiovascular disease and their nutritional determinants
- be aware of the clinical trials in which diet has been modified to reduce cardiovascular risk
- have an understanding of how information from epidemiological studies may be translated into practical dietary advice for individuals and populations.

19.1 INTRODUCTION

Cardiovascular diseases account for an appreciable proportion of mortality and serious morbidity in adults throughout the world. The different conditions assume varying degrees of importance in different countries. This chapter describes the cardiovascular diseases in which nutritional factors have been shown to play an important role in aetiology and management. Thus, the emphasis is on coronary heart disease (CHD) and cerebrovascular disease (stroke). The disease process primarily affects the arteries with symptoms and signs resulting from the consequent reduction in blood supply. It is important to appreciate the terminology used to describe the pathological process and clinical entities.

Atherosclerosis is the basic pathological lesion which tends to occlude the arteries to a varying

© 2010 Elsevier Ltd/Inc/BV
DOI: 10.1016/B978-0-7020-3118-2.00019-X

extent. A superimposed *thrombus*, or clot, may produce further narrowing to the extent that the artery is totally blocked. A variety of cells and lipids are involved in the pathogenesis of the atherosclerotic plaque and the arterial thrombus, including lipoproteins, cholesterol, triglycerides, platelets, monocytes, endothelial cells, fibroblasts and smooth muscle cells. Nutrition may influence the risk of CHD or stroke by modifying either atherogenesis or thrombogenesis or both processes. Two major clinical conditions may occur when atherosclerosis, with or without a superimposed thrombus, affects the coronary arteries (arteries supplying the heart muscle itself). *Angina pectoris* is characterised by pain or discomfort in the chest which is brought on by exertion or stress, and which may also radiate down the left arm and to the neck. It results from a reduction or temporary block to the blood flow through the coronary artery to the myocardium. The pain usually passes with rest and seldom lasts for more than 15 minutes. A *coronary thrombosis* or *myocardial infarction* results from prolonged total occlusion of the artery, which causes infarction or death of some of the heart muscle and is associated with prolonged and usually excruciating central chest pain. The terms coronary thrombosis and myocardial infarction are used to describe the same clinical condition, although they really describe the two pathological processes which underlie the disease. Together these two conditions are referred to as *coronary heart disease* or *ischaemic heart disease*. The terms are regarded as synonymous and relate to the two different pathological processes, the former to the disease of the coronary arteries which provide the heart with its blood supply whereas the latter describes the effects of reduced blood supply on the myocardium or heart muscle. When a similar disease process influences the blood supply to the brain a *cerebral thrombosis* or *stroke* occurs. A typical consequence of the effect on brain tissue is weakness or paralysis of one side of the body though the precise nature of the abnormality will depend upon where the block has occurred in the arterial system. This condition is comparable with a coronary thrombosis or myocardial infarction. A less than total block may produce short-term consequences (less than 24 hours) involving weakness on one side and difficulty with speech, known as a *transient ischaemic attack*. Such a clinical event is akin to angina. These conditions are referred to as *cerebrovascular diseases*. Reduced blood supply to the muscles of the legs resulting from atherosclerosis to

Table 19.1	Risk factors for coronary heart disease
Irreversible	• Masculine gender • Increasing age • Genetic traits, including monogenic and polygenic disorders of lipid metabolism • Body build
Potentially reversible	• Cigarette smoking • Dyslipidaemia: increased levels of cholesterol, triglyceride, low density and very low density lipoprotein and low levels of high density lipoprotein • Oxidisability of low density lipoprotein • Obesity, especially when associated with high waist circumference or waist/hip ratio • Hypertension • Physical inactivity • Hyperglycaemia, diabetes and insulin resistance • Increased thrombosis: increased haemostatic factors and enhanced platelet aggregation • High levels of homocysteine • High levels of inflammatory markers (e.g. CRP, IL-6, TNFα) • Impaired fetal nutrition
Psychosocial	• Low socioeconomic class • Stressful situations • Coronary-prone behaviour patterns: type A behaviour
Geographic	• Climate and season: cold weather • Soft drinking water

the arteries most distant to the heart (iliac and femoral arteries) causes pain on exercise in the muscle group(s) supplied by the affected arteries. The symptom of this peripheral vascular disease is known as intermittent claudication. Peripheral vascular disease is less clearly linked to nutrition than is CHD or stroke.

This chapter describes the epidemiology of cardiovascular disease, the risk factors (Table 19.1), nutritional determinants and the potential for dietary modification to reduce cardiovascular risk.

19.2 PREVALENCE OF CORONARY HEART DISEASE

In most industrialised countries CHD is the commonest single cause of death. Overall rates are higher in men than women, though as women age CHD contributes a greater proportion of total mortality. In recent years, in addition to the deaths, there are probably at least as many hospital discharges. This is still an appreciable under-estimate of the total morbidity resulting from CHD. Some cases of myocardial infarction, especially in older people, are not admitted to hospital and there are no statistics regarding the far greater number of people who are debilitated by angina pectoris even though they may not have suffered an acute myocardial infarction. Thus the cost to the health care services, to society as a whole and to individuals and their families is enormous. It should be noted that in more than half of all fatal myocardial infarctions, death occurs in the first hour after the attack. Most CHD deaths, therefore, occur too rapidly for treatment to influence the prognosis. Therefore in the medium and long term risk reduction rather than treatment of established disease provides the only means of reducing the burden of CVD.

There are marked international differences in rates of CHD (Fig. 19.1). Mortality rates are more than seven times higher in some Eastern European countries than they are in Japan. In Europe there is an almost three-fold difference between France,

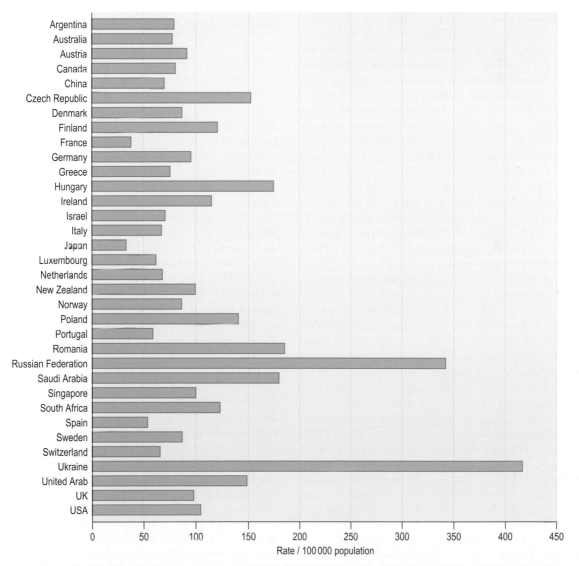

Fig. 19.1 International differences in coronary heart disease (CHD) rates. League table for 2002: mortality in men and women aged 40–69 years. *Source: WHO (2002) Death and DALY estimates. http: www.who.int/healthinfo/en/*

Spain and Portugal on the one hand and such countries as Finland, Scotland and Northern Ireland on the other. Some of the variation between countries is undoubtedly due to differences in diagnostic practice and coding of death certificates, but numerous studies using comparable methods have confirmed that real differences do exist in the frequency of the disease.

These international comparisons have played an important part in the search for causes. The experience of migrants suggests that these variations between countries are likely to be the result chiefly of environmental and behavioural differences. People who have migrated from a low-risk country (e.g. Japan) to a high-risk country (e.g. the USA) tend to have rates of CHD approaching that of the host country. There is also some evidence for the reverse: Finns living in Sweden have appreciably lower rates than those in their country of origin. In the UK, where CHD rates are appreciably higher in Scotland and Northern Ireland than in England, CHD risk depends upon country of residence at the time of death rather than country of birth.

Further evidence for the role of potentially modifiable factors comes from the major changes in the CHD rates of many countries (see Fig. *evolve* 19.1). Among men these include the increase in many European countries, North America, Australia and New Zealand during most of the third quarter of the twentieth century. Thereafter there was a continuing increase in most of Eastern Europe whereas in nearly all western European countries, North American and Oceania rates have shown an appreciable decline. In most countries except for Eastern Europe the rates in women also declined over the same period (Beaglehole 1999). More recently there has been a decline in some of the countries in Eastern Europe (Zatonski et al 2008). In general the decline has been most marked in countries where the attempt to reduce cardiovascular risk factors has been most effective. The situation is particularly complex in some countries where affluence and poverty tend to coexist and which are said to be in a state of nutrition transition. In such countries (e.g. India, South Africa) coronary heart disease and diseases of undernutrition tend to coexist, with rapidly escalating rates of CHD amongst some sections of the population. This change over a relatively short period of time encourages the belief that the disease is preventable if the causes can be found and modified. The hope is to reduce morbidity and mortality from CHD in those who are in the prime of life. Unfortunately there are only very limited data regarding trends in morbidity and it has been suggested that the reduction in mortality has not always been paralleled by a reduction in morbidity, suggesting that different mechanisms may be operating.

19.3 EPIDEMIOLOGICAL AND EXPERIMENTAL EVIDENCE LINKING DIET WITH CORONARY HEART DISEASE

THE ORIGINAL DIET–HEART HYPOTHESIS: THE LINK WITH SATURATED AND n–6 POLYUNSATURATED FATTY ACIDS

Much of our current understanding of the link between nutrition and coronary heart disease stems from the classical study of Ancel and Keys and coworkers in seven countries, selected because of their widely varying rates of coronary heart disease and mortality. Measured food consumption by people in 16 defined cohorts in these seven countries, and 10-year incidence rates of CHD deaths, form the basis for the correlations tested in the Seven Country Study (Keys 1980). The strongest correlation was noted between CHD and the percentage of energy derived from saturated fat (see Fig. *evolve* 19.2). Weaker inverse associations were found between percentages of energy derived from monounsaturated and polyunsaturated fat and CHD. Total fat was not significantly correlated with CHD death. Of the other well-known risk factors for CHD (see next section and Table 19.1) investigated in this study, only cholesterol and blood pressure appeared to be related to the geographical variation, leading to the suggestion that it is principally the nutrition-related factors which determine whether countries are likely to have high CHD rates. This study also provides evidence that the degree of risk conferred by factors not specifically related to nutrition is strongly influenced by nutrition-related factors. This is well illustrated by the more powerful relationship between cigarette smoking and CHD in the USA and northern Europe than in southern Europe (see Fig. *evolve* 19.3). Saturated fat intake and mean cholesterol levels were higher in the USA and northern Europe than in southern Europe. Saturated fat was believed to increase coronary heart disease risk because of its ability to elevate cholesterol levels and the modest protective effect of polyunsaturated fat (chiefly n-6 fatty acids) to act via cholesterol lowering. The epidemiological associations between cholesterol and fatty acids was confirmed by Keys in experimental studies, and an equation was developed some 50 years ago which demonstrated that when considering groups of individuals, change in serum cholesterol could be predicted from changes in dietary saturated and polyunsaturated fatty acids, and to a lesser extent dietary cholesterol:

$$\Delta \text{ plasma cholesterol in mmol/l}$$
$$= 0.035\,[2\Delta S - \Delta P] + 0.08\sqrt{\text{chol/MJ}}$$

Where chol/MJ = cholesterol intake in mg per megajoule, ΔS and ΔP = changes in percentages of dietary energy derived from saturated and polyunsaturated fatty acids (Keys et al 1965).

These findings have been repeatedly corroborated and extended (Kris-Etherton et al 2001). It is now clear that dietary saturated and n-6 polyunsaturated fatty acids predominantly influence low-density lipoprotein (LDL) cholesterol for which total cholesterol is a surrogate measure, and that the effects of myristic and palmitic acids in elevating total and LDL cholesterol are more marked than lauric acid. Stearic acid, the other major dietary saturated fatty acid, appears to have little effect on levels of lipids and lipoproteins. High intakes of saturated fatty acids are also associated with relatively high levels of high-density lipoprotein (HDL), but the effect on HDL is less marked than the effect on LDL.

Recent meta-analyses confirm the potential of n-6 polyunsaturated fatty acids to reduce LDL cholesterol and reduce cardiovascular risk. However very high intakes of n-6 polyunsaturated fatty acids (10% total energy) may reduce HDL as well as LDL. The effect of altering dietary cholesterol on LDL is much less than the effect of changing the nature of dietary fat. Despite the consistency of lipoprotein response to manipulation of dietary fatty acids when considering groups of individuals, there is considerable individual variation which cannot be explained by variation in compliance to dietary advice. Although ApoE polymorphisms have been associated with extent of lipoprotein response to changes in dietary fatty acids and cholesterol, genetic variation has not thus far been able to meaningfully distinguish responders from non-responders. A range of candidate genes have been examined but it seems likely that extent of response to diet is influenced by many different genes.

More recently it has become clear that saturated and n-6 polyunsaturated fatty acids may influence cardiovascular risk by mechanisms other than the effects on lipoproteins. Epidemiological and experimental evidence suggests that high intakes of saturated fatty acids reduce sensitivity to the action of insulin and so can increase cardiovascular risk via the range of abnormalities associated with the metabolic syndrome. There is also evidence that saturated fatty acids may enhance thrombogenesis. A mechanism may be via increased platelet aggregation as a result of inhibition of anti-aggregatory prostacyclin. Similarly n-6 polyunsaturated fatty acids may reduce platelet aggregation.

Despite this body of evidence suggesting a link between high intakes of saturated fatty acids and CHD, predominantly via an LDL-elevating mechanism, some inconsistencies have emerged. In particular, it has been noted that the French had relatively high intakes of saturated fatty acids and lower than expected rates of CHD. This has been attributed to the mitigating effects of protective factors (see below) and has sometimes been referred to as the 'French Paradox'. A similar phenomenon has been observed in other countries. It is also noteworthy that some within-population prospective studies have not demonstrated an increased cardiovascular risk associated with high intakes of saturated fatty acids nor a protective effect of n-6 polyunsaturated fatty acids. This is probably due to the range of intakes in a single population being too narrow to demonstrate an association.

CARDIOVASCULAR RISK FACTORS

Risk factors for CHD have principally been identified in prospective epidemiological studies. Like the Seven Country Study, the Framingham Study (Stykowski et al 1990), one of the earliest such cohort studies, confirmed increasing levels of cholesterol, blood pressure and cigarette smoking as important determinants of cardiovascular risk. The presence of diabetes and impaired glucose tolerance, obesity and lack of physical activity were also identified as cardiovascular risk factors at a relatively early stage of the research in this field. All these factors are associated with a graded increase in risk and in the case of cholesterol and blood pressure there is convincing evidence from randomised controlled intervention trials that lowering the risk factor reduces risk, thus providing robust evidence that the association is a causal one and that benefit is likely to accrue in populations as well as in individuals if the risk factor is modified. More recent analyses from the Framingham Study as well as very many more recent prospective studies have identified a host of physico-chemical as well as psychosocial risk factors some of which are potentially modifiable and some not (Table 19.1). Several are potentially amenable to modification by lifestyle changes. The role of individual dietary factors has been directly studied in only relatively few prospective studies since reliable dietary data are difficult to gather in studies of this type, usually involving tens of thousands of subjects. Most of the recent data regarding food and nutrients are derived from the various studies of health professionals studied by Willett and colleagues from Harvard. The section which follows describes dietary determinants of cardiovascular risk which, like saturated and n-6 unsaturated fatty acids, discussed earlier, have been identified in prospective epidemiological studies and investigated further using various experimental approaches.

NUTRITION–RELATED DETERMINANTS OF CARDIOVASCULAR RISK

Most of the early attempts to study dietary determinants of CHD rates were based on food or nutrient data derived from national food consumption data, the balance sheets of the Food and Agriculture Organization or, in the UK, more reliably, on household food surveys and on the national mortality statistics before 1970, during which time CHD was increasing (at least in men) in most affluent societies. The studies have either been cross-cultural comparisons at a single point in time, or an examination of increasing trends in relation to changing food consumption data in one or more countries. Positive associations with saturated fat, sucrose, animal protein and coffee, and negative correlations with flour (and other complex carbohydrates) and vegetables are some of the best described.

Perhaps more interesting are relatively recent studies from the USA, the UK, Eastern Europe, Australia, New Zealand and Iceland, which have examined the downward trend of CHD rates in relation to dietary change (Tuomilehto et al 1986, Pietinen et al 1996, Zatonski et al 2008). There are certainly associations between falling CHD rates apparent in these countries and changes in some foods and nutrients, but in view of the strong correlations (positive and negative) among different

dietary constituents it is difficult to be sure which dietary factor is principally involved, or indeed whether dietary change is simply occurring in parallel with some other more important environmental factor, e.g. increasing physical activity and reduction in cigarette smoking (Stykowski et al 1990). Furthermore, population food consumption data are notoriously unreliable (they are usually derived from local production figures, imports and exports, often with an incomplete account of quantities not utilised as food), and the accuracy with which mortality is recorded varies from country to country. Consequently, such data do not provide direct evidence concerning aetiology, only clues for further research. However some associations have been demonstrated as a result of direct measurements and corroborated in experimental situations.

Fish and n–3 polyunsaturated fatty acids

The Eskimo people (Inuit) of Greenland appear to have low rates of CHD despite a high intake of fat. The fat in the diet of the Greenland Eskimo is derived almost exclusively from marine foods, which contain large quantities of the n-3 fatty acids eicosopentaenoate (EPA, C20:5) and docosahexaenoate (DHA, C22:6). This observation was largely responsible for a considerable body of experimental and epidemiological research which suggested that regular consumption of fish, especially oily fish and fish oil, is protective against CHD. Reduced platelet aggregation appears to explain the reduced cardiovascular risk. The n-3 fatty acids (C20: 5 and C22: 6) form the anti-aggregatory prostanoid PGI_3. Platelet aggregation is largely controlled by a balance between the pro-aggregatory compound thromboxane A_2 (synthesised from arachidonic acid released from the platelet membrane after injury to the blood vessel wall) and the anti-aggregatory substance prostacyclin PGI_2 (also synthesised from arachidonic acid in the endothelial cells of the arterial wall). C20:5 and C22:6 inhibit conversion of arachidonic acid to thromboxane A_2 as well as facilitating the production of the additional anti-aggregatory substance PGI_3 (Fig. 19.2). The n-3 fatty acids may also reduce cardiovascular risk via effects on cardiac electrophysiology, arterial compliance, endothelial function, blood pressure, vascular reactivity and inflammation. It has been suggested that vegetable sources of n-3 fatty acids (α-linolenic acid) may

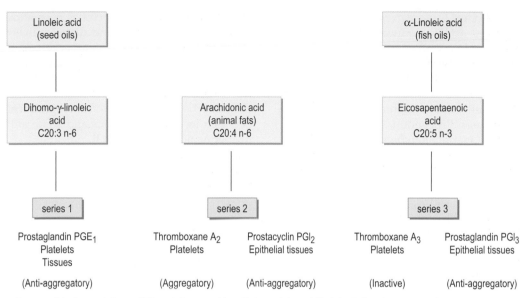

Fig. 19.2 Prostanoids formed from different fatty acids. *(Adapted from Ulbricht & Southgate 1991)*

similarly confer cardioprotection and explain at least to some extent the recent reduction in CHD mortality in some Eastern European countries (Zatonski et al 2008).

n–6 Unsaturated fatty acids

In addition to their potential to reduce LDL, polyunsaturated fatty acids of the n-6 series may also reduce CHD risk by reducing platelet aggregation by providing the series 1 prostanoid PGE$_1$, which is anti-aggregatory. Oleic acid may also act as an inhibitor of platelet aggregation, though the effect is less than for polyunsaturated fatty acids.

Trans-unsaturated fatty acids

Trans-unsaturated fatty acids are geometrical isomers of *cis*-unsaturated fatty acids that adopt a saturated fatty acid-like configuration. Partial hydrogenation, the process used to increase shelf-life of polyunsaturated fatty acids (PUFAs), creates *trans* fatty acids and also removes the critical double bonds in essential fatty acids. Metabolic studies have demonstrated that trans fatty acids render the plasma lipid profile even more atherogenic than saturated fatty acids, by not only elevating LDL cholesterol but also by decreasing HDL cholesterol and increasing lipoprotein (a). Several large cohort studies have found an increased risk of CHD associated with an increased intake of *trans* fatty acids.

Most *trans* fatty acids in the diet are derived from industrially hardened oils. Even though *trans* fatty acids have been reduced or eliminated from retail fats and spreads in many parts of the world, deep-fried fast foods, confectionery products and baked goods are a major and increasing source.

Antioxidant nutrients, flavonoids

Low-density lipoproteins appear to be atherogenic primarily when the constituent lipid is oxidised. Many experimental studies have shown that several dietary antioxidants, notably β-carotene, vitamin E and vitamin C, reduce LDL oxidation in vitro. Prospective epidemiological studies confirm these observations, the findings being particularly consistent for vitamin E as well as a group of biologically active substances known as flavonoids in berries, fruits and some vegetables. It is of interest to note that more recent cross-country comparisons similar to those undertaken in the original Seven Country Study have suggested that CHD risk may be predicted more accurately when antioxidant nutrient status is considered in addition to the conventional major risk factors. A high intake of nutrients and other substances with antioxidant activity may be at least a partial explanation for the 'French Paradox', the term used to describe the apparently paradoxical observation that the French have a remarkably low rate of CHD despite cholesterol levels that do not differ markedly from those in other European countries with much higher rates of CHD. Reduced susceptibility of LDL to oxidation may offset the detrimental effects of this potentially atherogenic lipoprotein. However, intervention trials involving antioxidant nutrients given as supplements have not generally been shown to be effective at reducing CHD risk (see 'Heart Outcomes Prevention Evaluation (HOPE) Study' and 'Overall perspective of the trials', below).

B vitamins

Case-control and prospective cohort studies have shown that an elevated plasma homocysteine concentration is associated with an increased risk of cardiovascular disease (Mangoni & Jackson 2002). Folic acid, vitamins B_2, B_6 and B_{12} all act as coenzymes for the metabolism of homocysteine and many studies have shown an inverse relationship between folate intake (and to a lesser extent, other B vitamins) and plasma homocysteine concentration. The consumption of folate-fortified foods (especially breakfast cereals) has been shown to lower plasma homocysteine (Venn et al 2002), but when folate is consumed in naturally occurring foods, the consumption of large quantities of folate-rich foods seems to be necessary to achieve appreciable homocysteine-lowering. Whether elevated plasma homocysteine concentration is a cause of cardiovascular disease or whether it is simply behaving as a biomarker of risk has not yet been fully resolved.

Wholegrain cereals and dietary fibre (non–starch polysaccharides)

The suggestion that unprocessed or lightly processed carbohydrate-containing foods might be protective against coronary heart disease as well as diabetes first received prominence in the 1970s when Trowell drew attention to the low rates of both conditions in Uganda where such foods provided a very high proportion of total energy. Of course there were many potentially confounding variables but high intakes of wholegrain cereals have now been repeatedly shown to confer cardioprotection in prospective studies (Truswell 1995). There are many possible explanations. High intakes of carbohydrates may be associated with reduced intakes of total and saturated fat. Wholegrain cereals are rich in dietary fibre (non-starch

polysaccharide; NSP), which has been shown to be protective against CHD and diabetes in some prospective studies. Soluble rather than insoluble forms of NSP reduce total and LDL cholesterol, and these carbohydrates occur to a greater extent in legumes, pulses and certain vegetables and fruits than in wholegrain cereals. Wholegrain cereals are also rich in unsaturated oils and some antioxidant nutrients, notably vitamin E.

Sodium and potassium

High blood pressure is a major risk factor for CHD and both forms of stroke (ischaemic and haemorrhagic). Of the many risk factors associated with high blood pressure, the dietary exposure that has been most investigated is sodium intake. It has been studied extensively in animal experimental models, in epidemiological studies and in controlled clinical trials. Data from these studies show convincingly that sodium intake is directly associated with blood pressure. An overview of observational data obtained from population studies suggests that a difference in sodium intake of 100 mmol (2.3 g) per day is associated with average differences in systolic blood pressure of 5 mmHg at age 15–19 years and 10 mmHg at age 60–69 years). Diastolic blood pressures are reduced by about half as much, but the association increases with age and magnitude of the initial blood pressure. It is estimated that a universal reduction in dietary intake of sodium by 50 mmol (1.5 g) per day would lead to a 50% reduction in the number of people requiring antihypertensive therapy, a 22% reduction in the number of deaths resulting from strokes and a 16% reduction in the number of deaths from CHD.

Cutler et al (1997) carried out a systematic review of the effects of dietary salt reduction on blood pressure levels. Based on an overview of 32 methodologically adequate trials, Cutler et al concluded that a daily reduction of sodium intake by 70–80 mmol was associated with a lowering of blood pressure in both hypertensive and normotensive individuals, with systolic and diastolic blood pressure reductions of 4.8/1.9 mmHg in the former and 2.5/1.1 mmHg in the latter. Clinical trials have also demonstrated the sustainable blood pressure lowering effects of sodium restriction in infancy as well as in the elderly in whom it provides a useful non-pharmacological therapy. One low sodium diet trial showed that low sodium diets, with 24-hour sodium excretion levels around 70 mmol, are effective and safe. Some individuals appear to be more sensitive to the blood pressure raising effects of sodium, but there is no clearly defined method of identifying such individuals.

A meta-analysis of randomised controlled trials reported that potassium supplements, typically 60–100 mmol/day (median 75 mmol/day) reduced mean blood pressures (systolic/diastolic) by 1.8/1.0 mmHg in normotensive subjects and 4.4/2.5 mmHg in hypertensive subjects (Whelton et al 1997). Several large cohort studies have also found an inverse association between potassium intake and risk of stroke. While potassium supplements have been shown to have protective effects on blood pressure and cardiovascular disease (CVD), there is no strong argument for their long-term use to reduce the risk for CVD. The levels of fruit and vegetable intake recommended by the World Health Organization and many national bodies should ensure an adequate intake of potassium. The DASH trials, which have examined dietary approaches to reduce blood pressure, found the maximum effect to be achieved by a high intake of vegetables, fruit and low fat dairy products in conjunction with a low sodium intake.

Nuts

Several large epidemiological studies have demonstrated that frequent consumption of nuts is associated with decreased risk of CHD. Most of these studies considered nuts as a group, combining many different types of nuts. Nuts are high in unsaturated fatty acids and low in saturated fats, and may contribute to cholesterol lowering by altering the fatty acid profile of the diet as a whole. However, because of the high energy content of nuts, advice to include them in the diet must be tempered in accordance with the desired energy balance.

Alcohol

There is evidence that low to moderate alcohol consumption lowers the risk of CHD. In a systematic review of ecological, case-control and cohort studies in which specific associations were available between consumption of beer, wine and spirits, and risk of CHD it was found that all alcoholic drinks were linked with lower risk. The beneficial effect may result from an HDL-raising effect of alcohol or the antioxidant content of some alcoholic beverages. However, other cardiovascular and health risks associated with alcohol do not favour a general recommendation for its use as a preventive measure against cardiovascular disease.

Boiled, unfiltered coffee

Boiled, unfiltered coffee raises total and LDL cholesterol because coffee beans contain a terpenoid lipid called cafestol. The amount of cafestol in the cup depends on the brewing method: it is zero for paper-filtered drip coffee, and high in the unfiltered coffee still widely drunk, for example, in Greece, the Middle East and Turkey. Intake of large amounts of unfiltered coffee markedly raises serum cholesterol and has been associated with CHD in Norway. A shift from unfiltered, boiled coffee to filtered coffee may have contributed to the decline in serum cholesterol in Finland.

Soya protein

Soya protein has been shown to inhibit atherosclerosis in animals. While there is no conclusive evidence of such an effect in humans, soya protein undoubtedly has a favourable effect on several cardiovascular risk factors. The beneficial effect on plasma lipoproteins (LDL cholesterol, triglyceride and possibly HDL cholesterol) has been the basis of the US Food and Drug Administration's approval of a health claim that '25 g of soya protein a day, as part of a diet low in saturated fat and cholesterol, may reduce the risk of heart disease'. Soya isoflavones have been shown to lower blood pressure. There is also some evidence of beneficial effects on vascular and endothelial function, platelet activation and aggregation, LDL oxidation and smooth muscle cell proliferation and migration. Several trials indicate that soya has a beneficial effect on plasma lipids (see Additional references section on the *evolve* website).

Obesity

Obesity is a major risk factor for CHD. While increasing body mass index (BMI) shows a modest and graded association with myocardial infarction, increasing waist circumference and waist/hip ratio show a more striking relationship. The effect is not surprising given the association between excess adiposity and several other risk factors, notably dyslipidaemia, hypertension, insulin resistance and type 2 diabetes. Weight loss corrects most of the clinical and metabolic derangements seen in overweight and obese individuals.

Impaired fetal nutrition

Robinson and Barker (2002) in Southampton observed some time ago that low-birthweight babies, especially those who tended to gain weight rapidly in early life, were more prone than those of normal weight to a range of clinical and metabolic abnormalities (including obesity, hypertension, dyslipidaemia, insulin resistance) that predispose to the increased risk of CHD and diabetes in later life. The fetal origins hypothesis (Barker) suggests that maternal malnutrition at critical stages of fetal development leads to intrauterine growth retardation, including decreased pancreatic islet β cells, decreased number of nephrons, insulin resistance and a range of other abnormalities which are not associated with later chronic diseases if the child remains in a relatively deprived nutritional environment. However, problems are proposed to occur if the malnourished fetus is born into conditions of adequate nutrition or overnutrition and rapid catch-up growth occurs. Much debate and research centres on the explanation for the observation, but the hypothesis has been offered as an explanation for the massive increase in cardiovascular disease and type 2 diabetes that has occurred with increasing affluence in some developing countries. The main message to be taken from this research at this stage is the importance of adequate and appropriate nutrition for women of childbearing age. There is insufficient evidence to recommend altering current advice regarding infant feeding practices.

Strength of evidence

The 2003 WHO/FAO report *Diet, nutrition and the prevention of chronic diseases* has classified each of the nutritional factors that have been related to cardiovascular disease according to level of evidence. Table 19.2 summarises the findings of this report (Joint WHO/FAO Expert Consultation 2003).

Table 19.2   Summary of the findings of the WHO/FAO report *Diet, nutrition and the prevention of chronic diseases* relating to lifestyle factors and risk of developing cardiovascular disease

EVIDENCE	DECREASED RISK	NO RELATIONSHIP	INCREASED RISK
Convincing	Regular physical activity Linoleic acid Fish and fish oils (EHA, DHA) Vegetables and fruits (including berries) Potassium Low-moderate alcohol intake (for CHD)	Vitamin E supplements	Myristic and palmitic acids *Trans*-unsaturated fatty acids High sodium intake Overweight High alcohol intake (for stroke)
Probable	α-Linolenic acid Oleic acid Non-starch polysaccharide Wholegrain cereals Nuts (unsalted) Plant sterols/stanols Folate	Stearic acid	Dietary cholesterol Unfiltered boiled coffee
Possible	Flavonoids Soy products		Fats rich in lauric acid Impaired fetal nutrition β-carotene supplements
Insufficient	Calcium Magnesium Vitamin C		Carbohydrates Iron

EPA, eicosapentaenoic acid.
DHA, docosahexaenoic acid.

Cardioprotective dietary patterns

It should be clear from the above that a range of dietary patterns may be protective against CHD. The Mediterranean diet has probably received the most attention, with populations consuming the traditional diets of countries surrounding the Mediterranean Sea having low rates of CHD. Several attributes of such diets are associated with reduced levels of cardiovascular risk factors. However, it is important to emphasise that there are other equally cardioprotective dietary patterns including traditional Asian diets and indeed a modified typical Western diet. Attributes of cardioprotective dietary patterns are listed in Table 19.3. In a recent study, a 'portfolio' of such dietary changes, together with the use of plant sterol enriched margarine, was shown to be associated with a reduction in LDL cholesterol equivalent to that observed on a statin drug, known to have powerful cholesterol-lowering effects (Jenkins et al 2003). Furthermore, the experimental diet was associated with a reduction in C-reactive protein, an inflammatory marker now known to be associated with increased cardiovascular risk.

While the concept of potentially beneficial eating patterns may be useful as a preventive strategy against cardiovascular disease, it is important to bear in mind that adopting individual attributes of such patterns may not confer benefit. For example, consuming substantial quantities of olive oil in the context of an otherwise inappropriate diet may confer little or no advantage. Further it should be noted that traditional cardioprotective patterns have been altered by many of the people consuming them, so that modern Mediterranean or Asian diets may for instance be high in saturated fatty acids and thus have, at least to some extent, lost their health benefits.

19.4 CLINICAL TRIALS OF DIETARY MODIFICATION

While prospective epidemiological studies provide strong evidence of risk or protection associated with individual nutrients or foods, proof of causality and the ultimate level of evidence for dietary recommendations can only be derived from randomised controlled trials. The early trials all attempted to lower cholesterol levels, usually by increasing the dietary polyunsaturated:saturated ratio (P:S), i.e. they were single factor intervention trials. More recent trials have involved multifactorial interventions, including dietary change intended to improve all nutrition-related risk indicators as well as attempts to modify risk factors that are not diet-related (e.g. cigarette smoking). Dietary intervention trials have been undertaken in people with and without evidence of CHD at the time the study was started (i.e. secondary and primary prevention trials). This review describes briefly a few landmark trials (Table 19.4) and presents an overview of all the important investigations of this kind. For full references to the clinical trials see Additional references (related to Section 19.4 on the *evolve* website 🖱).

LOS ANGELES VETERANS ADMINISTRATION STUDY

This was the first of the major intervention trials, in which 846 male volunteers (aged 55–89 years) were randomly allocated to 'experimental' and 'control' diets taken in different dining rooms. The control diet was intended to be typical North American (40% energy from fat, mostly saturated). The experimental diet contained half as much cholesterol, and predominantly polyunsaturated vegetable oils (n-6 PUFA) replaced approximately two-thirds of the animal fat, achieving a P:S ratio of 2. The trial was conducted under double-blind conditions. During the 8 years of the trial, plasma cholesterol in the experimental group was 13% lower, and coronary events, as well as deaths due to cardiovascular disease, were appreciably reduced, compared

---

Table 19.3	Attributes of cardioprotective diets

Low intakes of saturated fatty acids

High intakes of raw or appropriately prepared fruit and vegetables

Lightly processed cereal foods and wholegrains are preferred

Fat intakes are derived predominantly from unmodified vegetable oils*

Fish, nuts, seeds and vegetable protein sources are important dietary components

Meat, when consumed, is lean and eaten in small quantities

Energy balance reduces rates of obesity

---

*Coconut oil and palm oil are not encouraged because they tend to elevate LDL.

Table 19.4   Results of selected intervention trials (confidence intervals are given in parenthesis)

TRIAL	NO OF SUBJECTS	% REDUCTION IN CHOLESTEROL	ODDS RATIOS (EXPERIMENTAL VS CONTROL)	
			Total mortality	*Fatal and non-fatal CHD*
Veterans Administration	846	13	0.98 (0.83–1.15)	0.77
Oslo	1232	13	0.64 (0.37–1.12)	0.56
DART				
Fat advice	2033	3.5	0.98 (0.77–1.26)	0.92
Fish advice	2033	Negligible	0.74 (0.57–0.93)	0.85
Lyons Heart	605	Negligible	0.30 (0.11–0.82)	0.24
CHAOS	2002	NA	1.30	0.60
GISSI-Prevenzione				
n-3 fatty acids	2836	NA	0.80 (0.67–0.94)	0.80
Vitamin E	2830	NA	0.86 (0.72–1.02)	0.88
HOPE	1511	NA	1.00 (0.89–1.13)	1.05

NA, not available.

with the controls (Table 19.4). The beneficial effect of the cholesterol-lowering diet was most evident in those with high cholesterol levels at the start of the study. Deaths due to other and uncertain causes occurred more frequently in the experimental group, though no single other cause predominated. This increase in non-cardiovascular mortality in the experimental group raised for the first time the possibility that cholesterol lowering might be harmful in some respects, despite the reduction in CHD. However, this has not been substantiated in subsequent studies.

OSLO TRIAL

Middle-aged men at high risk of CHD (smokers or those having a cholesterol in the range 7.5–9.8 mmol/l) were divided into two groups; half received intensive dietary education and advice to stop smoking, the other half served as a control group. An impressive reduction in total coronary events was observed (Table 19.4) in association with a 13% fall in serum cholesterol and a 65% reduction in tobacco consumption. There was also an improvement in total mortality and there were no significant differences between the two groups with regard to non-cardiac causes of death. Detailed statistical analysis suggested that approximately 60% of the CHD reduction could be attributed to serum cholesterol change and 25% to smoking reduction. The composition of the experimental diet was quite different from that used in the Veterans Administration trial: total and saturated fat were markedly reduced without any appreciable increase in n-6 PUFA, and fibre-rich carbohydrate was increased. These differences could have accounted for the different results with regard to non-cardiovascular diseases.

DIET AND REINFARCTION TRIAL (DART)

This was the first trial to examine the effects of diets high in n-3 PUFA. Burr et al randomised 2033 men who had survived myocardial infarction to receive or not to receive advice on each of three dietary factors: (i) a reduction of fat intake and an increase in the ratio of polyunsaturated to saturated fat, (ii) an increase in fatty fish intake, and (iii) an increase in cereal fibre. For those unable to eat fatty fish, a fish oil supplement was recommended. Within the short (2 years) follow-up period, the subjects advised to eat fatty fish or a fish oil supplement had a 26% reduction in all causes of mortality compared with those not so advised. The other two diets were not associated with significant differences in mortality, but in view of the fact that fat modification only achieved a 3–4% reduction in serum cholesterol, compliance with the fat-modified and high fibre diets may have been less than that on the fish diet. Furthermore, diets aimed to reduce atherogenicity (n-6 PUFA) are likely to take longer to show a beneficial effect than those aimed to reduce thrombogenicity (n-3 PUFA). These results are the first to find that very simple advice aimed to reduce thrombogenicity (at least two weekly portions, 200–400 g of fatty fish) appears to reduce mortality appreciably. Results of follow-up long after the completion of the intervention phase were inconclusive.

LYONS HEART STUDY

This study is the most recent in the series of multifactorial dietary intervention studies in the secondary prevention of cardiovascular disease. Six hundred and five individuals with clinical ischaemic heart disease received conventional dietary advice or advice to follow a traditional Mediterranean diet ('experimental diet'). The experimental diet was lower in total and saturated fat (30% and 8% total energy) than the control diet (33% and 12% total energy) and contained more oleic (13% versus 10% total energy) and α-linolenic acid (0.80% versus 0.27%). Dietary linoleic acid was higher in the control group (5.3% versus 3.6%). The Mediterranean diet included more bread, legumes, vegetables and fruit and less meat and dairy products. Those in the experimental group were also provided with a margarine rich in α-linolenate (C18:3 n-3). The marked reductions in risk ratios for cardiovascular events as well as total mortality associated with the experimental diet are difficult to interpret. The confidence intervals are wide and it is difficult to understand why cholesterol levels did not fall despite the reduced intake of saturated fatty acids. The latter observation has led to the suggestion that the beneficial effect must have resulted from an antithrombogenic effect of the diet or a reduction in the risk of dysrhythmias as a result

of the increase in n-3 fatty acids. The study has been widely quoted as providing strong evidence for the health benefits associated with the Mediterranean diet.

CAMBRIDGE HEART ANTIOXIDANT STUDY (CHAOS)

Several early clinical trials involving supplementation with antioxidant nutrients (vitamins C and E and β-carotene) without concomitant dietary change suggested no benefit in terms of cardiovascular risk reduction despite strong evidence of a cardioprotective effect in epidemiological studies. This study from Cambridge involved the randomisation of over 2000 participants with pre-existing cardiovascular disease to receive either placebo or α-tocopherol 400 iu or 800 iu daily (268 or 537 mg, respectively). After 1.4 years non-fatal myocardial infarction was substantially reduced in those receiving α-tocopherol at either dose (14 out of 1035) compared to the control group (41 out of 967). However, there were marginally more total deaths in the α-tocopherol than in the control group (36 out of 1035 compared with 26 out of 967).

GISSI–PREVENZIONE STUDY

This large study examined the effect of supplementation with very-long-chain n-3 fatty acids (eicosa pentaenoic and docosahexaenoic acids) or vitamin E (300 mg) or both in 2830 subjects who had had a myocardial infarction. The trial was not conducted in a double-blind manner, but was nevertheless interesting in view of its size. Supplementation with n-3 fatty acids was associated with a statistically significant 15–20% reduction in all the important end-points (non-fatal myocardial infarction, cardiovascular deaths and total mortality). A smaller reduction in event rate in association with vitamin E supplementation did not achieve statistical significance.

HEART OUTCOMES PREVENTION EVALUATION (HOPE) STUDY

Patients at high risk of cardiovascular events because they had cardiovascular disease or diabetes and one other risk factor were randomised to receive placebo, 400 iu vitamin E (268 mg) or drug treatment (an angiotensin-converting-enzyme inhibitor, ramipril) and followed for 4.5 years. A primary outcome event (myocardial infarction, stroke or death from a cardiovascular cause) occurred in 16.2% (772 of the 4761) patients assigned to the vitamin E group and 15.5% (739 of the 4780) assigned to placebo. Furthermore, there were no differences between the two groups when considering total mortality or indeed any other cardiovascular end-points.

OVERALL PERSPECTIVE OF THE TRIALS

It is noteworthy, but perhaps not surprising that there have been relatively few recent dietary trials which have involved clinical endpoints. They are immensely complex and costly and are clearly unlikely to attract commercial sponsorship.

It is inappropriate to aggregate the results of the existing dietary intervention trials in a meta-analysis in view of the wide range of interventions that have been employed. Nevertheless certain conclusions may be drawn from the results of the various studies. There is convincing evidence that cholesterol lowering by dietary means reduces coronary events in the context of both primary and secondary prevention. Indeed there is confirmation of the rule derived from observational epidemiology that a 2–3% reduction in coronary events results from each 1% of cholesterol lowering achieved. There would seem to be reasonably strong evidence that lowering of total cholesterol (reflecting principally a reduction in LDL cholesterol) should primarily be achieved by reducing total and saturated fatty acids. Increasing n-6 polyunsaturated fatty acids (chiefly linoleic acid C18:2 n-6) may further decrease LDL and reduce cardiovascular risk. Oleic acid (C18:1 n-9), carbohydrate from lightly processed cereals (wholegrains), vegetables and fruit as well as linoleic acid may all contribute replacement energy for saturated fatty acids. However, it should be noted that for those who are overweight, reduction of saturated fat intake facilitates a reduction in energy intake and overcompensation should be discouraged. Two trials provide some support for the suggestion that dietary modification has the potential to reduce cardiovascular risk by means other than cholesterol lowering. The DART trial achieved appreciable reduction in cardiovascular mortality with minimal change in cholesterol, presumably because the increase in C20:5 n-3 and C22:6 n-3 in the fish or fish oil supplements resulted in reduced

tendency to thrombosis or perhaps reduced the risk of dysrythmias. Similarly the experimental diet in the Lyons Heart Study was not associated with appreciable cholesterol lowering. It is impossible to identify which of the many nutritional changes might have been responsible for the beneficial effects. There was undoubtedly an increase in a range of antioxidant nutrients which may have reduced oxidisability of LDL despite minimal change in cholesterol. Non-starch polysaccharide (dietary fibre) as well as starch increased because of the increase in cereals, vegetables and fruit. Total saturated fatty acids decreased while oleic and α-linolenic acids increased. The authors of the study regarded the last-mentioned change to be of particular importance. However, it would seem more plausible that a combination of all these factors contributed to the overall risk reduction resulting from favourable modification of several of the risk factors listed in Table 19.1.

When attempting to extrapolate the findings of the various trials into practical recommendations it is important not to be seduced by the many 'experts' who advocate the Mediterranean diet or some other dietary pattern as the most appropriate means of cardiovascular risk reduction. On the basis of existing evidence it seems more appropriate to conclude that there are probably several dietary patterns which are associated with a low risk of cardiovascular disease. These include the Mediterranean diet, a traditional Asian or African diet or indeed a more conventional Western diet which has been modified to reduce levels of cardiovascular risk factors. A low intake of saturated fatty acids appears to be the most consistent feature of the various dietary patterns associated with low CHD risk. While a Mediterranean diet does offer one means by which this dietary modification can be achieved, it can also be achieved by other eating patterns (e.g. Asian, modified Western).

The trials of nutrient supplements have generally been disappointing, apart perhaps from the GISSI-Prevenzione Study, which suggests potential benefit of supplementation with modest amounts of fish oils. More recent trials of supplementation with folic acid and other B vitamins aimed at reducing cardiovascular risk by lowering homocysteine levels have also shown no beneficial effect. There is no clear explanation as to why antioxidant nutrient supplementation trials have been largely negative despite strong suggestions of benefit from epidemiological data. The most likely explanation would seem to be either that a longer time frame might be necessary in order to demonstrate benefit or that a blend of these nutrients in proportions similar to those found in foods might be required to produce benefit, rather than a pharmacological dose of a single antioxidant nutrient. It is also possible that the antioxidant nutrients may be acting as a marker for some other protective factor present in the foods that contain these vitamins or flavonoids.

19.5 CEREBROVASCULAR DISEASE (STROKE)

Cerebrovascular disease presents clinically as a stroke which, like the clinical manifestations of CHD, also has a major impact on public health because of its high frequency in most affluent and developing countries. There are several different types of stroke. One cause of stroke is a bleed from one of the cerebral arteries (haemorrhagic stroke). This may be associated with a congenital abnormality (aneurysm) and/or raised levels of blood pressure. Thus nutritional determinants of hypertension are contributory causal factors.

Ischaemic strokes are more common and result from thrombosis and atheroma, the process being similar to that which results in myocardial infarction. The clinical features of stroke (typically loss or slurring of speech and weakness of one side of the body) result from the loss of blood supply to a section of the brain. Although the nutritional determinants have been far less studied than is the case for CHD, the risk factors for the two sets of conditions are similar and therefore nutritional factors which predispose to CHD should also apply. However in the relatively limited number of studies of stroke which have been carried out, some food groups emerge as being particularly relevant. Most striking is the protective effect of fruit and vegetables demonstrated in six of the seven large prospective studies that have examined the relationship, Although it appears that most categories of fruit and vegetables may be protective, the effect is particularly striking for cruciferous vegetables, green leafy vegetables and citrus fruits. Blood pressure is also a particularly important risk factor for ischaemic stroke, so that, once again, all the nutritional determinants of hypertension can be regarded as

especially relevant. Of the remaining nutrients and food groups which have been identified as causal or protective in terms of CHD, n-3 fatty acids, regular fish consumption and intake of whole grains have been shown to be protective against ischaemic stroke.

Thus, although there have been no intervention studies which have specifically examined the effect on clinical outcome, implementing a cardioprotective dietary pattern (Table *evolve* 19.1) can be expected to reduce the risk of both haemorrhagic and ischaemic stroke.

19.6 IMPLEMENTATION OF DIETARY ADVICE

Cardioprotective dietary patterns are appropriate for patients with established cardiovascular disease, those with cardiovascular risk factors, and entire populations in order to reduce population risk or to maintain rates amongst groups which currently have low rates. While people at high risk of a first or subsequent cardiovascular event will clearly reap the greatest individual benefit, a population approach is essential to reduce the epidemic proportions of cardiovascular diseases in many countries, or to prevent escalating rates in other countries. The level of intensity of required dietary modification depends upon level of risk and nature of individual risk factors. Table 19.5 provides ranges of population nutrient intake goals which are particularly relevant to cardiovascular disease as recommended by the WHO and FAO and in the UK. However these are substantially modified according to risk factor status.

For example, those with markedly raised levels of total and LDL cholesterol should reduce saturated fatty acids to 8% or less of total energy. For those with high blood pressure emphasis may be on salt reduction and an increase in fruit, vegetables and low fat dairy products. Details of sample eating plans are provided in Table *evolve* 19.1 . The greatest challenge for the future will be to develop approaches that will facilitate compliance with nutritional recommendations amongst individuals and populations. Governments need to appreciate that appropriate food choices by individuals require a supportive environment which may in turn need regulation and legislation.

Table 19.5   Ranges of population nutrient intake goals recommended by the WHO and FAO[a] and in the UK[b] (unless otherwise stated, the goals are expressed as percentage total energy)

	WHO/FAO	UK
Total fat	15–30%	35%
Saturated fatty acids (SFA)	<10%	<10%
Cis-polyunsaturated fatty Acids (PFA)	6–10%	NSR
n-6 PUFA	5–8%	<10%
n-3 PUFA	1–2%	1.5 g/week[e]
Cis-monounsaturated fatty Acids	By difference[c]	NSR
Trans fatty acids (TFA)	<1%	<2%
Dietary cholesterol (mg/day)	<300 mg/day	Approx 245 mg/day
Total carbohydrate	55–75%	50%
Free sugars[d]	<10%	Fruits and vegetables encouraged
Dietary fibre (NSP)	From foods	Complex carbohydrates encouraged
Protein	10–15%	NSR
Sodium chloride	<5 g/day	6 g/day /100 mmol/day
Potassium		3.5 g/day
Fruit and vegetables	>400 g/day	Encouraged

[a]Joint WHO/FAO Expert 2003.
[b]Report of the Cardiovascular Review Group Committee on Medical Aspects of Food Policy. Nutritional aspects of cardiovascular disease, Department of Health Report on Health and Social Subjects 46, London, HMSO, 1994.
[c]Total fat – (SFA & PFA & TFA).
[d]All monosaccharides and disaccharides added to foods by manufacturer, cook or consumer, plus sugars naturally present in honey, syrups and fruit juices.
[e]Mainly from oily fish.
NSR, No specific recommendation.

KEY POINTS

- Geographic variation and time trends indicate the importance of environmental determinants of cardiovascular disease.
- Nature of dietary fat is an important determinant of CHD in populations, influencing lipoprotein-mediated risk and other risk factors.
- Saturated and trans-unsaturated fatty acids increase CHD risk; n-6 and n-3 polyunsaturated fatty acids are protective.
- Antioxidant nutrients, flavonoids, folate and other B vitamins, non-starch polysaccharides, wholegrain cereals, nuts, soya protein and alcohol appear to protect against CHD via an influence on several important risk factors for CVD.
- Randomised controlled clinical trials demonstrate the potential for dietary change to reduce CHD rates.
- A range of different dietary patterns are cardioprotective.
- There is adequate evidence to recommend dietary change in high-risk populations and individuals.

References

Beaglehole R: International trends in coronary heart disease mortality and incidence rates, *Journal of Cardiovascular Risk* 6:63–68, 1999.

Cutler JA, Follmann D, Allender PS: Randomized trials of sodium reduction: an overview, *American Journal of Clinical Nutrition* 65:643–651, 1997.

Jenkins DJA, Kendall CWC, Marchie A, et al: Effects of a dietary portfolio of cholesterol-lowering foods versus lovastatin on serum lipids and c-reactive protein, *Journal of the American Medical Association* 290:502–510, 2003.

Joint WHO/FAO Expert Consultation: *Diet, nutrition and the prevention of chronic diseases.* WHO Technical Report Series 916, Geneva, 2003, World Health Organization.

Keys A: *Seven Countries: a multivariate analysis of death and coronary heart disease,* Cambridge, MA, 1980, Harvard University Press.

Keys A, Anderson JT, Grande F: Serum cholesterol response to changes in diet. IV. Particular saturated fatty acids in the diet, *Metabolism* 14:776–778, 1965.

Kris-Etherton P, Daniels SR, Eckel RH, et al: Summary of the scientific conference on dietary fatty acids and cardiovascular health: conference summary from the nutrition committee of the American Heart Association, *Circulation* 103(7):1034–1039, 2001.

Mangoni AA, Jackson SH: Homocysteine and cardiovascular disease: current evidence and future prospects, *American Journal of Medicine* 112:556–565, 2002.

Mann JI, Chisholm A: Cardiovascular Diseases. In Mann JI, Truswell AS, editors: *Essentials of Human Nutrition,* ed 3, Oxford, 2007,

Oxford University Press, pp 283–312.

Pietinen P, Vartiainen E, Seppanen R, et al: Changes in diet in Finland from 1972–1992: impact on coronary heart disease risk, *Preventive Medicine* 25:243–250, 1996.

Robinson SM, Barker DJ: Coronary heart disease: a disorder of growth, *Proceedings of the Nutrition Society* 61:537–542, 2002.

Stykowski PA, Kannel WB, D'Agostino RB: Changes in risk factors and the decline in mortality from cardiovascular disease. The Framingham Heart Study, *New England Journal of Medicine* 322:1635–1641, 1990.

Tuomilehto J, Geboers J, Salonen T, et al: Decline in cardiovascular mortality in North Karelia and other parts of Finland, *British Medical Journal* 293:1068–1071, 1986.

Truswell AS: Dietary fibre and plasma lipids, *European Journal of Clinical Nutrition* 49(Suppl 3):S105–S109, 1995.

Ulbricht TVL, Southgate DAT: Coronary heart disease: seven dietary factors, *Lancet* 338:985–992, 1991.

Venn BJ, Mann JI, Williams SM, et al: Dietary counseling to increase natural folate intake: a randomized, placebo-controlled trial in free-living subjects to assess effects on serum folate and plasma total homocysteine, *American Journal of Clinical Nutrition* 76:758–765, 2002.

Whelton PK, He J, Cutler JA, et al: Effects of oral potassium on blood pressure. Meta-analysis of randomized controlled clinical trials, *Journal of the American Medical Association* 277:1624–1632, 1997.

Zatonski W, Campos H, Willett W: Rapid declines in coronary heart disease mortality in Eastern Europe are associated with increased consumption of oils rich in alpha-linolenic acid, *European Journal of Epidemiology* 23(1):3–10, 2008.

Further reading

Armstrong BK, Mann JI, Adelstein AM, Eskin F: Commodity consumption and ischaemic heart disease mortality with special reference to dietary practices, *Journal of Chronic Diseases* 28:455–469, 1975.

Kris-Etherton PM, Zhao G, Binkoski AE, et al: The effects of nuts on coronary heart disease risk, *Nutrition Reviews* 59:103–111, 2001.

Law MR, Frost CD, Wald NJ: By how much does salt reduction lower

blood pressure? III, Analysis of data from trials of salt reduction, *British Medical Journal* 302:819–824, 1991.

Sacks FM, Svetkey LP, Vollmer WM, et al: Effects on blood pressure of reduced dietary sodium and the Dietary Approaches to Stop Hypertension (DASH) diet, *New England Journal of Medicine* 344:3–10, 2001.

Vessby B, Uusitupa M, Hermansen K, et al: Substituting dietary saturated

for monounsaturated fat impairs insulin sensitivity in healthy men and women: the KANWU Study, *Diabetologia* 44:312–319, 2001.

Whelton PK, Appel LJ, Espeland MA, et al: Sodium reduction and weight loss in the treatment of hypertension in older persons, *Journal of the American Medical Association* 279:839–846, 1998.

EVOLVE CONTENTS (available online at: evolve.elsevier.com/Geissler/nutrition)

Chapter **20**

Obesity

Arne Astrup and Sue Pedersen

CHAPTER CONTENTS

© 2010 Elsevier Ltd/Inc/BV
DOI: 10.1016/B978-0-7020-3118-2.00020-6

OBJECTIVES

By the end of this chapter you should be able to:

- know the definitions and their rationale of overweight and obesity in adults and children
- describe their prevalence in Western countries
- compare with other countries and describe time trends
- summarise the health risks of obesity and their mechanisms
- discuss the relative importance of causal factors
- compare critically different approaches to prevention and treatment.

20.1 INTRODUCTION

Obesity has become the major nutrition-related disease of this decade, and is defined as a condition of excessive body fat accumulation to an extent that increases the risk of complicating diseases. Overweight and obesity cause the development of diabetes, and contribute to high blood pressure, adverse blood lipid profile, infertility, birth complications and arthritis, and amplify asthma and a poor health status. Obesity is largely preventable through changes in lifestyle, especially diet.

20.2 EPIDEMIOLOGY OF OBESITY

DEFINITION OF OBESITY

Obesity is not a single entity, but it is most commonly classified by a single measure, the body mass index (BMI), a ratio of weight and height (BMI =

Table 20.1   The classification of underweight, normal weight and classes of overweight white individuals according to the WHO

CLASSIFICATION	BMI	RISK OF CO-MORBIDITIES (KG/M²)
Underweight	<18.5	Low (but risk of other clinical problems increased)
Normal range	18.5–24.9	Average
Overweight[a]	≥25	
Pre-obese	25.0–29.9	Mildly increased
Obese	**>30.0**	
Class I	30.0–34.9	Moderate
Class II	35.0–39.9	Severe
Class III	>40.0	

[a]The term overweight refers to a BMI >25, but is frequently adapted to refer to BMI 25–29.9, differentiating the pre-obese from the obese categories.

weight (kg)/height² (m²)). The World Health Organization (WHO) classifies underweight, normal weight, overweight and obesity according to categories of BMI (Table 20.1). This height-dependent measure of weight allows comparisons to be made more readily within and between populations of the same ethnic origin. The definition of the 'normal' range of BMI was based primarily on North American mortality data, and the cut-offs are different for Asian populations. The suggested categories are: 18.5 kg/m² underweight; 18.5–23 kg/m² increasing but acceptable risk; 23–27.5 kg/m² increased risk, and 27.5 kg/m² or higher, high risk. BMI does not, however, distinguish fat from lean tissue or water, nor does it identify whether the fat is accumulated in particular sites such as the abdomen, where it has more serious metabolic consequences. Techniques such as bioelectric impedance to estimate body fat, and DEXA scans to separate body mass into fat-free mass and fat mass, are increasingly used. DEXA (dual energy X-ray absorptiometry), MR (magnetic resonance), and CT (computer tomography) scans are used for an accurate assessment of intra-abdominal adipose tissue, although simple waist circumference is increasingly recognised as an easy and valid measure of abdominal obesity. Waist–hip ratio and skin fold thickness may also be used to verify fatness in individuals.

The BMI is the currently accepted standard of measure of obesity in children age 2–18 years.

Because children grow in both height and weight, norms for weight and BMI vary by both age and gender. To circumvent this issue, BMI can be evaluated relative to reference standards which have been developed in the US and the UK, as well as on an international level by IASO's International Obesity Task Force. Using this methodology, children are classified as being normal weight if their BMI falls between the 5th and 85th percentiles, overweight between the 85th and 95th percentiles, and obese if ≥95th percentile. Alternatively, age- and sex-specific cut points for BMI for overweight and obesity in children have also been developed, using dataset specific centiles linked to adult BMI cut off points of ≥25 and ≥30 kg/m², respectively.

PREVALENCE AND TIME TRENDS OF OVERWEIGHT AND OBESITY

The prevalence of obesity is increasing worldwide in almost every country and in all age groups. The steep increase has prompted this development to be called an epidemic, and because it is worldwide, a pandemic. In 2001, 14% of adult men and 17% of women in Denmark were obese, and in the UK, 21% of men and 24% of women were obese, and a further 47% of men and 33% of women were overweight (BMI 25–30 kg/m²). In the USA, the situation is even worse: in 2006, the prevalence of overweight and obesity in adults was 68% and 34%, respectively. Encouragingly, however, the prevalence of obesity in the USA was unchanged between 2003/4 and 2005/6, based on National Health and Nutritional Examination Survey (NHANES) data. Southern European countries such as Greece have very high prevalence rates similar to those in the USA. Europe is following a similar course to that of the USA, but is about 10 years behind; thus, in 10 years, the prevalence of obesity in Europe can be expected to reach the same level that exists in the USA today, if preventive initiatives and treatment measures are not successful. There are trends that suggest that the increase in prevalence of obesity has levelled off in several European countries in the period 2003–09. The reason for this is still obscure.

Obesity is now apparent in even some of the poorest countries of the world. Normally the obesity problem first appears in a country in the more affluent parts of the population, but in recent decades obesity is characteristically higher among groups with low levels of education, low income and low social class.

The proportion of obese people increases with age until around the age of retirement. Beyond this age the impact of obesity-related premature death and disease-related weight loss leads to a modest decline in the proportion of obese adults. People who today are in their 60s or older were born at a time of austerity and limited food supplies. Younger people have largely grown up in a world where a greater variety of food than ever before has become available and at relatively low cost, and so are more prone to develop obesity at a younger age.

Attention is increasingly focused on young people, where the problem of overweight and obesity has become more pronounced. Among young Danish males attending draft boards, there has been a dramatic increase in the prevalence of obesity from 0.1% in 1955 to about 7.4% in 2004–9, corresponding to an almost 80-fold increase. In the UK in 1997 amongst 4–18-year-olds, 4% were obese and a further 15% were overweight, with a higher rate of obesity among young people in Scotland and Wales, relative to England. Rates of overweight and obesity range from 10% to 20% in northern Europe and are higher still in southern Europe – from 20% to as high as 36% in parts of southern Italy. The prevalence of paediatric obesity is most alarming in the USA, affecting 17% of children and adolescents age 5–17, and 12% of children age 2–5; further, nearly one-third of American children are overweight. However, NHANES data also reveals that the prevalence of overweight and obesity among American children and adolescents has not changed significantly between 2003/4 and 2005/6.

There is a higher than expected level of obesity among certain ethnic groups living in Europe, probably due to increased genetic susceptibility to the consequences of the European lifestyle. Obesity rates are highest among people of Indian, Pakistani and black Caribbean origin, and the prevalence of obesity in young people of Asian origin is 3–4 times higher than among whites.

KEY POINTS

- Body weight classes are defined based on body mass index (BMI): weight (kg)/height² (m²).
- Overweight is defined as BMI ≥25 kg/m², and obesity as BMI ≥30 kg/m².
- Overweight and obesity have become highly prevalent; obesity affects 15–35% of the adult

population in the developed countries, and the majority of the adult population in these countries have a BMI of more than 25 kg/m^2.

- The obesity prevalence is increasing in most countries, in both genders and all age groups, but there are trends to suggest that the prevalence has plateaued in the USA as well as several European countries.
- Even the developing countries are experiencing a major increase in obesity.

20.3 RISKS OF OBESITY

HEALTH AND SOCIAL RISKS

The risks and complications of obesity and abdominal overweight are poorly recognised, but can account for more than 5% of all health costs. Even a normal BMI, but with abdominal fat accumulation, can be responsible for hypertension, hyperlipidaemia, type 2 diabetes, and cardiovascular disease, which makes it important to identify increased fatness as the underlying cause of the condition or disease. The increase in obesity rates has an important impact on the global incidence of cardiovascular disease, type 2 diabetes mellitus, cancer, osteoarthritis, obstructive sleep apnoea, infertility, birth complications and work disability. Obesity has a more pronounced impact on morbidity than on mortality, but a BMI of 40 is associated with a decreased life expectancy of around 10 years. Increases in the prevalence of obesity will potentially lead to an increase in the number of years that subjects suffer from obesity-related morbidity and disability.

SYMPTOMS AND CONSEQUENCES

Most overweight subjects suffer from low self-esteem and self-loathing, and also commonly phobias. They are discriminated against, even in the health sector, and can experience heat intolerance, intertrigo (inflammation of skin folds due to heat, moisture, friction and lack of air circulation), difficulties with physical activity, and sexual problems of a psychological and physical nature. These social and psychological problems often tend to be more pronounced than the somatic complications associated with obesity.

TYPE 2 DIABETES (see Ch. 21)

Definition

Type 2 diabetes mellitus is a chronic condition that arises when the pancreas does not produce enough insulin to overcome the insulin resistance in the peripheral tissues. Inadequate insulin secretion, insulin action, or both, leads to hyperglycaemia. This hyperglycaemia is associated with long-term damage, dysfunction and failure of various organs and tissues, particularly small vessel complications affecting the eyes (retinopathy), kidneys (nephropathy) and nerves (neuropathy), and large vessel complications affecting the heart, brain, and peripheral circulation (cardiovascular disease). Type 1 and type 2 diabetes were previously known as insulin-dependent diabetes mellitus (IDDM) and non-insulin-dependent diabetes mellitus (NIDDM), respectively, but this is not an appropriate distinction as many patients with type 2 diabetes, particularly in the later stages of the disease, require insulin therapy. The terms type 1 and type 2 are now used to distinguish patients who have diabetes due to absolute failure of pancreatic insulin production of autoimmune aetiology (type 1), versus relative failure of insulin production in the face of insulin resistance (type 2).

Role of overweight and obesity

Overweight and obesity are the major causes of the development of type 2 diabetes in individuals with a high genetic susceptibility to the disease. Type 2 diabetes occurs 50–100-fold more frequently in obese subjects than in lean subjects. In observational studies, overweight, obesity, physical inactivity, smoking, and diet composition can account for almost all cases of type 2 diabetes (Hu et al 2001). The genetic make-up determines if an obese individual develops type 2 diabetes or not, and many morbidly obese subjects without the genetic predisposition maintain a normal glucose tolerance throughout life. Diabetes is the most important medical consequence of obesity because it is common, has serious complications, is difficult to treat, reduces life expectancy by 8–10 years, and is expensive to manage.

Obesity-related mortality caused by diabetes

Diabetes is not directly the cause of most of the excess mortality among obese subjects. However, the metabolic abnormalities underlying type 2 diabetes (see 'Metabolic syndrome', below) are clearly the result of obesity, which in itself predisposes to cardiovascular disease, a leading cause of death amongst the obese (see Ch. 21).

Prevention of type 2 diabetes by weight loss

Some of the metabolic defects accompanying impaired glucose tolerance (IGT) and type 2 diabetes are reversible with weight loss, unless the diabetes has persisted for too long a time, with irreversible damage to insulin secretion (Harder et al 2004). In high risk subjects, such as obese subjects with IGT, weight loss can prevent and almost eliminate type 2 diabetes. In a Swedish surgical weight loss intervention study on obesity, the 2-year incidence of diabetes was 6.3% in the control group and only 0.2% in the weight loss group (Astrup 2004). This intervention study shows that 95% of new cases of type 2 diabetes among obese individuals can be prevented by a major (20–25 kg) sustained weight loss. Most of the benefit was maintained at 10 years when the incidence of diabetes was still five-fold lower than in controls, which corresponds to an 80% protection against developing diabetes. A weight loss of this magnitude induced by gastric surgical procedures reduces mortality by ~30% over 15 years, and about half is due to fewer deaths due to ischemic heart disease, and half to obesity-related cancers. More recent intervention studies have very clearly demonstrated that even a modest weight loss of 3–5% achieved by diet and slightly increased daily physical activity is sufficient to prevent nearly 60% of all new cases over a 4–5-year period. Further analyses have shown that it is the weight loss per se, not a specific diet or the physical activity, that is important.

INCREASED BLOOD PRESSURE (HYPERTENSION)

The risk of developing hypertension is 5–6 times greater with obesity. Blood pressure is positively correlated with both abdominal circumference and with the degree of obesity. Insulin resistance and hyperinsulinaemia appear to be responsible for the hypertension. Insulin has an anti-natriuretic effect that results in an increase of both extracellular and intravascular volume. It is also possible that the hyperinsulinaemia has a direct trophic effect on the smooth muscle cells of the arterioles, which can lead to a chronically hyperactive sympathetic nervous system.

The hypertension associated with obesity is just as harmful as hypertension from other causes, and should be controlled and treated with the same vigour as in the normal weight patient. Even a small weight loss can result in a marked drop in blood pressure, and weight loss is a much more effective treatment than salt restriction.

ATHEROSCLEROSIS, ISCHAEMIC HEART DISEASE AND STROKE

Obesity, and abdominal obesity in particular, are associated with a significant increased risk of atherosclerotic manifestations. The risk of developing ischaemic heart disease or stroke is 2.5 and 6 times greater, respectively, with a pronounced abdominal fat distribution than with a low waist measurement, i.e. even distribution. The increased risk of abdominal obesity in particular is multifactorial, including significant tendencies towards an unfavourable lipid profile, hypertension, insulin resistance and type 2 diabetes, increased inflammatory markers such as CRP and fibrinogen, and reduced fibrinolytic activity, amongst others.

ARTHRITIS

Osteoarthritis is a frequent complication of obesity, and obesity represents perhaps the strongest modifiable risk factor for developing osteoarthritis. Obesity-related osteoarthritis most commonly develops in the knees and ankles, and has a significant negative impact on quality of life. A decrease in BMI of as little as 2 kg/m^2 in women has been shown to decrease the risk of developing osteoarthritis a decade later by over 50%.

Gout (arthritis urica) is also a frequent complication of obesity. Plasma urate is increased in the majority of patients, but clinical symptoms are observed in only a minority.

METABOLIC SYNDROME (see Chs 19 and 21)

A number of studies point to the existence of a particular metabolic syndrome encompassing insulin resistance, hypertension, increased plasma VLDL, reduced HDL cholesterol, and abdominal obesity. This syndrome is also known as insulin resistance syndrome, since the underlying patho-physiology is that of reduced sensitivity to the action of insulin. A variety of risk factors for the development of cardiovascular disease appear to be associated with this syndrome, which links obesity with the most significant health complications (type 2 diabetes, hypertension and atherosclerosis). In addition to the level of obesity, other factors are significantly associated with the metabolic syndrome – fat distribution, level of physical activity and genetic disposition. A suggested definition of the syndrome is given by the International Diabetes Federation and shown below:

Waist ≥94 cm for men or ≥80 cm for women
(For south Asian, Japanese and Chinese
patients, waist ≥90 cm (men) or ≥80 cm
(women))

And at least two of the following components:

1. Fasting blood glucose ≥5.6 mmol/l, or diagnosed diabetes
2. HDL < 1.0 mmol/l for men, <1.3 mmol/l for women, or drug treatment for low HDL
3. Triglycerides ≥1.7 mmol/l or drug treatment for high triglycerides
4. Blood pressure ≥130/85 mmHg or drug treatment for hypertension

The way in which overweight and obesity con-tribute to the metabolic syndrome is not entirely clear, but hormones and substrates secreted by the adipose tissue are thought to be the main cause. An increased metabolism of free fatty acids and reduced secretion of the fat tissue hormone adiponectin, as well as increased secretion of cytokines, appear to play an important role in the development of insulin resistance in the muscle tissue. Treatment of the metabolic syndrome is weight loss and physical activity, with close attention towards cardiovascu-lar risk reduction.

POLYCYSTIC OVARY SYNDROME

The polycystic ovary syndrome (PCOS) is a common endocrinological disorder affecting 6–8% of repro-ductive-aged women. It is characterised by irregu-lar or absent menses, impaired fertility, hirsutism and acne. The pathogenetic foundation of PCOS is that of insulin resistance, which causes an excess production of androgens by the ovaries. While there is clearly a genetic predisposition to develop-ing PCOS, the presence of obesity worsens the degree of insulin resistance, and consequently worsens the symptom complex of PCOS. The primary treatment for overweight or obese women with PCOS is weight loss, as this has been shown to improve the clinical features of PCOS, including improved fertility rates.

MALIGNANCY

Obesity portends an increased risk of several types of cancer, and also increases the risk of death from cancer. In men and women with a BMI ≥40, the risk of dying from cancer compared to normal weight subjects is elevated by 50% and 60%, respectively. In the US, it is estimated that overweight and obesity may be responsible for 14% of all cancer deaths in men, and 20% in women. Obesity is asso-ciated with many different types of cancer, although the mechanism by which obesity promotes tumori-genesis varies by site. Mechanisms include chronic hyperinsulinaemia, increased bioavailability of steroid hormones (particularly oestrogen), and localised inflammation. Epidemiological studies have found an association between obesity and cancer of the colon (particularly in men), oesopha-gus, endometrium, kidney, female breast, pancreas, liver, gallbladder and stomach.

OTHER COMPLICATIONS

Obesity is also associated with several other comorbidities including hypoventilation syndrome and obstructive sleep apnoea, liver and gallstone diseases, psoriasis and asthmatic disease. Surgery of any kind is associated with an increased risk of complications in the obese. The length of hospital admission time is also generally prolonged when obese patients are treated for other complaints. The nature of obesity makes many clinical and para-clinical studies difficult to perform, and creates ongoing challenges in endeavours to broaden our knowledge base in this field.

KEY POINTS

- The risks and complications of obesity and abdominal overweight can account for more than 5% of all health costs.
- Even a quite normal BMI with abdominal fat accumulation can be responsible for hypertension, hyperlipidaemia, type 2 diabetes and cardiovascular disease.

- The increase in obesity has an important impact on the global incidence of cardiovascular disease, type 2 diabetes mellitus, cancer, osteoarthritis, infertility, birth complications, work disability and sleep apnoea.
- Obesity has a more pronounced impact on morbidity than on mortality, but a BMI of 40 kg/m^2 is associated with a decreased life expectancy of around 10 years.
- Increases in the prevalence of obesity will potentially lead to an increase in the number of years that subjects suffer from obesity-related morbidity and disability.

20.4 CAUSAL FACTORS

GENETICS

In only a minority of cases is obesity caused by a chromosome abnormality, a mutation in a single gene or a classic endocrine disorder. Most cases of obesity are due to an inadequately functioning appetite regulation and energy metabolism, where the energy density and fat content of food and drink are too high, mealtimes are irregular, daily physical activity is limited, and inactivity has become a characteristic of everyday life. An unlimited supply of cheap, tasty foodstuffs and larger food portions also help to promote overweight and risk of obesity. The disposition towards obesity is not necessarily genetic, since other influences, for example, chemicals or hormones transferred from mother to fetus during pregnancy, may programme the offspring to be susceptible to an obesity-promoting lifestyle. It is possible that a number of environmental factors, currently unknown, play an important role in the development of obesity. For example, recent studies suggest that severe overweight or excessive weight gain during pregnancy increases the offspring's predisposition to obesity within an obesity-inducing lifestyle. Further evidence shows that an adenovirus infection in the central nervous system (CNS) can induce obesity in animals, although human studies are not conclusive.

Chromosome and gene abnormalities

Prader–Willi syndrome is the most common genetic obesity disorder. It is caused by absence of a paternally derived region on chromosome 15, manifested as either a deletion or a double maternally derived region. The syndrome is characterised by cognitive impairment, low stature, genital hypoplasia and infertility, neonatal and infantile hypotonia, distinctive facial features, and small hands and feet. Because of severe hunger, low energy metabolism and reduced intellect, dietary treatment is often impossible, and surgical treatment may instead be indicated. Other less frequent congenital obesity disorders include Bardet–Biedl, Alström's and Cohen's syndromes.

Single-gene mutations that cause obesity in humans are extremely rare, though they have led to an important understanding of the physiological mechanisms for appetite regulation (Hebebrand et al 2003). A deficit of the satiety hormone leptin, produced by adipose tissue, can be found in children in a few families with mutations in the leptin gene. These children are characterised by a severe hyperphagia and respond with considerable weight loss when treated with leptin injections. Obesity caused by mutations in the gene coding for the leptin receptor is also found in a few individuals. The most common form of obesity due to a single gene mutation involves mutations in the melanocortin-4 receptor, which occur in 3–4% of children with severe obesity. Other mutations, such as in the genes for pro-opiomelanocortin and the prohormone convertase 1, are similarly associated with obesity. Mutations in the systems involved in appetite regulation are extremely rare, and account for only a very small percentage of the total cases of obesity. Many of the genes on a number of chromosomes are currently being screened in connection with obesity, but no definite association with the most usual form of obesity has so far been found.

The increasing activity within the field of genome-wide association studies for disease susceptibility genes has led to the identification of a common variant of the fat mass and obesity associated gene *FTO*, which predisposes to type 2 diabetes through an effect on body fat mass. Subsequent studies of large European study populations have confirmed a highly significant association between different variants of *FTO* and fatness, both among children and among adults of both sexes. For all ranges of BMI, the effect of the variant seems to be a 3–5 kg higher body weight (Kring et al 2008).

Genetic disposition

It is commonly observed that obesity 'runs' in families, but it has been difficult to determine the difference between genuine genetic inheritance and inheritance of environmental/lifestyle factors, for example hormonal transfer from an overweight mother to the fetus, or inheritance or influence of the parents' dietary and exercise habits. Many Nordic studies of twins and adopted children have suggested that adult body weight, and particularly obesity, appear to have a significant genetic component. About half of the phenotypic variation of weight and fat mass in a given fat-inducing environment is thought to have a genetic basis, but it is difficult to determine the source of the inheritance even in these types of study, since an early influence, for example in the womb or during infancy, can be critical and be mistakenly interpreted as reflecting genetic inheritance.

The supposed genetic component is generally not perceived in such a way that the development of obesity is fixed in the genes from the outset and can therefore only be changed with difficulty. Rather, the genetic component is perceived as a predisposition, which is expressed only when certain environmental factors are favourable. The most important obesity-triggering environmental factors that are generally acknowledged are a high dietary fat content, energy-rich drinks, a low level of physical activity and irregular mealtimes, though smoking cessation and pregnancy also play a role. It is still not precisely known how the genetic component is expressed physiologically, although a number of studies suggest that an abnormal lipid metabolism (which promotes fat deposition and inhibits oxidation), a poorly regulated appetite at a low level of physical activity, increased taste preference for fatty foods, and a reduced ability to spontaneously increase physical activity during periods of overeating are the most important candidates.

CHANGES IN ENVIRONMENT AND LIFESTYLE

Diet composition and drinks

The prevalence of obesity rose slowly from about 1920, with a dramatic increase in the years after World War II. During this period the diet has changed from consisting mainly of carbohydrate-rich foods (potatoes and other root vegetables, legumes, vegetables, grains, wholemeal bread) with a modest amount of fat, to the recent diet, where the consumption of meat, cheese, butter, other rich milk products and alcohol has increased at the cost of more energy-poor, carbohydrate-rich foods. The fat content of the diet has risen considerably.

Obesity is seldom seen among people who traditionally live on a diet with moderate fat content and a high content of energy-poor vegetables and wholemeal products. A rich, energy-dense diet with plentiful supply of sugary drinks tends to increase energy intake. In people with no special disposition towards obesity, such a fat-promoting diet can result in a marked weight gain and overweight. When the predisposed individual is exposed to this type of diet, the weight increase can be considerable and eventually lead to obesity.

The weak satiating effect of a fat-rich diet is linked to the high energy density, whereas the stronger satiating effect of carbohydrate and protein is less dependent on energy density. Typical carbohydrate-rich foods with a low content of fibre are less satisfying than similar products with a high fibre content, but the quantitative significance for weight regulation is poorly defined. The same applies to the glycaemic index of the carbohydrate-rich foods (see Ch. 6). While there is no basis to suggest that sugar in solid form satiates less than starch, there is growing evidence that sugar in drinks satiates less than sugar in solid form and studies have suggested that a high consumption of sugary drinks leads to a marked weight increase (Raben et al 2002).

Alcohol

It is normally assumed that the energy content of alcohol is added to the energy from the diet, such that alcohol increases the total energy intake. However the Health Survey of England indicated that non-drinkers are more likely to be obese than those who consume alcohol. Among alcohol consumers there is a gender difference in the effect on body weight. Somewhat surprisingly, alcohol intake does not increase weight among men, and women seem to lose weight with increasing alcohol intake. In women the energy intake from food is displaced by alcohol; women who drink a couple of units per day appear to eat less. The problem, however, is that most of the current knowledge is based on observational population studies, where confounding effects are possible. Thus, other factors cannot be ruled out: for example, smoking tobacco while consuming alcohol could instead be responsible for the attributed 'slimming' effect. In small doses the thermogenic effect of alcohol is only 8%, but it is possible that larger daily doses have a more pronounced effect on energy metabolism, for instance hypermetabolism among alcoholics tends to prevent weight gain. Epidemiological and experimental studies have together given no definite indication as to possible differences between beer and wine in terms of fat-promoting potential, and it is therefore unclear to what extent the increasing use of alcohol in Denmark contributes to the obesity epidemic. For further information on alcohol and energy see Chapter 9.

Portion size

The increasing prevalence of obesity is paralleled by increasing portion sizes in the marketplace. In the USA, for example, portion sizes grew between 200–500% over a 25-year period to the point where they far exceed recommended portion sizes. The discrepancy between recommended and actual serving sizes results in significant confusion on the part of the individual in estimating caloric intake. In fact, research has indicated that most people are unable to accurately estimate portion sizes and therefore cannot accurately estimate their energy intake. Portion sizes are an important determinant of energy intake; the number of calories ingested by subjects at a meal is directly correlated with the serving size offered.

Physical activity

The level of physical activity has fallen dramatically in the last 50 years, with the replacement of manual labour with machines and the increased use of every imaginable physical aid possible for housework, transport and leisure pursuits. Low daily physical activity is a risk factor for weight gain and one to two short weekly walks are not sufficient to compensate for this (Saris et al 2003). Only by regular physical activity is the capacity for fat oxidation increased and appetite regulation improved, depending on the intensity, length and frequency of the bouts of activity (Astrup et al 2004). The 30-minute daily physical exercise currently recommended by the American Heart Foundation and WHO, for example, is not enough to prevent weight gain and obesity in individuals predisposed to obesity; 45–60 minutes of daily activity is required.

MACRONUTRIENT BALANCE

With respect to the classic energy balance equation, energy balance = energy intake − energy expenditure, it appears that, in the dynamic phase of weight gain, energy intake exceeds energy expenditure. In the stationary phase of obesity, where weight is stable, there is a new energy balance, at a higher value of energy intake and expenditure. It is certain that a low relative energy expenditure (kJ/kg FFM) can contribute to the development of obesity, but the positive energy balance is mainly caused by excessive energy intake, so-called hyperphagia. Hyperphagia is manifest in individuals with a genetic predisposition to obesity by a failure in appetite regulation, which in particular can be brought about by a fat-rich diet and low level of physical activity. Hyperphagia can also result from psychological perturbances such as depression, or as a perceived comfort in the setting of significant social stressors. It should be noted that an energy intake of 12 MJ/day may be normal for a person with a high level of physical activity, whereas the same intake would be characterised as severe hyperphagia in someone with a low level of activity. This example illustrates how difficult it is to differentiate the two components of the energy balance equation when considering how obesity originates, and it appears that the physiological regulation of energy expenditure during physical activity is strongly connected to appetite.

More recently it has become clear that carbohydrate and protein are not converted to fat under normal circumstances in humans. That is because de novo lipogenesis is an energetically expensive process, which is suppressed when the fat intake of the diet is greater than about 20% of an isocaloric energy intake. This means that the fat in adipose tissue almost completely originates from the fat in the diet, so that the fatty acid composition of the diet is reflected in the adipose tissue, and that the macronutrient balance of each macro component of the diet (alcohol, fat, carbohydrate and protein) is regulated separately.

The alcohol balance has the highest priority in the combustion hierarchy, since alcohol cannot be stored in the body and is oxidised at the expense of the other macronutrients in the diet. The balance of protein and carbohydrate have the next highest priority, due to the limited size of the glycogen depots in the liver and muscle, and the protein stores, which can only tolerate oxidation for 1–2 days. In contrast, fat depots will withstand a much longer negative balance (see Ch. 5). After intake of a mixed meal, even with a high fat content, carbohydrate oxidation and storage is increased, whilst fat oxidation is inhibited and storage promoted. The change in substrate use and storage causes a rise in blood insulin concentration. This induces uptake of glucose by the cells, and lipoprotein lipase stimulates the uptake of triglyceride and inhibits lipolysis in adipose tissue. Supplementing a mixed meal with fat will not increase fat oxidation; the extra fat will be stored. When the composition of the diet varies with respect to fat and carbohydrate content, oxidative autoregulation ensures that the substrate undergoing combustion is gradually modified to correspond to the composition of the diet.

The regulation of the macronutrient balance has significance for understanding how the body regulates combustion and storage of nutrients with respect to intake, but provides no explanation about how some macronutrients fatten more than others; it is the energy balance that determines whether a person will gain or lose weight.

Signals from adipose tissue: lipostatic regulation

Body fat mass is also regulated through a lipostatic mechanism, which consists of a negative feedback between the fat depots and the brain (see Ch. 5). The size of the adipose tissue store is signalled to an appetite regulatory centre in the brain by the adipose hormone leptin (*leptos*, Greek term for thin), which is released from the fat tissue in an amount proportional to its size. Leptin induces satiety in the CNS, and has several additional endocrinological effects necessary for normal growth and development. A mutation in the gene coding for leptin has been found to be the cause of obesity in the *ob/ob* mouse. The mouse produces a defective leptin molecule that has no effect on the CNS. Leptin injections normalise weight in these mice, partly by reducing food intake and partly by increasing the animals' physical activity. Another monorecessive gene for obesity found in rodents, *db/db*, is responsible for a defective leptin receptor in the CNS. Mutations in the genes that code for leptin and the leptin receptor lead only in extremely rare cases to severe obesity in humans, but in overweight and obese individuals the blood leptin concentration is 10-fold higher than in normal-weight people, which suggests a state of leptin resistance in the obese. This situation has not been clarified to date.

Central integration of energy balance

The integration of both short- and long-term regulation of energy balance is effected in the arcuate nuclei of the medial hypothalamus, where two different central neurons have opposing effects in a complex interplay involving several neurotransmitters and receptors (see Section *evolve* 20.4 and Ch. 5 for further discussion of this topic).

Energy metabolism

Energy metabolism is described in detail in Chapter 5. The main difference in daily energy expenditure between individuals is a result of differences in the amount of fat-free body mass (FFM) and physical activity. While absolute and proportional FFM (relative to fat mass (FM)) can be altered by a dedicated exercise regimen, for most people, physical activity is the only realistic way to change and particularly increase energy expenditure.

A low relative basal metabolic rate (BMR in kJ/kg FFM) is known to increase the risk of weight gain, but it is unclear whether this condition has an impact on more than a minority of obese people. With a positive energy balance leading to weight gain, it is not only fat mass that increases. The fat-free body mass also increases, accounting for about one-third of the weight gain. This gain in FFM is composed mainly of increased organ and tissue mass, and the energy expenditure will be increased in proportion with the weight gain. The BMR in MJ/day can be estimated as 0.09 MJ/kg FFM + 1.55 MJ. A person with an excess 35 kg more than their ideal weight, of which about 12 kg will be FFM, will have a BMR per day that is more than 1 MJ higher than before the weight increase. In obesity, the level of physical activity is reduced, but as a result of the increased body mass, the energy expenditure in carrying out a given activity actually increases, such that the energy metabolism during physical activity is not reduced with obesity. Overweight patients often claim that they eat next to nothing and their dietary records apparently verify that the patient ingests only 4–6 MJ/day, despite weight stability. Measuring energy metabolism in these patients using double-labelled water (see Ch. 5) reveals this phenomenon to be due to a systematic under-reporting, presumably not acknowledged by the patients themselves.

Satiating effect of macronutrients

In a mixed diet, fat and alcohol satiate less than protein and carbohydrate joule for joule, which can partly be attributed to energy density. The outcome is that in order to achieve a state of satiety, a larger quantity of a fatty, carbohydrate-deficient diet must be eaten compared to a low fat, high carbohydrate diet (measured in mass (g) or volume (ml)). For most individuals, an increase in dietary fat content from the recommended 30% energy to 45% only results in an increased fat mass of 1–5 kg, but can have a dramatic negative effect on blood lipids, insulin sensitivity and coagulation/fibrinolysis factors. The type of carbohydrate and content of water and fibre, bound or free, also play a role in determining satiety.

The weak satiating effect of fat appears to occur when fat reaches the intestine (pre-absorptive), presumably through release of gastrointestinal peptide hormones (cholecystokinin (CCK), gastric inhibitory polypeptide (GIP), peptide YY (PYY), glucagon-like peptide (GLP-1), for example), which have a satiating effect via the hypothalamic centre for appetite control. In contrast, carbohydrate appears to affect the appetite after absorption (post-absorptive), partly through a direct effect on the brain via blood glucose and insulin, and partly through a satiating effect mediated by oxidation in the liver when glycogen depots in the liver have become fully loaded. The extent to which the satiating effect of simple carbohydrates like sucrose can be differentiated from that of more complex sugars is not entirely clear. There is also no evidence that replacement of sugar with artificial sweeteners leads to weight loss, unless it occurs as part of a strict calorie-controlled programme.

TRIGGERING FACTORS

Obesity can present itself from earliest childhood to senility, slowly or suddenly, with or without triggering factors. Several factors can potentially disturb the energy balance to such an extent that a large weight increase is involved.

Pregnancy

Fifty per cent of overweight women cite pregnancy as the main cause of their obesity (Linne et al 2002). First-time pregnant, non-smoking, hypertensive and already overweight women are a special risk group for excessive weight gain. The normal weight increase from conception to birth is 10–14 kg (about 20%), and the average gain from conception to a year after birth is 2 kg. This average figure, however, hides the fact that 30% have lost weight whilst the majority have gained – 15% more than 5 kg and 2% more than 10 kg. For underweight women, a greater gestational weight gain is accompanied by increased birthweight and reduced perinatal mortality, while for normal and overweight women, a gestational weight increase of >12 kg simply indicates a greater risk of caesarean section and lasting increased fat mass. The energy expenditure during pregnancy is about 330 MJ, of which the cost of fat storage accounts for only 10%, and increased energy intake accounts for the rest. In cases of severe overweight (>60%), weight gain during pregnancy should be limited to 5 kg, and with lesser degrees of obesity, energy restriction during pregnancy is not contra-indicated, although greater attention should be given to the quality of the diet.

Relative immobility

Acute weight gain is often seen with a sudden cessation of a habitually high level of physical activity, due to a specific occupation or sport. Obesity frequently occurs in taxi and bus drivers, as well as in chronically immobilised patients.

Impaired sleep and stress

Parallel to the increase in obesity prevalence seen in recent decades, a reduction in sleep times has also been observed. Between 1960 and 2002 in the USA, the average amount of sleep amongst adults decreased by approximately 1.5 hours per night. The factors responsible for this decrease in sleep include longer work days, increased environmental light, an increase in television viewing time, and the advent of the home computer and the internet. There is a U-shaped relationship between sleep duration and BMI, type 2 diabetes, cardiovascular disease and all-cause mortality, with the nadir of the curve indicating the optimum duration of sleep associated with lowest risk of approximately 7.7 hours/night. While the mechanisms underlying these associations are not fully elucidated, sleep restriction has been shown to result in a hormonal milieu that favours weight gain, including increased cortisol concentrations, decreased leptin (a satiety hormone), increased ghrelin (a hunger-stimulating hormone), insulin resistance and elevated levels of inflammatory cytokines. Clinically, sleep-deprived individuals experience increased hunger, especially for calorie-dense foods. A decrease in core body temperature with acute sleep deprivation has also been noted, suggesting that sleep loss may impact energy expenditure through thermoregulation.

Stress can increase the risk of weight gain and obesity, particularly among individuals with increased genetic risk as a result of polymorphisms in the glucocorticoid receptor. Glucocorticoid excess has a powerful stimulating effect on appetite, and fat deposition is typically of the android pattern.

Psychological trauma

Serious psychological trauma is often accompanied by voracious hyperphagia and weight increase in some individuals, whilst others react with anorexia and weight loss. Both manifestations can occur with grieving due to the loss of a close family member or after divorce. The incidence of the phenomenon is overestimated, since weight increase has sometimes been brought about by the use of psychotropic drugs, the weight-stimulating effects of which have only been acknowledged in recent years.

Smoking cessation

Tobacco smoking suppresses appetite and nicotine stimulates the sympathetic nervous system, such that 15–20 cigarettes a day can increase the daily energy metabolism by 10%. Smokers tend to be slimmer than non-smokers, but have more abdominal fat distribution, which is a risk factor for cardiovascular disease and diabetes. The average weight gain after stopping smoking is 3 kg for men and 4 kg for women over a 10-year period. For some the weight gain is merely normalising, but for most it is excessive. Risk groups are heavy smokers, and younger slim women with sedentary employment. Even though the health consequences of weight gain are secondary compared to the benefits of giving up smoking, the phenomenon is nevertheless important, since weight increase is the most frequent reason for taking up smoking again.

Endocrine obesity

Many endocrine disorders can be linked to weight gain and result in obesity. In patients with obesity, however, they represent a minority of causes. Hypothyroidism is often accompanied by weight gain, which can be attributed to the fact that energy expenditure can fall by up to 40%, depending on the severity of hypothyroidism. Despite effective treatment the weight seldom normalises. Weight gain is even seen in subclinical hypothyroidism, which is otherwise asymptomatic and manifest by only a very slight increase in thyroid stimulating hormone, while thyroid hormone levels themselves are maintained in the normal range. With thyrotoxicosis, weight loss is most commonly seen, but increase in weight can also occur in patients treated with antithyroid medication or radioactive iodine as they return to a euthyroid state, particularly amongst younger overweight women. Return to a euthyroid state can result in a weight gain of 5–7 kg within a year, or more if the patient becomes transiently hypothyroid as a consequence of treatment.

Abdominal obesity is a frequent clinical trait of Cushing's syndrome, which is a condition of excess cortisol production. Other features of Cushing's syndrome can include type 2 diabetes, hypertension, dyslipidaemia and oligomenorrhoea. All of these can also be found in the patient with visceral obesity; consequently, it can be difficult to distinguish some obese patients from those with Cushing's syndrome, so much so that the term 'pseudo-Cushing's has been coined to identify patients who have the clinical phenotype of Cushing's syndrome but do not demonstrate excess cortisol production. It is important to make this distinction clinically, as the treatment of Cushing's syndrome is directed at the cause of the excess cortisol production (usually a tumour of the pituitary or adrenal gland).

Growth hormone deficiency is usually caused by a pathological disturbance of the pituitary gland, such as a tumour, infiltrative disease or damage from radiation therapy. Lean body mass is decreased and fat mass (particularly visceral fat) is increased in untreated adults who are deficient in growth hormone, compared with those who have normal growth hormone secretion. These parameters improve with exogenous growth hormone therapy.

Hypothalamic obesity is a rare syndrome which is a consequence of disruption of hypothalamic integration of metabolic information regarding nutrient stores with afferent sensory information about food availability. It can be caused by trauma, tumour, inflammatory or infiltrative disease, surgery in the posterior fossa, or increased intracranial pressure. Obesity is only occasionally seen with the insulin-secreting tumour insulinoma.

Drug–induced obesity

A number of prescription drugs are associated with weight gain, a phenomenon that is all too often neglected by doctors (Tardieu et al 2003). Lithium, neuroleptics, cyclic antidepressants and the epilepsy drugs valproate and carbamazepine are among the most potent. Oestrogen, glucocorticoids and insulin can also cause weight gain, as can the anti-cancer drugs tamoxifen and megestrol acetate. During the treatment of AIDS patients with antiviral agents, a condition called lipodystrophy is sometimes induced, which is associated with an increased risk of type 2 diabetes and cardiovascular disease.

KEY POINTS

- In only a minority of cases is obesity caused by a chromosome abnormality, a mutation in a single gene or classic endocrine disorder.
- Most cases of obesity are due to a disposition towards an inadequately functioning appetite regulation and energy metabolism.
- Weight gain and obesity may be triggered in susceptible individuals when the energy density and fat content of the diet's food and drink is too high, mealtimes are irregular and daily physical activity is limited.
- An unlimited supply of cheap, tasty foodstuffs and larger food portions also help to promote overweight and risk of obesity.
- The disposition towards obesity is not necessarily genetic, since other influences, for example chemicals or hormones transferred from mother to fetus during pregnancy, may programme the offspring to be susceptible to an obesity-promoting lifestyle. Obesity can be triggered by pregnancy, immobility, impaired sleep, stress, drugs, psychological trauma, smoking cessation or rarely endocrine disorders.

20.5 PREVENTION AND TREATMENT

PRINCIPLES TO ACHIEVE DIET-INDUCED WEIGHT LOSS

In almost every overweight and obese patient, the diet must be adjusted to reduce energy intake. Dietary therapy consists of instructing patients as to how to modify their dietary intake to achieve a decrease in energy intake while maintaining a nutritionally adequate diet. Due to their enlarged body size, obese subjects have higher energy requirements for a given level of physical activity than their

normal-weight counterparts (Fig. 20.1). Obese diabetics have slightly higher energy requirements than obese subjects without diabetes for a given body size and composition, due to increased hepatic glucose production. Reducing the total energy intake of the obese patient to that of a normal-weight individual will inevitably cause weight loss, consisting of about 75% fat and 25% lean tissue, until weight normalisation occurs at a new energy equilibrium. For patients with class I obesity this requires an energy deficit of 300–500 kcal/day (1.3–2.2MJ/day), and for patients with class III obesity 500–1000 kcal/day (2.1–4.2MJ/day). The desirable rate of weight loss for most people is 0.5–1 kg per week after the first month of dieting, with younger, taller and more overweight subjects aiming for the upper

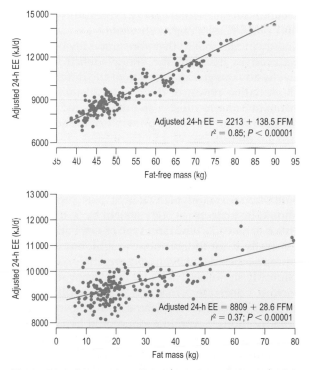

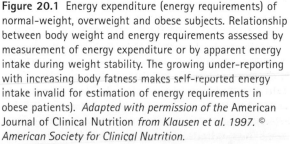

Figure 20.1 Energy expenditure (energy requirements) of normal-weight, overweight and obese subjects. Relationship between body weight and energy requirements assessed by measurement of energy expenditure or by apparent energy intake during weight stability. The growing under-reporting with increasing body fatness makes self-reported energy intake invalid for estimation of energy requirements in obese patients). *Adapted with permission of the* American Journal of Clinical Nutrition *from Klausen et al. 1997.* © *American Society for Clinical Nutrition.*

limit, and older, shorter and less overweight subjects for the lower rate. With higher rates of loss, there may be excessive loss of lean tissue. During the first month, weight loss will be more rapid because of the water diuresis associated with breakdown of glycogen stores.

There is evidence to support the idea that differences in diet composition exert some effects on energy absorption and energy expenditure, but these differences have less clinical importance compared with the major goal to reduce total energy intake. This can be achieved by setting an upper limit for energy intake. The larger the daily deficit in energy balance the more rapid the weight loss. A deficit of 300–500 kcal/day (1.3–2.1MJ/day) will produce a weight loss of 300–500 g/week, and a deficit of 500–1000 kcal/day (2.1–4.2MJ/day) will produce a weight loss of 500–1000 g/week. Greater initial energy deficits may produce even larger weight loss rates. Total energy expenditure declines and normalises along with weight loss, and total energy intake should therefore gradually be further reduced to maintain the energy deficit. Alternatively, advantage can be taken of the differences in the satiating power of the various dietary components in order to cause a spontaneous reduction in energy intake. This is the principle of the ad libitum low-fat diet.

CHOOSING THE DIETARY ENERGY DEFICIT

Initially, the target of a weight loss programme should be to decrease body weight by 5–10%. Once this is achieved a new target can be set. Patients will generally want to lose more weight, but it should be remembered that even a 5% weight is considered clinically significant, in that it improves cardiac risk factors, decreases risk of co-morbidities and decreases mortality associated with obesity-related complications. Several factors should be taken into consideration, e.g. the patient's degree of obesity, previous weight loss attempts, risk factors, co-morbidities, and personal and social capacity to undertake the necessary lifestyle changes.

To prescribe a diet with a defined energy deficit it is necessary to estimate the actual energy requirements of the patient. It would seem natural to estimate the patient's habitual energy intake from self-reported diet record over 3–7 days of weight stability. However, these estimates are invalid due to systematic under-reporting of energy intake by obese individuals amounting to 30–40% (Fig. 20.1).

Energy requirements should therefore be assessed indirectly by estimation of total energy expenditure. Resting metabolic rate (RMR) can be measured by indirect calorimetry or be estimated with great accuracy using equations based on body weight, gender and age (Table 20.2) or, even better, estimated from information on the size of fat-free mass and fat mass. Total energy expenditure (= energy requirement) is estimated by multiplication of RMR (kcal/day) by an activity factor (PAL; physical activity level) (Table 20.2). The energy level of the prescribed diet is defined as the patient's energy requirement minus the prescribed daily energy deficit.

THEORETICAL VERSUS CLINICAL OUTCOME

Translating the physiologically based considerations regarding energy balance and weight loss into clinical practice requires a high degree of compliance, which can be difficult to obtain. Weight loss results tend to be much better in clinical trials

Table 20.2	Estimating energy needs: revised WHO equations for estimating basal metabolic rate (BMR)
Men	
18–30 years	= (0.0630 × actual weight in kg + 2.8957) × 240 kcal/day
31–60 years	= (0.0484 × actual weight in kg + 3.6534) × 240 kcal/day
Women	
18–30 years	= (0.0621 × actual weight in kg + 2.0357) × 240 kcal/day
31–60 years	= (0.342 × actual weight in kg + 3.5377) × 240 kcal/day
Estimated total energy expenditure = BMR × activity factor	
Activity level	Activity factor
Low (sedentary)	1.3
Intermediate (some regular exercise)	1.5
High (regular activity or demanding job)	1.7

Reproduced with permission from: Astrup A (2004) Treatment of obesity. In: Ferrannini E, Zimmet P, De Fronzo R A, Keen H (eds) *International textbook of diabetes mellitus.* © John Wiley & Sons Limited.

conducted in specialised clinics than in trials conducted by non-specialists without sufficient resources and access to auxiliary therapists (dietitians, psychologists, etc.). Compliance and adherence to the diet are the cornerstones of successful weight loss and are the most complicated part of the dietary treatment of obesity. To improve adherence, consideration should be given to the patient's food preferences as well as to personal, educational and social factors. Great efforts should be made to see the patient frequently and regularly, as increased patient support is positively associated with the success of any weight loss programme. Furthermore, long-term weight reduction is unlikely to succeed unless the patient acquires new eating and physical activity habits. These behavioural changes should be an integral part of the treatment programme.

OPTIONS FOR WEIGHT LOSS DIETS

Therapeutic obesity diets distinguish between several recognised weight reduction regimens. Low-energy diets (LED) usually provide 800–1500 kcal/day (3.3–6.3MJ/day)and use fat-reduced foods, though weight loss occurs independent of the diet composition. Diets providing 1200 kcal/day (5MJ/day) or more have been classified as balanced-deficits diets, but this definition will not be used in this chapter. Very-low-energy diets (VLED) are modified fasts providing 200–800 kcal/day (0.8–3.3MJ/day) that replace normal foods. Ad libitum low-fat diets do not restrict energy intake directly, but target a restriction of ad libitum fat intake to 20–30% of total energy intake. Energy intake is spontaneously reduced because of the higher satiating effect of this diet, and a modest weight loss occurs.

Very-low-energy diets (VLED)

Starvation (less than 200 kcal/day, 0.8MJ/day) is the ultimate dietary treatment of obesity, but it is no longer used because of the numerous and serious medical complications associated with prolonged starvation. Starvation has been replaced by VLED (200–800 kcal/day; 0.8–3.3MJ/day), which aims to supply very little energy but all essential nutrients. Reducing the energy content of a diet requires an increased nutrient density. This can be difficult to obtain with natural foods if the diet is to be acceptable once the energy content of the diet becomes

lower than 800 kcal/day. This has led to the commercial production of VLEDs, supplemented with all nutrients in amounts that meet the recommended daily allowance (RDA) criteria. For decades, 250–400 kcal/day (1–1.7MJ/day) formula diets were extremely popular. The first VLEDs were clearly nutritionally insufficient, but reports of adverse effects and results from research have brought about a gradual increase in energy level. Some concern has been raised about the cardiac safety of the use of VLEDs with less than 800 kcal/day; in addition, patients using VLEDs have an increased risk of developing gallstones (Table 20.3). Their use without medical supervision has generally been abandoned and should not be recommended.

A number of studies have shown that VLEDs with energy levels of less than 800 kcal/day do not produce a greater weight loss and are less well accepted than those comprising 800 kcal/day. Today the 800 kcal/day VLED is the only version recognised as being both effective and safe. These VLEDs usually provide a ketogenic diet in the form of nutrition powders, or in the form of protein, mineral, trace element and vitamin-enriched meals or drinks. VLEDs can induce very rapid weight loss over a 2–3-month period, but do not seem to facilitate weight maintenance. This is not because a rapid initial weight loss causes poorer long-term weight maintenance per se, as initial weight losses are positively, not negatively, associated with long-term weight loss. It is because VLEDs are not educational and do not facilitate the gradual modification of the

Table 20.3	Adverse effects and complications of a VLED	
ADVERSE EFFECT	**OCCURRENCE**
Cold intolerance	~50%
Dry skin	~50%
Fatigue, dizziness, muscle cramps headache, gastrointestinal distress	10–20%
Hair loss	10%
Gallstones	10–30%
Bad breath	20–30%

Reproduced with permission from: Astrup A (2004) Treatment of obesity. In: Ferrannini E, Zimmet P, De Fronzo R A, Keen H (eds) *International textbook of diabetes mellitus.* © John Wiley & Sons Limited.

patient's eating behaviour, nutritional knowledge and skills, which seems to be required for long-term weight maintenance.

Low-energy diets (LED)

LEDs usually provide 800–1500 kcal/day (3.3–6.3MJ/day) and normally consist of natural foods. LEDs are also called 'traditional diets' and 'calorie-counting diets', because previously more emphasis was put on restricting the total energy level of the diet than on the macronutrient composition. Although macronutrient composition of the diet is of less importance for short-term weight loss, it is now usually modified in order to maximise the beneficial effect on cardiovascular risk factors and insulin resistance, to prevent cancers and to promote long-term weight maintenance.

For practical reasons, LEDs are low-fat, carbohydrate-rich diets, with a fixed energy allowance. An example of an appropriate nutrient composition for an LED is given in Table 20.4. It should be supplemented with daily vitamin and mineral tablets. A female patient may choose an energy level of 1000–1200 kcal/day and 1200–1500 kcal/day for men. LEDs produce a lower rate of weight loss than VLEDs (Fig. 20.2), but randomised clinical trials (RCT) demonstrate that the long-term (>1 year) weight loss is not different from that of the VLED. Furthermore, using LEDs for weight loss induction introduces healthy eating habits early in the weight reduction programme, giving a longer period in which to familiarise the patient with the dietary changes that are a central element in a weight maintenance programme. LEDs produce weight loss regardless of duration of treatment, and reduce body weight by an average of 8% over 3–12 months.

Ad libitum low–fat diets (<30% energy from fat)

Data from animal and experimental research, observational studies and numerous randomised control trials (RCT) have shown that a high dietary fat content plays an important role in the development of obesity. A high-fat diet promotes weight gain and obesity in sedentary individuals with little self-restraint who have a genetic predisposition to obesity. The main mechanisms are the passive over-consumption of energy promoted by the high energy density of fatty foods, and a reduced fat oxidation capacity in susceptible individuals. Low-fat diets are more satiating due to the high content of complex carbohydrates and protein. Restricting intake of dietary fat should be seen as a means to reducing the energy density of the diet and hence restrict the patient's total energy intake. Unfortunately, whereas the effect of fat-rich foods on weight gain and obesity is substantial, the ability of the ad libitum low-fat, carbohydrate-rich diet to induce weight loss is less pronounced. A systematic

Table 20.4	Example of the composition of a low-energy diet (LED)
NUTRIENT	RECOMMENDED ITAKE
Calories	500–1000 kcal/day below energy requirements
Total fat	20–30% of total calories
Saturated fatty acids	<10% of total calories
Monounsaturated fatty acids	<15% of total calories
Polyunsaturated fatty acids	<10% of total calories
Protein	15–20% of total calories
Carbohydrate	>55% of total calories
Fibre	20–30 g/day
Calcium	1000–1,500 mg/day
Other vitamins, minerals and trace elements	RDA. Full coverage should be ensured by a vitamin/mineral supplement daily

Reproduced with permission from: Astrup A (2004) Treatment of obesity. In: Ferrannini E, Zimmet P, De Fronzo R A, Keen H (eds) *International textbook of diabetes mellitus.* © John Wiley & Sons Limited.

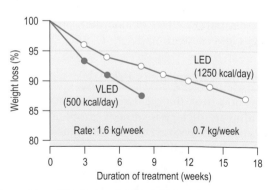

Figure 20.2 Weight loss in obese patients randomised to either a low-energy diet (LED) or a very-low-energy diet (VLED). Initial mean body weight was nearly 100 kg and mean weight loss 12.6 kg in both groups. *Adapted from Toubro & Astrup 1997.*

review of 28 ad libitum low-fat diet RCTs showed that a weight loss of 1.6 g/day was achieved for each percentage point reduction in energy from fat (Astrup et al 2000). A realistic reduction in dietary fat can result in a weight loss of 20–100 g/week, which becomes clinically significant when the total exceeds 5% of body weight. Interventions lasting >2 months have shown that ad libitum, low-fat diets produce a statistically highly significant weight loss difference of 3.3 kg compared to controls. The size of the weight loss is mainly determined by the reduction in dietary fat energy, but pre-treatment body weight is also positively associated with the weight loss. Obese patients with a mean body weight of 95 kg who reduce dietary fat from 45 to 25% energy under ad libitum conditions will reduce energy intake and will, on average, achieve a weight loss of 7.1 kg before a new equilibrium is reached. On the other hand, a normal-weight subject (60 kg) will lose only 0.5 kg with the same fat reduction. These weight loss predictions are probably under-estimated because the analysis relies on the reductions in dietary fat as reported by the patients, which tend to be exaggerated. Moreover, patients with better adherence also achieved better weight loss than those with poorer adherence. (See Section *evolve* 20.5(a) 🖱 for information on the effects on cardiovascular risk factors of low-fat diets.)

LED versus ad libitum low–fat diets?

Ad libitum low-fat diets produce a rate of weight loss of 100–200 g/week in unselected obese patients, whereas LEDs induce weight losses of 300–700 g/week. LEDs using low-fat diets are more effective in inducing weight loss than ad libitum low-fat diets, and they allow a better adjustment of the reduction in energy intake. LEDs are therefore the preferred dietary treatment for obesity. However, in an individually tailored treatment, the first step could be to prescribe an ad libitum low-fat diet to patients habitually consuming a high-fat diet, subsequently limiting energy intake if weight loss proves unsatisfactory.

Ad libitum low–carbohydrate diets (<25 g/day carbohydrate)

Diets that promote very low carbohydrate intakes have become very popular, as part of a popular physiological concept which links surges in blood glucose and insulin to weight gain and obesity

(Astrup et al 2004). The 'Atkins New Diet Revolution' is the most well known of these popular diets, and recommends a daily intake of <25 g carbohydrates. It is likely that such a 'ketogenic' diet in combination with a high protein intake possesses anorectic properties and produces weight loss in the short term, but it may be very problematic in the weight maintenance phase due to side effects, adverse effects on risk factor profile and an increased risk of developing type 2 diabetes in overweight and obese subjects. Very few controlled studies testing the low-carbohydrate diet have been published. One uncontrolled study found that an ad libitum low-carbohydrate diet (<25 g/day) produced a weight loss of 10.3% over 6 months in 51 obese subjects. Positive changes in blood lipids and blood pressure were also seen, but 68% of the participants experienced constipation, probably due to the low fibre intake. A fat-rich diet impairs the beneficial effects of physical training on insulin resistance. When the weight loss has slowed it is likely that the low-carbohydrate (high fat) diet will have very negative effects on most cardiovascular risk factors and, despite the weight loss, may increase insulin resistance and risk of type 2 diabetes. Low-carbohydrate diets cannot therefore be recommended.

DIETARY WEIGHT MAINTENANCE PROGRAMMES

In professional weight loss programmes, LEDs induce a 5% weight loss in almost all patients, and frequent clinical attendance during the initial 6 months of weight reduction appears to facilitate achievement of the therapy goals. Larger success criteria (>10% weight loss) can be met by the majority of patients if the treatment programme also includes group therapy and behaviour modification. The real challenge is to maintain the reduced body weight and prevent subsequent relapse (Fig. 20.3). In a systematic review of long-term (>3 years' follow-up) efficacy of dietary treatment of obesity, success was defined as maintenance of all weight initially lost, or maintenance of at least 9 kg of initial weight loss. Initial weight loss was 4–28 kg, and 15% of the followed up patients fulfilled one of the criteria for success, and the success rate was stable for up to 14 years of observation. Diet combined with group therapy leads to better long-term success rates (27%) than diet alone (15%), or diet combined with behaviour modification and active

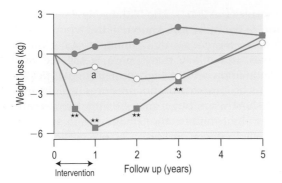

Figure 20.3 A 5-year follow-up of a 1-year randomised controlled trial of a reduced-fat ad libitum diet versus a usual diet (Swinburn et al 2001). Obese IGT patients were randomised to a reduced-fat diet (solid squares) or control (solid circles), and participated in monthly small-group education sessions on reduced-fat eating for 1 year. Weight decreased significantly in the reduced-fat diet group; the greatest difference was noted at 1 year (23.3 kg), best in the most compliant group, but diminished at subsequent follow-up. Glucose tolerance also improved in patients on the reduced-fat diet; a lower proportion had type 2 diabetes or impaired glucose tolerance at 1 year (47% versus 67%). This difference disappeared in subsequent years, but the more compliant 50% of the intervention group maintained lower fasting and 2-hour glucose at 5 years compared to control subjects. The line with open circles (a) stands for a subgroup of the reduced-fat intervention group with poor compliance. The asterisks denote statistically significant difference between the reduced-fat and the control group. *Copyright © 2001 American Diabetes Association. From* Diabetes Care, Vol. 24, *2001; 619–624. Adapted with permission from The American Diabetes Association.*

follow-up, though active follow-up produces better weight maintenance than passive follow-up (19% versus 10%).

Whereas the principle of energy restriction (LED) is successful for weight loss induction independent of dietary composition, the low-fat, high-protein/carbohydrate diet seems to be more effective for long-term weight maintenance and prevention of weight regain. In a study by Toubro and Astrup, patients were randomly assigned to two different weight maintenance groups, receiving either a low-fat diet ad libitum or a fixed-energy diet (LED) for 1 year after having lost a mean of 13.6 kg on energy-restricted diets. There was only a small weight regain during the weight maintenance

programme over 1 year. However, 2 years after the weight loss, the LED group had regained 11.3 kg, whereas the low-fat group had regained only 5.4 kg. Forty per cent of the patients in the LED group and 65% of the patients in the low fat group had maintained a weight loss of >5 kg.

DOES DIET COMPOSITION MATTER?

Numerous popular diet books promote changing diet composition in accordance with principles that are claimed to have a particularly favourable impact on weight loss and maintenance. Generally these claims are unsubstantiated and scientifically improbable, and some may even promote nutritionally insufficient diets. With LEDs, slightly more patients will be successful and fewer will drop out if the diet has a low (25% energy) rather than a high (45% energy) fat content (Petersen et al 2006). With ad libitum diets, and weight maintenance diets particularly, differences in the satiating effects of different macronutrients may have some importance (Makris et al 2008).

Carbohydrate types

The high carbohydrate content of low-fat diets stems mainly from the complex carbohydrates of different vegetables, fruits and whole grains, which are more satiating for fewer calories than fatty foods and are a good source of vitamins, minerals, trace elements and fibre. A high fibre content may further improve the satiating effect of the diet, and a diet rich in soluble fibre, including oat bran, legumes, barley and most fruits and vegetables, may be effective in reducing blood cholesterol and blood pressure levels. The recommended intake is 20–30 grams of fibre daily.

The role of simple carbohydrates in low fat diets remains controversial, mainly due to the lack of proper RCTs. Low-fat diets, high in either complex or simple carbohydrates, induce similar fat loss in overweight and obese subjects, and a diet high in simple carbohydrates has no detrimental effects on blood lipids. However, recent evidence suggests that a high intake of sugar from soft drinks may have a special fattening property.

Glycaemic index (GI)

Some scientists have warned against the fattening properties of high-GI foods such as potatoes, white bread, bagels and rice – foods that people are otherwise advised to eat as part of the currently recommended low-fat diet. Instead they advise people to eat more wholegrain products, and types of rice and potatoes characterised by a low GI. Low GI foods are beneficial for glycaemic control in diabetics and have a modest beneficial effect on cardiovascular risk factors, but their effect on body weight regulation is controversial (see Ch. 21).

The proponents of the GI hypothesis suggest that high-GI foods produce rapid and transient surges in blood glucose and insulin, which are in turn followed by rapidly returning hunger sensations and excessive caloric intake, but the scientific evidence is not conclusive. The effect of GI on weight loss seems to be in the order of 1 kg over 6–12 months when achieving a 10–15 GI unit difference between diets. Diets low in GI are also high in fibre and whole grain, and it is likely that fibre and whole grain are the key responsible dietary factors responsible for the assumed effect of GI.

These aspects prohibit issuing general dietary advice that low-GI foods are preferable to high-GI foods in preventing weight gain, although it appears likely that this dietary change will have beneficial effects on risk factors of cardiovascular disease and diabetes, and unlikely that it will exert any adverse effects. However, the GI concept is complicated for patients, and comprehensive tables are required in order to calculate the diet. Newer research shows that the GI of meals cannot be accurately calculated from the carbohydrate source alone but requires information about the energy, fat and protein content as well.

Protein content

A large body of experimental human data suggests that protein possesses a higher satiating power per calorie than carbohydrate and fat. The impact on weight loss of replacing carbohydrate with protein in ad libitum low-fat diets has been addressed in only one RCT. The protein-rich diet produced a larger weight loss than a high-carbohydrate diet, had no adverse effect on blood lipids, renal function or bone mineral density, and seemed to have a positive influence on the atherogenic risk factor profile in abdominally obese men. Replacement of some dietary carbohydrate by protein in ad libitum low-fat diets may improve weight loss. More freedom to choose between protein-rich and complex-carbohydrate-rich foods may encourage obese subjects to choose more lean meat and dairy products and hence improve adherence to low-fat diets in weight reduction programmes. Increased protein allowances in weight reduction diets should await confirmation of these results by other studies (Paddon-Jones et al 2008). The dietary principles promoted in recent popular diet books advocating high-protein, low-carbohydrate diets are not supported by the existing evidence.

Fat quality and high–MUFA diets

Although similar amounts of different fats contain nearly the same amount of energy, differences may exist in their satiating effects, which could influence total energy intake of ad libitum low-fat diets and weight maintenance diets. From a biochemical and physiological viewpoint, saturated fatty acids behave very differently from monounsaturated fats (MUFA), which seem to be more neutral than saturated or polyunsaturated fats in relation to cardiovascular disease, insulin resistance and cancer. However, animal studies suggest that MUFAs increase body weight more than polyunsaturated fatty acids (PUFA). In a cross-sectional, observational study in 128 males, the highest positive correlation was found between the intake of MUFAs and body fat mass, whereas no significant association was found between PUFAs and body fat, and only a weak association with saturated fat was seen. Two experimental appetite studies have concordantly shown that meals/infusions with MUFAs produce lower satiety, and that they suppress energy intake for the remainder of the day less than PUFAs. These preliminary reports suggest that a high MUFA content in the diet may promote passive overconsumption and obesity.

(For further information see Section *evolve* 20.5(b) 🖰).

Alcohol

Alcohol provides energy that displaces more nutritious foods. Alcohol suppresses fat oxidation, thereby allowing more dietary fat to be stored. The satiating effect of alcohol energy may be low, and alcohol consumption has been shown to promote passive over-consumption of fat. Alcohol has also been associated with obesity in epidemiological studies. High alcohol consumption also increases the risk of losing control over otherwise restrained behaviour. Consequently, energy from alcohol should be limited and needs to be assessed and appropriately controlled.

EXERCISE

Increased daily physical activity and exercise are important components of weight-control programmes. Physical activity is not as effective as a hypocaloric diet for inducing weight loss, which can easily be seen from the greater ability of diet compared with physical activity to produce a negative daily energy balance. However, patients should gradually increase their physical activity, and as patients lose weight, further increases in physical activity and exercise should be emphasised to help maintain lost weight. It is also helpful from a behavioural perspective to encourage patients to monitor their physical activity.

The impact of exercise for weight control is based on the ability of patients to engage in adequate levels of activity. The minimal level that should be recommended is at least 45–60 minutes of moderate-intensity physical activity on most days of the week (Saris et al 2003). This level of physical activity not only improves health-related factors, but also supports the recommendation of higher levels of exercise for weight-control purposes. The role of the clinician is to provide adequate guidance to patients regarding issues related to the intensity, duration and mode of exercise that may be most appropriate. When addressing these issues, it is also important to consider the barriers that individual patients may encounter that will have an effect on adoption and maintenance of exercise behaviours. For example, for patients who suffer from osteoarthritis as a consequence of their obesity, aerobic activities that minimise weight bearing such as swimming or cycling could be suggested. Medical centres can support patients by providing weekly or biweekly weigh-ins to track progress and provide ongoing feedback. Patients should be reminded that the ultimate goal of any weight management programme is gradual, incremental weight losses that are maintained over time. Sustainable and enjoyable changes in physical activity patterns must be made along with a lifelong commitment to health.

DRUGS FOR TREATMENT OF OBESITY

This section focuses solely on drugs currently available for the treatment of obesity, or drugs with weight-reducing properties used for the treatment of type 2 diabetes, depression or smoking cessation. For more detail see Section *evolve* 20.5(c) .

Lipase inhibitors (orlistat)

Mechanism of action and use

Malabsorption of dietary fat is an obvious drug target as high dietary fat intake plays a special role in promoting weight gain and obesity. A number of compounds that act as intestinal lipase inhibitors are currently being investigated for use in the treatment of obesity and related disorders, but only orlistat is currently approved and freely available. Orlistat is a specific inhibitor of intestinal lipase, the enzyme secreted from the exocrine pancreas and responsible for enzymatic fat digestion. At the recommended therapeutic dose (120 mg) taken immediately prior to or within 1 hour of each of the three daily main meals, the absorption of dietary fat is reduced by approximately 30%. Orlistat produces a negative energy balance resulting in weight loss.

Orlistat is recommended for use as the pharmacological support for modest caloric restriction and a diet providing less than 30% of energy from fat. The most frequent adverse effects of orlistat are flatulence, flatulence with discharge, oily spotting, faecal urgency and incontinence, oily stools and steatorrhoea. These adverse effects are generally self-limiting and transient, occurring within the first months of treatment and often triggered by the ingestion of high-fat meals. The unabsorbed fat binds some fat-soluble vitamins (A, D and E) and other nutrients (β-carotene, lycopene, flavonoids, etc.). A simple vitamin supplement and increased intake of fruit and vegetables counteracts this effect.

Orlistat is now available at a reduced dose of 60 mg as an over-the-counter preparation. It is taken with the same precautions as above, and has similar efficacy.

Treatment in simple obesity

The efficacy and safety of orlistat have been documented in several short- and long-term double-blind trials lasting for up to 4 years, involving a total of more than 30 000 patients, making orlistat the best investigated drug for the treatment of obesity. In most trials, orlistat induces a dose-dependent reduction in body weight, and the recommended dose induces a mean weight loss that typically exceeds that of the placebo group by 3–5 kg, to some extent independent of the degree of dietary energy restriction and other ancillary treatment.

Treatment in obese IGT and diabetics

Treatment of obese subjects with IGT using orlistat as an adjuvant to diet and lifestyle modification has been shown to decrease the incidence of progression to type 2 diabetes. The additional weight loss achieved by orlistat is sufficient to reduce the incidence of diabetes, even among less selected obese subjects.

Sibutramine

Sibutramine is a serotonin and noradrenaline (norepinephrine) reuptake inhibitor with only a weak inhibitory action on dopamine reuptake. It decreases food intake in humans by increasing meal-induced satiety. It also exerts a weak thermogenic effect both acutely and during long-term use. Sibutramine is generally well tolerated from a symptom perspective; and has few side effects, which include symptoms such as dry mouth, headache, insomnia and constipation. The adverse effects of sibutramine include increases in blood pressure and heart rate. Due to its cardiovascular side effect profile, sibutramine is not recommended for use in patients with a history of cardiovascular disease. Importantly, preliminary data from the Sibutramine Cardiovascular OUTcome (SCOUT) Trial suggests that there may be an increased risk of adverse cardiovascular events on this medication compared to placebo, in a population with a history of, or high risk for, cardiovascular disease. These findings highlight the importance of not using sibutramine in patients with coronary artery disease, but also raise concern for its use in patients without known cardiovascular disease, but who are at high risk based on comorbidities. Based on the SCOUT findings, in January 2010, the European Medicines Agency recommended suspension of marketing authorizations for sibutramine; the medication is still available for use in North America.

TYPE 2 DIABETES TREATMENTS

Metformin

Metformin is a biguanide that is considered to be first line therapy for the treatment of type 2 diabetes. It acts by decreasing peripheral insulin resistance, thereby targeting the underlying pathology of the disease. Metformin promotes a modest weight reduction in many diabetics, in contrast to most other treatment options, which cause weight gain.

GLP-1 analogues

Exenatide is the first clinically available analogue of glucagon-like-peptide-1 (GLP-1), and is approved in many countries for use in the treatment of type 2 diabetes. GLP-1 is a gastrointestinal incretin peptide which acts to potentiate insulin release and decrease glucagon release in response to a meal, as well as to slow gastric emptying and decrease food intake. Exenatide needs to be taken as two daily injections, whereas the newer GLP-1 analogue liraglutide only needs one daily injection. GLP-1 analogues also produce weight loss, but at higher dosages than required for glycemic control (Astrup et al 2009).

Antidepressants/smoking cessation agents

Although not indicated specifically for treatment of obesity, fluoxetine is a selective serotonin reuptake inhibitor that is used as a treatment for depression, and which may facilitate short-term weight loss in these patients. Thus, fluoxetine may be preferred over other antidepressants in obese patients, as many other antidepressive agents cause weight gain.

Bupropion is an antidepressant that is believed to act by enhancing noradrenergic and dopaminergic release in the central nervous system. However, because the efficacy of bupropion in a sustained release (SR) preparation for obesity management has been studied in only a small number of patients, it is not currently indicated specifically for treatment of obesity.

SURGICAL TREATMENT OF OBESITY

In light of the increasing prevalence and severity of obesity globally, bariatric surgery is being increasingly utilised as a treatment of obesity, with the number of procedures having increased more than 500% in the last 5 years in most developed countries. Bariatric surgery is indicated for adults with a BMI ≥ 40 kg/m^2, or ≥ 35 with obesity-related comorbidities such as type 2 diabetes, hypertension or obstructive sleep apnoea, who have failed intensive lifestyle and pharmacotherapeutic weight loss interventions.

Bariatric procedures can be classified as restrictive, in that they reduce food intake, or malabsorptive, in that they reduce food uptake from the gastrointestinal tract. The two most commonly performed procedures are laparascopic adjustable gastric banding and Roux-en-Y gastric bypass surgery (RYGB) (Fig. 20.4).

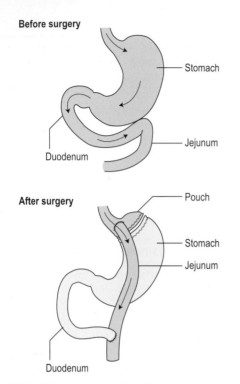

Figure 20.4 Before and after bariatic surgery.

Gastric banding is a purely restrictive procedure that compartmentalises the upper stomach by placing a tight, usually adjustable band around the entrance to the stomach. Advantages of gastric banding include the simplicity of the procedure and low rate of perioperative complications. The efficacy of gastric banding is variable; a weight loss of 20% can be seen by 1 year post procedure, but longer-term data suggest a significant (but highly variable) risk of weight regain.

RYGB employs a combined restrictive and malabsorptive approach to weight loss. It is characterised by the creation of a small gastric pouch, divided and separated from the stomach remnant. The small intestine is then divided, creating a proximal biliopancreatic limb that transports the secretions from the gastric remnant, liver and pancreas, and an alimentary (or Roux) limb that is anastomosed to the new gastric pouch to drain consumed food. The distal end of the biliopancreatic limb is then anastomosed to the alimentary limb, creating a common channel where digestive enzymes mix with ingested food. Weight loss following RYGB is impressive; in the landmark Swedish Obesity Study, weight loss was maximal at 38% at 1 year postoperatively. After 10 years, 74% of patients were able to maintain a weight loss of >20% compared to baseline, whereas a subset of patients regained weight.

In addition to eliciting weight loss, bariatric surgery is also highly effective in treating or reversing many complications of obesity, including type 2 diabetes, hypertension, dyslipidaemia and obstructive sleep apnoea, and also decreases the risk of overall mortality. RYGB has a particularly impressive effect upon type 2 diabetes; within 1 month postoperatively, over 80% of diabetes remits entirely. In addition to the mechanisms described above, RYGB also results in marked alterations in gastrointestinal hormone and incretin release, which is thought to be a significant contributor to the resolution rate of diabetes that is seen.

Long-term reductions in mortality in bariatric surgery populations as a whole have been documented to be as high as 29%, and as high as 40% post gastric bypass surgery.

For more information, see Section *evolve* 20.5(d) .

KEY POINTS

- Prevention and treatment of obesity requires a reduced energy intake and increased expenditure through physical activity.
- Energy intake should be reduced by a reduction in energy density and portion sizes of meals, and by avoiding drinks containing calories.
- To achieve weight loss, a reduced energy intake is pertinent, while both a changed diet composition and 30–60 minutes of daily physical activity are required for subsequent weight maintenance.
- Low-energy diets, either consisting of normal foods or meal replacements, are effective to induce a weight loss of 5–10% in most patients.
- The optimal diet is reduced in fat, with increased content of fibre-rich carbohydrates and protein from meat and dairy products. Many popular fad diets may produce transient weight loss, mainly by a high protein content and/or ketosis.
- Currently approved weight loss drugs improve the mean weight loss and increase the proportion of subjects who achieve more than 5–10% weight loss.
- Bariatric surgery is an option for treatment of patients with severe or comorbid obesity who have failed intensive lifestyle and/or pharmacotherapeutic interventions.

References

Astrup A: The effect of exercise and diet on glucose intolerance and substrate utilisation? In Allison SP, Go VLW, editors: *Metabolic issues of clinical nutrition,* Basel, 2004, Karger, pp 93–109.

Astrup A, Grunwald GK, Melanson EL, et al: The role of low-fat diets in body weight control: a meta-analysis of *ad libitum* intervention studies, *International Journal of Obesity* 24: 1545–1552, 2000.

Astrup A, Larsen TM, Harper A: Atkins and other low-carbohydrate diets: hoax or an effective tool for weight loss? *Lancet* 364: 897–899, 2004.

Astrup A, Rössner S, Van Gaal L, et al: Effects of liraglutide in the treatment of obesity: a randomised, double-blind, placebo-controlled study, *Lancet* 374: 1606–1616, 2009.

Harder H, Dinesen B, Astrup A: The effect of a rapid weight loss on lipid profile and glycemic control in obese type 2 diabetic patients, *International Journal of Obesity* 28: 180–182, 2004.

Hebebrand J, Friedel S, Schauble N, et al: Perspectives: molecular genetic research in human obesity, *Obesity Reviews* 4(3): 139–146, 2003.

Hu FB, Manson JE, Stampfer MJ, et al: Diet, lifestyle, and the risk of type 2 diabetes mellitus in women, *New England Journal of Medicine* 345(11): 790–797, 2001.

Klausen B, Toubro S, Astrup A: Age and sex effects on energy expenditure, *American Journal of Clinical Nutrition* 65: 895–907, 1997.

Kring SII, Holst C, Zimmermann E, Jess T, Berentzen T, Toubro S, Hansen T, Astrup A, Pedersen O, Sørensen TIA: FTO gene associated fatness in relation to body fat distribution and metabolic traits throughout a broad range of fatness, *PLoS ONE* www.plosone.org, 3(8):e2958, 2008.

Linne Y, Barkeling B, Rossner S: Long-term weight development after pregnancy, *Obesity Reviews* 3(2):75–83, 2002.

Makris AP, Foster GD, Astrup A: Diet composition and weight loss I. In Bray GA, Bouchard C, editors: *Handbook of obesity,* ed 3, New York. 2008, Informa Healthcare USA, pp 269–290.

Paddon-Jones D, Westman E, Mattes RD, et al: Protein, weight management, and satiety, *American Journal of Clinical Nutrition* 87: 1558S–1561S, 2008.

Petersen M, Taylor M, Saris W, et al: A 10 weeks randomised trial of hypocaloric low-fat versus medium-fat diet – the NUGENOB study, *International Journal of Obesity* 39: 552–560, 2006.

Raben A, Vasilaras TH, Møller AC, Astrup A: Sucrose compared with artificial sweeteners: different effects on ad libitum food intake and body weight after 10wk of supplementation in overweight subjects, *American Journal of Clinical Nutrition* 76: 721–729, 2002.

Saris WHM, Blair SN, van Baak MA, et al: How much physical activity is enough to prevent unhealthy weight gain? Outcome of the IASO 1st Stock Conference and consensus statement, *Obesity Reviews* 4(2): 91–100, 2003.

Tardieu S, Micallef J, Gentile S, Blin O: Weight gain profiles of new anti-psychotics: public health consequences, *Obesity Reviews* 4(3): 129–138, 2003.

Toubro S, Astrup A: Randomised comparison of diets for maintaining obese subjects' weight after major weight loss: ad lib, low fat, high carbohydrate diet v fixed energy intake, *British Medical Journal* 314: 29–34, 1997.

Further reading

Astrup A: Treatment of obesity. In Ferrannini E, Zimmet P, De Fronzo RA, Keen H, editors: *International textbook of diabetes mellitus,* ed 3, Chichester, 2004, John Wiley.

Astrup A, Toubro S: Drugs with thermogenic properties. In Bray GA, Bouchard C, James WPT, editors: *Handbook of obesity,* ed 2. New York, 2004, Marcel Dekker, pp 315–328.

Ayyad C, Andersen T: Long-term efficacy of dietary treatment for obesity: a systematic review of studies published between 1931 and 1999, *Obesity Reviews* 1(2): 113–120, 2000.

British Nutrition Foundation: *Obesity, The Report of the British Nutrition Foundation Task Force,* Oxford, 1999, Blackwell Science.

Goran MI, Astrup A: Energy metabolism. In Gibney MJ, Vorser HH, Kok FJ editors: *Introduction to human nutrition,* Oxford, 2002, The Nutrition Society, Blackwell Science, pp 30–45.

WHO Consultation on Obesity: Obesity: preventing and managing the global epidemic, *WHO Technical Report* 894, Geneva, 2000, World Health Organization.

Chapter 21

Diabetes mellitus

Gabrielle Riccardi, Brunella Capaldo and Angela A Rivellese

CHAPTER CONTENTS

OBJECTIVES

By the end of this chapter you should be able to:
- understand the aetiology and pathophysiology of diabetes mellitus
- distinguish between type 1 and type 2 diabetes mellitus
- demonstrate an insight into the link between diabetes and obesity
- understand insulin resistance and how to reduce it essentially through lifestyle modifications
- demonstrate a basic knowledge of how to prevent long-term complications of diabetes.

21.1 INTRODUCTION

Diabetes mellitus is a metabolic disorder of multiple aetiology characterised by chronic hyperglycaemia associated with impaired carbohydrate, fat and protein metabolism. These abnormalities are the consequence of either inadequate insulin secretion or impaired insulin action, or both. Diabetes has been classified by the World Health Organization into four distinct types (Table 21.1): type 1, type 2, gestational diabetes mellitus, other specific types (WHO 1999). Type 1 diabetes is characterised by a cell-mediated autoimmune destruction of pancreatic beta-cells that results in a partial or total inability to secrete insulin, and life-long need for insulin administration. Type 2 diabetes, until recently referred to as non-insulin-dependent diabetes, is characterised by disorders of insulin action and secretion, either feature being the predominant impairment. These individuals may not require

© 2010 Elsevier Ltd/Inc/BV
DOI: 10.1016/B978-0-7020-3118-2.00021-8

Table 21.1   Aetiological classification of diabetes mellitus

1. Type 1 diabetes
   A. Immune-mediated
   B. Idiopathic
2. Type 2 diabetes
3. Gestational diabetes
4. Other specific types
   A. Genetic defects in beta-cell function (MODY)
   B. Genetic defects in insulin action
   C. Disease of the endocrine pancreas
   D. Endocrinopathies
   E. Drug- or chemical-induced
   F. Infections
   G. Uncommon forms of immune-mediated diabetes
   H. Other genetic syndromes associated with diabetes

insulin treatment either initially or ever, although it may be undertaken in some cases as the most appropriate blood glucose-lowering treatment. The specific aetiologies of this form of diabetes are yet to be found, but it is known that most of these patients are obese or have increased body fat, predominantly in the abdominal region. Other specific types of diabetes include less common causes – where the underlying defect may be genetic, secondary to pancreatic disease, endocrine disorders, infections, drug or chemical toxins. Gestational diabetes is defined as any degree of glucose intolerance with onset or first recognition during pregnancy.

21.2 EPIDEMIOLOGY AND DIAGNOSIS OF DIABETES MELLITUS

The diagnostic criteria for diabetes mellitus have been modified based on the current classification. Diabetes can be diagnosed in three ways, and – in the absence of specific symptoms of the disease – each must be confirmed on a subsequent occasion: casual plasma glucose concentration >11.1 mmol/l (200 mg/dl), or fasting plasma glucose >7.0 mmol/l (126 mg/dl), or 2-hour plasma glucose >11.1 mmol/l (200 mg/dl) during an oral glucose tolerance test (OGTT) with 75 g of glucose.

Two other categories of impaired glucose metabolism are impaired glucose tolerance (IGT) and impaired fasting glucose (IFG), which can be considered a metabolic state halfway between normal glucose homeostasis and diabetes. IGT is diagnosed by the 2-hour plasma glucose after OGTT >140 and

<200 mg/dl with fasting value <126 mg/dl, while IFG is defined by fasting plasma glucose >110 and <126 mg/dl. These two categories are strong risk factors for future diabetes and/or cardiovascular disease. If untreated, approximately one-third of people with IGT develop type 2 diabetes within 5–10 years, one-third remain stable and one-third revert to normoglycaemia (Vaccaro et al 1999). In individuals with IGT, the mortality due to cardiovascular and cerebrovascular disease is approximately twice that of people with normal glucose tolerance.

IGT and type 2 diabetes are often associated with other metabolic disturbances and cardiovascular risk factors; this condition has been defined as the insulin resistance syndrome or metabolic syndrome. There is no internationally agreed definition of the metabolic syndrome, which is generally considered as an association of impaired glucose regulation (IGT or IFG) or type 2 diabetes, raised arterial pressure, raised plasma triglycerides, low HDL and central obesity (see Ch. 20). A statement from the US National Cholesterol Education Program (NCEP) attempts to define diagnostic criteria for the metabolic syndrome based exclusively on these clinical parameters (Expert Panel on Detection, Evaluation, and Treatment of High Blood Cholesterol in Adults 2001). Other abnormalities often associated with the metabolic syndrome are microalbuminuria, hyperuricaemia, non-alcoholic liver steatosis and coagulation disorders. There is growing evidence pointing to insulin resistance as the common aetiological factor of this condition, considered to be associated with increased risk for cardiovascular disease (Reaven 1988).

Type 2 diabetes mellitus accounts for almost 85–95% of all cases of diabetes. Its estimated prevalence is 2–6% of the population: half of these are diagnosed, while a similar number remain unrecognised. The prevalence is known to be much higher in older people and in some ethnic communities (up to 40% of Pima Indians). WHO has predicted that the global prevalence of type 2 diabetes will more than double, from 135 million in 1995 to 300 million in the following years. Long-term complications of type 2 diabetes include retinopathy with potential loss of vision, nephropathy leading to renal failure, peripheral neuropathy with risk of foot ulcers, and autonomic neuropathy which contributes to erectile dysfunction and cardiac arrhythmia. However, most of the morbidity and mortality associated with diabetes is attributable to macrovascular complications such as myocardial infarction, heart failure and acute stroke. Diabetes is associated with an age-adjusted cardiovascular mortality that is between two and four times that of the non-diabetic population, while life expectancy is reduced by 5 to 10 years in middle-aged patients with type 2 diabetes. Several observational studies suggest that diabetes is primarily a lifestyle disorder; the highest prevalence rates occur in developing countries and in populations undergoing 'Westernisation' or modernisation. Under such circumstances, it seems that genetic susceptibility interacts with environmental changes, such as sedentary lifestyle and overnutrition, leading to type 2 diabetes. Populations with the highest recorded prevalence of diabetes, such as Nauru or Pima Indians, share the common experience of change from a hunter-gatherer or agriculture-based lifestyle to one of sedentary living and a diet of energy-dense processed foods. A better understanding of the impact that lifestyle may have, not only on the risk of diabetes but also on its key mechanisms, should help implement more effective preventive measures focused on more specific targets.

21.3 AETIOLOGY AND PATHOPHYSIOLOGY OF DIABETES MELLITUS

TYPE 1 DIABETES MELLITUS

Type 1 diabetes is characterised by absolute insulin deficiency caused in most cases by immune-mediated destruction of the beta-cells (autoimmune type 1A). A minority of patients with type 1 diabetes, generally of African or Asian origin, have no evidence of autoimmunity although they are insulinopenic and ketosis-prone. This form of diabetes has been referred as type 1B. The pathogenesis of type 1 diabetes involves genetic, immunological and environmental factors.

Genetic Factors

Evidence for the involvement of genetic factors in the aetiology of type 1 diabetes comes from studies on animals, families and human twins. Studies on animal models of type 1 diabetes (NOD mouse, BB rat) have demonstrated that the susceptibility to disease is mostly linked to the major

histocompatibility system (HLA), although some non-HLA loci have also been found to be associated with the disease. A link between type 1 diabetes and the HLA system has been confirmed by population studies showing that genetic susceptibility to disease is related to HLA-DR and HLA-DQ genes located on chromosome 6. Studies on families with multiple members affected by type 1 diabetes have demonstrated that the risk of a sibling developing the disease is increased by up to 27 times by the age of 16. However, between monozygotic twins, the concordance rate for the disease is 35–70% (depending on the length of follow-up), indicating that genetic factors, although important, cannot completely explain the occurrence of the disease, which seems to be multifactorial in nature.

Immunological factors

The evidence that type 1 diabetes is an autoimmune disease rests on the evidence of lymphocytic infiltration of pancreatic islets, abnormalities of cell-mediated immune response and circulating autoantibodies (Bottazzo & Bonifacio 1991). Histological studies of pancreatic tissues from type 1 diabetic patients who died shortly after diagnosis revealed the presence of macrophages, T- and B-lymphocytes and other inflammatory cells that combine to give an inflammatory picture known as 'insulitis'. Abnormalities of circulating cell-mediated immunity consist of an increased number of activated lymphocytes CD4$^+$, which are known to play a major role in beta-cell destruction. Auto-antibodies against a variety of pancreatic islet components are commonly observed in patients with type 1 diabetes. These include antibodies to islet cells (ICA), insulin (IAA), glutamic acid decarboxylase (GAD), carboxypeptidase H, and several other minor antigens. Most of these antibodies appear shortly after diagnosis or even prior to the clinical onset of diabetes and tend to fall progressively thereafter. The early detection of these immunological markers paved the way to the possibility of predicting the disease in high-risk subjects, such as first-degree relatives of patients with type 1 diabetes. In these subjects the presence of multiple markers indicates a high risk (above 80%) of developing the disease within the subsequent 2 years. Based on this rationale, a number of clinical trials have been performed in an attempt to prevent the disease in high-risk subjects using different strategies, e.g. nicotinamide (Deutsche Nicotinamide

Intervention Study (DENIS) and European Nicotinamide Intervention Trial (ENDIT studies)) and subcutaneous insulin (Diabetes Prevention Trial 1). Unfortunately, none of these approaches has been shown to effectively reduce the risk of developing the disease.

Environmental factors

Environmental factors could contribute to the pathogenesis of type 1 diabetes mellitus through several mechanisms: (1) exerting a direct toxic effect on the beta-cells, (2) triggering an autoimmune reaction against the beta-cell, (3) damaging beta-cells so as to increase their susceptibility to autoimmune destruction. Environmental factors include drugs or chemicals (e.g. alloxan, streptozotocin, pentamidine), viruses and dietary factors. Among viruses potentially involved in human type 1 diabetes, clinical evidence points to mumps, coxsackie B, cytomegalovirus and rubella viruses as the most likely candidates. The viral aetiology is supported by seasonal variability in the incidence of the disease, with a peak in spring and autumn. In addition, clinical and epidemiological studies have shown a close relation between appearance of diabetes and preceding episodes of viral infections. However, despite its attractiveness, the viral hypothesis requires caution since clinical evidence is far from conclusive. Recently, growing attention has been focused on the potential role of dietary factors. In particular, there is evidence of a close relationship between cow's milk consumption and incidence of type 1 diabetes in childhood. The hypothesis is that antibodies produced against bovine seroalbumin may cross-react with antigens of beta-cells, triggering an autoimmune response. A multicentre trial is in progress to evaluate whether an early elimination of cow's milk from diet may prevent type 1 diabetes in infants with genetic risk for the disease.

Clinical manifestations

Because subjects who develop type 1 diabetes often have a rather abrupt onset of symptoms (polyuria, polydipsia (thirst), or even ketoacidosis), it was long assumed that beta-cell damage occurs rapidly. It is now accepted that type 1 diabetes gradually develops over many years. Some authors have proposed dividing the natural history of the disease into five stages: (1) genetic susceptibility, (2)

triggering events (environmental), (3) active autoimmunity, (4) gradual loss of glucose-induced insulin secretion, (5) appearance of overt diabetes. Thus, the presence of islet cell autoantibodies occurs long before the clinical appearance of the disease at a time when there is no elevation in blood glucose and glucose tolerance is near normal. When fasting hyperglycaemia develops, at least 80–90% of the functional capacity of beta-cells is irreversibly lost. Thus, the basic pathophysiological mechanism responsible for type 1 diabetes is the total and irreversible loss of beta-cell function. Insulin deficiency leads to multiple abnormalities of intermediary metabolism that culminate in hyperglycaemia and increased levels of ketone bodies with proneness to ketoacidosis (Fig. 21.1). Hyperglycaemia results from both increased glucose production by the liver and reduced glucose utilisation by peripheral tissue, mainly the skeletal muscle. Hepatic glucose production increases as a consequence of high rates of both glycogenolysis and gluconeogenesis. Under conditions of insulin deficiency, an accelerated flux of gluconeogenic substrates (alanine, lactate, glycerol) takes place from peripheral tissues to the liver, which fuels gluconeogenesis. Glucose utilisation decreases as a result of the lack of insulin stimulatory effect on glucose transport and the increased availability of free fatty acids, which are known to inhibit glucose transport across the muscle membrane through operation of the glucose–fatty acid (Randle) cycle. In uncontrolled type 1 diabetes, fatty acid mobilisation from adipose tissue is markedly increased. Normally, in the liver fatty acids

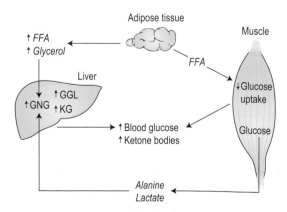

Fig. 21.1 Consequences of insulin deficiency in type 1 diabetes mellitus. GNG, gluconeogenesis; GGL, glycogenolysis; KG, ketogenesis.

undergo beta-oxidation to acetyl CoA, which is totally oxidised in the Krebs cycle to water and carbon dioxide. When there is an excessive breakdown of fatty acids, as occurs in an insulin-deficient state, the capacity of the liver to oxidise all acetyl CoA is exceeded and two carbon fragments combine to form acetoacetate. Hepatic ketone body synthesis is further enhanced by the low insulin to glucagon ratio that critically regulates the activity of key enzymes of ketogenesis. All these metabolic abnormalities account for the classic symptoms and signs of the disease, such as glycosuria, polyuria, polydipsia and weight loss. However, there is wide variability in clinical manifestations, with some individuals presenting acute signs of decompensation and others being asymptomatic thanks to good control with insulin therapy.

TYPE 2 DIABETES MELLITUS

Although type 2 diabetes has strong genetic components, modes of inheritance are largely unknown. One exception is the variant represented by MODY (maturity-onset diabetes of the young) that conforms to autosomal dominant inheritance with high penetrance. The role of heredity in type 2 diabetes is supported by familial aggregation, a concordance of 60–90% for the disease in identical twins, and marked differences in its prevalence in different ethnic groups.

For the more common forms of type 2 diabetes, it is believed that both genetic and acquired factors contribute to the disease. Genetic factors somehow confer susceptibility to develop glucose intolerance; the occurrence of diabetes will depend on the presence of non-genetic, environmental factors that disrupt the fine balance between insulin secretion and insulin action. Among environmental factors, obesity and sedentary lifestyle are the major factors known to impair glucose tolerance. Also of great interest is the recent evidence that dietary factors, especially a high intake of saturated fats, are associated with an increased risk of developing diabetes. Patients with type 2 diabetes have two major metabolic defects: (1) impaired insulin secretion, and (2) resistance to insulin action on target tissues, namely the liver, skeletal muscle and adipose tissue.

Defect of insulin secretion

In type 2 diabetic patients fasting insulin levels have been reported as low, normal or even elevated. This does not imply that insulin secretion is normal because, although fasting insulin is normal in absolute terms, it is inappropriately low for the ambient glucose level. At matched plasma glucose concentration, normal subjects would have a much higher insulin concentration. The main abnormality of beta-cell function in type 2 diabetes is the loss of glucose-induced insulin secretion. In normal subjects a rapid rise in plasma glucose elicits a biphasic insulin release: a first (early) phase lasting 5–10 minutes and a second (late) phase persisting for the duration of hyperglycaemia (Fig. 21.2). Although most of the insulin is secreted during the second-phase insulin response, the first-phase is recognised as serving an important physiological function, i.e. to stimulate glucose utilisation by peripheral tissues and to inhibit glucose production by the liver in order to prevent an exaggerated increase in plasma glucose in the postprandial state. In type 2 diabetic patients, the first-phase insulin response is characteristically lost while the late phase is preserved or only attenuated (Fig. 21.2). The main characteristics of this secretory defect have been extensively investigated over the last decades (Kahn 1996). They can be outlined as follows: (1) the defective insulin release is specific for glucose whereas insulin response to other secretagogues (arginine, isoproterenol, secretin) is substantially unaltered, (2) the potentiating effect of glucose on insulin response to secretagogues is reduced, confirming that in type 2 diabetes the beta-cell is selectively unresponsive to glucose; and (3) beta-cell glucose unresponsiveness may be partially restored by correction of hyperglycaemia, suggesting that it may be, at least in part, an acquired defect caused by the toxic effect of high blood glucose on the beta-cells (glucose toxicity hypothesis).

Other abnormalities of insulin secretion have been documented in type 2 diabetes and include disruption of the pulsatile insulin secretory pattern. In normal subjects, plasma insulin displays 5–10 minute oscillations, which disappear in diabetic patients. In addition, diabetic patients are characterised by increased levels of proinsulin and proinsulin:insulin ratio, indicating an abnormal processing of insulin precursors within the beta-cells. Recent studies utilizing post-mortem pancreas specimens have reported a 60% loss of islet beta-cell volume in patients with type 2 diabetes compared with weight-matched controls. The reduced volume was not a consequence of reduced beta cell proliferation but the result of an increased

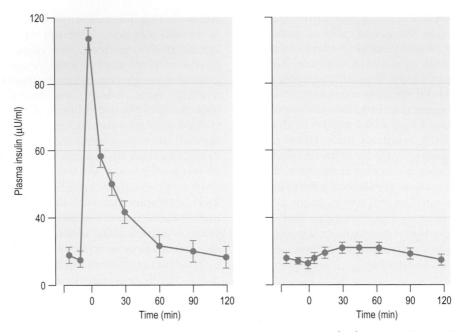

Fig. 21.2 Insulin release elicited by an intravenous glucose load in normal subjects (left) and in patients with type 2 diabetes mellitus (right).

rate of beta cell death by apoptosis. Autopsy studies have also shown qualitative alterations. The most characteristic morphological change is represented by amyloid deposition in the islets. These deposits consist of insoluble fibrils formed from a peptide designated 'islet amyloid polypeptide' (IAPP or amylin) that is co-secreted with insulin. The function of this peptide is unknown at present but its presence in secretory granules of the beta-cells suggests a regulatory role. Recently, some animal studies have demonstrated a relation between dietary fat intake and production and/or secretion of amylin in the beta-cells.

Most recently, great attention has been paid to certain peptides produced by the gastrointestinal tract in response to a meal, called incretins, which are able to stimulate insulin secretion. The two main incretins, glucose-dependent insulinotropic peptide (GIP) and glucagon-like peptide-1 (GLP-1), increase within minutes of food ingestion and potentiate the postprandial insulin release thus facilitating the rapid disposal of ingested nutrients. Interestingly, several studies have shown that the incretin effect is impaired in type 2 diabetic patients, due to a defect in incretin secretion/action. In particular, plasma levels of GIP appear normal but its effect on insulin secretion is blunted, whereas GLP-1 levels are significantly diminished both in the fasting and in the post-prandial state, thus contributing to the reduced postprandial insulin release (Nauck 2004) . Although the mechanisms underlying the reduced GLP-1 release remain unclear, recent clinical studies have shown that the infusion of GLP-1 analogues in diabetic patients is able to increase insulin release and to reduce glucose levels. Hence, new therapeutic strategies have been focused on the use of GLP-1 agonists for the treatment of type 2 diabetes.

Insulin resistance

Insulin resistance is a major pathogenic component of type 2 diabetes. Insulin resistance is a state in which a given concentration of insulin produces a less than normal biological response. As known, insulin exerts its biological effects by initially binding to its specific cell-surface receptors. After this, a number of signals are generated that interact with a variety of effector units (enzymatic systems) leading to multiple metabolic effects. Insulin promotes the storage of nutrients by stimulating glycogen synthesis, protein synthesis and lipogenesis and by inhibiting lipolysis, and glycogen and protein breakdown. In addition, insulin regulates water and electrolyte balance and stimulates cell growth and differentiation. This complex hormonal activity involves different intracellular pathways and mediators, which explains why some effects of insulin may be impaired (e.g. glucose metabolism) whereas others may not be (e.g. cellular growth). The cellular mechanisms underlying insulin resistance have been extensively investigated and all the receptor and post-receptor events that mediate insulin action have been carefully analysed. Defects in insulin signalling, glucose transport and metabolic pathways of intracellular glucose utilisation have been documented in type 2 diabetic patients (De Fronzo 1997). However, it is still unclear what the primary defect is, which defect is genetically determined and which is secondary to acquired factors, such as hyperglycaemia itself.

With regard to glucose metabolism, it is known that insulin lowers blood glucose through two mechanisms: (1) by suppressing glucose production from the liver, and (2) by promoting the uptake of glucose by peripheral tissues, especially the skeletal muscle. Under conditions of insulin resistance, as occurs in type 2 diabetes, the effect of insulin on the liver and peripheral tissues is impaired, thus producing the two major metabolic abnormalities observed in diabetic patients; i.e. fasting and postprandial hyperglycaemia.

Liver

As a result of impaired insulin action on the liver, type 2 diabetic patients tend to have abnormally increased glucose production in the post-absorptive state, which contributes to fasting hyperglycaemia. A strong positive correlation has been found between hepatic glucose production, measured by isotopic techniques, and fasting blood glucose level. The excess of hepatic glucose production is almost entirely accounted for by an increased rate of gluconeogenesis, which is ~40% higher in diabetic patients than in normal subjects. Such an increase is due to an increased supply of 3-carbon compounds (lactate, alanine, glycerol) from peripheral tissues to the liver as well as to a more efficient hepatic conversion of these substrates into glucose. Not only is hepatic glucose production increased in the basal state but it is less suppressed after glucose ingestion. This failure of the liver to adequately suppress its glucose production in response to insulin contributes to the impairment of postprandial glucose homeostasis. In addition, the ability of the liver to take up and dispose of dietary glucose also seems to be reduced.

Skeletal muscle

Skeletal muscle is another important site of insulin resistance in patients with type 2 diabetes. By means of a number of different techniques, it has been demonstrated that the ability of insulin to stimulate glucose uptake by the skeletal muscle is reduced by 40–50% in diabetic patients as compared with normal subjects. Subsequent studies employing ^{13}C magnetic resonance spectroscopy have established that the defect responsible for impaired muscle glucose uptake involves the glucose transport step. In vitro studies have demonstrated a defect in the translocation and/or activity of GLUT-4, the glucose transporters located in skeletal muscle. In addition, the activity of two of the key enzymes that regulate non-oxidative (glycogen synthase) and oxidative (pyruvate dehydrogenase) glucose metabolism is reduced in diabetic patients. However, this defect is likely to be secondary to the reduced glucose transport.

Adipose tissue

Insulin profoundly influences adipocyte metabolism by stimulating glucose transport and triglyceride synthesis (lipogenesis), as well as inhibiting lipolysis. In type 2 diabetes, particularly when associated with obesity, the ability of insulin to suppress lipolysis is markedly impaired. In addition, because glucose transport in the adipocyte is reduced, less glycerophosphate is formed through glycolysis and made available for triglyceride synthesis. The consequence is an increased flux of free fatty acids (FFA) from adipose tissue and a rise in their plasma concentration. It is important to consider that not only are FFA concentrations elevated in the fasting state, but they fail to be appropriately suppressed after meals. The result is a chronic elevation of FFA and triglyceride levels together with excessive deposition of fat in various tissues (including the skeletal muscle) in patients with type 2 diabetes, particularly when associated with obesity. In addition, there is evidence that a chronic elevation in FFAs has detrimental effects on insulin secretion and on the action of insulin in peripheral tissues (lipotoxicity).

What are the defects causing beta–cell dysfunction and insulin resistance?

It is widely accepted that beta-cell dysfunction and insulin resistance in type 2 diabetes are due to both genetic and acquired factors. An inherited defect in any part of the complex cascade that leads from glucose elevation to insulin processing and release could be a potential cause of beta-cell dysfunction. Mutations in the glucokinase gene, in the beta-cell glucose transporter (*GLUT 2*) gene, in mitochondrial DNA and in the insulin gene itself have been identified in some diabetic patients. However, the importance of these alterations in the common form of type 2 diabetes is questionable as these mutations have not been detected in populations with high prevalence of diabetes (e.g. Pima Indians). Other emerging factors associated with insulin secretory dysfunction include low birthweight (attributed to poor fetal development of the pancreas because of malnutrition) and deficiencies of some amino acids that seem to exert trophic effects on the beta-cells.

With regard to genetic factors responsible for insulin resistance, a number of candidate genes have been identified. Some mutations of the insulin receptor gene lead to altered insulin receptor biosynthesis; others impair the binding of insulin to its own receptor or insulin signalling. However, these mutations produce rare syndromes of severe insulin resistance but do not explain the insulin resistance associated with the common form of type 2 diabetes. The current view is that insulin resistance is not due to a few 'major' genes but to a large number of 'polygenes', each with a relatively minor effect.

The role of acquired factors in deteriorating insulin secretion and insulin action is well expressed by the concept of 'glucose toxicity' and 'lipotoxicity'. According to the glucose toxicity hypothesis, a chronic increment in plasma glucose concentration leads to progressive impairment in insulin secretion and insulin sensitivity. This hypothesis is mainly based on animal studies showing that rats made diabetic by partial pancreatectomy develop hyperglycaemia and, concomitantly, a progressive impairment in insulin secretion and insulin action. Interestingly, when chronic hyperglycaemia is corrected by phlorizin, a substance that increases glucose urinary loss without any effect on the beta-cell, both the first and second phase insulin secretion are restored to normal. In parallel, peripheral insulin sensitivity substantially improves with correction of hyperglycaemia. In addition, clinical studies in diabetic patients have shown that a tight glycaemic control, independent of the method by which it is achieved (diet, insulin or hypoglycaemic agents), ameliorates considerably insulin secretion and insulin action.

Like hyperglycaemia, the chronic elevation of FFAs may impair beta-cell function and contribute to the decreased uptake of glucose into peripheral tissues. This phenomenon has been referred to as 'lipotoxicity'. Studies in diabetic patients have shown that FFAs exert adverse effects on insulin sensitivity by interfering with the activity of GLUT-4, the glucose transporter located in skeletal muscle. This mechanism is likely to play a role in the impaired glucose tolerance associated with a high fat diet. The damage produced by glucolipotoxicity at both islet beta cell and peripheral tissues is responsible for the progression of the disease and the deterioration of glucose control over time.

Natural history of type 2 diabetes

A major question, and one that continues to be the subject of considerable debate, is which of the two defects, insulin resistance or insulin secretory dysfunction, comes first. An important advance in understanding the natural history of diabetes comes from longitudinal studies that have followed for several years people who progressed from the stage of normal glucose tolerance to impaired glucose tolerance to frank diabetes. Collectively, these studies show that defects in both insulin secretion and insulin action occur at an early stage during the development of diabetes and progressively worsen over time. These defects are likely to be genetically determined. The progressive deterioration is caused by the detrimental effects of some environmental factors, mainly obesity (particularly visceral fat accumulation), sedentary lifestyle, high fat intake, glucose toxicity and lipotoxicity. To compensate for reduced peripheral insulin sensitivity, the beta-cell usually increases its insulin secretion so as to prevent persistent hyperglycaemia. In this way, a near-normal blood glucose is maintained at the expense of increased insulin levels. However, when pancreatic beta-cells are no longer able to compensate with an appropriate increase in insulin secretion (because of a genetic defect or a progressive functional exhaustion), frank diabetes will develop (Weyer et al 1999). Understanding the temporal sequence of changes in insulin secretion and insulin action as well as their interaction in the progression of diabetes may have important implications for prevention of diabetes and suggests that lifestyle modifications should preserve both insulin secretion and insulin sensitivity.

21.4 VASCULAR COMPLICATIONS

MICROANGIOPATHY

Microangiopathy or microvascular complications of diabetes mellitus include retinopathy, nephropathy and neuropathy, although the contribution of microangiopathy to neuropathy is still not completely understood. The incidence of retinopathy increases with duration of diabetes in type 1 diabetic patients: after 20 years of diabetes, over 95% of patients have background retinopathy, although mostly without visual impairment. The risk of proliferative retinopathy, the main cause of blindness in type 1 diabetic patients, increases rapidly between 10 and 15 years after the onset of diabetes, then remains remarkably constant, reaching a cumulative risk of about 60% after 40 years of diabetes. In type 2 diabetic patients retinopathy can be present at the onset of the disease (from 7% to as many as 38%) perhaps due to the fact that this condition sometimes remains unrecognised for years. It then increases, reaching, after 20 years, a prevalence of about 60% for any kind of retinopathy and 20% for proliferative retinopathy.

Diabetic nephropathy affects 20–40% of patients with type 1 diabetes, while it is rarer in those with type 2. Diabetic microvascular complications result from the interaction of multiple genetic and metabolic factors, among which hyperglycaemia is almost certainly the most important one (Walker & Viberti 1991). In fact, all these complications are specific to diabetes and do not occur in the absence of long-lasting hyperglycaemia. The importance of hyperglycaemia in the determination and progression of microvascular complications has been proven beyond any doubt by the results of some intervention trials performed in the last few years in both type 1 and type 2 diabetic patients. These studies have clearly shown that improving blood glucose control significantly reduces the onset and progression of retinopathy, nephropathy and neuropathy. Besides hyperglycaemia and genetic factors, which determine a variable degree of susceptibility and which have not been fully identified, other factors are important in determining microvascular complications, such as hypertension, smoking and hyperlipidaemia. Hypertension has been shown to play a very important role, especially in the genesis of diabetic nephropathy. Intervention trials in type 2 diabetic patients have clearly shown that improving blood pressure control significantly reduces the onset and progression of both nephropathy and retinopathy.

How all these factors might lead to diabetic microangiopathy is still a matter of debate. Many hypotheses have been put forward and only partly proven. One possible pathway is illustrated in Figure *evolve* 21.1 🖱. Hyperglycaemia, together with other factors, may lead, through different mechanisms, to abnormal endothelium function, haemodynamic effects and changes in blood rheological characteristics. All these abnormalities may induce a thickening of basement membrane and an increased permeability with subsequent occlusive angiopathy, tissue hypoxia and organ damage.

MACROANGIOPATHY

Atherosclerotic arterial disease may manifest clinically as coronary heart disease, cerebrovascular disease or peripheral vascular disease. In diabetic patients atherosclerotic lesions are qualitatively similar to those present in the non-diabetic population, except that their progression appears to be accelerated. Both mortality and morbidity for all cardiovascular diseases are significantly increased in diabetic patients. In particular, both coronary heart disease and cerebrovascular disease mortality is increased from two to four fold in diabetic patients compared to the non-diabetic population. Moreover, about half of all lower limb amputations occur in diabetic patients.

The high prevalence of arterial disease in diabetes is explained partly by the increased frequency of the most important cardiovascular risk factors, and partly by other factors closely associated with diabetes (Table 21.2). LDL cholesterol remains one of the most important cardiovascular risk factors in diabetic patients. Recent intervention studies performed in diabetic patients with hypolipidaemic drugs, particularly statins, have clearly shown that LDL cholesterol reduction significantly decreases cardiovascular events and mortality. Beside LDL cholesterol, other lipid abnormalities, more typical of type 2 diabetes, such as increased triglycerides, VLDL and IDL particles, and decreased HDL cholesterol, may have an important role in determining the high cardiovascular risk of diabetic patients.

With regard to the role of high blood pressure, the data are very consistent and similar to those for LDL cholesterol. There is strong evidence that

Table 21.2	Main risk factors for cardiovascular disease in diabetic patients
GENERAL RISK FACTORS	**DIABETES-RELATED RISK FACTORS**
Smoking	Hyperglycaemia
Hyperlipidaemia	Hyperinsulinaemia/insulin resistance
Hypertension	Microalbuminuria/proteinuria
Hypercoagulability	
Obesity	
Physical inactivity	
Family history	

Table 21.3	Optimal goals for cardiovascular disease prevention in patients with diabetes
• BMI < 25 kg/m^2	
• Physical activity: 1/2 hour of brisk walking every day	
• Abstinence from smoking	
• Optimal blood glucose control (HbA1C < 7%)	
• LDL cholesterol < 100 mg/dl	
• HDL cholesterol > 45 mg/dl	
• Plasma triglycerides < 150 mg/dl	
• Blood pressure < 130/80 mmHg	

reducing blood pressure significantly decreases cardiovascular events in diabetic patients. The data concerning the role of hyperglycaemia in explaining, at least in part, the excess cardiovascular risk of diabetic patients, are somewhat more controversial. Epidemiological data, as a whole, support the relationship between hyperglycaemia and cardiovascular disease, even if the association is not as strong as for microvascular complications. Moreover, intervention studies show that improvement in blood glucose control reduces the incidence of cardiovascular events in type 2 diabetic patients, if the improvement is part of a multifactorial intervention that also includes targets for optimal plasma lipid and blood pressure levels (Gaede et al 2003).

Insulin resistance and/or hyperinsulinaemia, typical features of type 2 diabetic patients, are associated with an increased cardiovascular risk. It is not completely clear if this association is fully explained by the clustering of other cardiovascular risk factors with insulin resistance, such as lipid abnormalities, high blood pressure, coagulation abnormalities, high uric acid levels, low-grade inflammation and so on, or whether there is also a direct link between insulin resistance and/or hyperinsulinaemia and the atherosclerotic process. In any case, all these risk factors, together with others less well identified, may induce, through different mechanisms, endothelial injury. Different and repeated injuries increase the permeability of the endothelium to lipids as well as its adhesion to monocytes and platelets. This in turn increases the procoagulant activities of the endothelium and increases the expression of vasoactive molecules, cytokines and growth factors, which promote the migration of monocytes and proliferation of smooth muscle cells. In this way the atherosclerotic process starts and will continue until the formation of the atherosclerotic plaque, with progressive narrowing of the arterial lumen and arterial stenosis or plaque rupture, thrombus formation and acute ischaemia.

In conclusion, many factors may contribute to the excess cardiovascular risk typical of both type 1 and type 2 diabetic patients. Therefore, in order to reduce this risk, it is necessary to act not only on blood glucose control, but also on plasma lipids, blood pressure, hypercoagulable state, obesity, physical activity and smoking habits, to try to reach the goals indicated in Table 21.3 (ADA 2009).

21.5 MANAGEMENT OF DIABETES MELLITUS

DIET

Nutritional management is the cornerstone of therapy for diabetes mellitus. In many patients with type 2 diabetes it may be the only therapy required; in the others (type 1 and 2) it allows a more accurate blood glucose control with lower doses of oral hypoglycaemic drugs or insulin. In any case, the aims of nutritional management must be not only the optimisation of blood glucose control but also, and perhaps more importantly, the reduction of risk factors for cardiovascular diseases. Dietary recommendations for people with diabetes are very similar to those given to the general population for the promotion of good health. Of course, since diabetes mellitus is a chronic disease, diet therapy has to be considered as a lifelong practice and therefore it is essential that all nutritional programmes be adapted to the specific needs of the individual.

Total dietary energy

Most patients (60–70%) with type 2 diabetes are overweight or obese, and the frequency of moderate overweight has increased over the last years also in type 1 diabetic patients, especially those following intensive insulin therapy. All these patients should be encouraged to reduce their calorie intake and increase their energy expenditure. There is a very large body of evidence showing that body weight reduction, even if modest (5–10% of basal body weight), is able to improve blood glucose control, reduce insulin resistance and favourably affect the other cardiovascular risk factors, such as blood pressure and lipid abnormalities, often present in diabetic patients.

Two intervention trials, one in the USA (Diabetes Prevention Program Research Group 2002) and the other in Finland (Tuomilehto et al 2001), have clearly shown that a moderate weight reduction (about 5% of initial body weight), together with increased physical activity and changes in the composition of the diet (reduction in saturated fat, increased consumption of dietary fibre), is able to prevent type 2 diabetes, reducing its incidence in high-risk individuals by 60%. From a practical point of view, weight reduction may be achieved by reducing the consumption of energy dense foods, especially those rich in fat, to achieve a caloric deficit of 300–500 kcal/day. To be effective also in the long run this advice should be incorporated into structured, intensive lifestyle education programmes. The prescription of a very-low-energy diet should be restricted to special cases (BMI >35) and administered only in specialised centres.

Composition of the diet

According to the recommendations for the nutritional management of patients with diabetes mellitus (Mann et al 2004), the most important aspect in relation to the composition of the diet is the consumption of saturated fat, <10% of total energy or even <8% for patients at higher cardiovascular risk. This strong recommendation is supported by the high rates of cardiovascular diseases in people with diabetes and by the fact that saturated fat intake has very unfavourable effects on lipid metabolism

(increase in LDL cholesterol), insulin resistance and blood pressure. Together with saturated fat, cholesterol intake should also be reduced to less than 300 mg/day for all people with diabetes and less than 250 mg/day for those with raised LDL cholesterol. Taking into account the fact that protein intake should range between 10 and 20% of total energy (0.8 g/kg body weight/day) for those with incipient or established nephropathy, the remaining 80–90% of the total energy should be provided by a combination of carbohydrates and unsaturated fat (especially monounsaturated fatty acids) according to clinical circumstances and local or individual preferences (Table 21.4). As to carbohydrates, foods

Table 21.4	Dietary Recommendations for Diabetes (Mann et al 2004)
DIETARY FAT	
Saturated Fat + *trans*	<10% TE*; <8% TE if LDL cholesterol high
Monounsaturated fat (*cis*)	10–20% TE
n-6 polyunsaturated fat	<10% TE
n-3 polyunsaturated fat	2–3 servings of fish/week and plant sources of n-3 fatty acids
Cholesterol	<300 mg/day
Dietary carbohydrates	
Carbohydrates	• 45%–60% TE according to metabolic characteristics of patients
Dietary fibre	• Ideally <40 g/day (or 20 g/1000 kcal), half of which soluble, but beneficial effects obtained also with lower and more acceptable amounts • Cereal-based foods should, whenever possible, be wholegrain and high in fibre
Glycaemic index	• CHO-rich, low-glycaemic-index foods are suitable as CHO-rich choices provided other attributes of the foods are appropriate
Dietary protein	
Protein	• 10–20% TE • For patients with T1DM and established nephropathy 0.8 g/kg normal body weight/day
*TE, total energy (Mann et al 2004).	

rich in dietary fibre (legumes, vegetables) and/or with low glycaemic index are recommended, while high-glycaemic-index foods must be restricted and replaced with unsaturated fat. Fibre-rich foods (legumes, vegetables, fruit, cereal-derived foods) have been shown to improve blood glucose control and lipid profile in both type 1 and type 2 diabetic patients (Riccardi 2008). Therefore, an intake of dietary fibre of 15–20 g/1000 kcal, is recommended for diabetic patients as well as for the general population.

Dietary fibre is only one of the factors able to modulate the glycaemic response to carbohydrate-rich foods, which can be influenced also by other factors (physical state of foods, type of starch, presence of antinutrients). Due to the variety of factors that influence the impact of a meal on blood glucose, it is not possible to predict the postprandial glycaemic response of each food on the basis of its chemical characteristics. Therefore, it is necessary to examine the glycaemic response of foods in vivo and calculate their so-called glycaemic index. This index is based on the increase in blood glucose concentrations (the incremental area under the curve of blood glucose concentrations) after the ingestion of a portion of a test food containing 50 g of carbohydrates, divided by the incremental blood glucose area achieved with the same amount (50 g) of carbohydrates present in an equivalent portion of a reference food (glucose or white bread). According to this index, carbohydrate foods can be divided into broad categories characterised by a high or low glycaemic index. Fibre-rich foods have a low glycaemic index, although some foods with low fibre content (pasta, parboiled rice) may also have a relatively low glycaemic index.

It is now well documented that a diet containing mainly low-glycaemic-index foods improves metabolic control in diabetic patients and may have favourable effects on other cardiovascular risk factors. Therefore foods with a low glycaemic index (e.g. legumes, oats, pasta, parboiled rice, certain raw fruits) should replace, whenever possible, those with a high glycaemic index. Moreover, the diet for diabetic patients, in accordance with general guidelines for the promotion of good health, should be moderately restricted in salt intake (<6 g/day) and alcohol intake (20–30 g per day, 250 ml red wine, less for those who are overweight, hypertriglyceridaemic or have high blood pressure).

PHYSICAL EXERCISE

Aerobic physical exercise of moderate intensity but performed on a regular basis (daily or at least not less than four times/week) has been shown to improve blood glucose control, reduce insulin resistance, induce favourable effects on other cardiovascular risk factors, prevent the incidence of type 2 diabetes and, finally, reduce cardiovascular and total mortality (see Section evolve 21.5(a); Table evolve 21.1). Therefore, half an hour of brisk walking every day, or at least, four times a week, is strongly recommended not only for diabetic patients but for everyone. This kind of exercise may be carried out by any diabetic patient without particular precautions. Of course diabetic patients may wish to take more strenuous exercise (necessarily aerobic); in these cases some precautions must be taken and some advice should be given (see Table evolve 21.2). In type 2 diabetic patients, exercise increases peripheral glucose uptake but decreases insulin secretion; therefore, hypoglycaemia is rare and extra carbohydrate is generally not required. In type 1 diabetic patients, glycaemic changes during exercise depend largely on blood insulin levels and, therefore, on insulin administration. Hyperinsulinaemia may cause hypoglycaemia, while hypoinsulinaemia, combined with counter-regulatory hormone excess, may lead to hyperglycaemia. The risk of hypoglycaemia may be reduced by consuming 20–40 g extra carbohydrate before and hourly during exercise and/or by reducing pre-exercise insulin dosages (see Table evolve 21.3).

ORAL HYPOGLYCAEMIC AGENTS

When optimal blood glucose control (glycated haemoglobin, HbA_{1c} <7.0%, fasting and pre-meal blood glucose 80–120 mg/dl; 2-hour postprandial blood glucose 100–140 mg/dl) is not achieved in type 2 diabetic patients by non-pharmacological approaches (nutritional management and physical exercise), oral hypoglycaemic drugs should be added, if specific contraindications are not present (see Section evolve 21.5(b)). Drugs commonly used in the treatment of diabetes are listed in Table evolve 21.4 . Following the results of the UK Prospective Diabetes Study (UKPDS), showing that metformin significantly reduces cardiovascular risk in overweight type 2 diabetic patients, metformin is considered the first-choice drug in the treatment of type 2 diabetic patients, generally overweight. Therapy with metformin is also useful in these patients because of the weight loss that is generally associated with use of this drug (2–3 kg). Indications for the use of other drugs are based more on a pathophysiological basis than on their effects on cardiovascular end-points. A possible flow-chart for the pharmacological treatment of type 2 diabetic patients is shown in Figure *evolve* 21.2 : metformin is indicated as first choice; if optimal blood glucose control is not achieved, other drugs (sulphonylureas/glinides or pioglitazone or incretins) should be added; if the target values for blood glucose control are still not reached, bedtime insulin can be added or insulin therapy (3–4 administrations/ day) can replace oral drugs. For each of these points α-glucosidase inhibitors, which slow down carbohydrate absorption, may be added; pioglitazone and incretins may be added also to sulphonylureas + metformin or may be used instead of metformin; insulin therapy may be also considered as earlier therapy, especially in patients with very poor blood glucose control (i.e. HbA1c > 9%).

New hypoglycaemic oral drugs have been introduced in the last few years for the treatment of type 2 diabetic patients. These are: (1) thiazolinediones, which act especially on peripheral insulin action and are therefore useful instead of metformin or in addition to metformin and/or sulphonylureas, in the attempt to further reduce insulin resistance and its associated metabolic abnormalities; within this class of drugs pioglitazone should be preferred to rosiglitazone for the possible adverse effects of the latter on cardiovascular disease; (2) glinides (GND) (regaglinide, nateglinide), which increase insulin secretion, especially the first phase, with a very short time of action; these drugs may be useful in place of sulphonylureas when it is necessary to reduce postprandial blood glucose; 3) incretins, glucagon-like-peptide-1(GLP1) analogues (exenatide) and inhibitors of dipeptidyl peptidase 4 (DPP4), the enzyme that rapidly decreases GLP1. Both of these drugs improve blood glucose control, potentiating glucose-stimulated insulin secretion. Therefore they should not cause hypoglycaemia and the GLP1 analogues have the added advantage of reducing body weight. In any case, since incretin-based therapy has been introduced very recently, their long-term safety has not been completely established. In the use and choice of oral hypoglycaemic drugs it is important to consider the possibility of side effects, specific for each drug (see Table *evolve* 21.4) and the absolute contraindications (hepatic, renal and heart failure), which are valid for all drugs with some exceptions for α-glucosidase inhibitors and glinides.

INSULIN THERAPY

Insulin therapy is an essential lifesaving drug for type 1 diabetic patients, and can be used also in the treatment of type 2 diabetic patients when non-pharmacological therapy plus oral hypoglycaemic drugs is no longer able to achieve optimal blood glucose control (see Section *evolve* 21.5(c)). The types of insulin available today are generally based on human insulin, produced by DNA recombinant techniques, and, according to their time of action, may be divided into short-, intermediate- and long-acting insulin (see Table *evolve* 21.5). In the last few years other types of modified insulin molecules have been introduced in clinical practice. These are the so-called insulin analogues, one type with a very short time of action (lispro, aspart, Apidra) and the other type with a very long time of action (glargine, detemir) (see Table *evolve* 21.5). The first is very rapidly absorbed subcutaneously and therefore are particularly useful in reducing postprandial blood glucose. The second seems able to produce quite stable basal insulin concentrations for up to 24 hours. Insulin therapy must be tailored to the individual patient and adjusted on the basis of blood glucose control. Therefore, there are no strict rules for its dosage and type of administration. However, some schemes of insulin therapy are more commonly utilised than others, the most common being that based on three injections of short-acting insulin before breakfast, lunch and dinner plus an injection of intermediate insulin at bedtime. In place of short-acting insulin, rapid-acting analogues may be used, adding, if necessary, a few units of intermediate insulin before breakfast and lunch. Moreover, long-acting insulin analogues may be used instead of intermediate insulin at bedtime or before dinner. Whatever the type and the scheme of insulin therapy utilised, doctors and patients must always try to reach and maintain optimal blood glucose control (HbA$_{1c}$ <7%; fasting and pre-meal blood glucose 80–120 mg/dl; postprandial blood glucose 100–140 mg/dl). To achieve this, frequent blood glucose self-monitoring by patients is essential.

KEY POINTS

- Diabetes mellitus is a major cause of morbidity and mortality. Its prevalence is increasing all over the world due to increased prevalence of obesity and low levels of physical exercise.
- Type 1 diabetes is characterised by severe insulinopenia and absolute need of exogenous insulin to prevent ketoacidosis and death.
- Type 2 diabetes is frequently associated with obesity. Pathogenic mechanisms are: a defect in beta-cell function and a decrease in insulin action at the level of peripheral tissues (insulin resistance).
- The incidence of diabetes can be reduced by about 60% through lifestyle modifications, such as weight reduction, increased physical activity and reduced saturated fat consumption.
- Microangiopathic complications can be prevented or delayed by good glycaemic control.
- Cardiovascular complications can be reduced by about 50% through multifactorial treatment of the major cardiovascular risk factors.

References

ADA Standards of Medical Care in Diabetes 2009, *Diabetes Care 2009* 32:S13–S61, 2009J.

Bottazzo GF, Bonifacio E: Immune factors in the pathogenesis of insulin-dependent diabetes mellitus. In Pickup J, Williams G, editors: *Textbook of diabetes*, Oxford, 1991, Blackwell Scientific Publications.

De Fronzo RA: Pathogenesis of type 2 diabetes: metabolic and molecular implications for identifying diabetes genes, *Diabetes Reviews* 5(3):177–269, 1997.

Diabetes Prevention Program Research Group: Reduction in the incidence of type 2 diabetes with lifestyle intervention or metformin, *New England Journal of Medicine* 346:393–403, 2002.

Mann I, De Leeuw K, Hermansen B, et al: Evidence-based nutritional approaches to the treatment and prevention of diabetes mellitus, *Nutrition, Metabolism and Cardiovascular Diseases* 14(6):373–394, 2004 Dec.

Gaede P, Vedel P, Larsen N, et al: Multifactorial intervention and cardiovascular disease in patients with type 2 diabetes, *New England Journal of Medicine* 348:383–393, 2003.

Kahn SE: Regulation of beta-cell function in vivo: from health to disease, *Diabetes Reviews* 4(4):372–389, 1996.

Reaven GM: Role of insulin resistance in human disease, *Diabetes* 37:1595–1607, 1988.

Riccardi G, Rivellese AA, Giacco R: Role of glycemic index and glycemic load in the healthy state, in prediabetes and in diabetes, *American Journal of Clinical Nutrition* 87(1):269S–274S, 2008.

Tuomilehto J, Lindstrom J, Eriksson JG, et al: Prevention of type 2 diabetes by changes in lifestyle among subjects with impaired glucose tolerance, *New England Journal of Medicine* 344:1343–1350, 2001.

Vaccaro O, Ruffa G, Imperatore G, et al: Risk of diabetes in the new diagnostic category of impaired fasting glucose, *Diabetes Care* 22:1490–1493, 1999.

Walker JD, Viberti GC: Pathophysiology of microvascular disease: an overview. In Pickup J, Williams G, editors: *Textbook of diabetes*, Oxford, 1991, Blackwell Scientific Publications.

Weyer C, Bogardus C. Mott DM, Pratley RE: The natural history of insulin secretory dysfunction and insulin resistance in the pathogenesis of type 2 diabetes mellitus, *Journal of Clinical Investigation* 104:787–794, 1999.

WHO: Definition, diagnosis and classification of diabetes mellitus and its complications: report of a WHO consultation, Geneva, 1999, World Health Organization.

Further reading

Flechter GF, Balady G, Amsterdam EA, et al: Exercise standards for testing and training: a statement for health care professionals from the American Heart Association. *Circulation* 104:1694–1740, 2001.

Nauck MA, Baller B, Meier JJ: Gastric inhibitory peptide and glucagon like peptide-1 in the pathogenesis of type 2 diabetes. *Diabetes* 53(Suppl 3):S190–S196, 2004.

Riccardi G, Rivellese A, Williams C: The cardiovascular system in nutrition and metabolism. In Gibney M J, Macdonald I A, Roche HM, editors: *Nutrition and metabolism*. The Nutrition Society Textbook Series, Oxford, 2003, Blackwell Publishing.

Tanasescu M, Leitzmann MF, Rimm EB, et al: Physical activity in relation to cardiovascular disease and total mortality among men with type 2 diabetes. *Circulation* 107:2435–2439, 2003.

EVOLVE CONTENTS (available online at: evolve.elsevier.com/Geissler/nutrition)

Chapter 22

Cancers

Elizabeth A Spencer and Timothy J Key

CHAPTER CONTENTS

OBJECTIVES

By the end of this chapter you should be able to:
- describe the incidence of cancers worldwide and in the UK
- understand the pathophysiology of cancer
- appreciate the difficulties of linking environmental factors with cancer
- discuss the epidemiological data linking diet with cancer.

© 2010 Elsevier Ltd/Inc/BV
DOI: 10.1016/B978-0-7020-3118-2.00022-X

22.1 INTRODUCTION

Cancer is defined as a disease in which the normal control of cell division is lost, so that an individual cell multiplies inappropriately to form a tumour. The tumour may eventually spread through the body and overwhelm it, causing death (Stewart & Kleihues 2003).

Cancer has been recorded since the beginning of history, and was well known to the ancient Egyptians several thousand years ago. Until about a hundred years ago, however, cancer was a relatively minor cause of illness and death because it occurs mostly at old ages, and few people formerly lived long enough to be at significant risk of developing cancer. Thus concern about cancer as a major health problem has grown recently with the ageing of the population in developed countries, where cancer now accounts for approximately a quarter of deaths (see Section 22.2).

Cancer can arise from the cells of different tissues and organs in the body; thus there are many different types of cancer. The vast majority of human tumours are of epithelial origin, and cancers of connective tissues or haematopoetic cells are rarer. Cancer is caused by both external factors, including tobacco, alcohol, ionising radiation and ultraviolet light, and internal factors such as inherited mutations, immune conditions and hormones. The causes of cancer in different parts of the body vary – for example, tobacco causes cancer of the lungs, upper gastrointestinal tract, bladder and kidney but has almost no effect on the risk for developing cancers of the breast and prostate. Dietary factors are thought to be very important in determining the risk for developing cancer, but establishing the exact effects of diet on cancer risk has proved difficult, and currently relatively few dietary factors have been clearly shown to be important (WCRF/AICR 2007, Doll & Peto 2003).

22.2 DISTRIBUTION OF CANCERS THROUGHOUT THE WORLD

CANCER RATES WORLDWIDE

Worldwide, there were an estimated 10.8 million new cancer cases and 6.7 million deaths from cancer in the year 2002 (Ferlay 2002; see Section *evolve* 22.2 🖱). The most common cancers in terms of new cases were lung (1.4 million), breast (1.2 million), colorectal (1.0 million), stomach (934 000) and prostate (679 000).

Figure 22.1 shows age-standardised incidence rates for the common cancers in more developed and less developed countries. Lung and prostate cancers are the most common among men in more developed countries, but in less developed countries the most common cancers in men are lung and stomach cancers (Fig 22.1a).

Among women, breast cancer is by far the most common in more developed countries, and is also the most common among less developed countries, though by a much smaller margin (Fig. 22.1b). After breast cancer, the most common cancers among women in more developed countries are cancers of the colorectum and lung, whereas the second and third most common cancers among women in less developed countries are cancers of the cervix and stomach.

Table *evolve* 22.1 🖱 shows the age-standardised incidence rates for the common cancers in nine countries, selected to be representative of different parts of the world with good quality data on cancer incidence. Stomach cancer rates are high in Japan, Russia and China. Colorectal cancer rates are high in the USA, Japan, Italy and the UK. Liver cancer rates are very high in Japan and China, especially among men. Lung cancer rates are high in men in all selected countries except India, and relatively high in women in the USA, the UK and China. Breast cancer rates are high in the USA, Italy, the UK and Argentina. Prostate cancer rates are very high in the USA and high in South Africa, Italy and the UK. The large variation in rates suggests that environmental factors, such as diet, are important in the aetiology of cancer.

CANCER RATES IN THE UK

The four most common cancers in the UK are cancers of the breast (41 000 cases per year), lung (40 000 cases per year), colorectum (36 000 cases per year) and prostate (27 000 cases per year), and these four types of cancer together account for over half of all new cases (see Section *evolve* 22.2 🖱).

Figure 22.2 shows the trends in incidence for the four most common cancers among men and women in England and Wales between 1971 and 2005. In men, the most common cancer is now prostate cancer, diagnosis of this cancer having shown a

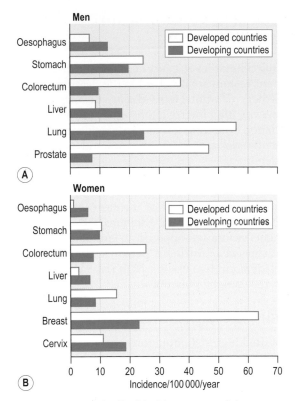

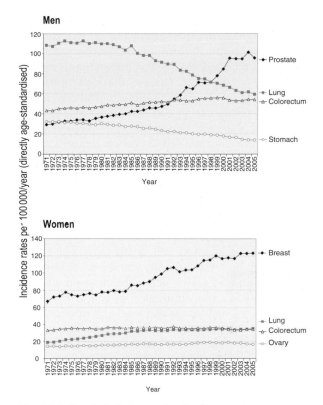

Fig. 22.1 Age-standardised incidence rates of the most common cancers in men (a) and women (b) in developed and developing countries.

Fig. 22.2 Trends in incidence for the four most common cancers among men (top) and women (bottom) in England and Wales 1971–2005. Data from Cancer Statistics: Registrations Series MB1, available from National Statistics Online at http: //www. statistics.gov.uk/StatBase/Product.asp?vlnk=8843

steep increase over the last five years, probably due to increased and earlier detection of this cancer. Lung cancer was the most common among men for many years, with very high rates at a maximum in the 1970s, and a steady fall since then due to reductions in cigarette smoking. Colorectal cancer rates increased moderately during this period, while stomach cancer rates fell substantially.

In women, breast cancer is by far the most common cancer, and the incidence is still increasing. The steep increase in incidence observed around 1990 is partly due to increased and earlier detection by the national breast cancer screening programme. Rates of colorectal cancer in women have not changed dramatically in the last 30 years, whereas lung cancer has increased substantially due to increases in cigarette smoking. The incidence of ovarian cancer has overall increased moderately since 1971, but data for recent years suggest that the incidence may be falling.

22.3 PATHOPHYSIOLOGY OF CANCER

Most cancers develop from a single cell that grows and divides more than it should, resulting in the formation of a tumour (growth). Cancers growing in most tissues take the form of a lump that grows, invades local non-cancerous tissue or adjacent tissues/organs, and may spread to other distant parts of the body through the bloodstream or lymphatic system. Cancers arising in the cells of the blood, such as leukaemia, do not form a lump because the cells are floating freely throughout the bloodstream.

The change from a normal cell into a cancer, termed carcinogenesis, is a multistage process. Cancers represent a form of dedifferentiation that is associated with the loss of growth control and disturbances in the regulation of the cell cycle. Hanahan and Weinberg (2000) suggested that most cancers acquire the following capabilities: self-sufficiency in growth signals, insensitivity to anti-growth signals, evasion of apoptosis, limitless replicative potential, sustained angiogenesis, tissue invasion and metastasis. The fundamental changes that determine carcinogenesis are mostly alterations (mutations) in the DNA; therefore cancer can be viewed as a genetic disease at the level of somatic cells. Typically the change from a normal cell to a cancer requires mutations in several different genes, perhaps five to ten (Stewart & Kleihues 2003). Mutations in many different genes can result in cancer, but certain genes are especially important and are very frequently involved; in particular, cancer usually results from changes in the function of genes that control cell division (mitosis) and cell death (apoptosis). The key genes in carcinogenesis can be considered in two classes: oncogenes, genes that when over-activated lead to over-stimulation of cell growth and cell division, such as *ras* and *myc*; and tumour suppressor genes such as *p53*, which normally limit the rate of cell division but, if inactivated by a mutation, allow uncontrolled cell division.

The genetic mutations that lead to an originally normal cell giving rise to a cancer can result from various causes. Some mutations are inherited, while others are caused during the lifetime of an individual by factors such as replication errors, ionising radiation, chemical carcinogens, viruses, and endogenous damage due for example to oxidants. The development of cells into a new cancer is strongly influenced by various growth-promoting agents, especially hormones.

Chance plays an important role in determining the occurrence of cancer. In very simplified terms, if mutations in several important genes occur in several different cells then the behaviour of all these cells could remain normal, but if the same mutations all occur together within one cell, then this cell could give rise to a cancer. Chance, however, plays no role in determining the cancer rates of populations (Doll & Peto 2003).

The process of carcinogenesis in humans usually extends over many years or even decades. Individuals who inherit a mutation in a key gene could be regarded as being born with the first step of carcinogenesis already present in all their cells. Mutations in cells accumulate throughout life. Most deaths due to cancer are caused by the spread of the cancer from its site of origin into adjacent areas and to other parts of the body (metastasis).

22.4 GENETIC FACTORS IN CARCINOGENESIS

At the cellular level, cancer is a genetic disease, and genetic factors are involved in the determination of whether or not individuals develop cancer. However, the interrelationships between genetic variation, the role of dietary factors, and other potential risk factors are complex and as yet poorly understood.

For the common types of cancer, current estimates are that inherited genetic factors contribute to around 5% or fewer of the cases of cancer in a population (Stewart & Kleihues 2003). Inherited genetic factors (as opposed to mutations in genes that can occur during a person's lifetime) can be considered in two classes: high risk mutations, and low risk genetic polymorphisms.

HIGH RISK MUTATIONS

Inherited high risk mutations confer a high risk for developing cancer, perhaps 10 to 50 times higher than the risk in individuals who do not have the mutation. The prevalence of these mutations, however, is low, generally around 1 in 1000 or less (Stewart & Kleihues 2003). As a consequence of the high risk conferred, these mutations cause clusters of cancers within families of closely related individuals that can be readily recognised by the medical profession and then studied by genetic epidemiologists. Well-known examples of genes which when mutated confer a high risk for common cancers are mismatch repair genes *MLH1* and *MSH2*, associated with hereditary non-polyposis colorectal cancer; and *BRCA1* and *BRCA2*, which give high risks for both breast and ovarian cancer. At present, there is no evidence that dietary factors can modulate the effects of genes such as these on cancer risk.

LOW RISK POLYMORPHISMS

Low risk polymorphisms are genetic variants that are termed polymorphisms (rather than mutations) because they occur at a prevalence of more than 1% in a population. Such polymorphisms appear to confer a risk of cancer only moderately higher (around 20–50%) than the risk in individuals with the 'wild type' allele (the most common phenotype in the population). Since the increase in risk is small to moderate, this class of genetic factor is less likely to cause obvious clustering of disease in families, and can more easily be identified by population-based epidemiological studies that compare the prevalence of a particular allele in individuals affected by cancer with the prevalence in unaffected controls. In fact, despite considerable interest and research activity in this area in the last decade, establishing relationships between genetic polymorphisms and cancer risk has proved difficult, with many false-positive reports from small studies. However, polymorphisms remain of great interest and potential importance, because, although they may only cause a moderate increase in the risk for an individual, their high frequency in populations means that they could contribute to an important proportion of cancer cases. The proposed mechanism of effect for some putative low risk polymorphisms is that they may modify the impact of environmental factors such as diet on cancer risk, for example by affecting the rate of detoxification or activation of mutagenic chemicals present in some foods.

22.5 NON–DIETARY CAUSES OF CANCER

The proportions of cancer due to avoidable causes have been estimated by Doll and Peto (2003; see Table *eolve* 22.2 (📖)). These estimates apply to Western countries such as the USA or the UK. In less developed countries the overall ranking of factors would be broadly similar, but the proportion of cancer due to infective factors would be higher and therefore some of the other factors correspondingly lower, due particularly to much higher rates of cancers of the liver (caused by hepatitis B virus and hepatitis C virus) and cervix (caused by human papillomavirus).

TOBACCO

Worldwide, the most important preventable cause of cancer is tobacco, which causes approximately 30% of cancers in Western countries. Tobacco causes cancers of the mouth, pharynx, oesophagus, larynx, lung, pancreas, kidney (pelvis) and bladder.

INFECTIONS

Infectious agents are responsible for about 9% of cancers worldwide, with the proportion being higher in less developed countries and lower in more developed countries. The most important numerically are cancer of the liver (hepatitis B virus and hepatitis C virus), cancer of the cervix (human papillomavirus) and stomach cancer (*Helicobacter pylori*). In some parts of the world parasites are important causes of cancer; for example, major causes of liver cancer (cholangiosarcoma) in China, Thailand and other parts of Asia are the liver flukes *Clonorchis sinensis* and *Opisthorchis viverrini*, and a major cause of bladder cancer in Egypt and Tanzania is the trematode worm *Schistosoma haematobium*.

HORMONAL AND REPRODUCTIVE FACTORS

Hormonal and reproductive factors are important determinants of three types of cancer in women, cancers of the breast, ovary and endometrium (lining of the womb). Childbirth reduces the risk for all three of these cancers; probably through inducing terminal differentiation of the epithelial cells in the breasts, and stopping, for the duration of pregnancies, ovulation in the ovaries and cell division in the susceptible cells in the endometrium. Hormonal factors are also important in cancer of the prostate and may be important in the aetiology of cancers of the testis.

ALCOHOL

Alcohol, if considered separately from diet, is responsible for about 6% of cancers in Western countries such as the UK. High alcohol consumption causes cancers of the mouth, pharynx, larynx, oesophagus, colorectum and liver, and even moderate alcohol intake causes a small increase in the risk for breast cancer (see 'Mechanisms for dietary factors predisposing to or protecting against cancer', below and Ch. 9).

IONISING RADIATION

Ionising radiation is estimated to cause about 5% of cancers in Western countries. In the UK, for example, approximately 5% of lung cancers are due to naturally occurring radon gas inside buildings.

OTHER FACTORS

Other factors including ultraviolet light, medical drugs, occupational exposures and pollution are each estimated to account for around 2% or less of cancers.

22.6 DIET AND CANCER

INTRODUCTION

Research problems

Research into the effects of diet on cancer is difficult. Different dietary factors may increase or reduce the risk for developing cancer, and the size of the effect on risk may be small or moderate (usually less than twofold), compared to the very large effects of some other agents (e.g. heavy smoking increases the risk for lung cancer by about 30-fold, persistent HPV infection increases the risk for cervical cancer by about 100-fold). But probably the biggest challenge in conducting research into diet and cancer is the difficulty in obtaining accurate estimates of dietary intake, compounded by the interrelations of intakes of most foods and nutrients, the relatively narrow range in food choices within many populations, and the biases in recall of food intake.

Types of evidence available

Much of the evidence for the potential role of lifestyle and environmental factors in the determination of cancer risk comes from descriptive epidemiology, which looks at the variations of cancer rates with place and time (Doll & Peto 2003). These studies have shown that, for all the common cancers, rates vary widely (by at least five-fold) between populations in different parts of the world, and that these variations are mostly not solely due to genetic make-up because rates change when people migrate from one country to another, and also change with time within populations.

Many of the prominent hypotheses for effects of diet on cancer risk have been derived from so-called ecological studies, where population-level averages of food intakes in different populations are compared with cancer rates. For example, this type of study led to the hypotheses that high intakes of meat may increase the risk for colorectal cancer, and that high intakes of fat may increase the risk for breast cancer. Observations in ecological studies do not constitute evidence of a causal relationship, because the diets of the individuals who actually develop cancer are not measured, and

many dietary and non-dietary factors vary between populations and could explain the variations in cancer rates.

Testing of hypotheses requires research on individuals, including observational studies that compare the diets of individuals who develop cancer with the diets of those who remain cancer free, and randomised trials that test the effect of dietary supplements or dietary change on cancer incidence. Observational studies that attempt to retrospectively assess the diets of people who have already developed cancer can be relatively cheap and rapid to conduct, but the results are subject to biased recall of previous diet by cancer patients, and biased participation in the research by healthy controls; thus small to moderate effects observed in this type of 'case-control' study should be interpreted very cautiously. More reliable are prospective (or 'cohort' studies), in which diet is assessed among healthy people who are then followed to relate diet at recruitment to cancer incidence; this type of study largely avoids the biases in case-control studies but is slow and expensive, and the reliability of the results can be compromised by substantial errors in estimation of usual dietary intake, and by the difficulties of identifying which of several correlated dietary and non-dietary factors is most closely related to cancer risk (see Section *evolve* 22.6(a) on the EPIC study).

Biomarkers of nutritional intake such as concentrations of micronutrients and fatty acids have begun to be investigated in large prospective cohort studies, but such studies are expensive and difficult to perform. Biomarkers can provide an estimate of dietary intake, avoiding errors due to self-reporting, and can help elucidate biological mechanisms by which dietary factors may influence cancer risk. However, the stability of blood biomarkers over time is often unknown, and the relationship between dietary intakes and the biomarker may not be clear.

Where biological samples are available it is also possible to investigate the relationship of genetic variants related to the intake, absorption and metabolism of nutrients, with disease risk. One recently developed approach is the genome-wide association study, in which the entire genome is scanned for variants which might relate to the risk of disease. The challenge is to identify the biological role of the variants identified, many of which are in non-coding portions of the genome.

Randomised controlled trials eliminate bias, and positive results provide clear evidence that the intervention has caused the change in cancer risk. However, such trials have to be very large and therefore expensive, and can only test one or two interventions over a few years; it is relatively simple to test the effect of nutritional supplements, but much harder to test the effects of changes in food intake. Thus few results are available from trials of dietary factors and cancer risk, and negative results do not rule out the possibility that there could be an effect at a different dose or if the intervention had been at a different age or had continued for longer (see Section *evolve* 22.6(b) on cancer prevention trials).

Experimental data can demonstrate effects of dietary factors on cancer risk in animals or in cultivated human cells, and provide the basis for hypotheses of effects in humans and plausible mechanisms to explain associations observed.

MECHANISMS FOR DIETARY FACTORS PREDISPOSING TO OR PROTECTING FROM CANCER

Dietary factors may be associated with cancer development in various ways. At the cellular level, these may be via DNA damage and repair, cell proliferation, carcinogen metabolism, apoptosis and cell differentiation. Hormonal regulation, inflammation and immune responses can also all be affected by dietary constituents. In epigenetic modulation, gene expression is influenced without changes to the DNA sequence. A single food component may influence multiple steps in the development of cancer.

Dietary mutagens

Diet may increase risk by supplying mutagens that directly damage the host DNA, but there are very few well-established examples of this mechanism. Two important examples are aflatoxin and Chinese-style salted fish. Aflatoxin is a food contaminant produced by the fungus *Aspergillus*; high levels of aflatoxin can occur in foods such as grains, oilseeds, nuts and dried fruit stored in hot and humid conditions, and, together with active hepatitis due to HBV, can cause liver cancer (see next section). Chinese-style salted fish increases the risk for nasopharyngeal cancer (see next section): this fish is usually allowed to partially decompose during processing and can contain high levels of nitrosamines.

Other food components are also hypothesised to increase cancer risk due to their mutagenic effects, but evidence as to whether this does in fact occur is not yet conclusive; for example, nitrites and their related compounds found in smoked, salted and some processed meat products may be converted to carcinogenic N-nitroso compounds in the body, and this may explain the probable carcinogenic effects of processed meats. Meat and fish cooked at high temperatures can contain moderately high levels of heterocyclic amines and polycyclic aromatic hydrocarbons, which might increase risk in particular for colorectal cancer. Starchy foods like bread, breakfast cereals and fried potatoes cooked at high temperatures contain moderate levels of acrylamide, which is carcinogenic when administered at high doses to experimental animals. Data on whether high dietary intakes of acrylamide cause cancer in human populations are inconclusive.

Alcohol

Alcohol is one of the best-established dietary factors that increase cancer risk, but the mechanisms by which chronic alcohol ingestion stimulates carcinogenesis are not certain. Studies in experimental animals support the concept that ethanol may act as a co-carcinogen. Alcohol may facilitate or enhance the role of other carcinogens via its ability to increase the absorption of carcinogens, or make mucosal cells more susceptible to chemical carcinogens. The metabolism of ethanol also leads to the generation of acetaldehyde within the oesophageal mucosa, which can form DNA adducts and may thus promote tumour growth. In addition, the effects of alcohol ingestion on metabolism in the liver may lead to impaired immunity, and the increase in breast cancer risk due to alcohol intake may be due to effects on oestrogen metabolism, leading to increases in blood levels of oestrogens.

Energy balance

The most striking finding that emerged from studies on diet and cancer in experimental animals conducted during the twentieth century was that energy restriction can substantially reduce the incidence of cancer. The implications of this observation for human populations are not clear, in particular because many of these experiments were carried out on weanling animals exposed to severe energy restriction that resulted in restricted growth.

Obesity in humans increases the risk for several types of cancer (oesophagus, colorectum, pancreas, breast, endometrium and kidney). The mechanisms by which obesity raises the risk for cancers of the colorectum, pancreas and kidney are not well understood. The increased risk for cancer of the oesophagus may be due to increased reflux of gastric contents, while for cancers of the breast and endometrium the mechanism is almost certainly increased production of oestrogens. Adipose tissue is a major source of oestrogen production among postmenopausal women, and obese women have much higher blood levels of endogenous (natural) oestrogens than thin women, causing an increase in the risks for cancers of the breast and endometrium because oestrogens stimulate the growth and division of the cells in these tissues (Key et al 2002).

Dietary fibre

Diets high in fibre have generally been associated with a reduction in the risk of colorectal cancer in both animal and human studies, although it is difficult to identify whether the 'dietary fibre' itself or other substances found in high fibre foods such as cereals, pulses, vegetables and fruits are associated with the beneficial effect. Given the effects of fibre on the luminal characteristics and function of the bowel, several mechanisms have been proposed through which dietary fibre may reduce the risk for colorectal cancer. High intakes of fibre increase stool bulk, reduce transit time through the colon and may thus minimise the absorption of carcinogens by the colonic mucosa. Dietary fibre may also reduce exposure to carcinogens through dilution of the gut contents and/or by binding the carcinogens for faecal excretion. Finally, fermentation of fibre in the large bowel produces short-chain fatty acids, such as butyrate, which may protect against colorectal cancer through the ability to promote differentiation, induce apoptosis and inhibit the production of carcinogenic secondary bile acids by lowering the intraluminal pH.

It has also been suggested that dietary fibre may reduce the risk of hormone-dependent cancers by regulating sex hormone levels. A diet high in fibre can reduce the enterohepatic circulation of steroids and this might ultimately reduce serum hormone concentrations by causing increased faecal excretion; however, the importance of this potential mechanism is not established (see Ch. 6).

Vitamins and minerals

Consumption of adequate amounts of certain vitamins and minerals may help to reduce the risk for many cancers. Indeed, it has been suggested that the relatively high incidence of cancers of the oesophagus and stomach in some developing countries is partly due to micronutrient deficiencies. Micronutrient deficiencies may increase susceptibility in several ways. Research in the 1990s explored the possibility that antioxidant nutrients might protect against cancer, but trials of antioxidant nutrients have so far been almost entirely negative. More recently interest in folate has increased. Low folate intakes may increase the risk of mutations and allow inappropriate DNA promoter methylation to take place, whereas evidence from supplementation trials suggests that high folic acid intakes might promote the growth of colorectal adenomas (see Section 10.5).

Possible plant anti-carcinogens

In addition to vitamins and minerals, many compounds in plants that are not nutrients are under investigation for possible anti-carcinogenic properties. Examples include: flavonoids such as quercetin found at high levels in apples, onions and tea; carotenoids such as lycopene and lutein found in tomato products and green vegetables, respectively; isothiocyanates, predominantly found in cruciferous vegetables; sulphur-containing compounds found predominantly in the *Allium* species, garlic, onions and leeks; and phytosterols, found in a wide variety of fruit and vegetables, which are established cholesterol-lowering agents and may also exhibit anti-cancer properties via several pathways such as regulation of signal transduction pathways that regulate tumour growth and apoptosis. Phytoestrogens such as isoflavones derived from soybeans, and lignans derived from wholegrain products, have received particular attention because of their possible anti-oestrogenic effects that could reduce risk for breast cancer in women and prostate cancer in men. However, research so far has not established a protective effect of any of these compounds for any type of cancer in humans.

Insulin-like growth factor

The cancer protective effect of energy restriction in animal models may be partly mediated by a reduction in circulating levels of the growth factor insulin-like growth factor-I (IGF-I). IGF-I is probably associated with the risk for some types of cancer in humans. Currently data suggest that blood levels of IGF-I in humans are related to intake of protein and dairy products.

Epigenetic regulation

Control of gene expression without altering the DNA sequence is known as epigenetic regulation, the most well known example is DNA methylation. In many genes, clusters of cytosine adjacent to guanine bases (CpG) sequences are found in the promoter regions that normally act to promote expression of the gene. DNA methylation is the addition of a methyl group (CH_3) to cytosine residues in these CpG sequences. When these sites are methylated, transcription factors cannot bind to these sites and the gene is not expressed. DNA methylation can be used in the differentiation of normal cells, by permanently switching off genes.

Dietary folate and other constituents which can act as methyl group donors (e.g. choline, methionine, betaine) are essential for this epigenetic control (as well as for DNA synthesis). Dietary components which do not themselves provide methyl groups may also influence the methylation process. Other types of epigenetic processes include genomic imprinting, the deacetylation and methylation of histones involved in the mechanism that regulates promoter transcription, and chromatin modifications.

Inflammation

Inflammation is a protective physiological response to infection or trauma but in the long term inflammation can lead to DNA damage and promote the development of cancer by increasing cell proliferation, inhibiting apoptosis and inducing the generation of new blood vessels. Dietary components can influence inflammatory processes. For example, heavy alcohol consumption may alter metabolic processes in the liver to impair immune function and increase the chances of developing liver cancer. It has been proposed that obesity is accompanied by generalised inflammation, contributing to increased cancer risk at a number of sites in the body.

OVERVIEW OF THE ASSOCIATIONS OF DIETARY FACTORS WITH THE RISK FOR THE COMMON TYPES OF CANCER

Oral cavity, pharynx and oesophagus

Cancers of the oral cavity, pharynx and oesophagus were estimated to account for 947 000 cases and 648 000 deaths in 2002. Incidence rates of these cancers vary widely between populations; for example, oesophageal cancer is over a hundred times more common in parts of central Asia, China and southern Africa than in most parts of Europe, North America and West Africa. In developed countries the main risk factors are alcohol and tobacco, and up to 75% of these cancers are attributable to these two lifestyle factors. The mechanism of the effect of alcohol on these cancers is not known, but may involve direct effects on the epithelium. Overweight/obesity is an established risk factor specifically for adenocarcinoma (but not squamous cell carcinoma) of the oesophagus. It has been proposed that a substantial proportion of cancers of the oral cavity, pharynx and oesophagus in some developing countries are due to micronutrient deficiencies related to a restricted diet that is low in fruit and vegetables and animal products. It should be noted, however, that the evidence for a protective effect of fruit and vegetables is largely derived from case-control studies and there are few data yet from prospective studies. The relative roles of various micronutrients are not yet clear, but deficiencies of riboflavin, folate, vitamin C and zinc might be involved. There is also consistent evidence that consuming drinks and foods at a very high temperature increases the risk for these cancers. The results of trials in Linxian, China, aimed at reducing oesophageal cancer rates with micronutrient supplements, have been promising but not definitive. These trials were set up on the basis of epidemiological evidence showing that the people of Linxian had low intakes of numerous nutrients and the world's highest rate of oesophageal cancer. They showed that individuals taking a combination of β-carotene, vitamin E and selenium had reduced mortality from cancer overall including a reduction in mortality from oesophageal cancer (Blot et al 1993). The role of such supplementation on risk in a population without micronutrient deficiencies is not known.

One type of cancer within this classification, nasopharyngeal cancer, is particularly common in

Southeast Asia, and has been consistently associated with a high intake of Chinese-style salted fish, especially during early childhood, as well as with infection with the Epstein–Barr virus (Doll & Peto 2003). Chinese-style salted fish is a special product that is usually softened by partial decomposition before or during salting; other types of salted fish have been studied and not found to be convincingly associated with the risk for developing nasopharyngeal cancer.

Stomach cancer

Stomach cancer was estimated to account for 934 000 cases and 700 000 deaths in 2002. Until about 20 years ago stomach cancer was the most common cancer in the world, but mortality rates have been falling, particularly in Western countries, and stomach cancer is now much less common in Europe or North America than in Asia. Infection with the bacterium *Helicobacter pylori* is an established risk factor, but not a sufficient cause, for the development of stomach cancer. Dietary changes are implicated in the recent decline in stomach cancer incidence and mortality rates in many countries. The worldwide decline in rates has occurred without a *Helicobacter pylori* eradication programme, but the introduction of refrigeration has been associated with decreased risk and has probably reduced intakes of pickled and salt-preserved foods and facilitated year-round fruit and vegetable availability. Substantial evidence suggests that risk of stomach cancer is increased by high intakes of some traditionally preserved salted foods, and that risk is decreased by sufficient intakes of fruit and vegetables.

Some research has shown that vitamin supplementation can inhibit *Helicobacter pylori* infection and there is evidence from case control studies, that dietary vitamin C is associated with decreased risk of stomach cancer. More recent prospective studies have reported that high plasma levels of vitamin C are related to lower risk. In Linxian, China, combined supplementation with β-carotene, selenium and α-tocopherol resulted in a significant reduction in stomach cancer mortality, but no significant benefit was obtained from vitamin C (Blot et al 1993). A trial in Colombia showed increased regression of precancerous gastric dysplasia both in subjects given β-carotene and in subjects given vitamin C (Correa et al 2000). Five year follow-up of a trial in Japan demonstrated protection from the progression of gastric mucosal atrophy with high dose vitamin C supplementation but longer follow-up would be needed to determine whether there is an effect on risk of gastric cancer (Sasazuki et al 2003).

Further prospective data are needed, in particular to examine whether some of the dietary associations may be partly confounded by *Helicobacter pylori* infection and whether dietary factors may modify the association of *Helicobacter pylori* with risk.

Colorectal cancer

Colorectal cancer is the third most common cancer in the world and was estimated to account for 1 023 000 cases and 529 000 deaths in 2002. Incidence rates are approximately ten-fold higher in developed than in developing countries. Colorectal tumours may develop relatively slowly, probably over a period of 10 or 20 years. Most arise from a precursor lesion, the adenomatous polyp, and prevention of colorectal adenomas may decrease the occurrence of colorectal cancer. Diet-related factors may account for up to 80% of the between-country differences in rates of colorectal cancer. The best established diet-related risk factor is overweight/obesity. Alcohol causes a small increase in risk. Adult height, which is partly determined by the adequacy of nutrition in childhood and adolescence, is weakly positively associated with increased risk, and physical activity has been consistently associated with a reduced risk. These factors together, however, do not explain the large variation between populations, and there is almost universal agreement that some aspects of a Western diet are a major determinant of risk. These include the following:

Fibre, fruit and vegetables
Burkitt suggested in the 1970s that the low rates of colorectal cancer in Africa were due to the high consumption of dietary fibre, and there are several plausible mechanisms for a protective effect. Many case-control studies of colorectal cancer have observed moderately lower risk in association with high consumption of dietary fibre, and/or fruits and vegetables, but the results of recent large prospective studies have not been consistent. Furthermore, results from randomised controlled trials have not shown that interventions with supplemental fibre or a diet low in fat and high in fibre and fruit and vegetables can reduce the recurrence of colorectal adenomas. It is possible that some of the

inconsistencies are due to differences between studies in the types of fibre eaten and in the methods for classifying fibre in food tables.

In the Pooling Project of Prospective Studies of Diet and Cancer, data on dietary fibre intakes and risk for colorectal cancer from 13 prospective cohort studies including 725 628 men and women among whom 8 081 colorectal cancer cases were identified, were pooled and analysed together. The main results showed no significant association; however, further analyses in the report showed a significantly increased risk for colorectal cancer among participants with a very low intake of fibre. Results from the European Prospective Investigation into Cancer and Nutrition (EPIC) showed a significantly lower risk for colorectal cancer associated with high fibre intake (see Section *evolve* 22.6(a)). Neither the Pooling Project nor the EPIC study showed clear differences in the association with risk according to fibre source (Bingham et al 2003; Park et al 2005).

Meat

International studies show a strong association between per capita consumption of meat and colorectal cancer mortality, and several biological mechanisms have been proposed through which meat may increase cancer risk. Mutagenic heterocyclic amines and polycyclic aromatic hydrocarbons can be formed during the cooking of meat at high temperatures, and nitrites and related compounds found in smoked, salted and some processed meat products may be converted to carcinogenic N-nitroso compounds in the colon. In addition, high iron levels in the colon may increase the formation of mutagenic free radicals. The recent WCRF/AACR report on diet and cancer concluded that the evidence that red and processed meat cause colorectal cancer is convincing. However, death rates for colorectal cancer are similar in Western vegetarians and comparable non-vegetarians. More evidence on dose response and the biological mechanisms of action will be informative.

Fat

As with meat, international correlation studies show a strong association between per capita xconsumption of fat and colorectal cancer mortality. One possible mechanism is that a high fat intake increases the level of potentially mutagenic secondary bile acids in the lumen of the large intestine.

The Women's Health Initiative Dietary Modification Trial evaluated the effects of a low-fat eating pattern on risk of colorectal cancer in postmenopausal women (Beresford et al 2006). Although the intervention group achieved a moderate reduction in their fat intake and increased their grain and fruit and vegetables intake, there was no evidence that the intervention reduced the risk of invasive colorectal cancer during the 8-year follow-up period (see Section *evolve* 22.6(b)).

Folate

In observational studies, high dietary folate intake has usually been associated with reduced risk of colorectal cancer risk. Diminished folate status may contribute to carcinogenesis by altering gene expression or by increased DNA damage. However, trials of supplementation with folic acid did not reduce the risk of colorectal adenomas (Cole et al 2007; Logan et al 2008). It has been suggested that, whilst a higher folate intake might be protective against initiation of colorectal neoplasia, it might promote the growth of existing tumours.

The finding that a common polymorphism in a key gene involved in folic acid metabolism (methylene tetrahydrofolate reductase) may also be associated with colorectal cancer strengthens the hypothesis that dietary folate may be an important factor in colorectal carcinogenesis, but the details of these associations are complex and not yet well understood (see Section *evolve* 22.6(c)).

Calcium and vitamin D

Relatively high intakes of calcium may reduce the risk for colorectal cancer, perhaps by forming complexes with secondary bile acids and haem in the intestinal lumen and thus inhibiting their damaging effects on the epithelium. Several observational studies have supported this hypothesis, and two trials have suggested that supplemental calcium may have a modest protective effect on the recurrence of colorectal adenomas. There is also evidence that relatively high blood levels of vitamin D are associated with a reduction in the risk for colorectal cancer.

Cancer of the liver

Liver cancer was estimated to account for 626 000 cases and 598 000 deaths in 2002, worldwide. Approximately 75% of cases of liver cancer occur in developing countries, and liver cancer rates vary over 20-fold between countries, being much higher in sub-Saharan Africa and southeast Asia than in Europe and North America. The major risk factor for hepatocellular carcinoma, the main type of liver cancer, is chronic infection with hepatitis B, and to a lesser extent, hepatitis C virus. Ingestion of foods contaminated with the mycotoxin aflatoxin is an important risk factor among people in developing countries with active hepatitis virus infection. Excessive alcohol consumption is established as the main diet-related risk factor for liver cancer in Western countries, probably via the development of cirrhosis and alcoholic hepatitis (Tomatis et al 1990, Doll & Peto 2003). Recent evidence shows that moderate alcohol intakes also slightly increase risk. Little is known about possible nutritional cofactors for viral carcinogenesis, but this may be an important area for research.

Cancer of the pancreas

Cancer of the pancreas was estimated to account for 232 000 cases and 227 000 deaths in 2002 and is more common in Western countries than in developing countries. Time trends suggest that both incidence and mortality for cancer of the pancreas are increasing in most parts of the world, although some of this apparent increase may be due to improvements in diagnostic methods. Overweight/obesity increases the risk, but this association is relatively small. Some studies have suggested that risk is increased by a high glycaemic load, high intakes of meat or dairy products or reduced by high intakes of fruits or vegetables, but data from prospective studies have been inconsistent and no associations with dietary intakes have been conclusively demonstrated.

Lung cancer

Lung cancer is the most common cancer in the world and was estimated to account for 1 352 000 cases and 1 179 000 deaths in 2002. Heavy smoking increases the risk by around 30-fold, and smoking causes over 80% of lung cancers in Western countries. The possibility that diet might also have an effect on lung cancer risk was raised in the 1970s following the observation that, after allowing for the effect of smoking, increased lung cancer risk was associated with a low dietary intake of vitamin A. Since then, numerous observational studies have found that lung cancer patients generally report a lower intake of fruits, vegetables and related nutrients (such as β-carotene) than controls. However,

the only one of these factors to have been tested in controlled trials, namely β-carotene, has failed to produce any benefit when given as a supplement for up to 12 years.

The possible effect of diet on lung cancer risk remains controversial. Several recent observational studies have continued to observe an association of fruits and vegetables with reduced risk, but this association has been weak in prospective studies. This apparent relationship may be due to residual confounding by smoking, since smokers generally consume less fruit and vegetables than non-smokers. In public health terms, the overriding priority for reducing lung cancer rates is to reduce the prevalence of smoking.

Breast cancer

Breast cancer is the second most common cancer in the world and the most common cancer among women. Breast cancer was estimated to account for 1 151 000 cases and 411 000 deaths in women in 2002. Incidence rates are about four times higher in Western countries than in less developed countries. Much of this international variation is due to differences in established reproductive risk factors such as age at menarche, parity and age at birth, and breastfeeding, but differences in dietary habits and physical activity may also contribute. In fact, age at menarche is partly determined by dietary factors, in that restricted dietary intake during childhood and adolescence can lead to delayed menarche. Adult height is weakly positively associated with risk, and is partly determined by dietary factors during childhood and adolescence in that restriction in food supply during growth can reduce adult height. Oestradiol and perhaps other hormones play a key role in the aetiology of breast cancer, and it is possible that any further dietary effects on risk are mediated by hormonal mechanisms (Key et al 2002).

Overweight/obesity

Obesity increases breast cancer risk in postmenopausal women by around 50%, probably by increasing serum concentrations of free oestradiol. Obesity does not increase risk among premenopausal women but obesity in premenopausal women is likely to lead to obesity throughout life and therefore to an eventual increase in breast cancer risk.

Physical activity

Physical activity may protect against weight gain and as such be protective against breast cancer among postmenopausal women. The evidence for an effect independent of body size or adiposity is so far inconclusive. Different assessment methods between studies, biases in reporting and lack of demonstrated mechanistic explanations contribute to the uncertainty.

Alcohol

The only other established dietary risk factor for breast cancer is alcohol. There is now a large amount of data from well-designed studies that consistently show a small increase in risk with increasing consumption, with about a 10% increase in risk for an average of one alcoholic drink every day. The mechanism for this association is not known, but may involve increases in oestrogen levels. It has been suggested that the adverse effect of alcohol may be exacerbated by a low folate intake, but the evidence for this is weak.

Fat

Much research and controversy has surrounded the hypothesis that a high fat intake increases breast cancer risk and the results of observational studies have varied. In the Women's Health Initiative Dietary Modification Trial, the effect of a low-fat eating pattern on risk of breast cancer in postmenopausal women was tested (Prentice et al 2006). 48 835 postmenopausal women, aged 50–79 years, without prior breast cancer were randomly assigned either to the dietary modification intervention, in which women were given dietary advice to reduce fat intake and increase grains, fruit and vegetables consumption, or to the comparison group. Over the follow-up of 8 years, during which 1 727 invasive breast cancers were identified, there was no evidence that the intervention significantly reduced breast cancer risk (see Section *evolve* 22.6(b)).

Other dietary factors

The results of studies of other dietary factors including meat, dairy products, fruit and vegetables, fibre and phytoestrogens are inconsistent and no associations with these factors have been established.

Cancer of the endometrium

Endometrial cancer was estimated to account for 199 000 cases and 50 000 deaths in women in 2002, with the highest incidence rates occurring in Western countries. Endometrial cancer risk is about three-fold higher in obese women than lean women. As with breast cancer, the effect of obesity in postmenopausal women on the risk for endometrial cancer is probably mediated by the increase in serum concentrations of oestradiol and the reduction in serum concentrations of sex hormone-binding globulin; in premenopausal women, the mechanism probably involves the increase in anovulation and consequent increased exposure to oestradiol unopposed by progesterone.

Cancer of the cervix

Cancer of the cervix was estimated to account for 493 000 cases and 274 000 deaths in women in 2002. The highest rates are in sub-Saharan Africa, Central and South America, and southeast Asia. The major cause of cervical cancer is infection with certain subtypes of the human papillomavirus. Fruits, vegetables and related nutrients such as carotenoids and folate tend to be inversely related with risk, but these associations may be entirely due to confounding by papillomavirus infections, smoking and other factors.

Cancer of the ovary

Cancer of the ovary was estimated to account for 205 000 cases and 125 000 deaths in women in 2002, with the highest incidence rates occurring in Western countries. Risk is reduced by high parity and by long-term use of combined oral contraceptives. Some studies have suggested that risk is increased by high intakes of fat or dairy products, and a high glycaemic load diet, and reduced by high intakes of vegetables, but the data are not consistent.

Prostate cancer

Prostate cancer was estimated to account for 679 000 cases and 221 000 deaths in 2002. Prostate cancer incidence rates are strongly affected by diagnostic practices and therefore difficult to interpret, but mortality rates show that death from prostate cancer is about ten times more common in North America and Europe than in Asia. Little is known about the aetiology of prostate cancer, although ecological studies suggest that it is positively associated with a Western-style diet. The data from prospective studies have not established any associations for specific nutrients or dietary factors. Diets high in red meat, dairy products and animal fat have frequently been implicated in the development of prostate cancer, but the data are not entirely consistent. Randomised controlled trials have provided substantial, consistent evidence that supplements of β-carotene do not alter the risk for prostate cancer. A recent trial has shown no benefit of supplementation with selenium and vitamin E (Lippman et al 2009) and another recent trial demonstrated no effect of vitamins C or E on risk of prostate cancer (Gaziano et al 2009). Lycopene, primarily from tomatoes, has been associated with a reduced risk in some observational studies, but the data are not consistent.

Hormones control the growth of the prostate, and interventions that lower androgen levels are moderately effective in treating this disease. Whereas prospective studies have not shown associations for serum sex hormones and prostate cancer risk, there is evidence that risk is increased by high levels of IGF-I. Diet might affect prostate cancer risk by affecting IGF-1 levels, and recent data suggest that high intakes of animal or dairy protein may increase circulating levels of IGF-I.

Bladder cancer

Cancer of the urinary bladder was estimated to account for 357 000 cases and 145 000 deaths in 2002. The geographic variation in incidence is about ten-fold, with relatively high rates in Western countries. Tobacco smoking increases the risk for bladder cancer, accounting for between a third to two-thirds of all bladder cancers. Occupational risk factors, such as exposure to aromatic amines and poly-aromatic hydrocarbons, also play an important role. Studies suggest that high intakes of fluid might reduce risk, but this is not established and more prospective data are needed.

Kidney cancer

Cancer of the kidney was estimated to account for 208 000 cases and 102 000 deaths in 2002. The range of geographic variation in incidence is moderate, with the highest incidence in Scandinavia and among the Inuit. Overweight/obesity is an established risk factor for cancer of the kidney, and may account for up to 30% of kidney cancers in both men and women. There are only limited data on the possible role of diet in the aetiology of kidney cancer. Some studies have observed an increase in risk with high intakes of meat and dairy products and a reduced risk with high intakes of vegetables, but the data are inconsistent.

22.7 RECOMMENDATIONS FOR REDUCING CANCER RISK

Table *evolve* 22.3 summarises the associations of the common cancers with dietary factors 🖰.

Recently, the World Cancer Research Fund and the American Institute for Cancer Research together conducted a major review of the available evidence on food, nutrition, physical activity and the prevention of cancer. The review gave a series of general recommendations for cancer prevention. These were qualified with further information for their application in public health and by the individual. The summary recommendations are:

1. Be as lean as possible within the normal range of body weight.
2. Be physically active as part of everyday life.
3. Limit consumption of energy-dense foods. Avoid sugary drinks.
4. Eat mostly foods of plant origin.
5. Limit intake of red meat and avoid processed meat.
6. Limit alcoholic drinks.
7. Limit consumption of salt.
8. Aim to meet nutritional needs through diet alone.

Special recommendation 1. Mothers to breastfeed; children to be breastfed.

Special recommendation 2. Cancer survivors: follow the recommendations for cancer prevention.

In developed countries, the highest priorities for cancer prevention are to prevent smoking, reduce the prevalence of overweight and obesity and reduce the consumption of alcohol. In developing countries, these diet-related cancer prevention recommendations need to be considered in the context of the diets and lifestyle of each population.

KEY POINTS

- Most cancers develop from a single cell.
- The change from a normal cell to cancer requires mutations in several genes.
- The accumulation of enough mutations in a single cell to cause cancer depends on endogenous processes, exogenous mutagens, and chance.
- Diet-related factors may account for about 30% of cancers in developed countries.
- Obesity increases the risk for cancers of the oesophagus, colorectum, pancreas, breast (postmenopausal), endometrium and kidney.
- Alcohol causes cancers of the oral cavity, pharynx, larynx, oesophagus, colorectum and liver, and causes a small increase in the risk for breast cancer.
- High intakes of red and processed meat probably increase the risk for colorectal cancer.
- High fibre intakes probably reduce the risk for colorectal cancer.
- Adequate intakes of fruit and vegetables probably reduce the risk for several types of cancer of the gastrointestinal tract.
- Micronutrient deficiencies might increase cancer risk in malnourished populations.
- Micronutrient supplementation trials have shown some benefit in reducing cancer risk in populations with dietary deficiencies
- In more developed regions, dietary intervention trials have not shown benefit in reducing cancer risk; high dose micronutrient supplements can be harmful.
- For many cancers the importance of dietary factors is not clear.

References

Beresford SA, Johnson KC, Ritenbaugh C, et al: Low-fat dietary pattern and risk of colorectal cancer: the Women's Health Initiative Randomized Controlled Dietary Modification Trial, *JAMA* 295(6):643–654, 2006.

Bingham SA, Day NE, Luben R, et al: European Prospective Investigation into Cancer and Nutrition. Dietary fibre in food and protection against colorectal cancer in the European Prospective Investigation into Cancer and Nutrition (EPIC): an observational study, *Lancet* 361(9368):1496–1501, 2003.

Blot WJ, Li JY, Taylor PR, et al: Nutrition intervention trials in Linxian, China: supplementation with specific vitamin/mineral combinations, cancer incidence, and disease-specific mortality in the general population, *J Natl Cancer Inst* 15; 85(18):1483–1492, 1993.

Byers T, Nestle M, McTiernan A, et al: Nutrition and Physical Activity Guidelines Advisory Committee. American Cancer Society guidelines on nutrition and physical activity for cancer prevention: Reducing the risk of cancer with healthy food choices and physical activity, *CA: Cancer Journal for Clinicians* 52:92–119, 2001.

Cole BF, Baron JA, Sandler RS, et al: Folic acid for the prevention of colorectal adenomas: a randomized clinical trial, *JAMA* 297(21):2351–2359, 2007.

Correa P, Fontham ET, Bravo JC, et al: Chemoprevention of gastric dysplasia: randomized trial of antioxidant supplements and anti-*Helicobacter pylori* therapy, *J Natl Cancer Inst* 92(23):1881–1888, 2000.

Department of Health: *Report on Health and Social Subjects 48. Nutritional aspects of the development of cancer. Report of the Working Group on Diet and Cancer Committee on the Medical Aspects of Food and Nutrition Policy,* London, 1998, The Stationery Office.

Doll R, Peto R: Epidemiology of cancer. In Warrell DA, Cox TM, Firth JD, Benz EJ Jr, editors: *Oxford textbook of medicine,* 4th edn, Oxford, 2003, Oxford University Press, pp 193–218.

Ferlay J, Bray F, Pisani P, et al: *GLOBOCAN 2002: Cancer incidence, mortality and prevalence worldwide.* IARC CancerBase No. 5. version 2.0, Lyon, 2004, IARC Press.

Gaziano JM, Glynn RJ, Christen WG, et al: Vitamins E and C in the prevention of prostate and total cancer in men: the Physicians' Health Study II randomized controlled trial, *JAMA* 301(1):102–103, 2009.

Hanahan D, Weinberg RA: The hallmarks of cancer, *Cell* 100(1):57–70, 2000.

Key TJ, Allen NE, Spencer EA, Travis RC: The effect of diet on risk of cancer, *Lancet* 360:861–868, 2002.

Lippman SM, Klein EA, Goodman PJ, et al: Effect of selenium and vitamin E on risk of prostate cancer and other cancers: the Selenium and Vitamin E Cancer Prevention Trial (SELECT), *JAMA* 301(1):39–51, 2009.

Logan RF, Grainge MJ, Shepherd VC, et al: Aspirin and folic acid for the prevention of recurrent colorectal adenomas, *Gastroenterology* 134(1):29–38, 2008.

Park Y, Hunter DJ, Spiegelman D, et al: Dietary fiber intake and risk of colorectal cancer: a pooled analysis of prospective cohort studies, *JAMA* 294(22):2849–2857, 2005.

Prentice RL, Caan B, Chlebowski R, et al: Low-fat dietary pattern and risk of invasive breast cancer: the Women's Health Initiative Randomized Controlled Dietary Modification Trial, *JAMA* 8; 295(6):629–642, 2006.

Sasazuki S, Sasaki S, Tsubono Y, et al: The effect of 5-year vitamin C supplementation on serum pepsinogen level and *Helicobacter pylori* infection, *Cancer Sci* 94(4):378–382, 2003.

Stewart BW, Kleihues P, editors: *World cancer report*, Lyon, 2003, World Health Organization.

Tomatis L, Aition A, Day NE, et al, editors: *Cancer: causes, occurrence and control.* Lyon, 1990, World Health Organization.

WHO *Diet, nutrition and the prevention of chronic diseases.* WHO Technical Report Series 916, Geneva, 2003, World Health Organization.

World Cancer Research Fund (WCRS)/American Institute for Cancer Research (AICR): *Food, nutrition, physical activity, and the prevention of cancer: a global perspective*, Washington DC, 2007, AICR.

Further reading

Boyle P, Autier P, Bartelink H, et al: European Code Against Cancer and scientific justification: third version (2003), *Annals of Oncology* 14(7):973–1005, 2003.

Boyle P, Boffetta P, Autier P: Diet, nutrition and cancer: public, media and scientific confusion, *Annals of Oncology* 19(10):1665–1667, 2008.

Ebrahim S, Davey Smith G: Mendelian randomization: can genetic epidemiology help redress the failures of observational epidemiology? *Hum Genet.* 123(1):15–33, 2008 Feb.

Gann P: Randomized trials of antioxidant supplementation for cancer prevention: first bias, now chance – next, cause, *JAMA* 301(1): 2009.

IARC Handbook of Cancer Prevention: *Weight control and physical activity*, Lyon, 2002, World Health Organization.

Mathers JC: Nutrition and cancer prevention: diet-gene interactions, *Proceedings of the Nutrition Society* 62(3):605–610, 2003.

Peto J: Cancer epidemiology in the last century and the next decade, *Nature* 411(6835):390–395, 2001.

Prentice RL, Willett WC, Greenwald P, et al: Nutrition and physical activity and chronic disease prevention: research strategies and recommendations, *J Natl Cancer Inst* 96(17):1276–1287, 2004.

Riboli E, Lambert R, editors: *Nutrition and lifestyle: opportunities for cancer prevention.* Lyon, 2002, World Health Organization.

Stein CJ, Colditz GA: Modifiable risk factors for cancer, *British Journal of Cancer* 90(2):299–303, 2004.

Thiébaut AC, Kipnis V, Schatzkin A, Freedman LS: The role of dietary measurement error in investigating the hypothesized link between dietary fat intake and breast cancer–a story with twists and turns, *Cancer Invest* 26(1):68–73, 2008.

Chapter 23

Diseases of the gastrointestinal tract

John O Hunter and Jenny L Lee*

CHAPTER CONTENTS

OBJECTIVES

By the end of this chapter you should be able to:
- describe the most common chronic diseases which affect the intestinal tract, their epidemiology and clinical presentation
- understand current views on their aetiology and what is understood of their pathophysiology
- discuss the role of diet in their management.

23.1 INTRODUCTION

As the prime function of the gastrointestinal tract is the ingestion, digestion and absorption of food it is perhaps surprising that the medical profession has often underplayed the importance of diet in gut disorders. Although coeliac disease was first

---

*Updated and modified from the previous edition chapter written by V A Chudleigh and J O Hunter

© 2010 Elsevier Ltd/Inc/BV
DOI: 10.1016/B978-0-7020-3118-2.00023-1

described in 1888, it was not until the 1950s that the importance of gluten in its pathogenesis was realised. The role of diet in irritable bowel syndrome is still disputed by some physicians. Certainly the gut may be damaged by a wide range of external factors including bacteria and other microorganisms, trauma, radiation and chemicals. Nevertheless food items may be related to the cause of some diseases, nutritional deficiencies are frequently prominent amongst the effects of gut disorders and diet is often the only practicable therapy which patients may be offered. Nutrition is thus a key factor in the understanding of diseases of the gastrointestinal tract.

23.2 EPIDEMIOLOGY OF GASTROINTESTINAL DISEASES

COELIAC DISEASE

Coeliac disease is a disorder caused by intolerance to the protein gluten found in wheat, barley and rye. Ingestion of the gluten causes villous atrophy of the small bowel and subsequent malabsorption. It was until recently considered classically to be a disease of childhood, developing when the infant is weaned on to gluten-containing foods. A second peak of incidence occurs in adults in the third to fourth decades. Due to improved diagnostic techniques, however, a wider spectrum of the disease has been uncovered. In addition to the classical presentation of symptomatic disease there are also patients in whom it has developed but where no symptoms are present (silent) and many more who have the genetic predisposition to develop coeliac disease, but have yet do so (latent). This phenomenon has been called the iceberg effect and makes it difficult to be certain of the true incidence. The recent introduction of reliable serological markers has facilitated population screening and it has been suggested that the incidence in England is as high as 1:300. Significant variations have been reported in the prevalence of the disease throughout Europe in both time and place, ranging from 1:100 to 1:2000 (Trocone, Greco, & Auricchio, 2002; Bingley et al 2004). These variations may relate to environmental factors such as breast feeding patterns and early gluten exposure.

INFLAMMATORY BOWEL DISEASE

Inflammatory bowel disease (IBD) comprises two main diseases, Crohn's disease (CD) and ulcerative colitis (UC). Both are chronic inflammatory disorders with similar clinical features, but whereas CD may occur anywhere in the gastrointestinal tract UC is confined to the colon. CD and UC occur predominantly in the northern hemisphere throughout North America and northern Europe (Loftus 2002; Shiviananda et al 1996). Ethnicity is a key factor, with Jewish populations being particularly prone. Ulcerative colitis has a greater incidence in white Americans, rarely occurring in South America, Asia and Africa. Urban populations have an increased risk of CD but in UC the majority of studies demonstrate no distinguishable difference between urban or rural communities, except in Great Britain and Scandinavia. The age of diagnosis has two peaks for both diseases. CD tends to present in adolescence or during the third decade. For UC the age of onset is slightly later occurring around the fourth to fifth decade. The second peak for both occurs around the eighth decade. In Crohn's disease there is equal incidence for men and women. The evidence is not clear for UC but it has been suggested that women have a marginally greater risk. The incidence of CD has risen markedly during the 20th century. The epidemiology of inflammatory bowel diseases indicates the involvement both genetic and environmental factors in its development and this is discussed later.

IRRITABLE BOWEL SYNDROME

The most frequently encountered disorder of the gastrointestinal tract is irritable bowel syndrome (IBS). In the Western world it accounts for up to 50% of referrals to gastroenterologists. The variations in diagnostic criteria for IBS make epidemiological data hard to translate but estimates indicate a prevalence of 10–15% (Muller-Lissner et al 2001). It is more likely to occur in women than men (2:1) and is not age-dependent.

23.3 COELIAC DISEASE

Coeliac disease produces atrophy of the small bowel mucosa, which leads to impairment of the digestion and absorption of nutrients. The atrophy and subsequent malabsorption of nutrients can be corrected by a gluten-free diet.

PATHOLOGY

Jejunal biopsy in coeliac disease reveals characteristic changes. Intestinal crypts are elongated and

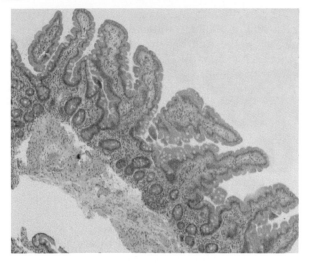

Fig. 23.1 Normal jejunal mucosa.

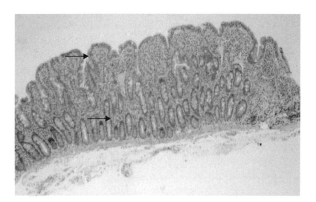

Fig. 23.2 A typical section of jejunal mucosa found in coeliac disease showing flattened mucosal surface with villous atrophy (top arrow) and elongated crypts (lower arrow).

open out on to a flattened mucosal surface where there is villous atrophy (Figs 23.1 and 23.2). The structural changes decrease the amount of epithelial surface available for digestion and absorption. The appearance of the mucosa in latent disease may appear superficially normal with residual villous structure; however the absorptive surface is less than the normal population. The length of intestine involved varies and correlates with the severity of clinical symptoms. Coeliac disease usually affects the jejunum, but in some cases lesions may extend as far as the distal ileum.

CLINICAL FEATURES

The classic features of symptomatic disease in childhood include weight loss, or failure to thrive, anaemia, lassitude and diarrhoea and may be accompanied by abdominal pain, steatorrhoea, blood loss and dehydration. Adult disease may also present with more subtle and variable symptoms such as anaemia, bone disease, neurological abnormalities and abnormal liver function. As stated previously, latent and silent cases of coeliac disease show no symptoms whatsoever. A suspicion of coeliac disease may be confirmed by the presence of serum antibodies to gliadin, endomysium or transglutaminase. However definitive diagnosis demands a jejunal biopsy confirming total or partial villous atrophy. The biopsy should be repeated after 6 months on a gluten-free diet to confirm histological improvement

AETIOLOGY

The cause of coeliac disease was unknown until 1950 when the Dutch paediatrician Dicke reported significant improvement of symptoms in patients with the condition during war time famine in the Netherlands, when supplies of wheat were scarce. He identified the toxic fraction in wheat as gluten. Gluten is the insoluble mass that remains when wheat dough is washed to remove starch granules and other soluble constituents. The major protein fractions of gluten are gliadin and glutenin and all forms of gliadin have been shown to be toxic to coeliac patients. It is believed that a small bowel mucosal enzyme, tissue transglutaminase (tTG), is important in modifying peptides derived from gliadin so that they become capable of forming autoantibodies.

Genetic factors are important in the pathogenesis of coeliac disease and it has now been shown that subjects who have human leukocyte antigen (HLA) DQ2 and DQ8 are at much greater risk of developing the disease. The physical role of the HLA system is to present peptide fragments of antigens to T cells. A 33 amino acid peptide derived from gliadin has been shown to be remarkably stable and found in foods toxic to coeliac patients including wheat, barley and rye but not in oats, rice and maize. It is an excellent substrate for tTG and the deamidated peptide had a much higher affinity for DQ2. When incubated with T cells from coeliac patients it caused a marked increase in lymphocyte proliferation. This might lead to release of cytokines and mucosal damage. Thus an autoantibody is formed by the action of tTG on gliadin and coeliac disease is associated with other autoimmune disorders including type I diabetes, thyroid disease, rheumatoid arthritis and dermatitis herpetiformis. This is important because certain cases of coeliac disease may only be diagnosed by the appearance of the other autoimmune conditions; in addition many believe that a gluten-free diet improves the control of the associated disease.

NUTRITION

As a result of damage to the gastrointestinal mucosa there is reduced production of digestive enzymes and subsequent reduction in digestive capability. Secondary to intestinal villous atrophy there may be significant reduction of mucosal surface area causing malabsorption of macro and micronutrients. Nutritional deficiencies will depend on the length and severity of small intestine affected. Iron deficiency anaemia is common. The duodenum is the primary absorption site for iron and the region in which lesions occur. Albumin concentrations may be reduced secondary to leakage into the gut lumen. In cases where there is prolonged, severe diarrhoea, levels of serum sodium and potassium may be decreased. Malabsorption severe enough to cause steatorrhoea may impair calcium and fat-soluble vitamin absorption by binding unabsorbed fats to form insoluble soap complexes. Calcium absorption may also be reduced by defective calcium transport mechanisms. Low bone mineral density and osteoporosis are subsequently common chronic features of the disease. Low serum folate concentrations are frequent in untreated disease but are not usually severe enough to cause megolablastic anaemia but may be associated with elevated plasma homocysteine, which is considered to be a risk factor for cardiovascular disease. Vitamin B_{12} deficiency is not as common, but may develop secondary to folate deficiency or if the disease affects the distal ileal mucosa. Increased loss of endogenous zinc may occur irrespective of disease severity. Serum copper concentrations may also be affected. Improvement of nutritional status may require adjunctive therapy in severe cases. In less severe presentations significant improvement may be achieved following introduction of a gluten-free diet and may not require replacement therapies.

The treatment of coeliac disease is the lifelong exclusion of gluten from the diet. The avoidance of gluten in the diet has traditionally required the strict exclusion of the prolamins in wheat (gliadin), barley (hordein), rye (secalin) and oats (avenin). The toxicity of avenin is now considered controversial. Recent research suggests that it may not be as toxic as previously thought, as it occurs in much lower concentrations than the other prolamins present in wheat, barley and rye.

The 33 amino acid polypeptide mentioned earlier is not found in oats and it is now believed that pure oats are not toxic to coeliac patients. Guidelines for professionals on inclusion of oats in the gluten-free diet advise that oats uncontaminated by wheat rye or barley may be consumed daily by coeliac patients without risk, although not in severe cases. However commercial oat products may be contaminated with gluten during manufacturing, transport and storage and should therefore be avoided.

Sources of gluten may be obvious or hidden in manufactured products making the diet difficult to follow (see Table *evolve* 23.1). By European law, foods are required to list cereals containing gluten on their ingredients lists. The national charity, Coeliac UK (see useful web links on the *evolve* website) produces a regularly updated list of manufactured foods that have been declared by their manufacturers to be gluten-free. The international CODEX standard which food products are required to meet to be gluten free was set at 200 ppm (parts per million) up until January 2009. Now, only foods which contain less than 20 ppm of gluten can be labelled 'gluten free'. Products which contain between 21 and 100 ppm gluten can be labelled 'very low gluten' and include specialist substitute products which contain CODEX wheat starch. Manufacturers have until 2012 to comply with the new legislation.

In addition to following the gluten-free diet, recommendations by the British Society of Gastroenterology and Coeliac UK suggest that all patients with coeliac disease should be advised to take 1000 mg of calcium per day using supplements if required, increasing to 1200 mg in males over 55 and post-menopausal women.

Some patients may fail to respond to the GF diet. This may be due to poor compliance or inadvertent inclusion of gluten in the diet. In patients who are successfully avoiding gluten, transglutaminase antibodies become negative. Dietary education with regular input from a dietitian is essential in order for the individual to establish and maintain a diet that is gluten-free and nutritionally complete. Complications of undiagnosed coeliac disease or failure to comply with dietary exclusion of gluten increases risk of intestinal lymphoma, carcinoma of the oesophagus or colon, osteoporosis and general malnutrition. Coeliac disease is associated with reduced splenic function and patients should be immunised to reduce the consequent increase risk of infections such as pneumonia and meningitis.

23.4 CROHN'S DISEASE

PATHOLOGY

Crohn's disease is a chronic inflammatory disorder of the alimentary tract, characterised by episodes of relapse and remission. It most commonly affects the terminal ileum and colon. Segments of intestine that are affected by inflammation are often separated by apparently normal areas; known as 'skip' lesions, they may occur throughout the length of the bowel. Inflammation may extend through the layers of the gastrointestinal wall (transmural). Ulceration of the mucosal wall, and oedema and inflammation of the bowel in between, give the mucosal surface the cobblestone appearance that is typical of this disease (Fig. 23.3) Fistulas, abnormal communications between two internal organs, or any part of the gastrointestinal tract and the skin,

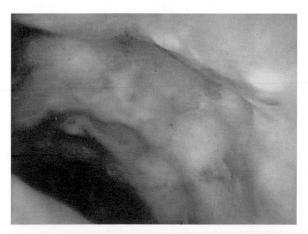

Fig. 23.3 Ulceration of the mucosal wall with oedema and inflammation of the bowel in between give the mucosal surface the 'cobblestone' appearance that is typical of this disease.

may arise in areas of the bowel that are severely affected. If the condition is given opportunity to become well established the bowel wall may thicken and the lumen narrow, predisposing the individual to strictures and intestinal obstruction.

CLINICAL FEATURES

Presentation varies according to the site and the extent of the disease. Symptoms associated with Crohn's disease are abdominal pain, diarrhoea, (defined as an increase in the number of stools with a loose or watery consistency, which may contain blood), weight loss or in children failure to thrive, fever and lethargy. Other organ systems may also be affected especially the eyes (iritis), the skin where painful nodules develop on the front of the legs (erythema nodosum) and joints, especially sacroiliac joints, knees and ankles.

Biochemical characteristics include raised inflammatory markers such as C reactive protein (CRP) or other acute phase proteins and a raised platelet count. Patients become anaemic and albumin concentrations in the blood are reduced. Increased migration of white cells through the bowel wall into the intestinal lumen occurs at sites of active disease where they accumulate in large numbers. White cells contain a protein known as calprotectin, and in active disease, the faecal concentration of this is increased, providing a means of assessing the degree of inflammation present. If white cells are labelled with radio-isotopes areas of active disease are clearly identified on scans taken with a gamma camera. This is known as white cell scanning, and the diagnosis may be confirmed by characteristic changes on radiographs with contrast media such as barium, or by endoscopy and biopsy.

AETIOLOGY

The aetiology of Crohn's disease is unknown. Both genetic and environmental factors are believed to contribute to the development of the disease. Individuals who have a first-degree relative with Crohn's disease have a risk of developing the disease two to three times greater than the rest of the population. Recent research has suggested that genes conferring susceptibility to CD exist. A specific gene, *NOD2*, is present in 20% of cases of CD. Intensive research continues in this field and other genes increasing susceptibility have recently been identified.

Environmental factors linked to Crohn's disease include smoking and diet. Smoking increases the risk of CD by a factor of two- to five-fold, in contrast to ulcerative colitis where it appears to be protective.

Prompted by epidemiological evidence the role of diet in the aetiology of Crohn's disease has been examined. Refined sugar consumption, fat, dietary fibre, fruit and vegetable intake, cereals (cornflakes), 'fast food', margarine and baker's yeast have been investigated. The data are generally difficult to interpret because of the inconsistency of results and limitations of the methodologies. Aspects of study design such as dietary recall of foods eaten years previously, effect of disease state on appetite and food choice (important in cross-sectional studies) and trial design, affect the validity of the research. A number of studies have reported that patients with Crohn's disease consume greater quantities of refined sugar foods than controls, but attempts to link this to the onset of CD is hampered by limitations in study design. In addition intervention trials have demonstrated that disease activity is not influenced by low-sugar diets (Riordan, Ruxton & Hunter, 1998).

Fats have also been implicated in the pathogenesis and clinical course of CD. Epidemiological data from Japan (Shoda et al 1996) show the incidence of CD has increased, displaying a strong correlation with increased fat consumption, and increase in the ratio of n-6 to n-3 fatty acids in the national diet, implicating altered lipid metabolism as a factor (Fig. 23.4). Replacement of n-6 arachidonic acid by other polyunsaturated fatty acids diverted from the n-3 pathway may reduce prostaglandin and thromboxane production, suppressing inflammation and maintaining immunocompetence.

The role of nutritional factors in the pathogenesis of CD is supported by studies on the importance of the faecal stream. This is composed of gastrointestinal secretions, but also food residues and bacteria. It has been known for many years that diversion of the faecal stream away from the colon by performing an ileostomy allows CD in the lower bowel to heal. Rutgeerts and his colleagues in Belgium performed endoscopic examinations of the colon in patients who had been given temporary ileostomies after gastrointestinal resections for CD to allow the anastomosis to heal. No evidence of CD was found in any patient. The ileostomies were then reversed so that the faecal stream returned to the lower bowel. After 6 months, all the patients had endoscopic evidence of Crohn's recurrence (Rutgeerts et al 1991).

The beneficial effects which antibiotics frequently produce suggest that the bacteria of the faecal stream are important in CD. Furthermore, there is an immune response to the gut bacteria, as in active CD over 80% are coated with immunoglobulin. The equal importance of food residues is suggested by finding that such immunoglobulin coating of bacteria falls back to normal (20%) when patients with CD are fed an enteral feed, containing virtually no fermentable residue, for 2 weeks (van de Waaij et al 2004). Enteral feeds where nitrogen may be presented as either amino acids, oligopeptides or single proteins, are all effective in producing remission in CD, with reduction of pro-inflammatory cytokine mRNA and healing of mucosal ulcers.

NUTRITION

Dietary therapy in CD may be used to correct nutritional deficiencies or as primary treatment for the condition.

Aetiology of nutritional deficiency

Nutritional deficiency is a common complication of Crohn's disease affecting both macro- and micronutrients (see Table *evolve* 23.2 ⬛). Because of its relapsing and remitting nature, deficiency states may develop insidiously over a number of years remaining undetected until they are multiple and severe.

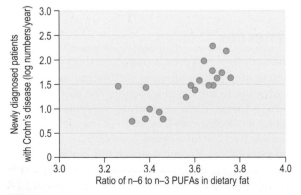

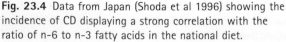

Fig. 23.4 Data from Japan (Shoda et al 1996) showing the incidence of CD displaying a strong correlation with the ratio of n-6 to n-3 fatty acids in the national diet.

Nutrient deficiency may arise by a number of different mechanisms, discussed below.

Although some conventional measures of nutritional status would suggest specific deficiencies in patients with CD there is limited evidence that deficiencies arise through inadequate dietary intake. On the other hand, the pathology of the disease and the associated medication do appear to limit absorption and handling of some nutrients.

Reduced dietary intake

Many patients eat inadequately because they develop anorexia or sitophobia (fear that eating may produce symptoms). Changes in taste may be caused by deficiency of trace elements such as zinc, copper and nickel or as a result of drug therapy. Strictures may cause abdominal pain and vomiting resulting in a reduction in dietary intake.

Malabsorption

The absorptive area of the small intestine may be considerably reduced as a result of inflammation or following surgery. A fistula may cause a short circuit, reducing the length of gastrointestinal tract available for digestion and absorption. Damage to the ileum frequently reduces absorption of vitamin B_{12}. Loss of the terminal ileum prevents re-absorption of bile salts whose deficiency may cause malabsorption of fat-soluble vitamins. The small intestine is normally sterile but Crohn's disease may allow colonisation by bacteria, which compete for nutrients.

Intestinal losses

Extensive intestinal ulceration leads to loss of albumin and iron as a result of leakage of blood and plasma from inflamed mucosa. Rapid intestinal transit may lead to loss of fluid and electrolytes and may hamper absorption. Fistulae from the upper intestine to the skin in particular may lead to significant deficiencies of nutrients, fluid and electrolytes.

Increased metabolic requirements

Protein requirements in patients with IBD are usually increased. Inflammation leads to increased production of cytokines, eicosanoids, catecholamines and glucocorticoids which gives rise to a catabolic response producing protein breakdown and negative nitrogen balance.

Drug–nutrient interactions

Corticosteroids are commonly used in the treatment of active Crohn's disease. Steroids reduce calcium absorption and increase its urinary excretion. Sulfasalazine causes competitive inhibition of folate absorption and cholestyramine binds many nutrients in the gastrointestinal tract, especially fat-soluble vitamins.

Protein–energy malnutrition

Reduced intake, increased metabolism and intestinal losses may cause protein–energy malnutrition (PEM) in the acute phase of the disease. A reduced serum level of albumin (hypoalbuminaemia) is common but should be used as a marker of disease activity rather than a measure of nutritional status for which determination of pre-albumin is more suitable. Low albumin may be a result of the inflammatory response on the acute phase plasma proteins as well as increased intestinal losses.

Assessment of nutritional deficiency

Although assessment of nutritional status is often made by measuring circulating concentrations of nutrients such values may not reflect long-term dietary intake and therefore data should be interpreted with caution.

Fat-soluble vitamins

Serum concentrations of the fat-soluble vitamins A (retinol) D (calciferol), E (alpha-tocopherol) and K (phyllquinone) are affected by Crohn's disease. Serum retinol may be decreased secondary to reduced concentrations of circulating retinol binding protein, and negative acute phase protein. Plasma levels of circulating retinol binding protein fall as part of the acute phase response and therefore low serum retinol concentrations may not be reflective of a deficiency state. Vitamin K produced endogenously by bacteria fermenting non-starch polysaccharides (NSP) in the colon may be reduced because of altered concentrations of gastrointestinal flora arising from antibiotic therapy or extensive large bowel resection.

Vitamin D and calcium

Low serum levels of 25-hydroxycholecalciferol have been reported in 23–75% of inpatients probably due to malabsorption in Crohn's disease. Vitamin D metabolism and calcium homeostasis are closely linked (Ch. 24) and many patients with Crohn's disease develop osteoporosis. Various mechanisms are thought to be involved including reduced dietary intake of calcium, malabsorption and the direct effect of pro-inflammatory cytokines on bone metabolism. However, long term corticosteroid treatment appears to be the most important. Bone mineral density measurements in patients whose Crohn's disease was treated by diet were similar to control values and significantly higher than patients who had been treated predominantly with corticosteroids (Dear et al 2001). Thus bone density appears to be affected predominantly by steroid usage and not disease activity.

Vitamin C

Measures of vitamin C (ascorbic acid) status may fall because of reduced dietary intake or possibly as a direct response to disease activity.

Mineral deficiencies

Iron-deficiency anaemia is a frequent complication in Crohn's disease and may develop secondary to gastrointestinal blood loss, reduced dietary intake and small bowel malabsorption or resection. Serum magnesium levels are kept constant at the expense of body stores, whereas serum zinc may be reduced in the presence of inflammation reflecting reduced albumin concentrations, despite normal tissue levels. Deficiencies of either may arise as a result of persistent diarrhoea, small bowel malabsorption or resection and reduced intakes. Selenium deficiency in CD has been reported in the literature, and various potential mechanisms have been proposed including use of corticosteroids and bowel resection.

The role of diet as a primary treatment

Dietary therapy may also be used as a primary treatment although its use remains controversial. However, comparisons show that the remission rate with elemental diet overall is equal to that achieved with corticosteroids and is greater when compliant patients alone are considered (King et al 1997). Up to 20% of patients are unable to comply with enteral feeds. This is unfortunate because the side effects of dietary therapy are much less serious than those for steroid use and diet has the additional benefit of correcting poor nutritional status.

The first stage of diet therapy involves the use of enteral feeding to achieve remission, which may be successful in up to 85% of compliant patients (O'Morain, Segal and Levi, 1984). The second stage involves the maintenance of remission. There is still disagreement as to whether a second stage involving dietary manipulation to detect food intolerances is necessary (Riordan et al 1993).

Elemental diet (ED) is a liquid containing a mixture of essential and non-essential amino acids, glucose, lipid, vitamins, minerals and trace elements. Other liquid diets shown to induce remission in Crohn's disease are semi-elemental (peptide-based) and polymeric diets (PD). Polymeric diets are whole protein feeds. Trial results of these feeds indicate varying degrees of success. Several advantages of PD over ED include palatability, cost, lower osmolarity, which reduces the incidence of diarrhoea, and greater concentration of energy per millilitre; however, these may be outweighed by the effectiveness of ED in achieving remission. The long chain triglyceride (LCT) content may be important. Feeds where less than 15% energy is derived from LCT appear to be more effective (Middleton et al 1995)

Efficacy of enteral diet may be influenced by duration of treatment and formula concentration. The mode of action of enteral feeds as a primary therapy remains unclear. Hypotheses include reduced antigenicity of the diet, immunomodulatory effects, improvement of nutritional status and alteration of the metabolic activity of the intestinal microbial flora. As yet no consensus has been reached and this remains a focal point for ongoing clinical trials.

Once remission is achieved there are a number of methods used in clinical practice to ensure against further relapse. Although this remains a controversial area, there is a general consensus that remission rates are disappointingly short if normal diet is resumed as soon as symptoms have cleared. Many paediatricians use enteral feeds for extended durations of up to 3 months and claim patients may subsequently return to a normal diet. Other authorities advise a search for food intolerance once remission is achieved. A low-fibre, fat-limited exclusion diet (LOFFLEX) has been developed for use in Crohn's patients by the gastroenterology research unit at Addenbrooke's Hospital, Cambridge (Woolner et al 1998) (see Table *evolve* 23.3). The LOFFLEX diet is used as an alternative to elimination diets, which are time-consuming, complicated and require considerable patient motivation. Developed from data gathered from patients completing the elimination diet, the core diet excludes foods that are most likely to cause symptoms. If patients maintain remission on the LOFFLEX diet, food reintroduction follows. During this phase, patients are able to identify and exclude foods that may trigger symptoms, ensuring remission is maintained. A comparison of the elimination diet with the LOFFLEX diet showed no significant difference in length of remission at two years in compliant, non-strictured patients with CD (Woolner et al 1998). The percentage of patients still in remission at 2 years was 59.4% and 55.6% respectively. Two-year remission rates following steroid treatment only were 31–35%. Other maintenance diets have been suggested by various centres but these have not yet been scientifically validated.

23.5 ULCERATIVE COLITIS

PATHOLOGY

Ulcerative colitis (UC) is an inflammatory disease that affects the mucosa of the colon starting from the anus and extending proximally. Mild cases may affect merely the rectum (proctitis) but commonly inflammation extends as far as the splenic flexure of the large intestine (left-sided colitis) and severe disease may affect the whole colon (pancolitis). Unlike Crohn's disease, UC does not affect the small intestine.

The biochemical characteristics are similar to those of CD. However, if inflammation is limited to the rectum a rise in C-reactive protein is unusual, unless the disease is particularly severe.

CLINICAL FEATURES

The characteristic symptoms of UC are diarrhoea and rectal bleeding with the passage of mucus. Blood loss may lead to anaemia and hypoalbuminaemia, which may be severe enough to cause peripheral oedema. Abdominal pain is common and is usually worse after meals. Anorexia leads to weight loss. Severe diarrhoea may cause loss of water and electrolytes leading to dehydration, hypomagnesaemia and hypocalcaemia. The development of megacolon, dilatation of the large intestine with thinning of the gastrointestinal wall and a high risk of perforation, is a medical emergency requiring surgery. As in Crohn's disease drugs used in the treatment of UC may also contribute to nutritional deficiency.

AETIOLOGY

The cause of UC is not known. Although its onset often appears to follow gastroenteritis no specific pathogen has yet been discovered. In contrast to normal individuals, the bacterial flora of the colon in patients with UC is highly unstable and may vary considerably over short periods of time. It has been reported that in UC a higher percentage of bacteria in the colon are coated with immunoglobulin than in normal controls and it has been suggested that mucosal inflammation may arise from an immune reaction to the resident colonic microflora. As in Crohn's disease there is a strong genetic tendency but so far no specific gene has been identified that increases susceptibility to UC.

Butyrate is a short-chain fatty acid which is the main fuel of the colonocyte and is obtained primarily as a result of fermentation in the colonic lumen. It has been suggested that in UC butyrate uptake may be impaired by hydrogen sulphide and mercaptides, compounds produced by bacterial fermentation, which may be found in the bowel in higher concentration in patients with UC. This effect is more marked in colonocytes taken from the distal colon where colitis is more common. Sulphide is produced by sulphate-reducing bacteria, which are present more frequently in UC than in controls. However, there is as yet no convincing evidence that butyrate supplementation via enemas helps in UC (Brauer 1995) and the therapeutic value of reducing colonic sulphide concentrations by low-sulphate diets remains unproven. However attempts to increase colonic butyrate content by dietary fibre supplements have shown more promising results. Several studies have reported the beneficial effects of germinated barley foodstuff (GBF), which promotes butyrate production in the colonic lumen in UC (Galvez et al 2005). *Plantago ovata* husk, however, appears to reduce the risk of relapse by normalising intestinal transit rather than by increasing butyrate production. Inulin or oligofructose may prove helpful in this situation.

The colonic mucosa in UC is inflamed and swollen with an increased blood flow. In more severe cases ulceration arises. Ulcers are initially small and discrete but may coalesce and enlarge, extending more deeply into the lamina propria. The colonic wall may become completely denuded, increasing the risk of perforation or leading to the dilated bowel known as a megacolon. Healing may result in scarring and stricture formation or the development of inflammatory pseudopolyps from isolated islands of mucosa. Although long-term UC carries a markedly increased risk of the development of colon cancer these pseudopolyps are not pre-malignant. It is believed that the development of colonic cancer in UC is a consequence of chronic inflammation rather than the development of the adenomatous polyps, which may arise in uninflamed bowel.

The pharmacological treatment of UC is similar to that of CD with prednisolone and other corticosteroids being the cornerstone of the management of many cases. In proctitis and left-sided disease these may be given by enema, but systemic administration is necessary in severe cases. Drugs releasing 5-amino salicylic acid are very helpful and patients who become steroid-dependent or resistant may require immunosuppressive agents such as azathioprine, ciclosporin or infliximab.

NUTRITION

There is little place for diet as primary therapy. Wright & Truelove (1965) reported relapse in patients when cows milk was reintroduced into the diet of patients with UC but a subsequent trial concluded that only 20% of patients with UC improve on a milk-free diet and that many of these suffer from unrelated hypolactasia. Milk exclusion carries a risk of calcium deficiency. Enteral feeds may be used to improve nutritional status but unlike Crohn's disease they do not reduce colonic inflammation. Supplementation with n-3 or n-6 fatty acids in the hope of reducing inflammation has not proved successful. Attempts to reduce colonic sulphide formation by following diets low in sulphate have yet to prove successful. It is crucial to avoid constipation, particularly in patients with left-sided colitis and proctitis and in these, poorly fermented

bulking agents such as sterculia and linseed may prove helpful.

23.6 IRRITABLE BOWEL SYNDROME

PATHOLOGY AND CLINICAL FEATURES

The Rome III criteria for IBS demand a 6-month history of abdominal pain accompanied by a change in bowel habit, which may be diarrhoea or constipation. Other symptoms include flatulence, bloating, a feeling of incomplete evacuation, urgency, straining and mucus. No abnormality, however, can be found to account for these symptoms after radiology and endoscopy of the gastrointestinal tract and standard haematological and biochemical screening. Stool culture reveals no pathogens. The diagnosis therefore is by negative exclusion of other pathology.

AETIOLOGY

Irritable bowel syndrome is the single most common condition referred to gastroenterologists in the Western world. It has been estimated that as many as 15% of westernised populations suffer from the condition at some time in their lives. This figure also includes fast-developing eastern European countries such as Russia. Prevalence in China, including Hong Kong, remains lower and is estimated at 3.6%. The high level of incidence makes it all the more frustrating that it is the least well understood of all gastrointestinal conditions. Treatment is often ineffective and symptoms may continue for years. Many patients seek treatment from homeopaths and alternative practitioners.

Confusion about IBS is compounded because it is not a single discrete entity but a syndrome made up of several quite separate conditions that may produce abdominal pain with or without a change in bowel habit. The lack of pathological findings has led many authorities to believe IBS is primarily a psychological condition. Approximately 20–25% of IBS patients suffer from an anxiety state. Anxiety in this group of patients may lead to hyperventilation and air swallowing; patients commonly present with pain, bloating and flatulence, which may be accompanied by other anxiety symptoms such as breathlessness, palpitations and dizziness. The Nijmegen questionnaire (see Table *evolve* 23.4) is invaluable in detecting those IBS patients whose symptoms are predominantly caused by anxiety. Depression may also cause gastrointestinal symptoms. Abdominal pain may arise from musculoskeletal causes or menstrual disturbances, which need to be distinguished from cases presenting with food-intolerant IBS. Under the influence of progesterone, the metabolic activity of the gut flora increases, which may lead to exacerbation of IBS symptoms premenstrually. Apart from gastrointestinal disorders, it is also important to exclude gynaecological problems such as endometriosis or ovarian cancer.

Painter & Burkitt (1971) proposed that IBS might be the result of insufficient intake of dietary fibre. They demonstrated whole gastrointestinal transit times in native Africans, who rarely suffer IBS, considerably shorter than those encountered in the British population. Fibre can be classified according to its ability to absorb water. Soluble fibre (e.g. pectin, guar, ispaghula) forms a viscous solution accessible to bacterial enzymes which rapidly ferment it with production of gases such as hydrogen and methane and other compounds such as short-chain fatty acids (SCFA). Generally little soluble fibre is recoverable from faeces. Insoluble fibre (e.g. cellulose) can bind water but does not form a solution. It is more resistant to fermentation and is thus excreted in larger amounts producing a greater laxative effect. The main sources of fibre in the diet are non-starch polysaccharides (NSP) although fibre supplements such as ispaghula, methylcellulose and sterculia are frequently used as laxatives. About 10–20g of NSP reaches the caecum daily, the rest of the fibre in the diet coming in the form of resistant starch. Most starch in the diet is digested by amylase but 1–5% is resistant, reaches the caecum and is fermented. Starch may be resistant because it is physically inaccessible in grains or seeds, because it is present in resistant granules as in raw banana and potato or following cooking. Cooking may disrupt the crystalline structure (gelatinisation). On cooling the crystals reform (retrogradation) a process which increases resistance to digestion by amylase.

However there appears to be little discernible difference in the fibre intake of healthy individuals and IBS sufferers. Furthermore in a review examining the outcome of 13 trials in which fibre was used to supplement the diet of IBS patients, only one out of six trials using bran reported an improvement in symptoms (Hammonds & Whorwell 1997). Indeed supplements of insoluble fibre, particularly wheat bran, may make IBS worse because they lead to increased fermentation and gas production. Nonfermentable fibre supplements (e.g. linseed, sterculia) are now generally reserved for cases in which IBS is associated with constipation.

Other forms of IBS may involve food intolerance. Twenty five unselected IBS patients were invited to follow an extremely restricted diet of lamb, rice and pears for 7 days. Twenty one agreed to do so and 14 reported that gastrointestinal symptoms had satisfactorily cleared. Reintroducing foods back singly and avoiding any that provoked symptom recurrence enabled the establishment of diets on which patients gained long-term symptom relief (Alun-Jones et al 1982). Double-blind placebo-controlled (DBPC) challenges were performed in 11 of the 14 and revealed increased prostaglandin E_2 release in the rectum after active challenge. Prostaglandin production correlated significantly with faecal weight.

A number of researchers have repeated this work and all have found IBS patients with objectively demonstrable food intolerance (Farah et al 1985). The incidence varied between 10% and 67% and depended on patient selection and the stringency of diets used.

The gastrointestinal tract is continuously exposed to a wide range of foreign bacteria, chemicals and foods, many of which have the capacity of acting as antigens and provoking immune responses (see Section 26.7). The gastrointestinal immune system is a major factor in the defence of the organism against these agents. Luminal antigens taken up by specialised cells in the Peyer's patches of the small intestine pass to the lymphatic system and stimulate the formulation of specific lymphocytes which migrate to reside in the intestinal mucosa. These lymphocytes are of two types, B and T. B lymphocytes in the gastrointestinal tract produce antibodies which are predominantly immunoglobulins A and M (IgA an IgM). T-helper lymphocytes may be Th1, which are primarily involved in cell-mediated protection against infection, or Th2, which may be involved in producing immunoglobulin E (IgE) – responsible for allergic responses. If the balance between Th1 and Th2 is upset, excessive IgE production may lead to the development of food allergies. Genuine IgE-mediated food allergy is relatively uncommon, probably occurring in only 1% of the population. It is now believed that non-IgE-mediated reactions to food may also be clinically important. These may be mediated by many different mechanisms, including direct pharmacological effects (e.g. caffeine, ethanol) and enzyme deficiencies (e.g. alactasia, monoamine oxidase inhibitors). These are referred to as food intolerances rather than food allergies, as no immune mechanism is involved.

No evidence of classical food allergy has been demonstrated in IBS. Serum IgE concentrations in these patients are normal. The radioallergoabsorbent (RAST) tests, which measures the amount of specific IgE antibodies in blood to various environmental and food allergens, and skin prick tests, which rely on the presence of circulating IgE antibodies are therefore of no value in identifying the foods concerned.

In contrast to classical IgE-mediated allergy, where small quantities of allergens provoke symptoms of pain, diarrhoea and vomiting within an hour, food reactions in patients with IBS are provoked by much larger quantities of food and may take several hours or days to begin. This has prompted a search for other mechanisms of food intolerance. Some foods such as coffee, tea and wine may provoke symptoms because of chemicals which they contain such as caffeine and ethanol. This is not true of the vast majority of food intolerances in IBS and it has now been suggested that abnormal colonic fermentation may underlie these reactions.

Prospective studies have shown that development of IBS is much more likely after bacterial gastroenteritis or a course of antibiotics. The relative risks are 11.9 and 3.9 respectively (Madden & Hunter 2002). These events may damage the colonic flora. It is now known that the colonic flora in IBS contains reduced numbers of *Lactobacillus* and *Bifidobacter* with overgrowth of facultative anaerobic organisms such as *Streptococcus*, *Proteus* and *E. coli*, which, although normally requiring oxygen for growth, are able to survive in the colon, where oxygen concentrations are very low. Such a gastrointestinal flora may produce abnormal fermentation of food residues entering the caecum.

A study of fermentation was performed in previously untreated IBS patients and normal controls who were asked to follow a standard British diet for 2 weeks. At the end of that time they were spent 24 hours in a purpose built calorimeter. Hydrogen and methane, both products of bacterial fermentation, were measured in air drawn from the calorimeter and compared to that of the surrounding room. Hydrogen production and the maximum rate of gas production were significantly increased in IBS patients compared to controls. The subjects were then invited to follow a standard exclusion diet which was carefully matched to contain the same amounts of substrates for fermentation as the standard diet and after 2 weeks calorimetry was repeated. Whilst there was no significant change in gas production in controls, hydrogen and maximum gas excretion fell dramatically in the patients with symptomatic improvement (King et al 1998; Fig. 23.5). Subsequent studies have confirmed increased colonic gas production and when this was reduced by antibiotics or after an enteral feed, symptomatic improvement again followed.

TREATMENT – NUTRITION

There is no evidence to suggest that nutritional deficiencies occur as a result of untreated IBS. However, nutrient deficiencies may develop secondary to individuals excluding specific foods or food groups from their diet. Reviews of dietary intakes have identified calcium and vitamin D as commonly occurring deficiencies and this is often secondary to individuals avoiding dairy products. In the case of IBS a thorough investigation of the diet is essential to establish if the individual may be at risk of developing a deficiency state. This review will be limited to the value of diet and nutritional supplementation in the management of IBS.

Manipulation of fibre in the diet may provide significant relief to individuals with IBS. The use of a high-fibre diet in IBS is limited to treatment of simple constipation. Fibre is an important substrate for fermentation. Reducing the fibre content of the diet to less than 10 g per day may reduce gas production and symptoms in patients who present with diarrhoea, bloating urgency and pain (Woolner & Kirby 2000). In many cases the patient may experience constipation or an alternating bowel habit instead of diarrhoea. The low-fibre diet supplemented by a synthetic, non-fermentable fibre provides a diet that can increase stool bulk without the side effects of excess fermentation often experienced with a high-fibre diet.

A specific exclusion diet has been developed for the treatment of food intolerant IBS (Table 23.1) (Parker et al 1995). Before any therapeutic dietary manipulation is undertaken, a thorough review of eating habits is essential to detect and correct any abnormal eating patterns or food aversions. The core exclusion diet is followed for a period of 2 weeks, after which patients whose symptoms significantly improve may reintroduce a food every 2

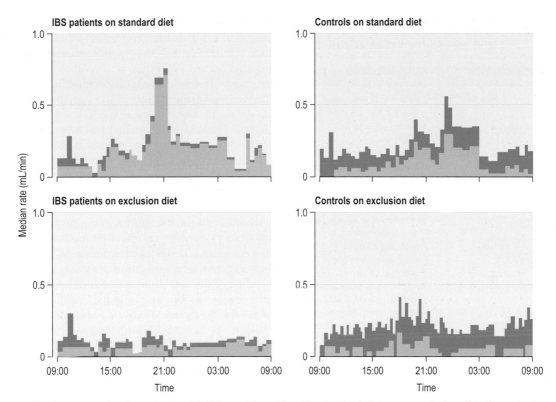

Fig. 23.5 Total gas excretion in patients with IBS receiving either the standard diet or an exclusion diet. Area charts showing median rate of total excretion (hydrogen: filled; methane: unfilled; ml/min (standard temperature and pressure)) at 30 min intervals during 24-h measurement on standard and exclusion diets. Excretion was maximal in late evening, diminished during sleep and increased again on waking (King et al 1998).

days with the exception of wheat, which should be tested over 7 days as its effects may come on slowly and insidiously. Foods that have not triggered symptoms may be reintroduced into the diet. Exclusion diet studies at Addenbrooke's Hospital, Cambridge, UK, have shown that approximately 50% of compliant patients respond successfully to the exclusion diet. However, although the exclusion diet may be an extremely successful intervention it is not without problems. Patients may experience symptoms of headache, nausea and fatigue 2–4 days after commencing the diet. Lifestyle implications may mean it is not a realistic treatment option for some.

In veterinary medicine, it is known that fermentation of simple sugars, whether in the rumen or in the colon, may lead to disease. There is however no evidence as yet to suggest that malfermentation in IBS is due to increased malabsorption of such sugars in the small intestine. Nevertheless, in humans, the handling of monosaccharides such as fructose and disaccharides such as lactose can cause difficulties.

Approximately 25% of Europeans with symptoms of IBS test positive for lactose intolerance. In a recent study fewer than 40% of patients with IBS who had a positive hydrogen breath test for lactose intolerance responded to a low-lactose diet. Of those who failed to respond several went on to trial an exclusion diet, identifying milk as the cause of symptoms. It has therefore been suggested that there is little value in treating IBS patients for hypolactasia as many appear to be upset by constituents of cow's milk other than lactose (Parker et al 2001). It follows that the management of IBS patients with hypolactasia should not differ from that of other food-intolerant patients with IBS.

Fructose is a monosaccharide sugar found in three forms in the diet: as free fructose (present in fruit and honey); as a constituent of the disaccharide sucrose; or as fructans, a polymer of fructose usually in oligosaccharide form (present in some vegetables and wheat). Polyols are sugar alcohols commonly added to foods as a sweetening ingredient. Reducing dietary fructose in its various forms and polyols may help reduce IBS symptoms.

Table 23.1   Addenbrooke's Hospital exclusion diet for IBS (Parker et al 1995)

FOODS NOT ALLOWED	FOODS ALLOWED
Pork and meat products	All other lean meat and poultry
Fish in batter/crumb, fish tinned in oil/tomato	All other types of fish, shellfish
Cow's, sheep's and goat's milk, dairy products, eggs and chocolate	Soya milk and products; soya margarine in moderation
Wheat, rye, barley, corn, oats, yeast	Rice, rice cakes, Rice Krispies, tapioca, sago, arrowroot
Corn oil, vegetable oil	Sunflower, olive oil, etc.; oils in moderation
Pulses, onion, tomato, sweetcorn	Potato and all other vegetables, two portions per day, no skins or seeds
Citrus, apple, banana, dried fruit	All other fruit, two portions per day, no skins or seeds
Tea, coffee, alcohol, squash, cola, etc.	Fruit and herbal teas, tap and mineral water, blackcurrant squash, non-citrus fruit juice
Gravy mixes, salad dressings, etc.	Salt, pepper, herbs and spices
Nuts, seeds	Sugar, jam, honey, mint cake (glucose)

Fructose malabsorption is reported in more than one in three IBS patients (Shepherd 2006). Studies in which fructose loads have been given to patients with fructose malabsorption induce bloating, pain, nausea and discomfort more readily in patients with IBS than those without. One study has demonstrated an improvement in all types of IBS symptoms in 74% of IBS patients found to have fructose malabsorption, following a diet low in fructose and polyols (Shepherd and Gibson 2006). In a follow-up double-blind randomised quadruple-arm placebo-controlled re-challenge trial, patients who responded to a low-fructose and polyols diet were challenged blindly with graded dose introduction of fructose, fructans and glucose (placebo) (Shepherd et al 2008). Significantly more patients reported inadequate symptom control and more severe symptoms when given fructose or fructans compared to glucose (placebo), demonstrating that dietary restriction of fructose was likely to be responsible for the symptom improvement on a low-fructose diet. The effectiveness of a low-fructose diet in the wider IBS population, i.e. without fructose malabsorption, is not known. Furthermore, fructose malabsorption is also common in healthy populations so testing for this in IBS patients may have limited value. Whether a low-fibre diet, a low-fructans diet or an exclusion diet is the best to correct malfermentation in IBS remains uncertain.

As diets are always restrictive and difficult to follow, considerable interest has arisen in the possibility of improving symptoms in IBS by manipulating the gastrointestinal tract directly. Probiotics are living microorganisms which, when consumed, exert health benefits beyond basic inherent nutrition. It has been suggested that restoring the 'normal' colonic microflora using probiotic supplementation may be an effective method of treating the condition. Unfortunately, because of a phenomenon known as colonisation resistance, it is not easy to change the intestinal microflora and most probiotic bacteria, like pathogens, disappear rapidly from the gastrointestinal tract when their administration ceases. Although some patients have reported benefit, there is no conclusive evidence that any bacterial preparation is consistently effective, and further research is needed to clarify the role of probiotics in the treatment of IBS. Thus the symptomatic benefit derived from a 4-week course of *Bifidobacterium infantis* 35624 in women with IBS was in the order of 20% (Whorwell et al 2006), whereas a 50% improvement is generally considered necessary for dietary treatment of IBS to be considered successful. The difficulties with colonisation resistance might in theory be overcome by promoting the growth of lactic acid bacteria by the administration of prebiotics such as inulin or oligofructose, which are known to promote the growth of bifidobacteria. However, it remains unclear whether or not prebiotics will also promote the growth of the facultative anaerobes that characterise IBS.

KEY POINTS

- Chronic disorders of the intestine are associated with complex interactions between diet, the intestinal microflora and intestinal mucosal immunity
- Diet may be of significant value in modifying intestinal damage and the clinical course of these diseases
- Manipulation of the gastrointestinal flora may provide a future means of treating these disorders.

References

Alun-Jones V, Mclaughlin P, Shorthouse M, et al: Food intolerance: a major factor in the pathogenesis of irritable bowel syndrome, *Lancet* 2:1115–1117, 1982.

Bingley PJ, Williamas AJK, Norcross A, et al: Undiagnosed coeliac disease at age seven: population-based prospective birth cohort study, *British Medical Journal* 328:322–323, 2004.

Brauer M, Al-Momen AK, Faller DV: Butyrate treatment in beta-hemoglobinopathies, *New England Journal of Medicine* 333(19):1287–1288, 1995.

Dear KL, Compston JE, Hunter JO: Treatments for Crohn's disease that minimise steroid doses are associated with a reduced risk of osteoporosis, *Clin Nutr* 20(6):541–546, 2001.

Farah DA, Calder I, Benson L, et al. Specific food intolerance: its place as a cause of gastrointestinal symptoms, *Gut* 26:164–168, 1985.

Galvez J, Rodríguez-Cabezas ME, Zarzuelo A: Effects of dietary fiber on inflammatory bowel disease, *Molecular Nutrition and Food Research* 19(6):601–608, 2005.

Hammonds R, Whorwell P: The role of fibre in IBS, *International Journal of Gastroenterology* 2:9–12, 1997.

King TS, Woolner JT, Hunter JO: Dietary treatment of active Crohn's disease. Diet is the best treatment, *British Medical Journal* 314(7097):1827–1828, 1997.

King TS, Elia M, Hunter JO: Abnormal colonic fermentation in irritable bowel syndrome, *Lancet* 352:1187–1189, 1998.

Loftus E: The epidemiology and natural history of Crohn's disease in a population-based patient cohort from North America: a systematic review, *Alimentary Pharmacology and Therapeutics* 16:51–60, 2002.

Madden JAJ, Hunter JO: A review of the role of the gut microflora in IBS and the effects of probiotics, *British Journal of Nutrition* 88(Suppl 1):S67–S72, 2002.

Middleton SJ, Rucker JT, Kirby GA, et al: Long-chain triglycerides reduce the efficacy of enteral feeds in patients with active Crohn's disease, *Clinical Nutrition* 14(4):229–236, 1995.

Muller-Lissner, SA, Bollani S, Brummer RJ, et al: Epidemiological aspects of irritable bowel syndrome in Europe and North America, *Digestion* 64(3):200–2004, 2001.

O'Morain C, Segal AH, Levi AJ: Elemental diet as a primary treatment of acute Crohn's disease: a controlled trial, *British Medical Journal* 288:1859–1862, 1984.

Painter NS, Burkitt DP: Diverticular disease of the colon: a deficiency disease of western civilisation, *British Medical Journal* 2:450–454, 1971.

Parker TJ, Naylor SJ, Riordan AM, et al: Management of patients with food intolerance in irritable bowel syndrome: the development and use of an exclusion diet, *Journal of Human Nutrition and Dietetics* 8:159–166, 1995.

Parker TJ, Woolner JT, Prevost, AT, et al: Irritable bowel syndrome: is the search for lactose intolerance justified? *European Journal of Gastroenterology and Hepatology* 13(3):219–225, 2001.

Riordan AM, Hunter JO, Cowan RE, et al: Treatment of active Crohn's disease by exclusion diet: East Anglian multi centre controlled trial, *Lancet* 342(8880):1131–1134, 1993.

Riordan AM, Ruxton CHS, Hunter JO: A review of associations between Crohn's disease and consumption of sugars, *European Journal of Clinical Nutrition* 52:229–238, 1998.

Rutgeerts P, Goboes K, Peeters M, et al: Effect of faecal stream diversion on recurrence of Crohn's disease in the neoterminal ileum, *Lancet* 338(8770):771–774, 1991.

Shepherd SJ, Gibson PR: Fructose malabsorption and symptoms of irritable bowel syndrome: Guidelines for effective dietary management, *JAMA* 106:1631–1639, 2006.

Shepherd SJ, Parker FC, Muir JG, Gibson PR: Dietary Triggers of Abdominal Symptoms in Patients with Irritable Bowel Syndrome: Randomized Placebo-Controlled Evidence, *Clinical Gastroenterology and Hepatology* 6:765 771, 2008.

Shiviananda S, Lennard-Jones J, Logan R, et al: Incidence of inflammatory bowel disease across Europe: is there a difference between north and south? Results of the European collaborative study on inflammatory bowel disease (EC-IBD), *Gut* 39(5):690–697, 1996.

Shoda R, Matsueda K, Yamamoto S, et al: Epidemiological analysis of Crohn's disease in Japan: increased dietary intake of n-6 polyunsaturated fatty acids and animal protein relates to the increase incidence of Crohn's disease in Japan, *American Journal of Clinical Nutrition* 63(5):741–745, 1996.

Trocone R, Greco L, Auricchio S: The controversial epidemiology of coeliac disease, *Acta Paediatrica* 89(2):140–141, 2002.

Van der Waaij LA, Kroese FG, Visser A, et al: Immunoglobulin coating of faecal bacteria in inflammatory bowel disease, *European Journal of Gastroenterology and Hepatology* 16(7):669–674, 2004.

Whorwell PJ, Altringer L, Morel J, et al: Efficacy of an encapsulated probiotic Bifidobacterium infantis 35624 in women with irritable bowel syndrome, *Am J Gastroenterol* 101(7):1581–1590, 2007.

Woolner JT, Kirby GA: Clinical audit of the effects of low-fibre diet on irritable bowel syndrome, *Journal of Human Nutrition and Dietetics* 13:249–253, 2000.

Woolner JT, Parker TJ, Kirby GA, et al: The development and evaluation of a diet for maintaining remission in Crohn's disease, *Journal of Human Nutrition and Dietetics* 11:1–11, 1998.

Wright R, Truelove SC: A Controlled therapeutic trial of various diets in ulcerative colitis, *British Medical Journal* 2(5454):138–141, 1965.

Further reading

Brostoff J, Challacombe S: *Food allergy and intolerance*, 2nd edn, London, 2002, Saunders.

Camilleri M, Spiller R: *Irritable bowel syndrome diagnosis and treatment*, Edinburgh, 2002, WB Saunders.

Feldman M, Scharschmidt B, Sleisenger M: *Sleisenger & Fordtran's Gastrointestinal and liver disease: pathophysiology/diagnosis/management*, 6th edn, London, 1998, WB Saunders.

Forbes A: *Inflammatory bowel disease, a clinician's guide*, London, 2001, Arnold.

Gibson P: *Baillière's clinical gastroenterology, ulcerative colitis*, Vol 11, No 1, London, 1997, Baillière Tindall.

Howdle P: *Baillière's clinical gastroenterology, coeliac disease*, Vol 9, No 2, London, 1995, Baillière Tindall.

Hunter JO: *Irritable bowel solutions*, London, 2007, Vermillion.

Roy H: Making Gluten easier to stomach, *American Journal of Gastroenterology* 98:249, 2003.

Thomas B: *Manual of dietetic practice*, 3rd edn, Oxford, 2001, Blackwell Science.

Chapter 24

Nutrition and the skeleton

Margo E Barker and Aubrey Blumsohn

CHAPTER CONTENTS

© 2010 Elsevier Ltd/Inc/BV
DOI: 10.1016/B978-0-7020-3118-2.00024-3

OBJECTIVES

By the end of this chapter you should:
- understand the dynamic nature of skeletal metabolism
- be able to define osteomalacia, rickets and osteoporosis
- be able to discuss the role of vitamin D and calcium nutrition in skeletal health
- appreciate the role of other nutrients in skeletal health.

24.1 INTRODUCTION

Osteoporosis and osteomalacia or rickets are the two main skeletal disorders that can be related to nutrient supply. Of these osteoporosis has the greatest public health importance in contemporary society. This chapter examines the evidence for the importance of nutritional factors in the pathogenesis of these disorders. Dietary deficiencies of calcium and vitamin D deficiency have been implicated as causative in the development of osteoporosis, but recent research has implicated lack of or excess of many other nutrients and food components. Deficiency of vitamin D is the most frequent cause of osteomalacia (adults) and rickets (children).

Although the primary role of the skeleton is to provide mechanical support and protection for internal organs, bone also serves several other functions. The skeleton is involved in the homeostatic regulation of several minerals, plays a role in acid–base homeostasis and serves as an important defence against some toxins such as lead, which can be adsorbed to bone. Bone marrow is involved in haematopoiesis (production of blood cells).

The chapter begins with a review of bone structure and skeletal remodelling and how bone mineral mass changes throughout the life-course. Some appreciation of bone physiology is necessary to understand how diet may impact on skeletal health. An awareness of the strengths and weaknesses of different designs of nutritional studies, and the value of different end-points as indices of skeletal health, is also important in evaluating the role of diet in influencing skeletal health.

24.2 BONE STRUCTURE AND REMODELLING

BONE COMPOSITION AND CELLS

The human adult skeleton weighs approximately 3–4 kg and consists of an organic matrix, minerals and bone cells. By weight, bone comprises about 10% water, 60% inorganic material, and 30% organic matrix. The organic matrix consists largely (95%) of a single protein, type I collagen. Other organic components include non-collagenous proteins, lipids and proteoglycans. The mineral phase of bone consists chiefly of calcium, phosphate and carbonate in a crystalline form called hydroxyapatite. Bone also serves as a reservoir for other minerals (Table 24.1). Deficiency or excess of these components in bone may contribute to loss of bone strength and to fractures. The two main types of bone cells, osteoclasts and osteoblasts, have opposite functions. Osteoclasts are multinucleated cells responsible for bone resorption. These cells attach to the mineralised bone surface and secrete protons and enzymes. Osteoblasts produce bone matrix and are responsible for bone formation. Other cells called osteocytes are found embedded within the bone and may function to regulate changes in bone structure in response to mechanical loading.

TYPES OF BONE

The skeleton is composed of two types of bone:

1. Cortical bone (sometimes called compact bone). This dense form of bone comprises about 80% of skeletal mass.

Table 24.1	Some important minerals in bone	
ELEMENT	TOTAL BONE CONTENT (g)	% BONE WEIGHT
Calcium	1000	25
Phosphate	400	10
Sodium	200	5
Magnesium	80	2
Zinc	8	0.2
Potassium	4	0.1
Strontium	0.8	0.02
Boron	1.6	0.04
Aluminium	0.8	0.02
Lead	0.4	0.01
Copper	0.08	0.002

2. Trabecular bone (also called spongy or cancellous bone). This type of bone consists of an intricate structural mesh of trabeculae that form the interior scaffolding of bone. The spaces between the trabeculae and the centres of the bones (marrow cavities) contain red and yellow marrow and other tissue. Red marrow is responsible for the formation of blood cells (haematopoiesis).

Although trabecular bone accounts for only 20% of total bone mass, it accounts for as much as 70% of bone surface area and metabolic activity. Trabecular bone constitutes most of the bone tissue of the axial skeleton (skull, ribs and spine). The ends of long bones also contain a variable proportion of trabecular bone. Regions of the skeleton which contain a high proportion of trabecular bone such as the hip, spine and wrist are most susceptible to fracture in patients with osteoporosis.

BONE REMODELLING

Bone is a metabolically active tissue. In the adult skeleton most metabolic activity occurs by the process of bone 'remodelling' or bone turnover. This metabolic activity serves to maintain the structure and homeostatic functions of the skeleton. Although the total amount of bone tissue in an adult is relatively static, there is a continuous turnover of bone mineral and organic matrix. About 5–10% of existing bone is replaced through remodelling each year. Remodelling involves a defined sequence of events (Fig. 24.1). The process of bone formation occurs at sites at which bone resorption has recently occurred. This integration between bone formation and bone resorption is termed 'coupling'.

In the long term, a change in bone mineral content reflects an imbalance between the processes of bone formation and resorption. Incomplete refilling of resorption cavities will result in a net loss of bone, and overfilling of these cavities will result in a net gain of bone. In the short term (<1 year) changes in bone mass can arise simply from a change in the rate of remodelling and hence the amount of 'remodelling space' (space taken up by remodelling cycles currently in progress). Therefore, short-term changes in bone mass do not necessarily reflect an imbalance between the fundamental rates of bone formation and resorption. Bone growth and change in bone shape in children occurs by a different mechanism called 'modelling'. In

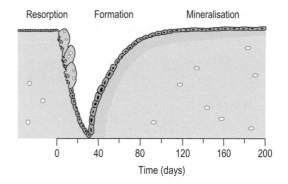

Fig. 24.1 Schematic view of bone remodelling. Activated osteoclasts attach themselves to the bone surfaces, and tunnel into the bone. Osteoblasts are attracted to the new cavities and secrete collagen strands (fibrils), which combine to form unmineralised matrix called osteoid. This osteoid is subsequently mineralised.

contrast to remodelling, the processes of bone formation and resorption are dissociated in time and space, so that a change in shape or size of the bone can occur.

A variety of so-called 'calciotropic hormones' regulate the process of bone formation and resorption. These include parathyroid hormone (PTH), vitamin D and its metabolites, sex steroids, glucocorticoids, growth hormone, insulin-like growth factors and many more. PTH stimulates bone resorption, but can also stimulate bone formation (anabolic action). Vitamin D metabolites affect bone metabolism directly and indirectly by influencing mineral supply. Sex steroids (oestradiol and testosterone) decrease bone remodelling. The effect of testosterone in men is mediated mainly by peripheral conversion to the female sex steroid, oestradiol. Growth hormone, insulin-like growth factor 1 (IGF-1) and thyroid hormones increase bone remodelling. The predominant effect of glucocorticoids is to inhibit bone formation.

BONE MINERAL CONTENT DURING GROWTH, AGEING, PREGNANCY AND LACTATION

By 10 weeks of gestation the human fetal skeleton is composed mainly of unmineralised cartilage. Mineralisation of the fetal skeleton occurs mainly during the last 10 weeks of pregnancy, and by late pregnancy calcium accrual by the fetus is more than

100 mg/day. Rapid accumulation of mineral in the skeleton continues after birth, and this is accompanied by change in the size and shape of bones during growth. Skeletal mass increases from about 100 g in the neonate to about 3000 g in an adult (peak bone mass). Peak bone mass is achieved at about age 35. The rate of change in bone mass increases during puberty, and more than 90% of peak bone mass is achieved by age 18. Bone mineral content declines in the elderly, and is particularly rapid in women after the menopause. It is important that adequate amounts of bone mineral are acquired during growth because that contributes to bone mineral content later in life. Because much of peak bone mass is attained by age 20, children and adolescents are a particularly important target for interventions to increase bone mass.

With ageing, individuals tend to maintain their ranking within the population distribution of bone mineral content. In other words peak bone mass is the most important predictor of bone mineral content in later life. Although some individuals do lose bone faster than others, these differences are less important, although rapid bone loss may be important in some people. After attainment of peak bone mass, there is a gradual loss of bone mineral in both men and women. Bone remodelling increases after the menopause in women and this is associated with accelerated loss of bone mineral. This is caused in large part by a reduced ovarian production of oestradiol. Oestrogen production is also an important determinant of bone mineral loss in older postmenopausal women as well as in men.

Genetic and lifestyle factors influence bone mineral accrual during growth. Lifestyle factors influencing peak bone mass include exercise, calcium intake, general nutritional status, smoking and use of medications such as corticosteroids and some contraceptives. Many studies comparing bone mineral content in members of the same family or in twins have shown that up to 75% of the difference in peak bone mass between individuals might be explained by genetic factors. In general, peak bone mass is greater in Blacks than in Whites. Although interventions such as exercise and calcium supplementation may increase bone mineral accrual during puberty, it is not clear whether these interventions will result in greater bone mineral content in adult life. Genetic factors are likely to be relatively less important as determinants of bone loss with ageing.

Pregnancy and lactation increase calcium requirements, and these demands are met by a combination of increased efficiency of maternal calcium absorption from the diet as well as maternal bone mineral loss. The amount of calcium required by the fetus is relatively small, approximately 30 g, in comparison with the much greater calcium demand imposed by lactation, up to 1 g of calcium per day for milk production. This additional calcium requirement for milk production is largely obtained as a result of skeletal mineral loss. Lumbar spine bone mineral content decreases by about 4% during pregnancy, and decreases progressively during lactation. Despite the substantial short-term impact of pregnancy and lactation on the skeleton, these physiological changes do not appear to have any long-lasting effect on bone mineral content or on later fracture risk.

BONE REMODELLING AND DISEASE

A wide variety of genetic and acquired diseases such as collagen disorders, cancer and infections can influence the skeleton directly. Other diseases may affect the skeleton by altering the normal regulation of bone remodelling. For example, endocrine disorders may involve excessive or defective secretion of a calciotropic hormone resulting in loss of bone mineral. The two most common diseases affecting the skeleton are (a) osteoporosis and (b) osteomalacia or rickets due to vitamin D deficiency. Nutrient supply plays a role in the pathogenesis of these disorders.

Disorders that influence intake or gastrointestinal absorption of nutrients, such as anorexia nervosa, coeliac disease and inflammatory bowel disease, may also cause skeletal disease. Low bone mineral content is common in patients with newly diagnosed coeliac disease, and bone mass improves in most patients when started on a gluten-free diet. Although these diseases influence nutritional status, the loss of bone mineral in these disorders is due to many factors in addition to deficient nutrient supply. These factors include drug therapy, immobility, endocrine disturbances and the response to inflammation. In anorexia nervosa, bone mineral loss is due not only to deficient supply of substrates required for bone function, but also to excess cortisol secretion and deficient production of oestradiol.

24.3 TYPES OF EVIDENCE LINKING DIET TO SKELETAL HEALTH

STUDY DESIGN

Individual case reports

There are many reports of individual patients or groups of patients who have developed skeletal disease due to markedly excessive or deficient intake of a particular nutrient. For example, individuals with vitamin A toxicity develop hypercalcaemia (elevated concentration of calcium in plasma) and skeletal disease. However, it is usually not possible to conclude from these studies that the nutrient is either harmful or beneficial to the skeleton within the general population. These case reports are, however, of considerable scientific interest and may help to guide further research into the role of the nutrient.

Cross-sectional studies of fracture risk

It is possible to relate the intake of a particular nutrient to fracture risk within the general population. It is also possible to relate a biomarker of nutrient exposure to fracture risk. For example, it has been found that consumption of carbonated beverages is associated with a substantially increased risk of fracture in adolescent girls. There are a number of pitfalls associated with cross-sectional observational studies. Intake of different nutrients may be strongly related to one another, and it may be difficult to be certain that any particular nutrient is important. It is also likely that nutrient intake is strongly related to other lifestyle and social factors such as smoking, exercise and social class. It is also possible that fracture risk could be associated with past intake of the nutrient rather than current intake.

Effect of dietary intervention on fracture incidence

Experimental studies relating a change in intake of a nutrient to fracture incidence provide very strong evidence that the nutrient is of relevance to skeletal health. Ideally such studies require appropriate placebo controls with randomisation to nutrient or placebo. However, placebo-controlled designs may be difficult for food interventions as well as some nutrients, and participants may not be blind to the treatment allocation. The nutrient dose is also important. If the magnitude of supplementation is greater than could be achieved by alterations in diet, then the study is pharmacological rather than nutritional.

Unfortunately, because fractures are infrequent, it is necessary to study a large number of people for a long period of time in order to demonstrate an effect where one exists. For example, to demonstrate a 50% reduction in the rate of fracture it may be necessary to study several thousand individuals for several years. Since the effect of individual nutrients may be small, randomised fracture intervention trials are not feasible for most nutrients. When trials are carried out, the results cannot be assumed to apply to individuals who are very different from those studied. For example, nutritional interventions shown to be beneficial in elderly institutionalised women may not be beneficial in younger women or in men.

SURROGATE INDICATORS OF FRACTURE RISK

Nutrient intervention trials with a fracture as an end-point are very difficult and expensive to carry out. In the case of most nutrients, such trials would be impossible. Therefore, much attention has been paid to the use of other 'surrogate' end-points, which might be presumed to relate to fracture risk. However the relationship between these surrogates and long-term fracture risk is not necessarily straightforward. These surrogates include bone mineral content, structural analysis of bone using imaging techniques, and biochemical assessment of bone turnover.

Nutrient intake may in part influence fracture risk through mechanisms that are not reflected by these skeletal surrogates. For example, nutrition might influence balance, the risk and severity of falling, muscle bulk and fat mass.

Bone densitometry

Bone mineral content (BMC) or bone mineral density (BMD) can be assessed by measuring the attenuation of X-rays by a skeletal region of interest. By using two different energies of X-ray beam it is possible to distinguish between X-ray attenuation due to fat, lean tissue or bone (dual energy X-ray absorptiometry, DEXA). The precision of DEXA (reproducibility typically about 2%) is poor in comparison with the rate of change in bone mineral content in response to nutrient intervention. It is therefore necessary to study the response to intervention for at least one year, but preferably for several years in many individuals.

Bone mineral density measured by DEXA is strongly related to fracture risk. However, bone densitometry cannot serve as a sole surrogate for fracture risk in studies of nutrition. Change in body weight can cause spurious underestimation or overestimation of BMD depending on the instrument used. This may confound nutritional studies. Other pitfalls have been brought to light by examination of change in BMD with drugs, such as bisphosphonates, which are designed to prevent fracture. In these studies, change in BMD does not appear to explain all of the reduction in fracture risk. Some of the reduction in risk might be explained by other factors such as a change in the rate of turnover of bone.

Other techniques for assessing bone structure

Several enhanced radiographic techniques may add to information provided by traditional densitometry. These include ultrasound assessment, generally at the heel, radiographic 'texture' analysis of bone or quantitative tomography. It is even possible to assess fracture risk using detailed mathematical analysis of three-dimensional computer reconstruction of whole bones from individual patients.

Measurement of bone remodelling

The rate of bone formation and resorption can be assessed using several techniques including histology (microscopic examination of removed bone), radiotracer kinetics and measurement of biochemical markers in blood or urine. Most of these biochemical markers reflect the synthesis or degradation of bone collagen. Differences in the rate of bone remodelling between individuals might be related to fracture risk, although these relationships are very weak. The change in bone remodelling with some drugs used to treat osteoporosis can be helpful to predict the reduction in fracture risk with treatment. Some drugs reduce fracture risk by reducing bone turnover (antiresorptive drugs) whilst others reduce fracture by increasing bone

turnover (anabolic drugs). Long-term reduction in bone turnover with some drugs might increase the risk of some fractures. The relationship between these measurements and fracture risk is therefore complicated, and the same principles that apply to prescription drugs may not apply to nutritional interventions, or to other populations, such as children. However, in adults, lower bone turnover is generally associated with lower fracture risk.

24.4 OSTEOPOROSIS, OSTEOMALACIA AND RICKETS

THE EPIDEMIOLOGY OF SKELETAL FRACTURE

Fractures are most common in children and in the very elderly. Fractures in children involve mainly long bones, tend to be more common in males than in females, and are only weakly associated with bone mineral content. By contrast, osteoporotic fractures in the elderly most commonly occur in bones which have a high proportion of trabecular bone (the wrist, hip and spine), are more common in women, and are strongly associated with low bone mineral content. The healthcare costs and morbidity associated with these fractures is substantial. The rate of osteoporotic fracture increases with age. About 30% of women and about 10% of men will experience an osteoporotic fracture at some point in their lifetimes.

The lifetime risk of hip fracture in North America and Europe is approximately 15%. The incidence of hip fracture differs substantially between countries for reasons that are not fully explained. X-ray screening studies of populations in these countries have shown that about 15% of women between the age of 50 and 80 have one or more vertebral (spine) fractures. Many vertebral fractures are not associated with back pain or other symptoms. In general, fracture rates are higher in northern European countries than in southern European countries. These differences may reflect differences in race and ethnicity, habits such as smoking, nutrition, body weight, exercise, and risk of falling.

The incidence of osteoporotic fractures is also increasing with time, due in part to increased life expectancy. However, the risk of fracture also appears to be increasing for reasons unrelated to increased lifespan. The most important reason for this is likely to be reduced physical activity, which could influence both bone mineral content and the risk of falling. It has been estimated that the number of hip fractures will increase approximately three-fold in European countries over the next 50 years.

OSTEOPOROSIS

Osteoporosis used to be thought of as a rare disease. It has been defined as a condition characterised by low bone mass and 'microarchitectural' deterioration of bone, resulting in an increased risk of fracture. Included in this definition is the concept that bone mineral content is not the only skeletal factor resulting in increased fracture risk. Changes in the internal 'microarchitecture' of bone (such as the way in which trabeculae in cancellous bone are connected) can also influence fracture risk without influencing bone mineral content.

Although many factors influence fracture risk, bone mineral density (BMD) is a predictor of fracture. Fracture risk in adults is approximately doubled for each standard deviation reduction in BMD at a variety of measurement sites (spine, hip and wrist). What this means is that fracture risk in individuals with BMD in the lowest 20% of the population is at least five times higher than that of other individuals of the same age and sex in the highest 20%.

The World Health Organization (WHO) has emphasised the role of BMD measurement in the definition and diagnosis of osteoporosis. The WHO define an individual as having osteoporosis at a BMD value 2.5 standard deviations below the young adult mean and osteopenia when BMD is between 1 and 2.5 standard deviations below.

Because BMD is not a perfect indicator of fracture risk, many osteoporotic fractures occur in individuals who do not fulfil these criteria for a diagnosis of osteoporosis. At least 30% of post-menopausal women in Western countries are defined as having osteoporosis according to WHO criteria. Some suggest that pressure from the pharmaceutical industry has led to an unhelpful definition of osteoporosis, as well as the overuse of drug treatments in patients where treatment benefit does not clearly outweigh risk.

Differences in skeletal geometry (length and width of bones) as well as non-skeletal factors, such as frequent falling, poor muscle strength, low body mass and poor vision, also influence fracture risk. Many of these risk factors may be influenced by nutritional status. Previous osteoporotic fractures greatly increase the chance of subsequent fractures irrespective of BMD. It is possible to estimate fracture risk given information about these clinical risk factors, BMD and age.

Risk factors for osteoporosis can be divided into those resulting in low peak bone mass, and those resulting in an increased rate of bone loss. Genetic factors are likely to play an important role in determining peak bone mass, but non-genetic factors during childhood are also likely to be important. These non-genetic factors include intake of calcium and other nutrients, exercise and delayed puberty. Risk factors for age-related bone loss include early menopause in women, low body mass, a low residual concentration of serum oestradiol after the menopause, poor nutritional status and lack of exercise. A variety of other diseases can result in loss of bone mineral, and it is important to exclude these secondary causes of osteoporosis in patients.

The aim of treatment in osteoporosis is to reduce the risk of fracture. This can be achieved by increasing BMD, by reducing bone remodelling and by decreasing the risk of falls. Lifestyle measures include avoidance of smoking, increasing dietary intake of calcium, ensuring adequate vitamin D status, and exercise. A variety of drugs such as bisphosphonates, oestrogens, selective oestrogen receptor modulators and intermittent parathyroid hormone have been shown to reduce fracture risk in some patients.

OSTEOMALACIA

Osteomalacia is a skeletal disorder resulting from defective mineralisation of bone matrix (osteoid). This results in accumulation of unmineralised osteoid. The commonest cause of osteomalacia is vitamin D deficiency. However, osteomalacia does have a number of other causes such as disorders of phosphate metabolism, genetic defects and excessive intake of nutrients such as fluoride.

RICKETS

Historically vitamin D deficiency was predominantly a disease of childhood. Where osteomalacia occurs in children prior to skeletal maturity, this results in deformities and the clinical features of rickets. Rickets is osteomalacia that occurs when bones are still growing. Rickets has been an important cause of childhood illness and deformity for many centuries. Following the industrial revolution, the combination of urbanisation, pollution and poor diet resulted in increased prevalence of the disease in the UK. Rickets continues to be an important disease in the developing world, and is still seen in developed countries, particularly in non-Whites.

Whistler described the clinical features of rickets in 1645. Children with rickets classically present with knock-knees or bowed legs, muscle weakness and short stature. In breastfed infants, rickets can develop within the first few months of birth, particularly when the mothers of these infants have vitamin D deficiency. These infants may have craniotabes (soft areas of the skull causing a 'ping-pong' ball sensation on pressure), thickening of the wrists and ankles, and enlargement of the costo-chondral junctions (rachitic rosary). Fractures and other deformities can occur. Children with rickets also have poor muscle development and tone. The skeleton is poorly mineralised, and the growth plates are widened (cupped) and irregular on X-ray. As in adult osteomalacia, there is an excess of unmineralised osteoid. The concentration of alkaline phosphatase is elevated in the blood of children with rickets, and the concentration of phosphate may be lower than expected. The concentration of calcium in the blood is generally maintained within the normal range. Infants with rickets may develop respiratory infections, and are more likely to have tuberculosis. Many of the clinical features of rickets resolve within a short period after administration of adequate amounts of vitamin D. Rickets may result in pelvic deformities that can lead to difficulties during labour and increased perinatal morbidity in subsequent generations (see Figs *evolve* 28.19, 28.20).

The importance of sunshine and diet in the aetiology of rickets was not defined until the early part of the twentieth century. It was discovered that a fat-soluble nutrient or sunshine exposure could cure the condition. An unfortified infant diet contains a very small amount of vitamin D, although there are small amounts in milk and egg yolk. A vegetarian diet or a high intake of phytate also predispose to the development of rickets.

Although rickets is commonly due to vitamin D deficiency, this is not the only cause. Since sunshine is plentiful in tropical countries, other factors are likely to explain the high prevalence of rickets in some of these countries. Increased skin pigmentation or traditional dress may account for some cases of vitamin D deficiency in sunny countries.

However, studies in South Africa and Nigeria have suggested that calcium deficiency alone may cause rickets. Genetic or acquired disorders of phosphate metabolism or vitamin D metabolism, and deficiency of the enzyme alkaline phosphatase can also cause osteomalacia and rickets.

24.5 CALCIUM AND VITAMIN D

EVOLUTIONARY PERSPECTIVES

Although the genetic constitution of modern humans has changed little over the past 10 000 years, environmental and nutritional influences on the skeleton have altered markedly over that time. It has been argued that human skeletal metabolism has adapted to conditions which are very different from those encountered by most modern humans. Cultivated plant foods such as cereal grains have far less calcium than do other vegetable food sources. Dietary calcium intake was probably twice as great in pre-agricultural humans, and this was largely of vegetable origin rather than of dairy origin. In most modern humans in Western industrialised countries about half of dietary calcium is derived from dairy foods. Cereals and cereal products provide up to 25% of dietary calcium. Other sources of calcium include green leafy vegetables such as spinach and broccoli, but the oxalate content of these foods may limit calcium bioavailability. Calcium fortification of some foods such as fruit juice and white bread differs between countries.

Modern humans get less exercise and far less sunshine exposure than did our evolutionary ancestors. Dietary sources of vitamin D in prehistoric humans are likely to have been minimal in comparison with the abundant supply from sunshine. There is very little vitamin D in the unsupplemented diet of most modern humans.

BODY WEIGHT AND THE SKELETON

Body weight is a strong predictor of osteoporotic fracture. Many factors contribute to excess fracture risks in lean individuals. Fractures may relate in part to an increased incidence of falls due to poor muscle strength. In individuals with more body fat, fracture may be prevented by fat 'padding' during falls. Obese individuals also have higher bone mineral density. This is related in part to increased production of oestrogens in fatty tissue, and to mechanical strains induced by excess body weight.

Extreme weight loss associated with anorexia nervosa results in marked loss of bone mineral content due to nutritional deprivation and amenorrhoea. Patients with anorexia nervosa are at increased risk of fracture during later life.

CALCIUM AND DAIRY FOODS

An acute effect of oral calcium on bone metabolism is well recognised. A reduction in bone resorption is observed within 2 hours of a single oral calcium dose. Studies using dairy foods show a similar effect. Longer-term studies have also shown that calcium or dairy supplementation for several weeks decreases serum PTH and bone resorption.

Numerous studies have addressed the effect of calcium intake on bone mineral density and fracture risk. The extent to which the skeletal effects of dairy foods can be attributed to increased calcium intake is not certain. A variety of calcium-supplemented food products are also available, but the skeletal benefits of these supplements cannot necessarily be assumed from their calcium composition. Several other components of dairy foods may have beneficial or deleterious effects on the skeleton. These include protein, phosphate, other minerals or specific proteins such as milk basic protein. Dairy foods may also result in modulation of endocrine systems such as the growth hormone–IGF-1 axis.

There have been many observational studies, incorporating cross-sectional, case-control and cohort designs, which have shown a positive association between calcium intake and bone mineral density or fracture risk. However, a substantial number of studies have found no association.

Randomised controlled trials of calcium or dairy food supplementation provide a better insight into the relationship. The participants investigated in studies fall into two age groups: (a) older men and women and (b) growing children. The results of randomised controlled trials of calcium supplementation are summarised in the sections below.

Calcium bioavailability

Bioavailability is the proportion of ingested calcium that is absorbed from the diet. This can vary between individuals and depends on the food source of calcium. Lactose in milk may increase calcium bioavailability from dairy foods. Dietary protein and non-digestible oligosaccharides may increase calcium absorption. Several other components of the diet such as phytates and oxalic acid can inhibit calcium absorption. Supplemental calcium can also alter the absorption of other nutrients such as iron, phosphorus and zinc.

Calcium and dairy intervention studies in postmenopausal women and men

Older people may have a greater calcium requirement than young adults. This greater need may result from impaired intestinal calcium absorption because of an age-related decline in intestinal mucosal mass, decreased dermal synthesis of vitamin D and a decline in renal synthesis of 1,25-$(OH)_2$ vitamin D. At least five studies have addressed whether non-dairy calcium supplementation reduces risk of osteoporotic fracture. The classic study of Chapuy et al (1994) in elderly women stands out by virtue of study size and the large number of fracture cases over the 3-year study period. This trial of over 3000 institutionalised women with a mean age of 84 years reported a substantial (29%) reduction in hip fracture with supplementation in comparison with placebo. The supplement in this trial was 1200 mg of calcium, as calcium phosphate, combined with 20 µg of vitamin D. The results of this study cannot necessarily be applied to other populations, younger women or men. The women studied were institutionalised, with generally poor mobility, and had low dietary calcium intake (mean 500 mg/day). However, Dawson-Hughes et al (1997) showed a reduction in incidence of non-vertebral fractures in elderly men and women living at home with a combined calcium and vitamin D supplement (500 mg/day calcium, 17.5 mg of vitamin D), and calcium and vitamin D combined are generally thought to have anti-fracture efficacy for hip fracture in older women who comply with taking the supplement (Bonjour et al 2009). There have been a few small supplementation trials using calcium alone with fracture as an end-point. Whilst these have shown a positive effect of calcium in reducing fracture risk, the small number of fractures in these studies limits interpretation. The effects of increasing consumption of dairy foods on fracture incidence have not been tested in older men or women.

A larger number of studies, reviewed by Heaney (2000), have examined the effect of supplemental calcium, with or without vitamin D, using BMD as a surrogate end-point. Almost all studies show a positive effect on BMD, although the size of effect is modest. The response to calcium supplementation may depend on habitual calcium intake. For example, one 3-year study observed no effect of supplemental calcium and vitamin D (1000 mg calcium, 25 µg vitamin D) on bone loss in men (Orwoll et al 1990). However, these men had high habitual calcium intakes (1160 mg/day) and were heterogeneous in age.

Several controlled trials of dairy supplementation in older women have also demonstrated a reduction in the rate of bone loss. A recent 2-year study of milk supplementation in postmenopausal Chinese women on a low calcium intake (about 400 mg/day) showed that women receiving a milk powder supplement (calcium content about 1 g/day) had a lower rate of bone loss at the total body, lumbar spine and total hip compared to a control group (Lau et al 2001). Calcium supplementation appears to have less influence on bone loss in the years immediately after the menopause. This may be due to the overriding importance of oestrogen deficiency during this time.

Calcium and dairy intervention studies in children and adolescents

Since a large proportion of peak bone mass is attained during childhood and puberty, children and adolescents are a particularly important target for interventions to increase bone mass. To this end, there have been a number of randomised controlled trials of calcium or dairy supplementation in children (see Table *evolve* 24.1 for a summary of studies 🖱). The level of daily supplementation varied from 500 to 1000 mg of calcium for periods up to 3 years. These studies found that calcium supplementation resulted in greater bone mass accrual. The magnitude of the increase in bone acquisition has been of the order of 1–7%. The increase in bone mineral content with calcium supplementation during childhood may be due in part to a reduction in the rate of bone remodelling and reduced remodelling space.

Although calcium or dairy supplementation has been shown to accelerate bone mineral accrual in children and adolescents during the period of supplementation, the long-term effects of supplementation are unclear. The possible beneficial effects of nutritional supplementation during puberty may relate to an effect on skeletal size rather than bone mineral density. Some studies have examined whether the benefits of supplementation are maintained after the intervention is withdrawn. The majority have failed to show a persistent effect, although larger studies are necessary to confirm this.

Concerns have been expressed that policies to increase intake of milk and dairy products could result in cardiovascular disease and obesity. However, recent studies have shown that milk supplementation is likely to result in a lowering of body mass and body fat rather than an increase.

The role of calcium supplementation in management of osteoporosis

Low calcium intake is only one factor contributing to loss of bone mass in patients with osteoporosis. Although calcium supplementation is important in many patients with osteoporosis, ensuring adequate protein intake is also likely to be of benefit. Maintenance of body weight is critical, since moderate weight loss and low body weight are associated with loss of bone mass and risk of fracture. Although a number of micronutrients, such as vitamin D and K and antioxidant vitamins, have been linked with increased risk of bone mineral loss, only vitamin D has recognised therapeutic value. Combined supplements of calcium and vitamin D are often recommended to patients with osteoporosis and dietary advice to increase intake of dairy products is commonplace. Excessive calcium intake may occasionally result in hypercalcaemia, may result in renal insufficiency or renal stones, and may impair absorption of other nutrients such as iron, phosphorus and zinc.

Recommended calcium intakes

The UK reference nutrient intake (RNI), which is the intake deemed sufficient to satisfy 97% of the population's requirements, is set at 700 mg per day for adults including elderly people. The reference nutrient intake for teenagers is 1000 mg/day for males and 800 mg/day for females, and 550 mg/day for children aged 7 to 10 years. In the USA recommended calcium intake is greater. For children and teenagers aged 9 to 18 years the reference intake is 1300 mg/day, whilst for adults it is 1000 mg/day and for the elderly 1200 mg/day. Most calcium supplementation studies which have shown a skeletal effect have used intakes of at least 1000 mg per day.

VITAMIN D HORMONE

Vitamin D and its metabolites play an important role in calcium and phosphate homeostasis and skeletal development. Vitamin D also plays a role in muscle function, control of cell proliferation and in the immune system.

The unfortunate designation of vitamin D as a 'vitamin' is derived largely from the important findings of Mellanby in 1919. He showed that oral administration of cod liver oil was able to cure rickets. Vitamin D is a sunlight-derived hormone precursor, and is not an essential nutrient in sunlight-exposed humans. Fatty fish such as sardines contain vitamin D, and there is also some vitamin D in eggs. Interesting experiments involving sailors in submarines have shown that individuals who are not exposed to ultraviolet light rapidly develop vitamin D insufficiency despite consuming a usual diet.

The main causes of vitamin D deficiency (Table 24.2) can be understood based on an appreciation of vitamin D metabolism (Fig. 24.2). Vitamin D is derived in large part from conversion of 7-dehydrocholesterol (provitamin D_3) to vitamin D_3 when skin is exposed to ultraviolet B (UV-B) irradiation from sunlight. Vitamin D generated in skin is termed vitamin D_3 (cholecalciferol). Some vitamin D supplements are of plant origin (ergocalciferol or vitamin D_2). Production of vitamin D in skin is reduced in wintertime, and in individuals with increased skin pigmentation. Individuals who do not venture out of doors, who wear clothing that covers a large proportion of body surface, or who live in countries with limited sunshine are also predisposed to vitamin D deficiency.

Endogenous vitamin D_3 and dietary D_3/D_2 are converted to 25-(OH) vitamin D (25-(OH)D) in the liver. 25-(OH)D is the main storage form of vitamin D and is commonly measured in serum to assess vitamin D status. The concentration of 25-(OH)D in serum shows a seasonal variation (Fig. 24.3). Anticonvulsant drug therapy is a risk factor for vitamin D deficiency because of increased conversion of 25-(OH)D to inactive metabolites in the liver.

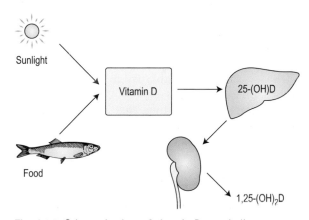

Fig. 24.2 Schematic view of vitamin D metabolism.

Table 24.2	Factors contributing to vitamin D hormone insufficiency
1. Deficiency of sunlight–derived vitamin D	
Failure to go out of doors Limited UV-B exposure in wintertime Countries with limited UV-B exposure Decreased skin exposure due to traditional dress Use of sunscreen creams Ageing Darker skin colour	
2. Gastrointestinal disease	
Pancreatic disease (fat malabsorption) Coeliac disease Other malabsorption syndromes	
3. Anticonvulsant drug therapy	
4. Defective renal production of 1,25–(OH)₂D	
Renal insufficiency Genetic vitamin D pseudodeficiency rickets	

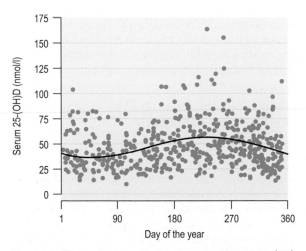

Fig. 24.3 Effect of season on the concentration of 25-(OH) vitamin D in serum of postmenopausal women in five European cities. *(Adapted from blumsohn et al J Bone Miner Res 2003; 18: 1274–1281 with permission of the American Society for Bone and Mineral Research.)*

25-(OH) vitamin D is converted to the hormone 1,25-dihydroxy vitamin D (1,25-$(OH)_2D$) in the kidneys. Renal conversion to 1,25-$(OH)_2D$ is stimulated by PTH and suppressed by phosphate. In patients with chronic renal failure, the ability of the kidney to synthesise 1,25-$(OH)_2D$ is reduced.

The physiological actions of 1,25-$(OH)_2D$ are mediated by binding to specific nuclear vitamin D receptors (VDR). In the gastrointestinal tract the action of 1,25-$(OH)_2D$ results in increased intestinal absorption of calcium and phosphorus. In severe vitamin D deficiency fractional dietary calcium absorption is generally less than 20% and occurs through a vitamin-D-independent mechanism. When vitamin D supply is sufficient, fractional calcium absorption is generally greater than 35%. The overall effect of 1,25-$(OH)_2D$ is to increase the concentration of calcium and phosphate in the plasma, and this allows mineralisation of newly formed bone matrix. 1,25-$(OH)_2D$ also acts via the VDR to activate osteoblasts, to stimulate bone resorption by osteoclasts.

It is commonly assumed that 25-(OH)D is biologically inert, and that the physiological actions of vitamin D are mediated only via renal production of 1,25-$(OH)_2D$. This dogma has been increasingly questioned. Although 1,25-$(OH)_2D$ is far more potent as an activator of the VDR, the concentration of 25-(OH)D is at least 100-fold greater. Plasma 25-(OH)D is an important determinant of skeletal disease in patients with renal failure in whom renal 1,25-$(OH)_2D$ production is impaired. Several tissues other than the kidney express the enzyme required to convert 25-(OH)D to 1,25-$(OH)_2D$ and this local conversion may be important. For further discussion of vitamin D metabolism see Section 11.2.

Skeletal consequences of vitamin D deficiency

In children, severe vitamin D deficiency causes rickets. Although vitamin-D-deficiency rickets is becoming less common in Western industrialised countries, childhood vitamin D deficiency remains a significant problem, particularly in Black and Asian children, and in children who are exclusively breastfed. Breast milk contains only small amounts of vitamin D. The clinical features of osteomalacia in adults are often more subtle. Patients with severe vitamin D deficiency often have generalised bone pain, muscle pain and muscle weakness. This may be misdiagnosed as 'chronic fatigue' or a rheumatological disorder.

Defining vitamin D deficiency and toxicity

It is generally accepted that the serum concentration of 25-(OH)D is the best indicator of vitamin D status. Serum 1,25-$(OH)_2D$ may be low, normal or increased in vitamin D deficiency, and measurement of 1,25-$(OH)_2D$ is not a useful indicator of vitamin D status. However, it has been difficult to define precise thresholds of plasma 25-(OH)D associated with deficiency, insufficiency or toxicity. It is possible to define thresholds by examining the relationship between plasma 25-(OH)D and fracture risk. However, plasma 25-(OH)D may be low in individuals with other risk factors for fracture (such as lack of exercise or poor general health), and the relationship between low 25-(OH)D and fracture may therefore not be causal.

Vitamin D insufficiency results in an elevated concentration of PTH in plasma (secondary hyperparathyroidism). Serum PTH is a sensitive indicator of vitamin D deficiency. It is possible to define thresholds for vitamin D deficiency based on cross-sectional studies of association between plasma 25-(OH)D and plasma PTH.

Individuals with plasma 25-(OH)D less than 50 nmol/l tend to have elevated serum PTH in comparison with vitamin-D-replete individuals. This secondary hyperparathyroidism is responsive to modest doses of exogenous vitamin D. It has therefore been suggested that individuals with plasma 25-(OH)D below 50 nmol/l should be regarded as vitamin-D-insufficient. Approximately half the population in most Western industrialised countries would be regarded as vitamin-D insufficient using this criterion. Plasma 25-(OH)D below 15 nmol/l is often associated with overt osteomalacia or rickets.

Vitamin D toxicity is unusual. Individuals regularly exposed to intense sunlight may have plasma 25-(OH)D concentrations up to 200 nmol/l throughout the year, and these individuals do not have any disturbance in skeletal metabolism. Plasma 25-(OH)D greater than 250 nmol/l may be consistent with vitamin D toxicity. The symptoms of vitamin D toxicity include nausea, vomiting, anorexia, fatigue and changes in mental state, such as confusion and nervousness. Serum calcium levels are elevated, which may result in calcium deposition in soft tissues such as arteries, kidney and heart. Heart arrhythmias may be a consequence of raised serum calcium.

Vitamin D and fracture risk

There is an association between plasma 25-(OH) vitamin D and bone mineral density in older people. Several studies have shown that combined calcium and vitamin D supplementation reduces fracture incidence particularly in elderly subjects with a low calcium intake. The independent role of vitamin D deficiency as a determinant of fractures in older people is less certain. In one important study, Trivedi et al (2003) examined the effect of vitamin D supplementation (2500 mg every 4 months for 5 years) in non-institutionalised elderly men and women. They found that there was a 22% reduction in the incidence of first fracture in comparison with placebo. However, some other randomised trials of vitamin D alone have not shown benefit in terms of fracture. The efficacy of vitamin D may depend on habitual calcium intake and the dose of vitamin D used. If vitamin D does prevent fracture, it is very likely that some of the benefit could be due to a reduction in the incidence of falls rather than increased bone mineral content. Vitamin D deficiency is common in elderly people who fall, and is associated with poor muscle strength and impaired motor function in the elderly.

Vitamin D status may also influence skeletal growth and bone mineral density during childhood and puberty. There is also some evidence to support the idea that vitamin D status during fetal development and the first year of life may result in long-lasting changes in skeletal function by 'programming' physiological function.

Recommended vitamin D intake

Vitamin D is only an essential nutrient in the absence of sunshine exposure. It is also difficult to determine the amount of vitamin D normally obtained from diet and from sunshine. This depends on a large number of variables including sunshine exposure, latitude and skin pigmentation. Foods containing vitamin D (such as oily fish and egg) may contain very different amounts depending on their source. For adults living a normal lifestyle, the panel on dietary reference values in the UK did not therefore recommend an RNI for oral vitamin D intake in adults. For adults confined indoors, the panel agreed an RNI of 10 µg/day. This amount of

vitamin D is, however, not sufficient to prevent vitamin D deficiency in the absence of any sunshine exposure, although it is likely to prevent overt osteomalacia. For infants up to 6 months of age, the panel recommended an intake of 8.5 mg/day. For individuals not exposed to sunshine, the United States Food and Nutrition Board recommended daily allowance (RDA) of vitamin D is 5 µg/day for infants, children and adults. The RDA is set at 10 µg/day for older adults (age 50 to 70 years) and at 15 µg/day for those over the age of 70.

24.6 PROTEIN, AND ACID–BASE BALANCE

PROTEIN INTAKE AND SKELETAL HEALTH

Bone matrix is composed largely of protein, and amino acid supply is therefore an essential requirement for bone formation. Early studies in humans and animals found that a diet high in protein results in increased urinary calcium excretion. This effect was thought to reflect increased bone resorption, possibly as a result of skeletal buffering of the net acid load associated with protein catabolism. Catabolism of plant protein results in less acid production; and plant protein has been suggested therefore to be less harmful. More recent studies suggest that the increased calcium excretion with high intake of animal protein may be due in large part to increased efficiency of dietary calcium absorption, rather than bone resorption, and that increasing the dietary acid load through augmenting protein intake has no effect on overall calcium balance or bone mineral loss. Evidence that intake of animal protein is harmful to the skeleton is not strong, and in fact, increasing protein intake may increase bone mineral density and decrease the risk of falls in some populations, particularly in the elderly.

Protein intake may alter skeletal health through several mechanisms in addition to the well-described effect on net acid intake. These mechanisms include improved dietary calcium absorption, increased serum IGF-1, and possible beneficial effects of specific proteins on the skeleton. IGF-1 stimulates osteoblast proliferation and differentiation, and enhances bone collagen and matrix synthesis. It is also possible that particular milk proteins, such as milk basic protein (MBP), may have a direct antiresorptive effect on the skeleton. Low serum IGF-1 has been associated with increased fracture risk. It is overly simplistic to consider animal protein as a single nutritional entity. Although many early studies showed that intake of purified protein products (such as casein) results in increased urine calcium loss, these proteins may not reflect the effect of common food proteins Studies using meat as a protein supplement have shown little effect on urinary calcium excretion.

Cohort studies relating protein intake to bone mineral density and fracture have also not provided consistent evidence of a harmful effect of dietary animal protein (see Table *evolve* 24.2 for summary references 📖). The majority of studies have shown a protective effect of animal and total protein on bone loss and fracture risk, whilst a couple of studies have indicated that high-protein diets are associated with increased risk of fracture when calcium intake is low.

The relevance of protein intake may also vary by age and nutritional status. Elderly persons with osteoporotic hip fracture are often undernourished, particularly with respect to protein, and tend to have a reduced concentration of albumin in serum. Low body weight is an important risk factor for fracture. Randomised controlled trials of patients who have already sustained a hip fracture have shown that protein supplementation improves clinical outcome, increases muscle strength and improves BMD. In these trials the protein supplement was given in conjunction with calcium. Correction of protein undernutrition could reduce fractures by increasing muscle mass, increasing bone mineral density, and by reducing the risk of falls. No controlled studies have investigated the effect of protein supplementation on fracture risk.

FRUIT AND VEGETABLE INTAKE

There is substantial observational evidence that a diet high in fruit and vegetables may be associated with a slightly reduced fracture risk. The relationship between the alkalinising effect of fruit and vegetable intake on the one hand and the acidifying effect of meat intake on the other hand has received considerable attention. However, as discussed above, the effect of animal protein on bone is controversial. Conclusions relating to the beneficial effect of fruit and vegetable intake currently rely on observational cross-sectional studies and a few cohort studies. Some studies use indirect indices of fruit and vegetable intake, such as potassium intake, magnesium intake, intake of various carotenoids or estimated net dietary acid load. These studies suggest that individuals who consume a diet rich in fruit and vegetables relative to animal protein have less bone mineral loss and lower fracture risk. Some cohort studies have failed to find such an association, and in other studies the effects are not gender-consistent. For example, one study reported that men with a high intake of fruit and vegetables had less bone loss at one site, but this did not apply to women. Most studies have not shown significant differences in skeletal health or fracture risk between vegetarians and meat-eaters.

The evidence relating to a possible beneficial role of fruit and vegetables is of variable quality and is potentially confounded by correlations between fruit and vegetable intake and intake of other foods and nutrients. For example, people who consume few fruit and vegetables may have poor overall dietary patterns high in nutrients that may be harmful and conversely deficient in nutrients that might benefit the skeleton. Intake of fruit and vegetables is also associated with lifestyle factors such as smoking, alcohol consumption and exercise. Adequate statistical correction for these confounders may not be possible. Even if fruit and vegetable intake is beneficial, the effect size is likely to be modest. One meta-analysis showed that less than 1% of the variance in bone mineral density was attributed to potassium intake, although this was statistically significant. It is premature to draw conclusions about the role of fruit and vegetables in the prevention of fracture risk until the results of randomised intervention trials are available.

24.7 OTHER VITAMINS

Several other vitamins have been studied in relation to bone health, including vitamins A, B, C and K. These are discussed in Section *evolve* 24.7 📖. The evidence of associations is not strong.

24.8 MINERALS

SODIUM

Numerous studies have shown that a diet high in sodium increases urinary calcium excretion. An increase in sodium intake equivalent to one teaspoon of salt increases urinary calcium excretion by about 1.5 mmol per day. However, this calciuria may be offset by increased calcium absorption with no detriment to overall calcium balance. Short-term experimental studies in postmenopausal women have shown that a low-sodium diet reduces bone remodelling. However, studies of dietary sodium intake in relation to BMD are less convincing, and there are no data to suggest that altering sodium intake would reduce fracture risk. Nevertheless, given the important effect of sodium intake on renal calcium handling, avoidance of excessive sodium intake does seem prudent in individuals at increased risk of fracture.

PHOSPHORUS

Bone mineral consists largely of calcium phosphate, and phosphorus supply is therefore essential for skeletal development. Phosphorus is the sixth most abundant element in the body. Bone mineral consists largely of calcium phosphate, and phosphorus supply is therefore essential for skeletal development. A reduced concentration of inorganic phosphorus in the extracellular fluid results in impaired skeletal mineralisation. Phosphorus is found in most common foods, and dietary phosphorus deficiency is therefore unusual. Phosphorus is also added to many processed foods and cola drinks as polyphosphates or phosphoric acid. Typical dietary intake of phosphorus is about 1500 mg/day. It is sometimes claimed that phosphorus intake in the typical adult diet is excessive, and that the molar ratio of dietary calcium to phosphorus should be about 1:1 for optimal skeletal health, although there is little evidence to support this.

Excess phosphorus intake lowers urinary calcium excretion and impairs absorption of calcium from the diet. The effect of high phosphate intake on the skeleton has been assessed by measuring bone mineral density, and by calcium balance studies. Some studies have shown an inverse relationship between phosphorus intake and bone mineral density. However, phosphorus intake is closely associated with intake of other nutrients, such as protein and calcium, as well as lifestyle factors, which may affect the skeleton. Cross-sectional studies of dietary phosphorus in relation to skeletal health are likely to be misleading. The possible harmful effect of a high-phosphorus diet on the skeleton may be more relevant when calcium requirements are high during puberty and calcium intakes are inadequate. The form of ingested phosphorus is also important. Polyphosphates may have

a greater deleterious effect on calcium balance than orthophosphates. There is little information on the independent relationship between phosphorus intake and fracture risk.

MAGNESIUM

Severe magnesium (Mg) deficiency results in disturbed calcium homeostasis, impaired PTH secretion, end-organ resistance to PTH, and hypocalcaemia. The implications of more subtle Mg deficiency are less clear. Some studies have shown that Mg intake is positively correlated with bone mineral density or quantitative ultrasound properties of bone in both adults and children. Intervention studies have also shown benefit of magnesium supplementation on bone mineral accrual in adolescents and on bone loss in postmenopausal women.

FLUORIDE

Fluoride increases the activity of osteoblasts. A number of studies have addressed the effect of fluoride in drinking water on fracture risk. These studies have shown a small increase in risk, a small beneficial effect, or no detectable effect. However, fluoride in drinking water accounts for a relatively small proportion of total fluoride intake, and these studies do not imply that the effect of dietary fluoride is unimportant. Substantially increased fluoride intake is associated with severe skeletal disease (fluorosis). Tea contains variable quantities of fluoride, with instant tea having particularly high concentrations; there have been occasional case reports of fluorosis associated with long-term consumption of vast quantities of instant tea. Fluorosis is also common in regions of Asia where drinking a particular type of fluoride-rich tea, brick tea, is popular. High-dose fluoride therapy in patients with osteoporosis increases trabecular bone mineral density, but this is associated with an increased rate of fracture rather than a decrease.

ZINC

There is very limited evidence that dietary zinc is important for the skeleton. Most empirical research has been orientated towards investigation of the effect of dietary zinc on bone growth in undernourished children. Some studies of children and adolescents have reported that zinc supplementation increases linear growth. The effects of dietary zinc on growth may be mediated through changes in serum IGF-1. Zinc undernutrition has been proposed as a risk factor for osteoporosis, especially since many elderly people consume zinc-deficient diets. Several studies have reported that women with postmenopausal osteoporosis had elevated urinary zinc levels compared to healthy controls, and poor zinc status has been associated with high bone turnover. However, the links between zinc status and osteoporosis risk are tenuous.

OTHER MINERALS

The possible role of other minerals, copper, boron, aluminium, chromium and strontium, is discussed in Section evolve 24.8 🖱. The evidence for associations is not strong.

24.9 OTHER DIETARY COMPONENTS

PHYTOESTROGENS

Phytoestrogens are widely promoted as a 'natural' alternative to oestrogen replacement therapy. Isoflavones are phytoestrogens which are found in high concentrations in foods such as soya. These compounds have weak oestrogen-like properties. It is important to distinguish between the nutritional effects of dietary phytoestrogens and pharmacological intake of these compounds.

A possible beneficial role of phytoestrogens for skeletal health has been demonstrated in several animal studies but the doses used have been very high and the relevance of these to human nutrition is uncertain. Human studies of isoflavone supplementation are conflicting. It has been argued that the dose of isoflavone in these human studies relative to body weight is only about 10% of that used in animal studies. Several studies have reported a positive association between BMD and intake of soya foods in Chinese and Japanese postmenopausal women. However, the association between soya food intake and bone mass has not been easy to demonstrate in populations with lower habitual soya intake.

ALCOHOL

Alcohol abuse and dependence may compromise bone quality and increase risk of fracture. The skeletal effects of excess alcohol intake are due to a direct toxic effect of alcohol on bone osteoblasts, insufficient intake of other nutrients, vitamin D deficiency, decreased sex hormone secretion and increased risk of falls. There is less evidence that moderate alcohol consumption is associated with fracture risk. Some studies have shown that modest alcohol intake is associated with increased BMD rather than a decrease.

CAFFEINE

Many observational epidemiological studies have investigated the association between intake of caffeine-containing beverages and fracture risk. The majority have found no association or a weak increase in risk with excessive consumption. The largest prospective study of caffeine intake and fracture risk showed that there was a three times greater risk of hip fracture for women consuming more than 817 mg caffeine per day (approximately five cups of coffee). However, in this study the number of hip fractures was small. It is possible that the association may not be causal, and may be due to other confounding associations such as an inverse association between caffeine intake and calcium intake or a positive association between caffeine intake and smoking. High caffeine intakes have been associated with greater risk of fracture in women with low calcium intakes (less than 700mg/d). Although caffeine ingestion leads to a slight decrease in the efficiency of calcium absorption, it has been estimated that this would be offset entirely by addition of two tablespoons of milk to a cup of coffee.

In studies which separated tea-drinkers from coffee-drinkers the former were shown to have a better bone mass and a reduced odds for fracture. The protective effect of tea may arise because of its fluoride and/or polyphenol content.

CARBONATED BEVERAGES

Several observational studies in teenagers have reported that a high intake of carbonated cola-type drinks is associated with a low bone mineral density and a higher prevalence of fracture. There have been few reports in adults and these have been inconsistent – in one large cross-sectional study a high intake of cola, but not other carbonated beverages, was associated with low hip BMD in adult women. The mechanism for this is not clear; the association may be spurious and arise because consumption of carbonated beverages is associated with other lifestyle and dietary factors, such as low exercise levels or reduced consumption of milk. The phosphorus content and caffeine content of carbonated drinks may contribute to risk.

KEY POINTS

- The skeleton is composed of two types of bone: cortical bone, which is a dense form of bone comprising about 80% of skeletal mass, and trabecular bone, which consists of an intricate structural mesh of trabeculae that form the interior scaffolding of bone.
- Bone is a metabolically active tissue. In the adult skeleton most metabolic activity occurs by the process of bone 'remodelling' or bone turnover. This metabolic activity serves to maintain the structure and homeostatic functions of the skeleton.
- Osteoporosis is a disease characterised by low bone mass and microarchitectural deterioration of bone, which results in an increased risk of fracture.
- Observational studies relating fracture risk to intake of calcium and other nutrients have yielded conflicting results. Where relationships are shown in cross-sectional studies, these may not be causal. Surrogate measures of fracture risk, such as bone mineral density and measures of bone turnover, provide useful supportive information, but do not provide definitive evidence of either benefit or harm.

- Nutritional intervention studies with fracture as an end-point provide much stronger evidence, but are impractical for most individual nutrients.
- It seems possible that nutritional intervention during childhood and puberty could increase peak bone mass and reduce the risk of fracture in later life. Controlled studies of calcium or dairy food supplementation in children and adolescents show short-term benefit in increasing bone mineral mass. However, this benefit may be lost following the cessation of supplementation.
- The majority of observational studies report that low intakes of animal protein are associated with lower bone mineral density and increased fracture risk. However, protein supplementation has not been tested in a controlled study with fracture as an outcome. It is possible that extremely elevated protein intake could result in bone loss. The evidence for this is, however, not substantial.
- Randomised controlled trials of a combined supplement of vitamin D and calcium show a reduction in fracture incidence in elderly people. The independent effect of vitamin D status on risk of fracture is unknown, although vitamin D deficiency is common in older adults even in countries which have plenty of sunshine.

References

Bonjour J-P, Gueguen L, Palacios C, Shearer MJ, Weaver CM: Minerals and vitamins in bone health: the potential value of dietary enhancement, *British Journal Nutrition* 102(7):962–966, 2009.

Chapuy MC, Arlot ME, Delmas PD, Meunier PJ: Effect of calcium and cholecalciferol treatment for three years on hip fractures in elderly women, *British Medical Journal* 308(6936):1081–1082, 1994.

Dawson-Hughes B, Harris SS, Krall EA, Dallal GE: Effect of calcium and vitamin D supplementation on bone density in men and women 65 years of age or older, *New England Journal of Medicine* 337(10):670–676, 1997.

Heaney RP: Calcium, dairy products and osteoporosis, *Journal of the American College of Nutrition* 19:83S–99S, 2000.

Lau EM, Woo J, Lam V, Hong A: Milk supplementation of the diet of postmenopausal Chinese women on a low calcium intake retards bone loss, *Journal of Bone and Mineral Research* 16:1204–1209, 2001.

Orwoll ES, Oviatt SK, McClung MR, et al: The rate of bone mineral loss in normal men and the effects of calcium and cholecalciferol supplementation, *Annals of Internal Medicine* 112:29–34, 1990.

Trivedi DP, Doll R, Khaw KT: Effect of four monthly oral vitamin D3 (cholecalciferol) supplementation on fractures and mortality in men and women living in the community: randomised double blind controlled trial, *British Medical Journal* 326(7387):469, 2003.

Further reading

Department of Health: *Dietary reference values for food energy and nutrients for the United Kingdom. Report on Health and Social Subjects 41*, London, 1991, HMSO.

Dietary reference intakes for calcium, phosphorus, magnesium, vitamin D, and fluoride 1997. Available online at: http://www.nap.edu

Heaney RP: Effects of caffeine on bone and the calcium economy, *Food and Chemical Toxicology* 40(9):1263–1270, 2002.

EVOLVE CONTENTS (available online at: evolve.elsevier.com/Geissler/nutrition)

Chapter 25

Dental diseases

Paula Moynihan

OBJECTIVES

By the end of this chapter you should be able to:
- give definitions for dental caries, erosion, abrasion and periodontal disease
- describe the indices used for the measurement of dental caries
- describe the epidemiology and trends of dental caries in Western and other countries
- outline the structure of the tooth
- explain the mechanisms of the decay process
- summarise evidence for the role of dietary sugars and fluoride in the causation and prevention of decay
- compare the relative cariogenicity of various sugars and other carbohydrates
- summarise the interaction of protective effects of fluoride and destructive effects of sugars
- summarise recent evidence for a role of nutrition in the aetiology of periodontal disease.

© 2010 Elsevier Ltd/Inc/BV
DOI: 10.1016/B978-0-7020-3118-2.00025-5

25.1 INTRODUCTION

Teeth are important in enhancing facial appearance and for integration into society, as well as being important for eating and speaking. Despite being associated with low mortality rate, dental diseases inflict considerable pain and anxiety and are costly to healthcare services – the direct costs of treating dental diseases exceeding the cost of treating cardiovascular diseases and osteoporosis. Attitudes towards dental health have changed dramatically over the last few decades: in the 1950s a common 21st birthday present for young women was a set of dentures. Nowadays, people are retaining their teeth well into older age and it is a realistic expectancy that teeth are for life. Dentistry has moved away from a profession that was mainly concerned with the reactive treatment of dental diseases, i.e. drilling and extraction of teeth, to a profession that has a true preventive focus, an aspect in which diet plays an important role.

Human beings have two dentitions. The deciduous dentition begins to appear in the mouth at about 6 months of age, consists of 20 teeth and is shed by early adolescence: the permanent dentition consists of 32 teeth and supplements, and replaces the deciduous dentition between the ages of about 6 and 21 years.

Dental diseases include enamel developmental defects (e.g. hypoplasia and fluorosis), dental tissue loss (e.g. erosion, abrasion and attrition), periodontal disease (gum disease) and dental caries (see Fig. *evolve* 25.1). Defects to enamel may occur while the teeth are forming. There are two main types of enamel developmental defect: fluorosis and hypoplasia. The former is caused by an excess ingestion of fluoride during tooth development and is considered further in Section 25.4. Enamel hypoplasia has many causes including infections, drug side effects, congenital defects and dental trauma; dietary deficiencies are one cause, considered further in Section 25.4.

Dental erosion is perceived to be an increasing problem and is defined as the loss of dental mineralised tissues by acids in a process that does not involve bacteria, i.e. it is caused by extrinsic acids from diet and/or the environment and by intrinsic acids through regurgitation. Dental erosion often coexists with other forms of tooth wear including attrition due to grinding of the tooth surfaces and abrasion, often due to over-harsh brushing of the teeth. Some degree of tooth surface loss is inevitable as the dentition ages. However, the age-related loss of dental tissue is now thought to be accelerated due to elements of the modern lifestyle including an increase in consumption of acidic drinks. The 2003 Children's Dental Health Survey showed that 53% of 5-years-olds and 30% of 12-year-olds had tooth surface loss to their incisors (front teeth) and this included the dentine and pulp in 24% and 3% of the population respectively. There are data from many types of study that show an association between acidic drink consumption and dental erosion. There are some data to show that acidic foods such as fruits also have the potential to cause erosion; however, such cases in humans are usually associated with unusual eating habits and/or very high levels of consumption.

The most common periodontal diseases are gingivitis, which is inflammation of the gums, and periodontitis which is more extensive and involves the periodontal ligament and eventually the alveolar bone. Both gingivitis and periodontitis are chronic inflammatory diseases and the latter leads to increased mobility of the teeth and their eventual loss through exfoliation. Most people have some extent of periodontal disease and loss of dental supporting tissues is an inevitable part of ageing. However, in some individuals loss occurs earlier in life and/or at an accelerated rate: about 10–15% of the population in industrialised countries have severe chronic periodontitis.

The most significant factor in the aetiology of periodontal disease is the presence of plaque on teeth adjacent to the gingivae that initiates the host's inflammatory response in the connective tissue underlying the junctional epithelium (Fig. 25.1). If plaque is left to accumulate, marked collagen destruction occurs and anaerobic bacteria build up subgingivally. Periodontitis is characterised by the destruction of the periodontal ligament and bone which may occur due to an increase in the proportion of subgingival pathogenic microorganisms, impaired host resistance or both. Intrinsic factors which modify an individual's response to plaque and its products include both dietary and hormonal factors (e.g. pregnancy) as well as certain diseases such as diabetes.

The main causes of tooth loss are dental caries in children and periodontal disease in adults; a summary of the most recent evidence for nutrition and periodontal disease is given in section 25.5.

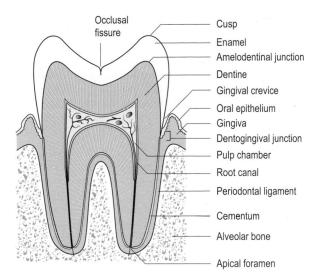

Fig. 25.1 Vertical section through a permanent molar tooth. Diagram drawn by D. S. Brown and reproduced with permission.

However, the main focus of this chapter is on diet, nutrition and dental caries.

25.2 EPIDEMIOLOGY OF DENTAL DECAY

Archaeological surveys have revealed that dental caries was rare until the nineteenth century when the prevalence and severity rose rapidly, 'poor teeth' being the most important cause of rejection of volunteers for service in the Boer War. The first surveys of the dental health of children in the UK were conducted between 1906 and 1908 and showed that 90% of children were affected by decay with an average of four decayed teeth per child. From this time, the general trend shows dental caries increased, as consumption of sugars increased, and reached its peak in the late 1950s and 1960s with interruptions to this trend occurring during the First and Second World Wars when the prevalence of dental caries fell by 40% and 30%, respectively, in the UK, due to a fall in sugars consumption. Decennial surveys of adult and child dental health have been conducted in the UK since 1968 and these, together with information from surveys conducted by the British Association for the Study of Community Dentistry, since 1985, provide information on more recent trends in dental health. Since the 1970s dental decay has declined dramatically, largely due to the introduction of fluoride,

especially in toothpaste. In 1983 the average number of teeth affected with dental caries per 12-year-old child was 3.1; this fell to 1.4 in 1993 and to 0.8 in 2003. The UK National Diet and Nutrition Survey (see Ch. 31.2) of children aged 4–18 years included an oral health survey that showed approximately 53% of young people had some decay to their teeth. Data on the levels of decay of the primary dentition show favourable trends between 1973 and 2003 but these improvements have now levelled off and in inner city populations levels are increasing slightly, since the 2003 survey of children's dental health in the UK. Regional prevalence in the UK is shown in Table *evolve* 25.1 .

INTERNATIONAL FIGURES. INDICES: DMFT, dmft

The severity of dental decay is measured using the dmft/DMFT (primary dentition/permanent dentition) index, which is a count of the number of teeth that are decayed, missing or filled. These indices are widely used throughout the world for monitoring levels of dental decay. In 1982 the World Health Organization (WHO)/Fédération Dentaire Internationale (FDI) established an oral health goal for the twenty-first century that DMFT of 12-year-olds should be less than 3. Table 25.1 shows figures from the WHO Global Data Bank on Oral Health, on levels of dental caries of 12-year-olds over the last half century (see also Table *evolve* 25.2). From these data two trends are observed: first the distinct fall in the severity of dental caries in developed countries and second the increase in caries levels in some developing countries that have increased sugars consumption. In some developing countries levels have subsequently fallen; however, there is still concern that, in countries undergoing nutrition transition, dental caries levels will rise due to increased consumption of free sugars. Despite improvement in dental health in many developed countries over the past 40 years, dental caries remains unacceptably high and in some countries the trend for improvement has now levelled off. Even in countries with low average DMFT scores, dental caries may still affect the majority of children.

Epidemiological data show quite high levels of decay in the primary dentition of children from many countries. In Africa, the prevalence of dental caries in young children is increasing in some parts and is associated with an increase in sugars consumption, while it stays low in countries where a

Table 25.1   Trends in dental caries levels of 12-year-olds in industrialised and developing countries

Country	MEAN DMFT PER PERSON AGED 12 YEARS					
	Year	DMFT	Year	DMFT	Year	DMFT
Highly industrialised countries						
Australia	1956	9.3	1982	2.1	2000	0.8
Finland	1975	7.5	1982	4.0	2000	1.2
Japan	1975	5.9	1993	3.6	2005	1.7
Norway	1940	12.0	1979	4.5	2004	1.7
Switzerland	1961–63	9.6	1980	1.7	1996	0.8
UK	1983	3.1	1993	1.4	2003	0.8
Romania	1985	5.0	1991	4.3	2000	2.8
USA	1946	7.6	1980	2.6	1999–2004	1.2
Developing countries						
Chile	1960	2.8	1978	6.6	1999	3.4
French Polynesia	1966	6.5	1986	3.2	1994	3.2
Iran	1974	2.4	1976	4.9	2003	1.2
Jordan	1962	0.2	1981	2.7	1995	3.3
Mexico	1975	5.3	1991	2.5–5.1	1997	2.5
Morocco	1970	2.6	1980	4.5	1999	2.5
Philippines	1967	1.4	1981	2.9	2005/6	2.9
Uganda	1966	0.4	1987	0.5	2002	0.9

Source: www.whocollab.od.mah.se/ accessed March 2009

poor economy restricts sugars consumption. Data on 5-year-old children from the UK, the Netherlands and Denmark suggest that the trend towards reduced prevalence of dental decay has halted. Low levels of decay in the primary dentition (dmft < 2.0) have been reported for Denmark, England, Finland, Italy, the Netherlands and Norway. Higher levels of decay (dmft >4.0) have been reported for Belarus, Hungary, Romania and Russia (WHO 2003).

Dental caries affects adults as well as children and the severity of the disease increases with age. The WHO oral health guidelines state that at age 35–44 years a DMFT of 14 or above is considered high. Current available data show high levels of caries in European adults, where DMFT values range from approximately 13 to 21 at 35–44 years. In most developing countries, the level of caries in adults of this age group is lower.

GEOGRAPHIC AND SOCIAL CLASS DIFFERENCES

Dental decay is very strongly related to social class, with highest levels in the most socially disadvantaged. In the UK and many other countries there are marked differences in caries prevalence and severity between social classes and in some instances between geographical regions. Information from the UK Children's Dental Health Surveys has shown that dental caries is strongly linked to social class with higher levels of dental caries, poorer oral hygiene practices and non-attendance all being more common in those from lower social classes. The UK National Diet and Nutrition Surveys (NDNS) of children aged 1.5–4.5 years and 4–18 years included an oral health survey that also provide information on levels of dental caries and other dental conditions in different age groups, social class groups and regions. These surveys have shown that, for preschool and school-aged children up to 18 years, levels of dental caries are highest in children from households headed by a manual worker. Higher levels of dental caries have also been reported in children of mothers with no formal qualifications, children from families in receipt of benefits and, for preschool children, children from lone parent families. The National Diet and Nutrition Survey also showed that preschool children from manual social classes were more likely to be frequent consumers of confectionery and sugared soft drinks and more likely to be users of dummies and reservoir feeders. In contrast to this, there is less of a relationship between levels of dental erosion in children and socio-demographic variables.

Dental health status may be assessed by looking at the proportion of a population that have no natural teeth, i.e. are edentulous. Older adults from manual worker backgrounds are more likely to be edentulous: the UK National Diet and Nutrition Survey showed that 59% of those from manual working backgrounds were edentulous compared with 38% of those from non-manual backgrounds. Dentate older adults from manual working backgrounds are also more likely to have unsound roots (root caries) than dentate older adults from non-manual working backgrounds.

UK dental health surveys have also indicated considerable regional differences in levels of decay. The most recent Children's Dental Health Survey published in 2003 showed that in 5-year-old children, the percent with decay was lower in England than in Wales and Northern Ireland and in England there was distinct regional variation. The highest prevalence of dental decay was seen in Yorkshire and Humber (52%) and London (51%) with the lowest prevalence in southeast England (30%) and eastern England (33%). For 12-year-old children the highest prevalence of decay was again seen in Yorkshire and Humber (59%) and the lowest prevalence in eastern England (25%). The oral health component of the National Diet and Nutrition Survey showed that in children aged 7–18 years those from the north of England are more likely to have dental erosion than those from London and the southeast. Likewise, the oral health component of the NDNS of persons aged 65 years and over showed those living in London and the southeast are more likely to retain their natural dentition than are those from the north of England and Scotland (63% dentate compared with 36% dentate, respectively). For dentate older adults, those from Scotland and the north of England are more likely to have unsound teeth compared with older adults from other regions. Additional data on caries levels by region are given in Table *evolve* 25.1 [image].

KEY POINTS

- The prevalence and severity of dental caries in industrialised countries has decreased since the late 1970s but improvements have now halted in younger age groups.

- In developing countries, where sugars intake has increased/is increasing, the prevalence of decay has increased/is increasing.
- Dental caries is strongly related to social class, with a higher prevalence in lower social classes.
- Dental decay is lower in England than in Wales, Scotland and Northern Ireland. In England the lowest levels are seen in the east with the highest levels in Yorkshire and Humber and London.

25.3 THE DECAY PROCESS

Today, the aetiology of dental caries is well established: dental caries is the localised loss of dental hard tissues as a result of acids produced by bacterial fermentation of sugars in the mouth. However, in the past, several theories for the causation of dental caries have been postulated, which are summarised below. It is now known that dental caries requires the presence of bacteria in dental plaque and a sugars substrate to occur, but its development is influenced by the structure of the tooth, the salivary flow rate and composition, and the presence or absence of fluoride.

THEORIES OF CAUSATION

Most research to support the theories of causation of dental caries favours the chemo-parasitic theory of W. D. Miller, although there were many earlier proposals. Ancient civilisations in China, Mesopotamia and Greece believed that dental caries was caused by worms – the treatment for which was fumigation. The extent to which the diet influenced these worms was unknown. The worms were thought to drink on the blood of the teeth and feed on the roots in the jaw.

W.D. Miller was an American working in Berlin when he published his chemo-parasitic theory in 1890. The principal feature of this theory is the three-way interaction between the tooth surface, bacteria and carbohydrate, i.e. the dissolution of enamel mineral by acids produced by plaque microorganisms through the fermentation of dietary sugars. During the last half of the nineteenth century, Pasteur had shown that sugars could be fermented to acids by microorganisms and Magitot showed that these acids were capable of destroying tooth tissue in vitro. W.D. Miller, in combining this information, showed that carbohydrate-containing foods, when incubated with saliva, caused demineralisation of teeth in vitro and he also showed that several types of oral bacteria were capable of fermenting carbohydrate foods. His experiments showed that lactic acid was the main acid produced during fermentation and that the centre of carious lesions was acidic. In view of this, Miller and other researchers viewed *Lactobacillus* as the main class of cariogenic bacteria. In 1924, Clarke, a scientist working in London, isolated *Streptococcus mutans* (*S. mutans*) from pre-carious lesions (areas of demineralisation that occur prior to the formation of a cavity) and determined the importance of *S. mutans* in caries initiation. What was originally described as '*S. mutans*' is now known to be a group of bacteria with similar properties referred to as 'mutans streptococci'. It is now thought that mutans streptococci initiate caries and that lactobacilli become involved at a later stage when the low pH conditions produced by mutans streptococci favour their growth.

In the 1950s Kite and co-workers from the USA demonstrated that dental caries was caused by foods in the mouth. They fed rats a cariogenic diet either by the normal oral route or by stomach intubation – dental caries only occurred in the rats fed orally. A few years later Orland and co-workers, also from America, developed a system for rearing germ-free rats. When these rats were fed a cariogenic diet dental caries did not develop. By contrast, rats fed the same diet but not reared in germ-free conditions developed caries, thereby illustrating that microorganisms are necessary for dental decay to occur.

In the 1920s and 1930s, dental caries was thought to be a deficiency disease. Lady May Mellanby (wife to Edward Mellanby who discovered vitamin D) believed that vitamin D deficiency was a major cause of dental caries due to its role in calcification. Her work was overshadowed by later work in the 1940s and 1950s which indicated that sugars in the mouth were the cause of decay.

In the mid twentieth century some scientists thought that the protein matrix was the site of initiation of dental caries and devised the proteolytic theory of dental caries (Gottlieb's proteolytic theory). This was subsequently elaborated on by Schatz and Martin, who postulated that the protein matrix was attacked initially by proteolytic enzymes and that the amino acids released dissolved the mineral of enamel by forming 'chelates' that would occur at neutrality (the 'chelation theory'). Later, in the 1960s, Jackson and co-workers proposed that dental caries was an autoimmune disease, another theory that never gained much credit. Of all the theories put forward, only the chemo-parasitic theory (also known as the 'acid theory') has persisted and is now widely accepted by dental scientists worldwide.

THE STRUCTURE OF THE TOOTH AND THE DECALCIFICATION PROCESS

In order to describe the action of bacterial acids on the teeth an appreciation of the tooth structure is required. The teeth are composed of three mineralised tissues – enamel, dentine and cementum (Fig. 25.1). Dentine forms the bulk of the tooth and is mesodermal in origin. The dentine forms the roots of the tooth and is covered by a thin layer of cementum. The outer layer of the crown of the tooth consists of enamel, a hard substance that is ectodermal in origin. The teeth are supported by the alveolar bone of the maxilla or mandible, covered in epithelium. The epithelium around the necks of the teeth is called the gingivae (gums). The teeth are held in the alveolar bone by the periodontal ligament, allowing the teeth to move slightly. Enamel contains no cells, nerves or blood vessels and is insensitive, but the dentine is very sensitive to many stimuli. The nerves and blood vessels supplying the dentine come from the pulp that forms the soft centre of a tooth and is in turn supplied by nerves and blood vessels from the alveolar bone via the apical foramen of the tooth roots. Dental enamel consists of crystals of hydroxyapatite, a crystalline compound composed of calcium and phosphate arranged in a characteristic way in a thinly dispersed organic matrix.

THE ROLE OF ORAL MICROORGANISMS IN DENTAL DISEASES AND THE ROLE OF DENTAL PLAQUE

An essential factor in the aetiology of dental caries is dental plaque, a white, slightly glutinous layer, which builds up on the surfaces of teeth when they are not cleaned. Dental plaque is composed of three main components: the pellicle, plaque microflora and extracellular plaque matrix. The pellicle is the first layer to form on clean enamel and consists of salivary proteins including glycoproteins that are adsorbed onto the enamel surface. Microorganisms then become attached to the pellicle and multiply, forming colonies and developing to form a continuous layer increasing in depth. The microorganisms make up 70% of plaque while the remaining 30% consists of the plaque matrix. The polymers that make up much of the matrix are derived from dietary sugar by enzymes secreted by the plaque microorganisms. Glucans (dextran and mutan) are formed mainly from dietary sucrose by glucosyl-transferase of plaque streptococci (see Fig. *evolve* 25.2 🖱). The glucans help maintain plaque integrity due to their glutinous nature but also form an energy store from which bacteria feed during long breaks between the host's meals. Sucrose can also be converted to fructans (levans), which are rapidly metabolised by plaque enzymes. Dental plaque can usually be found in areas around the teeth that are least easily cleaned, mainly in the pits and fissures of the occlusal (or chewing) surfaces, between adjacent teeth (proximal surfaces) or along the gingival margin of the tooth on the buccal (outer) or lingual (inner) surfaces of the teeth.

Dental caries arises as a result of an interaction between the host's diet, oral microflora and the host's tooth surfaces. Periodontal disease also occurs as a result of the presence of certain oral bacteria. It is therefore important to understand the composition of the oral microflora and how this alters in health and disease. The main concentration of bacteria in the mouth is in the dental plaque, contributing to the majority of plaque volume. It is estimated that dental plaque contains over 500 different types of bacteria. The majority play no direct role in caries development but the type of microorganism present will influence the properties of the plaque.

Mutans streptococci are the main bacteria associated with decay and they play a crucial role in the initiation and progression of dental caries. They readily produce acids from dietary sugars and can synthesise extracellular plaque polysaccharides from sucrose, creating ideal conditions for bacteria such as lactobacilli, bifidobacteria and some non-mutans streptococci, also associated with dental caries. Further information on cariogenic bacteria and bacteria associated with periodontal disease is given in Section *evolve* 25.3 🖱 and on the role of microorganisms in dental caries is given by Russell (2003) .

THE CARIES PROCESS

Dietary sugars diffuse into the dental plaque where they are metabolised by plaque microorganisms to acid. Most of the acid produced is lactic, with some acetic, formic and propionic acids also being produced. The acid produced reduces the pH of dental plaque, the mineral phase of enamel is dissolved by the plaque acids, and the caries process has begun. Enamel hydroxyapatite usually begins to dissolve around pH 5.5, which is sometimes referred to as the 'critical pH'. When the pH rises above this value, remineralisation of enamel may occur. Saliva promotes remineralisation as it contains bicarbonate which increases pH and encourages deposition of mineral in porous areas where demineralisation of enamel or dentine has occurred. A demineralised lesion may therefore be remineralised; however, this is a slow process that competes with factors causing demineralisation. If the pH in the mouth remains high enough for sufficient time then complete remineralisation may occur. However, if demineralisation dominates, the enamel becomes more porous until finally a carious lesion forms. The rate of demineralisation is affected by the concentration of hydrogen ions (i.e. pH at the tooth surface) and the frequency with which the plaque pH falls below the critical pH. Another relevant point is the amount of calcium and phosphate in plaque, since high levels of these minerals in plaque will help resist dissolution of the enamel. Overall, caries occurs when demineralisation exceeds remineralisation. The development of caries requires sugars and aciduric bacteria to occur, but is influenced by the composition of the tooth (the structure of the enamel can be altered by the diet while the teeth are forming), the quantity and composition of saliva (e.g. calcium and phosphate content and buffering power) and the time for which dietary sugars are available for fermentation.

THE STEPHAN CURVE: THE EFFECTS OF DIFFERENT FOOD COMBINATIONS ON PLAQUE PH

Stephan, in the 1940s, pioneered work on the pH of dental plaque using microelectrodes. This work indicated that the resting pH of plaque was around 6.5–7 but, on exposure to sugars (glucose or sucrose), fell rapidly within a few minutes, to around pH 5. The rapid fall was followed by a slow recovery to

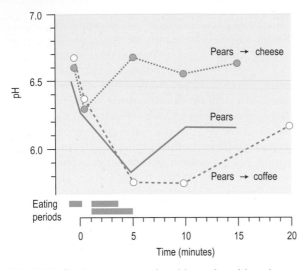

Fig. 25.2 Stephan curves produced by eating either cheese or sugared coffee after tinned pears in syrup. Adapted from Rugg-Gunn et al 1975, with permission.

baseline pH over the next 30–60 minutes. Stephan plotted pH against time and this time/pH graph is commonly referred to as a 'Stephan curve'. An example of a Stephan curve is shown in Figure 25.2. The Stephan curve has been commonly used to measure the acidogenic potential of a range of foods and this provides an indirect measure of the cariogenic potential of the food. However, it must be noted that measures of plaque pH alone must not be taken as a direct measure of cariogenic potential since these measurements take no account of protective factors in foods, the resistance of enamel and salivary factors that influence the caries process. In order to determine the cariogenic potential of a food, data from plaque pH studies need to be interpreted alongside data from other types of study including animal studies and epidemiological surveys.

Consumption of different food combinations results in different patterns in plaque pH. This was clearly illustrated in a study that looked at the effect on plaque pH of consuming a sugary snack followed by either sweetened coffee or a 15 g piece of cheese (Fig. 25.2). Consumption of cheese following a sugary snack almost abolishes the fall in plaque pH that usually results from sugars consumption. This effect of cheese is probably due to the stimulation of saliva by this highly flavoured food and its low carbohydrate (lactose) content. Other foods that are good stimuli to salivary flow include

peanuts and sugar-free chewing gum, and these also reduce the pH fall if consumed following a sugar-containing item. When sugars are consumed with other foods, the effect on pH is reduced, probably due to a diluting effect and the increased salivary flow due to mastication of other foods. This is one reason why it is often recommended to consume sugary foods at mealtimes only (another reason is that limiting sugars to mealtimes reduces the frequency of consumption). A study that examined the effect of consuming breakfast items in a different order on plaque pH illustrates this diluting effect. The breakfast items were sugar-containing coffee, a boiled egg and crispbread with butter. The smallest drop in pH was observed when all three items were consumed together and the largest drop in pH was observed when the sugared coffee was consumed alone. So consumption of one food may affect the acidogenicity of another.

Chewing sugar-free chewing gum following a sugars-containing snack has also been shown to increase the rate at which plaque pH returns to baseline. This has led to the advice to chew sugar-free gum following a sugary snack or meal.

KEY POINTS

- Dental caries occurs due to demineralisation of the dental mineralised tissues by acids derived from the bacterial metabolism of dietary sugars to acids.
- Plaque on the tooth surface is largely composed of bacterial cells and extracellular glucans.
- Mutans streptococci have an important role in dental caries since they can produce acid from sugars at a low pH.
- Changes in plaque pH on consumption of a food provide a measure of acidogenic potential, which is an indirect measure of cariogenic potential.

25.4 PROMOTING AND PROTECTIVE FACTORS

There are many factors that have the potential to promote dental decay: poor oral hygiene, high MS counts and an excess intake of dietary sugars among them. Likewise there are several factors known to be protective against decay, most notably fluoride exposure (both dietary and non-dietary) and restricted intake of sugars. However, there are also a number of other dietary factors that protect against dental caries, including milk, cheese and xylitol, and knowledge of these factors assists in making dietary advice for dental health more positive.

DIET

Diet can affect the teeth while they are forming, before they erupt into the mouth (a pre-eruptive effect) and, once erupted, by a local direct effect. Much research was undertaken in the first half of the twentieth century on the pre-eruptive effect of diet on tooth structure. Deficiencies of vitamin D, vitamin A and protein energy malnutrition (PEM) have been associated with enamel hypoplasia. This is an enamel developmental defect characterised by pits, fissures or larger areas of missing enamel that become stained post-eruption and which render the tooth more susceptible to decay. PEM and vitamin A deficiency also cause salivary gland atrophy, reducing the quantity and affecting the composition of saliva, ultimately reducing the mouth's defence against plaque acids. However, in developing countries, in the absence of dietary sugars, undernutrition is not associated with dental caries. Undernutrition coupled with a high intake of sugars results in levels of caries greater than expected for the level of sugars intake. Despite considerable past interest in the pre-eruptive effect of diet on tooth decay, today, the post-eruptive local effect of diet in the mouth is considered to be much more important. The aforementioned studies of Kite and colleagues showed that the presence of food in the mouth was a prerequisite for dental caries formation. There is a wealth of evidence for the association between diet and dental caries and most attention has focused on the important role of dietary sugars in the aetiology of caries.

The frequency of eating sugars, the amount eaten and the cariogenicity of different dietary sugars have all to be considered. The cariogenicity of starches, the relative cariogenicity of naturally occurring and 'free' sugars (sometimes called 'added' sugars), the possible effect of factors in foods that may protect against dental caries are important issues for health professionals and nutritional and dental scientists. The evidence relating diet to dental caries comes from a number of types of experiments, including human observational studies and human intervention studies, animal experiments, aforementioned plaque pH studies and in vitro laboratory experiments. The strongest evidence comes from human epidemiological studies; however, it is important to consider collative evidence from all types of study in order to obtain an overall picture regarding cariogenicity of a product.

THE ROLE OF DIETARY SUGARS

In the past, when sugar intake and levels of dental caries have been compared on an inter-country basis using food balance data and WHO data on caries levels of different countries, a positive correlation has been found. Today, the relationship is not so evident in countries that have a high sugars intake since the relationship between sugars intake and dental caries is thought to be sigmoid with countries having a high level of intake on the upper flattened part of the curve. However, sugar availability still accounts for over a quarter of the variation in dental caries levels.

Evidence for an association between sugars intake and dental caries also comes from observations of the marked increase in dental caries that has occurred in populations that have undergone the 'nutrition transition', that is they have moved away from their traditional diets that were low in free sugars and adopted a Westernised diet high in free sugars. The incidence of dental caries in Eskimos was very low before the introduction of a high sugars diet but dental caries subsequently increased rapidly. It is sometimes argued that in such populations the change in diet also included an increased consumption of refined starch and therefore increased sugars intake was not the sole cause of the change in caries. However, inhabitants of the island of Tristan da Cunha had a traditional diet that was low in sugars but high in cooked starch (potato) but had low levels of caries until sugar was introduced into the diet in the 1940s, which resulted in a marked increase in dental caries.

Other epidemiological studies have observed the level of dental caries in groups of people that habitually consume high or low amounts of sugars in their diet. Examples of high sugars consumers in which higher than average levels of dental caries have been reported include confectionery workers, sugar cane cutters and children taking long-term sugared liquid medicines. A low level of caries has been reported in groups of people with a low sugars intake, including children in institutions where strict dietary regimens low in sugars are followed and also in children with hereditary fructose intolerance, a condition in which fructose, and therefore sucrose, must be avoided.

During the Second World War there was a reduction in sugar availability in many countries. Data exist from 11 European countries showing that a reduction in caries accompanied reduced sugar availability. Takahashi studied levels of dental caries and sugar intake before, during and after the Second World War in Japan. Sugar consumption fell from 15 kg/year before the war to only 0.2 kg/year in 1946 and the annual dental caries increment in the first permanent molars mirrored the changes in sugar availability. More recent data on levels of dental decay in children in Iraq have shown that the dramatic fall in sugars consumption (from 140g/d to 33g/d) that resulted from the 1990 UN sanctions resulted in a sharp fall in levels of dental caries in children aged between 6 and 15 years. In the 14–15-years age group the mean DMFT fell from 10.7 to 2.9 between 1989 and 1995 (Jamel et al 2004).

Cross-sectional studies correlating sugars consumption with dental caries experience have been popular as they are easy to do, but they can be misleading. This is because simultaneous measurements of diet and dental caries levels may not provide a true reflection of the role of diet in the development of the disease. Dental caries takes time to develop and therefore it is the diet several years earlier that may be responsible for current levels of dental caries. Cross-sectional studies are of most use in young children where diet has not changed radically since the eruption of the teeth. Such studies have shown, for example, dental caries development to be closely related to prolonged and frequent use of sugar-containing soft drinks in bottles and use of sugared medicines by children.

When investigating the association between diet and the development of dental caries it is best to relate sugars consumption to changes in dental caries over time in a longitudinal design; however, this type of study is relatively rare. Two famous longitudinal studies are that of Rugg-Gunn et al (1984) in northeast England and Burt et al (1988) in Michigan, USA. In the study of caries and diet of over 400 English adolescents (aged 11–12 years) a small but significant correlation existed between sugars intake and caries increment over 2 years. The top 10% of sugars consumers developed significantly more dental caries than the 10% with the lowest sugars intake. The Michigan study (Burt et al 1988) investigated the relationship between

sugars intake and dental caries increment over 3 years in children initially aged 10–15 years and also found a significant relationship between the amount of dietary sugars and dental caries. Intake of sugars was generally high for all subjects in this study, with only 20 out of 499 children consuming less than 75 g/day. Stecksén-Blinks & Gustafsson (1986) conducted a longitudinal study of Swedish children aged 8 and 13 years and measured dietary intake of sugars and caries increment over 1 year. Those children who developed two or fewer decayed surfaces had a significantly lower sugars intake compared with children who developed three or more carious surfaces. More recent longitudinal studies support these earlier findings.

Ruottinen et al (2004) in a cohort study that monitored dental caries and diet from birth to age 10 years, found that those with the highest intakes of sucrose (top 5%) had a significantly higher level of dental caries compared with those with the lowest sucrose consumption (bottom 5%): the average dmft was 3.9 and 1.9 respectively, meaning those with lowest sugars consumption had half the level of dental caries.

Human intervention studies

There have been two historic human intervention studies of special importance. First, the Vipeholm study was conducted in a mental institution in Sweden shortly after the Second World War. The 964 patients (80% of whom were male) were divided by wards into one control group and six test groups. Groups were given high sucrose intakes at meals only, or at and between meals, in non-sticky (sucrose solution, chocolate) or sticky forms (caramels, toffees, sweet bread). The study was complicated but from the results it was concluded that: sugars consumption even at high levels is associated with only a small increase in caries increment if taken up to four times a day as part of meals; consumption of sugars between meals as well as at meals is associated with a marked increase in caries; and caries activity disappears on withdrawal of sugars from the diet. The highest caries increment was observed in the group that consumed 24 sticky toffees throughout the day. However, subtle differences between types of sugars were largely overridden by the effect of frequency. It would not be possible to repeat such a study today, as it would be unethical to prescribe high-sugars diets knowing of the association between sugars and dental caries.

The second human intervention study took place in Turku, Finland, in the 1970s. The aim of this 2-year study was to investigate the effect on dental caries of nearly total substitution of sucrose in a normal diet with either fructose or xylitol. When only cavities were counted the results showed 56% fewer cavities in the xylitol group than in the sucrose group but a similar number of cavities formed in the sucrose and fructose groups. The diet containing xylitol was therefore less cariogenic than the sucrose or fructose diets, but fructose was no less cariogenic than sucrose. The inability of plaque microorganisms to metabolise xylitol to acids probably explains this cariostatic effect.

More recently Rodrigues & Sheiham (2000) investigated the impact of introducing guidelines to reduce sugars intake in nursery schools in Brazil. Children attending nurseries that had not adopted the guidelines had sugars intake more than twice those that had adopted the guidelines (53 vs 22.9 g/day) and were almost five times more likely to develop dental caries.

Frequency and amount of sugars

The strong correlation between frequency and amount of sugars is clearly seen in many animal experiments (Table 25.2). The results of experiments in rats have shown caries severity to increase with increasing sugars concentration up to a concentration of 40% (see Fig. *evolve* 25.3). The frequency of intake was similar in the groups of rats so the weight and concentration of sugars eaten related to the severity of caries. Evidence from studies in humans also shows that the two variables are strongly associated (see Fig. *evolve* 25.4).

Some studies in humans have shown that frequency of sugars intake is related to caries development, including the aforementioned Vipeholm study. Studies conducted since the more widespread use of fluoride toothpaste have also shown caries development to be lower when intake of sugars does not exceed four times a day: for example, in a study of 5-year-old Icelandic children, those consuming sugars four or more times a day or three or more times between meals per day had significantly more caries compared with children who consumed sugars less frequently. Therefore it can be postulated that if intake of free sugars is limited to a maximum of four times a day, caries levels will be reduced. However, there is evidence from several longitudinal studies showing that the amount of sugars intake is more important than frequency, and epidemiological data show that as sugars intake exceeds 15 kg/year, frequency of intake of sugars increases. Therefore, there is evidence to show that both amount of sugars intake and the frequency with which they are eaten are important for caries development. However, as the two variables are strongly associated, reducing one of these variables will result in a reduction in the other.

STARCHES AND DENTAL CARIES

It has been suggested by some (e.g. the Biscuit, Cake, Chocolate and Confectionery Alliance) that all carbohydrate foods, sugars and starches should be considered cariogenic. This is because saliva contains amylase, which may hydrolyse dietary starch to form glucose, maltose and maltotriose that can then be fermented by plaque bacteria to acids. However, starch is heterogeneous in nature; it varies in botanical origin, may be consumed in its raw form as in fruits and vegetables or it may be cooked, and varies widely in degree of refinement and processing, and all these factors must be considered when assessing the cariogenicity of starches. Current dietary guidelines promote the consumption of starch-rich staple foods such as bread, potatoes, pasta, rice, other cereal grains and of fruit and vegetables. It is therefore important that the cariogenic potential of such foods is understood so that dietary advice for general health is not contraindicated in terms of dental health.

There is little evidence from epidemiological, animal and experimental studies of an association

Table 25.2	The mean number of carious fissure surfaces and daily food intake in four groups of rats fed at different frequencies per day; six animals per group		
GROUP	EATING FREQUENCY	NO. OF CARIOUS FISSURES	DAILY FOOD INTAKE (G)
1	12	0.7	6.0
2	18	2.2	6.0
3	24	4.0	6.0
4	30	4.7	6.0

(Reprinted from König et al 1968, with permission from Elsevier)

between intake of staple starchy foods and dental caries, and epidemiological studies have generally shown that populations with a high intake of starch-rich staple foods have low levels of caries. Further information on the cariogenic potential of starchy foods can be found in a thorough review of the evidence from epidemiological, animal and experimental studies (Rugg-Gunn 1993) and in Section *evolve* 25.4a.

FRUIT AND DENTAL CARIES

There is little evidence from epidemiological studies to show fresh whole fruit to be an important factor in the development of dental caries, and in fact apples have long been used as a symbol of oral health. Clinical trials of the effects of apple consumption on dental caries produced equivocal results; however, apples do contain polyphenols, which have an antibacterial nature. Fresh fruit contains 'intrinsic sugars', sugars that naturally form an integral part of the food and are not thought to be a threat to dental health (Department of Health 1989). Despite this, animal studies have shown that fruit causes caries when consumed at very high frequencies, often in a pulped form (i.e. extrinsic), and some plaque pH studies have found fruit to be acidogenic, but less so than sucrose. It is important to consider, however, that plaque pH studies take no account of the protective factors found in fresh fruits or of the fact that they provide a good stimulus to salivary flow. Based on the available evidence, it is probable that there is no relationship between whole fresh fruit and dental caries.

Many fruits are acidic, for example citric acid in citrus fruits, oxalic acid in rhubarb, tartaric acid in grapes and malic acid in apples. This has led to concern that fruit consumption may contribute to erosive tooth wear. Fruit juices are more erosive than whole fruits primarily because they are much more concentrated (1 × 200 ml portion of orange juice contains the juice of approximately three oranges). In addition, consumption of whole fruit provides a good stimulus to salivary flow which neutralises acid. Most data associating whole fruit consumption with dental erosion come from one-off case studies of unusual dietary habits, and the WHO report *Diet, nutrition and the prevention of chronic diseases* concluded that there was insufficient evidence to link whole fruit consumption to increased risk of dental erosion (WHO 2003).

In conclusion, fruit juices contain 'extrinsic sugars' and fruit acids along with fewer protective factors compared with whole fruits and they therefore pose a threat to dental health. By contrast, as habitually consumed, whole fruit does not pose significant risk to dental health and replacing foods high in free sugars with fresh fruit is likely to reduce dental decay.

OTHER CARBOHYDRATES AND DENTAL DECAY

Modern diets contain an increasing array of carbohydrates other than starches and sugars including maltodextrins, glucose syrups (collectively known as glucose polymers) and non-digestible oligosaccharides such as oligofructose and gluco-oligosaccharides. The latter are increasingly being used in foods as they are pre-biotics, encouraging the growth of favourable colonic bacteria. Relatively much less is understood on the cariogenic potential of these carbohydrates. However, the limited data that are available suggest that they are not safe for teeth.

THE ROLE OF FLUORIDE IN CARIES PREVENTION

Fluoride increases the resistance of the teeth to decay in several ways. First, if ingested during the development of the enamel, it becomes incorporated into the enamel crystal structure and replaces the hydroxyl groups in hydroxyapatite to form fluoroapatite, which is more stable and resistant to demineralisation. Second, remineralisation of enamel in the presence of fluoride results in the porous lesion being remineralised with fluoroapatite rather than hydroxyapatite; and thirdly, fluoride inhibits bacterial sugars metabolism, which results in less acid production. The inverse relationship between fluoride in drinking water and dental caries is well established and shows that fluoridation reduces dental caries by approximately 50% but does not eliminate dental caries. The benefits of water fluoridation have been observed even in populations where use of other sources of fluoride such as fluoride toothpaste is widespread.

Arguments for and against water fluoridation

The link between water fluoride content and dental caries prevention was first established in the USA in the early twentieth century and its effectiveness has now been demonstrated in over a hundred surveys in more than 20 countries including the UK. The first area in the UK to have an artificially fluoridated water supply was Birmingham in 1964, an area that consequently has seen a dramatic improvement in levels of dental caries. The reduction in dental treatment arising from fluoridation results in considerable savings to health costs, due to the fall in the number of extractions and general anaesthetics. There are examples where water fluoridation has been discontinued and subsequently levels of dental caries have increased, for example areas of Scotland including Kilmarnock, Wick and Stranraer where dental caries levels increased, despite the fact that fluoride toothpastes were available. A 25% increase in dental caries was observed in some areas of Scotland over 5 years after removal of water fluoridation.

Fluoridation of drinking water can substantially decrease dental caries but an excess of fluoride during the development of the teeth may cause 'dental fluorosis', an enamel developmental defect that manifests as small white diffuse opacities with severe pitting and staining of enamel in more severe cases. For permanent teeth the period when there is greatest risk from excess fluoride is between 2 and 6 years. Severe fluorosis is rare in the UK and cases have usually been linked with excessive fluoride ingestion from eating toothpaste or misuse of fluoride supplements. Severe fluorosis is observed particularly in countries that have very high levels of fluoride in water supplies. Enamel fluorosis as well as skeletal fluorosis are found in large areas of India, Thailand, in the Rift Valley of East Africa and in many Arab states. It is important to realise that fluoride is not the only cause of opacities in teeth.

The optimal level of fluoride in water is the level at which a substantial caries reduction is observed with a negligible prevalence of enamel fluorosis. In temperate climates including the UK the optimum concentration of fluoride is 1.0 mg/l, while in warmer climates it might be nearer 0.6 mg/l. Water fluoridation is endorsed by more than 150 science and health organisations including the International Dental Federation, the International Association for Dental Research and the WHO. Despite this expert endorsement, there are small groups of people who strongly oppose water fluoridation on the grounds of perceived health risks and imposed treatment of the water supply (see Section *evolve* 25.4b).

In conclusion, fluoridation of the water supply is a caries-preventive measure with the potential to reach the sectors of the population that are at highest risk of caries. One could argue that in some areas, where caries levels are very low, water fluoridation might not be a cost-effective measure. However, in some parts of the UK and other countries, including areas of social deprivation, prevalence of caries remains high and dental attendance, oral hygiene practice and dietary habits are poor. For such areas water fluoridation is a highly effective, economical public health measure.

Other sources of fluoride

The WHO report *Diet, nutrition and the prevention of chronic diseases* (WHO 2003) recommended that 'There should be promotion of adequate fluoride exposure via appropriate vehicles, for example affordable toothpaste, water, salt and milk'. Fluorides are widely found in nature in addition to being naturally present in some water supplies. Fluoride is found in seafood (when bones are eaten), tea leaves, some beers and in foods cooked in fluoridated water. In addition to water, suitable vehicles for artificial fluoridation are salt and milk although neither of these is used extensively. Salt fluoridation has been successfully implemented in Switzerland since 1955 and fluoridated salt sits alongside non-fluoridated salt in supermarkets, allowing the consumer choice, which is politically advantageous. In the UK a school milk fluoridation scheme was first introduced in the 1990s in Merseyside and its success has led to the growth of other schemes throughout the UK, which now involves over 42 000 children aged 3–11 in 16 local authority districts (see www.borrowfoundation.org). School milk fluoridation provides a useful means of conveying the benefits of fluoride to children living in socially disadvantaged communities where the water supply is non-fluoridated.

Dietary fluoride provides a local effect on the teeth whilst in the mouth and a systemic effect on the teeth after digestion and absorption. Fluoride in toothpaste and mouth rinse provides a mainly topical effect as these are not supposed to be swallowed.

Is refined sugar as strongly related to dental decay in the presence of fluoride?

Despite a marked effect of fluoride on caries prevalence, a relationship between sugars intake and caries still exists in the presence of fluoride. Longitudinal studies of the relationship between intake of dietary sugars and dental caries levels in children in the UK and USA have shown that the observed relationship between sugars intake and development of dental caries remains even after controlling for use of fluoride. Data from the National Diet and Nutrition Survey of children aged 1.5–4.5 years also shows a significant relationship between frequency of sugar-rich snacks and caries levels in young children even after controlling for use of fluoride. A study conducted in northeast England reported on the decrease in dental caries levels during the Second World War in 12-year-old children from areas with naturally high and low water fluoride. Caries levels were lower in the high fluoride area in 1943 but, following the wartime sugar restriction, dental caries levels fell further by approximately 50%, thus indicating that exposure to fluoride did not totally override the effect of sugar in the diet. A comprehensive literature review on changes in caries prevalence and associated factors (Marthaler 1990) concluded that even in modern societies that make use of preventive measures such as fluoride, a relationship between sugars consumption and caries still exists and free sugars remain the main threat for dental health in some developed and many developing countries. It is likely that, in industrialised countries where there is adequate exposure to fluoride, a further reduction in the prevalence and severity of dental caries will not be achieved without a reduction in the intake of free sugars. For example in fluoridated areas in the Republic of Ireland 30% of 5-year-olds and 46% of 12-year-olds still have decay. Furthermore, a systematic review (Burt & Pai 2001) that addressed whether in the era of extensive fluoride exposure individuals with a high level of sugars intake have greater caries severity compared with those with lower sugars intake concluded that, where there is good exposure to fluoride, sugars consumption is a moderate risk factor for caries in most people, but sugars consumption is likely to be a more powerful indicator for risk of caries in persons who do not have regular exposure to fluoride. Overall it was concluded that, where there is adequate use of fluoride, reduction of sugars consumption still has a role to play in the prevention of caries but this role is not as strong as it is without exposure to fluoride.

OTHER DIETARY FACTORS

Other minerals

Apart from fluoride there are other trace elements that influence dental caries although the influence is of relatively small importance. Dietary molybdenum, strontium, boron and lithium are related to a lower caries experience in humans while higher selenium intakes are related to higher caries prevalence.

Other factors that protect against dental caries

The protective effect of some food components against dental caries has been recognised for decades. In the 1930s Osborn and Noriskin suggested that foods provided substances that protect against decay. Apart from the well-recognised role of fluoride, other dietary components such as phosphates, calcium, casein and polyphenols may also have cariostatic properties. Milk, despite containing approximately 4% sugars as lactose, was one of the first foods to be described as cariostatic. Although lactose may be fermented to acid, it has been shown to be the least cariogenic of the common dietary sugars. Milk also contains high concentrations of calcium and phosphate and is also rich in casein. Many studies of several types have all indicated that milk is not cariogenic and may even protect against dental caries. The cariostatic nature of cheese is also well established with evidence from animal and human experimental and intervention studies demonstrating its cariostatic nature. Cheese is a strong gustatory stimulus to salivary flow which conveys protection to the teeth. However, cheese has been shown to be cariostatic in animals that have had their salivary glands removed and so the cariostatic effect is not due to saliva alone. A high concentration of calcium and phosphate and the formation of casein phosphopeptides are thought to convey a strong anti-caries effect.

Inorganic phosphates protect against dental caries by increasing the availability of phosphate in plaque so that demineralisation is resisted and remineralisation encouraged. Organic phosphates protect mainly by binding to the tooth surface and reducing enamel dissolution. Phytates are the most effective of these compounds. Despite promising results from incubation and animal experiments for a cariostatic effect of phosphates, studies in humans showed them to be less effective, possibly due to the higher phosphate concentration of human compared with rat saliva. Phytates also reduce the absorption of some micronutrients, e.g. iron and zinc, and are therefore unsuitable as caries-preventive food additives.

Recent interest is focusing on the cariostatic properties of polyphenolic compounds found in plant foods. Apples contain polyphenols yet clinical trials of the impact of apples on dental caries have shown equivocal results. Polyphenolic compounds in cranberries have antimicrobial effects and have been shown to reduce the adhesion of mutans streptococci. Both green and oolong teas contain polyphenolic compounds that have been shown to suppress mutans streptococci and reduce extracellular glucan formation. Other foods such as honey, chocolate and liquorice all contain factors that protect against dental caries but the benefits of these factors is overridden by the negative effect of the high sugars content of these foods or in the case of liquorice the dark staining effects.

Sugar-free foods that stimulate salivary flow can be classed as caries protective and include sugar-free chewing gum. Plaque pH studies have shown that chewing sugar-free gum increases plaque pH (see Fig. *evolve* 25.5). Results of several clinical trials have shown that sugared gums are cariogenic when compared with sugar-free gum or no gum and sugar-free gums are caries preventing compared with no gum. The most impressive results have been obtained with gums containing the non-sugar sweetener xylitol.

KEY POINTS

- Diet influences the teeth while forming but this effect is of less importance than the local intra-oral effect of diet on the teeth.
- Evidence from many different types of study has shown that both the frequency and the amount of intake of sugars are related to dental caries.
- Free sugars are the main culprits and should be the target for reduction. Starch-rich staple foods, fresh fruit and vegetables are not a threat to dental health and their intake should be increased, in line with numerous, non-commercial, authoritative reports.
- Some foods protect against decay. These include milk, cheese, some plant foods and foods that stimulate salivary flow.

- Fluoride, both dietary and non-dietary, is a highly effective caries-preventive measure but it does not eliminate dental caries. In populations exposed to fluoride, further reductions in caries levels will not occur without dietary modification.

25.5 NUTRITION AND PERIODONTAL DISEASE

Historically, periodontal disease has been seen to have little association with nutrition as earlier epidemiological studies failed to show associations between nutrition and disease levels. However, a more comprehensive knowledge of the disease at the cellular level and improved means of assessing nutritional status have resulted in refreshed interest in the role of nutrition in the aetiology of periodontal diseases. There is some evidence that certain forms of periodontal disease progress more rapidly in undernourished populations. The impaired immune response that occurs in undernutrition increases the vulnerability of the periodontal tissues to inflammatory stimuli from plaque (Enwonwu 1994). Assessing the importance of specific nutrient deficiencies on indices of periodontal disease may be difficult in population studies because periodontal disease usually develops slowly, and nutritional evaluation rarely reflects lifelong nutritional conditions. Individual nutritional deficiencies which may be strongly related to periodontal disease may affect only a few individuals; the problem is hidden in a large epidemiological survey. However, interestingly, a recent analysis of data from the USA National Health and Nutrition Examination Survey (NHANES) III Survey has found an inverse relationship between the intake of dietary calcium and periodontal disease. Risk of periodontal disease increased in females by 27% and 54% when intake of calcium was below 800 and 499 mg per day respectively (Nishida et al 2000). The gingival epithelium has a high requirement for folate due to these cells having a rapid turnover. Experimental studies in humans have shown that topical application of folate is effective in preventing gingivitis in pregnant women. Further analysis of NHANES III data has shown low serum folate to be independently associated with periodontal disease in older adults after controlling for confounding factors (Yu et al 2007).

A deficiency of vitamin C has been historically associated with periodontal disease since destruction of the dental supporting tissues is a symptom of scurvy. More recent studies have shown a weak but significant association between vitamin C status and indices of periodontitis. Vitamin C is essential for collagen formation, which is important for structural integrity of the periodontal ligament, blood vessel walls and alveolar bone matrix and is also a powerful antioxidant.

Dietary antioxidants may play an important role in protecting the tissues of the gingival from reactive oxygen species generated by plaque bacterial pathogens in periodontal disease. An association between ROS and periodontal inflammation exists. Several studies indicate antioxidant status is compromised in periodontal disease and a recent analysis of data from the NHANES III survey in the USA showed an inverse relationship between serum total antioxidant capacity and periodontitis (Chapple et al 2007). The impact of improving antioxidant status through dietary means on risk and progression of periodontitis remains to be determined. Despite interesting recent developments in the field of nutrition and periodontal disease, the main focus for prevention or treatment of periodontal disease is plaque removal.

KEY POINTS

- Historically periodontal disease was seen to have little association with nutrition with the exception of the established link between severe vitamin C deficiency and the oral symptoms of scurvy
- Recent analysis of epidemiological studies has shown a weak but signficiant association between vitamin C status and adult periodontitis
- Periodontal disease progresses more rapidly in the presence of undernutrition.
- Recent data from the USA NHANES survey has shown periodontitis to be associated with low dietary intakes of calcium and folate
- Periodontitis is associated with a decreased antioxidant vitamin status but it has not been established as to whether this is causal.

References

Burt B, Pai S: Sugar consumption and caries risk: a systematic review, *Journal of Dental Education* 65(10):1017–1023, 2001.

Burt BA, Eklund SA, Morgan KJ, et al: The effects of sugars intake and frequency of ingestion on dental caries increment in a three-year longitudinal study, *Journal of Dental Research* 67:1422–1429, 1988.

Chapple ILC, Milward MR, Dietrich T: The prevalence of inflammatory periodontitis is negatively associated with serum antioxidant concentrations, *Journal of Nutrition* 137:657–664, 2007.

Department of Health: *Dietary sugars and human diseases.* Report on Health and Social Subjects No 37, London, 1989, HMSO.

Enwonwu CO: Cellular and molecular effects of malnutrition and their relevance to periodontal disease, *Journal of Clinical Periodontology* 21:643–657, 1994.

Jamel H, Plasschaert A, Sheiman A: Dental caries experience and availability of sugars in Iraqi children before and after the United Nations sanctions, *International Dental Journal* 54:21–25, 2004.

König KG, Schmid P, Schmid R: An apparatus for frequency-controlled feeding of small rodents and its use in dental caries experiments, *Archives of Oral Biology* 13:13–26.A, 1968.

Marthaler T: Changes in the prevalence of dental caries: how much can be attributed to changes in diet? *Caries Research* 24:3–15, 1990.

Nishida M, Grossi SG, Dunford RG, Ho AW, Trevisan M, Genco RJ: Calcium and the risk for periodontal disease, *Journal of Periodontology* 71:1057–1066, 2000.

Rodrigues CS, Sheiham A: The relationships between dietary guidelines, sugar intake and caries in primary teeth in low income Brazilian 3-year-olds: a longitudinal study, *International Journal of Paediatric Dentistry* 10:47–55, 2000.

Rugg-Gunn AJ: *Nutrition and dental health,* Oxford, 1993, Oxford Medical Publications.

Rugg-Gunn AJ, Edgar WM, Geddes DAM, Jenkins GN: The effect of different meal patterns upon plaque pH in human subjects, *British Dental Journal* 139:351–356, 1975.

Rugg-Gunn AJ, Hackett AF, Appleton DR, et al: Relationship between dietary habits and caries increment assessed over two years in 405 English adolescent schoolchildren, *Archives of Oral Biology* 29:983–992, 1984.

Ruottinen S, Karjalainen S, Pienihakkinen K, et al: Sucrose intake since infancy and dental health in 10-year old children, *Caries Research* 38:142–148, 2004.

Russell RRB: Microbiological aspects of caries prevention. In Murray JJ, Nunn JH, Steele GJ, editors:

Prevention of oral disease, Oxford, 2003, Oxford University Press.

Sreebny LM: Cereal availability and dental caries, *Community Dentistry and Oral Epidemiology* 11:148–155, 1983.

Stecksén-Blicks C, Gustafsson L. Impact of oral hygiene and use of fluoride on caries increment in children during one year. *Community Dentistry and Oral Epidemiology* 14:185–189, 1986.

WHO: *Diet, nutrition and the prevention of chronic diseases.* Technical Report Series 916, Geneva, 2003, World Health Organization, Food and Agricultural Organization.

Yu Y–H, Kuo H-K, Lai Y-L: The association between serum folate levels and periodontal disease in older adults: data from the National Health and Nutrition Examination Survey 2001/02. *Journal of the American Geriatrics Society* 55:108–113, 2007.

Further reading

Fejerskov O, Kidd E: *Dental caries: the disease and its clinical management*, ed 2, Oxford, 2008, Blackwell Munksgaard.

Moynihan: Update on the nomenclature of carbohydrates and their dental effects, *Journal of Dentistry* 26:209–218, 1996.

Moynihan P: Foods and Factors that prevent dental caries, *Quintessence International* 38:130–134, 2007.

Moynihan PJ: Dietary advice in dental practice, *British Dental Journal* 93:563–568, 2002.

Murray JJ, Nunn JH, Steele JG: *Prevention of oral disease*, Oxford, 2003, Oxford University Press.

Rugg-Gunn AJ, Nunn JH: *Nutrition, diet and oral health*, Oxford, 1999, Oxford University Press.

Sheiham A: Dietary effects on dental diseases, *Public Health Nutrition* 4:569–591, 2001.

WHO: *Fluorides and oral health*. WHO Technical Report Series No 846, Geneva, 1996, WHO.

EVOLVE CONTENTS (available online at: evolve.elsevier.com/Geissler/nutrition)

Chapter 26

Immune function, food allergies and food intolerance

Stephan Strobel*

CHAPTER CONTENTS

*Updated and modified from the previous edition chapter
written by Stephen Strobel and Anne Ferguson, and with a
contribution by Andrew Tomkins

© 2010 Elsevier Ltd/Inc/BV
DOI: 10.1016/B978-0-7020-3118-2.00026-7

OBJECTIVES

By the end of this chapter you should:

- understand major aspects of the immune system and its regulation with particular reference to food allergies
- be able to discuss factors and mechanisms involved in immunological sensitisation and tolerance
- appreciate the effects of AIDS on immunity and the public health implications
- be familiar with the broad spectrum of food allergic diseases, food intolerances and their diagnosis, and principles of therapeutic management
- be familiar with and understand the effects of protein or micronutrient deficiencies on host immunity and immune responses
- be able to contribute to discussion on nutritional strategies related to diagnosis and management of adverse reactions to food.

26.1 INTRODUCTION

The science of immunology arose from the study of human resistance to infection. It was appreciated that after recovery from a particular infectious disease, the same disease rarely occurred again. This altered reactivity is what we call specific immunity and is mediated by T- and B-lymphocytes, antibodies, and by a broad range of immunological mechanisms. Immunology also encompasses non-specific antimicrobial protective mechanisms. These are innate in that they are not affected by prior contact with the infectious agent(s). Close relationships between innate and adaptive immunity are becoming better understood and specific receptors provide interfaces between these integrated defence systems. This chapter discusses features of the immune system and explores the relationships between nutrition, immunodeficiencies and interactions between micronutrient status and immune function. Finally, aspects of diagnosis and management of food allergy and food intolerance are discussed, with specific examples.

26.2 STRUCTURE AND FUNCTION OF THE IMMUNE SYSTEM

Cells which participate in immune responses are collected together in the lymphoid organs: thymus, spleen, lymph nodes, and Peyer's patches. In this environment they can perform their functions very effectively and they also disseminate immunity by migrating throughout the body. There are many other sites, particularly the mucosae, where cells of the immune system are dispersed between other cells, for example within the gut epithelium and lamina propria and other mucosal sites such as the respiratory tract, the breast and urogenital tract (Brandtzaeg 2007) (Fig. 26.1).

CELLS INVOLVED IN IMMUNITY

A wide range of cells participate in non-specific and specific immunity and many of these fulfil several different functions. *T (thymus-dependent) lymphocytes* perform important immunoregulatory functions via their secreted products and also act as effector cells, capable of killing other cells. Many immunological diseases, both immunodeficiency and abnormally enhanced reactivity, can ultimately be attributed to defects of T-cell regulatory function. In terms of protective immunity, T-cells are particularly important in defence against intracellular bacterial and protozoal pathogens, viruses and fungi.

Natural killer (NK) cells, which can develop without thymic influence, provide an important link at the interface of innate and adaptive

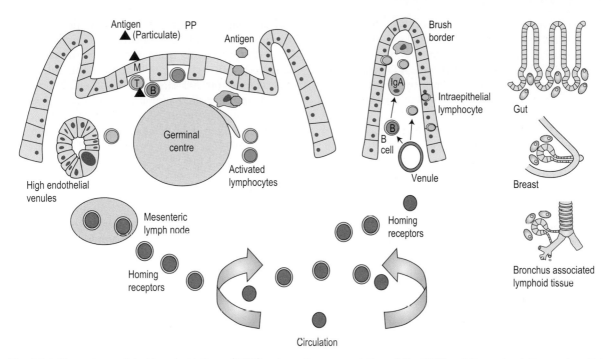

Fig. 26.1 The gut–associated lymphoid tissue (GALT): schematic representation of the GALT and the recirculation and partial homing pathway of activated lymphocytes. Once the T-lymphocytes in the Peyer's patches have become activated by gut-derived antigens they leave the mucosa and reach the systemic circulation via high endothelial venules, the mesenteric lymph nodes and the thoracic duct. From here, some home back to the lamina propria, others (T-lymphocytes) may reach other mucosal sites and in this way distribute gut-derived 'information' throughout the mucosa-associated lymphoid tissues (after Brandtzaeg 2003).

immunity. They are large granular lymphocytes which do not express markers of conventional T- or B cell lineage. These cells exhibit low affinity Fc receptors for IgG (FcRg) and can kill target cells by using antibody-dependent mechanisms or may, for example, kill virus-infected cells without prior sensitisation through perforin, which is a cytolytic protein stored in secretory granules of NK cells.

B-lymphocytes are independent of the thymus and in humans probably complete their early maturation within the bone marrow. When appropriately stimulated, B-lymphocytes undergo proliferation, maturation and differentiation to form immunoglobulin-producing plasma cells. Eventually there are many identical daughters derived from a single B-cell, forming a clone. The enormous diversity of antibodies that an individual can produce is explained partly by rearrangements of nucleic acid within precursor B-cells and partly by random mutation.

Antigen-presenting cells are found mainly in the lymphoid organs and the skin, and their main role is to present antigen in a particular way to lymphocytes

so as to start off the antigen-specific immune responses. They include interdigitating cells in the thymus, the Langerhans cells of the skin, interdigitating cells in the T areas of lymph nodes and follicular dendritic cells in B areas of lymph nodes.

MOLECULES OF THE IMMUNE SYSTEM

Immunoglobulins

Immunoglobulin (Ig) molecules are the effector products of B-cells and, although they all have a broadly similar structure, minor differences within the main immunological classes (IgG, IgM, IgA, IgD and IgE) are associated with a range of important biological properties. Molecules almost identical to secreted immunoglobulins are incorporated in the cell membranes of B-cells (surface Ig) and there are many related molecules concerned with antigen recognition and cell–cell communication.

In healthy adults, IgG accounts for more than 70% of the immunoglobulins in normal serum and is distributed equally between the blood and extracellular fluids. Infants receive the immunoglobulin of the G class via placental transfer from around 32 weeks of gestation. Other immunoglobulin classes (IgA, IgM, IgE, IgD) are usually produced after birth and are not transmitted transplacentally. Increased IgM levels at birth can indicate an intrauterine infection.

IgA accounts for about 20% of the total serum immunoglobulins. However, its function within the bloodstream and tissues is thought to be less important than its role as a secretory antibody. IgA is produced in two subclasses, IgA_1 and IgA_2. IgA_2 is usually found in areas of greatest bacterial exposure (gastrointestinal tract) and is more resistant to bacterial proteases. In the blood, IgA_1 is the predominant class. The major sites of IgA_2 synthesis are the laminae propriae underlying the respiratory tract, the gut and other mucosae. Secretory IgA as a dimer linked by a joining 'J' chain confers immunity to infection by enteric bacterial and viral pathogens and may also be involved in the regulation of the commensal gut flora. Oral immunisation strategies are used to induce protective immunity to intestinal infections such as cholera and others.

IgE concentration in serum is generally very low. This is partly because it has a considerable affinity for cell surfaces and binds to mast cells, eosinophils and basophils via low- and high-affinity receptors. Specific IgE antibodies are usually required for immediate hypersensitivity reactions, such as occur in atopic individuals, for instance in hay fever and food allergic reactions of the anaphylactic type. The physiological function of IgE antibodies in humans is unclear but they appear to be important in defence against helminth parasites (worms) and may have a role in targeting allergens to antigen-presenting cells.

Molecules on cell membrane

Various cells exhibit characteristic cytological features, but it must be appreciated that, particularly within the population of lymphocytes, cells which appear morphologically identical may be functionally very different. Many techniques are available to detect cell membrane molecules, which indicate the stage of differentiation and activation of lymphocytes, macrophages and other cells and thus allow subdivision of the main morphological categories.

Identification of CD (cluster of differentiation) surface markers on lymphocytes is valuable in clinical diagnosis (e.g. of immunodeficiency syndromes) and in the classification of malignancies. CD testing is usually done on a FACS (fluorescence-activated cell sorter) with monoclonal antibodies and well over 300 distinct human CD markers have been described. For a list and more detailed information see http://www.hlda9.org/Molecule-Information/tabid/54/Default.aspx, or http://www.ebioscience.com/ebioscience/whatsnew/humancdchart.htm.

Cytokines

In the late 1960s it was recognised that lymphocytes mediated their effects not only through direct cell-to-cell contact but also through soluble factors such as cytokines or both. Over 20 of such cytokines have now been described and various tests of antigen-specific cell-mediated immunity are available, based on the secretion of these factors by cells of the immune system. (See Figure *evolve* 26.1 for a scheme showing Th differentiation in mice and humans).

Interleukin-1 (IL-1)

IL-1 is secreted by many cell types in the presence of antigen or tissue injury. Cells that produce IL-1 are also able to present antigen to T-cells: stimulation of T-cells simultaneously with processed antigen and IL-1 is required for initiation of a specific immune response. IL-1-producing cells include circulating monocytes, macrophages, fibroblasts, B-cells and epithelial cells.

Interleukin-2 (IL-2)

IL-2 is secreted by activated T-cells and is responsible for amplification of the population of responding T-cells and for inducing the production of other cytokines from many cell types.

Tumour necrosis factor-alpha (TNF-α)

TNF-α is produced by mononuclear phagocytes in vitro when they are stimulated with bacterial endotoxin. TNF-α has effects on general cellular metabolism; it causes weight loss, fever and acute phase reaction (associated with infection or neoplasia). It activates other mononuclear cells and granulocytes and increases their non-specific killing capability. New members of this large family emerge regularly.

Interferon-gamma (IFN-γ)

IFN-γ is produced mainly by activated T-cells of the Th1 (T-helper cell) population following exposure to antigens or macrophages and natural killer (NK) cells. It increases class II expression on epithelial cells (among other cell and tissue types). This leads to increased antigen-presenting activity. It also activates macrophages for antitumour activity, in synergy with TNF-α.

Interleukin-4 (IL-4)

IL-4 is secreted by another functional subgroup of T-helper cells, the so-called Th2 cells. This cytokine affects T- and B-lymphocytes, NK cells, macrophages and others. IL-4 is particularly involved in cell growth and IgE isotype selection. Allergic patients have a tendency to respond to allergens with IL-4 secretion whereas non-allergic patients predominantly secrete IFN-γ under these conditions.

Interleukin-10 (IL-10)

Interleukin-10 is produced primarily by lymphocytes and monocytes. It has many effects in immunoregulation and inflammation. It downregulates the expression of Th1 cytokines, MHC class II antigens, and co-stimulatory molecules on macrophages and acts in a tolerance-inducing fashion. It also enhances B-cell survival, proliferation, and antibody production.

Interleukin-17 (IL-17)

Interleukin 17 is part of a large, recently described cytokine family and can regulate innate immunity and activities of phagocytes. It is secreted by a distinct Th-lymphocyte population (Th17) and promotes autoimmunity and has antiviral activity; it is also probably involved in the generation of oral tolerance phenomena.

Transforming growth factor beta (TGF-β)

TGF-β is a regulatory cytokine secreted by T-lymphocytes and affects B- and T-lymphocytes, macrophages and other cells. It has anti-inflammatory, suppressive (IgG, IgM) and stimulatory (IgA) effects and is thought to play a major role in oral tolerance induction.

Cells and interleukins do not act in isolation and subsequent responses such as tissue damage/repair are the result of an immunological cascade.

The major histocompatibility complex

Although the major histocompatibility complex (MHC) was originally identified through its role in transplant rejection, it is now recognised that proteins encoded by this region of the genome are involved in many aspects of immunological recognition. These include interactions between different lymphoid cells as well as between lymphocytes and antigen-presenting cells.

The MHC gene cluster is located on chromosome 6. It contains genes coding for the 'human leukocyte antigen' (HLA) cell surface glycoproteins, which are found on many cells, not only leukocytes.

Patterns of immune responses to fed antigen

The immune system of the gastrointestinal tract (gut-associated lymphoid tissue, GALT) has a number of different roles. When the route of entry is through the intestinal epithelium or follicle-associated epithelium of Peyer's patches of immunologically normal and mature mammals, the general trend is towards suppression of immunity, in other words, *oral tolerance*. However, active immunisation may also follow the feeding of antigen and this is typically in the form of harmless secretory IgA antibody. In some circumstances there is, however, induction of potentially pathogenic immune reactions when antigen is fed, for example IgE, IgG antibody or T-cell-mediated immunity. Thus there may be either induction or suppression of a particular immune response, whether antibody- or T-cell-mediated, when antigen is encountered via the gut (Fig. 26.2).

Regulation of gut immunity

T-lymphocytes are dispersed in the mucosa as well as in the organised lymphoid tissues of the GALT and, just as in the systemic immune system, gut T-lymphocytes have two main types of function: immunoregulatory and effector functions (Bischoff & Crowe 2004, Strobel & Mowat 2006).

Gut lymphoid cells generate protective immunity to infectious microorganisms and parasites. However, immune responses may disrupt intestinal anatomy and function by the 'innocent bystander' phenomenon. This occurs when substantial tissue damage occurs as an unavoidable by-product of a specific immune response to an infectious agent. The classical example of this is tuberculosis or leprosy. Inappropriate immune responses, developing in response to harmless antigens such as foods, are well recognised and

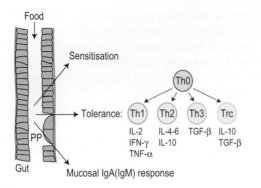

Fig. 26.2 Schematic diagram of the basic principles of oral tolerance induction to protein antigens. Single or multiple feeds will induce systemic tolerance and in some cases a mucosal immune response. This response may be favoured particularly if antigen gains access via the Peyer's patch. Under certain conditions, depending on the nature of the antigen and poorly understood host factors, systemic priming after oral antigen may also result. PP, Peyer's patch; Trc, T-regulatory cell.

are sometimes primarily responsible for the disease.

Oral tolerance (OT)

Oral tolerance describes a state of antigen-specific hyporesponsiveness or unresponsiveness after prior mucosal exposure. Breakdown of this homeostatic process is considered to be one cause of food hypersensitivity. The mechanisms by which tolerance is mediated include T-cell deletion, anergy (lack of immune response) and suppression. Cell-mediated delayed hypersensitivity reactions (Th1-type), which are implicated as pathogenetic mechanisms in the development of food-related gastrointestinal inflammation are particularly well suppressed. Regulatory events during the induction of tolerance are not well characterised. The balance between tolerance (suppression) and sensitisation (priming) is dependent on diverse factors including genetic background, nature of antigen, frequency and extent of administration, maturity of the immune system, immunological status of the host (e.g. affected by virus infections), maternal dietary exposure and antigen transmission via breast milk (Strobel & Mowat 2006, Berin & Mayer 2009).

Antigen administration during an ill-defined 'vulnerable' postnatal period is thought to have sensitising effects on individuals. Larger antigen doses may cause T-cell deletion and anergy, whereas smaller doses lead to suppression through induction of IL-4/IL-10-secreting Th2 cells and cells secreting IL-10 and TGF-β. Thus food allergic diseases can be envisaged as being due to a breakdown in the usual physiological downregulation of immunity to dietary and other gut-derived antigens. It is still unresolved whether early postnatal antigen exposure or delayed introduction are likely to prevent or reduce allergic sensitisation in the infant. Clinical studies that explore early antigen avoidance or increase exposure are currently underway. Major confounding variables in these studies are the genetic make up of the population studied, general eating habits, maternal food intake during and after pregnancy, duration of breast feeding and mode of delivery.

Allergic sensitisation

Patients are clinically sensitised when they have generated high enough specific IgE levels that permit elicitation of an allergic reaction. A number of individuals may have circulating antigen-specific IgE antibodies without clinical symptoms on ingestion of this particular food. This is one of the reasons why it is not possible to establish clinical diagnoses on the level of antigen-specific IgE alone. IgE antibody binds to high-affinity receptors on the surface of mast cells and basophils in such a manner that contact between only a few membrane-associated molecules and the inducing antigen will trigger the release of highly active mediators of inflammation, including histamine, proteolytic enzymes, leukotrienes and prostaglandins.

Aberrant immunity, malabsorption and infection

A range of dietary antigens, eaten every day, reach the organised lymphoid tissues in sufficient amounts to induce a variety of mostly harmless humoral and cellular immune responses. If a sensitisation has occurred, the entry of that same antigen in a further meal may result in a local immune reaction, which may cause immediate or delayed reactions including tissue damage.

Severe immunodeficiency states, where infants lack all or most important aspects of their immune system (e.g. X-linked severe combined immunodeficiency), do not cause primary nutritional deficiencies or morphological mucosal abnormalities. However, some intestinal and systemic infections resulting in failure to thrive states are common in these children and may secondarily lead to mucosal damage and nutritional deficiency states.

26.3 AN APPROACH TO CLINICAL INVESTIGATION OF THE IMMUNE SYSTEM

Protocols for the clinical evaluation of systemic immunity are widely used for the investigation and management of patients with primary, acquired, iatrogenic and nutrient-related immunodeficiency syndromes. Primary immunodeficiencies often present with bacterial, fungal or viral infections dependent on the underlying functional defect and microbiological investigations form a major part of clinical diagnostic workup. Genetic and functional tests are continuously evolving with the discovery of new immunodeficiency states and a better understanding of existing ones. About 150 primary immunodeficiencies that affect an extensive range of innate and adaptive immunity have been identified (Chinen & Shearer 2005, Geha et al 2007).

COMMONLY USED DIAGNOSTIC PROCEDURES FOR IMMUNODEFICIENCY STATES

Responses to immunisation, particularly with live vaccines (BCG), are valuable and can indicate normal or impaired cell-mediated immunity. An aberrant immune status can also be deduced from a history of atopy, for example rhinitis, eczema and asthma. Severe cell-mediated primary immunodeficiencies (SCID) usually present before 18 months of age. Isolated defects of immune function such as phagocytic and antibody deficiencies or combined immunodeficiencies may present during late childhood or adult life.

Blood examination

Examination of blood films should be the first investigation, with total white cell count, an accurately performed differential analysis and inspection of cell morphology. The absolute lymphocyte count in peripheral blood is an important but often neglected test. The final diagnosis of an immunode-

ficiency is based on specialised laboratory tests that must be interpreted by specialists in this area.

Genetic analysis forms an important part of the investigation of primary immunodeficiencies (Geha et al 2007).

Lymphocytes and specific cell-mediated immunity

Evidence of the existence of specific cell-mediated immunity (implying both normal afferent and efferent limbs) can be obtained by in vivo tests of delayed-type hypersensitivity, using a range of antigen to which the body will usually have been exposed. These 'recall' antigens include tuberculin, tetanus antigen and candida.

Many in vitro tests of antigen-reactive T-cell function are available, ranging from antigen-driven blast transformation to antigen-specific secretion of cytokines in culture. These tests are carried out using blood lymphocytes in specialised laboratories.

Immunoglobulins and antibodies

Assays of total immunoglobulins can be readily carried out on serum samples. Immediate skin prick tests and serum RAST tests are used for the in vivo and in vitro detection of IgE antibodies. More precise information on the induction and expression of humoral immunity is obtained by studying the primary and secondary immune responses to defined killed vaccine antigens.

Gastrointestinal mucosal immunity

It is difficult to study the immune system of the gastrointestinal tract in detail. Clinical tests of gastrointestinal immune function have been slow to develop and require mucosal biopsies and often short-term organ culture systems. Some guidelines for investigation of patients in whom intestinal mucosal immunodeficiency or hypersensitivity states may be present are given below.

Attention must also be paid to the potential roles of non-immunological digestive factors. These may act not only as alternative mechanisms of disease, mimicking immunological disorders (e.g. certain infections), but also as factors that will alter immunity in general (e.g. malnutrition, micronutrient deficiencies) or change intestinal antigen patterns (e.g. pancreatic insufficiency).

Mucosal hypersensitivity reactions

Normally it appears that pathogenic antigen-specific immunity of T-cell origin does not develop in the intestine to enterically encountered antigens such as bacteria and foods. The three jejunal mucosal histopathological features of villous atrophy, crypt hyperplasia and high intraepithelial lymphocyte count may imply the existence of a cell-mediated inflammatory immune reaction within the mucosa.

26.4 NUTRITION AND IMMUNODEFICIENCY DISORDERS

Virtually any component of the immune system, specific or non-specific, can be affected; the consequent immunodeficiency states vary in severity from trivial to fatal. Immunodeficiency can also result from acquired diseases. This is well illustrated in severe form in the acquired immunodeficiency syndrome (AIDS). Acquired immunodeficiency may also be iatrogenic, for example as a result of corticosteroid or other immunosuppressive treatment for autoimmune diseases. In addition to causing susceptibility to infection, immunodeficiency may be associated with abnormally regulated immune reactions, as in allergy or autoimmunity.

In general, an uncomplicated immunodeficiency itself has no effect on the nutritional capacity of the gut. Secondary effects often occur on the basis of diarrhoea and malabsorption when immunodeficiency is complicated by infections.

PRIMARY IMMUNODEFICIENCIES

Abnormalities of polymorph function and deficiencies of complement components or antibodies may all result in susceptibility to bacterial infection. A severe combined immunodeficiency syndrome can be caused by several different gene defects, which are autosomal or X-linked and which mostly lead to a deficiency affecting both humoral and cell-mediated immunity. The affected infants are susceptible to commonly occurring, normally benign viral infections and may die from generalised chickenpox, measles, cytomegalovirus or other viral infections.

Selective deficiency of the B-lymphocyte (antibody) system occurs in X-linked recessive hypo- or agammaglobulinaemia. The lack of immunoglobulins is not absolute, but the patient fails to respond to antigenic stimuli. Most patients with immunoglobulin deficiency suffer from 'acquired' or 'late-onset' hypogammaglobulinaemia known as 'common variable immunodeficiency'. This is associated with an unusually high incidence of autoimmune disease.

SECONDARY IMMUNODEFICIENCIES

Immunoglobulin deficiency may result from abnormal losses of serum proteins, for example in lymphangiectasia. Drugs may also depress the immune system; for example drugs used for treatment of epilepsy such as phenytoin or drugs used in rheumatoid arthritis such as penicillamine may induce IgA deficiency or even hypogammaglobulinaemia (low IgG).

Secondary T-cell defects can occur in Hodgkin's disease or sarcoidosis and following infections such as leprosy, miliary tuberculosis or measles. They may also result from loss of lymphocytes from the gut in protein-losing enteropathy or due to thoracic duct fistula, and can also be caused by treatment with cytotoxic drugs. Clearly one of the most important causes of secondary immunodeficiencies, infection and malnutrition is HIV infection and AIDS. (See http://www.unaids.org/en/KnowledgeCentre/).

26.5 NUTRITION AND IMMUNITY

Hunger and malnutrition remain among the most devastating problems worldwide, although obesity (BMI >35) and its associated co-morbidities such as heart disease, hypertension, stroke and maturity-onset diabetes have reached alarming dimensions worldwide and are not limited to high-income countries.

OVERNUTRITION AND IMMUNITY

It has been predicted that by 2030 86% of adults in the USA will be overweight or obese, and 51% obese (Wang et al 2008). Predictions for the UK paint a similar, although less dramatic picture. By 2010, 38% of adult men and 29% of women are expected to be obese (BMI >35) (Department of Health: Forecasting obesity to 2010; available online at http://www.dh.gov.uk/en/Publicationsandstatistics/Publications/PublicationsStatistics/

DH_4138630; (see also Figure *evolve* 26.2 for a projected incidence of childhood obesity according to parental obesity 🖱).

Obesity is correlated with increased concentration of the hormone leptin, often associated with leptin resistance. Leptin is produced by fat tissue and secreted into the bloodstream. It is distributed to the brain and other tissues physiologically regulating normal fat loss and appetite (see also Ch. 4). Furthermore, individuals with obesity present with increased secretion of the inflammatory cytokine TNF-α, reduced T-lymphocyte responses and an increased incidence of infectious diseases (Table 26.1). Obesity also affects the intestinal microbiota and is associated with the development of type 2 diabetes mellitus and associated complications. Most associated risks and immunological changes are reversible with weight reduction and increased physical activity.

UNDERNUTRITION AND IMMUNITY

The consequences of malnutrition include death, disability and stunted physical and mental development. Inadequate nutrition adversely affects many aspects of immune function and is the most common cause of secondary immunodeficiencies worldwide.

Protein calorie malnutrition (PCM), also termed protein energy malnutrition (PEM), can occur in two clinical extremes – kwashiorkor and marasmus, with gradual transitions between these two extremes (Keusch 2003; see also Ch. 28). Marasmus usually occurs early in infancy where children are wasted and grossly underweight but without oedema and skin changes. Patients with kwashiorkor, mostly in their second year of life or older, are growth-retarded and suffering from oedema, skin changes, abnormal hair, hepatomegaly and apathy.

Undernutrition which leads to the impairment of the immune function can be due to insufficient intake of energy, of macronutrients or of micronutrients (Cunningham-Rundles et al 2005, Lesourd 2006). These deficiency states often occur in combination. PCM and micronutrient deficiencies related to iodine, vitamin A, iron and zinc can present together. Proteins are essential for both cell replication and production of immunologically active molecules and receptors, and it is therefore not surprising that nearly all forms of immunity are affected by PCM (Table 26.1).

Clearly the level and impact of undernutrition is most pronounced in low and middle-income countries. In high-income countries, although moderate deficiencies can be present in any age-group, low income is an important determinant of undernutrition in the general public. Additionally, undernutrition is prevalent among the institutionalised elderly, patients with eating disorders, substance users, individuals on unsupervised elimination diets and in those recovering from major surgery.

Table 26.1   Effects of malnutrition on immunity and host defence functions

DEFICIENCY STATE	FUNCTIONS AFFECTED OR ENHANCED	INFECTIONS
Protein–energy malnutrition (acute)	Innate immunity: phagocytosis, macrophage activation, Adaptive immunity: T-cell activation, memory, antibody production, cytokine secretion, leptin levels decreased	Opportunistic, viral and helminth infections, including measles, tuberculosis and influenza Respiratory infections
Protein–energy malnutrition (chronic)	Thymic and T-cell development, innate immunity: complement, macrophage activation, adaptive immunity: immunoglobulins (IgG, IgA decreased) vaccine efficacy reduced, leptin levels decreased	Respiratory + skin + intestinal infections, other organisms: helminths, malaria, HIV, measles, influenza BCG, malaria, encapsulated organisms
Overnutrition	Innate immunity: leukocytes preactivated (interferon-γ, TNF-α increased), NK function + phagocytosis decreased Adaptive immunity: T-cell activation reduced Leptin concentrations increased (often with leptin resistance combined)	Opportunistic and fungal infections

Adapted from Schaible & Kaufmann 2007.

Undernutrition during pregnancy may result in a low birth weight, and may have effects in adult life.

Non-specific host defence and barrier functions

Skin, mucous membranes and epithelial surfaces act as non-specific host defence mechanisms and are adversely affected in children with kwashiorkor. Skin lesions found in these compromised children enhance penetration and adhesion of infectious organisms. This leads to mucosal and gastrointestinal infections, further impairing the absorption of essential nutrients.

INFLUENCE OF MICRONUTRIENTS ON IMMUNE FUNCTION

The developing child

There is very little reliable information on the effects of vitamins, saturated and unsaturated fatty acids, trace minerals and other food constituents on the infant's developing immune system (Kapil & Bhavna 2002). Most reports examine effects of corrections of moderate or severe deficiencies on immune responses in children (and animals). Very little is known of the effects of supplementation at the level of or above dietary reference values (DRVs) in a non-deficient population.

Vitamin A

Vitamin A deficiency is the second most serious nutritional deficiency worldwide. It is associated with increased morbidity in children, particularly in those suffering from respiratory tract infections and measles. Vitamin A is important for both innate and adaptive immune responses, including cell-mediated immunity and antibody responses. Vitamin A deficiency leads to a reduced integrity of mucosal epithelia that leads to an increased susceptibility to ocular, respiratory and gastrointestinal inflammatory and diarrhoeal diseases with subsequent malnutrition. Vitamin A deficiency has also been associated with diminished innate immune responses affecting phagocytic activity and NK cell function (Pesonen et al 2007, Uauy et al 2008). Several studies have shown a marked decline in measles-related deaths in vitamin-A-deficient children orally supplemented with vitamin A. Vitamin A supplementation has also been shown to enhance serum antibody responses to common vaccines. Adverse effects of vitamin A deficiency (Table 26.2) are usually restored to normal after supplementation. Vitamin A supplementation in deficiency states generally reduces morbidity and mortality from infectious disease, especially in children.

Vitamin C

Vitamin C is a water-soluble antioxidant and appears to affect most aspects of the immune system. High concentrations are found in white blood cells and reduced plasma levels are associated with reduced immune function, especially those affecting the bacterial killing efficiency of white blood cells. Vitamin C regulates the immune system via antiviral and anti-oxidant properties. Reactive oxygen species (ROS), which can be scavenged by vitamin C, play important roles in killing intracellular bacteria. Vitamin C has been shown in some studies to reduce inflammatory processes in vivo and in vitro, although the results are inconsistent.

Positive effects of vitamin C on the common cold have been disputed. Vitamin C levels in leukocytes fall rapidly during upper respiratory tract infections and return to normal during recovery, suggesting that supplementation during this phase might be beneficial. Vitamin C supplementation (600mg/day) in ultra-marathon runners decreased the incidence of upper respiratory tract infections but a recent Cochrane review concluded that vitamin C supplementation may affect symptoms

Table 26.2	Vitamin A deficiency – non-specific and specific effects on immunity
PARAMETER OR TEST	RESPONSE
Functional integrity of skin and mucosal surfaces	↓
Lysozyme production	↓
Phagocytosis	↓
Natural-killer-cell-mediated lysis	↓
Lymphocyte stimulation	↓
Interleukin-2 production	↓
Delayed hypersensitivity	↓

Above-normal intakes of vitamin A can cause immunological disturbances similar to those seen in vitamin A deficiency and may also decrease resistance to infection.

but does not reduce the incidence of common colds in the general population (Hemila et al 2008).

Vitamin D

The physiological function of vitamin D is to maintain serum calcium and phosphorus concentrations that maintain neuromuscular function, bone ossification and immunity. Vitamin enhances the efficiency of the small intestine to absorb dietary calcium and phosphorus. The active metabolite of vitamin D, $1,25(OH)_2D$, regulates the transcription of a large number of genes through binding to the vitamin D receptor (VDR) (Martineau et al 2007, Hewison 2008).

A deficiency of vitamin D, through dietary inadequacy or inadequate exposure to sunlight or both, leads to rickets and seems to interfere with natural killer cell function, resulting in increased infections. Vitamin D plays a role in the immune system and may help prevent infections, autoimmune diseases, cancer and diabetes.

In the immune system, $1,25(OH)_2D$ modulates synthesis of interleukins and cytokines. It has been shown to downregulate the immunostimulatory IL-12 while increasing secretion of the immunosuppressive IL-10. Besides stimulating monocytes and macrophages, $1,25(OH)_2D$ may act as an immunosuppressive agent by decreasing the rate of proliferation and the activity of both T- and B-cells while inducing suppressor T-cells (White 2008). The VDR is expressed in a number of human tissues, including muscle tissue, liver, intestine and reproductive organs – $1,25\text{-}(OH)_2D_3$ exerts most of its actions after it has bound to its specific receptor, which is present on monocytes and activated lymphocytes. The hormone inhibits lymphocyte proliferation and immunoglobulin production in a dose-dependent fashion and may interfere with T-helper cell (Th) function, reducing Th-induction of immunoglobulin production by B-cells and inhibiting the passive transfer of cellular immunity by Th. Vitamin D appears to be a protective factor in colon carcinogenesis and autoimmunity.

There is little information on the effects of vitamin D or its metabolites on the developing human immune system.

Vitamin E

Vitamin E is a major lipid-soluble antioxidant and deficiency states or supradietary levels affect immune cell function. Groups most likely to develop a deficiency of vitamin E include premature infants, elderly people living in sheltered accommodation, individuals on selective diets, alcohol and drug users, patients with gastrointestinal or hepatic disorders with malabsorption syndromes and individuals with abetalipoproteinaemia.

Vitamin E maintains cell membrane integrity by limiting lipid peroxidation by reactive oxygen species (ROS). Deficiencies are associated with reduced antibody production and T-cell proliferation following mitogen stimulation.

Vitamin E supplements in the elderly ranging from 60 mg to 800 mg/day for 30 days showed significant improvements in cytokine production (IL-2), enhanced NK-cell function, delayed hypersensitivity responses and enhanced hepatitis B vaccination antibodies. Supplementation of vitamin E in moderately deficient elderly people resulted in increased resistance to infection. High dose supplementation (above 400 mg/day) may lead to the inhibition of neutrophil function and a potential increase in the risk of developing cancer of the lung or prostate (Kilkkinen et al 2008, Lippman et al 2009).

Trace element deficiencies

Iron deficiency

Iron deficiency is the most common nutritional deficiency among children and especially women of childbearing age throughout the world. 2 billion people – over 30% of the world's population – are anaemic, many due to iron deficiency, and in resource-poor areas, infectious diseases frequently exacerbate this. Malaria, HIV/AIDS, hookworm infestation, schistosomiasis and other infections such as tuberculosis are particularly important factors contributing to the high prevalence of anaemia in some areas (http://www.who.int/nutrition/topics/ida/en/).

The relationship between iron status and immunity is complex and methodological problems in many studies make their interpretation uncertain. Iron is essential for electron transfer reactions, gene regulation, binding and transport of oxygen and regulation of cell differentiation and cell growth. It is involved in the neutrophil killing of bacteria through generation of toxic hydroxyl radicals. A deficiency leads to impaired cellular immunity with a CD4/CD8 T-lymphocyte inversion. However, even though iron deficiency leads to impairment of the immune system (Cunningham-Rundles et al 2005), the fundamental question is whether the incidence of infections is increased in the presence of iron-deficiency anaemia or during iron supplementation. Some bacteria need iron for their multiplication and iron supplementation during this period could worsen the clinical situation.

Taking together a number of studies in iron-deficient individuals, it seems that T-lymphocyte numbers and function and bactericidal activity of neutrophil can be adversely affected through a deficiency and restored to normal by iron supplementation.

Copper deficiency

Copper deficiency is rare in humans. Copper is a cofactor for several enzymes, including cytochrome C oxidase and superoxide dismutase. Copper is required for infant growth, host defence mechanisms, bone strength, red and white cell maturation, iron transport, cholesterol and glucose metabolism (Munoz et al 2007). Copper homeostasis is maintained over a wide range of intakes, mainly through changes in excretion. Deficiencies have been described in premature infants and in patients receiving total parenteral nutrition. Children with a complete absence of the copper-carrying protein ceruloplasmin in the blood and subsequent severe copper deficiency suffer from impaired T-cell immunity, increased bacterial infections and diarrhoea. A 90-day human study examining the effects of a low copper intake on immunity reported a reduced in vitro mitogen responsiveness of T-lymphocyte activation and circulating B-lymphocytes (Kelley et al 1995) and study participants exhibited an increased incidence of infections. High copper intake (7–8mg/day) may impair immune function, such as neutrophil numbers, serum interleukin-2 receptors and production of anti-viral antibodies (Turnlund et al 2004).

Zinc deficiency

Dietary zinc deficiencies are rare, although low plasma zinc levels can be found in a individuals in resource-poor countries. Zinc is important for highly proliferating cells of the immune system and deficiency affects both innate and adaptive immunity. Zinc has antioxidant activity and is involved in the cytosolic defence against ROS generated by activated macrophages through its role as a cofactor for superoxide dismutase (SOD). Normal zinc levels support Th1 responses and maintain skin and mucosal membrane integrity. Due to its major effects on the immune system and direct antiviral effects, zinc supplementation in children and adults with borderline zinc status can decrease lower respiratory and diarrhoeal illnesses (Brooks et al 2005). However the results of intervention trials have been inconsistent (Chang et al 2006). Among the factors which may account for this variability is the genetic background, extent of deficiency, co-administration of other micronutrients and the availability of zinc ions as gluconate or acetate.

Infants with acrodermatitis enteropathica, a rare inborn error with a reduced ability to absorb dietary zinc, show failure to thrive and show impaired lymphocyte proliferation and response to mitogens, decreased/inverted CD4/CD8 ratios, impaired NK activity and cytotoxicity. Children also demonstrate thymic atrophy and deficient thymic hormone activity (Table 26.3).

Selenium

Selenium is an essential trace element and concentrated in tissues involved in the immune response, such as lymph nodes, liver and spleen. It is required for an optimal immune response and deficiency states affect innate and adaptive immunity. Selenium plays a key role in antioxidant function, though a cofactor role for glutathione peroxidase, which may be important for macrophage activation. Selenium is a cofactor of a number of important transcription factors involved in cell-to-cell signalling during the normal immune response.

Immune functions possibly affected by selenium deficiencies are numerous and listed in Table 26.4.

Table 26.3	Zinc deficiency and effects on immunity
OBSERVATION/INVESTIGATION	**RESPONSE**
Thymic size	↓
Lymphocyte development	Impaired
Delayed hypersensitivity	↓
T-lymphocyte proliferation	↓
Cytokine production (IL-2, IFN-γ, TNF-α)	↓
CD4/CD8 ratio	↓
T-helper cell function (Th)	↓
Natural killer cell activity	↓

Table 26.4 Selenium deficiency	
OBSERVATION/INVESTIGATION	RESPONSE
Platelet aggregation and leukotriene synthesis	↑
IgG and IgM titres	↓
Antibody production by lymphocytes	↓
Neutrophil chemotaxis	↓
CD4+ cells	↑
CD8 cells	↓
CD4/CD8	↓
Effects described on immune cells after Se supplementation	
Neutrophil migration and bactericidal activity	↑
High-affinity IL-2 receptor	↑
T-cell function following age-related decline	↑
Natural killer cell activity	↑
Cytotoxic T-cell activity	↑
Lymphokine-activated killer cell activity	↑
Enhanced delayed-type hypersensitivity response	↓
UV-induced skin cancers and mortality	↓
Erythema following UV exposure	↓

Se supplementation, even in borderline deficiency states, has been shown to boost cell-mediated immune responses, protect cells against oxidative damage and downregulate inflammatory processes (Rayman et al 2008).

26.6 THE ROLE OF PROBIOTICS

The 'hygiene hypothesis' suggests that an increase in atopic diseases may have arisen over the last decades from a lack of microbial exposure and stimulation of the infant's immune system at an early age. The infant's immature 'naïve' intestinal immune system develops as it is exposed to dietary and microbial antigens in the gut. The evolving indigenous intestinal microbiota have a significant impact on the immune system and there is accumulating evidence indicating that an intimate interaction between gut microbiota and host defence mechanisms is important for the development and maintenance of a balance between tolerance to innocuous, mostly food antigens and the capability of mounting an inflammatory response towards potential pathogens.

Probiotics are defined as live bacteria, with a proven beneficial effect on the health of the host. Observed effects are associated with temporary mucosal colonisation thus (potentially) affecting the overall microbiota composition. *Prebiotics* are defined as non-digestible oligosaccharides, which beneficially affect the health of the host through effects on the microbiota. *Synbiotics* are a combination of the above.

Early studies in infants suggest that administration of strains of lactobacilli and *Bifidus* bacteria (i.e. probiotics) in early life might prevent the development of atopic dermatitis in high-risk children. These bacteria may also have a role in the treatment of cow's-milk-allergy-related diarrhoea. Clinical study results are, however, inconsistent most probably because of a large number of confounding variables such as study population, study design, bacterial strain and length of administration (Lahtinen et al 2006). To be effective, normally active live cultures need to be administered; however, optimal doses are still unknown and concerns over potential adverse effects such as systemic bacteraemias need further investigation. The immune stimulatory effects are currently not fully understood, but may be related to effects of specific bacterial components, which may modulate cellular transcription factors needed for T-lymphocyte and other immune cell activation (Strobel & Mowat 2006). Similar bacterial strains may display widely varying activities for enzymes such as β-galactosidase or may affect immunity in different ways (Medina et al 2007).

26.7 FOOD INTOLERANCE AND FOOD ALLERGY

The increased public awareness of the relevance of diet to health and the absence of simple and reliable diagnostic tests have also enhanced the idea that 'allergy', broadly defined as adverse reaction to foods and food additives, may cause a wide range of distressing physical and psychological problems and chronic, disabling symptoms (Bischoff & Crowe 2004, Nowak-Wegrzyn & Sampson 2006, Eigenmann et al 2008).

Many claims for effective in vitro diagnostic tests for food sensitivity have been made; a reliable diagnosis of either food intolerance or allergy, however, relies on clinical methodology and supportive laboratory investigations. Recent advances in understanding the mechanisms of food intolerance help distinguish these from psychologically based aversion reactions to foods.

SCOPE AND DEFINITIONS

Adverse reactions to ingested food cause a wide variety of symptoms, syndromes and diseases for which the general descriptive terms 'sensitivity', 'allergy' and 'intolerance' are often used. Except for immediate, IgE-mediated allergic reactions, these terms do not imply specific mechanisms for their pathogenesis and can be applied to a reaction with an unknown mechanism as well as to a clearly defined metabolic, pharmacological or as yet undescribed immunopathological process (Fig. 26.3)

Adverse reactions not based on an immunological mechanism can be due to such factors as enzyme deficiencies, pharmacological effects (e.g. due to caffeine), non-immunological direct histamine-containing or-releasing effects (e.g. certain shellfish and cheeses) and direct irritation (e.g. through gastric acid (oesophagitis) and spices).

Food intolerance and *food sensitivity* are often used in a general sense for all reproducible, unpleasant (i.e. adverse) reactions to a specific food or food ingredient that are not psychologically based. The reaction may have a clearly defined metabolic, pharmacological or immunopathological basis, or the mechanism may be unknown or disputed. The majority of adverse reactions to foods fall into this category. The provoking agent may be a single food or ingredient, but sometimes – particularly in IgE-mediated food allergy – many different foods are involved.

IgE-mediated food allergic reactions are generally reproducible and there is evidence of an abnormal immunological reaction to the food and a plausible mechanism implicating immunological processes (Table 26.5).

Psychologically based food reactions (food aversions) comprise both psychological avoidance, when the subject avoids food for psychological reasons, and psychological intolerance, which is an unpleasant bodily reaction caused not directly by the food but by emotions associated with the food. Psychological intolerance normally does not occur when the food is given in an unrecognisable form.

DIAGNOSTIC APPROACHES

No single laboratory or in vivo test allows the definite clinical diagnosis of an immediate IgE-mediated or delayed adverse reaction to food (Hill et al 2004, Sicherer & Leung 2008). A careful history and often a double-blind placebo-controlled food challenge are necessary to confirm or refute the diagnosis of a food allergic reaction (Strobel 2002) (Table 26.6).

Allergic reactions to a given food may not appear with absolute regularity and can be affected by the fat content of the meal, exercise, alcohol, medications or other factors. This needs to be kept in mind when a clinical history does not correspond with the results of diagnostic tests.

Elimination diet and challenge

Experienced clinicians, dieticians and patients may have difficulties in elucidating the exact

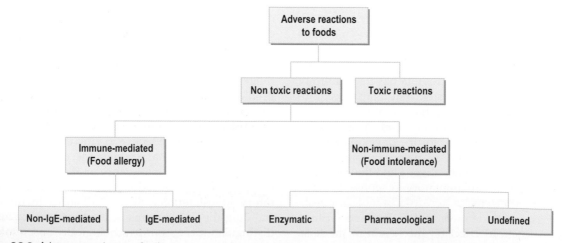

Fig. 26.3 Adverse reactions to foods.

Table 26.5 Clinical features of adverse reactions attributed to food and food ingredients

SYSTEM AFFECTED	CLINICAL FEATURES THAT COULD BE CAUSED BY ADVERSE REACTIONS TO FOODS
Skin	Urticaria Atopic dermatitis Angio-oedema
Gastrointestinal tract	Oral allergy syndrome (burning, itching of the lips and mouth and sometimes the larynx and pharynx) Pain, colic Nausea Vomiting Change in stool habit, e.g. looseness, frequency, blood, mucus Abdominal distension, flatulence Heartburn (gastro-oesophageal reflux) Failure to thrive
Respiratory tract	Asthma Rhinitis
Eyes	Watering eyes Conjunctivitis Peri-ocular pruritus
Cardiovascular system	Symptoms and signs of hypo- and hypertension
Blood	Symptoms and signs of haemolytic anaemia (rare)
Central nervous system	Headache Abnormal behaviour in children (including attention deficit hyperactivity disorder (ADHD)) Fatigue Lassitude
Generalised systemic	Anaphylaxis (circulatory collapse, wheeze, inability to swallow and other symptoms)

Table 26.6 Diagnosis of food allergy and intolerance

History

Frequency, type, severity, seasonality of reactions, interval since food ingestion, coexisting intestinal disease

Clinical examination

Entity, degree, extension, overlap of symptoms
In vivo tests
Skin prick tests
Elimination diet
Open challenge
Double-blind placebo-controlled challenge
Gastrointestinal procedures
Intestinal permeability evaluation with and without challenge
Endoscopy before and after challenge
Biopsy
In vitro tests
Food specific IgE antibodies
Food-specific IgG antibodies[a]
Cellular tests (lymphocyte proliferation)
Mediators in biological fluids after food challenge
Histological examination of intestinal biopsy

[a]Only suitable in some cases for monitoring of dietetic compliance.

In young children with atopic eczema, for example, appropriate elimination and challenge protocols have shown that around 60% respond positively to specific food challenges with dermal, gastrointestinal and respiratory reactions. The most common foods associated with these reactions are cow's milk, egg, wheat, peanuts and tree nuts, soya and, less often, fish and shellfish.

Problems with placebo responses

Experience of elimination diet and open challenge protocols has revealed that patients' perceptions and doctors' diagnoses of food intolerance are not invariably accurate. In patients with clear and convincing histories of adverse reactions, less than half of individuals can normally be confirmed as intolerant on objective testing. For this reason, double-blind placebo-controlled food challenges (DBPCFCs) should be used and if negative the food item should be introduced openly into the diet.

Coeliac disease, a special case of food intolerance

Coeliac disease is a particular form of food intolerance which affects around 1 in 200 individuals and

relationship between dietary constituents and the clinical reactions experienced or observed. It has become established practice to use as diagnostic criteria the objectively monitored effects of exclusion diets, blinded exposure and provocation tests. Some ingenuity may be required to define and record symptoms and signs during elimination and provocation studies.

is defined as lifelong gluten intolerance which responds normally to gluten withdrawal. The diagnosis is made with a small bowel biopsy with the help of measuring specific serum antibodies such as tissue-transglutaminase. Coeliac disease has a genetic basis and is thought to be an autoimmune process triggered by a toxic gliadin fraction (see Ch. 23).

Laboratory diagnostic procedures
(Table 26.7)

Skin prick (puncture) tests
In cases of suspected IgE-mediated immunological reactions to food, a skin prick test may be performed. In it a small amount of an allergen in solution is placed on the skin and then introduced into the epidermis by gently puncturing the skin surface to facilitate allergen–gE interaction. A positive reaction is manifested as the development of a weal, the diameter of which can be measured to grade the reaction. A positive test can confirm that the patient is atopic and can strengthen suspicions about probable precipitants. The diagnostic accuracy of a skin test varies according to the offending food. Negative reactions have a high (95%) accuracy of there *not* being an IgE-mediated reaction. However, positive tests have only a 50–60% predictive accuracy.

Radioallergosorbent test (RAST)
The radioallergosorbent test (RAST) demonstrates food-specific serum IgE antibodies. These tests correlate only variably with the correct diagnosis of a particular allergy in individuals with eczema and often suggest a state of immunological sensitisation without clinical reactivity. Overall, 10–15% of individuals exhibit skin test or RAST sensitisation and may tolerate exposure to those allergens without an adverse clinical reaction.

Atopy patch test (APT)
Atopic eczema in infancy and childhood is often caused or aggravated by common food allergens such as milk, egg and wheat. In order to test for these conditions, an APT has been described as a diagnostic tool with a high specificity. During the APT, suspected allergens are applied to the patient's back under a dressing and allowed to remain in contact with the skin for 48 hours. The area is then visually examined for reddening or evidence of infiltration. Prospective clinical studies in children have cast some doubt on the specificity and sensitivity of this test system (Mehl et al 2006). A combination of skin prick tests and the APT may increase diagnostic accuracy in some gastrointestinal diseases.

Endoscopic studies and intestinal biopsy
This test involves swallowing a thin tube or an endoscope which is passed through the stomach into the small intestine where a small piece of the intestinal lining is removed by a cutting device. This procedure is often used in patients with a variety of slow-onset gastrointestinal symptoms, such as frequent loose stools or features of unexplained iron deficiency, osteoporosis, weight loss, slower than expected gain in height, and other features of malnutrition. Intestinal biopsy is normally not indicated for the diagnosis of acute IgE-mediated gastrointestinal disease. In these conditions a biopsy may show degranulated IgE-positive mast cells or an eosinophilic infiltration on conventional histology.

Hydrogen breath test (lactase deficiency)
The hydrogen breath test measures the amount of hydrogen in a person's breath. Normally, very little hydrogen is detectable. However, undigested lactose in the colon is fermented by bacteria, and various gases, including hydrogen, are produced. The hydrogen is absorbed from the intestines and

Table 26.7	Clinical tests and procedures for food allergies	
VALIDATED	**UNVALIDATED OR BOGUS**
Double-blind placebo-controlled food challenge (DBPCFC)	Food-specific IgG and IgG subclass antibodies
Skin prick tests	Cytotoxicity test
Allergen-specific IgE measurements (RAST, radioallergosorbent test)	Sublingual subcutaneous and intradermal provocation and neutralisation tests
Endoscopic studies ± histological examination	Immune complex measurements
	Electro-acupuncture
Intestinal permeability test	Vega testing
Respiratory function test	Applied kinesiology (DRIA) test
Allergen patch test	Hair analysis

exhaled. In the test, the patient drinks a lactose-loaded drink, and the breath is analysed at regular intervals. Raised levels of hydrogen in the breath indicate impaired digestion of lactose. This test is available for children and adults.

Lactose tolerance test (lactase deficiency)

Normally, when lactose reaches the digestive system, the lactase enzyme (β-galactosidase) breaks it down into glucose and galactose. The liver then changes the galactose into glucose, which enters the bloodstream and raises the person's blood glucose level. If lactose is not or incompletely broken down, the blood glucose level does not rise and a diagnosis of lactose intolerance is confirmed.

Non-validated tests for the diagnosis of food allergies

IgG antibodies

Currently the determination of IgG antibodies to food has no or little predictive value for diagnosis and dietary management of patients with food allergic diseases. However, in non-IgE-mediated immunological adverse reactions to food, determination of IgG and possibly specific IgG_4 may be a helpful adjunct for monitoring adherence to diet. Measurement of food-specific IgG_4 is not sufficient for a diagnosis of food allergy (Stapel et al 2008).

SYMPTOMS, SYNDROMES AND FEATURES OF FOOD-INDUCED DISEASES

A wide range of factors determine the route to a state of allergic sensitisation and allergic disease. The factors are often interlinked and modulated by the host's genetic disposition and health status. (See Figure *evolve* 26.2 🖱️).

Food allergies and intolerance in children

A wide range of conditions in childhood have been associated with food allergies and intolerance; these include eczema, wheeze, urticaria, mood changes, angio-oedema, epilepsy, failure to thrive, diarrhoea, vomiting and gastrointestinal blood loss (Bischoff & Crowe 2004, Burks et al 2008). There is some evidence that a small number of hyperactive children, often boys, respond to dietary measures with improvement of symptoms related to attention deficit hyperactivity disorder (ADHD). Possi-

ble adverse effects of food colourings and preservatives on normal children's behaviour have been reported (Bateman et al 2004, McCann et al 2007).

Milk-induced colitis, mainly in breastfed children under 2 years of age, differs from ulcerative colitis in many clinical and pathological features. Small intestinal mucosal damage with malabsorption is best documented for cow's-milk-protein-induced enteropathy but can also occur with other food protein intolerance.

Food intolerance in adults

The incidence of adverse reactions to foods in adults is estimated to be 2–4% of the population and as such is lower than in childhood. Classic food allergic symptoms of asthma, urticaria and anaphylaxis can be found in adults (Sicherer & Sampson 2008). Adults with food allergic reactions often have a history of adverse reactions to foods in childhood. Assuming a lower food allergy incidence in adults, this indicates that there is some 'growing out of allergies' in childhood, often for milk and egg allergies. De novo sensitisation to foods in adults is less frequent. Adverse reactions to foods can affect all organ systems and examples are summarised in Table 26.5.

A number of patients report rather ill-defined symptoms in relation to food intake. This feature makes it often difficult to establish a sound diagnosis without resorting to elimination and challenge studies. The relationship between food intolerance and migraine is complex but its existence is well supported by clinical studies.

Migraine can be triggered by direct pharmacological actions of substances on the vessel wall or by as yet unresolved immunological mechanisms. The threshold for the development of a food-induced migraine is altered by many other factors such as fatigue, smoking, alcohol and the menstrual cycle.

There are anecdotal claims for an association between food allergy and *arthritis*, but there is little evidence that can withstand critical examination. *Psychiatric symptoms* such as irritability and depression may accompany other manifestations of food intolerance, but it remains to be established whether foods can provoke psychiatric disease directly.

Other food-provoked symptoms are *gastrointestinal* in origin. They include nausea, bloating, abdominal pain, constipation and diarrhoea. These features are similar to those of the irritable bowel syndrome. The symptoms may arise either because of abnormal motility or because an individual has a lower pain threshold to sensations accompanying normal contraction or distension of the gut. Not surprisingly, these symptoms are often closely related to foods. Many people who avoid specific foods and have an unsubstantiated self-diagnosis of food allergy suffer from irritable bowel syndrome. Their often self-imposed alterations in diet will influence gut motility, the composition of the stools and the production of gas, and in an introspective individual such physiological changes can reinforce the patient's concern. Recent studies explore the effects of anti-depressants and motility modulators in the treatment of irritable bowel syndrome.

Psychological food intolerance

There is no doubt that attitudes to food vary widely. Dieting, overeating and food fads are extremely common. Intolerance of food by proxy has been described, whereby in a patient with an eating disorder such as anorexia nervosa, the suggestion that the problem could be 'allergic' is seized upon to avoid the possible stigma of a psychiatric diagnosis. In childhood, perceived or imagined food intolerances can lead to severe failure to thrive and often form the background of induced illnesses (fictitious illness, Münchhausen by proxy) in children. Food fads and 'fashionable' dieting may lead to eating disorders in adolescents and adults.

PREVALENCE OF FOOD INTOLERANCE

Estimates about the incidence and prevalence are often based on studies that are not done prospectively, suffer from a selection bias, and diagnoses are usually not confirmed by DBPCFCs. Conservative estimates for adverse reactions to foods are around 3–5% in childhood and 2–4% in adults.

Considerably higher estimates in childhood (7.5%) and adults (8%) have been proposed. These estimates clearly indicate the scope of the problem and the importance of considering adverse reactions to foods in a sizeable number of patients. Table 26.8 depicts the most common foods encountered as allergens. (For detailed information relating to food allergy and intolerance in Europe and beyond refer to: http://www.europrevall.org/ and http://www.faan.org.)

Table 26.8	Most common foods encountered as allergens
FOODS MOST COMMONLY ENCOUNTERED AS ALLERGENS	OTHERS FOODS ALSO KNOWN TO TRIGGER ALLERGIC REACTIONS
Cow's milk	Fruits (kiwi, mango, banana)
Egg	Legumes (peas, lupine, lentils)
Soya	Seeds (sesame, sunflower)
Wheat	Spices (mustard, coriander)
Peanuts	Vegetables (celery, tomato)
Tree nuts	
Fish	
Shellfish	

APPROACHES TO DIETARY TREATMENT

Symptoms and clinical features may conform to well-recognised phenomena or to a disease associated with a specific food. This will be suspected from the history and confirmed by a small number of tests. Examples include asthma and rhinitis and flatus and diarrhoea induced by sugar alcohol such as sorbitol from dietetic foods.

In other patients, food intolerance will form part of a wider differential diagnosis. When symptoms are mild, simple symptomatic treatment, such as non-sedating antihistamines, antidiarrhoeals for occasional diarrhoea bouts or analgesics for headache, may be more appropriate initially than complex therapeutic diets, which tend to be time-consuming and difficult. If food intolerance is to be pursued, a baseline elimination diet is taken for some 3 weeks; if symptoms and signs disappear, relevant foods are identified during a planned period of reintroduction and should be confirmed by placebo-controlled challenges, especially in adults, if feasible. If the challenge is negative, it needs to be openly introduced into the diet to confirm the challenge results.

RELEVANCE OF FOOD ALLERGY IN DISEASE: THE EXAMPLE OF MILK

Patterns of antibody responses to cow's milk protein in humans

There have been many reports, using a wide range of techniques, of the titres and patterns of antibodies to cow's milk proteins in the sera of adults and children (Heine et al 2002). Milk-specific IgG antibodies are present in the serum of most children and also in 10–20% of healthy adults. Patients with diffuse small bowel disease and enhanced intestinal permeability from whatever cause tend to have high titres of serum antibody to many foods. IgE responses are thought to be of greater relevance than non-IgE responses in indicating the likely mechanism of food allergic diseases. Transient IgE antibodies to food proteins also occur in some healthy children and may be present in high titres in some individuals. IgE antibodies to food antigens are evidence of an atopic state in general (i.e. a predisposition to become allergic). If these food-specific IgE antibodies measured by a RAST are particularly raised, they are often combined with a positive skin test. Adverse allergic (immediate anaphylactic) reactions to this food under the above conditions are likely and must be confirmed or ruled out.

Allergy as a mechanism within the spectrum of food intolerance and disease

It is important to define the relevance of immunological mechanisms and of each particular foodstuff, as the cause of a symptom or disease, especially in atopic patients who may suffer from similar symptoms that can also be triggered by environmental allergens.

Goldman et al (1963) originally proposed the diagnosis of milk allergy in a patient if symptoms subsided after dietary elimination of milk and recurred within 48 hours after milk challenge. Reactions to three such challenges had to be positive with a similar onset, duration and clinical features before a diagnosis could be made. Such a repeated challenge can be too dangerous and too time-consuming for allergic infants. Clinical improvement on a 'blinded' elimination diet should be the first criterion for the routine diagnosis. However, the use of double-blind testing of triggering foods and placebo in children and adults and the use of objective indices of change, for example symptom score charts filled in by parents and teachers or carers, are preferred and greatly strengthen the clinical information likely to be obtained from a challenge test. If there is any doubt, a DBPCFC with the food in question needs to be performed, at times more than once. Eliminated foods need to be reintroduced into the children's diet at 6–12-month intervals – depending on clinical history, age and the eliminated food – to establish a potential development of tolerance and to avoid unnecessary long-term dietary restrictions.

The spectrum of food allergic reactions

Example cow's milk allergy

The wide clinical spectrum of food (cow's milk protein)-induced symptoms in childhood helps to illustrate these difficulties. Hill & Hosking (1997) assessed the relationship between clinical symptoms and serum antibody levels in children up to 5 years of age, shown by milk challenge to have adverse reactions to cow's milk. They found that the patients could be divided into three groups: first, those children who showed immediate symptoms with small amounts of milk, evidenced by anaphylaxis, angiooedema, urticaria and diarrhoea; secondly, those who developed symptoms often up to several hours after intake of moderate amounts of milk (approximately 200 ml) and in whom the skin test to the offending food was generally negative; and thirdly, those mostly older children suffering from a poorly defined multisystem involvement, including e.g. skin, lung, gastrointestinal tract, central nervous system (migraine), who often required larger amounts more frequently and in whom symptoms could take well over 24 hours to occur.

Atopic eczema

The incidence of atopic eczema is rising in Britain and foods are among the many environmental factors that contribute to aggravating this distressing skin disease. A lack of bacterial stimulation of the gastrointestinal tract through excessive cleanliness ('hygiene hypothesis') has been put forward as an additional hypothesis and made plausible through a number of prospective studies in children living on farms (Braun-Fahrlander 2003) (Fig. 26.4). The strongest evidence of a role for food in the pathogenesis of atopic eczema comes from studies in which children with atopic eczema have responded well to exclusion diets in double-blind controlled crossover trials. Eczema can occur in exclusively breastfed infants, and this can be due to the transfer of absorbed food antigens from the mother's diet to her milk. Food intolerance and enhanced immune responsiveness to foods are also features of atopic eczema in adults. The antigens concerned are usually in fish, shellfish, eggs, peanuts, tree nuts, wheat, soy and milk. A role of the skin and other immunological sites during primary food antigen sensitisation is possible.

Asthma

Clinical observations suggest that milk intolerance is an occasional trigger of asthma. Asthma overall

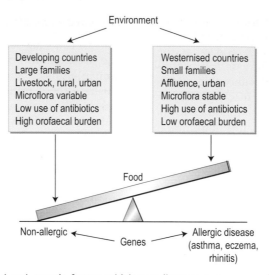

Fig. 26.4 Balance of environmental and genetic factors which contribute to or suppress allergic sensitisation – 'hygiene hypothesis'. *Administration of food proteins (allergens) at particular susceptible time points may tip the balance either way. After Wills-Karp et al 2001.*

is an important risk factor in patients suffering food allergic and in particular anaphylactic reactions. In about 5% of patients with asthma, foods may cause worsening of their symptoms.

Cow's milk intolerance with malabsorption syndrome

The classic milk-induced malabsorption syndrome with an abnormal (flat) intestinal mucosa and failure to thrive has become less frequent. More often infants and children suffer from vomiting, diarrhoea, eczema, urticaria and angio-oedema, recurrent otitis and also constipation (see Table 26.5). In the classic form, gastrointestinal investigations show malabsorption, and jejunal biopsy reveals abnormalities of the jejunal mucosa, ranging from moderate villous atrophy to pathology indistinguishable from coeliac disease. In children with less severe symptoms, as is currently the more common disease presentation, the only biological evidence may be a mild infiltration with eosinophils or mast cells within an otherwise normal mucosa. In vitro cellular tests may exhibit an increase in 'allergen-specific' cytokine response.

Cow's-milk-sensitive colitis

Typically, an infant with food-sensitive colitis presents before the age of 1 year, with the alarming picture of loose stools that contain mucus and blood. An elimination diet leads to quick resolution of symptoms. This is mirrored by a rapid histological recovery on rectal mucosal biopsy. The pathology of the rectum differs from classic ulcerative colitis in that there is preservation of the architecture of the mucosal crypts, with no crypt abscess formation and no depletion of goblet cell mucus. Additionally, there are substantial numbers of eosinophils and plasma cells in the infiltrate of the lamina propria. These infants respond well to elimination of cow's milk from their diet or from the mother's diet if they are still breastfed. Most children can tolerate cow's milk by the age of 2–3 years.

Principles of management

The treatment of cow's-milk-induced allergic systems is the complete elimination of milk and of milk-derived products. *Extensively* hydrolysed infant formulas are tolerated in most infants, who often suffer from the less severe form. These formulae are recommended for infants under 6 months of age. However, if symptoms do not subside within a week, amino-acid-based formulas should be used. In all children who do not receive sufficient amounts of formula feeds, calcium supplementation must be given. Occasionally lactose intolerance overlaps with the syndrome of cow's-milk-protein-sensitive enteropathy. Where there is extensive villous atrophy, loss of disaccharidase-containing mature enterocytes leads to a relative reduction in the disaccharidase activity of the small bowel mucosa.

In this case there may be a reversible lactose intolerance induced by the intestinal damage which itself has been caused by cow's milk protein intolerance. Lactose intolerance should not be generally accepted as a *primary* explanation of malabsorption, failure to thrive and gastrointestinal symptoms in infants since primary lactase deficiency is extremely rare and lactose intolerance states in a European population often indicates an underlying (mucosal) abnormality (see below).

LACTOSE INTOLERANCE

Lactose is a disaccharide (β-galactose-1,4-D-glucose) that is exclusively present in milk and milk products where it is the main sugar; its concentration is about 5% and 7% in cow's and human milk, respectively. It is a major source of energy in the young infant. Lactose is hydrolysed in the small intestine by a lactase (β-galactosidase) to give glucose and galactose. Galactose is then rapidly converted into glucose in the liver.

Lactase activity naturally falls from the infant level to adult levels (a 10- to 20-fold reduction) between the ages of 3 and 5 years in 75% of the world's population, while 25% of the population appear to maintain infant levels of lactase in adulthood. Both males and females are equally affected. In Europe 'lactase persisters' are in the majority. An individual with hypolactasia can exhibit lactose maldigestion in, for example, the breath hydrogen excretion test without displaying clinical symptoms of lactose intolerance.

Clinical features of lactose intolerance

Adverse reactions, which may develop 1–3 hours after a lactase-deficient, intolerant individual ingests lactose in food, include nausea, bloating, abdominal pain and diarrhoea. The clinical effects of lactose ingestion are closely related to the dose and there is a wide variation among individuals regarding the dose–response. The conventional lactose load, 50 g, used in tolerance tests, produces symptoms in 80–100% of lactose-intolerant individuals, whereas 10–15 g of lactose, equivalent to around half a pint of milk (~250 ml), will produce abdominal symptoms in 30–60%. Clinical reactions have been described after intake of less than 1g of lactose, although most lactase-deficient individuals tolerate 7–10 g of lactose without symptoms.

Clinical syndromes of lactose intolerance

Abdominal pain in children

Recurrent abdominal pain in children is almost as common as irritable bowel syndrome. The post-weaning drop in intestinal lactase activity may occur as early as 2 years in some ethnic groups, or at 5 years in white-background children, so that schoolchildren occasionally may be intolerant of lactose. Studies of recurrent abdominal pain in children in the USA have shown clinical lactose intolerance in a substantial proportion, particularly in black, Hispanic and Asian children. Lactose intolerance associated with abdominal pain is particularly relevant in children of ethnic groups with a high prevalence of hypolactasia.

Diarrhoea after gastric surgery

Gastric surgery and surgery of the small intestine radically alter the physiology of the upper gastrointestinal tract. As noted above, the rate of gastric emptying may affect the tolerance to lactose in a susceptible individual; with lactose feeding after surgery a lactase-deficient person may develop bloating, faintness and discomfort known as 'dumping' and diarrhoea.

Secondary, reversible lactose intolerance

Disaccharide intolerance may occur as a transient phenomenon associated with a wide variety of diseases of the small intestine in childhood including gastroenteritis, coeliac disease, giardiasis, protein calorie malnutrition, cow's milk protein intolerance, immunodeficiency syndromes and intestinal resections.

World Health Organization recommendations for management of children recovering from acute diarrhoea are that oral rehydration nutrition, including breastfeeding, should in general be introduced within 24 hours. Although many low-lactose and modified milk preparations are now available for nutrition of patients with acute and chronic diarrhoeas, these are likely to be more relevant in the management of immunologically based milk protein intolerance, or in chronic diarrhoeal disease, than during infectious acute gastroenteritis.

Treatment of lactose intolerance

As with other states of food intolerance, the strict diagnosis of lactose intolerance relies on objective measurements of the clinical effects of the withdrawal and reintroduction of lactose. Milk is such an important nutrient that before recommending a low-lactose diet with the avoidance of milk, milk intolerance should be formally confirmed. The only satisfactory treatment of lactose intolerance is a diet with low oral, tolerated, lactose content to avoid calcium- and vitamin-D-deficiency states. Foodstuffs high in lactose, such as fresh milk, powdered milk and milk puddings, should be avoided but most lactose-intolerant patients can tolerate about 10g of fermented milk products such as cheese and yoghurt, in which the lactose content has been reduced. Lactose-reduced milk and milk products are commercially available. Addition of external lactase enzymes to milk products with the aim of reducing the lactose content may be helpful in individual cases.

KEY POINTS

- Any component of the immune system may be absent or abnormal; the effect may range from trivial to fatal.
- Dysfunction of the immune system may be genetically determined or acquired from disease, drug treatment or radiotherapy.
- Immune deficiency may result in underactivity of the system and susceptibility to infection, or abnormal regulation as in allergy or autoimmunity.
- Poor nutrition compromises immune function not only in the malnourished of developing countries, but also in the undernourished of industrialised nations, such as those in hospital with infection, surgery, trauma or cancer, alcohol users, the elderly and food faddists.
- AIDS is a major cause of malnutrition and micronutrient deficiencies in resource-poor countries and in industrialised countries.
- Protein–energy malnutrition (PEM) in children causes atrophy of the lymph organs (thymus, tonsils, spleen, lymph nodes, Peyer's patches), which affects the overall immune status of the individual.
- Deficiency of vitamins A, E, B_6, pantothenic acid and folate all decrease cell and humoral immunocompetence, with an increased susceptibility to infections.
- Vitamin C enhances bacterial phagocytosis in vitro.

- Deficiency of the minerals Fe, Zn, Ca, Mg, Mn, Cu, Se, Cd, Cr, I, depresses immunocompetence as do toxic levels of the heavy metals Pb, Hg, Cd.
- Iron supplements should be given with caution to malnourished patients with infections as iron may stimulate bacterial multiplication.
- Zinc deficiency in fetal and early neonatal stages delays the development of the immune system.
- Food intolerance, food sensitivity and food allergy are terms often used for all reproducible adverse reactions to specific foods or ingredients.
- Food aversion, intolerance and allergy are sometimes difficult to distinguish, and can best be established by a blinded elimination diet and controlled reintroduction of the target foods (double-blind placebo-controlled food challenge).
- Lactose intolerance can be managed with a low-lactose diet. Fermented milk (yoghurt) and lactose-reduced milk products may be used to supplement small amounts of milk.
- Increased training opportunities for multiprofessional teams providing allergy services are needed to avoid patients resorting to unscientific methods and practitioners.
- The main foods incriminated in causing food allergic reactions are milk, egg, soya, wheat, peanut, tree nuts, fish, shellfish.

References

Bateman B, Warner JO, Hutchinson E, et al: The effects of a double blind, placebo controlled, artificial food colourings and benzoate preservative challenge on hyperactivity in a general population sample of preschool children, *Archives of Disease in Childhood* 89(6):506–511, 2004.

Berin MC, Mayer L: Immunophysiology of experimental food allergy, *Mucosal Immunology* 2(1):24–32, 2009.

Bischoff S, Crowe SE: Food allergy and the gastrointestinal tract, *Current Opinions in Gastroenterology* 20(2):156–161, 2004.

Brandtzaeg P: Mucosal immunity: integration between mother and the breast-fed infant, *Vaccine* 21:3382–3388, 2003.

Brandtzaeg P: Induction of secretory immunity and memory at mucosal surfaces, *Vaccine* 25(30):5467–5484, 2007.

Braun-Fahrlander C: Environmental exposure to endotoxin and other microbial products and the decreased risk of childhood atopy: evaluating developments since April 2002, *Current Opinions in Allergy and Clinical Immunology* 3(5):325–329, 2003.

Brooks WA, Santosham M, Naheed A, et al: Effect of weekly zinc supplements on incidence of pneumonia and diarrhoea in children younger than 2 years in an urban, low-income population in Bangladesh: randomised controlled trial, *Lancet* 366(9490):999–1004, 2005.

Burks W, Kulis M, Pons L: Food allergies and hypersensitivity: a review of pharmacotherapy and therapeutic strategies, *Expert Opinions in Pharmacotherapy* 9(7):1145–1152, 2008.

Chang AB, Torzillo PJ, Boyce NC, et al: Zinc and vitamin A supplementation in Indigenous Australian children hospitalised with lower respiratory tract infection: a randomised controlled trial, *Medical Journal of Australia* 184(3):107–112, 2006.

Chinen J, Shearer WT: Basic and clinical immunology, *Journal of Allergy and Clinical Immunology* 116(2):411–418, 2005.

Cunningham-Rundles S, McNeeley DF, Moon A: Mechanisms of nutrient modulation of the immune response, *Journal of Allergy and Clinical Immunology* 115(6):1119–1128; quiz 29, 2005.

Eigenmann PA, Beyer K, Wesley Burks A, et al: New visions for food allergy: an iPAC summary and future trends, *Pediatric Allergy and Immunology* 19(Suppl 19):26–39, 2008.

Geha RS, Notarangelo LD, Casanova JL, et al: Primary immunodeficiency diseases: an update from the International Union of Immunological Societies Primary Immunodeficiency Diseases Classification Committee, *Journal of Allergy and Clinical Immunology* 120(4):776–794, 2007.

Goldman AS, Anderson DW Jr, Sellers WA, et al: Milk allergy. I. Oral challenge with milk and isolated milk proteins in allergic children, *Pediatrics* 32:425–443, 1963.

Heine RG, Elsayed S, Hosking CS, Hill DJ: Cow's milk allergy in infancy, *Current Opinions in Allergy and Clinical Immunology* 2(3):217–225, 2002.

Hemila H, Chalker F, Treacy B, Douglas B: Vitamin C for preventing and treating the common cold (Review). Cochraine Library 2008, Issue 4, 2008.

Hewison M: Vitamin D and innate immunity, *Current Opinions in Investigative Drugs* 9(5):485–490, 2008.

Hill DJ, Hosking CS: Emerging disease profiles in infants and young children with food allergy, *Pediatric Allergy and Immunology* 8(10 Suppl):21–26, 1997.

Hill DJ, Heine RG, Hosking CS: The diagnostic value of skin prick testing in children with food allergy, *Pediatrics Allergy and Immunology* 15(5):435 441, 2004.

Kapil U, Bhavna A: Adverse effects of poor micronutrient status during childhood and adolescence, *Nutritional Reviews* 60(5 Pt 2):S84–S90, 2002.

Kelley DS, Daudu PA, Taylor PC, et al: Effects of low-copper diets on human immune response, *American Journal of Clinical Nutrition* 62(2):412–416, 1995.

Keusch GT: The history of nutrition: malnutrition, infection and immunity, *Journal of Nutrition* 133(1):336S–340S 2003.

Kilkkinen A, Knekt P, Heliovaara M, et al: Vitamin D status and the risk of lung cancer: a cohort study in Finland, *Cancer Epidemiol Biomarkers and Prevention* 17(11):3274–3278, 2008.

Lahtinen SJ, Gueimond M, Ouwehand AC, et al: Comparison of four methods to enumerate probiotic bifidobacteria in a fermented food product, *Food Microbiology* 23(6):571–577, 2006.

Lesourd B: Nutritional factors and immunological ageing, *Proceedings of the Nutrition Society* 65(3):319–325, 2006.

Lippman SM, Klein EA, Goodman PJ, et al: Effect of selenium and vitamin E on risk of prostate cancer and other cancers: the Selenium and Vitamin E Cancer Prevention Trial (SELECT), *Journal of the American Medical Association* 301(1):39–51, 2009.

McCann D, Barrett A, Cooper A, et al: Food additives and hyperactive behaviour in 3-year-old and 8/9-year-old children in the community: a randomised, double-blinded, placebo-controlled trial, *Lancet* 370(9598):1560–1567, 2007.

Martineau AR, Wilkinson RJ, Wilkinson, KA: A single dose of vitamin D enhances immunity to mycobacteria, *American Journal of Respiratory Critical Care Medicine* 176(2):208–213, 2007.

Medina M, Izquierdo E, Ennahar S, Sanz Y: Differential immunomodulatory properties of *Bifidobacterium longum* strains: relevance to probiotic selection and clinical applications, *Clinical and Experimental Immunology* 150(3):531–538, 2007.

Mehl A, Rolinck-Werninghaus C, Staden U, et al: The atopy patch test in the diagnostic workup of suspected food-related symptoms in children, *Journal of Allergy and Clinical Immunology* 118(4):923–929, 2006.

Munoz C, Rios E, Olivos J, Brunser O, Olivares M: Iron, copper and immunocompetence, *British Journal of Nutrition* 98(Suppl 1):S24–S28, 2007.

Nowak-Wegrzyn A, Sampson HA: Adverse reactions to foods, *Medical Clinics of North America* 90(1):97–127, 2006.

Pesonen M, Kallio MJ, Siimes MA, Ranki A: Retinol concentrations after birth are inversely associated with atopic manifestations in children and young adults, *Clinical Experimental Allergy* 37(1):54–61, 2007.

Rayman MP, Thompson AJ, Bekaert B, et al: Randomized controlled trial of the effect of selenium supplementation on thyroid function in the elderly in the United Kingdom, *American Journal of Clinical Nutrition* 87(2):370–378, 2008.

Schaible UE, Kaufmann SHE: Malnutrition and infection: Complex mechanisms and global impacts, *PLoS Medicine* 4(5):e115, 806–812, 2007.

Sicherer SH, Leung DY: Advances in allergic skin disease, anaphylaxis, and hypersensitivity reactions to foods, drugs, and insects in 2007, *Journal of Allergy and Clinical Immunology* 121(6):1351–1358, 2008.

Sicherer SH, Sampson HA: Food allergy: recent advances in

pathophysiology and treatment, *Annual Review of Medicine* 2008.

Stapel SO, Asero R, Ballmer-Weber BK, et al: Testing for IgG4 against foods is not recommended as a diagnostic tool: EAACI Task Force Report, *Allergy* 63:793–796, 2008.

Strobel S: Clinically validated diagnostic tests and non-validated procedures of unproven value. In Buttriss J, editor: *Adverse reactions to foods*, Oxford, 2002, Blackwell Scientific, pp 131–137.

Strobel S, Mowat AM: Oral tolerance and allergic responses to food proteins. *Current Opinions in Allergy and Clinical Immunology* 6(3):207–213, 2006.

Turnlund JR, Jacob RA, Keen CL, et al: Long-term high copper intake: effects on indexes of copper status, antioxidant status, and immune function in young men, *American Journal of Clinical Nutrition* 79(6):1037–1044, 2004.

Uauy R, Kain J, Mericq V, Rojas J, Corvalan C: Nutrition, child

growth, and chronic disease prevention, *Annals of Medicine* 40(1):11–20, 2008.

Wang Y, Beydoun MA, Liang L, et al: Will all Americans become overweight or obese? Estimating the progression and cost of the US obesity epidemic, *Obesity (Silver Spring)* 16(10):2323–2330, 2008.

White JH: Vitamin D signaling, infectious diseases, and regulation of innate immunity, *Infection and Immunity* 76(9):3837–3843, 2008.

Wills-Karp M, Santeliz J, Karp CL: The germless theory of allergic disease: revisiting the hygiene hypothesis, *Nature Reviews Immunology* 1, 69–75, 2001.

Zaninotto P, Wardle H, Stamatakis E, et al: *Forecasting Obesity*, Prepared for the Department of Health, Joint Health Surveys Unit, National Centre for Social Research Department of Epidemiology and Public Health at the Royal Free and University College Medical School, 2006, UCL London, pp 1–26.

Further reading

Lee IM, Cook NR, Gaziano JM, et al: Vitamin E in the primary prevention of cardiovascular disease and cancer: the Women's Health Study: a randomized controlled trial, *Journal of the American Medical Association* 294(1):56–65, 2005.

Newell ML: Antenatal and perinatal strategies to prevent mother-to-child transmission of HIV infection,

Transactions of the Royal Society of Tropical Medicine and Hygiene 97(1):22–24, 2003.

Schleithoff SS, Zittermann A, Tenderich G, et al: Vitamin D supplementation improves cytokine profiles in patients with congestive heart failure:a double-blind, randomized, placebo-controlled

trial, *American Journal of Clinical Nutrition* 83(4):754–759, 2006.

Tomkins A: Nutrition and maternal morbidity and mortality, *British Journal of Nutrition* 85(Suppl 2):S93–S99, 2001.

Chapter 27

Eating disorders

Zafra Cooper and Christopher G Fairburn*

CHAPTER CONTENTS

OBJECTIVES

By the end of this chapter you should be able to:

- define eating disorders and name the main types
- describe the main features of anorexia nervosa and bulimia nervosa
- outline the characteristics of other eating disorders.

27.1 INTRODUCTION

An eating disorder may be defined as a persistent disturbance of eating (or eating-related behaviour) which impairs physical health or psychosocial functioning, or both, and which is not secondary to any general medical disorder or any other psychiatric disorder. The best-recognised eating disorders are anorexia nervosa and bulimia nervosa, the two specific disorders recognised by the current psychiatric classificatory system (Diagnostic and Statistical Manual (DSM-IV) – see Section *evolve* 27.1 for full criteria for anorexia nervosa and bulimia nervosa). In addition, there are 'atypical eating disorders' also referred to as 'eating disorder not otherwise specified', which are disorders of clinical severity that do not meet the diagnostic criteria for anorexia nervosa or bulimia nervosa (see Section *evolve* 27.1). These are the most common form of eating disorder in outpatient settings and in community groups. These disorders share many features and together they are a major source of ill

---

*Updated and modified from the previous edition chapter written by C G Fairburn and A J Hill

© 2010 Elsevier Ltd/Inc/BV
DOI: 10.1016/B978-0-7020-3118-2.00027-9

health among young women in Western societies. In this chapter, the characteristics and management of these three groups of eating disorder will be described. Though important, the prevention of eating disorders is beyond the scope of this chapter. Suggested sources of further information are included in the further reading list and the list of useful websites on the *evolve* website 🖱. (See also Section 14.7 and Ch. 20.)

27.2 ANOREXIA NERVOSA

DEFINITION

Three features are required to make a diagnosis of anorexia nervosa:

1. An active maintenance of an unduly low weight. The definition of what constitutes low weight varies: 15% below a person's expected weight for their age, height and sex is the common cut-off or a body mass index of 17.5 or less is also used.

2. The over-evaluation of shape and weight; that is a tendency to judge self-worth largely, or even exclusively, in terms of shape and weight. Whereas it is usual to judge self-worth on the basis of performance in a variety of domains (such as relationships, work performance, sporting activities), people with anorexia nervosa evaluate themselves primarily in terms of their shape and weight. Thus, while low weight and emaciation are the most obvious features of anorexia nervosa, the most distinctive is the set of attitudes and values concerning body shape and weight. This cognitive disturbance is sometimes referred to as the core psychopathology of the disorder. It has been described in various terms, including 'relentless pursuit of thinness' and a 'morbid fear of fatness'. Thinness and weight loss are idealised and sought after, and strenuous attempts made to avoid weight gain and any possibility of fatness. This level of shape and weight concern is far more intense than the dissatisfaction regarded as normative for young women.

3. The third diagnostic feature is amenorrhoea (in postmenarcheal females not taking an oral contraceptive).

The defining low weight of anorexia nervosa is achieved in several ways, including strict dieting,

excessive exercising and, in some, self-induced vomiting or laxative misuse. The DSM-IV distinguishes between two subtypes of the disorder based on the presence of bulimic or purging symptoms (see Section *evolve* 27.1 for full DSM-IV criteria 🖱). The restricting subtype excludes regular binge-eating or purging behaviour. A person with anorexia nervosa can alternate between restricting and bulimic subtypes at different times in their illness, and can migrate into a different eating disorder such as bulimia nervosa (see below).

EPIDEMIOLOGY

Estimates of the incidence or prevalence of eating disorders in Western societies vary according to the assessment method, the population sample and the context of sampling. A typical estimate of the age-adjusted and sex-adjusted incidence rate of anorexia nervosa (the number of new cases arising) is 8 per 100 000 of the population per year (Hoek 2006). Incidence is highest in women aged 15–19 years.

The reported prevalence rates for anorexia nervosa vary between 0 and 0.9% with an average point prevalence (actual number of cases at a certain point in time) of 0.29% in young women (Hoek 2006). Since many patients deny or hide their eating disorder, the comparable community 1-year prevalence rate is estimated to be higher at 0.37% (Hoek 2006). In women the lifetime prevalence of anorexia nervosa ranges from 1.2% to 2.2% when strictly defined to around 4% for more broadly defined anorexia nervosa. Anorexia nervosa is more common in females than males with very few studies reporting incidence rates for males. Those that do suggest an incidence of less than 1.0 per 100 000 persons per year.

Some incidence figures have suggested an increase in young females with anorexia nervosa over recent decades (van Son et al 2006) but alternative explanations cannot be ruled out. These include changes in diagnostic practice, improved recognition of the disorder, wider availability of services and changes in the demographic structure of the population.

Certain groups in the population show higher than expected prevalence rates of anorexia nervosa. Female dancers and athletes, such as distance runners and gymnasts, are especially vulnerable. They share highly competitive subcultures where it may be common to manipulate eating and weight in an attempt to improve appearance and maximise performance.

Anorexia nervosa has long been thought to be confined to Western culture and in particular to Caucasians and has therefore been regarded as a 'culture-bound syndrome' (Grilo 2006). This view has been challenged by recent cross-cultural work and detailed examination of the historical reports of the disorder (Keel & Klump 2003, Attia & Walsh 2007). An alternative view is that eating disorders may simply vary in form from culture to culture (Franko 2007, Lee & Lock 2007).

DEVELOPMENT

The onset of anorexia nervosa is generally in adolescence, although childhood-onset or pre-pubertal cases are observed. In children, boys represent 20–25% of referrals. Occasionally, anorexia nervosa does not begin until adulthood. Usually it starts as unremarkable dieting which then gets out of control. As the dieting intensifies, body weight falls and the physiological and psychological features of semi-starvation develop. Additional methods of controlling shape and weight may also be used at any stage. The characteristic concerns about shape and weight may not be finally expressed until later. In some cases, the initial weight loss has some other origin such as a general medical illness. However, the low weight is then actively maintained.

CLINICAL FEATURES

Weight loss in anorexia nervosa is primarily achieved through a severe reduction in food intake. Some patients also fast at times. Although, diet histories are compromised by the over-reporting typical of anorexic patients, their diets are certainly inadequate in energy. Laboratory studies show that those with the restricting form of anorexia nervosa consume 60–70% less energy than age-matched controls. Interestingly, vitamin and mineral deficiencies are rarely seen. This may reflect a decreased metabolic need for micronutrients or an adequate intake of vitamins and minerals.

In most cases hunger persists and for this reason the term 'anorexia' is misleading. However, the perception and reporting of hunger are often distorted. Experimental investigations have revealed abnormal hunger–satiety curves relative to controls. It is also suggested that those with anorexia nervosa learn to control or suppress normal hunger signals. This denial of hunger may be experienced as rewarding and a mark of personal self-control. In addition, the physiological consequences of starvation, such as a slow rate of gastric emptying, can make normal food intake unpleasant as even small quantities of food may result in bloating. A return to a more normal pattern of eating and an increase in the amount eaten helps to rehabilitate the perception of hunger and satiety.

Frequent intense exercising is common and contributes to the low body weight. Laxative and diuretic misuse and self-induced vomiting may also be practised, especially by those patients whose control over eating occasionally breaks down. This is true of about a third of patients with anorexia nervosa, but the amount eaten during these binges is often not objectively large.

Accompanying the disordered eating is the disturbance of body image. This includes a perceptual component such that all, or parts, of the body may be seen as larger than their actual size, and the cognitive disturbance described earlier. Judging the body to be larger than it really is may justify the relentless pursuit of thinness. However, neither feature improves as weight is lost: indeed, both tend to get worse. Early in the course of illness, patients often have limited recognition of their disorder and experience their symptoms as ego-syntonic, meaning they are not viewed as a problem and patients therefore do not want to get rid of them.

A range of other psychological symptoms commonly accompany anorexia nervosa, many of which are known to result from semi-starvation. These include depressed mood, irritability, social withdrawal, loss of sexual libido, preoccupation with food, and eventually, reduced alertness and concentration. Dysphoria (unhappiness) is particularly important and often misunderstood by clinicians who make an inappropriate second diagnosis of a mood disorder. Similarly, severe obsessional symptoms, usually related to eating and food, are common in anorexia nervosa. Often, these symptoms improve with weight gain.

A wide range of physical complications is encountered in anorexia nervosa. Earlier last century the disorder was mistakenly attributed to pituitary insufficiency. More recently it was suggested there might be an underlying primary hypothalamic disorder. The balance of evidence, however, strongly suggests that the endocrine disturbance is secondary to abnormalities in eating and weight rather than being a cause of them.

On examination, the degree of emaciation is often striking. Growth may be stunted in patients with a pre-pubertal onset and there may be a failure of breast development. Often patients present with no physical complaints. However, systematic inquiry may reveal heightened sensitivity to cold and a variety of gastrointestinal symptoms such as constipation, fullness after eating, bloatedness and vague abdominal pain. Other symptoms include restlessness, lack of energy and early morning wakening.

In females who are not taking an oral contraceptive, amenorrhoea is (by definition) present. Amenorrhoea, if sustained, is associated with osteopenia, possibly progressing to osteoporosis and risk of bone fractures. Amenorrhoea that starts in early teenage years and persists into young adulthood presents the greatest risk to bone health as patients not only lose bone mass but fail to form bone at a critical phase of development. The resulting osteoporosis is often irreversible.

The physical complications of anorexia nervosa affect each main organ system of the body. Acute complications include dehydration, electrolyte disturbances (due to purging), cardiac compromise with various arrhythmias, gastrointestinal mobility disturbances, renal problems, infertility, hypothermia, and other evidence of hypometabolism.

CAUSATION

Dieting is a general vulnerability factor for both anorexia nervosa and bulimia nervosa. Longitudinal studies have shown that female teenagers who dieted were 5–18 times more likely to develop an eating disorder, depending on the severity of their dieting (Patton et al 1999). However, a simple linkage is problematic for two reasons. First, while many young women diet, relatively few develop an eating disorder. Second, dieting is more likely in those who are heavier and dissatisfied with their body. Dieting may therefore be a relatively nonspecific marker of other vulnerability factors.

Family studies indicate a 7–12-fold increase in the rates of anorexia nervosa and bulimia nervosa in relatives of eating-disordered probands compared with controls. Since first-degree relatives share both genes and environment, twin studies have been used to disentangle the two (Slof-Op 't Landt et al 2005). Such studies have implicated genetic factors showing that these contribute more than 50% of the variance to anorexia nervosa

(Klump & Gobrogge 2005). Clinic samples show concordance for anorexia nervosa of around 55% in identical twins and 5% in non-identical twins (Fairburn & Harrison 2003). These findings suggest a significant heritability for anorexia nervosa. There is also evidence of shared transmission between anorexia nervosa and bulimia nervosa. This suggests the existence of a broad eating disorder phenotype with possible shared genetic predispositions. Given the clear and possibly substantial genetic contribution to both anorexia nervosa and bulimia nervosa, molecular genetic studies have been conducted to identify the underlying loci and genes. Such studies are of two types. Genetic association studies have focussed in particular on polymorphisms in 5-HT (serotonin)-related genes because this neurotransmitter system is important in regulation of eating and mood, but a range of other polymorphisms have also been investigated. Despite this, no associations with eating disorders have been clearly replicated or confirmed in a family study or by meta-analysis. There has been one multi-centre genome-wide linkage study. It found linkage peaks for anorexia nervosa and bulimia nervosa on chromosomes 1, 4, 10 and 14. A further analysis, which covaried for related behavioural traits, identified a different locus on chromosome 1, as well as loci on chromosomes 2 and 13. All these findings await replication (Kaye et al 2008).

Accounts of the contribution of sociocultural factors to eating disorders seek evidence of the environmental transmission of pathology. Eating disorders appear to show some cultural specificity, being generally confined to countries that have an abundance of food, that hold a thin body shape as ideal, and in which dieting is commonplace (although, as noted above, this view has been challenged). The media are often blamed for their invariable use of extremely thin models and celebrities, driving others to achieve thinness themselves. However this probably overstates the influence of the media. Exposure to media images of thin bodies can induce body dissatisfaction, but mainly in those already dissatisfied. Equally the negative attitudes and behaviour towards fatness generally prevalent in Western society may also produce weight dissatisfaction. This dissatisfaction is a common precursor, and continuing accompaniment, of eating disorders. Thus sociocultural factors do appear to channel women's dissatisfaction and distress towards a focus on body shape and size, providing an outlet for individual pathology. The result is thinness being relentlessly pursued by those who see no better way to solve their problems (Polivy & Herman 2002).

Peers and family are also important contributors to the sociocultural context. Peers may be influential in victimising those not conforming to shape or weight ideals or aspirations. Family dynamics (enmeshment, intrusiveness, hostility) and abnormal attachment processes have been proposed as causes of eating disorders. However some of these features may be secondary to the presence of an ill family member. Despite this, research from retrospective case-controlled studies suggests that adolescents who perceive parental caring and expectations as low and those who report physical or sexual abuse are at risk for developing eating disorders. Maternal influence has been implicated as a negative contributory factor in some cases, the suggestion being that mothers may convey their own weight and shape concerns by acting as a role model, by directly making critical comments, or through inappropriate feeding interactions (Mazzeo et al 2005). Less attention has been paid to the potential role of other family members, nor have researchers looked closely at how families and peers may have a positive and protective function in respect of eating disorder vulnerability. Overall, it is difficult to conclude exactly how large a contribution to anorexia nervosa or bulimia nervosa is made by families or peers and there is uncertainty about the relative importance of their contributions.

Individual risk factors thought to be important in pathogenesis range from personality traits such as perfectionism, negative self-evaluation and obsessive features to premorbid psychiatric disorder and a variety of life stresses and difficulties. It is common for people to identify a single event that triggered their dieting or intensified their pursuit of thinness. Several of the changes characteristic of anorexia nervosa, in particular under-eating and low body weight act to perpetuate the disorder. The fullness and bloating resulting from the slowing in gastric emptying, even after eating small amounts of food, makes eating unpleasant. Similarly, the preoccupation with food and eating intensifies the difficulties with eating, encouraging social withdrawal. This isolates the person from his or her peers, encouraging further self-preoccupation. Weight loss may initially elicit compliments and social approval. In addition many patients report that exerting strict control over eating is in itself intensely rewarding. Nevertheless the most potent maintaining factor is likely to be cognitive disturbance, the extreme concerns about shape and weight and their control, which are characteristic of these disorders. Given its presence, most other features of the disorder are comprehensible.

ASSESSMENT

Few patients with anorexia nervosa refer themselves for treatment. Usually, they are persuaded to seek help by concerned relatives or friends, and as a consequence they may attend reluctantly. Careful history taking focused particularly on whether the low weight is being maintained through the patient's own efforts and whether it is associated with the characteristic core psychopathology, will make the diagnosis clear. Some patients will be unable to describe their behaviour accurately or truthfully, making assessment more difficult. Additional information from family and friends can often be revealing. Simple screening questions can help determine whether a formal evaluation of eating behaviour and attitudes is required (see Table *evolve* 27.1 for details of assessment methods).

Some of the presenting symptoms – loss of appetite, weight loss, amenorrhoea, unexplained vomiting – can be mimicked by a variety of medical conditions. Alternative diagnoses should be considered while recognising the possibility of denial or deception. Excluding the presence of coexisting depressive disorder can be difficult since many symptoms of depression are also consequences of semi-starvation. It is more straightforward to exclude the possibility of depression as the sole diagnosis as in this case the weight loss is not self-induced and the core psychopathology of anorexia nervosa is not seen.

Although physical tests are not required for diagnostic purposes, all patients with anorexia nervosa should have a thorough physical examination and whatever investigations are indicated as a result. Electrolytes should be checked in all those who frequently vomit or misuse significant quantities of laxatives or diuretics (see bulimia nervosa).

MANAGEMENT

Some patients with anorexia nervosa present with short histories and are willing and able to change. Others have an entrenched disorder and appear to resist all treatment attempts. Negotiating a plan of management is a complex procedure involving engaging the patient in the process of change, forging an effective therapeutic alliance, assessing risk, and exchanging information. The relationship between patient and clinician is critical and will have a profound impact on implementing the management plan.

In principle, there are two essential aspects to treatment. One is establishing healthy eating habits and a normal weight, and the second is addressing those factors liable to result in relapse. This generally involves the use of psychological treatments such as parental counselling, family therapy or cognitive behavioural therapy, each of which requires specialist training. Drugs have a limited role. There is no evidence to support the use of drugs in the treatment of anorexia nervosa. An initial report on young adults suggested that fluoxetine reduced the rate of relapse following inpatient treatment but a subsequent well-conducted two-centre study, again on young adults, failed to replicate the finding (Walsh et al 2006). However, if there is a co-existing clinical depression, antidepressant drugs can be prescribed.

Which treatments are the most effective?

Clinical services provided for anorexia nervosa fall into two types: those for children and adolescents and those for adults. It is worth noting that treatment outcome among adolescents with anorexia nervosa is generally good, in marked contrast with that amongst adults (Deter et al 2005). This may well be related to the nature of the disorder in these two groups. Adolescents with anorexia nervosa tend to have had the disorder for a very short time – often little more than a year – whereas adults generally have a history of 5 or more years of unremitting symptoms. Younger patients may be more responsive to treatment because many of the maintaining mechanisms that obstruct change in the more enduring cases may not yet be operating (Fairburn & Gowers 2008).

There is a range of treatment options for anorexia nervosa. A variety of interventions, both pharmacological (see above) and psychological are provided within a range of settings including outpatient, day patient (partial hospitalisation) and inpatient treatment. Patients may also move from one setting to another and within any one setting more than one treatment may be employed.

There is no empirical evidence to support the use of any one treatment setting over any other in terms of treatment outcome, nor is there robust evidence to support any specific psychological treatment. There has been one attempt to randomise patients to different treatment settings but the comparison was compromised by the finding that many patients did not want to be randomised to inpatient treatment. It is widely thought that there is good evidence to support the use of family therapy to treat adolescents with the disorder, with the most positive outcomes having been achieved using a specific form of family therapy (the Maudsley Model) with adolescent patients with disorders of recent onset (Wilson et al 2007). However only two studies have compared family therapy to another form of treatment and the findings of the one of these are difficult to interpret. Thus the case for favouring family therapy over other forms of treatment rests on a single study (Russell et al 1987) which involved a relatively small number of patients – all of whom had recently been discharged from a specialist inpatient unit. As regards the treatment of adults with anorexia nervosa, a recent systematic review concluded that the empirical evidence is sparse and inconclusive (Bulik et al 2007). Nevertheless one approach which appears promising is cognitive behaviour therapy (CBT). A variety of forms of enhanced CBT for both adults (Fairburn 2008, Dalle Grave et al 2008) and adolescents (Cooper & Stewart 2008) who are severely underweight have been described and are currently being evaluated.

Current treatment guidelines

There are four aspects to the initial stages of treatment:

- *Engagement*: in a collaborative therapeutic relationship
- *Education*: about clinical features of anorexia nervosa, and the importance of weight restoration
- *Agreeing the need for weight gain*: despite reluctance to change
- *Deciding on the treatment setting*: whether inpatient or outpatient.

For details of these initial stages of treatment see Section *evolve* 27.2 .

Inpatient treatment

Inpatient treatment programmes ideally have a mixture of elements. These include nutritional rehabilitation, medical rehabilitation, psychotherapy, family treatment and psychosocial rehabilitation. The precise mix of these will vary according to the age of the patient, their individual situation and local provision of facilities.

Nutritional therapy aims to achieve weight gain and the reinstatement of normal eating habits. Within a few days, patients should be introduced to eating regular meals and snacks amounting to 1000–1500 kcal/day. If possible, by the end of 2 weeks, these meals and snacks should be of a normal quantity and composition, consisting of about 2000 kcal/day. Early in the re-feeding process the patient should be monitored for re-feeding syndrome. This is characterised by sudden and sometimes severe hypophosphataemia, sudden drops in potassium and magnesium, hypokalaemia, gastrointestinal dysfunction and cardiac arrhythmias. Water retention should be anticipated and discussed with the patient.

A target rate of weight gain of 1 to 1.5 kg/week should be set, and the patient and staff should monitor the patient's weight each morning. The patient should be encouraged to be an active collaborator in the weight restoration process. Weighing gives the opportunity to discuss the patient's reaction to weight and to provide explanations for weight changes. Dietetic input in devising an individualised nutrition plan is important. Intakes of up to 3500 kcal/day may be needed to achieve the desired rate of weight gain, creating a need to use supplements in addition to meals and snacks. Energy-rich drinks are preferable to eating unusually large amounts of food since eating such quantities is hardly compatible with the goal of establishing healthy eating habits and may increase the risk of developing bulimia nervosa.

The target weight should be individualised, taking account of the patient's pre-morbid weight, and presented as a range since weight fluctuates naturally. Once patients enter the target weight range, dietary supplements should be phased out, leaving patients consuming a diet sufficient to maintain their weight. At this stage they should be given increasing control over their eating, and practice in shopping for and preparing food. Accordingly, a transitional period of day-patient treatment may be helpful. Unless considerable effort is put into this phase of treatment, the risk of relapse following discharge is considerable. Running concurrently with weight restoration will be the other forms of treatment. Psychotherapy may be most beneficial when weight is improved. Attention to cognitions typical of patients with anorexia nervosa and a focus on body image issues are common therapeutic components. Family treatment is seen as critical for younger patients and of value to older patients. For the latter patients, 'family' may include friends, partners and children. Attention to psychosocial issues is important for patients of all ages. Schooling will be a focus for younger patients. Issues relating to social relationships are almost always prominent among seriously ill patients with anorexia nervosa.

As the above suggests, inpatient treatment is a complex process involving specialist units with staff from a variety of disciplines including medical staff, nursing staff, dieticians, psychiatrists, clinical psychologists and occupational therapists.

Outpatient treatment

Often this is the sole form of treatment, although it may follow a period of inpatient or day-patient care. The choice of length and extent of outpatient treatment is increasingly based on an evaluation of medical risk and patient motivation. Family therapy and cognitive behavioural therapy are the psychological treatments most commonly available to outpatients (see above).

Day-patient treatment

There is increasing interest in the use of day-patient treatment instead of inpatient treatment for all but the most ill of patients. The programmes are for 4–7 days weekly and are intensive and multi-modal, including supervised meals, group and individual therapy. Day-patient treatment can be stressful and demanding for patients but is more cost-effective than inpatient treatment. Again, there are relatively few studies relating to effectiveness. The multi-modal nature of treatment makes it difficult to identify the most effective treatment components, and neither the optimum number of days per week nor the length of stay have been properly evaluated. This evidence should emerge as these programmes become more available.

COURSE AND OUTCOME

The proportion of adults with anorexia nervosa who fully recover is modest (Berkman et al 2007). The outcomes of less than 50% of cases can be rated as good. For about a quarter, outcome is poor, with weight never reaching the healthy range. Some residual features are common, particularly a degree of overconcern with shape, weight and eating and, in cases that persist, about a quarter develop bulimia nervosa. For adolescent cases, however, good outcomes have been reported in between half and three-quarters of cases (Fairburn & Gowers 2008).

Anorexia nervosa is the one eating disorder to be associated with a raised mortality rate (Berkman et al 2007), the standardised mortality ratio over the first 10 years from presentation being about 10 (Hoek 2006). The mortality rate among adolescents is low. Most deaths are a result of medical complications or due to suicide.

Few consistent predictors of treatment outcome have been identified. Poorer prognosis is associated with extremely low weight, vomiting, failure of previous treatment, disturbed family relationships and long duration of illness. In general, adolescents have better outcomes than adults, and younger adolescents better outcomes than older adolescents. It should be noted that some of these prognostic indicators have not been consistently replicated and may be more robust indicators of short-term rather than long-term outcomes.

KEY POINTS

- The judgement of self-worth primarily in terms of shape and weight is a core feature of anorexia nervosa.
- The disorder is much more common in females than males, with onset generally in adolescence.
- Weight loss is primarily achieved through a severe reduction in food intake.
- The goals of treatment are establishing healthy eating habits and a normal weight, and addressing those factors liable to result in relapse.
- A variety of treatment approaches are used but the proportion of adults who fully recover is modest.
- Outcome is generally good in adolescents

27.3 BULIMIA NERVOSA

DEFINITION

Three features also need to be present to make a diagnosis of bulimia nervosa:

1. The presence of recurrent binge-eating. A 'binge' is an episode of eating during which there is a sense of loss of control and an objectively large amount of food is eaten
2. The presence of extreme weight-control behaviour, such as strict dietary restriction, recurrent self-induced vomiting or marked laxative misuse
3. The over-evaluation of shape and weight, as in anorexia nervosa.

It is also specified that the diagnostic criteria for anorexia nervosa should not be met since otherwise some patients would be eligible to receive both eating disorder diagnoses. There are no weight criteria for bulimia nervosa, although body weight is often in the normal range as the effects of the overeating and weight control behaviour tend to cancel each other out. DSM-IV also distinguishes between the purging subtype of bulimia nervosa described above and a non-purging subtype. In the latter, the person uses compensatory behaviours such as fasting or excessive exercise rather than self-induced vomiting or laxatives (see Section *evolve* 27.1).

EPIDEMIOLOGY

People with bulimia nervosa are somewhat older than those with anorexia nervosa, most presenting in their late teens and early twenties. Bulimia nervosa was first described clinically in 1979 and viewed as an unusual variant of anorexia nervosa Initially there was a dramatic upsurge in the number of cases seen and the incidence of the disorder during the 1980s was reported as 13 per 100 000 of the population per year. However more recent evidence has suggested that this rise has now ceased and that there may even be a decline in the incidence rate. (Hoek 2006).

Using strict diagnostic criteria, the average point prevalence is about 1000 per 100 000 (i.e. 1%) (Hoek 2006) among young women. The comparable figure for men is a tenth of this, or 0.1%. The shame and secrecy associated with the disorder means that there is uncertainty about the true community prevalence of the disorder. It also results in a much poorer detection of bulimia nervosa in primary care (around 10% of cases, than of anorexia nervosa, 40% of cases (Hoek & van Hoeken 2003)) and while one-third of those meeting strict criteria for anorexia nervosa are treated in mental healthcare, the comparable figure for those with bulimia nervosa is only 6%. (Hoek 2006).

DEVELOPMENT

Bulimia nervosa has a slightly later age of onset than anorexia nervosa, usually in late adolescence or early adulthood. Many patients present with a history of disturbed eating stretching back into adolescence, and in around a quarter of cases they will have previously fulfilled diagnostic criteria for anorexia nervosa. Eventually episodes of binge-eating disrupt dietary restriction and body weight rises to normal or near normal levels. The disorder is self-perpetuating and patients often present with an unremitting history of disturbed eating of 8 or more years.

CLINICAL FEATURES

There are many similarities in the clinical features of bulimia nervosa and anorexia nervosa. The patients show the same concerns about shape and weight and engage in the same methods of weight control. Two important differences are in body weight and frequency of bulimic episodes. In bulimia nervosa, these binges are a source of great shame and they are kept hidden from others. This shame also leads to under-reporting, patients often unwilling to disclose the precise quantities or types of food consumed, or the pattern of binges and subsequent purging. Experimental studies show an eating pattern that includes long periods of deprivation, with most of the eating episodes occurring late in the day. The sense of lack of control over eating is reflected in the number of eating episodes that begin as meals or snacks but become binges that are followed by purging.

The characteristic alternation between severe restriction and episodes of binge-eating has led to the suggestion that restraint and binge-eating operate synergistically. Rigid control over eating is associated with multiple self-imposed dietary rules. These rules concern *when* food should be eaten (for example not before six in the evening), exactly *what* should be eaten (or rather not eaten; the result is a long list of 'forbidden foods'), and the overall *amount* of food that should be eaten (e.g. less than 4.2 MJ (1000 kcal) daily). Binges are often precipitated by breaking these rules. The other common trigger to binge-eating is the occurrence of events and circumstances that induce negative moods (depression, anxiety, anger or boredom).

Sustained depressive and anxiety symptoms are a more prominent feature of bulimia nervosa than anorexia nervosa. Impulsivity is also seen in a sub-group of cases, with self-harm and substance misuse noted.

The majority of patients have few physical complaints. The most commonly presented are irregular or absent menstruation, weakness and lethargy, and vague abdominal pain. Salivary gland enlargement may be present, a symptom associated with self-induced vomiting. Typically this involves the parotid glands and gives the patient's face a slightly rounded appearance. In addition, there may be significant erosion of the dental enamel on the palatal surface of the upper front teeth due to vomiting. A minority of patients, particularly those who take large quantities of laxatives or diuretics, have intermittent peripheral or facial oedema.

Nutritional abnormalities depend on the amount of restriction during non-binge periods. Purging behaviours do not completely prevent the digestion and absorption of food energy from the binge, which typically ranges between 4.2 and 8.4 MJ (1000–2000 kcal).

The most serious physical complications are apparent in those who frequently vomit or take laxatives or diuretics. Metabolic alkalosis, hypochloraemia and hypocalcaemia are the most common abnormalities and they may account for symptoms of weakness and tiredness. Severe electrolyte disturbance (particularly low potassium levels) is encountered occasionally, but even when it is longstanding there may be few accompanying symptoms. Despite concern about the consequences of low potassium levels, aggressive treatment is rarely appropriate. Instead, it should be monitored while the focus is on the treatment of the eating disorder itself.

CAUSATION

Many of the putative risk factors for anorexia nervosa (described earlier) have been shown to be risk factors for bulimia nervosa. There are some differences, however. For example, genetic studies show concordance of 35% in monozygotic twins and 30% in dizygotic twins, suggesting the disorder is less heritable than anorexia nervosa. Heritability estimates show a broader range (28–83%) than for anorexia nervosa, although this probably reflects the relaxation of diagnostic criteria to increase the number of affected twins for analysis (Fairburn & Harrison 2003). Despite this, the existence of a genetic component to this disorder is confirmed by heritability estimates of 46–71% for the key behaviours, binge-eating and self-induced vomiting (Klump et al 2001).

A variety of risk factors for bulimia nervosa have been identified. First there are demographic factors, with female gender, adolescence and living in a Western society (see above) all increasing risk. Second, exposure to an immediate social environment that encourages dieting has been implicated. Such exposure includes being brought up in a family in which there is intense interest in shape, weight and eating as a result of one or more members either having some degree of eating disorder or having a medical condition that affects eating or weight (e.g. diabetes mellitus), being under extreme occupational or recreational pressures to diet (e.g. ballet dancing) and the presence of parental and childhood obesity. The presence of obesity is likely to sensitise individuals to their appearance and weight, and thereby make them prone to diet. There is also some evidence that puberty occurs comparatively early which may also magnify concerns about shape. Third a range of factors have been identified that increase the risk of psychiatric disturbance in general and depression in particular. These include a family history of psychiatric disorder, especially depression, and a range of adverse childhood experiences including parenting deficits and sexual and physical abuse. It was thought that sexual abuse was especially common among those who develop bulimia nervosa, but the balance of evidence suggests that the rate is no higher than that among those who develop other psychiatric disorders. Fourth, the individual personality traits of perfectionism and low self-esteem are both common antecedents of bulimia nervosa as well as anorexia nervosa (as noted above). Typically they interact resulting in feelings of incompetence and ineffectiveness. Fifth, there is a raised rate of substance abuse in the families of patients with bulimia nervosa. It is not clear how this increases the risk of bulimia nervosa. Clinical observations suggest that some of those who develop bulimia nervosa learn to modulate their mood by engaging in self-harm (e.g. by cutting themselves) or by consuming large quantities of food, alcohol or psychoactive drugs.

An interesting issue is how those with anorexia nervosa are able to maintain strict control over their eating whereas this is not true of those with bulimia nervosa. While the explanation is unclear, several processes may be of relevance. Perfectionism, more pronounced in anorexia nervosa than bulimia nervosa, may enhance self-control whereas the vulnerability to obesity found in bulimia nervosa may undermine dietary restraint. Also, the mood lability found in bulimia nervosa may disrupt restraint

Certain cognitive and affective factors are important in the maintenance of bulimia nervosa. Dissociation, a changed state of consciousness that avoids unpleasant realities, is sometimes associated with binge-eating. Total immersion in the binge distracts the person from emotional distress. However, this relief is temporary, and negative affect plays an important role in binge-eating. Eating, especially when out of control, induces negative feelings, such as guilt. Purging relieves guilt but it evokes feelings of shame and self-disgust, lowering self-esteem and fostering the negative affect that triggers binge-eating.

ASSESSMENT

Most people with bulimia nervosa are ashamed of their eating habits, and keep them secret for many years. If they present for help they may complain of features associated with the disorder rather than the disorder itself. For example, they may present with gastrointestinal or gynaecological symptoms, depression or substance abuse. Under these circumstances, making the correct diagnosis can be difficult since there are rarely any pointers to the eating disorder itself. The best established measure of eating disorder features is the Eating Disorder Examination (Fairburn et al 2008). This interview is widely regarded as the 'gold standard' measure of eating disorders, but it is possibly too exhaustive to use on a routine clinical basis. There are several well-validated questionnaires for use in identifying cases of bulimia nervosa (see Table evolve 27.1). However, their precision is not perfect and the information they provide should be taken as suggestive that further enquiry would be useful.

Those patients who present directly complain of the binge-eating. Thus help seeking is more common than in anorexia nervosa as bingeing and purging have less perceived benefit than does food avoidance and low body weight. Consequently, they ask for help to control their eating. Assessment in such situations is generally straightforward. As with anorexia nervosa, no physical tests are needed to make the diagnosis, although electrolytes should be checked. The initial assessment should be broad enough to understand the potential causal and maintaining factors, and enable an individual case formulation.

MANAGEMENT

The treatment of bulimia nervosa, has been the subject of much research. Over 70 randomised controlled trials have been completed. This research has been reviewed by Wilson et al (2007) and several 'systematic reviews' have been conducted (National Collaborating Centre for Mental Health 2004, Shapiro et al 2007).

Which treatments are the most effective?

The NICE (National Institute for Clinical Excellence) review (2004) is particularly rigorous and, as with all NICE systematic reviews, it provides evidence-based guidelines for clinical management. In essence three main conclusions emerged from this systematic review. It is worth noting that the NICE conclusions are consistent with the most recently published systematic review (Shapiro et al 2007). First the leading treatment for bulimia nervosa is a specific form of (outpatient) cognitive behaviour therapy (CBT-BN). There is strong research support for this treatment and NICE recommended that it should be offered to adults with bulimia nervosa across the National Health Service. Second, a form of 'interpersonal psychotherapy' (IPT) offers an evidence-based alternative to cognitive behaviour therapy and involves about the same amount of therapist contact (Fairburn 1997) although it takes longer (about 8–12 months) for its beneficial effects to be realised. Third, antidepressant drugs and certain self-help programmes (preferably used with some form of professional support) both have some efficacy as treatments for bulimia nervosa and are relatively straightforward to implement. However, the evidence suggests that few patients make a full and lasting response with either treatment and these may be best considered first-line treatments. NICE further specified that fluoxetine was the antidepressant drug of choice (at a dose of 60 mg daily). It is worth noting that these recommendations apply to adults, as at the time of the systematic review, there were no published controlled trials focusing exclusively on the treatment of adolescents with bulimia nervosa. Two controlled trials of family-based treatments for adolescents have recently been published. In the first of these, family-based treatment was compared with a guided self-help form of cognitive behaviour therapy and included patients with bulimia nervosa and eating disorder NOS (Schmidt, et al 2007). In the second study family-based treatment was compared with supportive psychotherapy in adolescents with bulimia nervosa and sub-threshold bulimia nervosa strictly defined (Le Grange et al 2007). While family-based treatment showed an advantage over supportive psychotherapy, very few differences emerged when it was compared to cognitive behavioural self-help. Thus further work is required before firm evidence-based treatment guidelines can be proposed for adolescents. Thus the general conclusion is that there is a clear leading treatment for adults with bulimia nervosa, namely, CBT-BN. However, the research findings also indicate that this treatment is far from being a panacea since fewer than half the patients who start treatment make a full and lasting recovery.

Treatment guidelines

It is clear that the great majority of patients can be successfully managed on an outpatient basis. Inpatient or day-patient treatment is indicated in three circumstances, all of which are unusual. These are: first, if the patient is too depressed to be managed as an outpatient or there is significant risk of suicide; second, if the patient's physical health is a cause for concern; and third, if the eating disorder proves resistant to outpatient care. If hospitalisation is indicated, it should be brief and viewed as a preliminary to outpatient care.

Reducing and eventually eliminating binge-eating and purging are primary treatment goals. Nutritional or dietetic input has two components: dietary guidance and nutritional education. Dietary guidance includes meal-planning, assistance with regularising the pattern of eating, and discouragement of dieting. An eating plan of three meals per day with one to two snacks a day prescribed in a structured fashion helps break the chaotic eating pattern that supports the cycle of bingeing and purging. Nutrition education involves teaching about issues including body weight regulation, energy balance, the effects of starvation, misconceptions regarding dieting and weight control, and the physical consequences of purging behaviour. Both components are often delivered within the framework of treatment programmes such as cognitive behavioural therapy.

Specialised psychological treatment, such as CBT or IPT, is usually provided by clinical psychologists, although in principle there is no reason why it should not be administered by other health professionals so long as they have received the necessary training. CBT, the treatment with the most empirical support, aims to modify both the disturbed eating habits and the extreme concerns about shape and weight (the core psychopathology). It usually involves about 20 sessions over 5 months and can result in substantial improvement in all aspects of the disorder. The techniques used include the daily self-monitoring of relevant thoughts and behaviour (including food intake), binge-eating and purging; education about eating, shape and weight; the use of behavioural procedures to help establish a pattern of regular eating; the gradual reintroduction of avoided food; and cognitive procedures designed to identify and modify problematic thoughts and attitudes.

The effectiveness of self-help in some cases (see above) has led to the suggestion that a stepped care approach to treatment should be adopted. Step 1 is guided self-help (unless the patient has already followed such a programme). Those who do not respond are referred to a trained therapist to receive CBT (step 2). In this way trained therapists focus their efforts on those patients who truly need their help, while patients whose eating disorder is responsive to self-help procedures are saved from receiving an unnecessarily elaborate form of treatment. Step 3 may involve extending the cognitive behavioural therapy, an alternative psychotherapy, or the addition of medication. Such an approach has the advantage of apparent economy but runs the risk of increasing dropouts from treatment as patients feel they are failing.

COURSE AND OUTCOME

Bulimia nervosa has a chronic course tending to be self-perpetuating. Estimates of remission vary from 31% to 74% (Wilson et al 2007). Long-term follow-up studies (up to 10 years) suggest that between a third and two-thirds of those with bulimia nervosa continued to experience significant problems and

that 10–25% still had bulimia nervosa. There is also considerable flux within samples, with relapse being common (Berkman et al 2007). Over time bulimia nervosa may change into EDNOS. Given this background, the favourable outcome of properly administered CBT is striking. Predictors of poor response to treatment include childhood obesity, low self-esteem and personality disturbance.

Bulimia nervosa is associated with elevated psychiatric morbidity, particularly elevated levels of depression. Unlike anorexia nervosa, it is not associated with significantly elevated rates of mortality (Berkman et al 2007)

KEY POINTS

- While sharing many clinical features with anorexia nervosa, notably judgement of self-worth being primarily in terms of shape and weight, patients with bulimia nervosa differ with regard to body weight
- The prevalence of bulimia nervosa is higher than for anorexia nervosa, characteristically occurring in females in their late teens and early twenties living in Western societies
- Increased exposure to dieting, general risk for psychiatric disorder and certain individual personality traits contribute to the development of bulimia nervosa.
- Reducing and eliminating binge-eating and purging are primary treatment goals.
- Cognitive behavioural therapy is the evidence-based treatment of choice.

27.4 ATYPICAL EATING DISORDERS

It is often forgotten that the most common form of eating disorder in outpatient settings and the community is neither anorexia nervosa nor bulimia nervosa but eating disorder not otherwise specified (EDNOS) (see Section *evolve* 27.1). EDNOS, the residual category, is by far the most common presentation, constituting about 60% of cases seen in outpatient settings (Fairburn et al 2007) and around 75% of eating disorder cases in the community (Machado et al 2007) Within EDNOS is binge-eating disorder, a diagnosis not currently recognised as a separate disorder but listed in DSM-IV (see Section *evolve* 27.1). with research diagnostic criteria.

EATING DISORDER NOT OTHERWISE SPECIFIED (EDNOS)

Many patients with EDNOS have symptoms similar in form to anorexia nervosa and bulimia nervosa but fail to meet their diagnostic criteria either because a particular feature is missing (partial syndrome) or because they do not quite meet the specified level of severity (sub-threshold case). Nevertheless, the psychopathology of EDNOS closely resembles that seen in anorexia nervosa and bulimia nervosa. It is comparable in duration and severity to bulimia nervosa (Fairburn et al 2007) and it is likely that risk and maintaining factors are similar to those described above (Fairburn et al 2003). A recent controlled trial indicates that the response of those with EDNOS (with a BMI >17.5) to an enhanced form of CBT designed to be suitable for all forms of eating disorder (CBT-E) was no different from those patients with bulimia nervosa (Fairburn et al 2009).

A diagnosis of EDNOS should not be considered a low-grade disorder or one undeserving of treatment. Patients with eating disorders tend to migrate between the diagnostic categories of anorexia nervosa, bulimia nervosa and the atypical eating disorders (Fairburn & Harrison 2003). The main pathways are shown in Figure 27.1 (see Section *evolve* 27.1 🖱). This movement, together with the fact that they share the same distinctive and core psychopathology, suggests that common mechanisms are involved in their persistence. However,

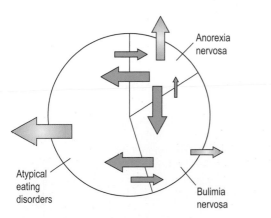

Fig. 27.1 The temporal movement between the eating disorders. The size of the arrow indicates likelihood of movement in the direction shown. Arrows that point outside the circle indicate recovery. *(Adapted from Fairburn & Harrison 2003).*

the fact that eating disorders do not evolve into other conditions shows the distinctiveness of the diagnostic category as a whole.

BINGE–EATING DISORDER (BED)

The research diagnostic criteria for binge-eating disorder differ from those of bulimia nervosa in several respects (see Section *evolve* 27.1 🖱). First, the frequency specification for BED is for binge episodes to occur on 2 days per week rather than 2 episodes per week. In bulimia nervosa a binge is normally terminated by some form of purging. In BED, binges are sometimes difficult to separate into discrete episodes. Indeed, some may last an entire day. Associated with this is an extended time frame: 6 months, rather than the 3 months for bulimia nervosa. This conservative requirement to show a key behaviour over a longer period is controversial but certainly acts to reduce the prevalence of BED. Second, BED does not include the core psychopathology of shape and weight overconcern, so important to understanding anorexia nervosa and bulimia nervosa. The only cognitive component in the diagnostic criteria is the significant distress over the binge-eating. Third, the regular use of inappropriate compensatory behaviours is an exclusionary criterion. Purging is 'recurrent' in the criteria for bulimia nervosa but no indication is available for how frequently the use of fasting or self-induced vomiting should be to define 'regular' for BED.

Estimates of the prevalence of BED vary widely, according to the implementation of these diagnostic criteria and the target sample. The better community studies suggest rates of 2–3% in the adult population (Grilo 2006). Not surprisingly, these figures are higher in obese samples, with BED present in 5–10% of those seeking treatment for obesity in the USA and rates between 5 and 8% in community studies of those with obesity (Berkman et al 2007). However, the association between BED and obesity is not invariable and many questions remain regarding the relationship. For example, in nearly half of patients with BED, the binge-eating preceded the first episode of dieting; these patients also report obesity at an earlier age than those who dieted before the eating disorder. Overall, the aetiology of binge-eating disorder has barely been studied. It would appear that these patients have lower exposure to the eating disorder risk factors noted above for anorexia nervosa and bulimia nervosa.

Most patients with binge-eating disorder are more concerned about their shape and weight compared with an obese control group although these concerns may not have the same intensity and personal significance as those seen in the other eating disorders. Another difference is that patients with binge-eating disorder eat relatively normally outside their binges, tending to over-eat rather than under-eat. Their binge-eating appears to be more of a habitual response to negative moods than a breakdown of rigid dietary restraint. In addition, binge-eating disorder is seen in an older age group (most presenting between age 30 and 50), and is more common in men than either anorexia nervosa or bulimia nervosa, with a ratio of women to men of 3:1 (Grilo 2006).

The treatment of binge-eating disorder has been the focus of a recent narrative review (Mitchell et al 2008) and two recent systematic reviews (National Collaborating Centre for Mental Health 2004, Brownley et al 2007). The NICE systematic review resulted in the following evidence-based recommendations: first, the leading treatment for binge-eating disorder is a form of cognitive behaviour therapy similar to that used to treat bulimia nervosa; second, other psychological treatments for binge-eating disorder including a variant of IPT (Wilfley et al 2002) and a simplified form of dialectical behaviour therapy (Telch et al 2001) are also efficacious, although the evidence supporting them is modest; and third, antidepressant drugs and certain self-help programmes (preferably used with some form of professional support) both have some efficacy as treatments for binge-eating disorder and are relatively straightforward to implement. These recommendations closely resemble those for bulimia nervosa.

Certain points need to be made about the management of binge-eating disorder. Binge-eating tends to be highly treatment-responsive. Many interventions seem to be helpful and there is a sizeable placebo response rate. Recent research suggests that guided cognitive behavioural self-help is almost as effective as full-scale cognitive behaviour therapy (Grilo 2006). Of particular note is that many patients with BED present with comorbid obesity and this is may be of more concern to them than the binge-eating. Perhaps surprisingly, eliminating the binge-eating has little effect on body weight. This is because these patients overeat in general (and under-exercise), and their binge-eating makes only a small contribution to their day-to-day energy surplus. The management of their accompanying excess weight is therefore a pressing clinical problem. At present it is not clear how best to combine weight management with treatment directed at the binge-eating. A new cognitive behavioural treatment for obesity has been designed to treat both problems in tandem (Cooper et al 2003) and emerging research findings suggest that this treatment is effective for the binge-eating and also produces short-term weight loss but that, in common with other treatments for obesity, the weight lost is regained in the longer term. There is also emerging evidence that drugs other than antidepressants benefit these patients. These include the appetite suppressant sibutramine and the anticonvulsant topiramate, both of which appear to produce concomitant weight loss in the short term. More rigorous and longer-term studies of these drugs are needed before they can be recommended.

There is little research on the course and outcome of EDNOS and BED. Retrospective accounts from patients with BED suggest long histories, but with periods which are symptom-free. Generally outcome for BED appeared to be better than for bulimia nervosa in earlier studies, but one recent 12-year follow-up reported few differences between the outcome of BED and BN (Fichter et al 2008). Similarly, outcome for EDNOS appears similar to bulimia nervosa.

KEY POINTS

- Many patients with EDNOS have symptoms similar in form to anorexia nervosa and bulimia nervosa but fail to meet their diagnostic criteria either because a particular feature is missing (partial syndrome) or because they do not quite meet the specified level of severity.
- The psychopathology of EDNOS is comparable in duration and severity to bulimia nervosa.
- Atypical eating disorders are by far the most common presentation constituting 60% of eating disorder cases in the community.
- Patients with eating disorders tend to migrate between the diagnostic categories of anorexia nervosa, bulimia nervosa and the atypical eating disorders.
- Patients with binge-eating disorder (BED) do not regularly use purging behaviours after bingeing.
- A variety of different approaches show success in treating BED.

References

Attia E, Walsh BT: Anorexia nervosa, *American Journal of Psychiatry* 164(12):1805–1810, 2007.

Berkman ND, Lohr KN, Bulik CM: Outcomes of eating disorders: a systematic review of the literature, *International Journal of Eating Disorders* 40(4):293–309, 2007.

Brownley KA, Berkman ND, Sedway JA, et al: Binge eating disorder treatment: a systematic review of randomized controlled trials, *International Journal of Eating Disorders* 40:337–348, 2007.

Bulik CM, Berkman ND, Brownley KA, et al: Anorexia nervosa treatment: a systematic review of randomized controlled trials, *International Journal of Eating Disorders* 40(4):310–320, 2007.

Cooper Z, Stewart A: CBT-E and the younger patient. In Fairburn CG, editor: *Cognitive behavior therapy and eating disorders*, New York, 2008, Guilford Press, pp 221–230.

Cooper Z, Fairburn CG, Hawker DM: *Cognitive-behavioral treatment of obesity*, New York, 2003, Guilford Press.

Dalle Grave R, Bohn K, Hawker DM, et al: Inpatient, day patient and two forms of outpatient CBT-E. In Fairburn CG, editor: *Cognitive behavior therapy and eating disorders*, New York, 2008, Guilford Press, pp 231–244.

Deter HC, Schellberg D, Kopp W, et al: Predictability of a favourable outcome in anorexia nervosa, *European Psychiatry* 20:165–172, 2005.

Fairburn CG: Interpersonal psychotherapy for bulimia nervosa. In Garner DM, Garfinkel PE, editors: *Handbook of treatment for eating disorders*, New York, 1997, Guilford Press.

Fairburn CG: *Cognitive behavior therapy and eating disorders*, New York, 2008, Guilford Press.

Fairburn CG, Gowers SG: Eating disorders. In: Rutter M, Bishop D,

Pine D, et al, editors: *Rutter's child and adolescent psychiatry*, Oxford, 2008, Blackwell.

Fairburn CG, Harrison PJ: Eating disorders, *Lancet* 361:407–416, 2003.

Fairburn CG, Cooper Z, Shafran R: Cognitive behavior therapy for eating disorders: A 'transdiagnostic' theory and treatment, *Behaviour Research and Therapy* 41(5):509–528, 2003.

Fairburn CG, Cooper Z, Bohn K, et al: The severity and status of eating disorder NOS, *Behaviour Research and Therapy* 45:1705–1715, 2007.

Fairburn CG, Cooper Z, O'Connor M: The Eating Disorder Examination, 16th ed. In Fairburn CG, editor: *Cognitive behavior therapy and eating disorders*, New York, 2008, Guilford Press, pp 265–308.

Fairburn CG, Cooper Z, Doll HA, et al: Transdiagnostic cognitive-behavioral therapy for patients with eating disorders: a two-site trial with 60-week follow-up, *American Journal of Psychiatry* 166(3):311–319, 2009.

Fichter MM, Quadflieg N, Hedlund S: Long-term course of binge eating disorder and bulimia nervosa: relevance for nosology and diagnostic criteria, *International Journal of Eating Disorders* 41(7):577–586, 2008.

Franko DL: Race, ethnicity, and eating disorders: considerations for DSM-V, *International Journal of Eating Disorders* 40: S31–S34, 2007.

Grilo CM: *Eating and weight disorders*, New York, 2006, Psychology Press.

Hoek HW: Incidence, prevalence and mortality of anorexia nervosa and other eating disorders, *Current Opinion in Psychiatry* 19:389–394, 2006.

Hoek HW, van Hoeken D: Review of the prevalence and incidence of eating disorders, *International Journal of Eating Disorders* 34:383–396, 2003.

Kaye HW, Bulik CM, Plotnicov K, et al: The genetics of anorexia nervosa collaborative study: methods and sample description, *International Journal of Eating Disorders* 41:289–300, 2008.

Keel PK, Klump KL: Are eating disorders culture-bound syndromes? Implications for conceptualizing their etiology, *Psychological Bulletin* 129(5):747–769, 2003.

Klump KL, Gobrogge KL: A review and primer of molecular genetic studies of anorexia nervosa, *International Journal of Eating Disorders* 37:S43–S48, 2005.

Klump KL, Kaye WH, Strober M: The evolving genetic foundations of eating disorders, *Psychiatric Clinics of North America* 24:215–225, 2001.

Le Grange D, Crosby RD, Rathouz PJ, et al: A randomized controlled comparison of family-based treatment and supportive psychotherapy for adolescent bulimia nervosa, *Archives of General Psychiatry* 64(9):1049–1056, 2007.

Lee HY, Lock J: Anorexia nervosa in Asian-American adolescents: do they differ from their non-Asian peers? *International Journal of Eating Disorders* 40:227–231, 2007.

Machado PP, Machado BC, Goncalves S, et al: The prevalence of eating disorders not otherwise specified, *International Journal of Eating Disorders* 40:212–217, 2007.

Mazzeo SE, Zucker NL, Gerke CK, et al: Parenting concerns of women with histories of eating disorders, *International Journal of Eating Disorders* 37(S1):S77–S79, 2005.

Mitchell JE, Devlin MJ, de Zwaan M, et al: *Binge eating disorder: clinical foundations and treatment*, New York, 2008, Guilford Press.

National Collaborating Centre for Mental Health: *Eating disorders: core interventions in the treatment and* management of anorexia nervosa, bulimia nervosa, and related eating disorders. National Clinical Practice Guideline CG9, Leicester, 2004, British Psychological Society, http://www.bps.org.uk/eatingdisorders/files/ED.pdf.

Patton GC, Selzer R, Coffey C, et al: Onset of adolescent eating disorders: population based cohort study over 3 years, *British Medical Journal* 318:765–768, 1999.

Polivy J, Herman CP: Causes of eating disorders, *Annual Review of Psychology* 53:187–213, 2002.

Russell GFM, Szmukler GI, Dare C, et al: an evaluation of family therapy in anorexia nervosa and bulimia nervosa, *Archives of General Psychiatry* 44:1047–1056, 1987.

Schmidt U, Lee S, Beecham J, et al: A randomized control trial of family therapy and cognitive behavior

therapy guided self-care for adolescents with bulimia nervosa and related disorders, *American Journal of Psychiatry* 164:591–598, 2007.

Shapiro JR, Berkman ND, Brownley KA, et al: Bulimia nervosa treatment: a systematic review of randomized controlled trials, *International Journal of Eating Disorders* 40:321–336, 2007.

Slof-Op 't Landt MC, van Furth EF, Meulenbelt I, et al: Eating disorders: from twin studies to candidate genes and beyond, *Twin Research and Human Genetics* 8:467–482, 2005.

Telch CF, Agras WS, Linehan MM: Dialectical behavior therapy for binge eating disorder, *Journal of Consulting and Clinical Psychology* 69:1061–1065, 2001.

Van Son GE, van Hoeken D, Bartelds AIM, et al: Urbanisation and the incidence of eating disorders, *British Journal of Psychiatry* 189:562–563, 2006.

Walsh BT, Kaplan AS, Attia E, et al: Fluoxetine after weight restoration in anorexia nervosa, *Journal of the American Medical Association* 295:2605–2612, 2006.

Wilfley DE, Welch RR, Stein RI, et al: A randomized comparison of group cognitive-behavioral therapy and group interpersonal psychotherapy for the treatment of overweight individuals with binge eating disorder, *Archives of General Psychiatry* 59:713–721, 2002.

Wilson GT, Grilo CM, Vitousek K: Psychological treatments for eating disorders, *American Psychologist* 62:199–216, 2007.

Chapter 28

Deficiency diseases

Maureen B Duggan*

CHAPTER CONTENTS

OBJECTIVES

By the end of this chapter you should be able to:
- describe the major deficiency diseases, where they occur, and their association with poverty and infection
- recognise the current and older terminology and classifications of malnutrition, and their limitations

---

*Updated and modified from the previous edition chapter written by Maureen Duggan and Barbara Golden

© 2010 Elsevier Ltd/Inc/BV
DOI: 10.1016/B978-0-7020-3118-2.00028-0

- discuss the immediate and underlying causes of the main deficiency diseases, recognising the importance of their interactions
- be aware of the deficiencies that may occur in situations of particular risk
- give examples of particular 'at risk' groups in different situations
- identify the long- and short-term consequences of simple and multiple deficiencies
- be aware of the general principles of treatment and prevention.

28.1 INTRODUCTION

The major deficiency diseases are here described in their global context, with emphasis on pathogenesis and principles of management. The epidemiology is covered in more detail in Chapter 33. Nutritional deficiency is common in poor regions of the world, where there is a vicious cycle of endemic food insecurity and structural injustice (see Ch. 32), and where the spread of infections such as malaria and diarrhoea is favoured by poverty and the tropical climate. Population movements forced by war and economic migration have also favoured the spread of HIV, which interacts with malnutrition to deadly effect.

Migrants and refugees are at increased risk of malnutrition, as are broken families, female-headed households and an increasing number of elderly, who may, in rural areas in regions affected by HIV, also be caring for orphaned grandchildren. In Western countries, the elderly are at increased risk of poverty and malnutrition as are immigrants, refugees, drug addicts, the homeless living in otherwise affluent cities, and some patients in hospital.

WHO (2003) reported that general nutritional status was improving in south and southeast Asia and in Central America and the Caribbean, but worsening in sub-Saharan Africa. Micronutrient status has generally improved for iodine and vitamin A, although the global iron situation is less good (WHO 2008). The strong correlation between nutrition and child survival justifies the use of child nutrition indicators as a proxy for public health adequacy.

The paradoxical association of obesity and micronutrient deficiency is more commonly reported among the poor in Western countries. The effects of detrimental fetal programming, first recognised in Western countries, are now evident in Asia and South America, in individuals underfed in fetal life and later exposed to high energy intakes at reduced levels of activity.

28.2 UNDERNUTRITION

DEFINITIONS

Malnutrition has been defined as a change in nutritional status that carries the penalty of illness, dysfunction or death. Strictly speaking, that definition includes dietary excess but in this section the term malnutrition is taken to mean undernutrition. Commonly used descriptive terms, e.g. chronic energy deficiency (CED) or protein energy malnutrition (PEM), may imply causality in a way that is now recognised as simplistic or false. Nevertheless they are preferable to the general term 'malnutrition', in common 'clinical' use, which ignores rather than excludes coincidental micronutrient deficiency. The archaic terms *marasmus* and *cachexia* are explained later. Since children are the earliest victims of food insecurity, many classifications were devised with childhood malnutrition in mind. For practical reasons these initially focused on growth, by measuring weight for age. Length measurement until the age of 2 years, and height thereafter, was introduced more recently. Growth failure is marked by 'thinness and shortness', which reflect the distinction between the ponderal and linear growth. 'Nutritional' growth faltering is not always due to simple under-feeding. Micronutrient deficiency and infection are major contributory factors. Not only does nutrient intake fall during infection, but nutrient requirements are increased to supply the costs of infection-related biosynthesis. Borderline malnutrition may be common enough to escape notice, but syndromes with clear physical signs and high fatality are well recognised. A stunted underweight child, living among similarly sized agemates, might well appear to be thriving.

In Section *evolve* 28.2(a) 🖱 we follow a typical village infant of a relatively short teenage mother through the nutritional experiences of her first year. This case study of an apparently healthy mother and baby being 'stunted' with reference to international 'standards' illustrates the conundrum of biological variability: how can we compare the nutritional status of the short, stocky Alaskan Inuit with that of a lanky east African cattle keeper? Following millennia of biological and cultural adaptation, the physique of each demonstrates 'good fit' with his environment. Adaptation takes other forms; e.g. metabolic adaptation to low protein and energy intakes respectively includes reduction in protein turnover and basal metabolic rate. Stunting has been described as an adaptation to long-standing underfeeding. In acute malaria, where host and pathogen compete for iron, an adaptive advantage has even been claimed for malnutrition though this is unproven (see Sections 28.5 and *evolve* 28.5(a) on iron and infection). Clearly there are limits to such adaptation beyond which health suffers. Height often falters in response to repeated infection as well as nutrient depletion. It is also true that variation in height, especially during the early years of life, owes more to nutritional and socioeconomic than to ethnic variability.

Biological variation in height and body build is generally accepted, with the proviso that extremes are likely to be detrimental. In practice we assume that anthropometric variables are normally distributed, the normal range extending from −2.0 to +2.0 standard deviations from the mean. Malnutrition is defined in terms of negative deviation >2.0 SD from the reference mean. However, a greater degree of deviation may be needed before the risk of an adverse outcome rises significantly.

ANTHROPOMETRIC INDICATORS, CLASSIFICATIONS AND REFERENCE STANDARDS

Indicators of nutritional status vary in their ability to predict functional outcome. There is a link between deficiency and malfunction that holds true for all nutrients. Lack of fuel compromises basal metabolism, activity and storage. Repair, growth and structural support fail in the absence of substrate, e.g. nitrogen and bulk minerals, as do enzymatic processes when micronutrients are deficient. The major fuel stores are in adipose tissue and lean body mass, with a minor contribution from glycogen. Anthropometry offers a simple way of estimating their magnitude. Weight for age in children and body mass index (BMI) in adults are commonly used indicators with body weight as a major component. Whereas total weight includes the weight of the skeleton and essential organs with slow tissue turnover, inclusion of height in the derived formula allows a better estimate of 'disposable' mass, i.e. lean and fat mass extra to that in essential structures.

An estimate of the partition of fuels between superficial adipose and fat-free mass may be made by measuring skinfold thickness. Indicators involving stature, e.g. weight for height in children, are better short-term prognostic predictors than weight for age alone, which was first used as a functional indicator by Gomez et al in 1956.

Deficiency of fuel stores, identified by anthropometry, is known in children as protein energy malnutrition (PEM), and in adults by the newer and less satisfactory term 'chronic energy deficiency' (CED). The term 'protein' is excluded from the descriptive term in adults on the basis that protein requirements are relatively less important after growth has ceased. We need to be aware of several archaic terms for PEM which are still embedded in the jargon of isolated field workers.

Marasmus is one example; it describes extreme thinness and was defined as weight <60% of the reference weight for age. However, if an underweight child is also severely stunted he may paradoxically appear plump. 'Wasting' is another confusing term. Its original meaning was similar to 'marasmic', but was defined as weight <80% of reference weight for a given height. 'Clinical wasting' and terms such as 'baggy pants' vividly describe severe fat loss over the buttocks. Wasting is held to indicate that malnutrition is recent, and does not distinguish between weight loss due to illness or underfeeding. The corollary that stunting indicates long-term malnutrition is open to simplistic misinterpretation.

The term 'kwashiorkor' indicates nutritional oedema which carries a poor prognosis, and all oedematous children are defined as severely malnourished (Table 28.1). The child with 'classical'

Table 28.1	Classification of malnutrition (WHO 1999)	
	MODERATE MALNUTRITION	**SEVERE MALNUTRITION**
Symmetrical oedema	No	Yes
Weight for height	SD score >−3.0 and <−2.0	SD score <−3.0
	≥70% and <80% reference	<70% reference
Height for age	SD score >−3.0 and <−2.0	SD score <−3.0
	≥85% and <90% reference	<85% reference

kwashiorkor also has variable underweight, 'psychosis' and dyspigmented skin and hair. (Figs *evolve* 28.2–28.8 ⬚ show examples of kwashiorkor and wasting; Fig. *evolve* 28.1 shows a healthy child for comparison ⬚). The typical history is of recent weaning or exposure to infection or other stress. Among other common features are dry or moist skin peeling, and enlargement of the liver. Nutritional oedema (kwashiorkor) is a complication of PEM rather than a different 'type' or part of a spectrum. Stunting is considered as distinct in aetiology and outcome from uncomplicated PEM (CED) due to reduced protein energy stores. Children with severe wasting plus oedema (marasmic kwashiorkor) or severe wasting plus stunting are particularly vulnerable.

Anthropometric assessment for undernutrition describes the appearance of individuals with reduced energy stores and quantifies that deficiency against reference standards to facilitate comparisons over time or between individuals,

groups or regions (see Ch. 31 and Section *evolve* 28.2(b) ⬚). Table 28.2 illustrates indicators used for assessment of children and adults, together with the cut-off points (COP) that define moderate malnutrition, and their validation or evidence basis.

THE PATHOGENESIS OF WEIGHT LOSS AND WASTING, KWASHIORKOR AND STUNTING

The main features of uncomplicated PEM and CED are weight loss and wasting caused by negative energy balance, in which available metabolisable energy is less than energy expenditure. Factors such as malabsorption, increased energy losses in urine and increased energy expenditure from the biosynthetic costs of infection or malignancy, and from fever, play a subsidiary role. The main cause of negative balance is an insufficient intake of food often of low energy density, exacerbated by infection-related anorexia. The energy shortfall is made

Table 28.2	Commonly used anthropometric indicators, the cut–off points for a diagnosis of 'moderate' malnutrition, and evidence base for use, where available	
INDICATOR	CUT–OFF POINT (COP) FOR DIAGNOSIS OF MALNUTRITION	EVIDENCE BASE FOR USE AS INDICATORS
Weight for age[a]	80% of reference mean ~SDScore-2.0	Risk of death rises when weight for age <70% and further at <60%[b,c]
Weight for height[a]	80% of reference mean ~SDScore-2.0	Risk of death rises at weight for height <70%[c]
Length or height for age	90% of reference mean ~SDScore-2.0	Risk of death rises at length for age <90%[b], rarely used as single index
Body mass index wt ÷ ht[2] (kg/m[2])	18.5 and 17 for men and women in developing countries[d]	Used in adults; borderline values usually supported by evidence of physical incapacity
Mid-upper arm circumference (MUAC) (see also Figs *evolve* 28.9, *evolve* 28.10 ⬚)	<12.5 cm[e]: the Shakir strip is coloured red, yellow and green to discriminate MUAC <12.5, 12–<14, and ≥14 cm respectively	Low MUAC <12.5 cm correlates with weight for age <80%, i.e. MUAC used as a swift screening test
Age 1 to <5 years		
MUAC in adults	<23 and <19 cm in men and women in developing countries	Evidence base less convincing, is used as a proxy for low BMI[f]
Height and MUAC	For heights between 70 and 130 cm COP for MUAC is 13.25–17.5	Screening in emergencies, RR death rises as MUAC falls[g]
Symmetrical oedema	At any weight for age or weight for height[h]	Associated with increased risk and therefore defines severe malnutrition

[a]Jelliffe & Jelliffe 1989, [b]Chen et al 1980, [c] Kielman & McCord 1978, [d]WHO 1990, [e]Shakir 1975, [f]James et al 1994, [g] Sommer & Loewenstein 1975, [h]WHO 1999. For full reference details see Further reading on the *evolve* website ('Anthropometric indicators, classifications and reference standards' section) ⬚.

up from energy stored in adipose and lean mass, usually muscle, leading to underweight and wasting. An increased intake is needed to restore lost weight and to provide the essential amino acids that are required to rebuild lost muscle mass. This is more difficult on a low-energy-dense diet.

Nutritional oedema is commonly triggered by infection. The body's protective response, particularly if it is already malnourished, is nutritionally costly (see Ch. 26). Reactive oxygen species, which are toxic, are generated during the cellular response to infection. Their adverse effect on intracellular metabolism is normally held in check by several antioxidant mechanisms, many of which require nutrients such as vitamins A, C and E, zinc, selenium and copper. Iron, especially free iron, may act as a pro-oxidant. In PEM, oxidative stress to structural lipids causes cell membranes to become permeable to sodium and potassium, which leak with water into the extracellular space, causing oedema. At the same time reduced hepatic synthesis of export proteins, due to an insufficient supply of amino acids from the diet or catabolism of endogenous protein, leads to a lower concentration of circulating plasma proteins including albumin and retinol-binding protein (Waterlow 1992). Hypoalbuminaemia, which lowers intravascular oncotic pressure, was considered to be the main cause of nutritional oedema until Golden and his co-workers demonstrated the importance in its genesis of imbalance between oxidative stress and protective antioxidants. Micronutrient deficiencies therefore play a critical role in predisposing the child with PEM to kwashiorkor, triggered by infection-related oxidant stress. Oedema may supervene at different degrees of wasting, even in apparently normal children.

Stunting, which affects up to 40% of children under 5 years in developing countries, is commonest in south Asia and sub-Saharan Africa. The nutritional determinants of linear growth act at the growth plate of long bones, together with growth hormone (GH) and insulin-like growth factor (IGF-1). Certain amino acids, specifically leucine, and various micronutrients such as zinc, copper, molybdenum and possibly vitamin A influence linear growth. Beneficial effects of zinc supplementation on stunted children have been widely reported. Interaction between micronutrients and possible confounding due to multiple concurrent deficiencies limit the conclusions from single nutrient supplementation studies. In a major multinational

growth study, dietary 'quality', implying dairy produce, fruits and green vegetables, had a greater positive influence on growth than any specific nutrient. Stunting and underweight have also been reported in young European children on alternative, macrobiotic, diets. Various cytokines produced in the acute phase response to infection may slow bone growth. Cohort studies have demonstrated cessation and faltering in growth due to frequent or chronic infections including HIV, or to worm infestation. Nutritional stunting is commonly multifactorial in origin. Catch-up in linear growth during nutritional rehabilitation rarely starts until weight recovery is well under way. It may occur immediately, after an interval, or never (Waterlow 1992).

GLOBAL TRENDS IN MALNUTRITION

Much of our information on the prevalence and trends in undernutrition comes from measurements in under-5 children who are both vulnerable and accessible. Comparative national data on underweight in adult women correlate strongly with low birthweight and underweight in children, emphasising the intergenerational effect of female malnutrition. Information on pregnancy weight gain, especially when combined with fetal birth weight, is important in identifying nutritional stress in pregnancy. General improvement in the ponderal and linear growth of young children has been observed over recent decades, except in sub-Saharan Africa.

There is little information on the community prevalence of severe or oedematous malnutrition. Community surveys in Africa show rates of severe PEM between 3% and 7%. The pattern of malnutrition seen in hospitals is biased towards more severe illness, although 'malnutrition' may be an unrecorded second diagnosis. Kwashiorkor, now rarely reported from Asia, is still common in African hospitals.

Kwashiorkor (plus marasmic kwashiorkor) constituted 51% (59%) of 5855 recent admissions with PEM to an urban unit in Malawi with an overall case fatality of 18% during the 4-year study period (Walford & Duggan, personal communication). A high prevalence of PEM persists in Africa although the under-5 death rate has fallen following various public health initiatives such as immunisation, oral rehydration and provision of vitamin A. Mortality rate is falling less rapidly in areas with high rates of malnutrition, which indicates that malnutrition is a marker for poor programme coverage in such areas. Oedematous malnutrition in hospital carries a persistently high case fatality of around 20%.

CAUSES OF MALNUTRITION

The risk of underfeeding begins in fetal life, and is commoner during the last trimester of pregnancy. Risk factors in the first few years of life include lactation failure, a low-energy-dense weaning diet, and infection. Maternal death increases risk at any age. Underfeeding may result from insufficient breast milk when the mother is ill, with HIV or another infection, or has twins. Breast milk substitutes may be unsuitable because of a high renal solute load, as with fresh cow's milk, or low energy density as with diluted cow's milk or incorrectly reconstituted formula (see Section *evolve* 28.2(c)). Water contamination is an important additional risk factor.

When kwashiorkor was first described, it was thought to be due to the low protein content of maize weaning porridge. The common history of infection was neglected. It later became clear that low energy intakes, from low-energy-dense foods, were also implicated. The current view is that nutrient density (energy density, protein energy % and micronutrient composition) plays a part in determining the adequacy of a weaning diet. A traditional weaning porridge often has much lower energy density than breast milk, with a low chemical protein score due to low levels of certain essential amino acids, virtually no vitamin A, and poorly available iron and zinc (WHO 1998). PEM is commonly seen in weanling children during the second year of life, children with kwashiorkor being somewhat older than children with simple wasting. Oedematous malnutrition is commonly triggered by infection, particularly by measles and diarrhoea accompanied by under-feeding. HIV has altered the pattern and now kwashiorkor is seen both in breast-fed babies and in older children. In these children, who may come from better-off families, PEM is associated with frank malabsorption and secondary infection which may be linked to HIV immune failure.

CED is often linked to HIV infection , the African nickname of which was 'slim disease'. HIV has an important cross-generational effect with high rates of orphans, who risk malnutrition and early death, even when seronegative. Malnutrition is highly prevalent in hospitals in developing countries, in association with other severe infections such as typhoid or tuberculosis, with malignancy, or lack of access to suitable feeds by postoperative or badly burned patients. In affluent countries toddlers with PEM usually present with faltering weight gain; oedema is extremely rare. The euphemism for the malnutrition of deprivation is 'non-organic failure to thrive'. Children refusing food or eating alternative diets may also present with marginal PEM. Anorexia nervosa and bulimia present in adolescence with weight loss which may be attributed to dieting and exercise (see Ch. 27). CED is also seen in the nutritionally vulnerable groups mentioned in the introduction.

The epidemiology of childhood malnutrition was reviewed by UNICEF in 1998. The many interacting causative factors include urban and rural poverty (see Ch. 32), which is linked to high fertility, land-hunger, insufficient and contaminated water, and persistent gender inequality, and exacerbated by HIV. The fundamental problem of food insecurity varies in magnitude in different regions. Other acute causes of insecurity are drought and war, which can lead to famine and malnourished refugees (see Section *evolve* 28.7(a)).

EFFECTS ON HEALTH AND GROWTH: SHORT AND LONG TERM

The magnitude of the effect of malnutrition on health depends on the timing and duration of nutritional stress. The immediate effects, when low birthweight is due to intrauterine growth retardation, are a high neonatal death rate, due to hypoglycaemia, hypothermia and infection. Malnutrition increases a child's vulnerability to other illnesses, especially infection. Even though it is rarely recorded as a cause of death, it contributes to the case fatality of many illnesses. Waterlow (1992) notes that 'child (1–5 years) mortality' rates give a better indication of the link with malnutrition than infant mortality (0–12 months), which includes birth hazards. Meta-analysis of Asian and African studies demonstrates that the relative risk of death due to diarrhoea, respiratory infection and malaria varies with nutritional status.

Severe malnutrition especially if accompanied by oedema has a high case fatality (from 20% for all severe PEM to >50% in kwashiorkor) related both to infection and to metabolic complications of the disease itself. It is difficult to disentangle the long-term effects of an episode of severe malnutrition from those of persistent socioeconomic deprivation. This applies both to PEM and to micronutrient deficiency. There is evidence of an adverse effect of prolonged stunting on cognitive development. In the longer term, the survivor of early malnutrition may recover completely, remain stunted, or have a delayed adolescent growth spurt. Delayed growth and final short stature in women contribute to obstruction in labour, and thereby to high maternal mortality. Adult female stunting is also associated with low birth weight. If the pendulum swings from early deprivation towards nutritional excess in adult life, the survivor is at increased risk of chronic diseases such as diabetes and heart disease. The effects of adverse fetal programming play a part in the diseases associated with the nutritional transition that is evident in a number of developing countries, characterised by rising intakes of fat, sugar and meat and by reduction in physical activity (see Chs 1 and 32; WHO 2003). Secular trends towards an increase in BMI, and increased prevalence of obesity, already evident in urban populations, are now affecting the rural poor in rapidly developing regions.

TREATMENT OF MALNUTRITION

Treatment of malnutrition is covered in Section *evolve* 28.2(c) 🖱.

PREVENTION OF MALNUTRITION

Healthy eating is easier to advocate than to achieve. Fetal nutrition, which is obviously important, depends not only on maternal energy intake but also on expenditure. Since pregnancy stress is greater during the planting season in agricultural societies, women should be encouraged to avoid heavy work, or be targeted for nutritional supplementation at this time. Exclusive breastfeeding is recommended for 6 months, except when milk supply fails to meet the growth requirements of the infant. The tradition of prolonged breastfeeding persists in developing countries, with 40–50% of mothers still breastfeeding 20–23 months after birth.

A current dilemma is the early infant feeding of babies whose mothers are HIV-positive or dead. The pros and cons of feeding with breast milk substitutes (BMS) are discussed in Section *evolve* 28.2(c) 🖱. In summary, although artificial feeding seems logical, in resource-poor situations where the risks

of contamination and other infection are high, there is a strong argument for 'safe suckling', even by an HIV-positive mother. Factors to be considered include the nutritional demands of breastfeeding, the possible risk of viral transmission if the fragile infant gut is damaged during mixed feeding, uncertainty about the infant's status, and the effects on transmission risk of short-term antiretroviral treatment. The present WHO/IATT 2006 guidelines encourage HIV-positive mothers to breastfeed uninfected babies exclusively for 6 months. The risks of mother to child transmission (MTCT) during mixed feeding suggest that weaning should then progress more swiftly in regions at risk than in the past. This also makes sense for mothers on antiretroviral treatment, even though the risks are less. Since general guidelines, based on operational research, are frequently revised, caution is advised in applying them to particular situations.

The aim during weaning is to ensure frequent intakes of palatable food of high nutrient density. Dietary diversification depends not only on access to a variety of foods, but also on willingness to adapt dietary and culinary traditions. Even if amylase-rich flour quadruples the energy density of porridge, there is often a time lag before such a technology is implemented. Local manufacture of commercial weaning foods in urban Kenya and Latin America has reduced their cost, and there is global interest in the preparation and social marketing of fortified convenience foods for poor developing countries. The success and expansion of efforts by the World Food Programme to provide healthy food for children attending school has contributed to their health and uptake of education. Access to sufficient healthy food for working and elderly adults depends on socioeconomic and educational advances and on improved social provision for the elderly.

KEY POINTS

- An important factor in the high prevalence of malnutrition in young children is the high nutritional requirement for growth.
- The nutritional determinants of weight gain and linear growth are distinct so that wasting and stunting (thinness and shortness) may be due to different deficiencies.
- Protein energy malnutrition (PEM) in children and chronic energy deficiency (CED) in adults are similar conditions.

- PEM and CED are typified by wasting (underweight for height); both may be complicated by oedema; in children this is known as kwashiorkor.
- Moderate malnutrition is common, oedematous malnutrition is rare but has a high case fatality.
- Nutritional status is improving in global terms except for sub-Saharan Africa, where a vicious cycle of poverty and infection, ineffective governance and war has hindered progress.

28.3 VITAMIN A DEFICIENCY

DEFINITION

Vitamin A deficiency (VAD) was previously graded qualitatively using the eye signs characteristic of grave deficiency. A public health problem of xerophthalmia was defined as a prevalence of >1% of night blindness, or >0.05% of corneal scarring. Its early nickname 'the anti-infection vitamin' still fits vitamin A, and we might now define VAD as an increased severity of infection attributable to failure of the normal protective role of vitamin A in epithelia, in the immune system, and as an antioxidant.

Technically sensitive biochemical indicators of status are now in general use. Direct measurement of serum retinol is preferred to measurements which depend on its binding to retinol binding protein, assessed either in terms of total or holo-RBP (WHO/FAO 2004). Although clinical eye signs of VAD rarely appear at retinol concentrations >0.35 μmol/l, a serum concentration <0.7 μmol/l is considered deficient, while a serum concentration of >1.05 is regarded as normal. Marginal deficiency, which is associated with depletion of hepatic stores of retinyl ester, is identified by a rise (of >15%) in the concentration of serum retinol after oral administration of a small dose of vitamin A. A positive relative dose response RDR indicates deficiency. The modified RDR measures de-hydroretinol in a single blood sample.

PREVALENCE AND TRENDS

VAD, both 'clinical' and subclinical (i.e. with and without eye signs) is widespread in the tropics, the most vulnerable group being preschool-age children. High rates of background infection both exacerbate and confuse the epidemiological picture, so that the impact of marginal VAD on morbidity and mortality due to simple childhood infections may

be underestimated. The International Vitamin A Consultative Group (IVACG) predicted that repletion would result in a 23–35% reduction in child mortality in areas of highly endemic deficiency,.

WHO/FAO 2004 estimated the total burden of VAD as follows; between 30% and 70% of preschool children are affected by VAD, the highest rates being seen in southeast Asia (~70%), with ~50% in Africa and 20–30% in the Americas, eastern Mediterranean and west Pacific, with no data from Europe. The geographical availability of vitamin A, after making adjustments for its dietary source, is also least secure in southeast Asia.

Vitamin A deficiency has been recognised as a public health problem in 100 countries, in many of which there is a vernacular word (e.g. 'chicken eye') for night blindness. Certain groups are at increased risk including refugees whose diet depends on relief supplies of micronutrient-deficient 'dry' foods and people suffering from cystic fibrosis, an inherited disease with mucosal malfunction and pancreatic fibrosis, who commonly malabsorb fat and can suffer from night blindness, so that vitamin A supplementation is a well-established part of their management.

CAUSES

Deficiency of vitamin A is likely when a low intake is further reduced by disruption of metabolic pathways due to disease or other concomitant deficiency, and where requirements are enhanced by infection. Poor people in many tropical countries have limited access to vitamin A as retinol and rely on its precursor, β-carotene, which is present in orange fruits, dark green leaves and some roots. Plant-derived β-carotene provides about three-quarters of dietary vitamin A, and the supply is markedly reduced in the long dry seasons.

Since the season of maximal availability of β-carotene may not coincide with the post-harvest season of plentiful energy and protein intake, which facilitates the childhood growth spurt, imbalance between supply and requirement may also influence the seasonality of VAD. The consumption of red palm oil, with its exceptionally high β-carotene content (83 mg of β-carotene per 100 g), was until recently limited to west Africa but is now more widespread. Other indigenous fruits have a high content of β-carotene (WHO/FAO 2004).

Past estimates of the bio-efficacy, the fraction of the nutrient converted to its active form, of β-carotene were too high, since its retinol equivalence (RE), estimated as 6, was assumed to be similar whatever the source. In fact, it is much less available in leaves and roots than in fruits, and the RE of β-carotene in a mixed African diet is now estimated at 21 (cf. 12 for fruits and 26 for green leaves). Consequently, many regional diets previously thought to be adequate may, on reassessment, be deficient in vitamin A.

Bioavailability of vitamin A is affected at other stages on its metabolic pathway. Loss during cleavage to retinol in the gut wall is increased in diarrhoeal disease; absorption of both retinol and β-carotene is dependent on luminal fat, low in impoverished diets and reduced by fat malabsorption. Retinol is released from liver stores bound to retinol binding protein and transthyretin. Synthesis of hepatic RBP is zinc-dependent, and its synthesis, together with that of other export proteins, is reduced in protein energy malnutrition. The action of vitamin A in the retina is also zinc-dependent.

Vitamin A requirements are enhanced during growth and in infections, demonstrated when chicken pox broke out in a cohort of Brazilian children with proven marginal deficiency who had been dosed with vitamin A. Repleted liver stores became exhausted significantly quicker in the children who developed chickenpox, indicating that infection increases requirements. Vitamin A supplementation has been shown to reduce case fatality and morbidity due to measles in several placebo-controlled studies in African children at risk of deficiency.

The effect of supplementation in other infections is variable. The severity of diarrhoeal disease is reduced in all children, but the severity of non-measles-related pneumonia is only reduced in children with coincidental PEM (WHO/FAO 2004). Relevant earlier studies demonstrated a higher incidence of diarrhoea and acute respiratory infection in Indonesian children with eye signs of deficiency than in normal controls, while animal studies demonstrated that experimental infection with the Newcastle disease virus exacerbated the signs of experimental VAD in chickens.

EFFECTS ON HEALTH

Vitamin A deficiency is largely responsible for the global annual toll of 0.5 million new cases of preventable blindness. The cumulative effects of retinol deficiency on the epithelia of the surface of the eye explain the progressive signs of xerophthalmia from dryness of the conjunctiva, Bitot's spots, thickening of the cornea, ulceration and scarring (for detail see Section evolve 28.3). Dryness of the eye, from which the term xerophthalmia is derived, is due to failure of tear production in the lachrymal ducts, exacerbated by reduced mucus production due to fewer goblet cells in the conjunctiva (see Figs evolve 28.11–28.14). Night blindness (XN), also an early sign, is only evident in children old enough to toddle about, although night blindness in their mothers may be a useful predictor. It is due to failure of conversion of retinol to retinal in the retina. The early signs of xerophthalmia, which are not easy to detect, may be more commonly seen in the Pacific than in Africa where rapidly progressive corneal disease, keratomalacia, is notoriously linked to measles.

The action of vitamin A in promoting mucus secretion in the respiratory tract and gut explains its protective effect in infections including measles and diarrhoeal disease. Vitamin A deficiency is also associated with a reduction in the number and cytotoxic activity of T-lymphocytes. Vitamin A both as retinol and as β-carotene acts as an antioxidant and deficiency may thus play a part in the development of oedema in children with PEM.

The observation that mother to child transmission (MTCT) of HIV was more common in vitamin-A-deficient women suggested the possibility that vitamin A might protect female genital mucosa. However recent work suggests that VAD is a marker for more advanced HIV disease, when the risk of MTCT is higher, and not a causal link.

The antioxidant action of vitamin A may also protect against diseases of ageing such as cataract and malignancy. In summary, the role of retinol in epithelial differentiation in the gut and respiratory tract as well as cornea, and its immune function, explains why VAD contributes to morbidity and mortality in many childhood infections. Other effects of deficiency are less well understood. Remodelling of bones during linear growth may be adversely affected by deficiency. The suggestion that VAD may reduce the availability of stored iron supports previous findings of occasional response of anaemia to VA repletion.

Toxicity is rare in situations where the main dietary source of vitamin A is β-carotene and when self-medication is rare. However, the risks of teratogenicity due to accidental overdosage have influenced public health policies in many countries. These risks may have been overstated, since such excessive intakes, in the region of 7500 µg RE compared with the recommended safe level of 800 µg RE or observed intakes of ~700 µg RE in a recent UK survey, must be very rare (WHO/FAO 2004). Despite the fact that many women of reproductive age are at risk of deficiency, women are rarely given prophylactic treatment with vitamin A except during lactation when the risks of teratogenicity are virtually absent. Studies in Nepal and India, using respectively low-dose medication and a 'dose' of red palm oil, have shown reductions in maternal mortality and anaemia respectively. WHO/FAO (2004) recommend a pregnancy increment of 100 µg RE in at risk situations. On the other hand, pregnant women with daily intakes of at least ~2400 µg RE, who would derive no benefit, are advised against supplements. Since β-carotene is safe in pregnancy, supplementation with the pro-vitamin or ensuring its adequate intake from natural foodstuffs are prudent options. WHO recommends the use of SI units, not IU: 0.3 µg retinol or RE is equivalent to 1.0 IU retinol or 3.0 IU β-carotene (WHO 2004).

TREATMENT AND PREVENTION

Acute and symptomatic vitamin A deficiency usually presents as keratomalacia. If the cornea is affected, e.g. by measles or exposure keratitis, the eye is kept closed and antibiotic and mydriatic ointment applied. Vitamin A is given by intramuscular injection when possible. Otherwise oral treatment with 15000 µg RE (50000 IU) is given on days 1, 2 and 28. It is now common policy to give 'prophylactic' supplementation to children at risk of exacerbating viral or other infection. All children with cystic fibrosis should receive daily multivitamin supplements.

Ideally, in countries with endemic vitamin A deficiency, healthy children are supplemented with vitamin A at 6-monthly intervals until the age of 5 years, and opportunistically during childhood infections. WHO recommends doses of 15000, 30000 and 60000 µg RE (50000, 100000 and 200000 IU) respectively for infants less than 6 months, 6–12 months and children 1–5 years. Lactating mothers are similarly supplemented with 60000 µg RE (200000 IU) within 2 months of delivery, reducing morbidity. In practice, however, it is not easy to achieve the intended coverage. Toxicity at these high doses is rarely reported.

Fortification is the most appropriate long-term preventive strategy in regions at risk, in view of the fact that sufficient intakes in industrialised countries are largely due to fortification. Fortification with vitamin A has been implemented successfully in Central America where fortified sugar, legally enforced for more than a decade, now provides more than 50% of the RDA for those over 2 years old. Various other vehicles have been assessed in pilot or voluntary programmes including noodle seasoning in Thailand, margarine in the Philippines, and maize and wheat flour in South Africa. Additional strategies include increasing agricultural production of high-β-carotene strains of cereals and tubers and increasing year round access by sun-drying of seasonal soft fruit with high β-carotene content (Allen 2003).

Social marketing strategies aim to increase consumption of vitamin-rich snacks and should encourage cooking practices which conserve vitamins and a prudent increase in fat intake to improve their absorption. Policies aimed at reduction of diarrhoeal and respiratory diseases are also relevant.

KEY POINTS

- β-Carotene, which is the major source of vitamin A in areas of endemic deficiency, is more bioavailable in fruit than leaves.
- Marginal deficiency, without clinical signs of xerophthalmia, is linked with increased morbidity in measles, and some other infections, especially diarrhoeal disease.
- Vitamin A requirements are increased in infection.
- Regular supplementation is generally given to young children at risk of deficiency.
- Global control of deficiency will depend on fortification of foods, plus new involvement of the commercial Global Alliance for Improved Nutrition (GAIN).
- WHO recommends replacement of IU by µg RE when reporting intakes and dosage and by µg retinol/dl or µmol/l for laboratory reporting of concentration in blood or milk.

28.4 IODINE–DEFICIENCY DISORDERS

DEFINITION

Iodine-deficiency disorders (IDD) occur where all food consumed is grown in iodine-deficient soil.

Since iodine is essential for the synthesis of thyroid hormone, deficiency results in hypothyroidism and, in severe form, in endemic 'cretinism', characterised by delayed motor and cognitive development and growth failure in children, and by a slow rate of general cellular metabolism at all ages. Milder deficiency, termed inadequate iodine nutrition (IIN) is becoming apparent, due to improved screening methods and also to persistence or re-emergence of iodine deficiency. In many areas goitre, due to reactive hyperplasia of an iodine-deficient thyroid gland, was a convenient marker for IDD (see Section *evolve* 28.4 and Figs *evolve* 28.15–28.16). The preferred method of biochemical screening of communities, using urinary iodine concentration, facilitates identification of milder degrees of iodine deficiency, with cut-off points of the concentration of urinary iodine in school age children for severe (<20 µg/l), moderate (20–<50 µg/l) and mild (50–<100 µg/l). Such surveys indicate that iodine deficiency is more widespread than previously thought.

PREVALENCE AND TRENDS

Recent changes in the global estimate of the prevalence and severity of iodine deficiency (WHO 2007) are explained by control measures resulting a fall in the prevalence of severe IDD, while improved techniques have uncovered more widespread milder deficiency (IIN). National survey data indicate that the number of countries in which iodine deficiency poses a public health problem had fallen between 1993 and 2007 from 126/130 to 47/130. Iodine deficiency, both moderate and severe, was still problematic in 14 countries (2003), six in Africa, and four in Europe (WHO 2004). Of 40 countries with mild deficiency, 19 were in Europe. Reasons for this paradoxical finding of a relatively high prevalence of a preventable nutritional deficit in a developed region are given in Section *evolve* 28.4 .

CAUSES

With the exception of seafood, the iodine content of all foods, animal or vegetable, depends on that of the soils in which they grew. Iodine deficiency occurs when people subsist on food grown on iodine-deficient soils and have no access to food from elsewhere. There is an iodine cycle in the environment in which iodine present in soil and sea water as iodide is oxidised to elemental iodine and then evaporates. Iodine is also leached out of soil

by heavy rain and flooding, and river water is often relatively high in iodine in the tropical rainy season. Iodine reaches the sea, increasing its iodine concentration, and that of marine plants and fish. Recycling of volatile iodine in rainwater is insufficient to replenish iodine-poor soils, which results in geographical variability of iodine in soils. Poverty and isolation are characteristic of areas of classical IDD. Up to 100 million people living in the highlands bordering the Rift Valley stretching from Ethiopia via Kenya, Tanzania, Uganda and the Democratic Republic of the Congo (DRC) south to Malawi are at risk of IDD. In such areas, notably the DRC, the problem is aggravated by consumption of the tuber cassava, which contains a toxin, linamarin. This goitrogen is hydrolysed to release cyanide, which, after further metabolism to thiocyanate, inhibits uptake of iodine by the thyroid gland, which hypertrophies further, increasing the size of the goitre. Other goitrogens occur in cabbage, bamboo shoots and bacteria in contaminated water. Goitre is not associated with the milder and more widespread iodine deficiency.

EFFECTS ON GROWTH AND HEALTH: SHORT AND LONG TERM

Failure to iodinate tyrosine, precursor to the active thyroid hormones tri- and tetra-iodothyronine (T_3 and T_4), has consequences which vary with the maturity of the affected individual. Iodine deficiency in fetal life results in failure to myelinate the central nervous system, especially the cerebellum. There is high fetal and neonatal loss, and survivors show hypertonia, poor coordination of movement and delay in cognitive development, 'learning difficulty', sometimes accompanied by deafness. The slowly growing infant is also slow to reach neurological developmental milestones.

Where IDD is complicated by consumption of goitrogens, goitre becomes visible in mid-childhood and more prominent in adult life, women being affected more than men. Biological variability in iodine requirements probably explains the varying expression of IDD in an affected community. The size and position of the goitre in relation to the trachea and mediastinum may produce debilitating and even life-threatening complications.

In areas where IIN is identified by biochemical screening for urinary iodine, the signs may only become apparent retrospectively after repletion, when communities 'come alive', with improvement in physical and intellectual performance by children and adults (WHO 2007). The implications for the general progress of a region are obvious.

Once supplementation or food fortification (see below) has started, goitre prevalence is no longer a valid proxy indicator for IDD, since goitre may persist for some time after iodine repletion (WHO 2007). Nor will the method serve when iodine deficiency is not accompanied by goitre. Reliance is therefore placed on measurement of urinary iodine, as well as surveillance to ensure that the chain of fortification is intact. Since median urinary iodine estimates the present dietary intake, and thereby the actual status of a community, it is used to monitor the progress and impact of control measures.

TREATMENT AND EVALUATION OF PROGRESS

Iodine supplementation was initially offered to affected individuals in communities at risk. Iodized oils were administered by intramuscular injection or orally, with the aim of 3-yearly dosage for women until the menopause and for men until 40 years, but compliance was a problem. Iodine supplementation of individuals gives way to universal salt fortification for both people and livestock but supplementation, in the form of iodized oil either daily or annually, for vulnerable groups such as pregnant and lactating women and children from 6 to 24 months may still be required during the interim period, before fortified salt is universally available (WHO 2007).

Periodic assessment of median urinary iodine concentration has replaced surveillance of goitre prevalence as an indicator of progress and impact. Ongoing assessment of the chain of salt fortification is of great importance. Further assessment of impact includes measurement of thyroid status in newborn and older children. Neonatal screening for thyroid-stimulating hormone (TSH), though easy to combine with other neonatal screening, may be too costly for use in poor countries. Thyroglobulin estimation, also using the dried blood spot method, has recently been adapted for field use in sentinel groups, such as school children (WHO 2007).

PREVENTION

Since re-iodination of deficient soils seems to be out of the question, and iodine deficiency does not respond to general socioeconomic development,

fortification of salt with iodine still appears to be the most effective method of management and is the preferred long-term strategy, salt being universally eaten and more often subject to large-scale processing than many other foods. The level of fortification is decided after determining the level of individual salt consumption in the region. Local small-scale manufacture may interfere with implementation as can cross-border smuggling of cheaper non-iodised salt. The success of fortification programmes in poor countries depends on effective health education, practical measures to reduce the cost to small-scale manufacturers, enforceable legislation, maintenance of the fortification equipment in working order, and sustained availability of testing kits. IIN, for example in Europe, occurs with low household uptakes of fortified salt, indicating that health education is also required. High salt intakes may result in high median levels of urinary iodine, and even in hyperthyroidism, especially in older people, when fortification is imperfectly supervised.

KEY POINTS

- Geographical deficiency of severe iodine deficiency tends to occur in mountainous regions where iodine is leached from the soil but milder degrees of iodine deficiency have wider distribution.
- Severe iodine deficiency is seen in isolated communities consuming their own produce , while milder iodine deficiency may occur in areas of marginal deficiency and inadequate uptake of iodised salt.
- IDD does not respond to measures aimed at improving general health and nutrition.
- Iodisation of salt is the preferred strategy and household uptake of fortified salt is a good indicator of the success of a national programme.
- Dosage with iodine-containing oil (lipiodol) is used as an interim measure and usually for vulnerable population groups.

28.5 IRON DEFICIENCY AND IRON-DEFICIENCY ANAEMIA

DEFINITION

Iron-deficiency anaemia (IDA) is defined by a haemoglobin concentration below the age-appropriate range for healthy individuals, due to iron deficiency

(ID) and responding to iron repletion. Anaemia is a late manifestation of iron deficiency. Although 50% of anaemia may be due to other causes, the term anaemia is often used incorrectly synonymously with iron-deficiency anaemia.

Since iron is essential to the synthesis of the oxygen carrier haemoglobin, the size and haemoglobin density of the red cell (*erythrocyte*) is reduced by deficiency. IDA is, therefore, characterised by small, pale (*microcytic, hypochromic*) red blood cells. These small corpuscles have a low mean volume (MCV) and lower mean concentration of haemoglobin (MCHC).The rate of production of red cells (erythropoiesis) is not affected by iron deficiency. By contrast, in deficiency of folic acid and vitamin B_{12}, which are both necessary for cell proliferation, the process of erythropoiesis is faulty and circulating red cells are fewer in number and unusually large (macrocytic). A disturbance in globin synthesis can occur in riboflavin deficiency, which is manifested by fewer circulating red cells of normal size and haemoglobin concentration. The rare anaemia of copper deficiency is microcytic and hypochromic. In multiple deficiency a mixed picture is common. (See Section *evolve* 28.5(b) for anaemias other than IDA et al).

The earliest sign of iron deficiency in an otherwise healthy individual is reduced stores, with low bone marrow iron, and low serum ferritin. As iron status deteriorates, the rate of iron transport falls, but red cell function remains satisfactory for a while. Uncomplicated iron deficiency produces an adaptive rise in transferrin synthesis and in total iron binding capacity (TIBC) due to a fall in saturation of circulating transferrin. Anaemia is evidence that iron has failed to reach the red blood cells. Physical signs such as reduced work capacity or breathlessness on exertion are seen in severe IDA.

Some indicators of iron status give confounding results. The ferritin apoprotein behaves like an acute phase protein so that in acute infection or inflammation its serum concentration may rise to normal or elevated levels, even when the body is iron-deficient. High values for serum ferritin may also coexist with anaemia in children with oedematous PEM. Ideally, combined indicators of iron metabolism and infection are recommended to assess iron status.By contrast, hepatic synthesis of the binding protein transferrin may fall in PEM. Hereafter we shall refer to iron deficiency as IDA implying severe ID.

PREVALENCE AND TRENDS

ID is the commonest nutritional deficiency worldwide, particularly affecting young children and women of reproductive age (WHO 1992, 2004, 2008). It is implicated in high rates of anaemia seen in many parts of the developing world. For example the prevalence of anaemia in preschool age children is 68%, 66% and 47% and in pregnant women 57%, 48% and 44% in sub-Saharan Africa, southeast Asia and the eastern Mediterranean respectively (WHO 2006). It is also the proven cause of poverty-associated anaemia in the USA and Europe.

CAUSES

Even when the adult diet is high in flesh foods and enhancers of iron absorption, the weaning diet may be deficient in iron unless cereals are fortified. ID in young children may be due to avoidance of commercial weaning foods containing meat for religious reasons. Vegetarian and vegan diets are associated with ID, in both adults and children, and dieting to lose weight is a risk factor in adolescent girls (Hercberg et al 2001).

As with other nutrients, iron status depends on the balance between intake and losses. Dietary ID is especially common where the main dietary source is non-haem iron in plant foods, which is absorbed less well than haem iron, and is exacerbated by blood loss. Avoidance of meat by adults is more commonly due to poverty than culture, flesh foods being eaten on special occasions. In meat-free diets, cereals, especially millet, are a major iron source with a small contribution due to contamination from soil or iron pots, and dark green vegetables and pulses are other main dietary source of iron. Regional diets have been classified by WHO according to bioavailability of iron, with nominal values of 5%, 10% and 15% for low, medium and high bioavailability respectively, according to their content of iron absorption inhibitors, such as phytate, calcium, tannin and oxalates, and enhancers, such as ascorbic acid, other fruit acids and a factor in flesh foods. ID is typically associated with diets of low bioavailability due to high phytate and little haem, and population differences in iron status are largely explained by differences in the dietary bioavailability of iron. The WHO/FAO (2004) has adjusted the RDA for iron according to its dietary bioavailability.

Blood loss, especially menstrual loss by healthy women, is an important cause of ID, explaining variation in status and iron requirements within populations. In the humid tropics, persistent low-grade blood loss due to intestinal parasites, such as hookworm and whipworm, also contributes to ID, as does blood loss due to urinary or intestinal schistosomiasis.

The major iron store in the newborn is in haemoglobin itself, and babies are born with a high haemoglobin concentration. A baby born with a low birthweight has a lower blood volume and a smaller iron store. Low-birthweight babies who are also born before term have even smaller stores. Catch-up growth, during the early months of suckling, on a diet that is naturally low in iron, leads to an increased risk of ID in infancy. This risk is increased if the baby is introduced early to unmodified cow's milk, which may cause microscopic intestinal blood loss. In practice such babies are ideally fed on breast milk, the low iron content of which is highly bioavailable, or on iron-fortified formulae. Weanling children with behavioural feeding problems, as well as those eating a low iron diet, are at risk of ID. Slow progression of weaning and use of unfortified cereals are also causally implicated in ID. Conditions such as coeliac disease, where the gut absorptive area is reduced, and chronic inflammatory bowel disease are also risk factors. IDA due to insidious blood loss may also be the mode of presentation of intestinal tumours.

EFFECTS ON HEALTH

At all ages IDA results in reduced oxygen carriage to the tissues with an adverse effect on oxidative metabolism. Reduction in the capacity for intense short-term and also endurance activity has been observed, the former associated with reduced oxidative capacity of muscle mitochondria and the latter with reduction in myoglobin and other iron-containing proteins in muscle. Diminished performance of standard tasks, which recovers on iron repletion, has been demonstrated in agricultural labourers suffering from longstanding ID. When ID in humans under-performing during exercise was treated, performance improved before muscle mitochondrial function had recovered, suggesting that reduced delivery of oxygen to muscle rather than reduced muscle function is the major limiting factor in humans. This may be independent of haemoglobin level since maximal oxygen consumption is also reduced in non-anaemic ID women.

In developing countries women are also engaged in hard physical work, even when pregnant. In these harsh environments anaemia in pregnancy is commonly associated with higher rates of low fetal birthweight and perinatal death. However, the importance of ID in severe anaemia is less certain because of the confounding effects of multiple deficiencies and malaria infection. Iron is also active in neurotransmitter systems in the brain and the effects of deficiency depend on the maturity of the affected individual. Animal studies suggest that different areas of the developing brain have different iron requirements and therefore different sensitivities to iron deprivation. The uptake of iron by the developing human brain is relatively slow, with 10% of adult values present at birth and 50% by 10 years. The results of studies on the long-term outcome of early ID or the benefits of repletion are conflicting: children with demonstrable delay in developmental milestones due to early-onset ID may 'catch up' after iron repletion; others indicate persistence of neurological defect, e.g. in memory or in speed of nerve conduction. Some of the more persistent neurological or cognitive effects may explained by defective nerve myelination and/or some functional 'disconnection' between external stimuli and the learning process. Studies in deprived communities risk confounding due to coincidental nutrient deficiencies or psychosocial disadvantage. On balance some damage is likely to be irreversible (Beard 2008).

The role of iron in infection is complex, since it is a nutrient for both host and pathogen, especially for intracellular organisms such as malaria, and also a potential toxicant. Animal studies of the interaction between ID and infection produce conflicting results, and human studies are hampered by the rarity of single nutrient deficiency and by the ethical imperative to treat illness. Nevertheless, studies in iron-deficient but otherwise healthy humans have shown effects of iron deficiency or cell-mediated immunity including reduced production of myeloperoxidase, a precursor to bacterial killing by neutrophils, reduced bactericidal activity of macrophages and also a reduction in number and proliferation of T-lymphocytes, whose rate of synthesis is catalysed by iron-containing enzymes. Such abnormalities can be corrected by iron repletion (Munoz et al 2007). The adverse effect of ID on the cellular response is more marked than its effect on humoral immunity. The body defends itself against the adverse effects of the redox capability of iron by means of a number of binding proteins, active in iron transport or storage. During the acute phase response to infection, these binding proteins also prevent access to iron by intracellular pathogens. Recent additions to the familiar list, including transferrin, lactoferrin and ferritin, etc., are hepcidin and NRAMP1. Effects of treatment are discussed below.

TREATMENT

The possibility that bacterial infection in young infants may be exacerbated by iron therapy, especially if given by injection, has long been recognised. The likely mechanism is that free iron becomes available to bacteria during the brief period of hyperferraemia. The side-effects of treatment are less clear-cut when iron is administered orally or as a fortificant in milk formula, or when subjects are followed up for longer, because immediate adverse effects may be outweighed by longer-term benefits. In view of the paucity of information on the infection-related effects of iron supplementation in breastfed babies further study is required . The situation with respect to malaria is completely different. In malarious areas iron supplementation is associated with an increased incidence of clinical malaria and sometimes of (linked) bacterial infection. However, iron supplementation does not affect the rate of malaria 'attack'.

Iron is not given currently by injection, and iron supplementation of formula milks is more modest. Prudence dictates that iron treatment of anaemic children be postponed until malaria has been treated, and community supplementation postponed until after the malaria season.

People with confirmed ID are generally treated with oral iron as a ferrous salt. Treatment should continue until stores are replete, estimated to be 3 months after normalisation of haemoglobin concentration.

Supplementation in pregnancy

Does every pregnant woman need supplemental iron? Supplementation of the ID mother reduces the risks of anaemia, preterm delivery and low fetal birthweight. On the other hand unnecessary supplementation may lead to maternal illness and low fetal birthweight. In areas with a high prevalence of ID, routine supplementation benefits the majority and is unlikely to do harm. Ideally, iron status should be checked early in pregnancy, before embarking on treatment. The WHO (2001) recommends daily supplements of 60 mg elemental iron and 400 µg folic acid in such areas, though dosage, frequency, formulation and timing of supplementation are all under review. The case for lower dosage is argued strongly in developed countries without a problem of ID. In the USA and Australia, doses ~20–30 mg are advised for healthy non-ID women (Cogswell 2003), while national policy in the UK encourages dietary measures unless ID has been proven.

Community supplementation programmes with iron, iron plus folate, or multiple micronutrients are widely promoted in developing countries. Multiple micronutrient supplementation (MMS) is an attractive option where multiple deficiency is likely. However, the causes of multiple deficiency are manifold, and when the situation is exacerbated by PEM and parasites, subjects may not respond to simple supplementation. The mechanism of response may also be uncertain; for example, growth attributed to zinc repletion may be due to non-specific appetite improvement. Furthermore, supplementation with a wide array of micronutrients may be no more effective than the 'old favourites', iron, folate, zinc and vitamins A and C.

PREVENTION

In areas at risk of ID, fortification of staple foods is a cost-effective strategy. The same principles apply as to fortification with other micronutrients – the level of need is assessed, a suitable vehicle is identified, ideally a cheap food with similar levels of consumption by all population groups. The iron should be in a bioavailable form, the product stable when stored, and with an acceptable taste. Central processing facilitates the technical process of fortification, though low-technology systems have been developed for fortification during small-scale milling of maize.

Food has been iron-fortified in the USA and UK for more than 50 years, cereals and commercial beverages being the vehicles commonly used. The redox action of the fortificant may affect the taste and colour of the vehicle, and iron may interact with other supplemental micronutrients. High-extraction, low-phytate wheat flour is a suitable vehicle, but maize and rice are less amenable to fortification. Considerable recent progress has been made in the fortification of cereal staples in Africa and Asia. Fortification practice varies considerably in the European Union: recent limited legislation (2007) resulted in some 'harmonisation'. With respect to vulnerable population groups, fortification of weaning foods is recognised as important, as is education about sources of iron, and enhancers of iron absorption in the vegetarian or halal weaning diet. Even when fortification appears to be successful and cost-beneficial, the long-term success of the strategy depends on legislation and active participation of an informed community.

KEY POINTS

- Iron deficiency is strongly linked with diets low in haem iron and high in phytate, which have low (~5%) bioavailability of iron.
- Variation in the magnitude of menstrual blood loss contributes to the variability of iron requirements of women in the reproductive age
- Dietary iron deficiency is exacerbated by blood loss due to intestinal parasites.
- Severe iron deficiency results in anaemia and is its major cause in deficient populations.
- Oxidative metabolism and therefore work capacity are reduced by iron deficiency.
- In young infants and children iron deficiency is also associated with motor and cognitive delay, though long-term sequelae are unclear.
- Routine iron supplementation of pregnant women prevents IDA in communities at risk, but policies are under review in Western countries
- Iron fortification of staple foods is a cost-effective preventive strategy.

28.6 OTHER DEFICIENCIES

Other fairly common micronutrient deficiencies – zinc, niacin and thiamine – are discussed in Section *evolve* 28.6 and the clinical signs of deficiencies are shown in Figs *evolve* 28.17–28.20 🖱.

28.7 SPECIFIC SITUATIONS AND POPULATION GROUPS AT RISK OF MALNUTRITION

FAMINES

(See also Section *evolve* 28.7(a) 🖱 and Section 32.4.)

Famine is defined as a sharp increase in mortality due to diseases related to acute starvation. Famine was thought to be a direct and inevitable consequence of sudden and severe crop failure, sometimes exacerbated by isolation and transport problems. This traditional paradigm was overturned when Sen (1982) demonstrated that widespread starvation could occur even when food was available. The present paradigm is based on his economic analysis, but includes other factors such as demographic, climatic or political disaster.

In the mid-nineteenth century, potato blight affected much of northern Europe, but Ireland alone was struck by famine. The potato had flourished in Ireland, giving high energy yields per cultivated area. Early warnings about rotting crops were met by a combination of forward planning and legislative inertia. Efforts were made to provide employment and hold down food prices, but a powerful political lobby strove to maintain high prices for wheat farmers. Ireland continued to export wheat, and imports remained subject to duty, until repeal of the Corn Laws. Even then, the release and distribution of unfamiliar 'Indian corn' (maize) imported as food aid were delayed. Prices soared, people left home or were evicted, and press reports of starvation, scurvy and famine oedema appeared. Many succumbed to louse-borne typhus and relapsing fever, or emigrated in conditions of appalling squalor. Death and emigration were together responsible for a major fall in population, although the actual death toll remains uncertain.

Famines in the twentieth and twenty-first centuries followed a similar pattern, and suppression of information was common. Sen studied famines in Bengal and Ethiopia in detail.

Floods and cyclones in wartime (1943) Bengal resulted in some crop losses. Meanwhile an urban boom, fuelled by armament production, had led to inflation of grain prices. Factory workers were little affected by this, but the service economy and food producers, specifically barbers and poor fishermen, found they could no longer buy sufficient rice for their needs. A sharp increase in price and some hoarding of rice further disrupted exchange conditions and there was widespread hunger. A similar natural catastrophe occurred in 1974 in (then) Bangladesh, resulting in rural unemployment plus an uncontrolled rise in rice price, although national statistics proved that per capita grain production actually peaked in the famine year. A drought in Ethiopia in the mid-1980s resulted in a failed harvest for subsistence farmers working exhausted land and using poor equipment. Their plight was exacerbated by a forced famine levy, plus continued pressure to remit a grain quota to the government as part of a strategy to hold down urban food prices. Farmers were forced to sell livestock, exacerbating the food shortage in drought-affected areas. Famine appears to be less likely in a functioning democracy, where the administration will be goaded by the media and political opposition into some effective response to an emergency.

Four stages of progression to famine have been identified: dearth or food shortage; privation and coping strategies; and social collapse with dispersal and migration. Communities familiar with food shortage are well practised in 'coping'. Coping strategies tend to 'protect' or 'modify' food consumption. The first is achieved by eating non-traditional staples, bought or donated, and the second by eking out existing stores by eating less, by 'diversifying', foraging for wild or 'famine' foods, or by reduction in the number fed from 'the same pot', as young men travel in search of work. Signs of failure to cope include falling attendance at work, markets, schools or immunisation clinics. Complete failure sees mass migration of the destitute, who arrive at camps or collection points already vulnerable to infectious disease, such that mortality soon rises.

Early intervention aims to interrupt this baleful progress before irrevocable damage has been done. In countries at risk, vulnerability mapping is undertaken, using satellite images, climatic and agricultural data including crop estimates, census and health information and anthropometric assessment. At the domestic level, information on food availability from production, labour or barter takes note of seasonal variation, of recent 'shocks' and traditional coping strategies. Baseline information is continually updated and re-analysed to compare predicted and actual outcome, and as part of a sophisticated warning system. This proactive data collation is an example of effective partnership between government and international agencies. There is a global and national responsibility to avert famine, by facilitating development, encouraging good governance and preventing war.

REFUGEES

Global statistics indicate that conflict has overtaken climatic disaster as the trigger for large-scale population movements. People migrate within their own or to another country, fleeing from danger or seeking food and security. The United Nations High Commission for Refugees (UNHCR 2007) estimates that around 16 million people are currently refugees and around 51 million are internally displaced by conflict (26 m) or natural disaster (25 m).

Nutritional support for refugees follows established guidelines. The type and level of intervention, decided after a needs assessment, is defined in descending order of priority as critical, severe and targeted. The first and second levels provide a general ration for everybody, plus targeted and or therapeutic feeding for vulnerable groups (see Section *evolve* 28.7(b) 🖱). Information on nutritional management is given on the websites of experienced international (UNICEF 2005) and non-governmental organisations.

MALNUTRITION IN HOSPITALS AND CARE HOMES

Undernutrition in patients is associated with prolonged stay in hospital. It may be estimated by anthropometry or by a nutrition risk assessment 'tool' or indicator. Such 'tools' provide a means of identifying at admission those at increased risk of malnutrition, for whom nutritional intervention is advisable (see Section *evolve* 28.2(b) 🖱).

Conditions such as mental illness and neurological incapacity, e.g. coma or stroke, interfere with eating; others, such as illness in the elderly, in the context of a poorly staffed ward, are also associated with reduced intake. The body's response to conditions such as infection, surgery or burns, and cardio-respiratory disease also has a 'nutritional cost' (Akner & Cederholm 2001).

The risk of nutritional deterioration is increased by existing malnutrition, inability to eat, underfeeding or an increased protein–energy requirement for infection or healing. Estimates of energy and protein requirements during illness were adjusted when research indicated that the high requirements of the acute phase do not apply throughout convalescence. Overfeeding, especially during total parenteral nutrition (TPN) was linked to the development of hepatic steatosis, an early sign of TPN-associated liver disease. Various preventive strategies are now advised to avoid nutrient deficits or excesses, to provide pro-active antibiotic treatment and to modulate the immune response by addition of nutrients such as n-3 fatty acids or arginine (McCowen & Bistrian 2003).

Patients with renal failure are at risk of negative energy and nitrogen balance and micronutrient deficiency due to uraemic anorexia, adaptive changes in protein turnover and loss of micronutrients during dialysis. Folate deficiency may present as failure of anaemia to respond to treatment with erythropoietin. Micronutrient supplementation, especially with the B vitamins, is recommended. Surgical patients are also at increased risk of deficiency when, for example, nutrient absorption has been compromised by gastric bypass or gut resection. Supplementation with B vitamins and some minerals may be indicated, allowance being made, in the latter case, for competition between minerals for absorption. Malnutrition may slow down the metabolism of drugs, and also affect the response to treatment of infection. Supplementation with antioxidant vitamins and minerals may act by repletion of deficiency or by immune modulation.

Prevention of malnutrition in the community and in care homes is one of the elements of primary care for the elderly and other vulnerable groups. Strategies to improve the nutrition of vulnerable patients include improving the choice and quality of meals, and identifying those who need help with feeding.

ALCOHOLISM

Alcoholism (see Ch. 9) is a global problem, the nutritional consequences of which are worse when superimposed on an already impoverished diet. A daily intake of around 10 units of alcohol will deliver 300 kJ energy, i.e 3–4% of the adult estimated average requirements (EAR), as 'empty calories'. The heavier drinker tends to eat less, and meals may be nutritionally inadequate or omitted due to forgetfulness or poverty. Signs of malnutrition CED will be evident when protein energy intake is compromised. Alcohol-related liver disease includes steatosis, hepatitis and cirrhosis, all of which may be associated with primary or secondary CED.

Micronutrient deficiency is common, only partly explained by dietary lack. Biochemical and clinical deficiency of the B vitamins may be accompanied by deficiency of magnesium, zinc and calcium, the latter partly due to excessive urinary loss and partly to vitamin D deficiency. Thiamin deficiency may be predicted from altered behaviour plus signs of CED. Chronic thiamin deficiency may result in polyneuropathy or the complexities of the Wernicke–Korsakoff syndrome (WKS). WKS may present acutely with signs mimicking those of acute alcohol toxicity such as unusual eye movements, an ataxic gait and finally stupor and coma. Memory tends to fail more gradually. Treatment with thiamine is effective if given in time, otherwise the changes are irreversible.

Cyanide toxicity due to consumption of cassava, in an otherwise deficient diet, is particularly prevalent in indigent alcoholics in west Africa. The condition, known as tropical ataxic neuropathy, presents with peripheral neuropathy accompanied by typical changes in the retina. There is biochemical evidence of deficiency of thiamine and riboflavin.

OTHER GROUPS AT RISK OF MALNUTRITION IN AFFLUENT COUNTRIES
Low socioeconomic groups

The demography of middle income and affluent countries is changing as a result of immigration and increased survival into old age, both of which may affect rates of poverty and malnutrition. The groups most vulnerable to poverty are single-parent families, the elderly, refugees and ethnic minorities. Isolation, depression and memory deficits associated with dementia or alcoholism may exacerbate the situation. Ethnic minorities, especially when isolated by language and educational disadvantage, are particularly prone to poverty and undernutrition. In the UK the ethnic groups most at risk of poverty originated in Bangladesh, Pakistan and sub-Saharan Africa. In the northern states of the USA, high rates of poverty are seen among unemployed urban African-Americans whereas Mexican Hispanics are the group most at risk in the south. In both the USA and UK at every educational level, an 'ethnic penalty' bars easy access to employment. Immigrants, especially recent arrivals unfamiliar with the 'bureaucratic systems' in the UK and USA, are at particular risk of food insecurity and actual hunger (Kasper et al 2000, Sellen et al 2002).

There is often a divergence between macro- and micronutrient status such that deficiency of iron and other micronutrients coexists with obesity in both children and adults. Failure to access healthy food is not the inevitable sequel of 'poverty and ignorance'. Among the poor of the southern USA, decisions about where to shop and what to buy are often determined by distance, or problems with urban transport. Isolation, depression and lack of autonomy have an adverse effect on the dietary intake and nutritional status of vulnerable people such as the elderly and refugees. Practical difficulties with food storage compound the problems of the homeless, as does dietary displacement by alcohol and drugs. Low income in the UK is a risk factor for similarly unbalanced dietary intakes, high in energy, deficient in micronutrients (Food Standards Agency 2007). However several strategies exist to deal with nutrition problems associated with poverty (see Section *evolve* 28.7(c) 🖱 and Ch. 33).

Vegetarian diets

Vegetarian diets (see Ch. 17) cover a wide range including vegan and macrobiotic diets and so cannot be considered as a single group. In general the diet of vegetarians, who form less than 5% of the population in Western countries, may be less restricted than is commonly thought. Plant-based diets are nutritionally adequate providing they are not restricted in variety or quality and the lower intake of saturated fatty acids and cholesterol and the higher intake of fruit and vegetables results in a lower risk of ischaemic heart disease. However deficiencies can occur as diets high in fruit and vegetables may be bulky and low in energy and therefore inadequate in young children. Vitamin B_{12} is the nutrient most likely to be lacking in vegan and to a lesser extent in vegetarian diets, leading to elevated plasma homocysteine concentrations and increased risk of neurological disorders. Vegetarians are at increased risk of iron-deficiency anaemia as iron from plant foods has low bioavailability. In vegan diets long-chain n-3 fatty acids are absent but intakes of linoleic acid are high, which may inhibit the synthesis of long-chain polyunsaturated fatty acids needed in fetal brain development. Vegans may have difficulty maintaining weight in old age.

Risks in pregnancy and early childhood

Poor nutrition linked to lack of education has cross-generational effects in all societies. Early onset of childbearing and short birth interval are associated with low maternal weight gain and low fetal birth-weight (LBW; King 2003). The immediate risks of LBW are reduced by effective neonatal care, but the sequelae of adverse fetal programming are not. If such babies are then 'overfed' in childhood, they are particularly prone to diseases of 'affluence' as adults. Adolescent mothers with poor diets are at particular risk due to the nutritional demands of their own growth and that of their baby. The risks of micronutrient deficiency during periods of rapid early child growth are greater among the poor and among those eating diets with low micronutrient bioavailability such as vegetarians and infants of some immigrant groups eating a halal weaning diet.

Elderly

The nutritional requirements of the elderly (see Ch. 16) reflect reduced energy expenditure, but sustained protein requirements (Millward 2008). Micronutrient deficiency may be due to dietary inadequacy, physical problems with eating, or malabsorption, sometimes associated with disease or bacterial overgrowth of the gut. Since oxidative stress is responsible for some of the effects of aging, antioxidant micronutrient status in the elderly has implications for health. Less skin exposure to sunlight, plus less effective skin metabolism of precursors of vitamin D, increases the risk of deficiency. The diseases associated with ageing such as coronary artery disease, Alzheimer's disease, poor cognitive functioning, and cancers all have nutritional components. The demographic shift gives impetus to studies aiming to establish the value of supplements including B vitamins, antioxidant vitamins and minerals, and EFA as a means of postponing the effects of ageing. Non-nutritional factors including physical activity and social integration also play a part in the nutritional health of the elderly. Joint or movement disorders such as tremor or ataxia reduce mobility, thereby contributing to obesity, which, when combined with sarcopenia and consequent muscle weakness, results in further reduction in activity. By contrast, physical fitness is associated with good nutritional health although it may not be clear which factor initiates the virtuous cycle (McNeill et al 2002).

KEY POINTS

- Famine occurs when people lose their entitlement (access) to food and may thus affect people who are not directly engaged in actual food production.
- Democracy, through early publication and exposure of problems, protects against famine.
- When refugees from war or famine congregate, safe management extends far beyond provision of food.
- Malnutrition occurs in hospitals in rich and poor countries.
- Malnutrition coexists with poverty, even in developed countries, e.g. among refugees, immigrants, the unemployed, the homeless and the elderly, and may be exacerbated by alcoholism

References

Akner G, Cederholm T: Treatment of protein energy malnutrition in chronic non-malignant disorders, *American Journal of Clinical Nutrition* 74:6–24, 2001.

Allen LH: Interventions for micronutrient deficiency control in developing countries: past present and future, *Journal of Nutrition* 133:3875S–3879S, 2003.

Beard JL: Why iron deficiency is important in infant development, *Journal of Nutrition* 138(12):2534–2536, 2008.

Cogswell ME, Parvanta I, Ickes L, Yip R, Brittenham GM: Iron supplementation during pregnancy, anemia, and birth weight: a randomized controlled trial, *American Journal of Clinical Nutrition* 78:773–781, 2003.

Food Standards Agency: In Nelson M, Evans B, Bates B, Church C, Boshier T, editors: *Low income diet and nutrition survey.* London, 2007, FSA.

Gomez F, Galvan RR, Frenk S, et al: Mortality in second and third degree malnutrition, *Journal of Tropical Paediatrics* 2:77–83; reprinted in *Bulletin of the World Health Organization* 78:1275–1280, 1956.

Hercberg S, Preziosi P, Galan P: Iron deficiency in Europe, *Public Health Nutrition* 4(2B):537–545, 2001.

Jelliffe DB, Jelliffe EFP: Direct Assessment of Nutritional Status. In *Community Nutritional Assessment*, Oxford, 1989, Oxford Medical Publications, pp 13–126.

Kasper J, Gupta SK, Tran P, Cook JT, Meyers AF: Hunger in legal immigrants to California, Texas and Illinois, *American Journal of Public Health* 90:1629–1633, 2000.

Kielman A, McCord C: Weight for age: an index of risk of death in children, *Lancet* i:1247–1250, 1978.

King JC: The risk of maternal nutritional depletion and poor outcomes increases in early or closely spaced pregnancies, *Journal of Nutrition* 133:1732S–1736S, 2003.

McCowen KC, Bistrian BR: Immunonutrition: problematic or problem solving? *American Journal of Clinical Nutrition* 77:764–770, 2003.

McNeill G, Vyvyan J, Seymour G, Hendry J, Macpherson I: Prediction of micronutrient status in men and women more than 75 years old, living in the community, *British Journal of Nutrition* 88:555–561, 2002.

Millward DJ: Sufficient protein for our elders? *American Journal of Clinical Nutrition* 88:1187–1188, 2008.

Munoz C, Rios E, Olivos J, et al: Iron, copper and immunocompetence, *British Journal of Nutrition* 98(Suppl 1):S24–S28, 2007.

Sellen DV, Tedstone AE, Frize J: Food insecurity among refugee families in East London; results of a pilot assessment, *Publ Health Nutrition* 5:637–644, 2002.

Sen A: *Poverty and famines; an essay on entitlement and deprivation*, Oxford, 1982, Oxford University Press, p 1–9, 45–51.

Sommer A, Loewenstein MS: Nutritional status and mortality; a prospective evaluation of the QUAC stick, *American Journal of Clinical Nutrition* 28:287–292, 1975.

UNICEF: *Emergency Field Handbook; a guidebook for UNICEF staff,* New York 2005.

UNHCR: *Report of the United Nations High Commissioner for Refugees*, 63rd Session supplement no 12, New York, 2008.

Waterlow JC: *Protein energy malnutrition*, London, 1992, Edward Arnold.

Waterlow JC, Buzina R, Keller W, et al: The presentation and use of height and weight data for comparing the nutritional status of children under the age of ten years, *Bulletin of the World Health Organization* 55:489–498, 1977.

WHO: *Second report on the world health situation*, Geneva, 1992, WHO, available online at: http://www.unsystem.org.scn/archive/rwn.

WHO: *Complementary feeding of young children in developing countries: a review of current scientific knowledge*, Geneva, 1998, WHO, available online at: http://www.who.nut/documents.

WHO: *The management of severe protein energy malnutrition: a manual for physicians and other senior health workers.* Geneva, 1999.

WHO: *Diet, nutrition and the prevention of chronic diseases*, WHO technical report Series 916, Geneva, 2003, WHO.

WHO/FAO: *Vitamin and mineral requirements in human nutrition*, ed. 2, Geneva, FAO Rome, 2004, WHO.

WHO: *Indicators for assessing iodine deficiency disorders and monitoring their elimination*, ed. 3, Geneva, 2007, WHO.

WHO/IATT: *Infant feeding consultation: Prevention of HIV infection in pregnant women mothers and their infants*, Geneva 2006.

WHO: In de Benoist B, McLean E, Egli L, Cogswell M, editors: *Worldwide prevalence of anaemia 1993–2005*, Geneva, 2008, WHO.

Further reading

Ashworth A, Burgess A: *Caring for severely malnourished children*, London, 2003, Macmillan.

Bothwell TH: Iron requirements in pregnancy and strategies to meet them, *American Journal of Clinical Nutrition* 72:257S–264S, 2000.

Devereux S: Famine in Africa. In Devereux A, Maxwell S: *Food security in sub-Saharan Africa*, Rugby, UK, 1999, ITDG Publishing, pp 117–148.

Medact: Famine and hunger. In: *Global Health Studies*, London, UK, 2001, Medact, available online at: http://www.medact.org.

WHO: Severe malnutrition. In: *Management of the child with a severe infection or severe malnutrition; guidelines for care at the first referral level in developing countries*, Geneva, 2000, WHO/FCH/CAH.

WHO/FAO: In Allen L, de Benoist B, Dary O, Hurrell R, editors. *Guidelines on food fortification with micronutrients*. Geneva/Rome, 2006, WHO/FAO.

(See also Further reading section on *evolve* website listed by subsection of the text. ⟨🖱⟩)

Chapter 29

Diet and genotype interactions – nutritional genomics

Paul Trayhurn and I Stuart Wood

CHAPTER CONTENTS

OBJECTIVES

By the end of this chapter you should be able to:
- understand the fundamentals of gene expression and how it is assessed
- understand the molecular basis for the ability of nutrients to influence gene expression and the ability of genotype to influence nutrient handling
- describe some common polymorphisms and their effects on nutrient metabolism
- appreciate the effects of specific genotypes on the susceptibility to disease.

29.1 INTRODUCTION

Since its origins in the 1950s, molecular biology has developed into the driving force behind much of modern biological science. The pervasiveness of molecular biology is such that the concepts and techniques that it represents have entered most other areas of the biological sciences. Molecular biological perspectives are also leading to a revolution in nutrition, and this is happening at several different levels. At the simplest level, it has for some years been possible to examine the effects of nutrients on the expression of specific genes, whether they encode enzymes, receptors, transporters or hormones. This means that we can increasingly construct a (reductionist) picture of dietary interaction from the level of body composition and whole body physiology, to substrate flux in metabolic pathways, to the amount and activity of enzymes, and through to the effects on gene expression.

© 2010 Elsevier Ltd/Inc/BV
DOI: 10.1016/B978-0-7020-3118-2.00029-2

Following from the developments in molecular biology and molecular genetics is the recent emergence of the field of nutritional genomics. This includes: (1) nutrigenomics, which investigates the effects of nutrients on the genome and proteome; (2) nutrigenetics, one of the key foci of which is to characterise the link between variations (polymorphisms) in particular genes and the individual response to nutrients – especially those relevant to disease (Ordovas and Mooser 2004). Interest in this area has developed rapidly and there is, for some, the long-term goal of being able to provide personalised dietary advice based on the predicted response to nutrients derived from the genetic profiling of an individual.

In this chapter we consider diet and genotype interactions and some of the early progress of nutritional genomics. General concepts are presented, together with selected specific examples.

29.2 A MOLECULAR APPROACH TO UNDERSTANDING NUTRIENT–GENE INTERACTIONS

FUNDAMENTALS OF GENE STRUCTURE

To understand the interaction between nutrients and the genome, it is first necessary to consider the fundamentals of gene action. The two key molecules involved in the transfer of genetic information are DNA and RNA. These polymeric macromolecules are composed of a chain of nucleotides each of which has a sugar moiety, a phosphate group and either a purine or a pyrimidine base (see Section 8.3). The key difference between RNA and DNA is that the sugar moiety in RNA is ribose while in DNA it is deoxyribose.

The nucleotides in DNA and RNA are linked by phosphate bridges to a sugar-phosphate backbone, each base being attached to the sugar moiety. DNA consists of two polynucleotide strands arranged in the double helix structure – a twentieth-century icon – discovered in 1953 by Watson and Crick, based on the work of Franklin and Wilkins. The sugar phosphate is on the outside of the helix with the bases in the centre. The two strands of the double helix are held together by hydrogen bonding between specific base pairs, each base pair consisting of a purine and pyrimidine, the pairings being A–T and C–G.

The information necessary for the synthesis of every individual protein in an organism is encoded

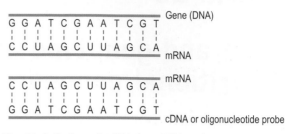

Fig. 29.1 Coding of mRNA from DNA and complementarity of cDNA, or oligonucleotide, probes in the detection of mRNAs.

by lengths of DNA – the genes. Large numbers of different genes are linked together and assembled with specific histoproteins to form chromosomes, the number of which varies from species to species. There are 46 chromosomes in humans. There has been much debate about the number of human genes, but a figure of around 23 000 – made of approximately 300 million base pairs – now seems probable following the sequencing of the human genome.

The human genome sequence, which is now available in fine detail, is a profound development – scientifically and culturally – and has underpinned the rapid emergence of nutritional genomics.

PRINCIPLES OF GENE EXPRESSION

The final protein product emanating from the expression of genes is reached through a complex, multi-step process (see Ch. 8 and Fig. 29.2), which begins in the nucleus with the transcription of DNA. The precision of base pairing allows DNA to act as a template for the synthesis of strands containing complementary sequences; this is the central element in the transfer of genetic information (Fig. 29.1). The sequence of four bases in DNA is therefore transcribed into a complementary strand of messenger RNA (mRNA). Genes consist of coding regions termed *exons*, regulatory sequences (*promoters*) and internal non-coding regions, or *introns*. In practice, only a small part (approximately 2%) of the mammalian genome actually codes for proteins and there is continuing debate on the significance of the large proportion of the genome which is without a direct coding function – sometimes referred to as 'junk DNA'.

Transcription produces an RNA molecule (the *primary* transcript) which is complementary to both

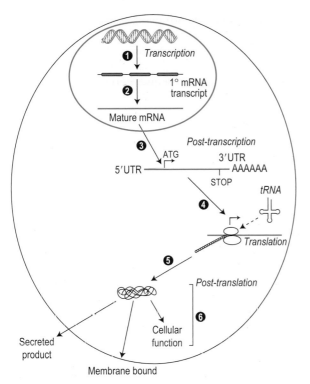

Fig. 29.2 Schematic overview of gene expression. Double-stranded DNA produces a single-stranded RNA molecule, the primary mRNA transcript, by the process of transcription (1). Non-coding segments of RNA – introns – are removed to form the mature transcript (2), which is transported from the nucleus to the cytoplasm (3). Ribosomes attach to the mature RNA transcript and initiate protein synthesis, or translation (4), from the start codon by the recruitment of tRNA molecules. Each tRNA molecule transports a specific amino acid, and this is determined from the codon sequence on the mRNA. On termination of protein synthesis, the nascent protein is released (5) and may undergo specific post-translation modification (6).

coding and non-coding regions of the gene, but the introns are removed to provide the mature transcript – the functional mRNA molecule. mRNA is transferred from the nucleus to the cytoplasm (in eukaryotic cells) where ribosome complexes are then formed on the mRNA transcript from which protein translation then commences through the mediation of transfer RNA (tRNA). Each amino acid of the 20 or so found in proteins is encoded by a sequence of three bases, and this triplet code is the same in all organisms – the concept of the universality of the genetic code. The genetic code has some degeneracy in that certain amino acids are

encoded by more than one triplet; for example, GCU, GCC, GCA and GCG all code for alanine. Once synthesised, a protein needs to fold into its appropriate three-dimensional structure and it may also undergo post-translational modifications (see below).

Regulation of gene expression by nutrients and other factors can, in principle, occur at any level from the initial transcription of genomic DNA through to the final modifications of the finished protein product.

TRANSCRIPTIONAL REGULATION OF GENE EXPRESSION

The primary control of gene regulation occurs at the level of transcription via modulation of the regulatory promoter region. The promoter consists of short lengths of bases (motifs) which are recognised by specific proteins, or transcription factors. These transcription factors bind to the DNA and exert their influence on transcriptional activity. Many motifs can be present within the promoter region and dictate where and when the gene is expressed. Furthermore, regulatory motifs affecting transcription can be found at a considerable distance from the start of the gene and are called enhancer regions. Nutrients can either have a direct influence on the transcription factors by acting as ligands, or indirectly by influencing the expression of other transcription factors, which in turn bind to the promoter of the target gene.

Retinol (vitamin A) provides a potent example of how a nutrient can influence transcription. Retinol is essential for vision, reproduction, growth and the differentiation of most cells. Once in its target cell, retinol is converted to isoforms of retinoic acid which are transferred to the nucleus and act as ligands for the transcription factors, retinoic acid receptor (RAR) and retinoic X receptor (RXR). These transcription factors bind to a motif, called the retinoic acid response element (RARE), found in a number of genes, and increase transcription of these genes.

POST-TRANSCRIPTIONAL REGULATION

Post-transcriptional regulation is evident where changes in the cytoplasmic levels of mRNA are observed without any corresponding changes in the transcription rates. This can occur at any one of a number of levels, including RNA synthesis, mRNA transport and mRNA stability. Processing of the primary RNA transcript requires the removal of intervening, non-coding regions to allow correct translation of the intended protein. Failure to do so would result in either degradation of the mRNA or non-translation of the functional protein. Alternative splicing of the primary transcript, where exons are placed together in a different order, results in different functional proteins being synthesised, i.e. one gene leads to several different mRNA transcripts and protein products. This is one reason why in the early stages of the Human Genome Project predictions of the number of human genes (over 100 000) were much too high.

Once processing of the mRNA transcript is complete, it is transported into the cytoplasm through pores in the nuclear membrane and this represents another point of regulation. The length of time the transcript remains in the cytoplasm determines the amount of protein that is translated. Hence, the stability of a particular mRNA can have a major influence on the production of the encoded protein. Those with short half-lives are able to respond quickly to external stimuli, as in the case of the rapid influx of nutrients in the post-absorptive state. The binding of regulatory proteins to recognition motifs on the mRNA transcript confers stability. One example of this is changes in transferrin receptor (TfR) expression in response to iron (see Figs *evolve* 29.1 and 29.2). When intracellular iron levels are low, iron regulatory proteins (IRPs) are up-regulated and bind to the mRNA of the transferrin receptor, thereby increasing stability and hence the synthesis of more protein. Conversely, when iron levels are high, the IRP complexes are released from the TfR mRNA, resulting in the mRNA being more susceptible to degradation and thus limiting cellular iron uptake.

TRANSLATIONAL REGULATION

Modulation of the translational apparatus to regulate gene expression can be regarded as operating at two levels – global and specific. As an example, global inhibition of protein synthesis can occur through the phosphorylation of an elongation initiation factor (e.g. eIF2) as a result of haem reduction. More common is the specific targeting of proteins in response to the metabolic status of the cell. Intracellular iron also plays a role in this mechanism. The same motifs found in the TfR used for

mRNA stabilisation are present in the iron binding protein, ferritin. But in this case, the ferritin–IRP complex is stabilised in the presence of low iron and this prevents translation of ferritin. Conversely, when iron is high and sequestration is required, the ferritin–IRP complex dissociates, allowing for ferritin synthesis.

As with post-transcriptional regulation, translational regulation is utilised when rapid changes in gene expression are required. In essence, while transcriptional regulation is seen as the major modulator of gene expression, the subsequent regulatory levels act as a fine-tuning mechanism.

POST-TRANSLATIONAL REGULATION

Once released from the ribosome, a nascent protein can undergo a series of chemical or processing modifications including proteolytic cleavage, polymerisation, glycosylation and phosphorylation. These result in changes in the biological function or activity of the protein. Glycosylation – the adding of carbohydrate molecules to specific amino acid residues at the protein surface – is required for the correct functioning of many membrane-bound (receptors) and secreted proteins. Phosphorylation is a major regulatory mechanism for many proteins within the cell, and provides for rapid changes in activity. The addition of phosphate groups to the amino acid residues serine, threonine and tyrosine is catalysed by kinases and removed by phosphatases. These opposing phosphorylation/ dephosphorylation reactions serve to activate and inactivate key enzymes involved in metabolic pathways, e.g. phosphorylase in the breakdown of glycogen. Other chemical modifications which modulate protein activity include demethylation, carboxylation, acetylation, palmitoylation, ubiquination and sulfation.

In some situations, a single polypeptide chain may be cleaved after the formation of disulphide bridges such that separate chains joined by those bridges are obtained. Thus the single chain of proinsulin becomes the two chains of insulin linked by two disulphide bridges. Many proteins also associate either with themselves to form a dimer or oligomer, or aggregate with others to form a subunit within a protein complex. For example, haemoglobin A consists of two alpha and two beta chains, while the enzyme pyruvate dehydrogenase is an aggregation of many different polypeptides.

29.3 METHODS AND TOOLS USED TO STUDY NUTRIENT–GENE INTERACTIONS

MEASUREMENTS OF GENE EXPRESSION

All genes are present in the nucleus of each cell of the body – but it is the 'which and when' of individual genes being 'switched on and off' or 'turned up or down' that ultimately determines cellular function. Thus, there are distinct tissue and cell-specific expression patterns. For example, the insulin gene is expressed in the β-cells of the pancreas and not in adipocytes or hepatocytes. Similarly, the pattern of genes expressed changes during development, and in response to environmental stress (such as hypoxia) as well as to diet and to other stimuli. The tissue specificity of gene expression is determined by the transcription factors which each cell type exhibits. Expression of a gene is determined by the detection and measurement of the corresponding mRNA. Tissues or cells may therefore be screened to assess whether a particular gene is expressed, or is being expressed at a particular point in time. In the case of a gene encoding a protein of unknown function, this can provide key information about its biological role. mRNA levels are also measured in order to determine the factors which regulate or influence the expression of a particular gene.

Three main techniques are available for detecting mRNAs, the first and until recently most widely used being northern blotting. In this case RNA (mRNAs and other RNAs) extracted from a tissue is separated on the basis of molecular size by electrophoresis on agarose gels. The various RNA species are then transferred onto a nylon membrane and the mRNA of interest is identified using a specific probe (labelled, for example with radioactivity, to allow detection) with sequences complementary to all or part of the sequence of the target mRNA (see Fig. 29.1). The probe may be a cDNA or a short (>25 bases) oligonucleotide.

In the ribonuclease (RNase) protection assay, extracted RNA is incubated in solution with a probe targeted to the specific mRNA and the enzyme ribonuclease A is used to destroy single chain strands of RNA. The duplex of probe and target mRNA is immune to digestion by the enzyme and is detected following gel electrophoresis. The RNase protection assay is more sensitive than northern blotting in the detection of mRNAs. However, the most sensitive technique is the reverse transcription polymerase chain reaction (RT-PCR), which is now generally regarded as the method of choice. RT-PCR employs short complementary sequences, or primers, to make a cDNA sequence specific to the mRNA of interest. The polymerase chain reaction is then employed to amplify the cDNA to in effect produce multiple DNA copies of the original mRNA. The PCR product, which will have a defined size, is separated by electrophoresis. RT-PCR is not, however, suitable for the accurate quantification of changes in mRNA level, the preferred method now being real-time PCR (or qPCR). In this technique, precise quantification of alterations of the level of an mRNA can be achieved over several orders of magnitude using specific probes or labels.

Northern blotting, the RNase protection assay and RT-PCR are each normally employed to detect a single mRNA at a time. Global gene expression, or the simultaneous expression of a large number of genes, can now be assessed, however, by the technology of DNA microarrays. In this procedure, large numbers (many thousands) of mRNAs can be detected at the same time using labelled probes (Moreno-Aliaga et al 2001). A further approach for simultaneously measuring the expression of a number of genes is that of PCR arrays. These allow from between a few dozen to several hundred mRNAs to be screened at the same time by employing the methodology of real-time PCR.

Each of these approaches for measuring gene expression involves the disruption of tissue and cell structures for the extraction of mRNAs. In situ hybridisation allows the expression of a particular gene to be localised to a specific region within a complex organ, such as the brain. Equally, the cell type in which expression of a gene takes place within a tissue can be determined. Examples include the initial localisation of the expression of the leptin receptor gene in regions of the hypothalamus.

PROTEOMICS

The genome provides a blueprint of the potential of an organism, but it does not tell us what actually takes place. Since proteins are the protagonists for cellular phenotype and the function of an organism, their presence represents an end point in realising the potential inherent in the genome (Tyers & Mann, 2003). Proteomics allows specific patterns of gene expression to be measured at the protein level. The proteome *(PROTein complement expressed by a genOME)* is normally defined as all the proteins that are present in a particular cell/tissue/organism at a particular time.

In proteomics, proteins extracted from tissue samples or from cells are resolved by high resolution two-dimensional gel electrophoresis and localised by staining and image analysis. Individual protein species can then be identified by mass spectrometry and database interrogation (Fuchs et al 2005).

Metabolomics

The metabolome represents the complement of metabolic reactions and metabolic products of an organism, the study of which has been widely utilised in the areas of toxicology and pharmacology. However, its application in the field of nutrition is still in its infancy (Gibney et al 2005). This technique offers considerable potential to investigate the complex interactions between nutrition and metabolism, particularly in disease states. The issues involved in adopting metabolomics as a nutritional research tool are challenging, but potentially highly rewarding. The human nutritional metabolome is influenced by a wide variety of both intrinsic (age, body composition, health status, etc.) and extrinsic (diet, colonic flora, stress, etc.) factors. The choice of the biofluids, which are central to metabolomic analysis, will also have to be carefully considered (saliva, blood and urine) and further adds to the complexity. A major challenge will be in the standardisation of nutritional metabolomics and, as with DNA microarrays and proteomics, dealing with the large volume of data generated from such studies.

In metabolomics, biofluids are subjected to either nuclear magnetic resonance (NMR) or mass-spectroscopy (MS), and the resultant spectra compared against a database for identification.

TRANSGENICS

Transgenics implies the integration of a gene from one species into the genomic DNA of another organism. Transgenic technology has enabled the effects of gene insertions on metabolic processes to be investigated. For example, the insertion and over-expression of the human gene for UCP3 (uncoupling protein-3) in the muscle of mice has shown that this uncoupling protein can, at least at very high levels, uncouple mitochondrial oxidative phosphorylation. In addition, the function of an extensive range of individual proteins has been investigated in mice by disabling or 'knocking-out' the parent gene. Such knock-outs have been employed to determine both the normal physiological role and the significance in disease processes of a given gene/gene product.

In the earlier phase of knock-out technology, a gene was disabled on a whole-body basis. However, techniques are now available so that genes can be knocked out selectively in individual tissues such as muscle. In this case, the effects of gene deletion can be studied in relation to the function of a particular tissue.

RNA INTERFERENCE

One of the recent techniques which is likely to impact strongly on the study of nutrient–gene interactions is RNA interference. Naturally occurring, short stretches of double-stranded RNA molecules are capable of regulating the expression of many genes within a cell and are involved in fundamental processes such as growth and development. The basis of RNA interference is that synthetic RNA molecules can be designed for specific genes to study the effects of preventing the expression of the target gene in a particular cell – termed gene knockdown. This technique, which is highly applicable to cell culture, provides a more robust and easier approach than gene knock-out in mice, potentially allowing hundreds of genes to be studied in a short time (Hannon 2002).

29.4 EFFECTS OF NUTRIENTS ON GENE EXPRESSION

As indicated earlier, the means by which nutrients can influence gene expression may be mediated at various levels. There is a complex interaction between the expression of genes elicited by nutrient uptake and how this expression profile affects the amounts of those nutrients required by the body (Table 29.1). The effects of nutrients on gene expression can be transmitted indirectly, such as via hormones, or directly – as in the effects of retinoic acid on transcription described earlier. Gene expression is ultimately dictated by a person's genotype and

Table 29.1   Examples of nutrient–gene interactions

NUTRIENT	GENE PRODUCT	EFFECT
Calcium	c-Fos, c-Jun, c-Myc	↑ Transcription
Iron	Metallothionein	↑ Transcription
	Ferritin	↑ Translation
Potassium	Aldosterone synthase	↑ Transcription
Zinc	Zinc fingers	Enhances specific transcription factor binding
	Metallothionein	↑ Transcription
Vitamin A (retinoic acid)	Retinoic receptor	↑ Transcription
Vitamin B_6	Steroid hormone receptor	↓ Transcription
	All genes	Purine and pyrimidine synthesis
Vitamin C (ascorbic acid)	Procollagen	↑ Transcription
	Lysyloxidase	↑ Translation
Vitamin D (cholecalciferol)	Calcium binding proteins	↑ Transcription
Vitamin E	All genes	Protects against free radical damage to DNA

differences between individuals are partly a result of which polymorphisms are present (see Section 29.5).

Nutrient requirements are influenced not only by genotype but also by the stage in the life cycle and the physiological status of an individual (e.g. pregnancy or illness). Many nutrients have been shown to influence gene expression, and several examples are presented here. The most obvious changes in response to nutritional state are those associated with fasting – the most extreme nutritional intervention – and subsequent refeeding. Thus the expression of many genes encoding transporters and hormones, as well as enzymes involved in metabolic pathways, may be altered on fasting and refeeding (e.g. the expression of leptin and of fatty acid synthase is suppressed on fasting and reactivated on refeeding). In addition, particular nutrients such as carbohydrates and lipids may have specific effects. Thus switching from a high-carbohydrate to a high-fat diet leads to the suppression of genes encoding proteins associated with fatty acid synthesis (e.g. fatty acid synthase), while the expression of genes involved in gluconeogenesis (e.g. phosphoenolpyruvate carboxykinase) is activated.

The intestine represents the foremost barrier between the environment and the body, across which nutrients must pass before they can be utilised. A complex interplay occurs between nutrient availability, absorption and gut microflora in adapting to short- and long-term changes in nutrient requirement. The mammalian intestine undergoes major adjustments during its development, and particularly at weaning when the high-protein milk diet of relatively constant composition is replaced by a diet of variable composition. Individual nutrients influence the expression of the genes encoding digestive enzymes and specific transporters to facilitate their uptake into the body. For example, monosaccharides such as glucose and fructose increase the number of specific transporter proteins present in the membrane of the cells lining the intestinal tract for maximal absorption via a combination of transcriptional and post-transcriptional events.

The fermentation of undigested dietary fibre by bacteria present in the lower intestine provides short-chain fatty acids including butyrate, which appears to be the preferred energy source for cells lining the large intestine. Additionally, the presence of butyrate has a pleiotropic effect on cellular gene expression and has been implicated as a protective factor against colon carcinomas. The varieties of species present in the gut microflora are sensitive to changes in dietary components. Major changes in the type of bacteria present may trigger the progression of intestinal disease.

Deficiencies in the levels of micronutrients – vitamins and minerals – result in many associated disease conditions, such as rickets and anaemia. The fetal demand for iron increases during gestation and failure to absorb adequate iron may lead to maternal iron-deficiency anaemia and an increased risk of premature birth. In recent years, evidence has accumulated to support a link between fetal nutritional status and adult morbidity and mortality. This is known as the 'fetal origins' or thrifty phenotype hypothesis which states that inappropriate levels of nutrition at critical times during fetal development can result in disproportionate growth, with the programming of the adult onset of several diseases including coronary heart disease, type 2 diabetes and hypertension. Such a phenomenon implies a long-term reprogramming of gene expression.

The amount of fat in the diet has been the focus of much attention in relation to the aetiology of major diseases such as coronary heart disease, cancer and obesity. There are strong associations between dietary fat intake, elevated levels of low-density lipoprotein (LDL) and the increased risk of cardiovascular disease (CVD). LDL is the main route for cholesterol delivery to peripheral tissues and contains the apoprotein B_{100} (apo-B_{100}) which acts as a ligand for the LDL receptor. Excess lipids in the liver divert apo-B_{100} from a degradation pathway to the assembly of very-low-density lipoprotein (VLDL), the precursor for LDL, by a post-transcriptional mechanism. Diets high in saturated fatty acids are associated with increased secretion of VLDL and elevated LDL levels. Furthermore, saturated fatty acids have also been shown to decrease the LDL receptor affinity, thus raising the levels of plasma LDL. The inclusion and replacement of saturated fatty acids with monounsaturated (MUFA) and polyunsaturated fatty acids (PUFAs) in the diet can reduce the risks of CVD by various direct and indirect mechanisms, including reduced apo-B_{100} secretion.

One of the additional health benefits from an increased intake of n-3 PUFAs, namely eicosapentaenoic (EPA) and docosahexaenoic (DHA) acids, is a reduction in cytokine synthesis, a mediator in the immune response. The release of the cytokines interleukin-1-beta (IL-1β) and tumour necrosis factor-alpha (TNF-α) from macrophages is decreased in the presence of n-3 PUFAs. Lymphocyte synthesis of interferon-γ (INFγ) and IL-2 is also decreased. The decrease in IL-2 synthesis can occur directly by the suppression of IL-2 transcription, or indirectly by (1) the reduction in IL-1 synthesis, and/or (2) suppression of the eicosanoid, leukotriene B_4 (LTB$_4$) synthesis. EPA inhibits the synthesis of LTB$_4$ at the expense of producing the less active LTB$_5$. The observed reduction in immune response by n-3 PUFAs has led to their therapeutic application in treating inflammatory diseases such as rheumatoid arthritis and psoriasis.

29.5 GENE POLYMORPHISMS AND THEIR EFFECTS ON NUTRIENT METABOLISM

Comparison of the genome of any two individuals will show genetic variation of some 0.1%. These differences underlie individual and population diversity in factors such as height, hair and skin colour, as well as disease susceptibility and the response to drug therapy. The most abundant and simplest form of variation is a result of mutations at individual points along the DNA sequence, termed single nucleotide polymorphisms (SNPs, pronounced 'snips'). Following completion of the draft of the human genome sequence, some 1.4 million SNPs were assigned to the genome map at an average density of 1 in 1000–2000 bases (Sachidanandam et al 2001). Now this figure is closer to 10 million common SNPs, which form the basis of the HapMap – a catalogue of common human genetic variations.

The location of SNPs within the genome dictates the extent of their influence on phenotype. Most SNPs are found in the non-coding regions of genes, some of which may be in the regulatory regions, and affect mRNA stability, or disrupt exon–intron boundaries. Of the SNPs that are found within the gene coding sequences, the resultant polymorphism can be either synonymous (no amino acid substitution occurs) or non-synonymous (amino acid substitution – which may alter the function of the encoded protein) (Fig. 29.3). This is because some polymorphisms do not alter the encoded amino acid, while others do (see 'Principles of gene expression', above).

Mutations that alter protein structure and function to a substantial extent generally result in an endpoint disease – an inborn error of metabolism.

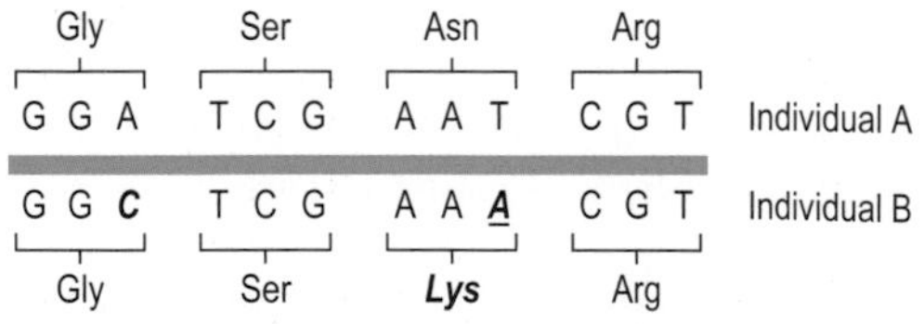

Fig. 29.3 Single nucleotide polymorphisms (SNPs) within a gene. The figure shows how a polymorphism within the coding region of a gene may result in either no change in the encoded amino acid or in an amino acid substitution – synonymous and non-synonymous polymorphisms, respectively.

These can range from single loss-of-function mutations, such as the rare condition glucose–galactose malabsorption (a defect in an intestinal glucose transporter), to loss of enzyme activity, for example of phenylalanine hydroxylase in the well-known inborn error of phenylketonuria. Both these cases may be alleviated by dietary intervention. By deciphering the association between genetic variation and disease, the possibility of designing specific diets, or providing dietary advice tailored to the genotype of an individual, can be envisaged. The ability to realise such a scenario depends upon appropriate technological advances so that SNPs can be readily identified. DNA microarrays or variant detector arrays have been developed to support the direct DNA sequencing approach to SNP detection, both being high-throughput technologies.

GENES AND DISEASE

Most common diseases such as diabetes, obesity and cardiovascular disease are a consequence of complex interactions between multiple genes and environmental/lifestyle factors – particularly diet and exercise. Such diseases can develop as the result of a mutation in a single gene, but this is rare (see section below on obesity). An individual's susceptibility to complex diseases is underpinned by the unique combination of SNPs distributed throughout their genome (Shastry 2002).

One strategy for looking at polygenic disorders is to perform an association study in which patterns of SNPs (haplotypes) are identified and compared between a disease-carrying population and a control group, termed genome-wide linkage analysis. A more recent advance in genetic analysis is the use of genome-wide association. These studies have led to a number of genetic advances, more recently in the field of nutrition (see below). Profiles of disease-related genes can be compiled to generate diagnosis and intervention strategies. There is now a considerable focus on the identification of SNPs and understanding their role in nutrition-related disease conditions.

Outlined below are some specific examples of SNPs in different genes and their consequences.

MTHFR

The enzyme 5,10-methylenetetrahydrofolate reductase (MTHFR) is involved in folate metabolism.

Its reaction product, 5-methyltetrahydrofolate, serves in the remethylation of homocysteine (Hcy) to the essential amino acid methionine, required for protein synthesis. A common SNP, resulting in a C to T change at position 677 (commonly referred to as C677T) causes an amino acid substitution of alanine to valine at position 222 (Ala222Val). The frequency of the homozygous *TT* genotype ranges from around 1% to 20% in different populations. This polymorphism has the effect of reducing the activity of the enzyme, which results in increased plasma levels of homocysteine, particularly in folate-deficient conditions (Ueland et al 2001).

The hyperhomocysteinaemia caused by the presence of the Ala222Val polymorphism increases the risk of neural tube defects (NTD) during pregnancy and may increase the risk of cardiovascular disease and modulate the risk of certain cancers, possibly to protect against colorectal cancer but increase the risk of some other cancers. Increasing the intake of folate appears to override deleterious effects of the *TT* genotype. During pregnancy, increasing the daily intake of total folate from 200 to 600 mg has been shown to half the risk of NTD.

A second common SNP has been described in MTHFR, A1298C, and this results in a glutamate to alanine substitution. Individually, the *CC* genotype has no effect on MTHFR activity. However, combined heterozygosity for both the C677T and A1298C polymorphisms can result in hyperhomocysteinaemia, although the presence of both mutations on the same allele is rare.

The UK Government's Scientific Advisory Committee on Nutrition (SACN) has recently recommended the mandatory fortification of flour with folic acid, a policy specifically aimed at reducing the incidence of pregnancies affected by neural tube defects (SACN 2006). The benefits of such a policy have been weighed against the possible adverse effects of high intakes of folic acid in some groups. It is well known, for example, that a high folate intake can lead to complications by masking the effects of vitamin B_{12} deficiency, particularly in the over-65 age group. This highlights the potential benefits of individualised nutritional assessments.

VITAMIN D RECEPTOR (VDR)

The steroid hormone 1,25-dihydroxyvitamin D_3 (cholecalciferol, $1,25(OH)_2D_3$), elicits its biological action through binding to the vitamin D receptor

(VDR). This receptor is a transcription factor and when it binds the vitamin D ligand in the nucleus transcription is activated in a wide range of tissues through responsive elements in the promoter regions of target genes. The principal action of vitamin D is to maintain calcium homeostasis to assist in the growth and integrity of bone. Other roles have been suggested, including roles in immune function and in cell differentiation. A number of loss-of-function mutations of the VDR gene have been identified which result in hereditary vitamin-D-resistant rickets.

Several subtle allelic polymorphisms have been identified in the VDR gene, which have been linked to diseases such as osteoporosis, a metabolic bone disorder characterised by reduced bone density (Uitterlinden et al 2002). However, the effects of these SNPs are not well understood. Many of the polymorphisms being studied are either found in intronic or non-coding regions (3'UTR) or are in the coding region but whose change has not resulted in an amino acid substitution, making it difficult to assign a functional role to the individual variations. Nevertheless, due to the large size of the VDR gene it is expected that many more SNPs will be identified and assessed for their contribution to susceptibility to disease states.

One polymorphism which does result in an amino acid change is found in exon 2. The T>C transition results in the removal of a start codon. Translation of this protein product begins at the next available start site, three amino acids further along. Whilst both protein products are known to exist, transcriptional activity appears to be higher for the shorter protein. The longer protein may be associated with lower bone mineral density. While it may be difficult at present to associate individual SNPs to bone disorders, the combination of different SNPs may produce varying levels of VDR protein and therefore account for variation in individual responses to levels of circulating vitamin D. Knowledge of the vitamin D response would consequently allow for the appropriate adjustment in dietary calcium intake.

GLUTEN SENSITIVITY (COELIAC DISEASE)

Gluten intolerance (coeliac disease) is one of the most common genetic diseases in Europe with between 1 in 130 and 1 in 500 of the population being affected (see Ch. 23). It is a digestive disorder in which the presence of gluten found in wheat and certain cereals causes damage to the mucosa of the small intestine, resulting in the malabsorption of nutrients from the diet.

Coeliac disease is an immune-mediated response associated with the major histocompatability complex (MHC) – one of the most gene-dense regions in the human genome, consisting of 264 human leukocyte antigen (HLA) genes. These genes are noted for their large number of polymorphisms (Table *evolve* 29.1). The broad range of symptoms presented with this disease implies that it is a multifactorial disorder with SNPs found on either HLA-related or other closely related genes (Guandalini & Gupta 2002).

Dietary intervention in this disease requires total exclusion of gluten-containing products. It is known that intolerance to gluten is highly variable between coeliac disease sufferers, implying that some individuals could accommodate small amounts of dietary gluten. However, no data are available to support this, so a total exclusion of dietary gluten is recommended. SNP typing and assignment of particular haplotypes to various symptomatic disease states is an achievable goal, potentially resulting in the safe reintroduction of small amounts of gluten back into the diet.

LACTOSE INTOLERANCE (LACTASE GENE)

Lactose (milk sugar) is broken down into its constitutive monosaccharides (glucose and galactose) by the intestinal brush border disaccharidase lactase (Ingram et al 2009, Lomer et al 2008). The ability to digest lactose declines in mammals after weaning, except for humans. It is now apparent that lactase non-persistence is the 'wild-type' condition and accounts for approximately 70% of the world's population. The variation in the ability to tolerate lactose into adult life has been attributed to the presence of polymorphisms within the gene. Several polymorphisms exist within the 50 kb lactase gene, distributed across only a very small number of haplotypes, such as the common northern European A haplotype. A SNP (C13910T) has been identified that controls lactase gene transcription. The SNPs identified thus far do not account for the wide global variation in lactose tolerance and it is likely that other important SNPs will be unveiled.

29.6 DIET, GENOTYPE AND SUSCEPTIBILITY TO DISEASE: THE EXAMPLE OF OBESITY

The susceptibility to a number of diseases involves an interaction between environmental factors and the genotype. Obesity is a good example of such a disease and one in which nutritional genomics has had some early successes. Although there is no doubt that the recent rapid escalation in the incidence of obesity in Western countries – and increasingly in the developing world – is the result of environmental factors, it is widely accepted that there is a genetic predisposition to the development of the disorder (Arner 2000). The environmental factors relate, of course, to diet (what and how much we eat) and to the level of physical activity. Easy access to cheap, palatable, high-fat 'fast foods' and increasingly sedentary lifestyles through the widespread use of cars and the substantial amounts of time being spent watching television, videos and computer screens are overwhelming our genetically determined regulatory mechanisms for energy balance.

There are several single gene mutations in laboratory animals which lead to frank obesity such as *ob, db, fat, tub* and *agouti* genes in mice, and the *fa* gene in the rat, which have proved invaluable in obesity research. These genes have now each been cloned and the protein product identified. There are also a number of transgenic models in which obesity, mild or substantial, has been identified as a consequence of the knock-out of a single gene, e.g. *UCP-1* knock-out (the *UCP-1* gene encodes the protein responsible for heat dissipation, or thermogenesis, in brown adipose tissue). The identification of the mutant genes in *ob/ob* and *db/db* mice and in the fatty *fa/fa* rat has revolutionised our understanding of the control of energy balance. A physiological regulatory loop has been identified, with the *ob* gene encoding the hormone leptin and the *db* gene encoding its receptor. The *fa* gene is the rat homologue of the *db* gene.

Leptin is synthesised in several tissues but the major site quantitatively, and the main source of the circulating protein, is white adipose tissue. This hormone is now recognised to have a very wide range of functions, but a central function is as a signal from adipocytes to the hypothalamus in the control of appetite (which is inhibited) and energy expenditure (which is stimulated). Mutations in the leptin gene or in its receptor result in either no protein product or a dysfunctional hormone, and a profound obesity of early onset ensues. There are human analogues to the mouse mutants; mutations in both the leptin and the leptin receptor gene have been identified in a handful of human subjects (Montague et al 1997). These individuals are obese and the adults show reproductive dysfunction, closely paralleling the phenotype of the mouse mutants. Although this demonstrates how a mutation in a single gene can lead to human obesity, its main significance lies in demonstrating that a functional leptin system is as important for the normal control of energy balance and body weight in humans as in rodents. Additional mutations causing obesity in humans include that reported for the melanocortin 4 receptor, now regarded as the most common monogenetic cause of human obesity.

However, overt mutations such as those for leptin and its receptor are rare in humans and do not inform the generality of obesity. Polymorphisms in specific genes or clusters of genes are, however, increasingly being linked to increased body fat and obesity. One of the most discussed such association is with the Trp64Arg polymorphism in the β_3-adrenoceptor. A number of studies have observed a linkage between this polymorphism and indices of fatness or fattening, while others, often in different populations or ethnic groups, have not. Similar associations have also been made with the Gln27Glu polymorphism in the human β_2-adrenoceptor and again there are apparent differences between studies or population groups.

This illustrates the problem in trying to find a consistent association between a single polymorphism and a complex phenotype such as body weight where many genes will be involved. Clearly, several different polymorphisms may have an additive effect, or different polymorphisms (linked to leanness) may have opposing effects thereby cancelling one another out. There is also the likelihood that dietary interactions modulate the effects of specific polymorphisms. The interaction between particular gene polymorphisms can be illustrated by the synergistic effect of the Trp64Arg polymorphism in the β_3-adrenoceptor gene with the A(-3826) G polymorphism in the uncoupling protein-1 gene. The two polymorphisms together strengthen the association with fattening.

The complexity of the number of genes involved in determining the amount of body fat is shown by reference to a study on the worm *Caenorhabditis elegans* (Ashrafi et al. 2003). 305 gene inactivations which cause reduced body fat and 112 which cause increased fat have been identified, there being a total of 16 757 genes in this worm. Many of these *C. elegans* genes have clear human homologues, thereby providing a focus for further studies on the genes underlying the predisposition to obesity.

One of the most recent advances has been the identification of the fat mass and obesity related gene (*FTO*). This discovery is the first of its kind utilising the genome-wide association scan (see earlier) as applied to the field of obesity genetics (Loos & Bouchard 2008). Initial findings suggest that this gene may encode a demethylation enzyme, or be involved in DNA repair, and that its effects may be mediated centrally and peripherally (such as in adipose tissue). A number of SNPs were identified in the first intron of the *FTO* gene and have shown to be associated with BMI, obesity and various obesity-related traits, but not lean mass or body height. Interestingly, the risk of obesity associated with the *FTO* SNPs is presently thought to be restricted to Caucasians, not having been found in populations of African or east Asian origin. As one might expect to find with a polygenic condition, having a particular SNP in the *FTO* gene only explains a small amount (around 1% in this case) of variance in BMI. However, this still represents the largest association to date, but it is clear that many other important gene polymorphisms are still to be unveiled. Overall, this provides a potent example of the integrative power of nutritional genomics.

KEY POINTS

- The concepts and techniques of molecular biology are being increasingly applied to nutritional science, and the interaction between an organism and nutrients, examined at the level of the genome and of gene products, constitutes nutritional genomics.
- It is now thought that there are just 23 000 genes in humans, most genes consisting of coding regions (*exons*), regulatory sequences (*promoters*) and non-coding internal regions (*introns*).
- The primary control of gene expression occurs at the level of transcription through modulation of the regulatory promoter region. Nutrients can influence gene transcription by interacting with transcription factors and by interactions at the post-transcriptional, translational and post-translational levels.

- New technologies allow global gene transcription, protein expression and metabolic profiling to be determined in a cell, tissue or organism, through DNA microarrays, proteomics and metabolomics.
- The genome of any two individuals shows approximately 0.1% variation and this is the basis for individual and population differences. The most common form of variation is the result of single base changes along the DNA sequence, termed single nucleotide polymorphisms (SNPs).
- Most common nutrition-related diseases such as coronary heart disease and obesity are the consequence of an interaction between the genome and the environment – only rarely do they result from a major mutation in a single gene, SNPs being central to determining the individual susceptibility to a disease.

References

Arner P: Obesity – a genetic disease of adipose tissue? *British Journal of Nutrition* 83(Suppl 1):S9–16, 2000.

Ashrafi K, Chang FY, Watts JL, et al: Genome-wide RNAi analysis of *Caenorhabditis elegans* fat regulatory genes, *Nature* 421:268–272, 2003.

Fuchs D, Winkelmann I, Johnson IT, et al: Proteomics in nutrition research: principles, technologies and applications, *British Journal of Nutrition* 94:302–314, 2005.

Gibney MJ, Walsh M, Brennan L, et al: Metabolomics in human nutrition: opportunities and challenges, *American Journal of Clinical Nutrition* 82:497–503,2005.

Guandalini S, Gupta P: Celiac disease: a diagnostic challenge with many facets, *Clinical and Applied Immunology Reviews* 2:293–305, 2002.

Hannon GJ: RNA interference, *Nature* 418:244–251, 2002.

Ingram CJ, Mulcare CA, Itan Y, et al: Lactose digestion and the evolutionary genetics of lactase persistence, *Human Genetics* 124:579–591, 2009.

Lomer MC, Parkes GC, Sanderson JD: Review article: lactose intolerance in clinical practice – myths and realities, *Alimentary Pharmacology and Therapeutics* 27:93–103, 2008.

Loos RJ, Bouchard C: FTO: the first gene contributing to common forms of human obesity, *Obesity Reviews* 9:246–250, 2008.

Montague CT, Farooqi IS, Whitehead JP, et al: Congenital leptin deficiency is associated with severe early-onset obesity in humans, *Nature* 387:903–908, 1997.

Moreno-Aliaga MJ, Marti A, Garcia-Foncillas J, et al: DNA hybridization arrays: a powerful technology for nutritional and obesity research, *British Journal of Nutrition* 86:119–122, 2001.

Ordovas JM, Mooser V: Nutrigenomics and nutrigenetics, *Current Opinion in Lipidology* 15:101–108, 2004.

Sachidanandam R, Weissman D, Schmidt SC, et al: A map of human genome sequence variation containing 1.42 million single nucleotide polymorphisms, *Nature* 409:928–933, 2001.

Scientific Advisory Committee on Nutrition (SACN): *Folate and disease prevention*, London, 2006, The Stationery Office.

Shastry BS: SNP alleles in human disease and evolution, *Journal of Human Genetics* 47:561–566, 2002.

Tyers M, Mann M: From genomics to proteomics, *Nature* 422:193–197, 2003.

Ueland PM, Hustad S, Schneede J, et al: Biological and clinical implications of the MTHFR C677T polymorphism, *Trends in Pharmacological Sciences* 22:195–201, 2001.

Uitterlinden AG, Fang Y, Bergink AP, et al: The role of vitamin D receptor gene polymorphisms in bone biology. *Molecular and Cellular Endocrinology* 197:15–21, 2002.

Further Reading

Berg JM, Tymoczko JL, Stryer L: *Biochemistry*, ed. 6. New York, 2007, Freeman.

Brigelius-Flohé R, Joost H-G: *Nutritional genomics: impact on health and disease*, Weinheim, 2006, Wiley-VCH.

Kaput J, Rodriguez RL: *Nutritional genomics: discovering the path to personalised nutrition*, Hoboken, NJ, 2006, Wiley.

Kendrew J, Lawrence E: *The encyclopaedia of molecular biology*, Oxford, 1994, Blackwell Science.

Lewin BM: Genes IX, ed. 9, Sudbury, MA, 2006, Jones & Bartlett.

Lodish HF, Berk A, Kaiser CA, et al: *Molecular cell biology*, ed. 6, New York, 2007, Freeman.

McLaren DS: *A colour atlas and text of diet-related disorders*, ed. 2, London, 1992, Wolfe.

PART 6

Public health nutrition

Chapter 30

The science of epidemiology

Annhild Mosdøl and Eric Brunner

CHAPTER CONTENTS

OBJECTIVES

By the end of this chapter you should be able to:
- define nutritional epidemiology
- summarise its aims and limitations
- outline the concepts of population, exposure, outcome and epidemiological effect
- define validity and repeatability
- interpret results of a study taking into account possible effects of bias, chance and confounding, and the question of generalisability
- summarise criteria for assessing evidence of causality
- explain the main features of different epidemiological study designs, including their strengths and weaknesses.

© 2010 Elsevier Ltd/Inc/BV
DOI: 10.1016/B978-0-7020-3118-2.00030-9

30.1 INTRODUCTION: WHAT IS EPIDEMIOLOGY?

Epidemiology is the study of the distribution and causes of disease in populations. It addresses the following types of question: Why is breast cancer more common in the USA than in Japan? Can diets rich in fruit and vegetables reduce blood pressure? Do dietary differences explain social gradients in cardiovascular disease mortality?

The word *epidemiology* comes from Greek and is made up of the words *epi* – upon, *demos* – the population, and *-logy* – the study of. The key word is population. Throughout the previous chapters, there have been numerous examples of studies at the cellular or organ level, and among selected groups of individuals. Epidemiology provides methodological tools for investigations of health and disease at the *population level*. It can be defined as (1) studies of the distribution of diseases and health-related conditions, (2) investigation into their aetiology and (3) analysis of how these diseases best can be prevented and controlled in a population. Nutritional epidemiology is one speciality of epidemiology applied to nutrition-related concerns including the role of nutrition in the causes and prevention of ill health (Margetts & Nelson 1997). Studies spanning from the molecular to the population level are complementary for understanding the nature of health and disease.

Knowledge of epidemiology is useful for all health practitioners. Most papers published in medical or nutritional journals use at least basic epidemiological terminology. To interpret what you read and understand the evidence, whether it is to update yourself on nutritional advances or to identify the best evidence-based treatments in a clinical setting, you will need epidemiology. In public health and health promotion, epidemiology is important both to provide knowledge for action and to evaluate the effect of interventions.

This chapter aims to be a first introduction to epidemiology to give the reader skills that enable them to critically read and interpret epidemiological studies. The first three sections describe the basic concepts of epidemiology (Section 30.2), important aspects to consider when interpreting results (Section 30.3) and the most common study types (Section 30.4) with examples from nutritional epidemiology. The last (Section 30.5) discusses some central issues that are particularly relevant in nutritional epidemiology.

30.2 IMPORTANT CONCEPTS IN EPIDEMIOLOGY

Epidemiology provides the framework for designing our own studies and evaluating the work of other scientists. It all starts by posing good questions. A good epidemiological question can be described in the same way as the definition of a hypothesis – any conjecture cast in a form that will allow it to be tested and proven false. A question like 'Is vitamin C good for health?' is too unspecific to be addressed in a scientific manner. 'Will taking 100 mg of vitamin C daily for 5 years reduce the risk of myocardial infarction?' on the other hand is a focused and clear question that can be answered. To formulate clear research questions you need to specify who you are interested in studying, *the population*, what you are interested in studying the effects of, *an exposure*, and what *outcome* you are interested in finding out about. The relation between the exposure and the outcome is evaluated by *measures of association and effect*. These are the essential elements of all epidemiological studies, no matter the study design used.

THE POPULATION AT RISK

In 2000 there were an estimated 10.6 million overweight pre-school children in Asia while there were 2.4 million in Latin America and the Caribbean (de Onis & Blössner 2000). In which region is overweight the most common? The limited information given above is not sufficient to answer this question since we lack a denominator. Since the total population of 0–5-year-olds is largest in Asia ($n = 367$ million) the proportion of overweight was 2.9% compared to 4.4% in Latin America and the Caribbean ($n = 54.5$ million). To describe the magnitude of disease at a group level it is necessary to take account of the relevant source population. Many of the measures in epidemiology are proportions, ratios and rates where the defined study population is the necessary denominator.

The population of interest for a particular question is called the *population at risk*. It can be defined in broad terms such as people living in world regions, countries or districts, but is often narrowed down by specific demographic characteristics such as age and gender. In some instances, the population of interest is defined by very specific characteristics such as the children of mothers who used vitamin A supplements during pregnancy. The phenomenon or event under study defines these boundaries. In a study of dietary effects on prostate cancer, women are irrelevant and should not be included in the study population. Thus, the population at risk is the group of people to whom an event can occur. The population at risk is also sometimes called the *target population*.

The concept of *risk* is fundamental in epidemiology. We are all accustomed to and use the word risk in everyday life setting. We have an intuitive feeling of some risks being either larger or smaller than other risks. In epidemiology, risk refers to a *probability* that a defined event is going to happen during a given population and time period. If we have a situation where an event can occur or not in a group of people, the risk of it happening will vary between 0 (it will never occur) and 1 (it will always occur). Probability is a concept related to the likely distribution of alternative events or outcomes. For example, the proportion of boys among all babies born is generally about 52% and we can say that the risk of having a boy is 0.52.

THE OUTCOME

In epidemiological studies, the term *outcome* refers to the disease or health-related variable being studied. Although the word presumably derives from clinical studies and implies some kind of follow-up, it is used in all kinds of epidemiological study designs to label the health-related phenomenon being studied. Endpoint is another word used to describe the study outcome.

Outcome measures are typically either binary (consisting of two categories) or continuous variables, although other types of outcome variable may be studied. A common binary outcome measure is mortality, when the population is divided into the dead and the alive at the end of a study. Likewise, disease status can be categorised as the diseased versus the non-diseased participants. When the outcome measure is binary as in these examples, the dead or the diseased respectively are called *the cases* as opposed to *controls* or *referents*. On the other hand, the outcome variable may measure a continuum of severity rather than an all or none phenomenon. Examples of continuous outcomes measures are plasma homocysteine concentration, systolic blood pressure or body weight. These measures may be presented and analysed as continuous measures, but it is often practical to

categorise them into a binary form based on a defined cut-off level. Body mass index (BMI) is a continuous variable, but can be analysed as the proportion of participants with BMI over 30 kg/m^2. Although such cutoff points can be useful, it is important to remember that in general they are arbitrary.

When a binary outcome is being studied, there are three important types of measurement: incidence, prevalence and mortality rates. *Incidence* is defined as the number of new cases appearing in the study population during a specified period of time. If the study population is roughly constant, the incidence is:

$$\frac{\text{Number of new events in a defined period}}{\text{The population at risk at the beginning of the period}}$$

In many cases, the assumption of a constant study population holds true, although birth, death, loss to follow-up or migration may be sufficiently large to cause difficulties. This estimate is typically used in routine health statistics. If a population of 100 000 people saw 190 cancer cases over a period of 1 year, the cancer incidence would be 0.0019 per person year. By convention this figure is often presented per 1000 person years in order to get a figure closer to 1, here giving 1.9 cancer cases per 1000 person years.

The most accurate way of measuring incidence is to divide the number of new cases by the *person time at risk*. Person time is calculated by summing up the time each individual is at risk during the measurement period. This measure takes into account that when a person becomes a case it is no longer part of the population at risk. To calculate person time at risk you need information about the date of each event when the individual ceases to contribute to the observation time.

$$\text{Incidence rate} = \frac{\text{Number of new cases}}{\text{Total person time at risk}}$$

The British Whitehall II study of civil servants recruited 10 308 participants between 1985 and 1988. In 1999, 355 of the participants had died (mean follow-up time of 12.7 years). A rough estimate of total observation time is 10 308 persons × 12.7 years – 130 912 person years. However, as no new participants entered the study after 1988 the total number of participants decreases as they drop out or die. The exact observation time is slightly lower than the estimate above and calculated to be 130 613 person years of follow up, giving an incidence rate of 355 deaths/130 613 person-years or 2.7 deaths per 1000 person years.

The *prevalence* is the proportion of a population that meets the definition of a case at a given point in time, for instance the percentage of a population who have type 2 diabetes mellitus at a given date. A prevalence figure is not at rate as it has no dimension of time. Prevalence may be used to estimate the disease burden in a population, for instance to plan health services.

The incidence and the prevalence describe different aspects of the disease burden in a population and their relationship depends on the nature of the disease and the effectiveness of its treatment. For a diseased person there are three prospects: they can continue being ill, recover from the disease or die. The risk of death among the diseased is described by the *case-fatality rate*, which is the incidence of death among the cases. When the duration of a disease is short, its prevalence in the population will be lower than if the duration of the disease is long, given the same incidence rate. It follows from this that efforts to improve the survival of a disease without curing it will increase its prevalence and consequently the burden on the health services. For instance, the treatment of diabetes patients has improved substantially, but the disease is rarely cured and patients may require medical care for the rest of their lives. Figure 30.1 illustrates how the prevalence pool is related to incidence, recovery and death.

Mortality rates are a type of incidence rate – the incidence of death. Crude mortality rates are calculated from the observed number of deaths and the size of the population of interest. Mortality rates of specific diseases can be calculated in the same way by using only deaths from the specific cause.

$$\text{Crude mortality rate} = \frac{\text{Number of deaths in a year}}{\text{Mid-year population}}$$

Crude mortality rates may hide useful information needed to understand the health and disease patterns of different populations. Crude cancer death rates are lower in Mexico than in the USA. It may look as if the Mexican population experiences fewer cancer deaths and is less exposed to risk factors for cancer. However, the difference in mortality rates is partly due to the different age distribution in the two countries. Cancer rates are higher in older people. A population with a high proportion of older persons will have higher crude cancer mortality rates compared to a young population given the same age-specific cancer death rates. Breaking down mortality rates for specific groups, most commonly by gender and age, will contribute to a better of understanding of death rates over time and between populations. Crude and adjusted rates may be applied to measures of disease incidence in the same way as measures of death. Box 30.1 provides definitions of the terms used in this section.

THE EXPOSURE

An *exposure* is any factor suspected to modify the risk of the outcome of interest. Exposures include a broad range of factors, from microbiological agents to all kinds of physical, social or psychological vari-

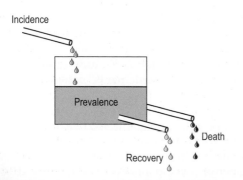

Fig. 30.1 The relationship between incidence, the prevalence pool and the duration of the disease.

BOX 30.1 Definitions of incidence, prevalence and mortality rates

Incidence

$$= \frac{\text{Number of new cases} \times 1000}{\text{Total person time at risk}}$$

Prevalence

$$= \frac{\text{Number of existing cases at one point in time}}{\text{Population at same place and time}}$$

Crude death rate

$$= \frac{\text{Number of deaths (defined place and time)} \times 1000}{\text{Mid period population (same place and time)}}$$

Age specific death rate

$$= \frac{\text{Number of deaths to people in a particular age group (defined place and time)} \times 1000}{\text{Mid period population (age group, same place and time)}}$$

Cause–specific death rate

$$= \frac{\text{Number of deaths to due to a particular cause (defined place and time)} \times 1000}{\text{Mid period population (same place and time)}}$$

ables. An exposure can either be based on observations of what happens naturally in a population or the study participants are assigned to a certain exposure in an experimental setting. Common exposures in nutritional epidemiology include intake of nutrients or foods, food patterns and socio-economic variables. You may have noticed that some of the examples of exposure variables could also be outcome variables. In a study of stroke, blood pressure may be the exposure variable of interest, but in another setting blood pressure can be the outcome of interest and we could be interested in studying how it is affected by exposure to high vegetable intakes. A factor or variable is designated as exposure or outcome depending on the objective of the study and the relationship being examined.

As with outcome variables, exposure variables may be presented in a binary form by dividing the population into the exposed and the unexposed. Exposure variables on continuous scales can be used as such or be categorised into two or more groups with graded levels of exposure using relevant cut-points. For instance vegetable intakes measured on a continuous scale in g/day can be categorised into three exposure levels defined as intakes <200 g/day, 200–400 g/day and >400 g/day. The way the exposure is measured depends on the question being asked. If the outcome is a food-borne disease, it may be sufficient to know whether the study participants have eaten shellfish from a certain shop in the last week or not. When studying thyroid cancer, the average shellfish consumption over time may be more relevant.

In experimental settings the exposure of interest is an *intervention*. Usually this is hypothesized to be a protective factor, such as a treatment or a drug, as it would be unethical to expose participants to suspected harmful factors. Exposures can also be called risk factors. When established, a risk factor is a characteristic that is suspected to increase the probability of a particular disease or malign condition to develop.

MEASURES OF ASSOCIATION AND EFFECT

In general, an *association* refers to the statistical link between two variables or factors. Several measures of association are used to summarise exposure–outcome relationships, each with its special applications. The choice of suitable measures for a given study will depend on the format of the exposure and outcome variables, whether they are binary or continuous.

Binary exposure – binary outcome

Relative risk (abbreviated RR) is the measure of effect most commonly used by epidemiologists when both the exposure and the outcome are binary variables. This is given by the ratio of risk, or incidence, in the exposed group to the risk in the unexposed group. If the risk of developing colon cancer during a follow up period of 10 years is 40 in a group of 1000 people exposed to a diet high in processed meat compared to a risk of 20 cancer cases in a group of 1000 with low intake (here considered the unexposed), the relative risk is $(40/1000)/(20/1000) = 2$. A relative risk of 1 indicates that there is no difference in incidence between the exposed and the unexposed. When the relative risk is higher than 1, as in the example above, the exposure poses a hazard; while a relative risk lower than 1 means that the exposure is protective. Another commonly used measure is the attributable risk (abbreviated AR), which is the incidence among the exposed minus the incidence among the non-exposed. Attributable risk estimates the size of the excess risk due to a particular exposure or risk factor.

The *odds ratio* (abbreviated OR) is frequently used to describe an association and is an alternative to relative risk outlined above. The term *odds* refers to a measure of likelihood based on a ratio rather than a proportion. The odds of throwing the number 3 with a dice is one to five, meaning that you are five times more likely to get one of the other five numbers. However, the *probability* that you will get number 3 is one in six (1/6 or 16.7% chance). In a case-control study (see Section 30.4), the odds ratio is calculated by dividing the odds of exposure among the cases by the odds of exposure in the non-cases. Consider the relationship between obesity (the exposure) and gestational diabetes (the outcome). If 50 of 100 women with gestational diabetes were obese compared with 20 of 100 non-diabetics, the odds of obesity among the diabetics are 50/50 (odds = 1), and the odds of obesity among the non-diabetics are 20/80 (odds = 0.25). In our example the OR is $(50/50)/(20/80) = 1/0.25 = 4$. The odds of being obese among the women with gestational diabetes are four times greater than among the healthy women. An OR of 1 indicates that there is no difference in the odds of being exposed among the cases as compared to the controls.

Table 30.1 shows a standard 'two by two'-table for studies where both the exposure and the outcome are in a binary form and give the formulas to calculate RR, AR and OR. The study participants

Table 30.1	Calculating relative risk, attributable risk and odds ratio		
	CASES	NON–CASES	TOTAL
Exposed	a	b	a + b
Non-exposed	c	d	c + d
Total	a + c	b + d	

$$PR = \frac{Risk_{exposed}}{Risk_{unexposed}} = \frac{(a/(a+b))}{(c/(c+b))}$$

$$AR = Risk_{exposed} - Risk_{unexposed} = (a/(a+b)) - (c/(c+b))$$

$$OR = \frac{(a/c)}{(b/d)} = \frac{ad}{bc}$$

will fall into four groups (denoted a–d) depending on whether they are either exposed or non-exposed combined with their status as a case or a control (alternatively referent or non-case). When the relative risk and odds ratio can be calculated on the same set of data, these will often be similar. How closely they match depends on the ratio of cases compared to the controls (See Box *evolve* 30.1).

Binary exposure – continuous outcome

If the exposure variable is binary and the outcome is a continuous variable, the effect due to the exposure can be expressed as the mean difference in outcome between the two groups. An example is the mean difference in serum homocysteine level at the start and the end of the study among participants given a supplement containing a vitamin B complex compared to the participants given placebo tablets.

Continuous exposure – continuous outcome

When both the exposure and the outcome variables are continuous, the observation pair for each individual in the sample can be plotted against each other. Statistical methods such as correlation and regression analyses are used to describe such relationships in numerical terms. When we compare the level of exposure versus the level of outcome, the most important characteristic is the relative position of each individual compared to other individuals in the sample. Thus, in many instances it is less important to know the exact exposure level of each respondent as long as the method used to measure the exposure manages to *rank* individuals correctly.

Continuous exposure – binary outcome

The combination of continuous exposure and binary outcome is seen frequently in nutritional epidemiology. The exposure is often a measure of nutrient intake or status, such as circulating serum homocysteine level, and the outcome is development of disease, such as myocardial infarction. The statistical technique used in these situations is logistic regression and the results are presented as OR. In this case the OR is obtained using a different technique from the 'two by two'-table described in Table 30.1, but is interpreted in the same way.

The approaches outlined above to the quantification and description of epidemiological associations are among the most commonly used measures to quantify associations and effects, but are not the only ones available.

QUALITY OF THE MEASUREMENTS

Poorly measured variables, either exposure or outcome, can lead to misleading results and incorrect conclusions. The word *validity* is used in different situations, usually to describe whether aspects of a study can be considered to represent the truth. The validity of a measurement is an expression of the degree to which it assesses the aspect it is intended to measure (Last 2001). The waist-to-hip ratio is commonly used to measure central obesity, but gives a rather crude estimate of intra-abdominal fat. A dual-energy X-ray absorption (DEXA) scan would give a more valid estimate of the true fat mass.

The reproducibility of a measurement is another quality marker. It indicates whether a method is capable of producing the same result when used repeatedly under the same conditions. Repeatability is both a feature of the variable itself, i.e. natural biological variation in the variable measured, and associated with the technical error of its measurement (how well is the measurement performed). A stable measure is adult height. We would expect to find the same value when measured repeatedly over some weeks and it is relatively easy to minimise errors in measurement. Blood glucose on the other hand varies naturally over the course of a day. To get a valid estimate of a person's blood glucose levels it is important both to decide the most relevant aspect of glucose metabolism and to standardise the measurement procedures. By deciding to measure fasting blood glucose, the amount of error due to fluctuations after meals is minimised. Repeat measurements of a variable may provide better estimates of the true average and will also give a quantification of its reproducibility.

Figure 30.2 uses target and bullet holes to illustrate the difference between the validity and reproducibility for measurements of a variable. The bull's eye is the true value we are aiming at. Picture A is our goal – high validity and reproducibility as the hits are positioned closely and the average is close to the truth. In Picture B, each shot arrives closely to each other, giving a high reproducibility, but the target is missed every time. Picture C shows a situation where the average of all the scattered hits is close to the bull's eye, meaning it is valid but not reproducible. Situation D has both poor reproducibility and poor validity.

Any measurement will to some extent deviate from the 'truth'. The most valid measurement methods are often relatively burdensome and expensive. Investigators may choose to use a less valid method for measuring the variables of interest, but it is important to assess the size of unavoidable errors so they may be taken into account when analysing and discussing the results. To establish the validity of a measurement we need to compare it with an absolute or gold standard method. The gold standard is usually the best existing/available test for the measure of interest. The more practical or cheaper measurement method is here called the test method while the gold standard is called the reference method.

For variables in a binary form, whether it is exposure or outcome, the validity of a measurement can be determined by classifying the subjects by the test method and by the reference method. Four quality measures for the test methods are commonly derived from such an assessment in a 'two by two' table: sensitivity, specificity, positive predictive value and negative predictive value. These measures are defined in Section *evolve* 30.2 🖰. For variables in a continuous form, the validity is estimated by comparing the degree of association between the test method and the standard reference method. Such data are often presented as correlations and contingency tables, for instance by cross-tabulation according to quartiles of the distribution for each of the methods. This gives a picture of how well the survey test method is able to rank values (i.e. low, medium-low, medium-high and high exposure) compared to the standard reference method.

KEY POINTS

- Population: the population of interest for a particular study question.
- Outcome: the disease or health-related variable being studied.
- Exposure: any factor that may influence the risk of the outcome.
- Measures of association and effect: the quantified relationship between exposure and outcome.
- Validity of measurements: the degree to which a measurement assesses the aspect it is intended to measure.
- Reproducibility of measurements: the degree to which a measurement produces the same result when used repeatedly.

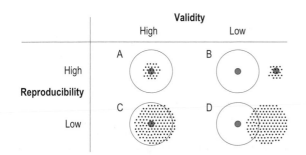

Fig. 30.2 Illustration of the terms validity and reproducibility by using a target where the gunshots, shown as bullet holes (the measurements), have been aimed at the bull's eye (the truth). When all the bullet holes are positioned close to each other, the shooting gives a highly reproducible result (A&B); if positioned over a wider area reproducibility is low (C&D). If the shooting is systematically drawn to one side of the target, the validity is poor (B&D), while bullet holes symmetrically around the bull's eye indicate high validity (A&C).

30.3 INTERPRETATION OF RESULTS

The survey is completed and the measures collected, but how should the results be interpreted? And how do you interpret studies reported in scientific journals? The epidemiologist is primarily interested in assessing and evaluating associations or effects, which address questions of disease cau-sality, prevention or treatment. In general, an observed association may the product of four dif-ferent influences: bias, chance, confounding or cause. Before we even start to consider the impor-tance of the results in question, the first three options should be considered carefully.

BIAS

Bias refers to measurement errors or misclassifica-tion that lead to results that consistently deviate from the truth. Many sources of bias have been identified, but they fit into two broad categories: selection bias and information bias. When study participants have been selected to the study in a way that distorts the results, we have *selection bias*. This can arise in many ways. In a clinical setting, the terminally ill patients may be more willing to try out a novel treatment with unknown risks attached to it than those with good prospects. If the new treatment performs badly it may be difficult to know whether the treatment really was poor or the patients would have died anyway. Important ques-tions to ask when assessing a study sample can be: In what way were participants selected for investi-gation and how representative were they of the population at risk with regard to the study question?

Another example applies to studies where people are invited to participate, but only a subset is willing to take part. The size of this sample relative to the original group is described by the *response rate*. Almost without exception, participants who volun-teer to take part in studies are likely to differ from the general population, for instance by being more highly educated or more health conscious. The prevalence of disease being studied can differ among responders compared to the population from which they came from. Faced with such studies you might ask: What was the response rate and are the responders and non-responders likely to have differed in important ways? It is easier said than done to make sure that study groups are rep-resentative of the population at risk. However, not all differences pose a problem; it depends on the study objective. If a study sample is not fully rep-resentative of the study population, the results may misrepresent the true disease burden. However, the relationship between an exposure and an outcome may be correctly estimated even when there is con-siderable selection bias.

If the quality of the information we have col-lected on either the exposure or the outcome varies systematically between groups, we have *information bias*. Dietary assessment studies repeatedly show that obese subjects tend to underestimate their energy intake more than non-obese subjects do (Maurer et al 2006). Thus, it is necessary to be cau-tious about self-reports of diet in a study of the causes of obesity. Information bias can also arise when asking people about past exposures. A mother who has recently given birth to a child with neural tube defects may ask herself what could have caused it. She may recall supplement use and diet more meticulously than a mother with a healthy baby. This type of information bias is called recall bias. As with selection bias, information bias is potentially important if its magnitude differs in relation to the presence or absence of the study outcome.

Bias is caused by imperfections in design or implementation of a study, and it is difficult or even impossible to remove its effects at a later stage. Almost all studies are somewhat biased. This does not mean that they are scientifically unacceptable or that their results should be disregarded. If a study has been analysed and interpreted carefully, the investigators will have addressed this question themselves. There are no simple formulas for meas-uring biases and quantifying their effects. Each study must be judged by assessing the probable impact of biases on the study question and then allowing for them when drawing conclusions.

THE ROLE OF CHANCE

When do we know that a numerical difference is meaningful? If a group of children who had been breastfed for at least 4 months had an average primary school reading test score of 67 while chil-dren who had never been given breast milk had a score of 65, are they really different? We need to enter the realm of statistics. Chance can be thought of as variation due to sampling variation, biological differences and other unknown factors. Statistical methods provide measures to quantify the element of chance and account for the uncertainty in the results of our study. It is important to recognise that a study utilizes a sample, but our primary interest lies in what the study sample tell us about the pop-ulation from which it is drawn.

Hypothesis testing is used to test for chance effects and is central to many statistical tests. If we estimate the mean level of a parameter in one sample, say mean fasting blood glucose, we would get a slightly different result by chance if the procedure was repeated in another sample from the same population. The procedure called hypothesis testing starts by defining a *null hypothesis*, which usually is a statement saying that there is no real difference (only differences by chance) between the two groups we are studying. The *p-value* gives the probability of getting the observed or a more extreme result if the null hypothesis is true, or rephrased: what is the likelihood that we observe this difference between two groups if they really are similar? Usually a p-value less than 5% ($p < 0.05$) is considered to give a statistically significant result leading to rejection of the null hypothesis.

Significance testing assesses whether a result, such as a difference between groups, is likely to be due to chance or some real effect. It cannot prove that it is one or another. Note that failing to reject the null hypothesis is not the same as saying that it is true. With a p-value of 0.05, the investigator runs a risk of falsely rejecting the null hypothesis on average 5% of the time. Two possible errors can be made when using the p-value to make a decision: to conclude that a difference exists when it does not, is called a *type I error* (false positive or alpha error). Conversely, concluding that a difference does not exist when in fact it does by failing to reject a false null hypothesis is called a *type II error* (false negative or beta error).

Confidence intervals provide a measure of the uncertainty in our data by giving a lower and upper confidence limit of the true value in question. The intervals have a given probability, usually 95% or 99%, that the true value in the underlying population is included. We want confidence intervals to be narrow because this means that the estimate is likely to be more precise than with a wide confidence interval. Since the confidence interval combines information about chance effects and precision, it is preferred against hypothesis testing alone. Thus, statistical methods are an important tool in epidemiology.

CONFOUNDING

A *confounder* is any factor that can cause or prevent the outcome of interest and at the same time is associated with the exposure in a way that distorts the observed exposure–outcome association. Confounding is therefore about the confusion that may

arise because two or more potential causal influences are mixed up with one another. Let us assume we have recorded the coffee-drinking habits in a study sample. During the observation period the heavy coffee drinkers have a higher rate of bladder cancer than the participants drinking little or no coffee (the observed association). Can the relationship between bladder cancer and coffee drinking be due to another risk factor for this type of cancer that is also associated with coffee intake? If smokers tend to drink more coffee than non-smokers there is a positive association between coffee drinking and smoking habits. Further, if smoking is a real risk factor for bladder cancer, the observed association between coffee and bladder cancer is confounded by smoking habits. A confounding factor may produce a spurious effect, as above, or can hide a real effect.

Confounding may be regarded as a type of bias, but unlike other biases confounding can often be adjusted for. In the example above, the association between coffee drinking and bladder cancer can be analysed separately in smokers and non-smokers in a *stratified analysis*. Age is a common confounder in many studies because the risk of most diseases increases with age. If we compare two groups with different age distributions, the risk estimates may be *standardised* to a common age distribution. Confounding can also be controlled for in statistical models, which simulate a stratified analysis. However, these modifications are possible only if the relevant confounding factor has been measured. If confounding is considered at the design stage, it can be controlled by *exclusion of sub-groups* which may cause interpretation problems. In experimental settings, random allocation of participants (*randomisation*) to two treatments minimises confounding as any such factors will tend to be equally distributed in the two groups by chance.

CAUSALITY

Smoking as a risk factor for lung cancer has one of the largest relative risks demonstrated for any non-communicable disease. Still, we have all heard about old men smoking 40 cigarettes a day living into their nineties. How can we regard smoking as a cause of lung cancer when many smokers never get the disease? Epidemiology is the science that takes a health-related hypothesis into the real world and attaches a probability to it. When considered together with other types of evidence, such as that derived from laboratory-based studies, epidemiology is a powerful tool for testing whether a proposed disease mechanism is important for population health.

What guidelines should be used for judging the evidence? Causation can rarely be proven without doubt, but if the possible presence of chance, bias or confounding has been assessed carefully the question of causality can be approached in different ways. Sir Austin Bradford Hill suggested a list of aspects to consider when judging whether an association between an exposure and an outcome could be causal (Hill 1974). None of these are absolute criteria for a causal relationship. The nine points are often referred to as the Bradford Hill criteria:

1. *Strength of the association:* A strong association, as measured by relative risks, increases the likelihood that it reflects a causal relationship. Confounding may also create strong associations, but if an association is to be completely explained by confounding the confounder must carry an even higher risk for the disease under study. However, weak associations may also be causal and important in understanding disease aetiology.

2. *Consistency:* Tabloid newspapers may make headlines of one study showing that eating carrots increase the risk of stroke, but the scientific community will judge such findings against the results of other studies. When a body of studies consistently point in the same direction over time and across populations, the evidence is strengthened. As studies giving null results often fail to be published, the available studies may not represent the full span of evidence concerning a given risk-factor–disease relationship. This is called publication bias.

3. *Specificity:* The concept of specificity is that one particular exposure leads to a specific disease and that one disease always is triggered by the same cause. This criterion is relevant in some situations, but increasingly we discover that many diseases can have multiple causes and some factors may contribute to more than one condition.

4. *Temporal sequence of cause and effect*: If a statistically significant association is found between two variables but the presumed cause occurs after the effect rather than before it, the association cannot be causal. A logical temporal sequence of events, with the exposure appearing before the outcome, is an absolute criterion for causality.

5. *Biological gradient:* A dose–response relationship where the risk increases progressively with higher exposure is generally strong support for a causal interpretation. However, a dose–response curve may have many different forms and we do not always know where on this curve the observed range of exposure is situated.

6. *Biological plausibility and coherence:* Biological plausibility and coherence with present knowledge will strengthen the confidence that an association is causal. Still, many epidemiological studies have pointed to possible risk factors for disease that could not be explained by biological knowledge at the time they were published. Such findings often spark off further studies to examine possible mechanisms in depth.

7. *Experiment (reversibility):* When an epidemiological association can be reversed it is strong confirmation that the link most likely is causal. Reversion appears when reduction in a factor shown to increase the disease risk gives a corresponding drop in disease risk. An example is patients who manage to lower their total serum cholesterol level through a controlled diet and who later present a reduced risk of coronary heart diseases.

There are clearly also different levels of cause. This is more comprehensively understood with many non-communicable diseases where several causal factors are involved. If a factor triggers a disease every time it is present, it is called a *sufficient cause*. Apart from some genetic abnormalities, there are very few conditions where this holds true. Even food poisoning or other infections will depend on the vulnerability of the person exposed. The bacteria are on the other hand a *necessary cause* of the food poisoning. If a necessary cause is absent, the disease cannot occur. We have already defined a *risk factor* as a characteristic that is known to increase the probability that a particular disease or malign condition will develop. Risk factors are neither sufficient nor necessary causes of disease. Smoking is a good example, as many smokers never get lung cancer while a small number of non-smokers do. Smoking is nevertheless the most important cause of lung cancer. Nutritional exposures are very often risk factors; they modify the likelihood of diseases occurring but are neither sufficient nor necessary causes.

Only in a very few cases, such as serious injuries, will a causal factor trigger a disease or a health outcome directly. For most health outcomes, there will be *causal pathways* between the exposure and the outcome. Fruit and vegetable intake is thought to exert part of its protective effect on development of cancers by increasing the circulating antioxidant level, which may protect DNA from oxidative damage and prevent cells from becoming malignant (WCRF/AICR Expert Panel 2007). For someone interested in the biochemical aspects of nutrition, the molecular actions of nutrients are the most interesting aspects of this causal pathway. For those giving specific dietary advice to individuals, the dietary aspects of preventing cancer are most relevant. Among public health nutritionists, there may be particular interest in the social, cultural and psychological determinants of food habits. Each level of this causal pathway contributes to a full understanding of the incidence of the disease at the population level.

KEY POINTS

- An observed exposure–outcome association can be due to one of four factors: bias, chance, confounding or a true causal relationship.
- Bias – systematic deviation of results from the truth – takes two main forms: selection bias (related to the sample) and information bias (related to the data).
- Chance – random variation may produce a plausible or implausible finding.
- Confounding – confusion between two processes – may distort study findings.
- Causality can rarely be proven, but if bias, chance and confounding have been considered and the Bradford Hill criteria are broadly met, then causal inference is appropriate.

30.4 EPIDEMIOLOGICAL STUDY DESIGNS

SOME ELEMENTS OF PLANNING AND DESIGNING STUDIES

When someone starts planning an epidemiological study, the most important task is to formulate the essential questions the study seeks to answer. These questions will guide the decisions that need to be taken regarding the study sample, how exposure and outcome are measured and the preferred study design. It is at this stage that potential biases best can be controlled or minimised. If a relevant variable is missed during the implementation, for instance a confounder, it can rarely be made up for after the data collection is completed.

Who should be included in the study sample and how many participants need to be included? These two questions are very important. The goal is usually to generate results that have a wider application beyond the study participants, in other words to get results that are *generalisable* to the whole target population or the population at risk. If we could include everyone from the target population in our study, the question of generalisability would not be an issue. This is rarely feasible or desirable. The generalisability of a study is closely related to the *external validity*. Validity has earlier been defined as the degree to which a measurement assesses the aspect it is intended to measure (see Section 30.2 under 'Quality of the measurements'). The external validity considers to what extent the study captures accurately the phenomenon as it exists in the target population.

Often the study sample is formed in two steps. A subset of the target population is selected on simple criteria to form the study population; it can for instance be through random selection from the general population or by choosing an accessible group that can be followed up over time. The study sample is the subset of the study population that actively participates in the study and is described by the response rate (see Section 30.3 under 'Bias'). It is usually desirable to get a sample which is representative of the target population in terms of age, sex and other demographic factors. Other important characteristics of external validity will differ with the study question. For instance, in a study exploring causal relationships it is important that the exposure–outcome relationship found in a study sample represents the association in the larger population. If prevalence is important, the level of risk factors or outcome should be captured with minimal bias.

The other crucial task when selecting a study sample is to determine the necessary number of participants. It is vital that the sample size is big enough to detect as statistically significant any true differences between the study groups.

Performing studies that are too small to answer the main objective is a waste of resources and can be considered unethical. It is possible to calculate the necessary sample size of a study that will achieve a specific statistical significance level if the true difference in the outcome is at a predefined level. Such *power calculations* are described briefly in Section *evolve* 30.4(a) 🖱.

The best study design in a particular situation depends on the question being asked. Figure 30.3 gives a schematic overview of the main study designs, and the following two sections will go through their features, strengths and weaknesses (see Section *evolve* 30.4(b) for examples 🖱). Study designs differ according to whether the researchers observe (*observational* studies) or attempt to influence the exposure (*experimental* studies). Studies differ according to the time order of collecting information in exposure and outcome. They are called *retrospective* when information is gathered about exposures in the past. They are *prospective* when exposure status is measured at the beginning of the study and the sample is followed over time to gather information on outcomes. The preferred design depends on characteristics of the main exposure and outcome variables, what is already known about the relevant question and the resources available (Table 30.2).

OBSERVATIONAL STUDY DESIGNS

Ecological studies

Many of the hypotheses regarding diet–disease relationships have originated from simple comparison of cause-specific death rates in different countries matched with exposures available at the population level. An example is death rates due to cardiovascular disease and average consumption of fruit and vegetables in different countries. In these ecological studies, the exposure and outcome measures are matched at a group level instead of the individual level. Ecological studies can be easy and inexpensive, as this type of information is readily available in many countries and from international organisations such as WHO and FAO. The comparison does not have to be between populations, but can also be the same population compared over time (i.e. percentage energy from fat over time compared with corresponding mortality of cardiovascular diseases). Another classic design is to compare disease rates of immigrants with the

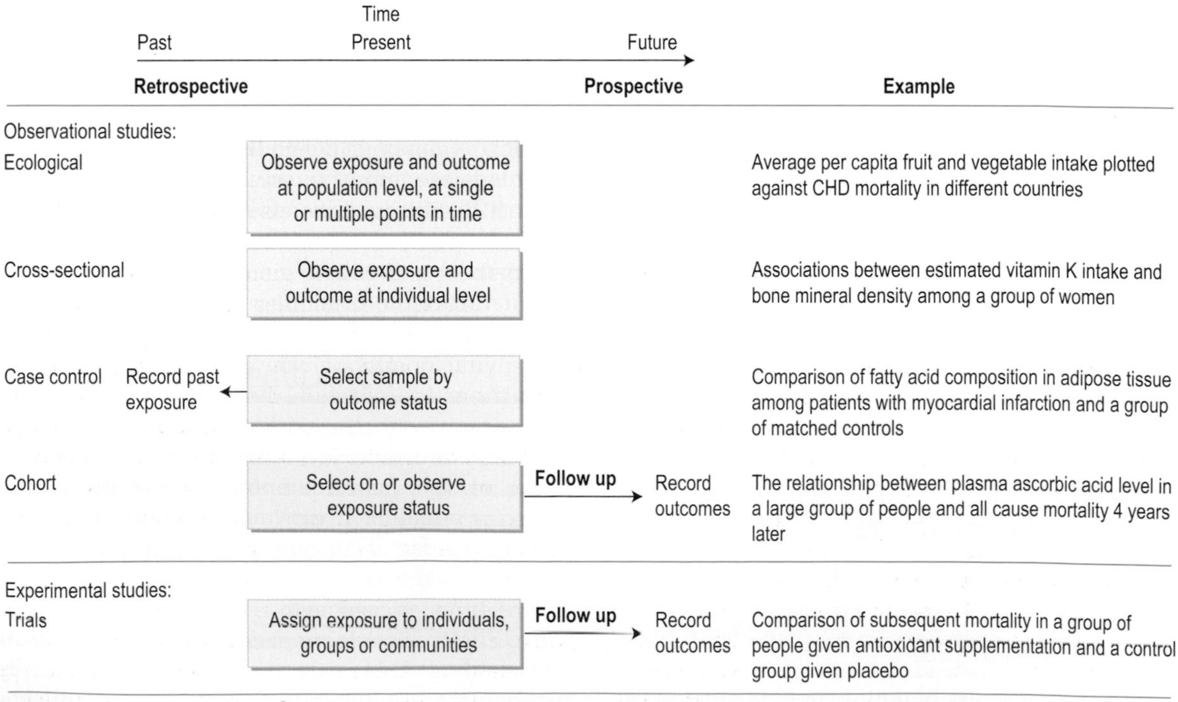

	Time			
	Past	Present	Future	
	Retrospective		Prospective	Example
Observational studies:				
Ecological		Observe exposure and outcome at population level, at single or multiple points in time		Average per capita fruit and vegetable intake plotted against CHD mortality in different countries
Cross-sectional		Observe exposure and outcome at individual level		Associations between estimated vitamin K intake and bone mineral density among a group of women
Case control	Record past exposure ←	Select sample by outcome status		Comparison of fatty acid composition in adipose tissue among patients with myocardial infarction and a group of matched controls
Cohort		Select on or observe exposure status	**Follow up** → Record outcomes	The relationship between plasma ascorbic acid level in a large group of people and all cause mortality 4 years later
Experimental studies:				
Trials		Assign exposure to individuals, groups or communities	**Follow up** → Record outcomes	Comparison of subsequent mortality in a group of people given antioxidant supplementation and a control group given placebo

Fig. 30.3 A schematic overview of epidemiological study designs and their main characteristics

Table 30.2   Advantages and disadvantages of different epidemiological study designs

STUDIES	ADVANTAGES	DISADVANTAGES
Ecological studies	▪ Quick and easy to carry out ▪ Hypothesis-generating	▪ Cannot be used for causal investigations since the data are on groups rather than individuals ▪ Not good for hypothesis-testing
Cross-sectional studies	▪ Quick and easy to carry out ▪ Gives prevalence of condition in population ▪ Hypothesis-generating	▪ Cannot differentiate temporal sequence ▪ Unsuited for rare conditions or conditions of short duration ▪ Not good for hypothesis-testing
Case-control studies	▪ Quick and easy to carry out ▪ Can study many risk factors ▪ Require relatively few participants ▪ Suited for studies of rare diseases	▪ Cannot provide measures of risk, only odds ratios ▪ Subject to recall bias, difficult to validate the measurements ▪ Poor differentiation of temporal sequences ▪ Only one outcome can be studied
Cohort studies	▪ Can provide measures of risk ▪ Can study many exposures and outcomes ▪ Permit quality control of the exposure measurements	▪ Time-consuming and costly, many participants required ▪ Can only examine the exposures that were measured at the onset of the study; factors relevant to study may change ▪ Can only be used for common outcomes ▪ It may be difficult to keep track of the study sample
Randomised controlled trials	▪ The gold standard for evaluating treatments or interventions ▪ Allow the investigators to have strong control of the parameters (minimises bias and confounding)	▪ Can be time-consuming and costly ▪ Only one exposure can be studied ▪ Can have problems with participants not complying or dropping out of the study ▪ The generalisability may be limited ▪ Unethical if exposure is suspected to pose a hazard

disease rates in their native country (*migrant studies*). Ecological studies must be interpreted with caution, as an association observed at a group level may not reflect a causal association at the individual level.

Cross-sectional studies

In cross-sectional studies, the outcome and exposure status are determined simultaneously. These studies are also called prevalence studies as they measure the proportion of people with a condition at given point in time as well as the frequency of exposure. This is useful information for planning health services and the results can usually be obtained quickly. The design is, on the other hand, poorly suited to studies of rare diseases or diseases of short duration as only a few in the population will have the relevant condition at any given time. Data from cross-sectional studies can be used to explore aetiological associations but there is one particular important limitation. Since both exposure and outcome are measured at the same time, it is impossible to know if one appeared before the other. You may observe that people with high blood cholesterol eat more low-fat foods than the general population, but this can be due to recent dietary changes if these people have been advised to reduce their cardiovascular risk.

Case–control studies

In a case-control study, patients who have developed a specific disease or condition (the cases) are compared with disease-free individuals (the controls) who are representative of the population the cases come from. The amount and frequency of past exposures are compared between the cases and the controls to determine if these are different. This type of study is relatively quick to conduct and is well suited for rare diseases. An example is assessment of wheat consumption before their first birthday among children who have developed coeliac disease compared to healthy children of the same age. Case-control studies allow for examination of several exposures suspected to be aetiological factors and adjustment for possible confounders. Odds ratios are used to present the results. The disadvantage of retrospective case-control studies is that the exposure measurements may rely on recall of past experiences which may cause recall bias. Biological measurements can also be biased, as these may change after disease onset. Prospective case-control studies can also be carried out by analysing sub-samples of a cohort study. Recall bias is not relevant in such studies.

Cohort studies

Cohort studies follow a group of people though time and record which individuals develop the outcome of interest, usually a disease or a cause-specific death. One of the important advantages is that the exposure is measured at the start of the study before disease appears. Information bias or behaviour changes due to emerging symptoms of disease will therefore not pose a problem. Several large cohort studies are in progress to investigate the dietary effects on cancer, including EPIC, a European multicentre study (see Ch. 22) and the Nurses' Health study in the USA. These studies follow thousands of people over several years before there are enough cases to analyse. The British Whitehall II study of civil servants is another large, ongoing cohort study with a main aim to study the causes of social inequalities in health, including the role of dietary differences.

The effect measure in cohort studies is usually relative risk, as the incidence of disease among those exposed to some factor is compared with the incidence in the unexposed members of the cohort. The main disadvantages of cohort studies are that a long follow-up time is often needed before there are a sufficient number of outcomes to analyse, and their high costs. Meanwhile some of the exposure variables may have become irrelevant or the researchers may wish other exposures had been included from the onset.

EXPERIMENTAL STUDY DESIGNS

Randomised controlled trials

Trials are studies that assess the effects of an intervention or treatment by comparing it with an established treatment or *placebo* (inactive treatment). The treatment could for instance be a medical intervention, a drug, a nutrient supplement, a particular food or an eating pattern. A trial can have one of two aims, to evaluate either *effectiveness* or *efficacy*. This essential distinction should always be explicit for the trial and the evidence user. An effective intervention is one which does what it is intended to do under routine circumstances (Does it work?). Efficacy, on the other hand, refers to the benefit of an intervention under ideal circumstances (Can it work?). Participants in trials should be randomly allocated to the intervention or the control group to minimise bias and confounding. Ideally, neither the participants nor the investigator should know who is in which group, meaning the study is double-blinded. Trials provide strong evidence that any observed effect or difference between the study groups is likely to be due to the intervention being tested.

There are several difficulties with trials. Trials depend on participants who give consent and they may not always represent the population of interest. There is less of a problem of errors in categorising the exposure correctly, but instead the challenge is compliance: to what extent do the participants follow the instructions they have been given? Blinding can sometimes be difficult, for instance when the treatment involves eating patterns or other behavioural factors that cannot easily be camouflaged. It may also be difficult to estimate a pure treatment effect in studies involving food because humans need a rather constant intake of energy and fluids. Any induced changes to the sources of these two variables are likely to be compensated for by changes in other sources. Trials may be expensive and require a long follow-up period. In most cases, a trial would be unethical if the treatment involves a potential hazard to the participants.

Community intervention studies

Community intervention studies involve interventions at group, community or population level. Interventions designed to promote health at the community level may take a number of forms, using mass media, supermarkets, workplaces and other settings believed to offer cost-effective means of influencing population behaviour. Preferably, but not necessarily, such intervention studies involve a control group, but community studies may also consist of an uncontrolled before-and-after design. Usually there is a quantitative evaluation of change or the consequences of change. Whereas a randomised controlled trial follows a fixed group of individuals over time, a community intervention may involve one or more surveys, not always with the same set of participants, in order to estimate the intervention effect within the community as a whole.

SYSTEMATIC REVIEWS

Systematic reviews were partly developed as a strategy to ease information overload with the ever-increasing flow of primary research articles. Systematic reviews summarise the results of similar studies by using explicit methods for selecting primary studies and criteria for assessing their quality. Instead of disregarding small studies that are underpowered on their own, the results can be combined. The results of the studies are summarised in meta-analyses, but the data are not statistically combined (Section *evolve* 30.4(c) 🖰). Meta-analysis can only be done if the variables in the different studies, both the exposure and outcome, are sufficiently similar to be combined. Well conducted meta-analyses provide a precise estimate of the effects of interest. It may also be possible to examine heterogeneity in results obtained from individual studies. Systematic reviews are potentially subject to selection and publication bias. Methods have been developed to investigate these sources of error.

A number of groups and organisations have been formed in order to promote systematic reviewing as a useful scientific activity and support those who wish to carry out such reviews. The Cochrane Collaboration (http://www.cochrane.org/) was founded in 1993 with an aim 'to help people make well-informed decisions about health care by preparing, maintaining and ensuring accessibility to systematic reviews'. The main emphasis of the Cochrane Collaboration is on the effects of health care interventions.

KEY POINTS

- The essential question a study seeks to answer guides the decisions regarding the nature and size of study sample, how exposure and outcome are measured and the preferred study design.
- Power calculations help to ensure that a new study will be able to answer the primary research question.
- The external validity (generalisability) of a study depends on its design and execution.
- Observational studies, study designs (ecological studies, cross-sectional studies, case-control studies and cohort studies) permit examinations of the world as it is, including its hazards.
- Experimental studies (trials) are powerful tools for testing health-related hypotheses (usually treatment or prevention).
- Systematic reviews are means of summarising existing evidence and reducing information overload.

30.5 NUTRITIONAL EPIDEMIOLOGY

Epidemiology has expanded from its early focus on infectious disease to the aetiology of chronic disease. Diet is a relevant exposure for many chronic diseases, and the challenges of nutritional epidemiology are active research topics. This section presents some of the important methodological issues.

MEASUREMENT OF DIETARY EXPOSURE

Unlike smoking, which is a relatively straightforward exposure to quantify, dietary intake is complex. Measurement can involve differing dimensions of food intake such as nutrients, non-nutrients, single food items and food groups. In general, diet varies considerably from day to day, and dietary habits may change over time. The composition of food items varies depending on where it was grown, the weather that season and production methods. Since we expect large day-to-day variations in intake, careful consideration of the most appropriate measurement for the given study objective is needed. If we want to study whether dietary factors modify the risk of developing chronic diseases, average diet over years is probably the most important aspect to capture.

The dietary exposure can be defined either as the food and drink entering the mouth, in other words the dietary intake, or as the dietary component taken up by the body. The assessment methods available to measure dietary intake are covered in Chapter 31, but it is fair to say that all methods have shortcomings in an epidemiological context. Section 30.2 (under 'Quality of the measurements') introduced validity and reproducibility as important concepts that define the quality of measurements. Most dietary assessment methods rely on some kind of self-report from the study participants, which has flaws in terms of capturing both the quality and quantity of foods actually eaten. It is well documented that most dietary data contain considerable misreporting, particularly underreporting of foods consumed, as reflected by estimated total energy intake (Maurer et al 2006).

One of the central purposes of epidemiology is to examine relationships between an exposure and an outcome. Therefore it is the degree of exposure relative to other members of the population that is the most relevant aspect to capture. It is less important to determine the absolute exposure level as long as each individual's exposure is correctly ranked relative to the other study participants. If all study participants underestimated their food intake to the same degree, it could still be determined who had low, medium and high intakes of a nutrient. This theoretical situation is, however, not observed in practice (Maurer et al 2006). The research community increasingly recognises that dietary data are less accurate and precise than it ideally would like to collect. We could say that these data contain large *measurement errors*. A considerable part of the research effort in nutritional epidemiology has been devoted to developing dietary assessment methods suitable for large observational studies involving thousands of people. Important aspects of the development process include documenting the validity and reproducibility of these methods, investigating the error-structure of dietary data and exploring ways to handle these errors in statistical analysis.

Measurement error is a problem in epidemiology because the observed effect of diet on disease risk can deviate considerably from the true effect. Epidemiologists find that if the exposure of interest is measured only with non-differential measurement error, meaning that the errors are similar among the diseased and non-diseased (or other health outcomes such as obesity), the effect estimate will be *biased towards null*. This means that the estimated size of the diet–disease association being studied will be under estimated. In some situations, such as in a small study, the association may be missed altogether. In more complex studies where two or more dietary exposures are included in the analysis at the same time, differences in respective amounts of measurement error, even when they are non-differential errors, can lead to under- or over estimation of the epidemiological effect being investigated.

Biomarkers of dietary intake are biochemical analytes in body fluids and tissues which are selected to be used as predictors for levels of nutrient intake and tissue status (see Section 31.4). Many biomarkers are available, and we can assess some but not all aspects of diet using this approach. The use of biomarkers may not be a practical alternative to dietary assessment in large epidemiological studies because of the substantial cost of collection and laboratory analysis. Biomarkers of nutrient intake are particularly useful in combination with self-reported dietary assessment methods (Bingham 2002). However, it is important to remember that although biomarkers can provide an objective estimate of some aspects of dietary intake, an observed diet–disease relationship based on a biomarker may still be subject to confounding. This is discussed further in the next section.

CONFOUNDING OF DIET–DISEASE RELATIONSHIPS

Rigorous understanding of nutritional epidemiology requires that one gets to grips with the issue of confounding. A prominent feature of dietary variables is that they are strongly correlated with each other, either directly or inversely. For instance, persons with a high intake of vitamin C tend to have high intakes of fibre, β-carotene and other antioxidants as a consequence of the combinations of nutrients in the chosen foods. Several studies also show that within populations there are patterns of food choices where high intakes of some foods are associated with other intakes. In a study of British adults, one out of four patterns identified was characterized by high intakes of white bread, butter, margarine, sugar/confectionery and tea, while another had high intakes of whole grain bread, fish/shellfish and fruits/nuts (Pryer et al 2000).

Possible confounding by total energy intake is an important aspect to consider in all studies of diet–disease relationships. This can be illustrated by comparing two people with the same fibre intake of 23 g/day. If one is a small woman with an energy intake of 7 MJ while the other is a large, physically active man with an energy intake of 14 MJ, the former has a fibre-rich diet while the other has a fibre-poor diet. Thus, dietary data will usually be energy-adjusted in epidemiological studies, either by the residuals method (Willett 1998) or by introducing an energy term in the statistical model. Confounding can also be caused if one food item tends to be interchanged with another in the population.

If people eating high amounts of fish also tend to have low intakes of meat and vice versa, fish and meat intakes are inversely correlated with each other in the study population. The latest summary of the evidence regarding diet and cancer concludes that eating fish may protect against colorectal cancer, but it cannot be ruled out that the observation is confounded by meat intake (WCRF/AICR Expert Panel 2007, p.285).

Dietary habits are also associated with a range of non-dietary health behaviours that affect health. Eating a healthy diet may for instance be associated with being physically active and a non-smoker. Socio-demographic variables such as education, work and income levels may also confound diet–disease relationships. Many aspects of confounding are illustrated by the case of β-carotene and risk of cardiovascular mortality. Several observational studies showed that people eating more fruit and vegetables rich in β-carotene and having higher circulating serum β-carotene levels have lower rates of cardiovascular disease. However, when β-carotene supplementation was tested in large randomised controlled trials, there was no beneficial effect (Figure 30.4) (Egger et al 1998). There are several possible explanations for these findings including: (1) the observed relationship between β-carotene and cardiovascular mortality was confounded by other nutrients or bioactive components in fruit and vegetables; (2) β-carotene was a marker of a 'healthy' dietary pattern, and thus confounded for instance by high polyunsaturated fat intake or the combined effect of several dietary practices; (3) the observed effect was due to a healthy lifestyle or higher socioeconomic position among those with high levels of circulating β-carotene.

In epidemiology, it is common to try to isolate the effect of a single exposure by holding others constant through statistical modelling techniques. This corresponds to the method of standardisation to control confounding as described in Section 30.3 under 'Confounding'. However, when variables are strongly correlated with the factor being studied, adjusting for the influence of other factors in statistical models may be difficult and potentially misleading. In summary, it is unlikely that the effect of a single nutrient on disease risk can be isolated from the effect of other, correlated aspects of diet and lifestyle in observational studies.

FUTURE PERSPECTIVES IN NUTRITIONAL EPIDEMIOLOGY

Some of the most important public health problems today are coronary heart disease, diabetes and cancers. These disease groups have multiple and complex causal pathways where dietary factors are

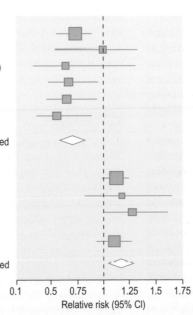

Fig. 30.4 Results from a systematic review on the effects of serum β-carotene (exposure) and rates of cardiovascular diseases (outcome).

part of a larger picture. Dietary determinants of disease often fall into the risk factor category: they increase the probability that a particular disease or malign condition will develop, but are not classified as sufficient or necessary causes. There are numerous studies of the role of diet in the aetiology in these diseases, but it takes considerable research effort to synthesise the evidence regarding a diet–disease relationship. The World Cancer Research Fund and American Institute for Cancer Research have published extensive reviews of the evidence regarding how food, nutrition and physical activity influence the risk of cancers. These reviews are based on explicit criteria for how to collect, discuss and judge the evidence (WCRF/AICR Expert Panel 2007, Ch. 3). A similar review regarding dietary prevention of chronic diseases has been published by the WHO (2003). Understanding of diet–disease relationships may change as evidence accumulates and systematic review methods become more sophisticated. An example is the lower level of certainty that fruit and vegetables protect women from breast cancer in the second extensive review of the evidence (WCRF/AICR Expert Panel 2007).

For many dietary variables, all individuals in a population are exposed and the range of exposure in that population may be rather narrow. This can pose a problem when we want to study how some dietary component affects risk of disease. In a population where everyone eats exactly the same amount of fruit and vegetables, we would not be able to show any positive or negative effects on the risk of cancer – no matter how strong the real effect is. It is more difficult to detect an association if the range of exposure in the study population is narrow compared to when it is wide. Some of the large cancer cohort studies, for instance EPIC, are designed to overcome this problem by studying diet–disease relationships across populations with diverse diets.

Many of the diseases we would like to study, particularly cancer, have a long lag between the start of the relevant exposure and the manifest stages of the disease. This is the *latency period*. It will normally take many years for healthy cells to turn malignant and then a single cancer cell may again take years to develop into a detectable tumour. The relevant dietary exposure affecting the risk of developing cancer may be between 10 and 60 years back in time (WCRF/AICR Expert Panel 2007). Exposures could also exert their effect during critical periods. When would be the correct point in time to get information about exposures? Researchers need to have a theory of the time dimensions relevant to the study outcome to handle these challenges properly.

Developments in genetics have added a new research dimension in epidemiology that is relevant in the nutritional context. After a food enters the mouth, there are several steps before the relevant nutrient is delivered to the site of action. One dimension of individual differences in biological responses to nutrients is common genetic variation. Individuals with a particular gene variant, or genotype, may have a different biological response to a nutrient exposure from those with the alternative genotype. This is called gene–environment interaction or, when the diet is involved, gene–nutrient interaction. It may be that knowledge of how common gene variants influence nutrient status could provide a novel method by which nutrient–disease effects can be investigated. Since genetic variation is usually randomly distributed between individuals, it may be possible to produce findings from observational studies that are free of the major problem of confounding.

It is likely that diet has an important influence on many if not all common non-communicable diseases. Narrow ranges of exposure, possible synergies among nutrients and small individual nutritional effects each present a challenge in studies of diet–disease relationships. Nevertheless, public health nutrition based on good science has a large contribution to make. Since everyone eats, a small change in diet at the population level may have a large positive effect on disease rates at a population level. The potential for dietary prevention of disease has yet to be fully understood.

KEY POINTS

- The effects of diet can be studied at a number of levels: nutrients, non-nutrients, foods and food patterns. This is a challenge of nutritional epidemiology.
- Dietary variables are strongly interrelated. It may be difficult to single out the relevant variable.
- Great care is needed in dietary assessment and in the capture of the relevant period of exposure.
- Between-population comparisons offer a useful means for investigating dietary effects on health by widening the range of exposures.

References

Bingham SA: Biomarkers in nutritional epidemiology, *Public Health Nutrition* 5:821–827, 2002.

De Onis M, Blössner M: Prevalence and trends of overweight among preschool children in developing countries, *American Journal of Clinical Nutrition* 72:1032–1039, 2000.

Egger M, Schneider M, Smith GD: Meta-analysis: spurious precision? Meta-analysis of observational studies, *British Medical Journal* 316:140–144, 1998.

Hill AB: *Principles of medical statistics,* ed 9, London, 1974, The Lancet Ltd.

Last JM: *A dictionary of epidemiology,* ed 4, New York, 2001, Oxford University Press.

Margetts BM, Nelson M: *Design concepts in nutritional epidemiology,* ed 2, Oxford, 1997, Oxford University Press.

Maurer J, Taren DL, Teixeira PJ, et al: The psychosocial and behavioral characteristics related to energy misreporting, *Nutrition Reviews* 64(2 Pt 1):53–66, 2006.

Pryer JA, Nichols R, Elliott P, et al: Dietary patterns among a national random sample of British adults, *Journal of Epidemiology and Community Health* 55:29–37, 2000.

Willett W: *Nutritional epidemiology,* ed 2, New York, 1998, Oxford University Press.

WCRF/AICR Expert Panel: *Food, nutrition, physical activity and the prevention of cancer: a global perspective,* London, 2007, World Cancer Research Fund/ American Institute for Cancer Research.

WHO: *Diet, nutrition and the prevention of chronic diseases.* Report of the joint WHO/FAO expert consultation. WHO Technical Report Series, No. 916 (TRS 916), Geneva, 2003, World Health Organization.

Further reading

Introduction to epidemiology:

Coggon D, Barker DJP, Rose G: *Epidemiology for the uninitiated,* ed 5, London, 1997, BMJ Publishing Group.

Rothman KJ: Epidemiology: an introduction, New York, 2002, Oxford University Press.

Nutritional epidemiology:

Margetts BM, Nelson M: *Design concepts in nutritional epidemiology,* ed 2, Oxford, 1997, Oxford University Press.

Willett W: *Nutritional epidemiology,* ed 2, New York, 1998, Oxford University Press.

Introduction to medical statistics:

Altman DG: *Practical statistics for medical research,* London, 1991, Chapman & Hall.

Kirkwood BR, Sterne JAC: *Essential medical statistics,* ed 2, Oxford, 2003, Blackwell Publishing.

EVOLVE CONTENTS (available online at: evolve.elsevier.com/Geissler/nutrition)

Chapter 31

Nutritional assessment methods

Christopher J Bates, Barry Bogin and Bridget Holmes*

CHAPTER CONTENTS

OBJECTIVES

By the end of this chapter you should be able to:
- summarise the purposes for which each of the currently used measures of nutritional status has been developed, the scope of their individual usefulness and their limitations
- outline the broad choices of different types of available measures, comprising (a) dietary estimation; (b) anthropometric measurements; (c) biochemical status indices; and, to a lesser extent, (d) functional and clinical evidence of adequacy
- summarise the common criteria for usefulness and reliability of these indices and measures, and list some of the common pitfalls that must be avoided during planning, practical work and interpretation.

*Updated and modified from the previous edition chapter by Christopher J Bates, Michael Nelson and Stanley Ulijaszek

31.1 INTRODUCTION

Christopher J. Bates

Measures of nutritional status are usually valuable inasmuch as they may be predictive of health outcomes. The practical requirements for assessment of nutritional adequacy arise from the need to intervene, either by advice or by more aggressive strategies, to improve the nutrition of individuals or populations, and thereby to reduce the risks and the burdens of those diseases that have, or may have, a nutritional component. Such diseases may range from the classical 'single nutrient' deficiency diseases such as beriberi or scurvy to multifactorial diseases such as vascular diseases or cancer, where nutrition is thought to play a modulating role as one of many aetiological factors.

The major categories of nutritional assessment strategies include: (a) dietary, (b) anthropometric, (c) biochemical status and (d) functional and clinical status (Gibson 1990).

Dietary assessment can be performed by weighed or household-measures-intake records, usually for 4 or 7 days. It can be done by diet histories or recalls, usually for the previous 24 hours, or by a food frequency questionnaire to probe the frequency with which specified food items are usually eaten, per week for instance.

Anthropometry measures typically include weight and height (with body mass index being calculated from these); mid-upper arm circumference, and perhaps others such as demispan and skinfold thicknesses.

Biochemical status measures or indices are selected and tailored for each nutrient, and are often the concentration of the nutrient or its derivatives in a body fluid such as serum or plasma. Thus plasma retinol is an index of vitamin A status; 25-hydroxy-vitamin D is an index of vitamin D status, and the activation of the flavin-dependent red cell enzyme erythrocyte glutathione reductase is an index of riboflavin (vitamin B_2) status.

Functional indices assess the integrity and efficiency of metabolic processes that are nutrient-dependent. Thus plasma homocysteine concentration is influenced by several B vitamins and is a functional index for their adequacy. Dark adaptation is influenced by vitamin A and zinc. Blood clotting is influenced by vitamin K.

Clinical indices comprise clinical signs or symptoms of nutrient deficiency: thus rickets is a sign of vitamin D deficiency and impaired blood clotting is a symptom of vitamin K deficiency. To some extent these indices may overlap: for instance, some biochemical indices are based on nutrient concentrations in body fluids which are, in turn, highly dependent on recent dietary intake, whereas others are based on related biochemical functions and metabolic-pathway adequacy, which are more dependent on tissue status and are more closely related to functional adequacy.

In this chapter, the main focus is on the first three categories, (a) to (c), although the importance of category (d) is always implicit in the discussion. The functional tests are most useful as research tools to investigate causal links, whereas the biochemical indices are most useful in population surveys and individual nutritional investigations. Clinical signs may be less specific for particular nutrients than are biochemical tests (see Ch. 28).

One of the most important growth areas in current nutritional research effort is the development of useful 'intermediate markers' between diet and health outcomes, since many of the latter may develop over long periods, and indeed over a lifetime. Where it is possible to demonstrate, experimentally, the influence of a change in dietary patterns on an intermediate marker, coupled with a strong relationship between that marker and a long-term health outcome, it is then possible to conduct population intervention studies, using the intermediate markers, to help identify those high-risk groups that could benefit from aggressive nutritional interventions.

In this chapter, the three assessment categories, (a) to (c), are compared and contrasted for their advantages and disadvantages, and their pitfalls and associated need for precautions. The contrasting approaches to the nutritional assessment of individuals and of populations will be considered, with respect to feasibility, validity and reproducibility (see Ch. 30). Validity measures the closeness of the estimate to the true value (its accuracy). Reproducibility measures the spread (or precision) of estimates. High validity and reproducibility means that a measure has a closer approximation to the truth. The requirements and precautions for reliable assessment methodologies will be discussed, together with the criteria for the choice of indices for different types of questions.

For some population studies, a single type of assessment may permit the deployment of resources to large numbers of participants. However, a combination of several categories of assessment may provide more reliable information, and help to avoid the pitfalls of confounders. Thus the balance between simplicity of design and robustness of conclusions is a challenge, requiring care and astuteness at the planning stage. (Many more references for this chapter are provided on the accompanying *evolve* website 🖱; see Additional references and further reading.)

31.2 METHODS OF DIETARY ASSESSMENT

Bridget Holmes*

OBJECTIVES

On completion of this section, the reader should:
- understand the purpose of dietary assessment
- be able to describe the various methods of dietary assessment used at national, household and individual level
- be aware of the strengths and weaknesses of the different approaches to dietary assessment at national, household and individual level
- recognise the contexts in which it is appropriate to use specific methods
- understand how to take into account the measurement errors associated with dietary assessment when interpreting results from dietary surveys.

The aim of this section is to explore the reasons for undertaking dietary assessment, to outline the different techniques that are available, to clarify which techniques are appropriate for specific purposes, and to consider the errors that arise when measuring diet and how to cope with them. Further information on the *evolve* website includes detailed definitions of different methods (see Section *evolve* 31.2(a) 🖱), how to describe the methods when reporting findings from dietary investigations (see Section *evolve* 31.2(b) 🖱) and an extended section on identifying and dealing with measurement error in dietary assessment (see Section *evolve* 31.2(c) 🖱).

---

*Updated and modified from the previous edition chapter section by Michael Nelson

THE OBJECTIVES OF DIETARY ASSESSMENT

Before undertaking any dietary assessment, it is necessary to consider the exact purpose of the assessment, what is to be measured, in whom, over what time period, and how the measurements are to be collected. This will determine which technique is most appropriate for a given purpose, and avoid wasting resources using a technique that does not provide an appropriate measure.

What is the underlying purpose?

All dietary assessments aim to measure food consumption or to estimate the intake of nutrients or non-nutrients in individuals or groups (Cameron & van Staveren 1988). There will, however, be an *underlying purpose*, which will dictate the level and nature of measurements to be made. For example, assessments vary from very precise estimates of a single nutrient in metabolic balance studies to broad estimates of the total quantity of food available for consumption for an entire country.

What is to be measured?

In a given culture, it is essential to know which substances constitute food or drink and which are taboo or unacceptable. In France, for example, horse meat is eaten commonly, whereas in England the consumption of horse meat is less acceptable. In societies where food is gathered in the wild, nuts, berries, mushrooms, insects and other foodstuffs may make important contributions to nutrient intake. Failure to identify all of the important food sources will lead inevitably to an underestimate of consumption.

The same is true of beverages; it is vital to identify fluid sources and composition. This is especially important where alcoholic beverages contribute to energy and nutrient intake (e.g. thiamin from beer).

It is also important to decide at the outset whether it is foods or nutrients (or both) that are to be assessed. Some studies may concentrate on patterns of food consumption and be less concerned with nutrient content (e.g. in relation to nutrition education). Others may require detail of nutrient intake that cannot be provided reliably by food composition tables (e.g. metabolic balance studies).

Whose diet is to be measured?

If diet is to be assessed for a country or region, and data are to be collected at an aggregate level, then the choice of method will be dictated largely by government decisions concerning information collected from growers, producers, importers, exporters, food processors and manufacturers, and those responsible for food storage. At the household and individual level, however, issues concerning literacy and level of education will be important in the choice of method. Age of subjects will also be important given that children under the age of 12 and some older people may have trouble remembering accurately what they ate over the previous days or weeks. Not all methods will be applicable to all groups.

When is diet to be assessed?

In individuals, diet on weekdays and weekends may differ. There are seasonal variations in food availability in every country, often very marked in countries that have extreme wet and dry seasons or variations in employment and income (e.g. fruit picking in itinerant labourers). The timing of administration of a dietary questionnaire (before or after a meal, for example) may influence the reported levels of consumption. A particularly difficult problem arises when the aim is to assess diet in the distant past because it is believed to relate to current disease state (e.g. the influence of past intakes of dietary calcium in relation to current risk of osteoporotic fracture).

How is diet to be assessed?

The choice of dietary assessment method will be largely influenced by the answers to the above questions – why? what? who? when? Of considerable importance, however, is the level of resource available to undertake the dietary assessment, in terms of financial resource/cost-effectiveness and available time. Consideration also needs to be given to who will be doing the measuring of diet (e.g. nutritionists, clinicians, interviewers), as this may also influence method selection.

METHODS OF DIETARY ASSESSMENT

There are five stages at which food availability and consumption can be measured (Fig. 31.1). These range from national statistics to individual con-

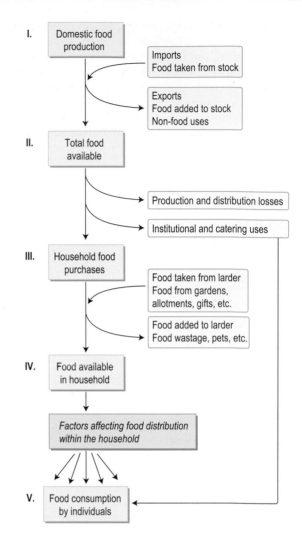

Fig. 31.1 Points in the food supply chain at which it is convenient to measure food availability or consumption

sumption. Information from the finer levels of measurement (individual, household or institution) can be built up to provide a picture of consumption at regional or national level.

Domestic food production (I)

Most governments require farmers and food producers to report how much food they produce. This is part of ongoing food surveillance which provides an overview of the adequacy of the national food supply. It also provides information about the levels of agricultural self-sufficiency (how much of a country's food supply is produced domestically).

It is useful in planning food supplies and meeting requirements.

This type of information is of limited value on its own, however. No country is entirely self-sufficient. Moreover, the quality of reporting varies between countries. Developed countries with large farms and highly mechanised means of production are likely to provide more complete and accurate information than countries in which a large part of the food production is based on subsistence agriculture with many smallholders and tenant farmers.

Total food available (II)

Of far greater usefulness in estimating a country's food supply are *food balance* data (or 'food disappearance data' or 'consumption level estimates') published quarterly by the United Nations Food and Agriculture Organization and then summarised in longer time series (Food and Agricultural Organization of the United Nations 2003). These values reflect domestic food production *plus* imported food (including food aid), food taken from storage, *minus* food exported or added to stocks or used for non-food purposes (e.g. sugar used in the brewing industry, grain fed to livestock). When the totals are divided by the number of people in the population, the result is expressed as food 'available' per person. It is also possible to estimate the nutrient content of the food available and to estimate the availability of energy and nutrients per person.

These data are widely used for making comparisons between countries to learn about the extent of hunger at the national level (see Chs 32 and 33) as well as the relationships between diet and disease. They are also useful for assessing time trends in diet within countries, although they are not direct measurements of diet.

Food balance data are limited in three important ways. First, they provide only an estimate for the country as a whole and therefore there is no information on distribution of consumption within the country, and no indication of any groups within the population that may be consuming amounts consistently above or below the average. Second, no account is taken of waste or losses of food from the system (e.g. domestic spoilage and plate waste or food given to domestic animals). This may lead to an overestimate of apparent availability. Third, the consumption estimates give higher values than those derived from other types of survey. In economically developed countries especially, the estimate of energy available for consumption may be as much as 25% above the estimated requirement of the population. This suggests that there may be biases inherent in the reporting system which may lead to a distortion in estimated differences in consumption between countries. The agreement in ranking of countries based on a comparison of food balance data and other types of dietary survey, however, suggests that the data may be useful for some epidemiological purposes.

Measurements at household level (III and IV)

There are four main techniques used to assess food consumption at the household level: food accounts, inventories, household recall and list-recall (Lagiou & Trichopoulou 2001). The strengths and limitations of the food account method (and the other methods described below) are summarised in Table *evolve* 31.2(a) 🖥.

Food accounts

In the food accounts method, the main food provider (the person in the household who does the food shopping and preparation) is asked to keep a record of either the quantity or cost (or both) of all household food acquisitions (purchases, gifts, food from gardens or allotments, payments in kind, take-away foods eaten at home, etc.). Typically, no information is collected on changes in larder stocks (see inventory method, below). Menu records of food and drink provided and the age and gender of the people present at meals served during the survey period may be used to estimate the proportion of diet consumed away from home. Additionally, individuals within the household may be asked to keep records of foods acquired and eaten away from home. Waste is usually estimated as a fixed amount, typically between 5% and 10%. The energy and nutrient content of the household diet can be estimated from appropriate food composition data that take into account storage and preparation losses and the relative proportions of foods making up aggregated categories (e.g. 'meat products'). Although changes in larder stocks are not taken into account, it is assumed that over a sufficient number of households (say about 20), the *average* change in larder stocks is zero (i.e. some households will consume more than they purchase, using food stored in larders, refrigerators and freezers, and others will consume less than they purchase, putting food into storage). Food account data can therefore provide reasonable estimates of average food consumption and nutrient intake per person.

In Britain, the National Food Survey (NFS) was conducted annually for over half a century (Department for the Environment, Food and Rural Affairs 2002) from 1950 to March 2001. Although in its original inception it included a larder inventory, it was felt that this distorted the picture of normal consumption by drawing respondents' attention to food in the larder which would otherwise have remained uneaten. Reporting of consumption of sweets, soft drinks, alcoholic beverages and foods eaten away from home was not included until 1992. Reports are published annually, and these provide an excellent unbroken record of British food habits since 1950. The published results afford opportunities to conduct time trend, social class and regional analyses in relation to epidemiological questions.

Since April 2001, the data have been collected in the Expenditure and Food Survey. This combines the former NFS and Family Expenditure Survey. The latter provided much more detailed socioeconomic and demographic data about each household than the NFS, and the new survey allows for better analysis in relation to variations in household characteristics. Key issues in the implementation and analysis of food account data are summarised in Table *evolve* 31.2(b) 🖱.

Inventory method

The inventory method is similar in nature to the food account method, in that respondents are asked to keep records of all foods coming into the house. In addition, a larder inventory is carried out at the beginning and end of the survey period. This was the method used by the NFS prior to 1952 including the first study on urban working class households. The ability of respondents to provide accurate inventory data is good.

The method has the advantages of providing a direct measure of the amount of food and nutrient available for consumption within a single household. However, because the inventory may draw respondents' attention to foods in the larder that might otherwise have remained unconsumed, it distorts typical purchasing patterns if maintained over a short period such as one week. Larder inventory surveys lasting several weeks or longer may not be subject to this weakness.

Household record

In the household record method, the foods available for consumption (whether raw or processed) are weighed, or estimated in household measures, allowing for preparation waste (e.g. discarded outer leaves, peel, trimmed fat, etc.). Any food consumed by visitors is estimated and subtracted from the total, and an allowance is made for food waste (food prepared but not consumed), either by collecting the waste directly (which is likely to underestimate the true waste) or by estimating the proportion of the total prepared food believed to be wasted.

The technique is a combination of recall and record. Typically, the interviewer calls in the morning, establishes the household composition, and asks the respondent to recall the quantities of food used to prepare breakfast. The foods to be used in the preparation of lunch are weighed or recorded in household measures. An afternoon interview allows the waste at lunch to be estimated, and the foods for the evening meal to be measured and recorded.

The technique is useful in countries where much of the diet is home-produced rather than pre-processed. Where the level of literacy is variable or low, the number of visits to each household can be tailored to obtain the required detail. Because the technique provides a direct measure of food available for consumption and makes no assumptions about changes in food stocks, it can be used, like the inventory method, to identify households with particular consumption characteristics.

The limitations to the method are similar to those of the food account method. In addition, the larder inventory and presence of an observer may distort usual patterns of food usage.

List–recall method

This is a structured survey in which the respondent is asked to recall the amount and cost of food obtained for household use over a given period, usually one week. In addition to food purchases and acquisitions, it takes into account the use of food. It can therefore be used to provide an estimate of food costs as well as net household consumption of both foods and nutrients. The technique was used in the United States Food Consumption Surveys.

The technique is well suited to populations in which most food is purchased rather than home-produced. It is relatively quick and cheap, as it requires only a single interview. It is helpful to notify the respondent of the study in advance, in order that he or she may keep records of purchases (such as supermarket receipts) to aid the recall, but this may have the effect of distorting food consumption patterns. The information on food use helps to overcome problems about movement of foods into and out of stock, but distortions in recall which are characteristic of any memory-based survey will inevitably influence the outcome. Problems persist concerning foods eaten away from home, consumption of food by visitors, and distribution of nutrients within families.

Measurement of food consumption in individuals (V)

There are two main approaches to individual dietary assessment, *prospective* and *retrospective*. Prospective methods involve subjects collecting or recording their current diet, while retrospective methods require subjects to recall their recent or past diet. Both types of assessment have strengths and limitations, and these are summarised in Table 31.1. Exact definitions of techniques in current use are given in Section *evolve* 31.2(a) 🖱.

Generally speaking, any measurement of diet will be biased in some way by the measurement process itself. There are therefore no entirely objective measures of an individual's food consumption or nutrient intake except in the controlled conditions of a metabolic unit. For example, the reported diet may not reflect the *actual* diet because subjects choose not to record or report certain items (especially 'unhealthy' foods such as sweets and alcoholic beverages for example). In addition, a record or recall of diet may not reflect the *usual* diet because, for example, a respondent may choose to report or consume more foods regarded as 'healthy' (such as fruits and vegetables) and fewer foods regarded as 'unhealthy' (such as crisps or sweets). Subjects may also simplify their diet or eat less than usual in order to make the recording process easier. These errors are independent of those due to poor memory or inaccurate recording. The main consequence of these processes is an underestimation of dietary intake and a misrepresentation of healthy versus unhealthy foods. Measurements of characteristics such as 'dietary restraint', 'social approval' and 'social desirability' help to identify subjects likely to misreport food consumption. Separating inaccurate reports of dietary intake as a result of under-recording and/or undereating from those

where subjects have consumed less than usual due to illness or dieting, for example, can be facilitated by asking whether or not the subject's intake was typical or not, and if not, why. The use of food composition tables to estimate the nutrient content of the diet will lead to further inaccuracies. Coding and data entry errors for computer analysis are common and the distortions that occur are often difficult to detect. The topic is discussed in detail in Section *evolve* 31.2(c) 🖱.

Prospective methods – advantages and disadvantages

The main advantage of prospective methods is that they provide a direct measure of current diet. Also, they can be carried out for varying lengths of time according to the level of accuracy of the estimate of food consumption or nutrient intake required. Dietary energy intakes in the UK, for example, are typically more variable from day to day than carbohydrate intakes. It therefore takes twice as long to achieve a given level of precision for estimates of energy (7 days) intake as it does for carbohydrate (3–4 days). In general, for a given food or nutrient, the more days of information collected, the better the precision of the estimate. However, there is a balance to be found between achieving precise estimates of intake and maintaining recording enthusiasm of the subjects so as to minimise changes in patterns of usual consumption.

The main disadvantage of prospective methods is that they are labour-intensive for both the respondent and the interviewer. The respondent needs good literacy, language and numeracy skills in order to provide an accurate record. This limits the usefulness of prospective methods in populations where literacy levels are low, unless trained recorders are present (but the presence of an observer may result in a distortion of usual diet). Good subject motivation and a commitment to complete the record accurately and objectively are needed.

Retrospective methods – advantages and disadvantages

Retrospective methods require subjects to 'recall' their current or past diet. This may involve remembering the type and amount of all individual items consumed over a specified period of time (e.g. 24-hour recall), or creating a mental construct of 'usual' consumption involving recollection of both the frequency of consumption of specific foods or food groups and the amounts consumed. The main advantages of the retrospective methods are that

Table 31.1   General features, strengths and limitations of prospective and retrospective individual dietary assessment methods

METHOD	STRENGTHS	LIMITATIONS
Prospective methods		
General features	Measures current diet Direct observation of what is eaten Duration of survey can be varied to meet requirements for precision Do not rely on subjects memory Generally more commonly used therefore allowing for comparison between studies	High level of respondent burden Require good literacy, numeracy and language skills Subjects need to be well motivated and committed High level of respondent burden and commitment may result in lower response rates Usual consumption pattern may change due to: inconvenience of recording; choice of foods which are easy to record; recording more foods which are believed to be more 'healthy' and less 'unhealthy' foods True consumption levels may be under-reported, particularly in overweight subjects Coding and data entry errors are common
Duplicate diet	Direct analysis of nutrient content of food (not dependent upon food composition tables) Required in metabolic balance studies	Very expensive Intense supervision needed Usual diet may not be consumed
Weighed inventory	Widely used, facilitates comparisons between studies Precise portion size assessment	Food composition tables used to estimate nutrient intake
Household measures	No scales needed Fewer recording skills required compared to weighed inventory	Loss of precision compared with weighed inventory
Retrospective methods		
General features	Measures current or past diet Lower respondent burden compared to prospective methods Effect on usual consumption pattern lower than prospective methods Quick to administer Expensive equipment not required Repeated measurements increases precision	Recording of true consumption may be affected by errors in memory, biases in perception and conceptualisation of food portion sizes; presence of observer Daily variation in diet not usually assessed Dependent on regular eating habits Food composition tables used to estimate nutrient intake
Diet history	Assesses 'usual' diet	Over-reporting of foods believed to be 'healthy' (e.g. fruit)
24-hour recall	Very quick to administer Suitable for those with low literacy and numeracy skills Can be repeated to gain measure of daily variation and improve precision	Prone to underestimate intake due to omissions Interviewer burden is high Single observation provides poor measure of individual intake
Food frequency and amount questionnaire	Suitable for large-scale surveys Can be posted Short version can focus on specific nutrients with few food sources	Requires validation in relation to reference measure Literacy and numeracy skills needed if self-completed

they are relatively quick to administer compared with prospective methods. They are also less expensive in terms of equipment and (except for repeat 24-hour recalls, see below) resources considering the time taken for interviewers to see subjects. A further advantage of retrospective methods is that, because there is a lower respondent burden than for prospective methods, the chances of obtaining a

more representative sample of all consumers is increased. They can also be used to assess diet in the past, which may be relevant to studies where the underlying causes of chronic diseases such as heart disease or cancer may lie in past rather than current diet.

The main disadvantage of retrospective methods relates to sources of bias. Errors in memory result in the omission of foods from the assessment. This may be a problem for some elderly subjects and for children under the age of about 12. Subjects *and* interviewers must have good skills relating to the perception and conceptualisation of food portion size (the ability to develop an accurate mental construct of the amount of food consumed and to translate that construct into a description or selection of an appropriate food portion photograph which corresponds to the amount actually consumed). Amongst respondents, this is a problem especially in children under 12 years of age. The presence of an observer (interviewer) may cause subjects to overemphasise what they perceive as the 'healthy' aspects of their diet and to minimise the 'unhealthy' aspects ('social desirability' and 'social approval' bias). Daily variation in diet is less readily assessed using retrospective methods (unless using repeat 24-hour recalls). Subjects who do not have regular eating habits will have difficulty describing the 'usual' frequency of consumption. And, as with most prospective methods, the use of food composition tables will introduce error into the estimates of energy and nutrient intake. (See Section *evolve* 31.2(b) for advantages and disadvantages of each method .)

Prospective methods

- *Duplicate diet method*. This technique requires subjects to weigh and record their food consumption at the time of eating. At the same time, they put aside an exact duplicate portion of each food consumed which is analysed chemically for energy and nutrient content. The main advantage of this method is that it is independent of errors associated with the use of food composition tables. It is best suited to metabolic balance studies in free-living populations.

- *Weighed inventory method*. The weighed inventory is one of the most widely used techniques. It was first described by Elsie Widdowson in 1936. Subjects keep a record of all food and drink consumed. Each food item is weighed prior to consumption using portable food weighing scales. Items left over are also weighed. In practice, most weighed inventories include a proportion of items recorded in household measures.

- *Household measures method*. The method is similar to the weighed inventory, except that subjects record portion sizes in household measures (cups, bowls, spoonfuls, etc.)

rather than weighing their food. In more recent times, sets of food photographs are provided to aid subjects with recording portion size. Records in household measures have the advantage of simplifying the recording process for subjects.

- *Food checklist method*. Respondents are provided each day with a pre-printed list of foods and asked to tick a box each time an item is consumed. A space is usually provided to record foods eaten but not listed. Standard portion sizes may be indicated, or portion descriptions entered. The method is simple to use and well liked by respondents, but the information collected is less detailed than with other prospective methods and food consumption and nutrient intakes are less precise as a result.

Retrospective methods

- *24-hour recall method*. The 24-hour recall (originally attributed to Wiehl in 1942) involves a trained interviewer asking subjects to recall and describe every item of food and drink consumed over exactly 24 hours. The information is obtained through systematic repetition of open-ended questions. Amounts may be described in household measures or using food photographs. Interviewers must be thoroughly familiar with both the local diet and the food composition tables to be used to estimate nutrient intakes, in order to probe subjects effectively and obtain adequate detail for subsequent coding of data. The 'multiple-pass' 24-hour recall is now in widespread use (consisting of several stages including an uninterrupted 'quick list' of items recalled; a detailed interview elaborating the quick list that determines detail and amounts; and a thorough review of the detailed interview). This multiple pass method minimises the opportunity for items to be forgotten.

- *Diet history method*. The diet history was originally described by Burke in 1947 and although used less frequently today, is one of the oldest approaches for assessing diet. It is used to assess 'usual' diet over the recent past. Typically, a trained interviewer begins by carrying out a 24-hour recall which is elaborated in an interview lasting up to 2 hours. For each meal, subjects are asked to describe the range of foods that would be likely to be consumed, the frequency of their consumption, and typical amounts. Differences between weekdays and weekends are clarified, and seasonal variations elaborated.

- *Food frequency questionnaire.* Food frequency questionnaires (FFQ) are pre-printed lists of foods on which subjects are asked to indicate the typical frequency of consumption and to state in household measures the average amount consumed on the days when the food is eaten. The number of foods on the list varies. Optically scannable questionnaires speed up the coding of information. An example of a segment of an FFQ is shown in Figure *evolve* 31.2(c) 🖱.

Brief dietary assessment methods are useful when total diet does not need to be assessed. For example, simplified FFQs that contain far fewer food items than would typically be included may be used in instances where a single nutrient or type of food is being estimated. Although such assessments can be made at a low cost with a low respondent and interviewer burden, they have several limitations including an inability to assess entire diet and provide quantitatively precise information (Thompson & Subar 2008).

Dietary assessment in population subgroups

The choice of dietary assessment method must be selected on the basis not only of the question to be answered but also the population group in which the assessment is to take place. Assessing the intake of population subgroups, such as minority ethnic groups, low-income groups, pregnant women or those at either end of life's spectrum (the youngest young or the oldest old) often presents specific problems.

- *Ethnic populations.* If the population to be assessed is composed primarily of, or contains a significant proportion of minority ethnic groups for whom foods consumed and cooking practices are not conventional, modifications to dietary assessment methods are required. If interviewers are not from the same ethnic background as subjects they should familiarise themselves with foods, recipes, differences in food names and portion sizes in order to facilitate the collection of accurate dietary data. Food composition databases may also require updating to represent ethnic foods and recipes (Thompson & Subar 2008).

- *Children.* The variable nature of children's diets and their rapidly changing eating habits present challenges for dietary assessment (Thompson & Subar 2008). Problems with recalling frequency as well as both the types and amounts of foods consumed and the ability to conceptualize portion size apply to younger children (Biró et al 2002). Since younger children are less able to participate in dietary assessment, the ability of parents or guardians to accurately report their children's food intake is vital. While cognitive abilities are developed by adolescence, older children capable of reporting are often uninterested in providing complete and accurate reports (Livingstone & Robson 2000).

- *Elderly.* Methods that require recalling past diet e.g. recall and FFQ methods, are inappropriate if memory is impaired, and sensory difficulties such as loss of hearing and vision, and physical difficulties including being chair- or bedridden affect the ability to record dietary intake. In some cases the subject may have little involvement in food acquisition or preparation thus limiting the subject's ability to accurately name or describe the foods consumed (Adamson et al 2009). Additionally, special diets (e.g. high-fibre, soft foods due to difficulties chewing) are common in this group and methods may require adaptation as a result.

- *Low income.* Studies in low-income groups often encompass several specific subgroups, including minority ethnic groups, elderly and families with large numbers of siblings. As a result, dietary assessment in such a diverse group is often problematic. Lower literacy, numeracy and language skills exist alongside physical problems of record-keeping amongst the elderly and disabled. Drug and alcohol abuse create problems that impact not only on the quality of the data but also on the safety and welfare of interviewers. Additionally a higher likelihood of domestic chaos and stress factors arise among low-income households which mediate against accurate record-keeping and the ability to undertake dietary assessment (Holmes et al 2008).

- *Pregnant women.* Dietary assessment during pregnancy is complex as a result of changes in energy and nutrient needs, appetite and meal patterns. Social desirability bias may affect reporting in this group, especially with regard to alcohol consumption and supplement intake. Validation of dietary assessment methods in pregnant women is limited (National Institutes of Health 2007).

Conclusions regarding individual dietary assessments

The wide variety of techniques for assessing individuals' diets reflects both the difficulties and frustrations associated with attempts to measure diet without bias, and the importance attached to the need to obtain accurate measurements in many different circumstances. Improvements in dietary assessment techniques have been hampered by the lack of a readily measured absolute standard or reference of intake against which to assess the precision of other measures. The situation has improved to some degree in recent years as a result of better understanding of how to identify misreporting (see 'Validity and measurement error', below). Nevertheless, many of the problems regarding objective assessment of individuals' diets remain. The need to measure diet requires us to appreciate the many limitations, and to continue to develop and improve methods of dietary assessment.

Appropriate uses of dietary survey methods

Techniques for dietary assessment are summarised in Table 31.2. It is clear that certain techniques are limited to particular applications. For example, food balance sheets are appropriate for assessing diet at the country level, facilitating comparisons between countries and mapping trends in consumption within a country over time. Weighed inventory data can be used to assess diet at individual level and to build up pictures of regional or national consumption based on representative samples, but they may be too labour-intensive for

Table 31.2   Appropriate uses of dietary survey methods (+++ very suitable, ++ moderately suitable, + limited suitability)

LEVEL OF DIETARY MEASUREMENT	DIETARY SURVEY METHOD							
	FOOD BALANCE SHEETS	HOUSEHOLD SURVEYS	SURVEYS OF INDIVIDUALS					
			PROSPECTIVE			RETROSPECTIVE		
			Duplicate diet[a]	Weighed inventory	Household measures	Diet history	24-hour recall	Questionnaires
National	+++	+++	+[b]	+[b]	+[b]	+[b]	++[b]	+[b]
Regional	–	+++	+[b]	+[b]	+[b]	+[b]	++[b]	+[b]
Institution/group	–	+++	+[b]	++[b]	++[b]	++[b]	++[b]	++[b]
Household	–	++[c]	++[d]	++[d]	++[d]	++[d]	++[d]	++[d]
Individual	–	+[e]	+++[f]	+++[f]	+++[f]	+++[f]	+++[f]	+++[f]
Type of study								
Epidemiological	+++[g]	+++[g]	+[h]	+++[h]	+++[h]	++[h]	+++[h]	+++[h]
Clinical	–	–	++	+++	+++	+++	+++[i]	+++
Metabolic	–	–	+++	+[j]	–	–	–	–

–Not suitable
[a]Includes other techniques of direct analysis (see text).
[b]Requires sample representative of population, institution or group, or analysis weighted to reflect balance of subgroups.
[c]Requires larder inventory. Short-term measures (e.g. one week) may not reflect usual diet in individual households.
[d]The need for data from all household members may distort usual household food consumption patterns.
[e]Requires complex mathematical modelling of within-household food and nutrient distribution.
[f]Important to screen out individuals whose responses may not be valid (see text).
[g]Appropriate for ecological studies.
[h]See Margetts & Nelson (1997) for detailed discussion of use of dietary survey methods in epidemiological studies.
[i]Requires repeat 24-hour recalls for valid classification of subjects according to levels of intake (see text).
[j]Useful only if range of foods is of limited variation in composition, allowing reliable use of food composition tables.

looking at distribution of food in families and cannot be used for metabolic studies. The footnotes given in Table 31.2 clarify the specific problems, limitations or advantages of using a particular technique in a particular setting.

Validity and measurement error

Despite the fact that techniques of dietary assessment have changed little since the 1970s, there has been a growing awareness of the sources of bias in measurements of diet. Not only is there now an acceptance of the fact that all dietary assessment methods are influenced by the reporting process itself but also a recognition of the need to separate subjects with valid records from those who are believed to have inaccurate records. Dieticians, clinicians, epidemiologists and researchers no longer accept that their particular measure of diet is 'good enough'. Instead, they seek to determine the biases in their measurements in order to adjust for them when assessing the relationships between diet and health. The main problems arising from inaccurate measurements are:

- incorrect *positioning* of a country, household or person in relation to the truth or some external reference measure (e.g. dietary reference values)
- incorrect *ranking* of countries, households or persons in relation to one another.

The first type of error can result in inappropriate investigations or actions being taken to remedy an apparent dietary deficit or excess that does not really exist. Alternatively, no action may be taken when some is needed (e.g. a true deficit is not detected because diet is overestimated). The second type of error tends to undermine the ability to assess relationships between diet and health (e.g. someone who properly belongs in the top quarter of the distribution of intake is classified in the bottom quarter, or vice versa). Again, this can lead either to inappropriate recommendations for improving health in the population or, more often, a failure to take action because the true relationship between diet and health is obscured by measurement error. Measurement error and their effects are described by Nelson & Beresford (2003).

Section *evolve* 31.2(c) 🖱 lists some of the sources of measurement error, their principal effects, some ways of taking errors into account in analysis, and

ideas for dealing with them in practice. A summary is given in Table *evolve* 31.2(c) 🖱.

KEY POINTS

- There is a wide variety of methods available for assessing diet. The method chosen should be appropriate for the purpose, the population and circumstances of the work being carried out.
- All methods for dietary assessment include errors. It is important:
  - not to take the measurements of food consumption and nutrient intake at face value;
  - to understand the likely sources of error; and
  - to appreciate how the errors may influence the interpretation of apparent associations (or apparent lack of association) between diet and health.
- When reporting findings on dietary assessment, it is important to provide a full description of the sample characteristics (e.g. age, height, weight, body mass index), number of subjects or households and number of days of measurement collected.

31.3 ANTHROPOMETRIC ASSESSMENT

Barry Bogin*

OBJECTIVES

- To understand the different uses of various anthropometric measures used to assess nutritional status.
- To appreciate how inaccuracies in their recording can be minimised.
- To be able to compare the measures to the most appropriate reference to estimate levels of under- and overnutrition.

Anthropometry is the scientific study of variation in the size and shape of the human body. Compared with the dietary, biochemical status, and functional and clinical status methods, anthropometry may provide a relatively quick and inexpensive means for the assessment of nutritional status. Anthropometric nutritional assessment involves the measurement of aspects of body size (e.g. height and weight).

---

*Updated and modified from the previous edition chapter section by Stanley J Ulijaszek

These are then related to references or standards, according to the age and sex of the subject, which reflect the body growth of healthy and well-nourished individuals (see Box 31.1). Differences from the reference values are taken to be outcomes of nutritional experience. The World Health Organization states that anthropometry 'reflects both health

---

BOX 31.1   Growth standards and references

The World Health Organization in 2007 published new standards of growth in length/height-for-age, weight-for-age, head-circumference-for-age, arm-circumference-for-age, triceps-skinfold-for-age and other anthropometric dimensions for infants and children (WHO 2007; see also *evolve* websites on Growth standards 🖥).

The standards describe normal child growth from birth to 5.0 years under optimal environmental conditions and can be applied to all children everywhere, regardless of ethnicity, socioeconomic status and type of feeding.

The new standards differ from any existing growth reference charts in a number of ways.

First, standards describe 'how children should grow', in contrast to reference charts, which describe how certain groups of children *do* grow. They are based on breastfed samples, making breastfeeding the biological 'norm' and establishing the breastfed infant as the normative growth model. The previous growth reference was based on the growth of artificially fed children.

The pooled sample from the six participating countries (Brazil, Ghana, India, Norway, Oman and the USA) allows the development of a truly international standard. In contrast, the previous international reference was based on children from a single country. The new standard emphasizes the fact that infant and child populations grow similarly across the world's major regions when their needs for health and care are met.

These standards also include growth indicators beyond height and weight that are particularly useful for monitoring the increasing epidemic of childhood obesity, such as the skinfold thicknessess.

The WHO and many individual nations publish growth references for people over the age of 5 years. The previously used British growth charts were replaced with the WHO growth standards and references in 2009. For recent British and US data on height, weight and body mass index see *evolve* websites 🖥. The WHO is in the process of developing growth standards for people over age 5.

---

and nutritional status and predicts performance, health and survival. As such, it is a valuable, but currently underused, tool for guiding public health policy and clinical decisions (WHO 2009).

USES, ADVANTAGES AND LIMITATIONS

The reasons why the WHO and other health authorities recommend anthropometry as the primary method of nutritional assessment is the relatively low cost and portability of equipment needed, the relatively low level of training required to use this equipment, and the high accuracy and precision relative to dietary methods. Some examples of anthropometric equipment are illustrated in Figures *evolve* 31.3(a) and *evolve* 31.3(b) 🖥. A range of anthropometric equipment may be seen on *evolve* websites on Equipment 🖥. Training is best done via an approved course, such as those run by the International Society for the Advancement of Kinanthropometry and with an anthropometric handbook, for instance that published by the International Fund for Agricultural Development (IFAD), a branch of the United Nations (see *evolve* websites on Training 🖥).

Although a wide range of anthropometric measurements can be made for ergonomic, anthropological, physiological, medical and sports purposes, a rather more limited list is appropriate to nutritional anthropometry (Table 31.3). All of the measurements given in this table are appropriate for the assessment of undernutrition at all ages. For older children, adolescents and adults, waist and hip circumference, in addition to weight, height, arm circumference and skinfolds, are useful in the assessment of overnutrition.

The following are instructions for the main anthropometric measurement techniques, height, length, weight, arm circumference and skinfolds (triceps skinfold), adapted from *evolve* websites on Techniques 🖥. Additional measurements may be useful, especially leg length in proportion to total body height. Please see Frisamcho (2008) and Bogin and Varela Silva (2010). All measurements should be taken by at least two people, one who is primarily responsible for positioning the subject and reading the measurement, and another who makes sure the positioning is correct and who records the measurement. The recorder must repeat the measurement aloud and receive confirmation before finalizing the record. Computerized anthropometric devices that automatically record measurements exist, but are not reviewed here (Lu & Wang 2008).

Table 31.3 Recommended measurements for anthropometric nutritional assessment

AGE GROUP (YEARS)	PRACTICAL FIELD OBSERVATIONS	MORE DETAILED OBSERVATIONS
0–1	Weight, length	Head and arm circumference, Triceps and subscapular skinfolds
1–5	Weight, length, height, arm circumference	Triceps and subscapular skinfolds
5–20	Weight, height, arm circumference	Triceps, subscapular and medial calf skinfolds, calf circumference
Over 20	Weight and height	Arm and calf circumference Triceps, subscapular and medial calf skinfolds Waist and hip circumferences (overnutrition only) Demispan (elderly subjects)

1. Height – The measurement of the maximum distance from the floor to the highest point on the head, when the subject is facing directly ahead, with shoes off, feet together, arms by the sides, and heels, buttocks and upper back in contact with the wall (see Figs *evolve* 31.3a and *evolve* 31.3(c) 🖰. The equipment required is a stadiometer, portable anthropometer or steel ruler placed against a wall. Experienced technicians achieve a reliability of ±3.0 mm on repeated height measurements of the same person. Height is greater in the morning, so it should be measured at the same time of day each time, especially if the same person is measured on two or more occasions.

2. Recumbent length – As infants under 2.0 years old cannot stand erect well enough for a useful measure of height, body length is measured lying down (recumbent). A measuring board is used, normally with a fixed headpiece and an adjustable footpiece (see Fig. *evolve* 31.3(c) 🖰). It is placed so that it is stable on a hard, flat surface, such as the floor. Place the record form beside the board (Arrow 1 in Fig. *evolve* 31.3d 🖰) and kneel at the base of the board (Arrow 2), to the right side of the child so that you can move the footpiece with your right hand (Arrow 3). With the help of the mother or an assistant, gently lower the child onto the measuring board. With your hands cupped over the child's ears (Arrow 4) and your arms straight (Arrow 5), place the child's head against the base of the board. The child should be looking straight up (Arrow 6) and lying flat in the centre of the board (Arrow 7). With your left hand on the child's shins (Arrow 8) press

them gently, but firmly against the board and check the position of the child (Arrows 1–8). When the child's position is correct, move the footpiece with your right hand until it is firmly against the child's heels (Arrow 9) and read the measurement to the nearest 0.1 cm.

3. Body mass/weight – The person stands (or sits) on the balance with minimal movement and with hands by his/her side, or a young child can be placed in a sling attached to a hanging spring scale. Shoes and excess clothing should be removed so that the subject is dressed in light gown, bathing suit or minimal clothing acceptable for the cultural situation (see Fig. *evolve* 31.3e 🖰). The spring scale, or a balance, is calibrated for accuracy using weights authenticated by a government department of weights and measures Weight measurements are generally reliable, with most errors due to mis-calibration or mis-reading of the equipment.

4. Arm circumference –The person stands with her/his back to the examiner (see Fig. *evolve* 31.3f 🖰) and the right arm flexed. The examiner locates the acromion process of the scapula (tip of the shoulder) and the olecranon process of the ulna (tip of the elbow) and measures the distance between these two points. A mark is placed on the triceps muscle at the mid-point between the shoulder and elbow. A flexible tape, made of steel or non-stretchable plastic, is wrapped around the arm at the level of the mark and tightened to just touch the skin in all places, without compression. The circumference is read from the tape measure.

5. Skinfolds – The measurement of skinfolds can use between three and nine different standard anatomical sites around the body. The right side or the left side of the body only is usually measured for consistency. The tester pinches the skin at the appropriate site to raise a double layer of skin and the underlying adipose tissue, but not the muscle. The skinfold calipers (see Figs *evolve* 31.3(b), *evolve* 31.3(g) 🖱), are then applied 1 cm below and at right angles to the pinch, the jaws of the caliper are released and a reading in millimetres (mm) is taken 2 seconds later, as fat tissue is compressible under continuous pressure. The mean of two measurements is calculated. If the two measurements differ by more than 10%, a third is taken and the median value used. The triceps site is the most commonly measured for nutritional assessment. (See Fig. *evolve* 31.3(g) for details of the triceps site measurement 🖱.)

The most common anthropometric measures of undernutrition in children are weight and height, either individually or combined, relative to reference values. The two preferred indices are height for age and weight for height, since they can be used to discriminate between acute and chronic undernutrition (Waterlow et al 1977). Table 31.4 summarises the usefulness of weight for age, height for age and weight for height in nutritional assessment in children. Weight for height can also be used to assess overnutrition in children, and the body mass index (BMI) (weight(kg)/height(m)^2) × 100) is now the most widely used measure for this purpose (e.g. Cole et al 1995), although it is a less sensitive marker of body fatness than are skinfold thicknesses.

For adults the most commonly used measure of undernutrition and overnutrition is the BMI. Adult undernutrition, called chronic energy deficiency (CED), is classified by the following BMI cut-offs: 17–18.5, grade I; 16–17, grade II; below 16, grade III CED. BMI cut-offs of 25, 30 and 40 are used internationally to define mild, moderate and severe obesity respectively (Shetty & James 1994), although various nations may have differently defined criteria. The cut-off of 25 is also called overweight. BMI is an appropriate index in the general population, especially in the wealthier nations of North America, western Europe, Australia and Japan. However, in these nations, people in better than average physical condition, especially athletes with considerable muscle mass, will have a higher BMI but not excessive fat. In many poorer nations, malnutrition and chronic disease can result in short stature due to relative stunting of the legs. Because the trunk of the body is more massive than the legs, such people will have a normal to high BMI but may have low fat, and may even be undernourished. Because of these limitations of BMI, waist and hip circumferences, and waist-to-hip ratio, are often preferred measures of the central distribution of body fatness.

TYPES OF ANTHROPOMETRIC MEASUREMENT

Height (or length) and weight, are fundamental to all nutritional anthropometric studies, since they give the simplest measure of attained skeletal size (height or length), and of soft tissue mass (weight). Height is a measure of accumulated size over time. Relatively low height for age indicates a chronic deficiency in growth, such as prolonged illness or undernutrition. In contrast, weight for height

Table 31.4   The usefulness of weight and height measures relative to reference data

	WEIGHT FOR AGE	HEIGHT FOR AGE	WEIGHT FOR HEIGHT
Usefulness in populations whose age is unknown or inaccurate	4	4	1
Usefulness in identifying wasted children	3	4	1
Usefulness in identifying stunted children	2	1	4
Sensitivity to weight change over a short time frame	2	4	1
Ease of accurate collection?	2	3	2

1: excellent; 2: good; 3: moderate; 4: poor. (After Gorstein et al 1994.)

reflects a more current indication of energy balance, as weight can be lost or gained relatively quickly. Height declines with increasing age in the elderly, a trend that has been noted in studies throughout the world. Also, some elderly people cannot stand erect or lie down in a fully stretched position. Demispan (distance between index–middle finger web and the sternal notch) has been shown to be a reliable and reproducible alternative measure of stature in the elderly (see Section *evolve* 31.3(e) 🖱).

Arm circumference (also circumferences of the calf or thigh) is used as a proxy for soft tissue mass and provides an indication of the total amount of bone, muscle, and fat at the mid-point of the upper arm. It is useful for assessing global nutritional status, especially the reserves of energy (adipose tissue) and protein (muscle tissue) of the body. The cross-sectional area of bone in the upper arm (or leg) is assumed to be standard across populations, and unaffected by acute undernutrition. This is broadly acceptable, as the size and relative proportions are largely inherited characteristics that vary within populations as much as between them. Skeletal growth, although responding both to nutritional circumstances and to physical activity, is less plastic than soft tissue mass. Estimation of body fat by skinfold assumes that subcutaneous fat is an indicator of total body fat, including the visceral fat around major body organs and the interstitial fat of many tissues. Although this assumption is not always true, variation in subcutaneous fat does correlate well with other methods for measuring total body fatness such as underwater weighing and bioelectrical impedance. Visceral fat and subcutaneous fat have biologically distinct metabolic activity. Total fat loss in obese subjects involves different reductions in the two tissues. This is hardly surprising, as at least several dozen genomic and proteomic systems influence glucose homeostasis, insulin action and lipid metabolism (Chen & Hess 2008). Waist and hip circumferences give a composite measure of fatness, both subcutaneous and visceral. Lower limb skinfold and circumference measures are valuable, since it cannot be assumed that measures of the upper body are also representative of the lower body as upper–lower body differences in fatness and muscularity are possible in individuals performing hard work on a regular basis. This may not be true for young children, and older children not engaged in child labour; in this case, upper body measures alone are useful in nutritional assessment. In practice, measurements of upper arm circumferences as the only indicator of body composition may be both accurate and useful only in children below the age of 6 years.

ACCURACY OF MEASUREMENTS

The major limitation of anthropometry is the extent to which measurement error can influence interpretation of nutritional status. Potential anthropometrists need good training, although the relative simplicity of measurement can encourage investigators to skimp on training. It is most important that anthropometrists achieve good levels of precision and accuracy. Details of quality control and training are given in Section *evolve* 31.3(d) 🖱.

REFERENCES AND STANDARDS FOR ANTHROPOMETRIC NUTRITIONAL ASSESSMENT

The definition of growth references and standards is given in Box 31.1. The historical development of these types of growth chart comes from large-scale anthropometric surveys associated with health insurance and public health surveillance in industrialised nations. The majority of these surveys were initiated in the first half of the twentieth century. They generated growth curves for children, and distribution curves for height and weight for adults, used for health monitoring, with a famous example being the weight-for-height tables of the Metropolitan Life Insurance Company, published in 1959 and updated in 1999 (see *evolve* websites on Growth standards 🖱. Such normative population-based constructs were later used in nutritional assessment globally as normative growth charts were generated from anthropometric surveys in several less developed countries. Indigenously produced growth references are useful, so long as the reference data fulfil the criteria given in Table 31.5. WHO growth standards may be preferred for the ages at which they are available.

To estimate nutritional status of children from anthropometry, the measurements must be related to normative values, by expressing individual values as percentiles, percentages of the mean or median reference values for age, and/or Z (standard deviation) scores (Box 31.2). Whichever of these comparators is used, the proportion of the population falling below cut-offs defining the normative range is calculated. Software to carry out these calculations is available for use with the WHO, US, UK and German growth standards (see *evolve* websites on Software 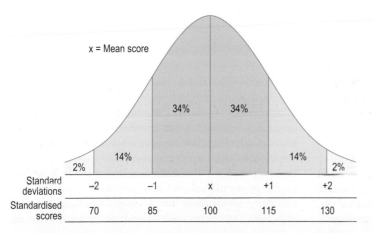). Software for use with the WHO standards and references and US references is also available in Frisancho 2008.

KEY POINTS

- Anthropometry is the most frequently used means of assessing nutrition status of a population.
- Each age group and sex has its own most appropriate anthropometric measures.
- The ease of collection of anthropometric measures should not mask the considerable potential for error in collection, but these errors are manageable if anticipated.
- The measurements are typically compared to measurements obtained for 'healthy' populations. These normative references or standards are continually being updated and reviewed and care must be taken to use the most appropriate one and to cite its use.

Table 31.5   Minimal criteria for anthropometric reference data in nutritional evaluation

1. The population should be well nourished
2. Each age/sex group of the sample should contain at least 200 individuals
3. The sample should be cross-sectional
4 Sampling procedures should be defined and reproducible
5. Measuring procedures should be optimal
6. Measurements should include all variables used in nutritional evaluation
7. Raw data and smoothing procedures should be available

From Waterlow et al., 1977

BOX 31.2   Using percentiles and Z-scores (standard deviation scores) for nutritional assessment of anthropometric data

Nutritional anthropometric data may be compared directly with growth standards or reference values, especially percentiles of growth, or be statistically standardised for age using standard deviation scores (also known as Z-scores) relative to reference data. Z-scores express the anthropometric values as a number of standard deviations above or below the mean value. The formula used to calculate the standard deviations is:

$$Z = \frac{\text{Observed value} - \text{mean value of the population}}{\text{Standard deviation of the population}}$$

The relationship between percentiles and standard deviation scores may be seen in Figure 31.2. In terms of growth in height, weight or any other anthropometric measure, the first percentile, corresponding to a standard deviation score of −2.2, represents the smallest person, the 50th percentile, a standard deviation of 0, represents the 'average person' and the 99th percentile, corresponding to a standard deviation score of +2.2, represents the largest person.

When anthropometric measurements are considered by age and sex, percentiles and standard deviations can be used for nutrition status surveillance. Examples of such uses are given in Table *evolve* 31.3(b) 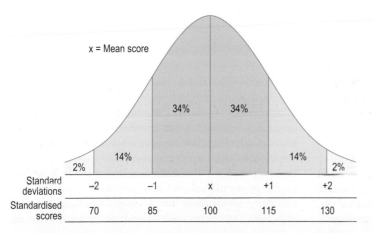. The cut offs of ⊥1, ±2 and ±3 Z-scores, or above or below a given percentile (such as above the 85th or below the 15th percentile of weight for age) can be used as estimates of the level of overnutrition or undernutrition in children and adults, at either individual or population level.

Fig. 31.2 Relationship between percentiles and standard deviation or Z-scores. A normal distribution curve, labelled with the percentage of cases in 6 portions under the curve, the corresponding standard deviations, also called Z-scores, from the mean (median) of the curve, and the standardized scores, or the percentage below or above the mean (median) for the distribution. (Reproduced with kind permission. NFER. http://www.nfer.ac.uk/research-areas/assessment/standardised scores-and-percentile-tanks.cfm.)

x = Mean score

| | 2% | 14% | 34% | 34% | 14% | 2% |

| Standard deviations | −2 | −1 | x | +1 | +2 |
| Standardised scores | 70 | 85 | 100 | 115 | 130 |

31.4 BIOCHEMICAL ASSESSMENT

Christopher J. Bates

OBJECTIVES

- To summarise the available choices of tissue and body fluid samples that may be selected and collected for biochemical status assessment.
- To summarise the necessary precautions to be taken during sample selection, storage and analysis, and to provide an outline of essential fieldwork and laboratory methodologies.
- To highlight some common problems of interpretation, and inter-relationships between the biochemical and other indices of nutritional status, for a composite and integrated picture of status and nutritional adequacy.

As explained in Section 31.1, biochemical assessment ideally forms part of a co-ordinated set of nutritional investigations that may also include diet estimates, anthropometry, functional and clinical investigations. These are used to distinguish between physiological deficiency, adequacy and overload of nutrients, and to assist in the diagnosis of nutrition-related factors that are relevant to the causation and treatment of disease states. The design of the biochemical part of the nutritional assessment depends on there being an available and suitable sample of body fluid or tissue for analysis and feasible biochemical tests to estimate the concentrations or functional adequacy of key nutrients. The results must then be interpreted in the light of established normal ranges. Therefore, it is essential to have access to suitable analytical equipment, suitable laboratory facilities and relevant expertise for sample collection, storage, sample analysis and interpretation. The use of an extensive range of different individual markers is, for instance, exemplified in the design of recent UK nutrition surveys such as the UK National Diet and Nutrition Survey Series, published by the Stationery Office between 1990 and the present time.

BIOCHEMICAL MARKERS OF NUTRITIONAL INTAKE AND STATUS

Biochemical markers are specific diagnostic analytes that can be measured in accessible human body fluids and tissues such as blood, urine, saliva, hair and nails, used as predictors for the different levels of nutrient intake and of tissue status adequacy that occur in human individuals and populations.

Biochemical markers are potentially useful for the following reasons:

- They can often be measured with high specificity and excellent accuracy and objectivity, and unlike diet assessments they can be obtained without reliance on the accuracy of information being provided by the individuals being studied
- They can represent the integral effect of dietary intakes of nutrients from food and supplements over a period of time, ranging from hours up to months or even years before the sample is taken
- Different types of index for each nutrient can specifically reflect either recent intakes or long-term intakes and status, and thus the accumulating risk of functional inadequacy and disease risk. 'Functional' indices, such as plasma homocysteine or dark adaptation, may provide links with the risk of disease or of physiological malfunction, which, in turn, can provide a goal for the definition of nutrient adequacy or optimal nutrition for individual nutrients
- Unlike clinical signs and symptoms of deficiency disease, biochemical markers can be nutrient-specific and can be rapidly and predictably responsive to the correction of nutrient deficiencies. Some, however, may reflect adequacy or deficiency of multiple nutrients, and should be interpreted accordingly
- In a few cases, dietary nutrient intakes can be predicted more accurately from biochemical indices than from diet assessment, especially urinary sodium, potassium and fluoride, used as markers for intakes of these elements, and urinary nitrogen and iodide, used as markers for protein and iodine intakes, respectively (Bates et al 1997, Zimmerman 2008).

Although biochemical marker measurements can be informative on their own, they are even more powerful when combined with nutrient intake estimates and clinical assessments of nutritional adequacy. These three approaches can be likened to different windows providing different but complementary viewpoints on a single landscape, or to different forensic tools combining to build an irrefutable legal case involving a single crime. In combination they can define both 'nutritional adequacy', i.e. freedom from deleterious effects of malnutrition which can threaten health and lead to deficiency disease, and 'optimum nutrition', for which the concept of minimum nutritional adequacy is modified by the concept of variable tissue stores, whose repletion can provide additional insurance against future dietary shortage or increased tissue demand.

The concepts of 'optimum nutrition' and 'normal ranges' are discussed further in Sections *evolve* 31.4a and *evolve* 31.4(b) 📱. The study of genetic subgroups, and how these can be affected differentially by nutrition, comprises the study of gene–nutrient interactions, which is at an early and very exciting stage of research. Recent studies of nutritional genomics, proteomics and metabolomics indicate the potential for new approaches to biochemical index development, provided that the challenges of interpretation can be overcome (see Section 13.4).

The relevance of biochemical status measurements to public health issues is illustrated by the fact that food supply planning and the regulation of fortification and food supplements rely on status measurements in population surveys and controlled intervention studies. A recent example has been the issue of whether to fortify flour with folic acid to reduce the prevalence of neural tube defects in developing embryos (see Chs 15 and 33).

NUTRIENT INDICES AND USEFULNESS FOR PREDICTING INTAKES

Biochemical status indices for individual nutrients

Protein and essential amino acids
There are no good indices for tissue protein status in the sense of reflecting the adequacy of dietary protein as distinct from metabolic processes. The most commonly used index is serum (or plasma) albumin. This is lowered in conditions such as kwashiorkor, attributable to low protein intakes or poor protein quality. However, serum albumin may also be lowered by the acute phase reaction (see Section *evolve* 31.4 📱), and indeed, severely malnourished children commonly also present with infections that affect their acute phase status.

Serum albumin is traditionally measured by a dye-based assay, or by a newer and more specific and reliable immunoassay. An alternative, possibly more reliable index of inadequate protein supply is the plasma amino acid profile, since the 'essential' amino acids, notably the branched-chain amino-acids, are lowered when dietary protein is inadequate. Protein intakes can be monitored fairly accurately by nitrogen excretion rates, although protein is not the only dietary contributor to urinary nitrogen (Bates et al 1997, Bingham 2002).

Essential fatty acid status (and fatty acid profiling)
Serum or plasma is frequently used for fatty acid profiling, and hence for monitoring of essential fatty acid (EFA) intakes. However, its interpretation is complicated by variability of lipoprotein profiles and by diurnal variation. More promising, but less explored, are new techniques for fatty acids in red cell membranes, fat biopsies (reflecting long-term fat store composition), etc. New research into relationships with alternative, 'critical', sites, such as nerve cell membranes, is needed.

Fat-soluble vitamins (see Table *evolve* 31.4(a) 📱)
- Vitamins A and E are commonly measured in serum or plasma, together with the carotenoid pigments, by high-performance liquid chromatography. A low level of plasma retinol is indicative of poor status *only* when acute phase status is normal. A high level may be indicative either of adequate or of marginal status; a low level may be indicative of low status or it may be the consequence of acute-phase infection/inflammatory processes.
- Plasma vitamin E (tocopherol) levels are usually expressed as a ratio to cholesterol or total lipids, since the vitamin E content of plasma is highly dependent on its lipid content, and this ratio is a reasonably reliable indicator of vitamin E status, although it is not ideal in terms of its specificity and sensitivity. Alpha-tocopherol is controlled in a different manner from gamma-tocopherol, so the minor gamma-tocopherol component in plasma (differing from the alpha-form by just one methyl group on the aromatic ring of the vitamin) may give different nutritional information from the major alpha-tocopherol component.
- Vitamin D status is usually assessed by the concentration of 25-hydroxyvitamin D in serum or plasma (Prentice et al 2008). Levels may vary enormously between the seasons and with variable sunlight exposure. Older people in the

UK, especially those in institutions such as nursing homes, are especially vulnerable to inadequate vitamin D status. Their reference nutrient intake (RNI), intended to achieve adequate status, is 10 µg/d, but few people of any age-group in the UK have been found to achieve, or even approach, this intake. Poor vitamin D status is also found in many people from the Indian subcontinent and other (e.g. dark-skinned) people from tropical countries who are now living in the UK.

● Vitamin K status is measured crudely by the rate of blood clotting, or more sensitively and specifically by 'PIVKA' (protein induced by vitamin K absence or antagonism) and recently by vitamin K serum or plasma levels or the degree of under-carboxylation of osteocalcin, a bone-related peptide, in plasma. There is a need for more research on vitamin K indices and their functional interpretation.

Water–soluble vitamins (see Table *evolve* 31.4(b) 📱)

● Vitamin C status is usually measured by serum or plasma vitamin C concentrations or in older studies by the vitamin C content of buffy coat (i.e. unfractionated white cells). The latter index is more closely related to body stores and long-term status for vitamin C, but it requires a cumbersome assay, creating heavy demands for fieldwork. Like the plasma index, it is subject to several ambiguities of interpretation. Despite confounding influences of acute phase processes in some studies, plasma vitamin C has been found to correlate relatively well with recent intakes (the most recent 1–2 weeks) of this vitamin, from foods and supplements.

● Of the B-vitamins, thiamin (B_1), riboflavin (B_2) and pyridoxine (B_6) levels are commonly assessed by the activation coefficients of specific erythrocyte enzymes that require these vitamins as part of the essential cofactors, such as transketolase for thiamin; glutathione reductase for riboflavin, and certain erythrocyte amino acid aminotransferases for the vitamin B_6 coenzymes. For vitamin B_6, direct measurement of plasma or red cell pyridoxal phosphate concentration is often preferred. Folate, vitamin B_{12}, biotin and pantothenic acid status are commonly assessed by serum or plasma concentrations. Red cell folate is a better index of long-term folate intakes and body-stores than plasma or serum folate, but it is more difficult to measure accurately. Niacin status is usually asessed by its urinary breakdown products: *N*-methyl nicotinamide (NMN) or pyridones. Several B vitamins can be assessed by their erythrocyte concentrations, which some investigators now prefer, since they are relatively free from acute phase effects. Unfortunately there is a dearth of published normal ranges and of quality control materials. Several B vitamins have associated functional indices (e.g. homocysteine or methylmalonic acid), which are discussed below.

● Non-vitamin dietary organics, e.g. polyphenols, phytoestrogens, pterins, carnitine, choline, etc., will not be discussed, because studies of their status indices are at a very early stage of development.

● Carotenoids in serum or plasma can be measured by high-performance liquid chromatography in the same assay run as vitamins A and E (see above) and their biological properties are being explored. Alpha and beta-carotenes and beta-cryptoxanthin can be converted in the body to vitamin A; all carotenoids have anti- or pro-oxidant (i.e. redox-modulatory) properties, as do vitamins E, C and several other micronutrients. This has sparked much recent research into their putative roles in modulating chronic disease processes.

Mineral nutrients (see Table *evolve* 31.4(c) 📱)

Macro-essential elements include sodium, potassium, calcium, phosphorus, magnesium and chlorine (Na, K, Ca, P, Mg and Cl). Some of these (notably Na, K) can be monitored by 24h urine collections (Bingham 2002), or, less accurately, by spot urine samples with creatinine as the denominator; others (e.g. Mg) are best studied in blood serum or plasma; yet others (e.g. Ca, P) are best studied in relation to their functional effects – e.g. on bone-related enzymes and bone turnover markers. Micro-essential elements include iron, zinc, copper, selenium, chromium, manganese and iodine (Fe, Zn, Cu, Se, Cr, Mn and I). Zinc can be assessed by plasma zinc levels (Gibson et al 2008) but this index is strongly (negatively) affected by acute phase effects (see Section *evolve* 31.4(e) 📱) and by any reduction in plasma protein concentration, notably albumin. Copper can, albeit with caveats, be assessed by the copper–zinc erythrocyte enzyme superoxide dismutase – however there are no robust status indices for this element. Se can be assessed by serum, plasma or red cell Se levels, or by the selenium enzyme glutathione peroxidase, usually in whole blood or red cells. Chromium and manganese have been assayed in blood fractions, but interpretation is difficult. Direct iodine measurements are usually performed on urine samples; however there are also some plasma analytes (e.g. thyroid-stimulating hormone, thyroglobulin, T_4 and T_3 thyroid hormones and their ratios), which can be used as indirect indicators of iodine status (Zimmerman 2008).

Elements with uncertain physiological roles such as boron, silicon, vanadium, lithium (B, Si, V, Li), etc. have been studied in blood fractions, but little definitive status information is available.

Toxic elements

Aluminium, mercury, lead and cadmium (Al, Hg, Pb, Cd) can be measured in blood: Hg and Pb occur mainly in erythrocytes; Al and Cd occur mainly in plasma.

Functional assays

These are measures of the functional integrity of nutrient-dependent biochemical pathways, as distinct from straightforward concentration assays. There is a growing interest in nutrient-sensitive functional status indices such as plasma homocysteine (responsive to variations in folate, vitamin B_{12} and vitamin B_6 status); plasma methylmalonic acid (responsive to vitamin B_{12} status) and oxidative damage markers (such as malondialdehyde or F_2-isoprostanes) which are modulated by the so-called 'antioxidant' nutrients, e.g. vitamins E, C, the carotenoids and selenium. These physiological damage markers may sometimes be used to predict disease risk, or be used as intermediate end-points for intervention (e.g. supplementation) studies. They are sensitive to variations in nutrient status and may be complemented by physiological or pathological markers, e.g. blood pressure; rates of arterial restenosis; retinal maculopathy, intestinal polyposis, etc., all acting as intermediate indicators of disease risk, disease progression, etc. There are several major ongoing intervention studies that have been designed to determine whether micronutrient supplements, with or without prophylactic pharmaceuticals, can modulate the risk of disease appearance or progression, in high-risk population groups such as smokers, or people exposed to industrial toxins or having a history of or genetic propensity to disease processes such as myocardial infarct, cataract, etc.

VALIDITY, ACCURACY AND REPRODUCIBILITY

To be meaningful, biochemical assays must be valid, accurate and reproducible. However, achieving this goal is neither straightforward nor simple. First, the samples must be adequately collected, separated and stored. For blood samples, one must consider the stability of the analyte and its distribution between the blood components. For example, homocysteine leaches rapidly out of the erythrocytes at room temperature, and the level in plasma then steadily rises. Vitamin C may deteriorate rapidly, especially in separated plasma or serum, through oxidation. Red cell folate deteriorates if stored without a reducing agent (such as vitamin C). Carotenoids and some B-vitamins can be destroyed by light. One must also consider contamination: trace elements may be leached from blood containers, syringes, needles or skin surfaces. Urine samples may require an antimicrobial preservative if collected or stored at room temperature e.g. for 24 h or longer, and they may need a marker for completeness of the 24 h collection, e.g. divided oral doses of para-amino-benzoic acid (PABA) (Bingham 2002). Hair and finger- or toenail samples must be cleaned and must if possible represent a defined period of their growth. Saliva samples must be free of food contaminants. Blood samples for plasma, white cells, red cells, etc. must be treated with an assay-compatible anticoagulant, then separated under controlled conditions of time and temperature and stored, usually frozen at very low temperatures, for example −80°C. Vitamin C needs an acid preservative such as metaphosphoric acid.

The chemical assay or measurement selected must be sufficiently specific (i.e. capable of measuring just a single substance), it must be accurate, precise (i.e. reproducible) and sensitive (i.e. capable of measuring the very low concentrations that typically occur in body fluids). A wide variety of techniques is available, and the art of the analyst is to optimise cost, accuracy, precision and specificity. It may be desirable to measure more than one chemical form of a particular nutrient, e.g. folate or iron. Assays must be monitored by appropriate quality assurance procedures (see Section *evolve* 31.4(c) 🖰). These may include: (i) commercial control samples with assigned values or ranges of analytes, (ii) round robin interlaboratory sample exchange or external quality assurance schemes, which provide consensus values from several laboratories, and (iii) drift control samples monitoring precision and enabling rejection of runs that fall outside pre-determined performance limits. Drift is the tendency for an assay to alter its characteristics, e.g. its sensitivity, often imperceptibly but progressively, over a period of time, which can then give rise to false conclusions. The necessary precautionary measures vary between analytes and, in the absence of external quality assurance schemes, it is important to cross-validate the preferred assays, for example by comparing colorimetric or microbiological assays against 'gold-standard' high-performance liquid chromatography assays, or with mass spectrometric analyses.

When reporting the results of an assay, it is very important to ensure that the units are appropriate, correct and unambiguously stated. In the older literature, many concentration results were given in obscure, often in-house 'units' of concentration, or else in analyte weight per volume, e.g. mg/litre More recently, especially in European countries, molar or SI units (e.g. mmol/litre) have been preferred. The choice of a suitable comparison (i.e. 'normal') range of values is also critical (see Section *evolve* 31.4(b) 🖰). Different laboratories may use slightly different assay procedures, which have only rarely been harmonised between them. The 'population-comparison' or 'normal' range then needs to be laboratory-specific and locally (and frequently) generated and verified. Only where the assay has been well-harmonised between laboratories can a broadly accepted population comparison or normal range be used.

Another common pitfall is to assume that the only influences on blood nutrient levels are variations in intake and in tissue stores – however another powerful influence is the common acute phase reaction (caused by infection and inflammation), see below. Some blood nutrient concentrations increase, whereas others fall during an acute phase reaction (see Section *evolve* 31.4(e) 🖰); however, they usually return to their original levels when the condition improves. This is a very common cause of misinterpretation of 'abnormal' indices. Thus a high ferritin concentration may imply iron sufficiency, but it may also arise through inflammation, so that a combination of iron status markers, e.g. serum transferrin receptors and/or free erythrocyte porphyrin, will then be needed, so as to help avoid erroneous conclusions. The acute phase reaction can be monitored by variations in acute phase protein concentrations in plasma. Erythrocyte (i.e. red-blood-cell-derived) indices seem to be less vulnerable to this source of ambiguity than are many plasma nutrient concentrations.

Temporal variations

Many blood and urine nutrients exhibit 24-hour- and seasonal-cycles, which can be a source of misinterpretation. Thus a sample taken at one time of day or one season may yield a conclusion that is quite different from that at a different time-point. Therefore, representative surveys need to span a range of collection times, especially if there is a big seasonal variation in climate and food availability. There may be secular changes over longer time periods, attributable to changing climatic conditions or changing lifestyles, food imports, etc., which need to be monitored by periodic or regularly repeated surveys. The effects of public health interventions, such as the fortification of flour or the removal of lead from petrol, may be overlaid by natural fluctuations or drift over time. Therefore, the reliable monitoring of intervention effectiveness must take such fluctuations and drift effects into account.

Compartments and sample types

The fundamental aim of biochemical monitoring is to define whole body adequacy for specific nutrients. However, the practicalities of assessment usually limit the researcher to readily accessible fluids and surface tissues. The relationship between these and the critically vulnerable internal organs is complex, modulated by blood homeostasis or selective and controlled excretion. For example, it is futile to measure the iron content of urine, since urine does not reflect body stores or iron intakes. Certain mineral elements, notably calcium, copper and zinc (Bates et al 1997, Gibson et al 2008) lack satisfactory biochemical indices, partly because the most vulnerable tissues and compartments cannot easily be monitored. For most vitamins, on the other hand, there are blood indices that adequately reflect body stores and/or intakes. For some nutrients, notably the alkali metals (sodium, potassium) and iodine and fluorine, urinary excretion is a good measure of recent intake, but for most other nutrients, urine is useless as a source of status or intake information. Other potential sources of information for some nutrients include hair, nails, cheek cell scrapings, white blood cells and saliva (for further information on compartments and sample types see Section *evolve* 31.4(d) ⬛).

FACTORS AFFECTING THE RELATIONSHIP BETWEEN NUTRITIONAL STATUS INDICES AND INTAKES

Many unexpected pitfalls have been encountered when attempting to predict nutrient intakes from biochemical status indices. They have included:

1. Intakes and status indices having different time-courses from each other, and also differing responses to the effects of various confounding factors. To monitor a relationship between a nutrient intake and the corresponding biochemical status index reliably, it is advisable to estimate the diet immediately before the collection of samples for status analysis. The optimum diet estimation period may be a few hours or several weeks or months, depending on the rate of turnover of the compartment and the analyte.

2. Other confounding factors affecting the relationships between nutrient intake and status index values include:

   - Variable chemical forms and stabilities of nutrients in food and of analytes in status samples

   - Variable absorption efficiency and bioavailability; confounding effects of nutrient interactions. For instance, iron absorption is positively enhanced by vitamin C and by protein, but is negatively influenced by phytate, tannins, large quantities of other divalent metal ions, etc.

   - Variable rates of turnover, i.e. breakdown; variable distribution between body compartments; variable excretion rates and pathways. For instance, vitamin C and folate turnover rates are increased by smoking; vitamin A excretion is increased during infection

   - Effect of homeostatic mechanisms, especially in the blood and tissues. For instance, plasma calcium is maintained within narrow limits by hormonally controlled mechanisms which

extract it from, or deposit it in, calcified tissues such as bone; plasma retinol is maintained within narrow limits in adequately supplied individuals, mainly by homeostatic control of plasma retinol binding protein concentrations; plasma sodium and potassium levels are likewise homeostatically controlled by the adrenal mineralocorticoid hormones

   - Variable tissue growth rates at sites such as nails and hair, which affects the interpretation of hair or nail concentrations, e.g. of trace elements

   - Problems of sample contamination, especially for trace element work

   - Effects of age, gender, ethnic group, genetic polymorphisms, etc., on status index values and their normal ranges

   - Acute phase effects on biochemical status indices (see Section *evolve* 31.4(e) ⬛).

MARKERS OF NUTRIENT INTAKE

It is important to understand that, although many nutrient-related biochemical indices are influenced by corresponding nutrient intakes, some are not, for example because variable absorption, homeostatic control or nutrient turnover or excretion may perturb the predicted intake : status relationships. Therefore the following subdivision is proposed:

1. For a few nutrients there can be a relatively reliable prediction of intakes from status measurements: e.g. of nitrogen intake from nitrogen excretion in timed urine collections; of Na, K, I, F intakes from urinary Na, K, I, F excretion rates over a 24 h collection period (Bates et al 1997).

2. For a further set of nutrients the biochemical markers predict only approximate intake categories (e.g. high, medium or low) but cannot provide a precise quantitative estimate of intakes. These probably include plasma vitamin C, the plasma carotenoids, and plasma or blood levels of B vitamins. Some markers are capable of predicting intake categories only if other supply sources are minimal: for example, plasma 25(OH)vitamin D can predict vitamin D intake, provided that irradiation sources do not make a major contribution (Prentice et al 2008). Some indices can distinguish between inadequate and adequate intakes but not between adequate and high intakes: these

probably include plasma retinol and plasma zinc. Others can distinguish between adequate and high intakes but not between deficient and marginally adequate intakes: these probably include urinary thiamin, riboflavin and vitamin C (Bates et al 1997).

3. Markers that are essentially useless as indicators of intake, except under very strictly defined circumstances and with additional markers or precautions: these include plasma levels of many mineral elements, e.g. calcium, sodium, potassium and copper. By contrast, plasma iron, zinc, magnesium and selenium can provide both useful status information and

some prediction of nutrient intakes (Gibson et al 2008, Zimmerman 2008).

In conclusion, the biochemical markers of nutrient intakes and tissue status are potentially powerful tools, but are often subject to misuse and misinterpretation. They can provide valuable objective nutritional information, to help bridge the gap between diet on the one hand and diet-related disease on the other, but to do so they require careful choice, measurement and interpretation. There are thus many exciting and important opportunities for new research in this field. For further information on analytical techniques for blood vitamin and mineral status see Section *evolve* 31.4(d).

KEY POINTS

- Biochemical indices of nutrient status may, in certain cases, reflect recent intakes, or they may reflect body stores, or a combination of these. They can fulfil the need for objective assessments of nutrient adequacy, at the whole body level.
- However, confounding factors such as homeostatic mechanisms, acute phase effects, uneven distribution of nutrients between body compartments, etc. can confuse interpretation, unless these modulating factors are properly understood and allowed for.

- A lack of proper precautions during measurement can result in incorrect measurements and conclusions.
- Despite these caveats, carefully selected and properly validated biochemical indices provide a powerful and valuable adjunct to other evidence of nutritional adequacy or inadequacy for individuals and populations. They form an essential component of nutritional research and of public health surveillance programmes.

References

Dietary assessment

Adamson AJ, Collerton J, Davies K, et al, and the Newcastle 85+ study core team: Nutrition in advanced age: dietary assessment in the Newcastle 85+ study, *European Journal of Clinical Nutrition* 63:S6–S18, 2009.

Biró G, Hulshof KFAM, Ovesen L, Amorim Cruz JA, for the EFCOSUM group: Selection of methodology to assess food intake, *European Journal of Clinical Nutrition* 56(Suppl 2):S25–S32, 2002.

Cameron ME, van Staveren WA, editors: *Manual on methodology for food consumption studies*, Oxford, 1988, Oxford University Press.

Department for the Environment, Food and Rural Affairs: *National Food Survey 2000*, London, 2002, The Stationery Office.

Food and Agricultural Organization of the United Nations: *Food balance data*. Rome, 2010, FAO United Nations, available on line at: http://faostat.fao.org.

Gibson R: *Principles of nutritional assessment*, Oxford, 1990, Oxford University Press.

Holmes B, Dick K, Nelson M: A comparison of four dietary assessment methods in materially deprived households in England, *Public Health Nutrition* 11:444–456, 2008.

Lagiou P, Trichopoulou A, DAFNE contributors: DAta Food NEtworking. The DAFNE initiative: the methodology for assessing dietary patterns across Europe using household budget survey data, *Public Health Nutrition* 4(5B):1135–1141, 2001.

Livingstone MBE, Robson P: Measurement of dietary intake in children, *Proceedings of the Nutrition Society* 59:279–293, 2000.

Margetts BM, Nelson M: *Design concepts in nutritional epidemiology*, ed 2, Oxford, 1997, Oxford University Press.

National Institutes of Health: *National Children's Study dietary assessment literature review*. Applied research program and Westat, Rockville, MD, 2007, National Institutes of Health, ch 2. Available on line at: http://riskfactor.cancer.gov/tools/children/review/pdf/

Nelson M, Beresford S: Nutritional epidemiology. In Kohlmeier L, Margetts BM, editors: *Public health nutrition*, London, 2003, Nutrition Society.

Thompson FE, Subar AF: Dietary assessment methodology. In Coulston AM, Boushey CJ, editors: *Nutrition in the prevention and treatment of disease*, ed 2, San Diego, 2008, Academic Press.

Anthropometry

Bogin B, Varela-Silva MI: Leg Length, Body Proportion, and Health: A Review with a Note on Beauty, *International Journal of Environmental Research and Public Health* 7:1047–1075, 2010.

Chen X, Hess S: Adipose proteome analysis: focus on mediators of insulin resistance, *Expert Review of Proteomics* 5:827–839, 2008.

Cole TJ, Freeman JV, Preece MA: Body mass index reference curves for the UK, 1990, *Archives of Disease in Childhood* 73:25–29, 1995.

Frisancho AR: *Anthropometric standards: an interactive nutritional reference of body size and body composition for children and adults*, Ann Arbor, MI, 2008, University of Michigan Press.

Gorstein J, Sullivan K, Yip R, et al: Issues in the assessment of nutritional status using anthropometry, *Bulletin of the World Health Organization* 273–283, 1994.

Lu J-M, Wang M-JJ: Automated anthropometric data collection using 3D whole body scanners *Expert Systems with Applications, An International Journal* 35:407–414, 2008.

Shetty PS, James WPT: *Body mass index. A measure of chronic energy deficiency in adults.* FAO Food and Nutrition Paper No. 56, Rome, 1994, Food and Agriculture Organization.

Waterlow JC, Buzina A, Keller W, et al: The presentation and use of height and weight data for comparing the nutritional status of groups of children under the age of 10 years, *Bulletin of the World Health Organization* 55:489–498, 1977.

Biochemical

Bates CJ, Thurnham DI, Bingham SA, Margetts BM, Nelson M: Biochemical markers of nutrient intake. In Margetts BM, Nelson M, editors: *Design concepts in nutritional epidemiology*, ed 2, Oxford, 1997, Oxford University Press, pp 170–240.

Bingham SA: Biomarkers in nutritional epidemiology, *Public Health Nutrition* 5:821–827, 2002.

Gibson RS, Hess SY, Holz C, Brown KH: Indicators of zinc status at the population level, *British Journal of Nutrition* 99(Suppl 3):S14–S23, 2008.

Prentice A, Goldberg GR, Schoenmakers I: Vitamin D across the life cycle: physiology, and biomarkers, *American Journal of Clinical Nutrition* 88(Suppl):500S–506S, 2008.

Zimmerman MB: Methods to assess iron and iodine stastus, *British Journal of Nutrition* 99(Suppl 3):S2–S9, 2008.

Further reading

Dietary assessment

Margetts BM, Nelson M: *Design concepts in nutritional epidemiology*, ed 2, Oxford, 1997, Oxford University Press.

European Journal of Clinical Nutrition: Supplement on 'Dietary Assessment at the Ends of Life's Spectrum', February 2009.

Anthropometry

Bogin B: *Patterns of human growth*, ed 2, Cambridge, 1999, Cambridge University Press.

Gorstein J, Sullivan K, Yip R, et al: Issues in the assessment of nutritional status using anthropometry, *Bulletin of the World Health Organization* 273–283, 1994.

Margetts BM, Nelson M: *Design concepts in nutritional epidemiology*, ed 2, Oxford, 1997, Oxford University Press.

World Health Organization: *Physical status: the use and interpretation of anthropometry.* WHO Technical Report Series Number 854, Geneva, 1995, World Health Organization.

Biochemical

Bates CJ: Vitamins/fat-soluble; Vitamin/water soluble, analysis of. In Worsfeld P, Townshend A, Poole C, editors: *Encyclopedia of analytical chemistry: applications, theory and instrumentation*, ed 2, Oxford, 2005, Academic Press, pp 159–180.

Gibson RS: *Principles of nutritional assessment*, Oxford, 1990, Oxford University Press, p 691.

Hesketh J: Nutrigenomics and selenium: gene expression patterns, physiological targets and genetics, *Annual Review of Nutrition* 28:157–178, 2008.

Sauberlich HE: *Laboratory tests for the assessment of nutritional status*, Boca Raton, FL, 1999, CRC Press, p 486.

Chapter 32

Food supply, factors affecting production, trade and access

Marc J Cohen

CHAPTER CONTENTS

OBJECTIVES

By the end of this chapter, you should be able to:
- compare world food supply with population needs
- give examples of past scares about the adequacy of world food supply, and the reasons for their resolution
- discuss the socioeconomic, agroecological and health constraints on future food production
- explain the factors impeding access to food
- discuss the causes and impacts of increased food prices in the late 2000s
- show how globalisation relates to food security

© 2010 Elsevier Ltd/Inc/BV
DOI: 10.1016/B978-0-7020-3118-2.00032-2

- demonstrate the multiple functions of agricultural and rural development in achieving equitable and sustainable food security
- elucidate the role of various approaches to agricultural research, including biotechnology, in achieving food security
- make clear the relationship between sustainable natural resource management and food security
- define the terms food security, food insecurity, food supply, food demand, hunger, famine, Green Revolution and entitlements.

32.1 INTRODUCTION

At the 1996 World Food Summit, high-level representatives of 186 nations and the European Union, including over 100 heads of state and government, agreed to the Rome Declaration on World Food Security, which states:

> We consider it intolerable that more that 800 million people throughout the world, and particularly in developing countries, do not have enough food to meet their basic nutritional needs. This situation is unacceptable. Food supplies have increased substantially, but constraints on access to food, instability of supply and demand, as well as natural and man-made disasters, prevent basic food needs from being fulfilled.

Fourteen years on, food insecurity has worsened in the developing world, and there is serious doubt as to whether it will be possible to achieve the Summit's goal of halving the number of hungry people from 1990 levels by no later than 2015, or the related Millennium Development Goal of reducing hunger and poverty by half by that same year. Absolute food shortages are much less of a concern today than in the past, and food production and stocks remain more than adequate to meet everyone's minimum calorie requirements. Rather, *access* to food is the critical problem. Compounding low incomes and lack of productive resources among food-insecure populations is the more recent issue of the use of food and feed crops to produce energy; this contributed to higher food prices in 2007 and 2008.

Despite overall supply-side adequacy, many analysts continue to worry that human population growth will outpace the earth's ability to produce adequate food supplies. This concern, voiced by Thomas R. Malthus in 1798, remains a preoccupation over two centuries later (Brown 2003), notwithstanding the successful role of science, technology and public policy in addressing this dilemma. Growing demand for animal products in the developing world (World Bank 2007) further fuels concern about overburdening the earth's 'carrying capacity'.

A decade into the twenty-first century, the paradoxical nature of contemporary food insecurity is all too clear: the overwhelming majority of the world's hungry people live in rural areas and depend on food production and other agricultural activities for their livelihood. Growing integration of global markets, combined with revolutionary advances in transportation and communications, holds great promise for better matching food supplies and needs. But rich-country farm subsidies and trade barriers make it difficult for poor farmers in developing countries to reap potential gains.

This chapter examines whether technological and institutional innovation will continue to allow food production to keep pace with population growth and rising food demand, as well as the environmental costs that this will entail. It also focuses on access to food and the bearing that globalisation has on food security. The chapter concludes by looking at the policy actions needed to achieve food security in developing countries – particularly the importance of broad-based agricultural and rural development – while ensuring sustainable management of the natural resource base upon which food production depends. For a review of publications on food supply see Section *evolve* 32.1.

32.2 DEFINITION OF FOOD SECURITY

According to the Food and Agriculture Organization of the United Nations (FAO), '*Food security* exists when all people, at all times, have physical and economic access to sufficient, safe, and nutritious food to meet their dietary needs and food preferences for an active and healthy life'. This definition is in keeping with the principle that everyone has a right to adequate food, to be free from hunger and to enjoy general human dignity, enshrined in the International Bill of Human Rights. *Food insecurity*, then, is the absence of food security. *Hunger*, a condition in which people lack the basic food intake to provide them with the energy and nutrients for fully productive, active lives, is an outcome of food insecurity.

The availability of adequate food is a necessary condition for achieving food security, but it is not sufficient. Of equal importance are *access to food, appropriate utilisation of food* and the *stability* of both availability and access (FAO 2006). Thus, even when food supplies are satisfactory, food insecurity may persist because people lack access, whether by means of production, purchase, public social safety net programmes, private charity or some combination of these, to available food. In addition, people may fail to consume sufficient quantities of food or a balanced diet even when supplies are ample (see Section *evolve* 32.2 on food insecurity in sub-Saharan Africa 🖱). Sudden shocks (such as an economic or climatic crisis) or cyclical events (such as seasonal food insecurity) may cause a loss of access to food.

KEY POINTS

■ Food security requires more than just adequate food availability; it also is a matter of access to the food that is available, its appropriate utilisation and the stability of availability and access.

32.3 WORLD FOOD SUPPLY

PAST TRENDS AND CURRENT SUPPLY SITUATION

Scholars and policy-makers alike have long worried about how to balance food supplies with the demands of a rapidly growing population. Malthus claimed that population increases by a geometric ratio, whereas food production only increases by an arithmetic ratio, and thereby exerts a natural 'check' on population growth. Malthusian worries may have reached their apogee in the late 1960s and early 1970s. Then, analysts wrote off much of Asia as 'a hopeless basket case'. The threat of famine gripped West and Central Africa, Ethiopia and Bangladesh, and it seemed as though Malthus's 'check' had kicked in with a vengeance. The popular press in the industrialised countries turned out tomes on 'lifeboat ethics' and 'triage'.

The Green Revolution

In fact, food availability rose dramatically between 1961 and 2004, and by the latter year, global har-vests and stocks offered more than enough calories per person per day to meet minimum requirements, if the food were distributed according to need. Per capita production and agricultural productivity rose during this period, while prices for key food commodities fell (World Bank 2007). The key factor controverting Malthusian predictions was a rapid increase in the output of cereals, the main source of calories in developing countries, as farmers in Asia and Latin America widely adopted high-yielding varieties, and governments, especially in Asia, implemented policies that supported agricultural development. By 2002, developing-country cereal harvests, at 1.2 billion tonnes, were triple those of 40 years earlier, while the population was a little over twice as large. Daily per capita calorie supplies in the developing world jumped from 2140, barely above the minimum requirement for light activity of 2100, in 1970 to 2669 in 2003. However, calorie availability per person remained only minimally adequate in sub-Saharan Africa and barely above the threshold in south Asia (Rosegrant et al 2001; FAOSTAT database 2008). It is important to note that these figures say nothing about how the available food is actually distributed.

Yield gains – attributable to a great extent to farmer adoption of high-yielding cereal crop varieties bred at international agricultural research centres and adapted to local conditions at national agricultural research institutions – accounted for much of the increase in cereal output and calorie availability. Area expansion played a much less important role. Planting of these varieties coincided with expansion of irrigated area and fertiliser use; this process is called the *Green Revolution*. Production increased broadly in the developing world, especially in Asia, including South Asia, with sub-Saharan Africa lagging behind (Fig. 32.1) (World Bank 2007) (see Section *evolve* 32.3(a) on the Green Revolution 🖱).

This evidence tends to support the views of anti-Malthusians, who argue that population growth spurs technological and institutional innovations to address the problems of resource scarcity.

Socioeconomic and environmental impact of the Green Revolution

Initial studies of the socioeconomic impact of the Green Revolution suggested that large-scale farmers were the main adopters, while small farmers often lost out because larger harvests meant lower prices.

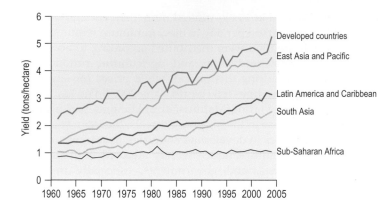

Fig. 32.1 Developing country cereal yields, 1960–2005. *Source: World Bank.*

Also, some analysts contended that the technology encouraged mechanisation, resulting in rural job losses. In fact, small farmers adopted high-yielding seeds after witnessing larger farmers' success with the new varieties. In Asia, new breeding efforts developed seeds more suitable to the needs of poorer farmers (e.g. with less need for purchased inputs), and policies sought to improve provision to small farmers of services such as extension, credit, marketing and access to inputs. Production gains generally created more non-farm rural employment opportunities than were lost. Cereal prices did decline substantially: between 1982 and 1997, world wheat prices dropped 28% in real terms, rice prices 29% and maize prices 30% (Rosegrant et al 2001). Food prices generally continued to fall in real terms through 2002. Lower prices benefited non-farm poor consumers in rural areas and cities alike, as well as poor farmers who were net purchasers of food (as most poor farmers are in many developing countries). Even farmers who produced more than they consumed gained, as technological advances reduced unit costs of production and hence increased profits. From 2002 to mid-2008, however, food prices rose steeply.

The Green Revolution had environmental benefits as well. Increased yields on existing farmland alleviated the need to clear new land in order to boost production. This is estimated to have preserved over 300 million hectares (equivalent to more than the combined total farmland of the USA, Canada and Brazil) of forests and grasslands, including considerable wildlife habitat, thereby conserving biodiversity and limiting atmospheric releases of carbon that can cause global warming.

At the same time, widespread planting of high-yielding varieties of cereal crops in some instances has contributed to environmental problems, such as increased soil salinity and lowered water tables in irrigated areas; water, air and soil degradation resulting from excessive agricultural input use; and human health problems due to heavy pesticide use. Harm to non-target species from pesticides offset some of the biodiversity gains (World Bank 2007, Rosegrant et al 2001).

Recent cereals supply trends

Between 2000 and 2007, demand for cereals exceeded supply, and stocks fell (Fig. 32.2). Partly in response to higher food prices in 2007 and 2008 (see below), global cereal production set a record in 2008, rising by an estimated 2.8%. Production was forecast to exceed utilization in 2008/9, allowing the rebuilding of global stocks.

Supply trend of non-cereal crops

There is some evidence that increased cereal output has come at the expense of pulses and vegetables that could improve dietary quality. In Bangladesh, real cereal prices declined by 40% between 1975 and 2000, thanks to widespread adoption of Green Revolution varieties, but prices for lentils, vegetables and animal products increased by 25–50%.

Related to this, there was concern in the 1960s and 1970s that protein deficiency was the main nutrition problem in developing countries. This led to a major plant breeding effort aimed at developing 'protein quality' maize in the early 1970s. However, by mid-decade, nutritionists came to agree that insufficient calorie intake was the cause of the apparent 'protein gap' rather than deficiency of protein per se (see Section *evolve* 32.3(b) on the 'protein gap'). Breeding thereafter focused on

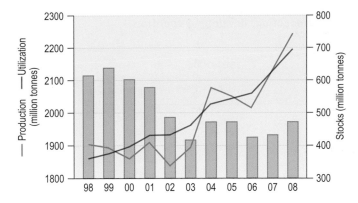

Fig. 32.2 Cereal production, utilization and stocks.
Source: FAO (Food Outlook Nov. 2008)

increasing the calorie supply by increasing the quantity of cereals available rather than their quality. Since the late 1990s, breeders have renewed their focus on nutritional quality with efforts to develop micronutrient-dense staples.

While cereals and livestock products are the main dietary staples, many poor people in developing countries rely on root and tuber crops such as cassava, yams and potatoes, either as their main staple or as a supplementary source of calories, vitamins and protein. In sub-Saharan Africa, root and tuber consumption accounts for 20% of caloric intake, and cassava is the staple of 200 million people, second only to maize as the leading source of calories. Roots and tubers are also a key part of the diet in the poorer western provinces of China, such as Sichuan, and in poverty-stricken northeast Brazil. These crops, particularly cassava, are viewed as 'crisis foods' by poor consumers, who may switch to consumption of these cheaper foods when cereal prices rise prohibitively. Poor farmers value cassava roots because they can be stored in the ground for up to 18 months (FAO 2008a). Cassava is vegetatively propagated and so requires no purchased inputs. Production was forecast to rise by 5% in 2008, following a record crop the previous year.

In contrast to cereals, there has been little research to develop yield-increasing technology for root and tuber crops. Yields grew only 1% per year between 1967 and 1997, compared to cereal yield growth of 2–3% in most developing regions during the same period, and the growth rate for roots and tubers slowed in the 1990s. However, potato yields and area planted both grew at about twice the rate for all root and tuber crops during the same period, given the larger commercial markets available, and commercial production of cassava for use

as starch and feed is increasing (Rosegrant et al 2001, FAO 2008a).

FUTURE SUPPLY OUTLOOK

Cereals output is expected to grow steadily through 2017, and aggregate global food supplies should remain adequate to meet minimum needs (OECD/ FAO 2008). However, stocks will not be replenished substantially between 2008 and 2017. Climate change is likely to lead to more variable weather and food production. Growth rates of cereal yields have slowed substantially since the early 1980s, falling to 1% per year for wheat and maize and even less for rice (Table 32.1). In the absence of major technological breakthroughs, even slower growth is expected during 2008–2017 (OECD/FAO 2008, World Bank 2007, Rosegrant et al 2001).

POPULATION GROWTH

Despite expansion of global food supplies, fears of an imbalance between population growth and food production endure. According to United Nations projections, world population is expected to increase by 37% between 2007 and 2050, from 6.7 billion to 9.2 billion. This represents a downward revision from past projections, due to the devastating impact of HIV/AIDS in severely affected countries, especially in sub-Saharan Africa (for expanded section see Section *evolve* 32.3(c) Population growth).

SUBSISTENCE AND COMMERCIAL AGRICULTURAL SYSTEMS

Farming systems in developing countries, and especially those in which low-income and small-

Table 32.1   Growth (%) of cereal yields, area and production, developing countries, 1970–2005

	1970–1990			1990–2005		
	Yield	Area	Production	Yield	Area	Production
Rice	2.35	0.49	2.84	0.92	0.31	1.23
Wheat	3.75	0.88	4.62	1.27	−0.35	0.91
Maize	2.65	0.97	3.61	1.64	0.66	2.3
All Cereals	2.68	0.73	3.41	1.2	0.21	1.41

Source: FAO.

scale farmers are engaged, can be conceptualised as lying on a continuum between pure subsistence agriculture, in which farmers produce exclusively for the farm family's consumption, and pure commercial farming, in which producers sell 100% of output on the market. In practice, most small-scale farms in developing countries undertake a mix of self-provisioning and production for the market. To the extent that farmers produce for the market and specialise, they take on additional market-related risks. Small farmers may address some of the problems they face by moving toward commercialisation through collective action, e.g. by forming cooperatives to gain access to inputs, markets or services. Commercial production frequently means gains in income, which in turn may lead to improvements in household nutrition. Realities on the ground in developing countries involve a vast variety of locations on the above subsistence to commercialisation continuum and an equal variety of outcomes in terms of profitability and food and nutrition security.

CONSTRAINTS TO PRODUCTION

Small farmers in developing countries face many problems in their struggle for sustainable livelihoods. These include socioeconomic, political, agroecological and health constraints.

Socioeconomic and political factors

Among the socioeconomic and political limitations on food production are public policies and investments that are biased against poor farmers and consumers, women and less-favoured areas; inadequate infrastructure; inequitable access to land and other critical resources; poorly functioning and poorly integrated markets; and lack of access to credit and technical assistance.

Whether or not people own assets, such as land or livestock, makes a critical difference to whether they will be poor and food-insecure, as well as whether they will be able to produce food for themselves or for sale. Rural land ownership is extremely unequal in Latin America, despite extensive land reform efforts, and in some countries in sub-Saharan Africa, such as Kenya, South Africa, Zimbabwe and Malawi. Worldwide, landless rural people who depend on wage income tend to be among those most likely to be poor, although in sub-Saharan Africa smallholder farmers are just as likely to be poor. When poor people do own land, it is generally of poor quality, with less certain access to water and less secure rights. When poor people have secure rights to assets such as land, water, credit, information and technology, they are more likely to invest in land management and sustainable natural resource use. Secure ownership or use rights over land mean that poor people have more stable incomes (either in the form of food directly consumed or the cash from selling their produce), and farm output often rises once secure property rights are in place (IFAD 2001).

Women play a central role as producers of food, managers of natural resources, income earners and caretakers of household food security and nutrition. In sub-Saharan Africa, women farmers produce about 75% of the domestically grown food, but have less access to education and to labour, fertiliser and other inputs than men do, and often face restrictions on their right to own or control land. In both Africa and Latin America, extension services and technical assistance focus primarily on male farmers. In Burkina Faso, men and children provide more labour to farm plots controlled by men than to women's plots, while women primarily contribute the labour on plots they control. Women's plots have 20–30% lower yields. Research confirms that total household agricultural output would increase if there were more equitable allocation of labour and inputs. Agricultural productivity increases dramatically when women get the same amount of inputs as men. When female African farmers obtain the same levels of education, experience, access to services such as extension and farm inputs that currently benefit male farmers, they increase their yields for maize, beans and cowpeas (all crops consumed by poor people) by 22% over current levels. In Kenya, a year of primary education provided to all women farmers would boost overall maize yields by 24%. In Burkina Faso, total household agricultural output could increase by 10–20% if currently used inputs were reallocated from men's to women's plots (Quisumbing 2003).

In addition, the social status and degree of empowerment of women has a direct bearing on the sustainability of natural resource management. To the extent that rural women enjoy ownership or control over land, the more likely they are to undertake natural-resource-conserving measures. Poor rural women also often expend much time and effort in fetching fuel, usually in the form of wood, for cooking, lighting and agricultural processing. Affordable technologies that reduce the time and effort women need to spend searching for fuel allow them to spend more time on other tasks, e.g. child care. At the same time, the development of affordable alternatives to wood as an energy source can reduce deforestation. In a similar 'win–win' approach, integrated pest management technologies can help protect natural resources while also reducing the time women and children must spend weeding crops (Quisumbing 2003).

Poor and food-insecure people frequently lack political voice and organisations that are accountable to them and capable of articulating their interests to policy-makers and other power holders. As a result, policies tend to benefit people who are already well off, and policy-makers tend to give low priority to the needs of poor and hungry people or programmes that would benefit them. A World Bank (2001) report based on extensive interviews of poor people in developing and transition countries found that they regard their situation as one where freedom and the power to control one's life are lacking. A low-income Jamaican woman compared poverty to 'living in jail, living in bondage, waiting to be free'.

Agroecological constraints

In many developing countries, poverty, low agricultural productivity and environmental degradation interact in a vicious downward spiral. This is especially pronounced in resource-poor areas that are experiencing high rates of population growth and are home to hundreds of millions of food-insecure people, particularly in south Asia and sub-Saharan Africa, as well as on the hillsides of Central America and southeast Asia. Agricultural growth, poverty alleviation and environmental sustainability are not necessarily complementary. Poor farmers throughout the developing world often face low soil fertility and lack of access to plant nutrients, along with variable weather and acid, salinated and waterlogged soils that contribute to low yields, production risks and natural resource degradation (Pender & Hazell 2000).

Less-favoured areas may be 'less-favoured' by nature or by humans. They include lands that have low agricultural potential because of limited and uncertain rainfall, poor soils, steep slopes or other biophysical constraints, as well as areas that may have high agricultural potential but have limited access to infrastructure and markets, low population density or other socioeconomic constraints. Although only 40% of the rural population of the developing world lives in these areas, in sub-Saharan Africa the figure is 67%. Low agricultural productivity and land degradation are severe and deforestation, overgrazing and soil erosion and soil nutrient depletion are widespread.

Some natural resource degradation in agricultural areas has been caused by the misuse of modern farming inputs (especially pesticides, fertilisers and irrigation water in high-potential areas). But a great deal of environmental degradation is concentrated in resource-poor areas that have not adopted modern technology.

Globally, degradation between 1945 and 1990 caused cumulative crop productivity losses of 5%, with mean reductions for sub-Saharan Africa of 6.2% (World Bank 2007, Rosegrant et al 2001, Pender & Hazell 2000). Losses to pests reduce potential farm output value by 50%. In developing countries, losses greatly exceed agricultural aid received.

Better management of farm inputs can reduce their negative environmental effects without a loss in farm yields. This includes integrated pest management, judicious use of synthetic pesticides and pest-resistant plant varieties, improved application of fertilizers and water and no- or low-tillage crop management.

Unless properly managed, fresh water may well emerge as the key constraint to global food production, particularly in central and western Asia, North Africa and much of sub-Saharan Africa, where population growth is expected to continue to be high and exploitable per capita water resources are quite low. While water supplies are adequate in the aggregate to meet demand for the foreseeable future, water is poorly distributed across countries, within countries, between seasons and among multiple uses. Agriculture accounts for 85% of water consumption in developing countries, and irrigated agriculture supplies about 40% of world food production. About 1.4 billion people live in river basins where water use exceeds minimum recharge levels; because of excessive withdrawals, a number of large rivers no longer reach the sea during a part of the year. Overuse of groundwater leads to falling water tables and saline intrusion, making further cultivation of large swaths of land impossible.

The International Food Policy Research Institute (IFPRI) projects that, between 1995 and 2025, developing countries will increase water withdrawals by 27%. Industrial and household water use will increase by 62%, largely at the expense of agricultural use, which will only grow by 4%. This will result in 300 million tonnes less irrigated cereal production, a volume equivalent to the entire 2000 US cereal harvest. As a result, developing-country cereal imports will more than double. If water use is even less efficient, a water crisis could result, with an additional 10% decline in worldwide cereal production, dramatic increases in cereal prices and a substantial increase in food insecurity.

There is now scientific agreement that climate change and variability will have substantial negative effects on food security and nutrition, particularly because of more frequent and intense droughts and floods, which will reduce dietary diversity and food consumption and increase the incidence of diarrhoeal and other infectious diseases. Deforestation and agricultural activities in developing countries account for over 20% of the greenhouse gas emissions that can cause climate change. Climate change is likely to exacerbate declining reliability of irrigation water supplies and competition for water. Agricultural output in developing countries is expected to decline by 10–20% by 2080 as a result. The United Nations projects that up to 50 million people will flee environmental deterioration by 2020, possibly leading to food and water emergencies, ill health and malnutrition and increased likelihood of conflict (World Bank 2007, Cohen et al 2008).

Appropriate agricultural practices can mitigate climate change by increasing soil carbon sinks and reducing greenhouse gas emissions, at low cost. These practices include reduced deforestation, more sustainable forest management and adoption of agroforestry which integrates tree and crop cultivation (Cohen et al 2008) (for expanded version see Section *evolve* 32.3(d) Agroecological constraints).

Health constraints

Infectious disease has a significant bearing on food production, especially in sub-Saharan Africa. Nearly 40 million people are currently living with HIV/AIDS, which causes about 3 million deaths annually. It has contributed to labour shortages (from those afflicted and those affected, i.e. caring for the afflicted), a decline in the transfer of farmer knowledge across generations, weaker collective action, weaker property rights, a declining asset base, breakdown of social bonds, loss of livestock, and reliance on crops that are easier to produce but less nutritious and economically valuable. A majority of the people affected by HIV/AIDS work in agriculture. Because malaria often strikes during harvest time, it also threatens food output; the disease kills around a million people a year.

In order to cope with the effects of HIV/AIDS on agriculture and food security, as labour becomes depleted, new cultivation technologies and varieties need to be developed that do not rely so much on labour, yet allow crops to remain drought-resistant and nutritious. Innovations such as farmer field schools can facilitate the transfer of community-specific and organisation-specific knowledge within and between generations. Making institutions, including agricultural research centres, more client-focused can help natural resource management remain effective in the presence of weakened social capital (i.e. the norms and networks that allow collective action, especially at the community level) and property rights. For example, where there are large numbers of women widowed by AIDS, gender-equitable land ownership rights are ever more important.

Agricultural practices also pose threats to health. Irrigation increases the spread of malaria, and pesticide poisoning results in 355 000 deaths per year. Large-scale livestock operations raise the risk that animal diseases, such as avian influenza, will spread to humans (World Bank 2007).

It is critical to explore integrated efforts to address development problems across sectors. For example, the use of drip irrigation can make agricultural water use more efficient while denying habitat to malaria mosquitoes.

KEY POINTS

- Technological and institutional innovation has permitted food production to more than keep pace with population growth.
- Projections to the year 2017 indicate that food supplies will remain adequate.
- Poor farmers frequently engage in a mix of subsistence and commercial activities.
- Small-scale farmers face many constraints, including lack of access to productive resources, natural resource degradation and health crises.
- Climate change will have severe impacts on agriculture and food security, especially in sub-Saharan Africa; the most vulnerable people will suffer earliest and the most.

32.4 WORLD FOOD DEMAND AND ACCESS TO FOOD

DEMAND FOR FOOD

Food demand derives primarily from income growth, population growth (see 'Population growth', above) and urbanisation. The World Bank projects annual growth in income per person in the developing world of 4.6% between 2010 and 2015, notwithstanding the prospects of a global recession during 2008/9. This is a considerably higher rate of income growth than in the 1980s and 1990s.

Urban population in developing countries is expected to more than double between 2007 and 2050, when two-thirds of the developing world's population will live in urban areas. The increase in the city-dwelling population of the developing

world will exceed its overall population increase, as some of the growth in the urban population will result from the arrival of migrants from the countryside.

When people move to cities, their lifestyles become more sedentary, and women experience higher opportunity costs on their time. As a result, urban dwellers tend to shift consumption to foods that require less preparation time (e.g. from sorghum, millet, maize and root crops to rice and wheat), and to more meat, milk, fruit, vegetables and processed foods.

Food and feed will remain the largest sources of demand growth in agriculture through 2017, but demand for feedstock for bioenergy will continue to rise rapidly. These competing demands for farm products will continue to exert upward pressure on prices, especially for maize. Demand for maize and other coarse grains to support developing-country livestock production will account for 75% of the global market in these cereals by 2017. Meat production is expected to rise by 2.5% annually in the developing world between 2008 and 2017. Rice consumption is expected to grow by nearly 10% in sub-Saharan Africa over the next decade. Developed countries are likely to remain the key global suppliers of coarse grains, while Asian developing countries will meet much of the demand for imported rice in Africa (OECD/FAO 2008). It is anticipated that cereal production will need to increase by 50% and meat production by 85% during 2000–2030 (World Bank 2007).

RISING FOOD PRICES

Between 1961 and 2002, real food prices declined steadily, with a sharp drop between 1975 and 1985. Beginning in 2002, real food prices began to rise, and by mid-2008 had climbed 64%. In nominal terms, wheat and maize prices were triple the level of early 2003, while the price of rice ballooned fivefold. Milk prices also tripled, while beef and poultry prices doubled (Fig. 32.3). A number of structural and conjunctural forces aligned to drive food prices up, including rising energy prices, subsidised biofuel production (see Section *evolve* 32.4 ▣), income and population growth, globalisation, urbanisation, land and water constraints, underinvestment in rural infrastructure and agricultural innovation, lack of access to inputs and weather disruptions. National trade policies aimed at easing

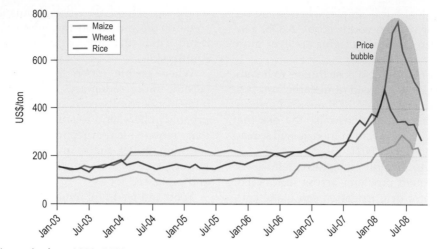

Fig. 32.3 Global cereal prices, 2003–2008. *Source: FAOSTAT.*

Table 32.2	Net buyers of staple foods (% of reference population)		
COUNTRY	ALL HOUSEHOLDS	URBAN POOR	RURAL POOR
Bangladesh	77	96	83
Guatemala	91	98	82
Malawi	93	99	95
Nicaragua	90	94	73
Pakistan	84	96	83
Tajikistan	91	97	77
Vietnam	46	100	41
Sources: FAO.			

the effects of the price increases, such as export bans and import subsidies, have contributed to volatility on international food markets. Depreciation of the US dollar since 2005 also pushed the dollar prices of commodities upwards and contributed to increased speculation as a hedge against further dollar depreciation (Timmer 2008).

Increased food prices benefit households that are net producers of food, but have an adverse impact on households that are net buyers. Most urban households (regardless of income level) are net buyers, as are many poor rural households in developing countries (Table 32.2). When food prices rise (or incomes fall), families will try to maintain staple consumption, often by purchasing cheaper staples and eliminating animal source foods, fruits and vegetables from the food budget. A food price increase of 50% in Bangladesh will lead to a 30% rise in iron deficiency among women and children, with negative effects on maternal mortality and children's physical and cognitive development and their productivity and earnings as adults. (FAO 2008b, World Bank 2007).

After peaking in mid-2008, cereal prices declined 30–40% in the third quarter of the year, due to the worldwide recession, good weather and farmers' favourable production responses to higher prices in many countries. However, most analysts do not believe that prices will return to the levels of the early years of the decade, due to continued strong demand for energy and for cereals for food, feed and fuel, as well as to structural land and water constraints. In addition, climate change poses a serious long-term constraint on food production (von Braun 2008).

Policies that enhance the productivity of small-holder farmers will help them to respond to higher prices with increased output, thereby eventually benefiting consumers with increased supplies and reduced prices. Private sector actors in food-processing and retail industries have an important role to play in ensuring supply response (von Braun 2008) (for expanded material see Section *evolve* 32.4(a) Rising food prices 🖰).

CURRENT STATE OF FOOD INSECURITY AND FUTURE OUTLOOK

According to the FAO, as of 2004, there were 832 million food-insecure people in developing

REGION	1970		1991		2004	
	Number	*%*	*Number*	*%*	*Number*	*%*
Developing world	959	37	823	20	832	16
Sub-Saharan Africa	88	34	169	34	212	30
West Asia and North Africa	45	25	15	7	33	8
Latin America and the Caribbean	54	19	53	12	45	8
East and southeast Asia	504	43	290	16	219	11
South Asia	267	37	283	25	314	21

Table 32.3   Food insecurity in developing countries, 1970, 1991 and 2004 (millions of people and percentage of population)

Source: FAO.

countries (Table 32.3). Food insecurity can be found in the countries in transition from centrally planned to market-oriented economies and even in the industrialised countries. However, the problems are more severe and affect a far greater proportion of the population in developing nations. The world made progress – albeit slowly and unevenly – in reducing hunger between 1970 and the mid-1990s. However, since then, the number of food-insecure people in the developing world has increased, and by 2004, the figure was just 13% less than in 1970, although the food-insecure percentage of the population of the developing world had dropped dramatically, from 37% to 16%. South Asia and sub-Saharan Africa are home to over three-fifths of all food-insecure people, and form hunger's centre of gravity. FAO estimates that rising food prices added 115 million people to the ranks of the food-insecure in 2007 and 2008, bringing the total to 963 million, or more than in 1970. This raises very serious doubts about the possibility of meeting the World Food Summit goal of reducing the number of hungry people to half of 1990–1992 level – i.e. to 420 million people – by no later than 2015 (FAO 2008b).

Real people with names and faces stand behind these hunger numbers (Box 32.1).

ACCESS TO FOOD

The large numbers of people who remain food-insecure and the slow progress in reducing hunger may seem paradoxical in the light of adequate food availability (see 'Past trends and current supply situation', above). However, current food availability is sufficient to provide everyone with their

---

BOX 32.1   A profile of hunger

Kone Figue is a mother of six in Ponoundogou in northern Côte d'Ivoire, West Africa. She and her husband farm six hectares of government-owned land. They grow cotton and groundnuts, mostly for sale, and maize (to eat and feed to their two cows) on about half the land, along with some yams and cassava. They plant the rest of the land with rice, their family's main staple food.

But the rice crop does not stretch out to provide a whole year's worth of meals, so the family ends up consuming the yams and cassava, even though they much prefer rice (preferably spiced up with some of the groundnuts).

Kone weeds and harvests the rice by hand, with the aid of simple tools like a hoe and a sickle. Her husband clears the land and sows the seeds. It is backbreaking work. Kone cannot afford to buy fertiliser or chemical weedkillers, and even with manure from her cows, her yields are meagre.

Adapted from Schiøler 1998.

---

minimum calorie requirements *if the food were distributed according to need*; food is *not* so distributed.

People obtain access to the food that is available through *entitlements*, i.e. the amount of food or other necessities that they can command based on their income and assets, given the legal, political, economic and cultural context in which they live. Thus, a farmer may produce food, but may have to deliver some of her harvest to a landlord before she can consume what remains. Likewise, a wage earner's income permits her to command a certain amount of food. Government programmes, private charity and gifts are other forms of entitlement (Drèze & Sen 1989).

Poverty drives food insecurity

Food insecurity persists primarily because of poverty. Low-income people cannot afford to buy all of the food they need, even though poor households typically spend 50–70% of their income on food. In addition, poor people frequently lack access to land and other productive resources, and so cannot produce food for themselves (IFAD 2001). According to the World Bank, as of 2005, 879 million people in developing countries (or about 16% of the population of the developing world) lived on the equivalent of less than US$1 per day, in a state of extreme poverty, and could not meet their needs for food and the other necessities of life on a sustainable basis (Table 32.4). The World Bank estimates that increases in energy and food prices in 2007/8 added at least 100 million additional people to the ranks of the poor, and that those who were already poor have fallen into even deeper poverty, especially in urban areas.

Despite rapid urbanisation in developing countries, 75% of people living in poverty remain in rural areas, and the majority of poor people in developing countries will remain rural for much of the 21st century, although a majority of the overall population will be urban by 2020. Urbanisation is expected to increase urban poverty and

food insecurity. Poor urban dwellers are more dependent on money income, may have fewer opportunities to grow their own food and require access to childcare in order to pursue income-earning opportunities. The needed resources to address food insecurity may not be land so much as economic opportunities, such as secure employment at a wage adequate to meet basic needs or the chance to own a business, as well as access to social safety net programmes (for an expanded section see Section *evolve* 32.4(c) Poverty drives food insecurity 🖱).

Transitory food emergencies

From time to time, natural disasters, violent conflicts, economic collapse, political crisis or some combination of these factors will create food emergencies. Whilst these emergencies are often transitory in duration, they may have long-lasting impacts on the affected people. Research in Africa and Asia indicates that drought can lead to child malnutrition that in turn causes poor school performance and reduced earnings over the course of a lifetime. In November 2008, the United Nations appealed for $7 billion in humanitarian assistance for 30 million people in 31 countries, mainly in sub-Saharan Africa. Needs are generally acute among refugees and internally displaced persons, who often live in camps and depend on humanitarian assistance for survival. Since the end of the Cold War, internal conflicts have proliferated in developing and transition countries, particularly in sub-Saharan Africa. At the end of 2007, 14 million refugees had crossed international borders to escape these struggles, which displaced another 26 million people within their own countries. Even after conflict ends, the costly burden of reconstruction may leave many people food-insecure for years. Landmines continue to maim and keep land out of production long after fighting ends. Not only does violent conflict cause hunger, but hunger can also contribute to conflict, especially when resources are scarce and perceptions of economic injustice are widespread, as in Rwanda in 1994 or Central America in the 1970s and 1980s.

Where armed conflicts and civil strife occur, governments and the international community must give priority to conflict resolution and prevention. It is essential to expand and strengthen early warning systems and response mechanisms for food and political crises, to include conflict

Table 32.4	People living on less than $1 per day, 1990 and 2005 (millions of people and percentage of population)			
	1990		2005	
	No.	*%*	*No.*	*%*
Developing world	1300	30	876	16
Sub-Saharan Africa	245	48	304	40
East Asia and Pacific	623	39	176	9
South Asia	381	34	351	24
Latin America and the Caribbean	29	7	31	6
West Asia and North Africa	4	2	5	2

Source: World Bank.

prevention in food security and development efforts and to link food security and long-term sustainable development to humanitarian assistance programmes. Savings from conflict avoidance should be calculated as returns to aid and development spending. Humanitarian assistance must include agricultural and rural development components that lead to secure livelihoods and build sustainable social and agricultural systems. Development programmes should be implemented so as to avoid competition and foster cooperation among groups or communities, especially in conflict-prone areas.

Famine is a catastrophic disruption of the social, economic and institutional systems that provide for food production, distribution and consumption. Contemporary famines stem less from crop failure than from the political and financial failures of governments to prevent famine and respond effectively. The emergence of 'new-variant famines', in which HIV/AIDS interacts with violence, natural disaster and/or political economic failure, means that the margin for coping and recovery has narrowed greatly among vulnerable people, especially in sub-Saharan Africa.

KEY POINTS

- Urbanisation and growth in population and income will drive increased demand for food, including animal products, through 2020.
- Developing-country cereal production will not keep pace with demand growth, meaning increased imports.
- Due to persistent poverty, rising food prices and competing demand for cereals, it will be nearly impossible to meet the World Food Summit goal of halving hunger by 2015.
- Food insecurity is concentrated in the rural areas of south Asia and sub-Saharan Africa.
- Discrimination, political disempowerment, violent conflict and natural disasters also contribute to food insecurity.

32.5 GLOBALISATION, INTERNATIONAL TRADE AND FOOD SECURITY

The volume of the global cereal trade more than doubled during 1967–1997, led by developing-country imports of wheat for food and maize for feed. Developed countries (mainly the USA, European Union and Australia) heavily dominate world export sales, along with a handful of developing countries (mainly Argentina, with India, Thailand and Vietnam lagging far behind) (Rosegrant et al 2001).

Globalisation – i.e. the growing integration of global markets for goods, services and capital resulting in part from technological developments in transportation, information and communications – offers significant new opportunities for economic growth in most developing countries, but it also carries significant risks: the inability of many developing-country industries to compete in the short term; the potential destabilising effects of uncontrolled short-term capital flows; increased exposure to price risk and worsening inequality as many poor people and backward regions may get left behind. Managing risks while exploiting growth opportunities will be a key challenge for developing countries in the years ahead.

The 1994 Uruguay round of trade negotiations under the aegis of the General Agreement on Tariffs and Trade (GATT) resulted in creation of the World Trade Organization (WTO) and the integration of agriculture into rule-governed trade for the first time (see Section *evolve* 32.5(a) on GATT and WTO 🖱). In response to the WTO Agreement on Agriculture and structural adjustment programmes enacted in the 1980s and 1990s with the strong encouragement of aid donors, many developing countries have liberalised food and agricultural trade (see Section *evolve* 32.5(b) on structural adjustment 🖱). The developed countries have not reciprocated, instead maintaining barriers to high-value imports from developing countries such as beef, sugar, groundnuts, dairy products and processed goods. Losses due to these trade barriers are not offset by developed countries' preferential trade schemes for specified quantities of certain developing-country exports. Developed countries' own domestic farm subsidies, which exceed US$300 billion per year (nearly three times the level of overall development assistance), have depressing effects on world prices, making developed-country exports cheaper than domestic produce and export crops in many developing countries. For example, European Union sugar subsidies under the Common Agricultural Programme (CAP) have secured a 40% world market share, at the expense of such non-subsidising developing-country exporters as Malawi, Thailand and Zambia (see Section *evolve* 32.5(c) on the Common Agricultural Policy 🖱)). When Haiti removed barriers to rice imports, highly subsidised US rice sales severely undercut local producers, accelerated migration to the cities as agricultural livelihoods collapsed and increased the population's exposure to volatile global rice prices. US subsidies to less than 25 000 cotton farmers exceed the gross national incomes of some of the poor West African cotton exporting countries that depend on cotton revenues for livelihoods and government budgets. The subsidies have helped the USA to capture 40% of the global cotton market, and the WTO has declared them to be in violation of trade rules. Coupled with developed-country trade barriers, these subsidies are a major impediment to developing-country agricultural development, depriving developing countries of $17 billion per year in export earnings, a sum five times greater than annual aid to agriculture and rural development. At the same time, many developing countries lack administrative, technical and infrastructural capacity to take full advantage of existing global trade rules or influence the creation of new ones (World Bank 2007, Pinstrup-Andersen et al 1999).

Africa's share of world agricultural trade continues to decline rapidly. The effect of current trade agreements is likely to be adverse for most African countries (Pinstrup-Andersen et al 1999).

More open global agricultural markets would increase developing countries' share of agricultural exports, but would also increase the cost of food imports, leaving net-food-importing countries worse off. Low-income net purchasers of food would be particularly adversely affected. It is therefore important to have safety-net programmes available to address the impact of anticipated trade liberalisation on these vulnerable groups (World Bank 2007).

In the Doha round of international agricultural trade negotiations, begun in 2001 under WTO auspices, developing-country delegates have proposed a 'development box' and a 'food security box'. Basically, these would allow developing countries to protect and subsidise efforts to achieve food security and agricultural and rural development. Developing countries have also sought increased access to developed-country markets. The Group of 20 (G20), composed of developing-country agricultural exporters and led by Brazil, China, India and South Africa, has pressed developed-country exporters to reform their trade policies, but disagreements between the USA and European Union

had created an impasse in the negotiations in 2007–2008.

Coalitions with certain groups of higher-income countries may help developing countries to improve their bargaining position in pursuing better access to industrialised countries' markets and other measures to ensure that trade supports food security. The Cairns Group, which includes both developing- and developed-country non-subsidising agricultural exporters, is an example of such a coalition. (The members are Argentina, Australia, Bolivia, Brazil, Canada, Chile, Colombia, Costa Rica, Guatemala, Indonesia, Malaysia, New Zealand, Paraguay, the Philippines, South Africa, Thailand and Uruguay.) Without appropriate domestic economic and agricultural policies, however, developing countries in general and poor people in particular will not capture fully potential benefits from trade liberalisation. The distribution of benefits will be determined largely by the distribution of productive assets.

Another aspect of food globalisation is the expansion of developed-country supermarkets in developing countries. Issues related to this development include whether poor farmers will be able to meet quality standards and whether large-scale food marketing will meet the needs of poor consumers in terms of both affordability and accessibility.

KEY POINTS

■ Unless developed countries reduce their agricultural subsidies and open their markets to developing-country exports, the potential of globalisation to contribute to food security will mostly go unrealised.

32.6 BROAD-BASED AGRICULTURAL AND RURAL DEVELOPMENT IS KEY TO FOOD SECURITY

Ironically, although food insecurity results more from problems of access to food than from lack of food availability, broad-based agricultural and rural development must be at the centre of any strategy to achieve food security in the developing world. In order for development to be broad-based, economic growth in rural areas generated by farm and non-farm activities is necessary, but not sufficient. Policies must ensure that small farmers and other rural poor people have political voice and access to the economic opportunities resulting from that growth.

Broad-based agricultural and rural development is essential to food security because the substantial majority of poor and food-insecure people will remain rural for most of the 21st century and because agriculture and associated rural activities will remain their main sources of income (Ravallion et al 2007, IFAD 2001). Low agricultural productivity in developing countries results in high unit costs of food, poverty, food insecurity, poor nutrition, low farmer and farm worker incomes, little demand for goods and services produced by poor non-agricultural rural households, and urban unemployment and underemployment. Research has shown that for every new US dollar of farm income earned in low-income developing countries, income in the economy as a whole rises by up to US$2.60, as growing farm demand generates employment, income and growth economy-wide. As agricultural production increases, it generates demand for inputs and implements. The need to process food and agricultural raw materials also stimulates rural non-farm activities, which offer employment, management and entrepreneurial opportunities for rural poor people, including women.

The development of well-functioning and well-integrated markets for agricultural inputs, commodities and processed goods, especially in rural areas, will contribute enormously to poverty alleviation, food security and the overall quality of life in developing countries. A *market* can be any context in which the sale and purchase of goods and services takes place. There need be no physical entity corresponding to the market; it might consist of a global telecommunications network on which company shares are traded. A *market economy* is an economic system in which decisions about the allocation of resources and production are made on the basis of prices generated by voluntary exchanges among producers, consumers, workers and owners of the factors of production (i.e. land, labour and capital).

Market performance improves and marketing costs fall when the government no longer monopolises trade and a competitive private sector emerges. Yet even as the government reduces its role, competent public administration will remain essential to enforce contracts, maintain grading and quality control standards, regulate market conduct and investment, maintain public safety and health, create infrastructure (roads, storage facilities and water works), provide agricultural research and extension services, implement credible and sustainable macroeconomic policies, and provide a favourable environment for savings and investment and accurate and transparent incentives for consumers and producers alike.

Markets alone cannot guarantee equity. Key public policies and investments must ensure that:

- poor farmers have access to yield-increasing crop varieties – including drought- and salt-tolerant and pest-resistant varieties – improved livestock, and other yield-increasing and environment-friendly technology
- poor farmers likewise have access to productive resources, including land, water, tools, fertilisers and pest management
- smallholders have opportunities to participate in production of export crops, as this will have spillover effects on input use and food crop productivity, increase access to markets, and have a beneficial impact on income and food security
- institutional barriers to the creation and expansion of small-scale rural credit and savings institutions are removed, and credit is accessible to small-scale farmers, traders, transporters and processing enterprises (see Section *evolve* 32.6(a) on Credit and other financial services 🐭)
- primary education, health care, clean water, safe sanitation and good nutrition are available for all.

To succeed, agricultural and rural development programmes must be implemented within an appropriate policy context. This includes good governance – the rule of law, transparency, sound public administration, democratic and inclusive decision-making and respect for human rights. Democratic governments are more likely to be responsive to the needs of all their citizens and to make food security a high priority. To ensure responsive policies, poor people need accountable organisations that articulate their interests. Farmer associations and cooperatives can help ensure that small farmers have access to inputs, credit, markets and opportunities to engage in more diversified, higher-value crop production. In addition, trade, macroeconomic and sectoral policies must not discriminate against agriculture, poor people, women or less-favoured areas (von Braun 2008, World Bank 2007, Kherallah et al 2002, Drèze & Sen 1989).

BOOSTING PUBLIC INVESTMENT

Developing-country governments underinvest in agriculture and rural development, despite their critical role in poverty alleviation and economic growth. Many policy-makers believe that agriculture is a declining sector, and have put resources instead into industry and urban development, which tend to have more politically potent constituencies. Long-term declines in real food prices have contributed to a sense of complacency about agriculture among both donor and developing-country governments. Also, in the 1980s and 1990s, there was a tendency in development circles to stress natural resource management, gender equality and democratisation without linking programmes to the agricultural context that remains central to the livelihoods of most poor people.

According to the FAO, African governments devoted just 4.5% of their budgets to agriculture in 2002, down from 5.2% in 1990. The World Bank estimates that sub-Saharan African governments devoted more than 2% of gross domestic product to military spending in the early 2000s (with all government spending accounting for 7.2%). In the 2003 Maputo Declaration, African heads of state pledged to raise agriculture's budget share to 10% by 2010.

AID TO AGRICULTURE

Official development assistance (ODA) donors, too, need to change their policies. In 2004, aid to agriculture and rural development from all donors was less than half the level of 25 years earlier in real terms. Agricultural aid accounted for just 4% of total ODA, compared to 18% in 1979. The value of aid to agriculture in Africa was about the same as in 1975, $1.2 billion (World Bank 2007). Aid donors also need to rethink their 20-year emphasis on reducing governments' economic role, which has contributed to developing-country underinvestment in agriculture.

AGRICULTURAL RESEARCH: A GLOBAL PUBLIC GOOD

Public agricultural research – i.e. agricultural research that is publicly funded and generally carried out by national government agencies or international organisations – played a crucial role in the success of the Green Revolution. More recently, it is the public sector that has carried out virtually all of the research on so-called 'orphan crops', i.e. crops widely consumed by poor people but for which markets are poorly developed and offer little profit potential, e.g. cassava, varieties of beans such as cowpeas and coarse grains such as millet. The private sector, in contrast, focuses on agricultural research for which there is a market and profit potential, e.g. hybrid maize, soybeans and fruits and vegetables that are traded internationally.

The private sector is unlikely to undertake much research needed by small farmers in developing countries because expected profits from disseminating the fruits of this research are unlikely to cover the cost of investment. However, between 1990 and 2000, donors' support for international agricultural research centres declined about 10% in real terms. Funding stabilised in the mid-1990s, but there have not been significant increases.

The average share of farm production invested in public agricultural research in developing countries is 0.6%, as compared to 2.6% in higher-income countries. Average annual growth rates of public agricultural research expenditures in developing countries in the 1990s were below those of the period 1976–1991, and in sub-Saharan Africa, the rate turned negative (Fig. 32.4) (Beintema & Stads 2008).

Pro-poor agricultural research must join all appropriate scientific tools and methods – including agroecology, conventional plant breeding and genetic engineering – with better utilisation of indigenous knowledge. It is important that poor farmers have access to insights into agricultural development from the full range of approaches to tackling their problems (for expanded material see Sections *evolve* 32.6(b) Agricultural research: a global public good ; and *evolve* 32.6(c), a case study on international agricultural research as a global public good).

Agroecology

Although high-yielding Green Revolution technologies have been responsible for enormous productivity increases among small-scale farmers in Asia, many farmers in the region's less-favoured areas have been bypassed. The desire to find ways of assisting these farmers, combined with concerns about excessive dependence on external inputs such as fertilisers, pesticides and irrigation water embodied in the first generation of Green Revolution technologies, has stimulated interest in alternative or

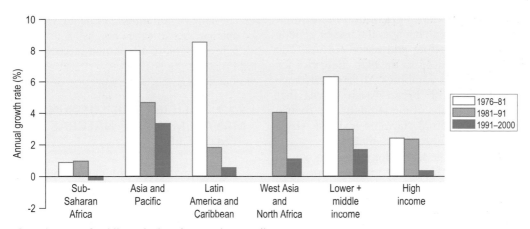

Fig. 32.4 Growth rates of public agricultural research expenditure, 1981–2000. *Source: IFPRI Agricultural Science and Technology Indicators initiative.*

complementary approaches, including the 'agroecological approach'. This aims to reduce the amount of purchased external inputs that farmers have to use. Instead, it relies heavily on available farm labour and organic material, as well as on improved knowledge and farm management.

One of the great strengths of the agroecological approach is that it promotes sustainable management of natural resources and active participation by farmers in identifying problems as well as designing and implementing appropriate solutions at the farm and community levels. Such participatory technology development can be extremely effective in finding the most appropriate solutions to production problems.

The market for organic produce in Europe and the USA totalled US$23 billion in 2003. If smallholders using agroecological methods are able to meet organic certification standards, they may be able to benefit from this rapidly growing market (World Bank 2007).

The potential of modern agricultural biotechnology for food security

(This section draws on ideas in Pinstrup-Andersen & Cohen 2001 and World Bank 2007. See also Section *evolve* 32.6(d) on Biotechnology .)

It is possible that the introduction of modern agricultural biotechnology into developing countries can contribute to increased productivity, lower unit costs and prices for food, preservation of forests and fragile land, poverty reduction and improved nutrition. This depends on whether the research is relevant to poor people, on the economic and social policy environment and on the nature of the intellectual property rights arrangements governing the technology. By raising productivity in food production, agricultural biotechnology could reduce the need to cultivate new lands and help conserve biodiversity.

Modern agricultural biotechnology offers many potential benefits to developing countries. It may help achieve the productivity gains needed to feed a growing global population, introduce resistance to pests and diseases without high-cost purchased inputs, heighten crops' tolerance to adverse weather and soil conditions, improve the nutritional value of some foods and enhance the durability of products during harvesting or shipping. Biotechnology research could aid the development of drought-tolerant and pest-resistant crops, to the benefit of small farmers and poor consumers. The development of cereal plants capable of capturing nitrogen from the air could contribute greatly to plant nutrition, helping poor farmers who often cannot afford fertilisers, and who experience low yields as a result. Biotechnology may offer cost-effective solutions to vitamin and mineral deficiencies, such as provitamin-A-rich rice, and be used to develop protein-enhanced crops or edible vaccines. By raising productivity in food production, agricultural biotechnology could reduce the need to cultivate new lands and help conserve biodiversity. Bioengineered products may reduce reliance on pesticides, thereby reducing farmers' crop protection costs and benefiting both the environment and public health.

Some forms of modern agricultural biotechnology are uncontroversial, such as the use of genetic markers in plant breeding and tissue culture. The latter approach was used to develop 'new rice for Africa', a variety that combines African resistance of harsh weather with broad Asian leaves that prevent weeds from absorbing sunlight and reduce the time that poor female farmers in West Africa must spend weeding their crops by hand.

However, transgenic technology, also known as genetic modification, has proved highly controversial. This technology involves the transfer of genes between species, and even across the boundaries of the animal, plant and microorganism kingdoms.

Except for limited work on rice and cassava, little research on genetically modified (GM) foodcrops has focused on the productivity and nutrition of poor people. In 2007, commercial farms in the USA, Canada, Argentina and Brazil accounted for 87% of GM crop plantings, with the USA alone accounting for 50%, and with most of the hectarage devoted to maize, cotton, soybean and canola that tolerate herbicides and/or are resistant to pests. To date, private firms have carried out most of the research on GM crops, so it is hardly surprising that they have focused on commercial markets. Moreover, they have subjected their research processes and products to intellectual property rights protection, which may create barriers to their use in pro-poor public sector research efforts, although there are some examples of public–private partnerships that have overcome these barriers. Additional public and philanthropic resources are needed in support of the appropriate research in developing countries, which also requires appropriate institutions and policies to manage public health and environmental risks (for an expanded section see Section *evolve* 32.6(e) on Potential of biotechnology for food security 🖱).

KEY POINTS

- Equitable agricultural and rural development is essential to achieve food security.
- The development of well-integrated markets is necessary but not sufficient.
- Public policies are also essential to ensure that rural poor people have access to resources and services.
- At present, developing-country governments and aid donors substantially underinvest in agriculture.
- Pro-poor agricultural research, engaging all

relevant scientific tools, including, where appropriate, biotechnology, has a critical role to play in efforts to attain food security.

32.7 POLICIES FOR SUSTAINABLE MANAGEMENT OF NATURAL RESOURCES

A high degree of complementarity amongst agricultural development, poverty reduction and environmental sustainability is more likely when agricultural development is broad-based and inclusive of small- and medium-sized farms, market-oriented, participatory and decentralised, and driven by technological change that enhances productivity without degrading natural resources. It is particularly important to 'get the incentives right', as subsidy policies may encourage unsustainable practices. Reforms may be politically difficult: for example, replacing generalized fertiliser subsidies with subsidies targeted to low-income farmers. Paying farmers to protect forests and watersheds can improve carbon sequestration (thereby mitigating climate change), biodiversity conservation and maintenance of flows for drinking and irrigation water. Policies aimed at achieving sustainable agricultural development must take into account the role of property rights and collective action in natural resource management. Many natural resource management technologies and practices take years to give full returns, e.g. terracing hillsides to prevent degradation. Without secure rights to resources, farmers lack incentives to adopt these approaches. Some technologies need to be adopted over a wide area to be effective, e.g. integrated pest management (IPM), so adopting farmers must cooperate with their neighbours in collective action.

PROMOTING SUSTAINABLE DEVELOPMENT IN LESS–FAVOURED AREAS

Although productivity is lower in less-favoured areas, these zones usually have comparative advantage in some agricultural production or non-farm activities if investment in infrastructure and institutions is adequate. Active engagement of communities, including women, is essential for sustainable management of both natural resources and conflicts over their use. Research has found that public investment in less-favoured areas of China and India results in high returns that sometimes exceed those of investment in favoured areas in terms of both economic growth and poverty reduction. Investments in agricultural research, education, roads and irrigation have greater incremental impact in less-favoured areas in these two countries, in part because opportunities for investment in these areas have been neglected. In sub-Saharan Africa, where overall agricultural public investment is low, additional investment is needed in both high-potential and less-favoured areas (World Bank 2007, Pender & Hazell 2000).

SOIL FERTILITY MANAGEMENT

Low soil fertility and lack of access to reasonably priced fertilisers, along with failure to replenish soil nutrients, must be rectified through efficient and timely use of organic and inorganic fertilisers and improved soil management. Chemical fertiliser use should be reduced where heavy application causes environmental harm. Fertiliser subsidies that encourage excessive use should be removed, but subsidies may remain necessary for less-favoured areas where current use is low and soil fertility is being diminished (Pinstrup-Andersen et al 1999).

INTEGRATED PEST MANAGEMENT

Until the 1990s, developing-country governments and aid donors alike encouraged use of synthetic pesticides. Now, consensus is emerging on IPM. IPM has a variety of definitions, but it is generally understood to mean a flexible approach to pest management that draws upon a range of methods to produce a result that combines the greatest value to the farmer with environmentally acceptable and sustainable outcomes. The techniques used for crop protection in IPM may include traditional crop management – crop rotation, intercropping, mulching, tillage and the like. IPM may also use pest-resistant crop varieties (developed through conventional breeding or genetic engineering), biological control agents, biopesticides and, as a last resort, judicious use of synthetic chemical pesticides. The options used by the farmer depend on the local context – agroecological needs, availability and affordability of the various alternatives (see Section *evolve* 32.7, which describes a case study on biological pest control 🖱).

WATER POLICY REFORM

Comprehensive water policy reform is needed to help save water, improve use efficiency and boost crop output per unit. Such reforms will be difficult, due to widespread practices and cultural norms that treat water as a free good and vested interests benefiting from current arrangements. Reforms might include secure and tradable rights for users, and subsidies targeted to poor water users in place of general subsidies. Devolving irrigation infrastructure and management to user associations, combined with secure access to water, will provide incentives for efficient use. Appropriate technology is needed to support conservation incentives. It can be difficult in practice to negotiate and enforce agreements allocating rights over groundwater or establishing the rights of upstream and downstream users, but agreements that are perceived as fair by all users have a greater chance of succeeding. It is essential to ensure that indigenous people, pastoralists and smallholder farmers, including women, have access to water (World Bank 2007).

KEY POINTS

- Efforts to achieve food security must take sustainable natural resource management, including the role of property rights and collective action, into account.
- Public investments in agricultural and rural development in less-favoured areas often lead to high returns in terms of both economic growth and poverty reduction.
- Policies must ensure that soil fertility is maintained.
- Policies should favour integrated pest management strategies, to ensure sustainability.
- Policies should promote efficient agricultural water use.

32.8 CONCLUSION

Implementing the policy changes outlined in this chapter will be expensive, and will require difficult political choices. But the task is far from impossible. IFPRI estimates that developing-country governments and aid donors will invest US$14.3 billion annually in agricultural research, irrigation and rural roads between 2008 and 2015. In order to achieve the first Millennium Development Goal – halving the proportion of people living in poverty and hunger from 1990 levels – developing countries and aid donors would need to invest an additional US$14.2 billion annually in these priority sectors, plus US$25 billion a year in female secondary education and access to clean drinking water. In sub-Saharan Africa, the additional investments would total US$11 billion (Fan & Rosegrant 2008). These sums are substantial, but the total annual investment requirements (US$54 billion) amount to just 4% of global military spending in 2007 (US$1.3 trillion). Accelerated progress toward sustainable food security will depend upon the willingness of developing- and developed-country governments, international aid agencies, non-governmental organisations, business and industry, and individuals to back their anti-hunger rhetoric with action, resources and changes in behaviour and institutions. The research community has a moral obligation to monitor the presence or absence of such changes.

References

Beintema N, Stads G-J: *Measuring agricultural research investments: a revised global picture*, ASTI Background Note. Washington DC, 2008, IFPRI. Accessible at http://www.asti.cgiar.org/pdf/global_revision.pdf.

Brown LR: *Plan B: rescuing a planet under stress and a civilization in trouble*, New York, 2003, W.W. Norton. Accessible at http://www.earth-policy.org/Books/PlanB_contents.htm.

Cohen MJ, Tirado C, Aberman N-L, Thompson B: *Impact of climate change and bioenergy on nutrition*, Rome/Washington, 2008, FAO/IFPRI. Accessible at http://www.ifpri.org/pubs/cp/cohen2008climate/cohenetal2008climate.pdf.

Drèze J, Sen A: *Hunger and public action*, Oxford, 1989, Clarendon Press.

Fan S, Rosegrant MW: *Investing in agriculture to overcome the world food crisis and reduce poverty and hunger*, 2008, Washington IFPRI Policy Brief 3. Accessible at http://www.ifpri.org/pubs/bp/bp003.pdf.

FAO (Food and Agriculture Organisation of the United Nations): *Food security brief*, Rome, 2006, FAO. Accessible at ftp://ftp.fao.org/es/ESA/policybriefs/pb_02.pdf.

FAO: *Food outlook*, November. Rome, 2008a, FAO.

FAO: *The state of food insecurity in the world 2008*, Rome, 2008b, FAO. Accessible at ftp: //ftp.fao.org/docrep/fao/011/i0291e/i0291e00.pdf.

FAOSTAT database, Rome, 2008, FAO. Accessible at http://faostat.fao.org/default.aspx.

IFAD (International Fund for Agricultural Development): *Rural poverty report 2001*, Rome, 2001, IFAD. Accessible at http://www.ifad.org/poverty/index.htm.

Kherallah M, Delgado C, Gabre-Madhin E, et al. *Reforming agricultural markets in Africa*, Baltimore, 2002, Johns Hopkins University Press for IFPRI.

OECD (Organisation for Economic Co-operation and Development)/FAO: *Agricultural outlook, 2008–2017. Highlights*, Rome and Paris, 2008, FOA and OECD. Accessible at http://www.agri-outlook.org/dataoecd/54/15/40715381.pdf.

Pender J, Hazell P, editors: *Promoting sustainable development in less-favoured areas*, 2020 Vision Focus No. 4. Washington DC, 2000, IFPRI. Accessible at http://www.ifpri.org/pubs/pubs.htm.

Pinstrup-Andersen P, Cohen MJ: Modern agricultural biotechnology and developing-country food security. In Nelson GC, editor: *Genetically modified organisms in agriculture: economics and politics*, London, 2001, Academic Press. pp 179–189.

Pinstrup-Andersen P, Pandya-Lorch R, Rosegrant MW: *World food prospects: critical issues for the early twenty-first century*. 2020 Vision Food Policy Report. Washington DC, 1999, IFPRI. Accessible at http://www.ifpri.org/pubs/pubs.htm.

Quisumbing AR, editor: *Household decisions, gender and development: a synthesis of recent research*, Baltimore, 2003, Johns Hopkins University Press IFPRI.

Ravallion M, Chen S, Sangraula P: *New evidence on the urbanization of global poverty*. World Bank Policy Research Working Paper No. 4199. Washington DC, 2007, World Bank. Accessible at http://www-wds.worldbank.org/external/default/WDSContentServer/IW3P/IB/2007/08/27/000158349_20070827111606/Rendered/PDF/wps419901update1.pdf.

Rosegrant MW, Paisner MS, Meijer S, Witcover J: *Global food projections to 2020: emerging trends and alternative futures*, Washington DC, 2001, IFPRI. Accessible at http://www.ifpri.org/pubs/pubs.htm.

Schiøler E: *Good news from Africa*, Washington DC, 1998, IFPRI.

Timmer CP: *Causes of high food prices*, ADB Economics Working Paper No. 128. Manila, 2008, Asian Development Bank.

Von Braun J: *High food prices: the what, who and how of proposed policy actions,* Washington DC, 2008, IFPRI. Accessible at http://www.ifpri.org/PUBS/ib/foodprices.asp.

World Bank: *Poverty trends and voices of the poor,* 2001. Accessible at http://www.worldbank.org/poverty/data/trends/scenario.htm.

World Bank: *World Development Report 2008: agriculture for development,* Washington DC, 2007, World Bank.

Further reading

Adato M, Meinzen-Dick R, editors: *Agricultural research, livelihoods and poverty: studies of economic and social impacts in six countries,* Baltimore, 2007, Johns Hopkins University Press for IFPRI.

Chen S, Ravallion M: *The developing world is poorer than we thought, but no less successful in the fight against poverty,* 2008. World Bank Policy Research Working Paper No. 4703. Accessible at http://www-wds.worldbank.org/external/default/WDSContentServer/IW3P/IB/2008/08/26/000158349_20080826113239/Rendered/PDF/WPS4703.pdf.

Eicher CK, Staatz JM, editors: *International agricultural development,* 3rd ed. Baltimore, 1998, Johns Hopkins University Press.

Fan S, editor: *Pubic expenditures, growth and poverty in developing countries: lessons from developing countries,* Baltimore, 2008, Johns Hopkins University Press for IFPRI.

Haggblade S, Hazell PBR, Reardon T, editors: *Transforming the rural nonfarm economy: opportunities and threats in the developing world.* Baltimore, 2007, Johns Hopkins University Press for IFPRI.

Knox A, Meinzen-Dick R, Hazell P: Property rights, collective action, and technologies for natural resource management: a conceptual framework. In Meinzen-Dick R, Knox A, Place F, Swallow B, editors: *Innovation in natural resource management: the role of property rights and collective action in developing countries,* Baltimore, 2002, Johns Hopkins University Press for IFPRI, pp 12–44.

Messer E, Cohen MJ, Marchione T: *Conflict: a cause and effect of hunger.* Environmental Change and Security Project Report No. 7. Washington DC, 2001, Woodrow Wilson International Center for Scholars, Smithsonian Institution, pp 1–16.

Nweke F, Haggblade S, Zulu B: Recent growth in African cassava. In Haggblade S, editor: *Building on successes in African agriculture,* 2020 Vision Focus No. 12. Brief 3. Washington DC, 2004, IFPRI.

Rosegrant MW, Cai X, Cline SA: *World water and food to 2025: averting an impending crisis,* Washington DC, 2002, IFPRI.

SIPRI (Stockholm International Peace Research Institute): *Recent trends in military expenditure,* Stockholm, 2008, SIPRI. Accessible at http://www.sipri.org/contents/milap/milex/mex_trends.html.

United Nations High-level Task Force on the Global Food Security Crisis: *Comprehensive framework for action,* New York, 2008, United Nations. Accessible at http://www.un.org/issues/food/taskforce/Documentation/CFA%20Web.pdf.

UN Population Division: *World population prospects: the 2006 revision,* New York, 2007, UN Department of Economic and Social Affairs. Accessible at http://www.un.org/esa/population/publications/wpp2006/wpp2006.htm.

UN Population Division: *World urbanization prospects: the 2007 revision,* New York, 2008, UN Department of Economic and Social Affairs. Accessible at http://www.un.org/esa/population/publications/wup2007/2007wup.htm.

Von Braun J: *Food and financial crises: implications for agriculture and the poor,* Washington, DC, 2008, IFPRI. Accessible at http://www.ifpri.org/PUBS/agm08/jvbagm2008.asp.

Von Braun J, Diaz-Bonilla E, editors: *Globalization of food and agriculture and the poor,* New Delhi, 2008, Oxford University Press.

EVOLVE CONTENTS (available online at: evolve.elsevier.com/Geissler/nutrition)

Chapter **33**

Food and nutrition policies and interventions

Catherine Geissler*

CHAPTER CONTENTS

OBJECTIVES

By the end of this chapter you should be able to:
- Make the case for public intervention in addressing malnutrition
- Describe the main types of malnutrition worldwide, their prevalence and trends
- Appreciate the types of factor involved
- Be able to analyse causes by level, such as immediate, underlying and root
- Appreciate the factors involved in matching cause of nutritional problems with appropriate interventions or preventative measures
- Describe the types of direct and indirect measure to improve nutritional status
- Explain the evolution of emphasis in types of policy intervention used over the last half century to reduce malnutrition
- Explain the current challenges to food and nutrition security

*Updated and modified from the previous edition chapter written by Lawrence Haddad and Catherine Geissler

© 2010 Elsevier Ltd/Inc/BV
DOI: 10.1016/B978-0-7020-3118-2.00033-4

33.1 INTRODUCTION

Nutrition policies and interventions are designed to reduce malnutrition in populations. In this chapter the term 'Malnutrition' encompasses both 'undernutrition' (due to some combination of food, care and health deprivations) and 'overnutrition' (due to a combination of the excess consumption of some macronutrient diet components, although there may be some deficiencies of others, e.g. micronutrients, and too little physical exercise). There are several reasons why governments have an important role to play in the elimination of malnutrition. First, many goods and services relevant for good nutrition status will not be provided by the private sector. Examples include nutrition education broadcast campaigns. The private sector is unlikely to engage in this type of activity because the costs of providing such services on a 'pay per view' basis are too high. Second, when private decisions generate large costs accruing to someone without a say in the decision, such as in the decision not to get immunised and the associated dangers of spread of infection, there is a role for the government to act. Third, when there is a large difference in information available to a user and a provider about the value of the product, for example the saturated fat content of a particular food, then the government is justified in acting to narrow the information gap. Fourth, when interventions are of particular importance for equity, such as in universal salt iodisation or the availability of primary health care, the public sector has a key role to play. Another rationale for public-sector involvement derives from a human rights perspective. Democratically elected governments have obligations with regard to many human rights, including the right to adequate nutrition, and are directly accountable to the populations they serve.

This chapter reviews some of the policy and intervention options available to governments and their partners for reducing malnutrition. The chapter briefly reviews the extent and causes of malnutrition using the food-care-health conceptual model of nutrition status, popularised by the United Nations (UN). The bulk of the chapter is spent examining currently used direct and indirect nutrition interventions and policies, identifying their strengths and weaknesses. Direct nutrition interventions have a stated objective of improving nutrition, and indirect interventions or policies may affect nutrition status in important ways but do not necessarily have this as their primary goal. Causes are examined at the immediate (e.g. infection), underlying (e.g. inability to purchase food) and root (e.g. poor government performance in formulating, enacting and enforcing legislation) levels. The chapter then traces the evolution of thinking in food and nutrition interventions and concludes by reviewing the new challenges facing food and nutrition security, today and in the future.

The extent of various types of malnutrition differs between developing and developed countries. For example general undernutrition and specific vitamin and mineral deficiencies are more prevalent in developing countries, whereas chronic diseases related to poor nutrition (here referred to as 'overnutrition' for brevity), such as obesity, coronary heart disease, diabetes and osteoporosis, are more prevalent in developed countries. However pockets of undernutrition exist in developed countries and chronic diseases related to overnutrition are expanding rapidly in the developing world, especially in the poor but lower-mortality countries. Undernutrition and overnutrition coexist (the 'nutrition transition') to the greatest extent in countries undergoing rapid socioeconomic and demographic transitions such as the countries of the former Soviet Union. The challenge of balancing interventions to address under- and overnutrition is particularly great for these countries.

33.2 EXTENT AND CAUSES OF MALNUTRITION

Descriptions of the extent, causes of (and responses to) malnutrition are usefully classified by stage in the life cycle. Typically, causes and hence intervention should begin with the infant. This is because dramatic growth failure most typically occurs between the ages of 12 and 18 months. When it does fail, typically measured as stunting (see Ch. 28), there is a low probability of meaningful catch-up growth. The impairments in cognitive function are also largely irreversible. Hence early infant malnutrition has consequences throughout the life-cycle. Malnourished babies become malnourished adolescents and adults who are less able to learn in school and less productive in the labour market. Malnourished female babies will be more likely to be malnourished girls and women who give birth to malnourished babies. Moreover the 'Barker hypothesis' or 'fetal programming hypothesis' (see Chs 14, 29) posits that maternal dietary imbalances at critical periods of development in the womb can trigger an adaptive redistribution of fetal resources (including low birthweight (LBW)). Such adaptations affect fetal structure and metabolism in ways that predispose the individual to chronic diseases later in life. Whenever possible, this section reviews the extent and causes of malnutrition by these stages in the life cycle.

ASSESSMENT OF EXTENT AND WORLDWIDE DISTRIBUTION OF MALNUTRITION

The data on the extent and distribution of malnutrition are beset with difficulties, particularly for the developing world. At the simplest level, different UN agencies have different regional grouping labels, and in some cases the same regional label has different country groupings by agency (ACC/SCN 2000). At a more basic level, the data are not collected in a comparable manner across countries, or are just not collected at all. Anthropometric data from the World Health Organization (WHO) for infants tend to be subject to the highest level of quality control and are hence the most comparable. Food deprivation data from the Food and Agriculture Organization of the UN (FAO) give the appearance of comparability across countries and time, but it is well known that comparability largely rests on the validity of some questionable statistical assumptions about the within-country distribution of food consumption. The data on adult anthropometry and micronutrient deficiency are also very patchy. Nevertheless, a rough approximation of the extent, pattern and trends of the malnutrition problem can be estimated using existing data. Until recently the international organisations concentrated on documenting only nutritional status in developing countries. However since about 2000 they have started to include the epidemiology of obesity and diet-related degenerative diseases (ACC/SCN 2004).

Stunting (low height for age) and underweight (low weight for age) of infants in the developing world is widespread. In south Asia over 30% of all children under the age of 5 are stunted. Africa has the highest prevalence of stunting, although the total number in Asia is almost twice that in Africa (Table 33.1). In terms of trends, the prevalence of stunting for the developing countries as a whole is

decreasing slowly over time, while the absolute numbers for Africa are increasing (Table 33.2).

Adult anthropometric data in the form of body mass index are not as comprehensive or as thoroughly screened for quality as are the infant data. Nevertheless, data from WHO show the percentage of adults with BMIs above the cutoff for obesity in selected countries (Table 33.3). Of these countries it can be seen that the USA has the highest prevalence (over 40% in both men and women), although Western Samoa, which is not shown as no data is available for recent years had even higher levels in 1991 (59% of men and 78% of women). In Europe the prevalence in the UK, Germany and the Czech Republic is similar, around 30%, but is much lower in France at around 10%, while in the Asian countries, China, India and Japan, it is still only around 2%, but growing.

The poorest countries are still grappling mainly with underweight, and the developed countries with overnutrition issues such as obesity. Despite the widespread efforts to reduce the extent of obesity and its associated diseases, their prevalence continue to increase. The trends for selected countries are shown in Table 33.4. For further details see Chapter 20.

An additional worrying trend is being exhibited by many developing countries – the coexistence of under- and overnutrition (Popkin et al 2001). We shall return to this co-existence issue in Section 33.5.

Micronutrient malnutrition data are also far from perfect, with patchy data on the prevalence of the major micronutrient deficiencies – iodine, iron and vitamin A (MI 2001) (see also Chs 11, 12, 28). In gross terms, WHO estimates that iron deficiency is one of the most prevalent disorders and affects approximately 4–5 billion people worldwide (http://www.who.int/nut/ida.htm) while anaemia affects 1.62 billion people, i.e. 25% of the population, with the highest prevalence in preschool children (47.4%) and the lowest in men (12.7%) (WHO 2008a), 1989 million are iodine-deficient (WHO 2004) and 140 million preschool children, and more than 7 million pregnant women are vitamin-A-deficient (WHO 2009). Regional and age group breakdowns are presented in Tables 33.5–33.8.

For iron deficiency, anaemia prevalence is used as a proxy. In industrialized countries this is likely to be a close approximation, but in the developing world anaemia can occur due to factors other than iron deficiency such as malaria, other parasitic

Table 33.1   Estimated prevalence and number of stunted children, 1995–2005

UN REGIONS AND SUBREGIONS	PREVALENCE OF STUNTING (%)			NUMBER STUNTED (MILLIONS)		
	1995	*2000*	*2005*	*1995*	*2000*	*2005*
Africa	36.1	35.2	34.5	44.9	45.1	48.5
Eastern	44.4	44.4	44.4	17.3	19.4	21.6
Northern	24.4	21.7	19.1	5.1	4.6	4.2
Southern	25.0	24.6	24.3	1.4	1.5	1.4
Western	33.8	32.9	32.0	11.8	12.7	13.9
Asia	35.4	30.1	25.7	130.8	109.4	92.4
Eastern	21.5	14.8	10.0	23.5	15.2	9.5
South central	45.2	39.7	34.5	81.0	71.5	63.5
South east	36.8	32.1	27.7	21.3	18.1	15.3
Western	21.7	18.7	16.1	5.0	4.5	4.1
Latin American and the Caribbean	15.9	13.7	11.8	8.8	7.6	6.5
Caribbean	9.6	7.4	5.7	0.4	0.3	0.2
Central America	23.0	24.0	18.0	3.7	3.3	2.9
South America	13.3	11.3	9.6	4.7	4.0	3.4
Oceania	n/a	n/a	n/a	n/a	n/a	n/a
All developing countries	33.5	29.6	26.5	181.5	162.1	147.5

Note: Stunting is defined as low height-for-age at < −2 standard deviations of the median value of the NCHS/WHO international growth reference.
n/a, not available.
Source: ACC/SCN 2004.

infections, current infectious diseases and other pathologies. Bearing this in mind, Table 33.5 shows that anaemia is a serious problem throughout the life cycle, both in industrialized and developing countries. It is a particular problem for pregnant women, who have particularly high haematinic needs (Table 33.5).

Table 33.6 presents prevalence data by WHO region. The rates are highest in Africa, followed by Southeast Asia (which includes India but not China, which is in the Western Pacific region). The next highest prevalence is in the Eastern Mediterranean region (which includes the Middle East, Pakistan and North Africa) and the lowest in Europe and the Americas. However, Southeast Asia has by far the greatest total numbers.

One of the most visible manifestations of iodine deficiency is goitre (see Chs 12, 28) and this is used as one indicator of deficiency although the current preferred method of detection is urinary iodine (UI) excretion as a measure of iodine intake. Iodine deficiency is very prevalent in most areas of the world apart from the Americas, with the highest prevalence in Europe and the Eastern Mediterranean region (Table 33.7). Data from 1993 to 2003 indicate

an increase goitre prevalence, which is inconsistent with UI data. This may be explained by the time lag in the disappearance of goitre following salt iodisation, and the fact that many of the surveys were carried out before 1998 and extensive implementation of such programmes. The number of countries with iodine deficiency as a public health problem decreased from 110 to 54 between 1993 and 2003. In the last decade there has been substantial progress towards elimination of iodine deficiency. Iodine intake is more than adequate in 24 countries, with the emerging risk of iodine-induced hyperthyroidism in susceptible groups following the introduction of iodised salt. Regional figures mask differences between countries; for example, in Europe no data are available for 14 countries, 15 have optimal iodine intakes, 19 mild deficiency and 4 moderate deficiency.

Severe vitamin A deficiency manifests itself clinically as night blindness and corneal xerosis (see Chs 11, 28). Subclinical vitamin A deficiency in preschool children is defined as serum retinol levels <0.7 μmol/L. Models have been constructed for small samples to model the relationship between the two indicators so that the more frequently

Table 33.2 Percentage of preschool children (under-5s) with low weight for age

REGION	% UNDER–FIVES UNDERWEIGHT	
	1990	*2006*
Developing countries	31	26
East Asia/Pacific	23	14
South Asia	54	46
Latin America/Caribbean	11	6
Middle East/North Africa	13	12
Sub-Saharan Africa	32	28
CEE/CIS*	11	5

Source: www.unicef.org accessed 13/7/09.
Estimated using NCHS/WHO/CDC reference data.
*CEE/CIS = Central and Eastern Europe/Commonwealth of Independent States.

Table 33.3 Percentage of obese adults in selected countries (2005)

REGION COUNTRY	BMI ≥ 30 (OBESE)	
	Men	*Women*
Europe		
UK	29.5	31.7
France	11.3	9.6
Germany	28.8	28.7
Italy	18.7	18.8
Czech Republic	26.8	30.9
North America		
United States	42.3	48.6
Canada	28.1	29.5
South/Central America		
Brazil	11.5	24.7
Mexico	30.3	44.2
Asia		
China	1.8	2.6
India	1.7	2.1
Japan	2.6	2.2
Africa		
Kenya	0.2	2.6
Nigeria	2.9	8.2
Senegal	2.0	13.0
Ghana	4.4	5.6
Oceania		
Australia	27.0	32.2

Source: WHO Global Infobase, available online at http://www.who.int, accessed on 13/7/09.

Table 33.4 Trends in obesity in selected countries

COUNTRY	YEAR	MEN	WOMEN
UK	1980	6	8
	1986/7	7	12
	1991/2	13	15
	1995	15	16.5
	2005	29.5	31.7
USA	1973	11.6	16.1
	1978	12	14.8
	1991	19.7	24.7
	2005	42.3	48.6
Brazil	1975	3.1	8.2
	1989	5.9	13.3
	2005	11.5	24.7
Japan	1982	0.9	2.6
	1987	1.3	2.8
	1993	1.8	2.6
	2005	2.6	2.2
China	1989	0.3	0.9
	1991	0.4	0.9
	1992	1.2	1.6
	2005	1.8	2.6

Sources: WHO 1998; 2005 data from WHO Global Infobase www.who.int accessed 13/7/09.

Table 33.5 The worldwide prevalence of anaemia by age group (1993–2005) based on haemoglobin concentration

POPULATION GROUP	PREVALENCE OF ANAEMIA	POPULATION AFFECTED
	Percent	*Number (millions)*
Preschool-age children	47.4	293
School-age children	25.4	305
Pregnant women	41.8	56
Non-pregnant women	30.2	468
Men	12.7	260
Elderly	23.9	164
Total population	24.8	1620

Source: WHO 2008a.

Table 33.6   Prevalence of anaemia (1993–2005) by WHO region

WHO REGION	PRESCHOOL-AGE CHILDREN[a]		PREGNANT WOMEN		NON-PREGNANT WOMEN	
	Prevalence (%)	Number affected (millions)	Prevalence (%)	Number affected (millions)	Prevalence (%)	Number affected (millions)
Africa	67.6	83.5	57.1	17.2	47.5	69.9
Americas	29.3	23.1	24.1	3.9	17.8	39
Southeast Asia	65.5	115.3	48.2	18.1	45.7	182
Europe	21.7	11.1	25.1	2.6	19	40.8
Eastern Mediterranean	46.7	0.8	44.2	7.1	32.4	39.8
Western Pacific	23.1	27.4	30.7	7.6	21.5	97
Global	47.4	293.1	41.8	56.4	30.2	468.4

[a]Population subgroups: Preschool-age children (0.00–4.99 years); Pregnant women (no age range defined); Non-pregnant women (15.00–49.99 years).
Source: WHO 2008a.

Table 33.7   Proportion of school age children (6–12 years) and general population (all ages groups) with insufficient iodine intake (UI < 100 µg/l) by WHO region, 2003

REGION	SCHOOL AGE CHILDREN (%)	GENERAL POPULATION (%)
Africa	42.3	42.6
Americas	10.1	9.8
Southeast Asia	39.9	39.8
Europe	59.9	56.9
Eastern Mediterranean	55.4	54.1
Western Pacific	26.2	24
Total	36.5	35.2

Source: WHO 2004.

Table 33.8   Estimated prevalence of subclinical vitamin A deficiency, defined as serum retinol level <0.7 µmol/L, among preschool children and pregnant women 1995–2005 by WHO region

REGIONS	PRESCHOOL CHILDREN (%)	PREGNANT WOMEN (%)
Africa	44.4	13.5
Americas	15.6	2.0
Southeast Asia	49.9	17.3
Europe	19.7	11.6
Eastern Mediterranean	20.4	16.1
Western Pacific	12.9	21.5
Global	33.3	15.3

Source: WHO 2009.

recorded clinical signs can roughly be projected to the subclinical level. The estimated prevalence of clinical (night-blindness) and subclinical (low serum retinol) vitamin A deficiency in countries at risk (1995–2005) is 0.9% and 33.3% respectively in preschool children and 7.8% and 15.3% in pregnant women (WHO 2009) While clinical signs of vitamin A deficiency are relatively rare, subclinical deficiency, which increases the likelihood of morbidity and mortality in preschool children, is estimated to be widespread in this age group in developing countries, especially in south Asia and Africa (Table 33.8). In pregnant women the estimated prevalence is lower than in preschool children. It is especially low in the Americas, but particularly high in the Western Pacific.

In developed countries certain other potential micronutrient deficiencies have become more of a concern in recent years. These include folate deficiency in women in relation to spina bifida in a small percentage of newborns, but also raised homocysteine levels related to the more prevalent coronary heart disease. Another is selenium deficiency. But research on these has not yet been sufficient to persuade all governments of the need for public health interventions.

In addition to anthropometric data and patchy micronutrient status data, food balance sheet data are available for most developing (and developed) countries for most years. These data are compiled by FAO from food production, food trade and food aid flows. The foods are converted into calories and divided by population size to give the dietary energy supply (DES) in calories per capita. The DES numbers are converted to estimates of the numbers of individuals without access to food using various distributional assumptions, and they are misleadingly called estimates of 'undernourishment'. These figures are most useful in describing trends. Table 33.9 shows that most of the 'undernourished' reside in Asia and the Pacific. But this is due mainly to the large population in this region. In fact the prevalence of 'undernourishment' is highest in sub-Saharan Africa at 30%. In most areas, apart from the Near East and North Africa, the prevalence has been decreasing since the early 1990s, but numbers have increased in Africa.

Figure 33.1 shows trends in the prevalence and numbers of undernourished from 1990–02 to 2003–05 in relation to the World Food Summit in 1996 goals and the Millenium Development goals for 2015. These goals were respectively to reduce the numbers of malnourished to 420 million, and to halve the proportion of people who suffer from hunger from the 1990 base by 2015. China shows a dramatic reduction in numbers but for many countries in the developing world the numbers and proportions are increasing. Similar to the stunting statistics, 'undernourishment' numbers have been getting worse in East and southern Africa.

In summary, we can say that on a worldwide basis undernutrition has been decreasing in terms of rates, although not numbers, but slowly, and from a very high base. In many of the regions of sub-Saharan Africa the numbers and rates are increasing. However food security is extremely vulnerable to economic fluctuations and the world economic crisis from 2006 onwards has led to sharp increases in the prices of fuels and staple foods, reduced incomes, and a substantial increase in the total numbers of malnourished people, announced by FAO in June 2009 to be 1020 million (FAO 2009).

The next sections describe the causes of malnutrition and highlight the particular situation in sub-Saharan Africa.

KEY POINTS

- Undernutrition is located largely in south Asia and sub-Saharan Africa.
- Undernutrition is declining slowly in south Asia, but increasing in sub-Saharan Africa.
- Overnutrition is located in all countries, in general more prevalent in developed countries and increasing rapidly both in the developed and developing world.
- Many of the databases to assess the extent of undernutrition are very weak.

ANALYSIS OF CAUSES

The causes of malnutrition are represented in the consensus conceptual diagram (Fig. 33.2) for child undernutrition but similar analysis can be applied

---

Table 33.9   The numbers of 'undernourished' from the FAO (more accurately 'estimated numbers of food deficit individuals from food supply data')

	NUMBER & PERCENTAGE OF PEOPLE UNDERNOURISHED (MILLIONS)					
	1990–92		1995–97		2003–05	
	No	%	No	%	No	%
World	841.9	16	831.8	14	848.0	13
Developed countries	19.1	–	21.4	–	15.8	–
Developing world	822.8	20	810.4	18	832.2	16
Asia and the Pacific	582.4	20	535.0	17	541.9	16
Latin America and the Caribbean	52.6	12	51.8	11	45.2	8
Near East and North Africa	19.1	6	20.6	8	33.0	8
Sub-Saharan Africa	168.8	34	194.0	34	212.1	30

Source: FAO 2008.

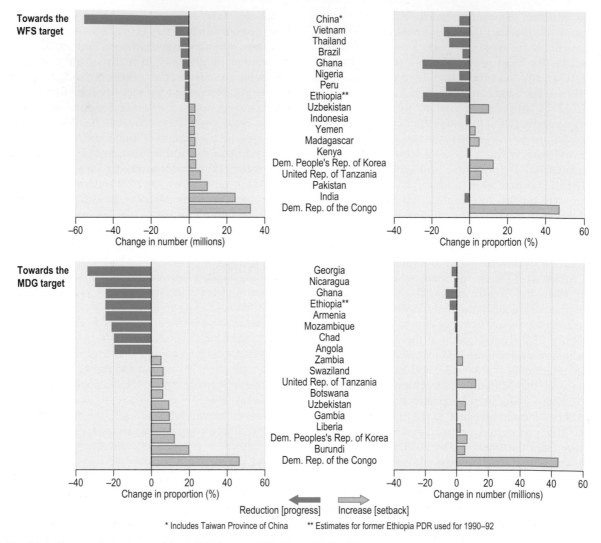

Fig. 33.1 Changes in 'undernourishment' between 1990–02 and 2003–05. *Source FAO 2008.*

to all age groups. The diagram indicates that the causes lie at many levels (immediate, underlying and basic) and in many sectors (agriculture, health, water, education and employment to name a few). It is important to understand the causes of malnutrition as this diagnosis guides the nature of the intervention needed to promote good nutrition status as well as the likelihood of success of the intervention. If, for example, food availability at the household level is adequate, but infant girls are not receiving enough food, then there are social inequalities that need to be recognised and addressed. If infants are receiving sufficient food in terms of energy but have many micronutrient deficiencies, then diet quality is a key constraint. If the infants

are having frequent bouts of diarrhoea due to poor water quality, then even a good diet will not prevent malnutrition. Finally, if food intake in terms of quality and quantity is sufficient, as is the health and sanitation environment, but the child is failing to thrive, it might be due to lack of quality interaction (e.g. psychosocial stimulation) between infant and parent or caretaker. Similar logic can be applied to other age or social groups. The examples described in the following paragraphs focus first on undernutrition, followed by examples related to over nutrition. The terms undernutrition and overnutrition are convenient simplifications but can be misleading. In reference to undernutrition, if people do not eat enough food they are likely to be

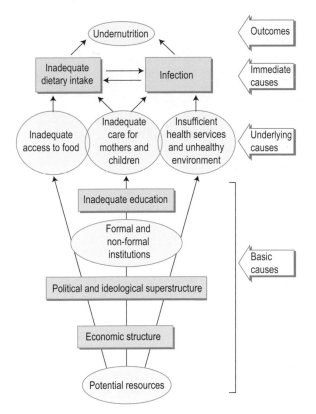

Fig. 33.2 The food-care-health model of undernutrition.
Source: UNICEF 1990.

deficient in most nutrients and susceptible to various deficiency diseases; however, for overnutrition people may consume excess energy, but depending on the quality of their food they may have a poor balance of macronutrients and also be deficient in certain micronutrients, eventually leading to the chronic diseases, commonly called the 'diseases of affluence'. With these caveats we shall continue to use here the terms undernutrition and overnutrition for simplicity

Immediate causes

The most immediate causes of malnutrition in young children (and also adults) are poor diet and infection (see Ch. 26). If the child is not able to ingest enough food, both in terms of quantity and quality that can be used for growth and development, then malnutrition occurs. Infection and an inadequate diet reinforce each other. Infection reduces the intake of nutrients by diminishing appetite, inhibiting nutrient absorption and increasing nutrient requirements for combating infection,

while poor diet reduces the effectiveness of the immune function.

Equivalent immediate causes of overnutrition are excess intake of energy, although not of all micronutrients, through bottlefeeding, high-fat foods, snacking, calorific drinks and also lack of exercise.

Underlying causes

Inadequate dietary intake and disease are in turn affected by underlying sets of factors, grouped as household food insecurity, poor care for mothers and children and the inadequate provision of health services and an unhealthy environment.

Food security 'exists when all people, at all times, have physical and economic access to sufficient, safe, and nutritious food to meet their dietary needs and food preferences for an active and healthy life' (FAO 1996, and see Ch. 32).

Essentially a food-insecure household cannot get reliable access to food, in terms of quantity and quality, consistent with good health, either from their own production or in the market. Household food insecurity has many interrelated causes: poor crop yields, low incomes, high food prices, low rates of exchange between food and non-food, and a lack of access to assets, including land, water, agricultural extension and credit. Extreme crop failure, especially if repeated over several years, sometimes exacerbated by civil conflict and AIDS, manifests itself as widespread food deprivation and death (see Ch. 32).

If a household is food-insecure, it is likely that infants and other vulnerable groups within the household are getting an inadequate diet. Poor health services, unclean drinking water and non-existent hygiene disposal systems all increase the likelihood of infection, particularly diarrhoea, which is the third leading cause of disability-adjusted life years (DALYs) lost in children under the age of 4, accounting for 17% of DALYs in this age group (Murray & Lopez 1996). Care is defined as the practices by care givers around care for women (e.g. time for resting and appropriate food during pregnancy), breastfeeding and feeding of young children, psychosocial stimulation of infants, food preparation and storage practices, hygiene practices and care for children during illness, including diagnosis and health seeking behaviour (Engle et al 1997). Care for mothers and infants is essential if food at the household level is to get to infants in the right form at the right time in the right quantities. Care is also essential if hygiene practices are performed that minimize exposure to the hazards of the health environment and minimize the need for health services. The provision of care requires accurate information about the best practices, and the time and authority to implement them. Emphasis is on young children and women as they are the most vulnerable sections of the community but of course older children and men can also be affected.

Underlying causes of overnutrition are mainly the converse, including overall food security, availability of plentiful, varied and relatively inexpensive food products (although not always the most healthy), food advertising, a sedentary lifestyle at work and leisure due to labour saving devices, transport, computers, work pressures, and increased perceptions of risk for children playing outside and walking or cycling to school.

Basic causes

The basic or root causes of malnutrition, both under- and overnutrition, are essentially political and economic. There are very few instances of high levels of undernutrition, as opposed to overnutrition, above gross domestic product (GPD) per capita levels of $4000 (Smith & Haddad 2002). Income growth is important for reducing undernutrition; however, the relationship is not as tight as one might think. Figure 33.3 uses survey data to model the effects of rapid income growth over a sustained time period for 12 countries.

Overall the study finds that a 10% increase in income produces a 5% reduction in the rate of undernutrition. Only in three countries does a rapid income growth rate alone achieve the Millennium Development Goal of halving the 1990 rate of undernutrition by 2015. So income growth is extremely helpful in decreasing undernutrition rates, especially when income distribution is more equal, but it is by no means sufficient, and given the wide range of levels of undernutrition at a given GDP per capita, some may say it is not necessary.

Other factors beyond income growth are obviously essential for good nutrition at all ages, such as good levels of education, social equity and enlightened government behaviour. Good governance – by which we mean institutions that give voice to all parts of society, respect for the civil, political, economic, social and cultural rights of its

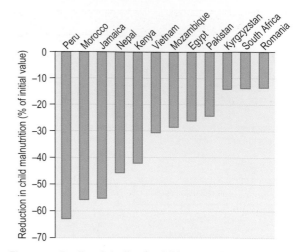

Fig. 33.3 Predicted decline in child malnutrition due to 2.5% growth in per capita income, 1990s to 2015.
Reproduced from Haddad et al. Reducing malnutrition: how far can income growth take us? World Bank Economic Review 2003; 7(1): 107–131 by permission of Oxford University Press.

citizens, and appropriate levels of investment in public goods such as safety, research, roads, health and education – is more likely to produce these conditions. Good education levels mean that individuals know how to access, assess, and use information that is helpful to the attainment of good nutrition status (such as the right types of foods to consume, what to do in the case of diarrhoea, and the optimal duration of exclusive breastfeeding). The status of women relative to men is a dimension of society and values that is crucial to the nutrition status of women and of infants. This is demonstrated in part by the fact that many of the underlying and basic causes of undernutrition are better in south Asia than in sub-Saharan Africa, and yet undernutrition levels, at least for preschool children, are worse in south Asia (see Table 33.2). Empirical work using nationally representative data from 36 countries (Smith et al 2003) shows that the poor status of women relative to men in south Asia plays an important role in explaining what has become known as the 'Asian enigma'. Yet, even if the status of women relative to men in south Asia does not improve, the rate of stunting in that region is at least declining, which is not the case in sub-Saharan Africa: the rate of stunting is on the increase. The special case of sub-Saharan Africa has been mentioned frequently. Some of the factors behind the tragic decline in nutrition status in sub-Saharan Africa are summarised in Box 33.1.

<table>
<tr><td>

BOX 33.1 Factors behind nutritional decline in sub-Saharan Africa

- Closed markets in the developed world (especially the European Union) for their exports
- HIV/AIDS – generating a health and development crisis and undermining the ability to respond to the crisis
- Wars and refugee movements
- Military expenditure
- Drought
- Crop and livestock disease
- Many ecosystems making technology diffusion and adaptation difficult
- Underinvestment in agricultural research
- No economy serving as regional driver (Nigeria and South Africa's underwhelming economic performance)
- Low levels of human capital in terms of literacy
- Declining terms of trade for natural resources on world markets
- Low population densities leading to thin infrastructure and market institutions

Source: Authors.
</td></tr>
</table>

The basic causes of overnutrition are also essentially political and economic, affecting many of the factors mentioned above and more particularly such factors as employment, incomes, work pressures hence time availability, food prices, taxation policies, advertising policies and environmental factors such as facilities for transport, including cycling, and for sport.

KEY POINTS

- The causes of undernutrition and overnutrition are at three levels – immediate, underlying and basic.
- The immediate causes of undernutrition relate to poor food intake and infection.
- The immediate causes of overnutrition relate to excess energy intake and/or inadequate energy expenditure.
- The underlying causes of undernutrition relate to household food insecurity, poor support for caring practices and a weak health and sanitation environment.
- The underlying causes of overnutrition relate to household food security, a plentiful, relatively

inexpensive and varied supply of energy dense food, and low levels of activity.
- The basic causes of both are economic and political in nature.
- The status of women is key in promoting good nutrition.
- Sub-Saharan Africa is beset by multiple factors at all levels that make progress in reducing malnutrition very difficult.

33.3 TYPES OF INTERVENTION

Much is known about how to combat the different forms of malnutrition. This is especially true for undernutrition but less so for overnutrition which is a more recent worldwide phenomenon with a shorter history of interventions on which to draw conclusions. However this clear distinction between under- and overnutrition becomes more blurred as knowledge of the effects of fetal programming increases, indicating that fetal and infant adaptation to nutritional stress increases susceptibility later in life to the chronic diseases associated with overnutrition. Therefore many interventions apply to both ends of the malnutrition spectrum. For direct interventions, such as micronutrient supplementation, or exclusive breastfeeding to 6 months, efficacy trials tell us what can work under controlled conditions, and effectiveness trials and cost-effectiveness estimates tell us what works under real-life conditions using scarce resources that have alternative uses. The interventions, when they work, produce benefit–cost ratios that are competitive with other investments (Gillespie & Haddad 2003). For indirect interventions – those that have an impact on nutrition, but do not have nutrition as a primary or even secondary goal – such as food price subsidies, agricultural commercialization or microfinance targeted to women, it is difficult to obtain a strong experimental design. For these interventions we have to rely more on plausibility assessments of impact on nutrition, usually working via the underlying determinants of nutrition.

Table 33.10 summarizes the direct and indirect interventions that are thought to work especially, but not solely, for undernutrition by type of problem being addressed. In general, the direct interventions focus on (a) improving breastfeeding rates up to 6 months of age, (b) improving the quality and quantity of foods that complement breastfeeding beyond 6 months of age, (c) improving the quality

Table 33.10   Direct and indirect actions to reduce malnutrition

OBJECTIVE	DIRECT INTERVENTIONS	INDIRECT ACTIONS
Improving Pregnancy Outcome	• Target supplements to undernourished women – preconception weight <40–45 kg, or low attained weight during pregnancy; low BMI or height are less useful indicators. • Trimester 3 most effective to improve birthweight but intervene as soon as possible, and for as long as possible • Provide energy – or encourage consumption of more of normal diet (if protein intake is adequate) • Improve dietary quality and provide multiple micronutrients • Provide iodine in areas with endemic deficiency • Other risk factors for low birthweight are young maternal age at conception, so target interventions at those still growing	• Improve the status of women to lower age at first marriage • Microcredit, targeted to women • More emphasis on education of girls • Improved maternity benefits
Improving Child Growth	• Improve breastfeeding with exclusive breastfeeding for 4–6 months • Continue breastfeeding during complementary feeding • Need national and international guidelines on complementary feeding; when, what/dietary quality, how much, micronutrients? • Energy intake improves weight, not length. Increases in energy density most often needed (via reductions in water content of food) • Protein: extra intake usually limited benefit • Animal: dried skim milk improved growth in 12/15 trials, but fewer impacts of fish and meat • Micronutrient fortification of cereal staples is important • Multiple micronutrient supplementation is promising	• Agricultural research to be more focused on diet quality and nutrition outcomes • Agricultural production systems more in tune with child-care needs • Improved water, sanitation and health service delivery (better quality, better targeted)
Preventing and Treating Anaemia	Pregnancy • Fe supplements increase maternal haemoglobin and iron status and increase infant Fe status for 6 months after birth • No conclusions as to benefits for maternal and infant health and function • Daily (as opposed to weekly) supplements during pregnancy are more effective Infancy • Supplement all LBW infants with Fe from 2 months • Other need for Fe supplementation is uncertain (Cut-offs? Morbidity? Benefits for function?) Children Daily or weekly Fe supplements give improved mental and motor function Adults • Fe supplements lead to positive work performance even for iron deficiency/mild anemia, and tasks with moderate effort • Increased ascorbic acid from local foods not effective • Fe fortification of wheat (Venezuela), salt (+iodine in India), dry milk (Chile) effective • NaFeEDTA (an iron fortificant) shows good potential and increased Fe status when added to salt, soy sauce, etc. • Multiple micronutrients may be more effective? • Plant breeding for iron-dense cereals shows some promise, but awaiting efficacy and effectiveness trials • Food-based solutions cannot rely on plant sources – animal sources are critical	• Agricultural research to be more focused on diet quality and nutrition outcomes • Improved status of women for improved intrahousehold food distribution • Improved legislation for fortification • Improved technology for fortification

Table 33.10 Direct and indirect actions to reduce malnutrition—cont'd

OBJECTIVE	DIRECT INTERVENTIONS	INDIRECT ACTIONS
Preventing and Treating Iodine Deficiency	• Salt iodisation is crucial • Prevent cretinism by iodine to the mother during first trimester but no later than second trimester Supplementation late in pregnancy may improve infant function • Not clear that iodine supplementation in deficient children improves cognition or growth • Iodised oil to 6-week-old infants reduces mortality in first 2 months by 72%	• Improved legislation for fortification
Preventing and Treating Vitamin A Deficiency	Pregnancy • Low-dose vitamin A or beta-carotene supplements in pregnancy decrease maternal mortality by 40%; also increases haemoglobin Infants and children • High-dose maternal supplementation at birth followed by breastfeeding leads to a 64% reduction in mortality under 12 months, 23% reduction in mortality 6–60 age group and major reduction (40%) in HIV mortality • Can also increase growth of malnourished children • Urgent need to (a) accelerate food fortification and (b) improve the availability of vitamin-A-rich foods • Continue genetically modified approaches, but with appropriate safety standards	• Improved legislation for fortification • Agricultural research to be more focused on diet quality and nutrition outcomes • Improved status of women for improved intrahousehold food distribution
Preventing Diet-Related Chronic Disease	Mass media may be able to play a role in nutrition education in developed countries but not enough experience of what will work e.g. in Asia. Dietary guidelines: used in developed countries to explicitly shift the diet towards healthy components, but difficulties when large pockets of undernutrition co exist. China is a good example. Food processing modifications (e.g. changes resulting in differing fat absorption); shifts in breeding, feeding and market trim practices in the livestock sector can contribute to lower levels of fat in meat over time School-based efforts: School-based initiatives offer important possibilities for improving diet and activity patterns; however, few initiatives have made a marked improvement in this area and surprisingly few have been carefully evaluated. Others, e.g. workplace interventions, social marketing campaigns, etc.	• Food price policy to encourage the consumption of healthier foods • Regulation relative to nutrient content of the diet • Environmental policies to facilitate increased activity • Education re levels of exercise

and quantity of food consumed by adolescent girls and pregnant and lactating women, (d) supplementing diets of all individuals with micronutrient capsules and/or fortifying foods with added micronutrients during processing, (e) improving the quality of nutrition information provided to parents and caretakers, and (f) increasing the diversity of diets consumed by all individuals via home-based production of small livestock, fruit and vegetables. Indirect interventions focus on (a) lowering the price of foods to consumers via subsidies or vouchers, (b) improving access to income (more work, higher productivity) and in more affluent countries social security, e.g. pensions, unemployment benefits, etc., (c) improving the ability to borrow and save to smooth consumption from one period to the next, (d) improving the ability of women to make decisions that improve nutrition, (e) improving education and the ability to acquire and use information, (f) improving access to water, sanitation and preventative and curative health services, and (g) raising the productivity and nutrient content of crops and livestock.

DIRECT INTERVENTIONS

Following are the main conclusions, based on an extensive literature review described by Allen & Gillespie (2001), on the efficacy of direct interventions targeting the main undernutrition outcomes in developing countries – low birthweight at term (or more precisely intrauterine growth retardation), stunting, and the three main micronutrient deficiencies – Fe, I and vitamin A. There is less information on the efficacy and effectiveness of approaches to overweight, obesity and diet-related chronic disease, beyond what is known about approaches to preventing or reducing the predisposing factors of IUGR and stunting (see Chs 19, 20, 21). Also, there is very little experience with policies and programs in this area anywhere in the developing world (World Bank 2006 annex 3.1). A fuller version of this section can be found in the accompanying Section *evolve* 33.3(a) .

Low birthweight at term (intrauterine growth retardation)

The following paragraphs outline conclusions that can be drawn from randomised, controlled efficacy trials of supplementary feeding of pregnant women.

- Only supplements that provide more energy cause a significant improvement in birth weight.
- Maternal supplementation can also increase maternal weight gain, infant head circumference and, when there is a serious energy shortage, the length of the newborn infant.
- For undernourished women or those who have a low body weight (<40 kg), these improvements in pregnancy outcome could be obtained by encouraging them to consume more of their normal diet where possible and/ or providing appropriate energy-containing supplements. The supplements should ideally be formulated from local foods.

- Where the normal diet is particularly low in protein or, as is often the case, low in micronutrients, it is important to ensure that these nutrients are also provided as supplements.
- If targeting is desired, women with the lowest weight (at conception through early pregnancy) and/or lowest energy intakes are most likely to benefit.
- There are conflicting data on whether supplementation is more effective during the second or third trimester for improving birth weight. However, it is clear that supplementation during either trimester can reduce the prevalence of LBW.
- Young maternal age at conception is an additional risk factor for poor pregnancy outcome; it is important to target interventions to those who are still growing.
- Whenever possible, attention should be paid to improving the quality as well as the quantity of food consumed during pregnancy.
- In areas of endemic iodine deficiency, adequate maternal iodine status is critical for the prevention of neonatal deaths, LBW and abnormal cognitive and physical development of the infant (see Iodine deficiency, below).
- Non-nutritional interventions that can improve pregnancy outcome include reducing energy expenditure in physical work, increasing age at conception, malarial prophylaxis and cessation of cigarette smoking.

Stunting

The main direct interventions aimed at preventing or reducing stunting comprise breastfeeding and complementary feeding promotion, supplementary feeding and micronutrient supplementation. Efficacy trials on these interventions suggest a number of conclusions and recommendations, outlined in the following paragraphs.

- Exclusive breastfeeding is strongly recommended for the first 6 months of life. Breastfeeding should be continued when other foods are added to the infant's diet. In general, the quality of complementary foods is poor compared to breast milk.
- There is probably no advantage to the infant of introducing complementary foods prior to 6

months, especially where the quantity and quality of such foods is inadequate.

- The energy density of many gruels, soups, broths and other watery foods fed to infants is often below the recommended 0.6 kcal/g. Energy intake can be increased by reducing the water added to foods where possible, and/or providing additional feedings. At present there is insufficient evidence to promote the use of amylases to lower the viscosity of cereals. Adding extra energy in the form of oil or sugar can adversely affect the density of protein and micronutrients in the diet.
- Even where breast milk intake is relatively low, in most situations the amount of protein in complementary foods will be more than adequate; adding protein alone or improving protein quality will not improve growth.
- Randomised controlled trials of the effects of processed complementary foods have shown a mixed impact on growth. Of nine trials, most included infants aged 6–12 months.
- Intervention after age 12 months was less effective than between 6 and 12 months. However, there was an increased risk of displacement of breast milk when intakes of complementary foods were high, especially before 6 months of age.

In most developing countries and even in wealthier regions, the micronutrient content of unfortified complementary foods is inadequate to meet infant requirements. It is particularly difficult for infants to consume enough iron, zinc or calcium; and vitamin A, riboflavin, thiamin and vitamin B_6 intakes are often low.

- Micronutrient intakes can also be improved by targeting animal products to young children. The consumption of higher amounts of animal products was associated with better growth and micronutrient status in several studies.
- Micronutrient fortification of cereal staples is especially important where these are major constituents of complementary foods.

Commercial ready to use foods (RTUF) enriched with micronutrients are being increasingly promoted and used in emergency situations and in community nutrition projects (see *evolve* 28.2 (c)), but should be used judiciously to avoid their potential to de-value continued breastfeeding and indigenous foods, to further commercialise infant feeding, and delay the gradual transition to family foods and sustainable meal patterns. There are concerns about their cost for poor families and about the medicalisation of food by health programmes).

Iron deficiency

Intervention trials have demonstrated a number of benefits from improving iron status and reducing anemia, as outlined below.

- Randomised, controlled clinical trials show that iron supplementation of pregnant women improves haemoglobin and iron status, even in industrialised countries. Efficacy increases with iron doses up to 60 mg/day. Where iron supplementation has not been effective, this has been due predominantly to programmatic constraints such as lack of available supplements and poor compliance.
- No conclusions can be made about the benefits of iron supplementation during pregnancy on maternal or fetal health, function or survival. Maternal iron supplementation during pregnancy can improve both maternal and infant iron status for up to about 6 months postpartum.
- A recent meta-analysis comparing the efficacy of daily and weekly randomized controlled iron supplementation trials concluded that daily iron supplementation is most effective for preventing anaemia – and especially severe anaemia – during pregnancy.
- LBW infants are born with very low iron stores, which are depleted by 2–3 months postpartum. Because breast milk cannot meet their iron requirements, they should be supplemented with iron starting at 2 months of age.
- Anaemia during infancy could result in long-term or permanent impairment of psychomotor function, although more studies are needed on this question. Iron supplementation of anaemic preschool children improves their cognitive and physical development. Improved growth of iron-supplemented preschool children and school children was observed in some studies but not in others.
- Anaemia is associated with lower productivity, even in tasks requiring moderate effort such as factory work and housework. Iron deficiency that has not yet progressed to anaemia may also reduce work capacity. Efficacy trials have

shown iron supplements to improve work performance of anaemic individuals.

- Except for iron fortification, there have been few attempts to assess the effectiveness of food-based strategies to improve iron status. Increasing ascorbic acid intake through local foods is probably an inadequate strategy to improve iron status where iron deficiency is prevalent. Targeting animal products to those with highest iron requirements, and supporting the production of small animals and fish, would increase the intake of absorbable iron and other micronutrients. There are strategies available to increase iron absorption through plant breeding but the efficacy and effectiveness of this approach have not been evaluated.

- Fortification of foods with iron has produced improvements in iron status in several countries. Iron fortification of maize and wheat in Venezuela is one such example.

- The search for better fortificants continues, and sodium-iron-EDTA has good potential. When added to sugar it increased haemoglobin and ferritin concentrations in a community trial in Guatemala. Iron added to soy sauce as sodium-iron-EDTA appears to be well absorbed and has been tested in large-scale production and fortification trials in the People's Republic of China. (These showed a drop in anaemia of one-third.)

- Weekly delivery of iron supplements does improve iron status, almost as well as daily delivery in the case of children and adolescents. (However caution is advised in malarial areas (WHO 2007.) This programmatic approach may be a cheaper, more effective way to prevent iron deficiency. Ways should be sought to deliver weekly iron through schools, community-based programmes and other situations. However, daily supplements are still more effective for pregnant women.

- Supplements containing multiple vitamins and minerals could be more effective for improving haemoglobin response than iron alone; multiple micronutrient deficiencies often occur simultaneously and several nutrients are required for haemoglobin synthesis. Multiple micronutrient supplements are now being formulated and tested by international organizations.

Iodine–deficiency disorders

Efficacy trials, summarized by Allen & Gillespie (2001), suggest the following:

- Salt iodisation is by far the most important population-based intervention for IDD control and has been shown to be efficacious in alleviating IDD, assuming that iodine concentrations in the salt are at appropriate levels at the time of consumption.

- Efforts toward establishing and sustaining national salt iodisation programmes have accelerated over recent years. Effective partnerships have been forged between relevant UN agencies, national and international non-government organizations (NGOs) and the salt industry.

- Cretinism, which results from maternal iodine deficiency during pregnancy, can be prevented by supplementing the mother during pregnancy, preferably during the first trimester but no later than the second trimester. Supplementation in late pregnancy, if that is the first time the mother can be reached, may provide some small benefits for infant function.

- Iodine deficiency during early life adversely affects learning ability, motivation, school performance and general cognitive function. It is not yet clear whether iodine supplementation benefits cognitive function if started during childhood. More studies are needed on this question. Neither is it clear whether supplementation improves growth of children.

- In an iodine-deficient region, iodine supplementation, even in the last half of pregnancy, substantially reduces infant mortality and improves birthweight.

- Giving iodised oil to 6-week-old infants caused a 72% reduction in mortality in the first 2 months. This suggests that it may be useful to administer iodized oil in WHO's Expanded Program on Immunization (EPI), in areas where iodine deficiency is prevalent.

Vitamin A deficiency (VAD)

Most countries where VAD is known to be a major public health problem have policies supporting the regular supplementation of children, an approach of known large-scale effectiveness that can reach the subpopulations affected by, or at risk of being affected by, VAD.

- Supplementation of women during pregnancy reduces the higher prevalence of night blindness that occurs in such women in areas of endemic VAD. Night blindness is associated with a higher risk of maternal morbidity and mortality.

- A high-dose supplement given on the day of birth lowered total infant mortality during the subsequent 4 months, but a multicentre trial of the efficacy of high-dose vitamin A given in the EPI programme failed to find an impact on mortality or morbidity during the first year of life. It is likely that the dose given was too low to improve infant vitamin A status for long. Maternal supplementation postpartum can improve both maternal and infant vitamin A status, the latter through higher breast milk content of the vitamin.

- A meta-analysis revealed that high-dose vitamin A supplementation reduced mortality from diarrhoea and measles by 23% in infants and children aged 6 months to 5 years. Severe diarrhoea was reduced by low-dose vitamin A in one study of severely malnourished children, but the reported benefits of high-dose vitamin A on diarrhoea-related outcomes have been variable. Little impact on recovery from acute lower respiratory tract infections has been found.

- Food-based strategies have good potential for preventing VAD. A number of food-based interventions have been implemented on a large scale but few have been evaluated adequately. Significant progress has been made in understanding how to effect behaviour change in such programmes, and about which food-based strategies are likely to be effective for improving vitamin A status. Food-based approaches need to be pursued more vigorously so that they become a larger part of the longer-term global strategy for alleviating VAD.

- The finding that the bioconversion of pro-vitamin A in dark-green leafy vegetables is less than one-quarter of that previously thought has raised doubts about the degree of efficacy of certain diet modification approaches to improving vitamin A status.

- Innovations include the promotion of egg consumption by small children in Bangladesh, which has shown promising results.

- Breastfeeding promotion, protection and support remain an essential component of control programmes for young children, as does infectious disease control, not only through immunisation, but also via complementary hygiene and sanitation interventions.

- There is an urgent need to expand efforts in fortification where foods reaching the target population groups are processed or where local fortification is feasible. Oil fortification with vitamin A is mandatory throughout most of South Asia although often not enforced.

- Control approaches based on improved availability of vitamin-A-rich foods and possibly genetic modification of staple foods to enhance vitamin A availability, as with iron, have been slower to develop and more difficult to implement, but progress is being made.

KEY POINTS

- A number of direct interventions exist that have shown to be efficacious, effective and cost-effective in reducing undernutrition.
- These interventions exist for all stages of the lifecycle and for specific micronutrient deficiencies–vitamin A, iron and iodine being the most common.
- Least is known in a practical nutrition intervention sense in a developing country setting about how to improve the birthweight of term newborns.

INDIRECT INTERVENTIONS

The discussion of indirect actions to reduce nutrition will not be as detailed as the discussion of the direct actions, because of the heterogeneity of indirect actions that can affect nutrition in a positive sense. Table 33.10 summarizes direct and indirect interventions, and ways in which indirect interventions can be strengthened for nutrition. This has relevance for both developed and developing countries. (For examples of such interventions in the UK see Section *evolve* 33.4(a) and Chs 19–21.) Recall that indirect actions are defined as ones that affect nutrition, even though improving nutrition outcomes is not a key goal of the intervention, such as:

- making agriculture more productive in ways that are consistent with improved nutrition
- making price policies more pro-poor and for the malnourished
- making income generation and income-transfer programs more pro-poor and for the malnourished
- improving the monitoring of food insecurity
- strengthening the role of women in society and in the home
- expanding the coverage of public health clinics
- strengthening the quality of health and sanitation service delivery
- improving access to water in sufficient quantity and quality
- improving access to good quality sanitation.

Is this too passive a role for these indirect actions? Might they not benefit in terms of their own goals from an explicit integration of direct nutrition components into their much larger indirect actions, for example integrating nutrition into the delivery of other health services?

The evidence that investments in nutrition can be a foundation for success in other areas is quite compelling. Not only should nutrition be viewed as a driver of intergenerational development, it should be viewed as a broad, non-exclusive investment opportunity. Because nutrition has a broad a etiology many different sectors can feasibly invest in it, and have a strong incentive to do so because of its broad developmental impact via such effects as cognitive development, child survival, income generation and reduced chronic disease, and also because added accountability has been thrust upon them by the international community's Millennium Development Goals. If these sectors did invest in nutrition, could they serve their own sectoral goals and allow nutrition investments to effect much larger resource flows, thereby accelerating reductions in malnutrition? This is an approach that seems to offer promise.

For example, in recent years such an approach is increasingly found in poverty interventions from South and Central America, and to a lesser extent in south Asia. The general idea behind them is to prevent economic or weather-related shocks from disrupting household asset accumulation (as happens, for example, when a child is pulled out of school or not taken to a health clinic: human capital accumulation is halted). Some interventions transfer cash (PROGRESA in Mexico, PRAF in Honduras, and Red de Protección in Nicaragua) or food (Food for Education in Bangladesh) in return for school attendance and health clinic attendance. See Section *evolve* 33.3(b) 🐭 for case studies on the PROGRESA experience in Mexico and on the Food for Education programme in Bangladesh.

These programmes are generally classified as development interventions but are motivated by a desire to keep chronic poverty and economic shocks from undermining the development process. They have worked well in the above countries. The expenditures underlying them are regarded as investments rather than transfers by the governments involved. They are probably more effective at preventing the impact of shocks rather than improving the response to shocks in that they rely on administrative targeting rather than self-selection (as opposed to public works programmes, for example). Large development interventions can become explicitly focused on both protecting and households and promoting their ability to deal with shocks as a means to a development end.

In order to effectively insert direct components into indirect actions to effect large resource flows for nutrition improvement, nutritionists and nutrition investors need to be more strategic in the use of opportunities created by the changing development context. Advocacy for nutrition is not just information dissemination – it requires a better understanding of the values, interests, motivations, beliefs, goals and constraints of all stakeholders (international organisations, national and local governments, communities, the private sector, the media, consumers and researchers) in order to shine light within the black box of the political economy of nutrition. An improved understanding of how decisions are made will help position nutrition better in this dynamic context, ultimately making it 'good politics' to act for nutrition.

Although no such overall review of the effectiveness of various interventions in reducing the chronic nutrition-related diseases has yet been carried out, some systematic reviews on interventions for specific diseases have been conducted, e.g. childhood obesity (Shaw et al 2006, Summerbell et al 2005, Hooper et al 2000, Thomas et al 2006). Interventions in the form of clinical trials are described for cardiovascular diseases in Chapter 19, prevention and treatment measures for obesity in Chapter 20 and the management and prevention of diabetes in Chapter 21 (Table 33.10).

KEY POINTS

■ Indirect interventions do not have improvements in nutrition as an explicit objective, but can have powerful indirect and supportive effects on nutrition status.

■ Indirect interventions relate to agriculture, income generation and maintenance, the status of women, education, water access (quality and quantity), sanitation and health services (preventive and curative) and environmental measures to moderate activity.

■ An increasingly popular (and so far effective) modality is the explicit insertion of direct intervention components into indirect interventions, e.g. the nutrition behaviour change component of the large cash transfer program PROGRESA in Mexico.

33.4 THE EVOLUTION OF THINKING ABOUT FOOD AND NUTRITION SECURITY AND NUTRITION–RELEVANT INTERVENTIONS AND POLICY

This section outlines the changes in thinking about food and nutrition concepts, causes, interventions and policy over the past 50 years or so, and highlights some of the contextual issues currently on the agenda or soon to be emerging.

THE 1950s TO DATE

The types of intervention that have been most strongly promoted by governments and international agencies have followed changes in perceptions of what were the most important problems, and their causes. In general, the perceptions around nutrition interventions and policy have moved from a 'food-production-only' perspective at the national level to rather sophisticated perspectives on food as a human right.

1950s

The 1950s focused on producing enough food at the national level to potentially feed all people.

Nutrition was considered to be primarily an issue of insufficient food quantity. The focus was on expanding agricultural output by bringing more land into cultivation. As the availability of good quality land for new production became limited, the returns to land expansion fell.

There was increased recognition that an integrated approach to improving nutrition was required and 'Applied Nutrition Programmes' were promoted by the international agencies (FAO 1972). These were broad-based community development programmes designed to improve the quantity and quality of local food production and use, and to improve income. Components included prevention against infections, nutrition education, horticulture, animal production, fish ponds, food storage, pest control, cottage industry cooperatives, fortification and improved transport. Some of these, e.g. Korea, were later evaluated and found to be successful, but because of their limited geographic outreach had little global impact (Geissler 1993).

1960s

In the 1960s, the focus – still on food production – switched to yield, or output per hectare. The 'Green Revolution', led by the newly formed Consultative Group on International Agricultural Research (CGIAR), was an effort to develop high-yielding varieties of crops that would help to meet the increasing demand fuelled in large part by rapid population growth in the 1960s. The 'Green Revolution' succeeded in preventing large-scale famine – yields increased sharply, especially for the farmers who could afford the complementary inputs for the new varieties. Consumers benefited from lower cereal prices, allowing them to diversify diets into foods richer in proteins and nutrients. However, the new techniques were not particularly environmentally friendly, relying on pesticides, herbicides, inorganic fertilizers and irrigation and dams (see Ch. 32).

1970s

In the 1970s, the idea of broad-based agricultural growth as a driver of economic growth more generally took hold. Agriculture was not just about producing food, but it was about producing income, both for farmers and for the rural non-farm entrepreneurs that farmers purchased goods from. The notion that income (or economic access) was very important for reducing malnutrition was promoted by Sen's analyses of famines as entitlement failures. There was also the increased recognition of the role that education played, especially women's education, and nutrition-specific education, in promoting nutrition status.

The concept of National Nutrition Policies/Planning also developed. It had been assumed in the development literature that, as countries became more affluent, there would be a 'trickle-down effect' into improved nutrition. In the 1970s Alan Berg in *The Nutrition Factor* (Berg 1973) developed the idea that specifically targeting nutrition would improve human resources by reducing mortality, morbidity, the use of health services, educational loss, etc. and so be a lever to economic development. An intersectoral planning approach was promoted, and adopted by the development agencies (Joy 1973, FAO 1975). The World Food Conference in Rome in 1974, following an international food crisis in previous years, was instrumental in stimulating widespread analyses of the world food supply. Resolutions from the conference included that countries should have a national nutrition policy, and technical support was provided to many countries to do so.

The 1970s also saw an increased interest in nutrition policy for developed countries, with the growing realisation that existing legislation, which was based on food purity and the prevention of adulteration as well as control of deficiencies, was not adequate to deal with the changing nature of nutrition problems towards chronic nutrition-related diseases. For further information about nutrition policy in developed countries (see Sections *evolve* 33.4 (a) 📱 and (b)). Several government advisory, professional and consumer bodies in the USA, UK and other countries recommended appropriate dietary goals with the common theme of reducing fat, sugar and salt intake and increasing the intake of dietary fibre, fruit and vegetables. In contrast to policies related to undernutrition that promote increased consumption of nutrients, the advice to reduce the intake of certain nutrients appeared to be a threat to some sectors of the food industry. There was considerable opposition to the advice and arguments about the validity of the evidence on which the recommendations were based. Additional constraints to updating food and nutrition policy included legislation designed to prevent adulteration and maintain quality as previously perceived, such as minimum fat levels

in milk and premiums on animals with high fat content. However the proposals were gradually accepted and incorporated into government policies, while industry recognised new opportunities in the production of high-fibre, low-fat, low-salt and low-sugar food products. Norway was the first developed country to have an integrated Food and Nutrition Policy as promoted in the World Food Conference. The UK and other European countries subsequently developed food and nutrition policies within their health and agriculture sectors (see the 1990s).

1980s

The 1980s saw greater recognition of the role that women play in child nutrition through their economic as well as their reproductive role (social access). The income that women control empower them to make decisions that benefit their own health and the health of children. The decade also saw the recognition of the role of diet quality in the promotion of nutrition status. The notion that micro-nutrients play a more general role in child survival (beyond deficiency diseases) emerged and led to the development in developing countries of small-scale home gardening, capsule distribution and fortification programmes that remain popular today. Such programmes had been in use for several decades in developed countries, such as providing land for kitchen garden allotments and the provision of supplements to children and mothers, during the world wars, and the fortification of white flour with vitamins and minerals from that period. Compulsory fortification of margarine with vitamins A and D has existed in the UK since the 1967 Margarine Regulations came into force in 1971.

The 1980s formalised the notion of food insecurity as being not just about lack of access to food today, but also about the risk of losing access to food tomorrow. The risk of losing access was debilitating and also led to actions fashioned to cope with that risk, but which had very high costs – such as short-termism on the issue of natural resource mining, the over-diversification of income sources and the uneconomic storage of food at the household level. Finally, in the 1980s the importance of the triumvirate of food, care and health for nutrition came to be accepted. Interactions became clearer: poor-quality drinking water could undermine household food security; without adequate care for mothers, children could not be breastfed; without time to undertake health-seeking behaviour, preventive (and often curative) health care would not be accessed.

1990s

In the UK explicit nutritional goals were set for the first time in the 1992 government health policy *The Health of the Nation* which focused on five key areas for action: coronary heart disease and stroke, cancers, mental illness, HIV/AIDS and sexual health, and accidents, the first two of which are diet-related. The diet and nutrition targets are shown in Box 33.2.

By concentrating on these targets it was expected that the associated dietary changes and reduction in obesity would have beneficial consequences on such diseases as cancer, osteoarthritis, diabetes, etc. A Nutrition Task Force was set up to oversee implementation of action, promote coordination and cooperation between interested parties, and establish mechanisms for monitoring and evaluating progress. On a regional basis, the WHO European Region prepared the first Action Plan for Food and Nutrition Policy 2000–2005, which included a Food and Nutrition Task Force. The second Action Plan for Food and Nutrition Policy 2007–2012 (WHO 2008b) lists the international agreements that have been drawn up to tackle the challenges described in

the first and adapts and renews the policy to take account of these developments.

Food safety became a major concern in the 1990s, particularly in the developed countries. European consumers in particular, having lost faith in the science establishment because of its initial assurances about the lack of danger to human health of BSE ('mad cow disease'), became extremely cautious about the safety of the food they purchased. And they were generally able and willing to pay a premium for assurances about the food production and processes used. In the UK this distrust also led to a revision of government structure via the Food Standards Act 1999, so that agricultural and consumer food interests, which had been combined within the Ministry of Agriculture Food and Fisheries (MAFF), were separated into the Food Standards Agency (FSA) (www.food.org) to champion consumer interests and the Department for the Environment Food and Rural Affairs to look after agriculture (www.defra.org). The role of the FSA is described in Section *evolve* 33.4(b) 🦶. A similar body was later established within the European Union, the European Food Safety Authority in 2002 (www.efsa.europa.eu). In the USA food and nutrition are regulated by the Food and Drug Administration (www.fda.gov). The capacity required to adhere to the new food safety expectations has made it harder for developing country exporters to gain market share in the developed world, harming their own food security through constraints to export opportunities.

Conflated with these new food safety expectations have been concerns about genetically modified (GM) foods. To date, GM foods have realised benefits largely for producers in terms of higher productivity and lower costs. Despite no obvious benefits to consumers other than perhaps lower prices, those in the USA have been consuming GM soybean products from early in the 1990s. But European consumers and many in the USA are concerned that the food safety and environmental safety issues related to GM foods have not been adequately researched. Difficult policy issues have been raised: will USA food aid shipments containing some GM foods not be admitted into hunger-wracked areas for fear of introducing GM seeds into the developing countries, agricultural systems that then prevent them from exporting to Europe and other countries? The mandatory labelling of foods as 'containing GM organisms, was put forward as one solution to such issues, allowing consumers to

---

BOX 33.2	**Diet and nutrition targets for the UK in 2005: *The Health of the Nation* 1992 (baseline 1990)**

To reduce the average % food energy from saturated fats by at least 35% (to no more than 11% food energy)

To reduce the average % food energy from total fat by at least 12% (to no more than about 35% food energy)

To reduce the % of men and women aged 16–64 who are obese by at least 25% and 35% respectively (to no more than 6% of men and 8% of women)

To reduce the % of men drinking more than 21 units of alcohol per week and women drinking more than 14 units per week by 30% (to 18% of men and 7% of women)

make informed choices, but this has been opposed by GM producers, who claim that it would be too expensive to keep the GM and non-GM crops separate throughout the food distribution chain. GMOs are also involved in nutrition from the health side (vaccines and other drugs), but here the issue is not so much safety as access – the drug companies are resisting differential pricing regimes for rich and poor countries, making the argument that such pricing schemes will diminish their incentive to innovate. There are some new institutional arrangements (e.g. public–private interactions such as GAVI on vaccines (at www.gavialliance.org) and GAIN on food fortification (at www.gainhealth. org) that are seeking to create incentives for the private sector to develop drugs and fortified foods for the benefit of the poor. Much rests on their success.

Also in the 1990s awareness increased that pockets of food poverty still existed in developed countries, following the increased economic inequality that developed in the 1980s in the UK and other countries, partly due to government cutbacks in welfare programmes. This led to reports and actions to relieve the constraints of the poor (Riches 1997) and echoed a similar period in the USA in the 1960s about 'Hunger in America' which resulted in new welfare programmes such as WIC (Kennedy 1999) (see Section *evolve* 33.4(a) 🖱).

Finally, the right to food, first formalised in the 1948 Universal Declaration of Human Rights, and then confirmed in milestones such as the 1966 Covenants on Civil and Political Rights and on Economic, Social and Cultural Rights, the 1989 Convention on the Rights of the Child, and the 1996 World Food Summit hosted by FAO, came of age from the 1990s. The concepts are that governments have a duty to respect, protect, facilitate and fulfil if necessary the rights of the individual to secure adequate food and nutrition. In a legal sense the right to food can be used by one branch of a country's government to compel other branches to promote food and nutrition security, as happened in India in 2003 (Box 33.3) or it can be used by the UN to 'name and shame' countries that do not give food and nutrition issues prominence. In an analytical and programmatic context it focuses us on the capacity of different actors to make claims and deliver on obligations, often in an interlocking sequence. In others words it helps focus on accountability via identification of roles and responsibilities, and on capabilities.

BOX 33.3   Supreme Court of India's ruling on right to food

On 23 July 2001, the court said: 'In our opinion, what is of utmost importance is to see that food is provided to the aged, infirm, disabled, destitute women, destitute men who are in danger of starvation, pregnant and lactating women and destitute children, especially in cases where they or members of their family do not have sufficient funds to provide food for them. In case of famine, there may be shortage of food, but here the situation is that amongst plenty there is scarcity. Plenty of food is available, but distribution of the same amongst the very poor and the destitute is scarce and non-existent leading to mal-nourishment, starvation and other related problems.'

On 28 November 2001, the court issued directions to eight of the major schemes, calling on them to identify the needy and to provide them with grain and other services by early 2002. For example, for the Targeted Public Distribution Scheme, 'The States are directed to complete the identification of BPL (below poverty level) families, issuing of cards, and commencement of distribution of 25 kgs grain per family per month latest by 1st January, 2002'.

PUCL Bulletin, July 2001. Supreme Court of India. Record of proceedings. Writ petition (civil) no. 196 of 2001.

CURRENT CONCERNS AND EMERGING ISSUES SINCE 2000

Obesity and related conditions

The main current nutrition issue in the developed countries is the continued increase in obesity, in both adults and children, with concomitant increases in related conditions such as diabetes. In the UK it has been recognised that this cannot be tackled only on the nutrition front, and already in 1992 the UK government included an activity task force associated with the first explicit nutrition policy. From the early 2000s the problem of obesity hit the political agenda strongly, resulting in much political and public debate, including the role of government, industry, parents and the individual, with contrasting views about the nanny state and the need for government to take more vigorous action. However, despite these policies and varied interventions, obesity continues to grow in the UK to 30% and 32% for men and women respectively in 2005 as compared to the *Health of the Nation* targets of 6% and 8% for that year. The situation is similar in many other countries.

Increasing research also refines the association between various food factors and aspects of health and so determines policy. For example the USA has already undertaken folate fortification of flour and the UK is poised to do so.

Environment

Other related emerging issues are environmental concerns, which include the growth of the organic food market, although set back by the recent economic downturn and a study commissioned by the UK Food Standards Agency published in July 2009 showing that organic foods had no nutritional benefits – pesticides and fertilisers were not included in the study. Other food-related environmental concerns include the ecological sustainability of the food supply, especially the trade of produce that could be supplied locally, and the effect on global warming. Food safety and GM foods continue to be important issues in both developed and developing countries (see Ch. 32).

Food and nutrition security

The context within which food security and nutrition status need to be enhanced is changing rapidly, presenting opportunities and threats. The recent sharp rise in food prices (see Section *evolve* 32.4(a)) is a clear threat to food security and nutrition (Shrimpton et al 2009). Globalisation, namely the rapidly increasing levels of global food trade, financial flows, labour flows and information flows, present opportunities to be seized and risks to be managed in the pursuit of improved nutrition. Governments have to invest in infrastructure and market institutions that allow them to take advantage of new opportunities and they have to design and implement safety net programmes such as Progresa in Mexico or the Food for Education programme in Bangladesh that protect and compensate those who stand to lose from more open markets.

Urbanization

Urbanization is progressing rapidly throughout the world. Not only are people shifting to urban areas, but so too is the concentration of under- and overnutrition. The poor in urban areas are equally at risk of undernutrition as are the poor in rural areas, perhaps more so since they have little access to the means to produce their own food. Interventions that work in rural areas cannot be assumed to work as well in urban areas without re-design. This is because the main differences in urban areas – a reliance on food purchase, the large numbers of mothers working away from home, and water and air pollution from waste and fuels – make nutrition more susceptible to loss of regular employment, food price fluctuations, the quantity and quality of child care for low-income working mothers, and illnesses caused from environmental contaminants.

Ageing population

The demographic profile of the developing world's population is changing rapidly. The aging of the populations of all countries, both developed and developing, is a result of lower infant mortality rates and lower birth rates. The shift in the demographic profile does, however, place new pressure on efforts to finance undernutrition efforts adequately through public finance due to the new demands for spending on overnutrition-related issues such as diabetes and heart disease, although the presence of older family members – if they live close by – should help parents to cope with the multiple demands of work and child rearing.

AIDs

In contrast to most of the world, where life expectancy is on the rise, in one area, sub-Saharan Africa, due to HIV/AIDS, it is on the decline, along with most indicators of malnutrition (ACC/SCN 2004). AIDS is also looming large over China, India, Cambodia and Russia. AIDS kills adults of working age and very young infants. Adult mortality, the chronic illness that precedes it, and the caring for the adult with AIDS all serve to undermine the ability of farmers to produce food and families to purchase it, mothers to care for children, and the provision of public goods such as safe water and health care. Good maternal nutrition status is also thought to minimise mother to child transmission via birthing, although breastfeeding does increase the risk if the mother is HIV-positive.

Nutrition transition

The diet transition in the developing world seems to be accelerating – for both rich and poor, rural and urban (see Ch. 1). It is a transition towards a coexistence of under- and overnutrition. It is driven by changing preferences fuelled by some of the factors discussed above – but in the context of undernutrition such as growing incomes, changing relative prices, urbanisation, ageing, changing food choice options fuelled by changes in food technology and changes in the food distribution systems, and by a legacy of low birthweights from the previous generation. What can food and nutrition policy do to make this transition healthier? Section *evolve* 33.4(c) 🐭 outlines some of the options. We should note that these options have had mixed success in the industrialized countries. The policy tradeoffs in the developing world are even more complicated. For example, price policy efforts to overcome overnutrition by making some foods with high saturated fat content more expensive might well undermine efforts to overcome undernutrition because those same foods may be rich in micronutrients. The public health anti-smoking policy model offers some insights, but it should not be leaned on too heavily – food is not tobacco. There are plenty of areas in which additional technical research is needed to assess competing risks and to help develop policy options. The need to understand the nutrition policy process will be even more critical in the crowded policy landscape occupied by the issue of the diet transition.

Millenium Development Goals

The Millennium Development Goals have once again brought into sharp focus the rate of progress or lack of it towards meeting the goals. For many years there has been international concern about the rate of progress in improving nutrition. In 1992 Alan Berg asked 'What is the reason for our failure to make large dents in malnutrition?' (Berg 1992). He concluded that the answer lay in imbalanced research emphasis and the lack of appropriately trained people. Most graduate nutrition students do increasingly narrow research, rarely broad-based applied research, so that they are not equipped for the broad role of designing and managing nutrition interventions. This is partly due to the pressure to publish in journals with high scientific ratings. He considered that what we need are nutrition engineers, i.e. 'a person who carries through a enterprise and brings about a result' through integrated programmes, and suggested the need for new institutions.

The World Bank has recently revived Alan Berg's seminal work on the role of nutrition in national development (Berg 1973) in the recent document entitled *Repositioning Nutrition as Central to Development* (World Bank 2006). The impetus for the report was the growing international awareness that many of the MDGs will not be reached unless malnutrition is tackled, and also that there is now 'unequivocal evidence that there are workable solutions and that they are excellent investments'. The May 2004 Copenhagen Consensus, in which a long list of development actions was reviewed by eminent economists, it was concluded that the returns of investing in micronutrient programmes are second only to fighting HIV/AIDS and other nutrition-related interventions were among the top dozen. They concluded that new partnerships are critical and urged development partners to extend their activities beyond responding to government requests. They should influence them to put nutrition higher on the agenda wherever it is holding back achievement of the MDGs, requiring a common view of the malnutrition problem, broad strategies to address it, and speaking with a common voice. (See Section *evolve* 33.4(d) on development partners supporting nutrition 🐭).

Nutrition Governance

This type of collaboration has in fact been the aim of the UN Standing Committee for Nutrition (SCN), a body set up to harmonise approaches to improving nutrition among the UN agencies, governmental and non-governmental partners, to have a greater overall impact on nutrition. This role is essential but unfortunately the partners have not been willing to provide adequate funding for the SCN to fulfil its function adequately.

An appeal for better governance has also been voiced again more recently in the *Lancet* series on malnutrition (Morris et al 2008). They observe that many transnational organisations work to support efforts to eliminate maternal and child undernutrition in high-burden countries and argue that the international system should serve four functions: stewardship, mobilisation of financial resources, direct provision of nutrition services at times of natural disaster or conflict, and human and institutional resource strengthening. But they find substantial shortcomings in the system due to fragmentation, lack of an evidence base for prioritised action, institutional inertia, and failure to join up with promising developments in parallel sectors because of systemic problems which affect most organisations working in the field. They make recommendations to overcome some of the most important problems, and propose five priority actions for the development of a new international architecture – a new global governance structure, a more effective UN, fewer parallel organisations but fewer mandate gaps, more investment in capacity strengthening in high-burden countries, and research leadership in areas that matter.

KEY POINTS

- Public policy for malnutrition reduction has moved from food production to food access to diet diversity to the food–care–health model.
- Human rights are increasingly being se.en as useful in putting pressure on governments to address malnutrition.
- Globalisation, urbanisation and ageing represent new challenges to the achievement of good nutrition status, being particularly important in the growth of overnutrition (i.e. diet-related chronic diseases) in poor countries.

- Ageing and overnutrition are important challenges in developed countries.
- For many countries in East and southern Africa, HIV/AIDS represents a huge challenge to the attainment of good nutrition.
- The international governance of nutrition needs to be strengthened to accelerate nutritional improvements.

References

ACC/SCN (United Nations Administrative Committee on Coordination/Sub-Committee on Nutrition): *Fourth report on the world nutrition situation*, Geneva, 2000, ACC/SCN in collaboration with the International Food Policy Research Institute, Washington DC.

ACC/SCN *Fifth report on the world nutrition situation*, Geneva, 2004, SCN.

Allen LH, Gillespie SR: *What works? A review of the efficacy and effectiveness of nutrition interventions.* ACC/SCN Nutrition Policy Paper No. 19. Nutrition and Development Series No. 5, Manila, 2001, Asian Development Bank.

Berg A: *The nutrition factor in national development*, Washington DC, 1973, The Brookings Institute,

Berg A: Sliding toward nutrition malpractice: time to reconsider and redeploy, *American Journal of Clinical Nutrition* 57:3–7, 1992.

Engle PL, Menon P, Haddad L: Care and nutrition: Concepts and measurement, *World Development* 27:1309–1337, 1999.

FAO: *Planning and evaluation of applied nutrition programmes.* FAO

Nutritional Studies 26, Rome, 1972, FAO.

FAO: *Food and nutrition planning.* Nutrition Consultants Report Series 35, Rome, 1975, FAO.

FAO *The World Food Summit FAO Rome, 1996.* Available online at http://www.tao.org/wfs/index_en.htm, accessed 1/8/09.

FAO. *The state of food insecurity in the world (SOFI)*, 2008 Available online at: http://www.fao.org/publications/sofi/index_en.htm accessed 25-7-09).

FAO 2009 *The state of food insecurity in the world (SOFI)* (in press).

Geissler C: Stature and other indicators of development: comparisons in Thailand and the Philippines, Korea and Iran. In Geissler C, Oddy DJ, editors: *Food, diet and economic change, past and present*, Leicester, 1993, Leicester University Press.

Gillespie S, Haddad L: *The double burden of malnutrition in Asia and the Pacific*, New Delhi 2003, Sage Publications.

Haddad L, Alderman HS, Appleton L, Song, Yohannnes Y: Reducing malnutrition: how far can income

growth take us? *World Bank Economic Review* 17(1):107–131, 2003.

Hooper L, Summerbell CD, Higgins JPT, et al. Reduced or modified dietary fat for preventing cardiovascular disease. *Cochrane Database of Systematic Reviews* 2000, Issue 2. Art. No.: CD002137. DOI: 10.1002/14651858.CD002137.

Joy L: Food and nutrition planning, *Journal of Agricultural Economics* 24(1), 1973.

Kennedy E: Public policy in nutrition: the US nutrition safety net – past, present and future. *Food Policy* 24:325–333, 1999.

MI (The Micronutrient Initiative): *The Micronutrient Report*, Mason JB, Lotfi M, Dalmiya N, Sethuraman K and M. Deitchler. Ottawa. 2001, The Micronutrient Initiative.

Morris SS, Cogill B, Vany R: Effective international action against undernutrition: why has it proven so difficult and what can be done to accelerate the progress? *Lancet* 371:608–621, 2008.

Murray C, Lopez A, editors: *The global burden of disease*, Boston, MA, 1996, Harvard School of Public Health on behalf of the World Health Organization and the World Bank.

Popkin BS, Horton, Kim S: *The nutrition transition and prevention of diet-related chronic diseases in Asia and the Pacific.* Nutrition and Development Series No. 6. Manila, 2001, Asian Development Bank.

Riches G, editor: *First world hunger: food security and welfare politics,* Basingstoke, UK, 1997, Macmillan.

Shaw KA, Gennat HC, O'Rourke P, Del Mar C. Exercise for overweight or obesity. *Cochrane Database of Systematic Reviews* 2006, Issue 4. Art. No.: CD003817. DOI: 10.1002/14651858.CD003817.pub3.

Shrimpton R, Prudhon C, Engesveen K: The impact of high food process on maternal and child nutrition, *SCN News* 37:60–68, 2009.

Smith LC, Haddad L: How Potent is economic growth in reducing undernutrition? What are the pathways of impact? New cross-country evidence, *Economic Development and Cultural Change* 51(Number 1):October, 2002.

Smith LC, Ramakrishnan U, Ndiaye A, et al: The importance of women's status for child nutrition in developing countries, *IFPRI Research Report* 1312, 2003.

Summerbell CD, Waters E, Edmunds L, Kelly SAM, Brown T, Campbell KJ. Interventions for preventing obesity in children. *Cochrane Database of Systematic Reviews* 2005, Issue 1. Art. No.: CD001871. DOI: 10.1002/14651858.CD001871.pub2.

Thomas D, Elliott EJ, Naughton GA. Exercise for type 2 diabetes mellitus. *Cochrane Database of Systematic Reviews* 2006, Issue 3. Art. No.: CD002968. DOI: 10.1002/14651858.CD002968.pub2.

UNICEF *Strategy for improved nutrition of children and women in developing countries,* New York, 1990, UNICEF.

WHO: *Iodine status worldwide. WHO database on iodine deficiency 1993–2003,* Geneva, 2004, WHO. Available online at http://www.who.int/vmins/iodine/status/en/index.html.

WHO: *Worldwide prevalence of anaemia 1993–2005. WHO global database on anaemia,* Geneva, 2008a, WHO. Available online at: http://www.who.int/vmins/anaemia/en.

WHO: *European Action Plan for Food and Nutrition Policy,* Copenhagen, 2008b, WHO.

WHO: Consultation on prevention and control of iron deficiency in infants and young children in malaria-endemic areas, *Food and Nutrition Bulletin* 28(Suppl 4):S621–S627, 2007. Available online at: http://www.ncbi.nlm.nih.gov/pubmed/18297899.

WHO: *Global prevalence of vitamin A deficiency in populations at risk 1995–2005,* Geneva, 2009, WHO. Available online at: http://www.who.int/vmins/vitamina/en.

WHO: Obesity – preventing and managing the global epidemic. Report of a WHO consultation on obesity, 3–5 June, 1997, Geneva, 1998, World Health Organization.

World Bank: *Repositioning nutrition as central to development: a strategy for large scale action,* Washington DC, 2006, World Bank.

Further reading

Government Office for Science: *Foresight. Tackling obesities: future choices,* London UK, 2007, GOS.

Lang T, Barling D, Caraher M: *Food policy. Integrating health, environment and society,* Oxford, 2009, Oxford University Press.

Millstone E, Lang T: *The atlas of food. Who eats what, where, why,* 2nd ed. Brighton, UK, 2008, Myriad Editions, for Earthscan.

SCN Reports on the World Nutrition Situation: 1st 1987, 2nd 1992, 3rd 1997, 4th 2000, 5th 2004, 6th 2009.

Available on line at http://www.unscn.org.

WHO: *Comparative analysis of nutrition policies in the WHO European region,* Geneva, 2006, WHO. Available online at: http://www.euro.who.int/document/Nut/instanbul_conf%20ebd02.pdf.

Glossary

Note: there is a list of abbrevations on page 729

abrasion – Tooth wear caused by brushing

acceptable daily intake (ADI) – The amount of a food additive that could be taken daily for an entire lifespan without appreciable risk. Determined by measuring the highest dose of the substance that has no effect on experimental animals, then dividing by a safety factor of 100

acetal – Product of addition of alcohol to aldehyde

acetomenaphthone – Synthetic compound with vitamin K activity; vitamin K_3, or menaquinone-0

achlorhydria – Deficiency of hydrochloric acid in gastric digestive juice

acid – Chemically, compounds that dissociate (ionise) in water to give rise to hydrogen ions (H^+); they taste sour

acid foods, basic foods – These terms refer to the residue of the metabolism of foods. The mineral salts of sodium, potassium, magnesium and calcium are base-forming, while phosphorus, sulphur and chlorine are acid-forming. Which of these predominates in foods determines whether the residue is acidic or basic (alkaline); meat, cheese, eggs and cereals leave an acidic residue, while milk, vegetables and some fruits leave a basic residue

acidogenicity – Ability to produce acid through bacterial metabolism

acidosis – An increase in the acidity of blood plasma to below the normal range of pH 7.3–7.45, resulting from a loss of the buffering capacity of the plasma, alteration in the excretion of carbon dioxide, excessive loss of base from the body or metabolic overproduction of acids

acrodermatitis enteropathica – Severe functional zinc deficiency due to failure to secrete an as yet unidentified compound in pancreatic juice that is required for zinc absorption

acrodynia – Dermatitis seen in animals deficient in vitamin B_6. There is no evidence for a similar dermatitis in deficient human beings

acrylamide – A chemical that can be generated when the amino acid asparagine is heated above 100°C in the presence of sugars

active transport – Energy-requiring transport of solutes across cell membranes, against the prevailing concentration gradient

acute phase proteins – A variety of serum proteins synthesised in increased (or sometimes decreased) amounts in response to trauma and infection, so confounding their use as indices of nutritional status

acute phase reaction – Increase or decrease in the concentration of certain proteins, or other substances, including micronutrients, in blood serum, following infections or tissue-inflammatory reactions. This reaction represents the body's normal response in counteracting the deleterious effects of a noxious stimulus, but the changes in distributions of proteins and nutrients between body compartments can confound attempts to measure nutrient status by blood assays in those situations where an acute phase reaction is present. Its presence can be monitored, e.g. by measuring C-reactive protein (CRP) or α_1-antichymotrypsin (ACT), both of which are increased by infections or inflammation, in serum or plasma

additive – Any compound not commonly regarded or used as a food which is added to foods as an

© 2010 Elsevier Ltd/Inc/BV
DOI: 10.1016/B978-0-7020-3118-2.00034-6

aid in manufacturing or processing, or to improve the keeping properties, flavour, colour, texture, appearance or stability of the food, or as a convenience to the consumer. The term excludes vitamins, minerals and other nutrients added to enrich or restore nutritional value. Herbs, spices, hops, salt, yeast or protein hydrolysates, air and water are usually excluded from this definition

adenine – A nucleotide, one of the purine bases of the nucleic acids (DNA and RNA). The compound formed between adenine and ribose is the nucleoside adenosine, and can form four phosphorylated derivatives important in metabolism: adenosine monophosphate (AMP, also known as adenylic acid); adenosine diphosphate (ADP); adenosine triphosphate (ATP) and cyclic adenosine monophosphate (cAMP)

adenocarcinoma – Cancer of the glandular epithelium

adenosine diphosphate (ADP) – *See* adenosine triphosphate; energy metabolism

adenosine triphosphate (ATP) – The coenzyme that acts as an intermediate between energy-yielding (catabolic) metabolism (the oxidation of metabolic fuels) and energy expenditure as physical work and in synthetic (anabolic) reactions. *See* energy metabolism

adequate intake – Where there is inadequate scientific evidence to establish requirements and reference intakes for a nutrient for which deficiency is rarely, if ever, seen, the observed levels of intake are assumed to be greater than requirements, and thus provide an estimate of intakes that are (more than) adequate to meet needs

adipocyte – A fat-containing cell in adipose tissue

adiponectin – Hormone secreted by adipose tissue that seems to be involved in energy homeostasis; it enhances insulin sensitivity and glucose tolerance, as well as oxidation of fatty acids in muscle

adipose tissue – Body fat storage tissue, distributed under the skin, around body organs and in body cavities – composed of cells that synthesise and store fat, releasing it for metabolism in fasting. Also known as white adipose tissue, to distinguish it from the metabolically more active brown adipose tissue, which is involved in heat production to maintain body temperature. The energy yield of adipose tissue is 34–38 MJ (8000–9000 kcal) per kg

adiposis – Presence of an abnormally large accumulation of fat in the body – also known as liposis

adipsia – Absence of thirst

adulteration – The addition of substances to foods, etc. in order to increase the bulk and reduce the cost, with intent to defraud the purchaser

aerobic – (1) Aerobic microorganisms (aerobes) are those that require oxygen for growth; obligate aerobes cannot survive in the absence of oxygen. The opposite are anaerobic organisms, which do not require oxygen for growth; obligate anaerobes cannot survive in the presence of oxygen. (2) Aerobic exercise is physical activity that requires an increase in heart rate and respiration to meet the increased demand of muscle for oxygen, as contrasted with maximum exertion or sprinting, when muscle can metabolise anaerobically

agalactia – Failure of the mother to secrete enough milk to feed a suckling infant

ageusia – Loss or impairment of the sense of taste

agricultural biotechnology – The application of molecular biology to agriculture, including but not limited to transgenic techniques, in which scientists develop plant and animal varieties that contain genes from other species

AIDS – Acquired immune deficiency syndrome; *see* HIV

alactasia – Partial or complete deficiency of the enzyme lactase in the small intestine, resulting in an inability to digest the sugar lactose in milk, and hence intolerance of milk

alanine – A non-essential amino acid

albumin (albumen) – A group of relatively small water-soluble proteins: ovalbumin in egg-white, lactalbumin in milk; plasma or serum albumin is one of the major blood proteins, which transports certain metabolites including non-esterified fatty acids in the bloodstream. Serum albumin concentration is sometimes measured as an index of protein–energy malnutrition. Often used as a non-specific term for proteins (e.g. albuminuria is the excretion of proteins in the urine)

alcohol – Chemically, alcohols are compounds with the general formula $C_nH_{(2n-1)}OH$. The alcohol in alcoholic beverages is ethyl alcohol (ethanol, C_2H_5OH)

alcohol units – For convenience in calculating intakes of alcohol, a unit of alcohol is defined as 8 g (10 ml) of absolute alcohol

aldosterone – A steroid hormone secreted by the adrenal cortex; controls the excretion of salts and water by the kidneys

alkali (or base) – A compound that takes up hydrogen ions and so raises the pH of a solution

alkaline tide – Small increase in blood pH after a meal as a result of the secretion of gastric acid

alkaloids – Naturally occurring organic bases which have pharmacological actions. Many are found in plant foods, including potatoes and tomatoes (the *Solanum* alkaloids), or as the products of fungal action (e.g. ergot), although they also occur in animal foods (e.g. tetrodotoxin in puffer fish, tetramine in shellfish)

alkalosis – *See* acidosis

allele – One of two or more alternative forms of a gene located at the corresponding site on homologous chromosomes

allergen – A chemical compound, commonly a protein, which causes the production of antibodies, and hence an allergic reaction

allergy – Adverse reaction to foods caused by the production of antibodies

allotriophagy – An unnatural desire for abnormal foods; also known as cissa, cittosis and pica

alpha helix (α-helix) – Common secondary structure in proteins

alpha linkage (α-linkage) – Bond formed by ring closure of a sugar with the hydroxyl group to the right of the chain in the Fischer projection formula (q.v.)

alveolar bone – Spongy part of jaw bone that supports the teeth

amenorrhoea – Cessation of menstruation, normally occurring between the ages of 40 and 55 (the menopause), but sometimes at an early age, especially as a result of severe under-nutrition (as in anorexia nervosa) when body weight falls below about 45 kg

Ames test – An in vitro test for the ability of chemicals, including potential food additives, to cause mutation in bacteria (the mutagenic potential). Commonly used as a preliminary screening method to detect substances likely to be carcinogenic

amines – Formed by the decarboxylation of amino acids. Three are potentially important in foods: phenylethylamine (formed from phenylalanine), tyramine (from tyrosine) and tryptamine (from tryptophan), because they stimulate the sympathetic nervous system and can cause increased blood pressure. In sensitive people they are one of the possible dietary causes of migraine

amino acid profile – The amino acid composition of a protein

amino acids – The basic units from which proteins are made. Chemically compounds with an amino group ($-NH_3^+$) and a carboxyl group ($-COO^-$) attached to the same carbon atom

aminoaciduria – Excretion of abnormal amounts of one or more amino acids in the urine, usually as a result of a genetic disease

aminogram – A diagrammatic representation of the amino acid composition of a protein. A plasma aminogram is the composition of the free amino acid pool in blood plasma

aminopeptidase – An enzyme secreted in the pancreatic juice which removes amino acids sequentially from the free amino terminal of a peptide or protein (i.e. the end that has a free amino group exposed). Since it works at the end of the peptide chain, it is an exopeptidase

aminotransferase – Any enzyme that catalyses the reaction of transamination

amylases – Enzymes that hydrolyse starch. α-Amylase (dextrinogenic amylase or diastase) acts to produce small dextrin fragments from starch, while β-amylase (maltogenic amylase) liberates maltose, some free glucose and isomaltose from the branch points in amylopectin. Salivary and pancreatic amylases are α-amylases

amylodyspepsia – An inability to digest starch

amylopectin – The branched chain form of starch, with branches formed by α1–6 bonds. About 75–80% of most starches; the remainder is amylose

amylose – The straight chain form of starch, with only α1–4 bonds. About 20–25% of most starches; the remainder is amylopectin

anabolic hormones – Natural or synthetic hormones that stimulate growth and the development of muscle tissue

anabolism – The process of building up or synthesising

anaemia – A shortage of red blood cells, leading to pallor and shortness of breath, especially on exertion. Most commonly due to a dietary deficiency of iron, or excessive blood loss. Other dietary deficiencies can also result in anaemia, including deficiency of vitamin B_{12} or folic acid (megaloblastic anaemia), vitamin E (haemolytic anaemia), and rarely vitamin C or vitamin B_6

anaemia, haemolytic – Anaemia caused by premature and excessive destruction of red blood cells; not normally due to nutritional deficiency, but can occur as a result of vitamin E deficiency in premature infants

anaemia, megaloblastic – Release into the circulation of immature precursors of red blood cells, due to deficiency of either folate or vitamin B_{12}

anaemia, pernicious – Anaemia due to deficiency of vitamin B_{12}, most commonly as a result of failure to absorb the vitamin from the diet. There is release into the circulation of immature precursors of red blood cells (megaloblastic anaemia) and progressive damage to the spinal cord (subacute combined degeneration), which is not reversed on restoring the vitamin

anaerobes – Microorganisms that grow in the absence of oxygen. Obligate anaerobes cannot survive in the presence of oxygen, facultative anaerobes grow in the presence or absence of oxygen

anaerobic threshold – The level of exercise at which the rate of oxygen uptake into muscle becomes limiting and there is anaerobic metabolism to yield lactate

aneuploidy – An abnormal number of chromosomes, usually associated with miscarriage, or developmental abnormalities such as Down's syndrome where there are three copies of chromosome 21 instead of two

aneurysm – Local dilatation (swelling and weakening) of the wall of a blood vessel, usually the result of atherosclerosis and hypertension; especially serious when occurring in the aorta, when rupture may prove fatal

angina (angina pectoris) – Paroxysmal thoracic pain and choking sensation, especially during exercise or stress, due to partial blockage of a coronary artery (blood vessel supplying the heart), as a result of atherosclerosis

angio-oedema – Presence of fluid in subcutaneous tissues or submucosa, particularly of the face, eyes, lips and sometimes tongue and throat; may occur during an anaphylactic reaction

angiotensin-converting enzyme (ACE) – Enzyme, in the blood vessels of the lungs, which activates angiotensin. Many of the drugs for treatment of hypertension are ACE inhibitors

angular stomatitis – A characteristic cracking and fissuring of the skin at the angles of the mouth, a symptom of vitamin B_2 deficiency, but also seen in other conditions

anion – A negatively charged ion

anomers – Isomers of a sugar differing only in configuration at the hemiacetal carbon atom

anorectic drugs (anorexigenic drugs) – Drugs that depress the appetite, used as an aid to weight reduction. Apart from sibutramine (Reductil), most have been withdrawn from use; diethylpropion and mazindol are available but not recommended

anorexia – Lack of appetite

anorexia nervosa – A psychological disturbance resulting in a refusal to eat, possibly with restriction to a very limited range of foods, and often accompanied by a rigid programme of vigorous physical exercise, to the point of exhaustion. The result is a very considerable loss of weight, with tissue atrophy and a fall in basal metabolic rate. It is especially prevalent among adolescent girls; when body weight falls below about 45 kg there is a cessation of menstruation

anosmia – Lack or impairment of the sense of smell

anovulation – Failure to ovulate spontaneously

antacids – Bases that neutralise acids, used generally to counteract excessive gastric acidity and to treat indigestion: sodium bicarbonate, aluminium hydroxide, magnesium carbonate and magnesium hydroxide

anthocyanins – Violet, red and blue water-soluble colours extracted from flowers, fruits and leaves

anthropometry – Body measurements used as an index of physiological development and nutritional status; a non-invasive way of assessing body composition. Weight for age provides information about the overall nutritional status of children; weight for height is used to detect acute malnutrition (wasting); height for age to detect chronic malnutrition (stunting). Midupper arm circumference provides an index of muscle wastage in undernutrition. Skinfold thickness is related to the amount of subcutaneous fat as an index of over- or undernutrition

antibody – Immunoglobulin that specifically counteracts an antigen or allergen (*see* allergen)

antidiarrhoeal – Drug used to treat diarrhoea by absorbing water from the intestine, altering intestinal motility or adsorbing toxins

antidiuretic – Drug used to reduce the excretion of urine and so conserve fluid in the body

antiemetic – Drug used to prevent or alleviate nausea and vomiting

antienzymes – Substances that inhibit the action of enzymes. Many inhibit digestive enzymes and are present in raw legumes. Most are proteins, and therefore inactivated by heat

antigen – Any compound that is foreign to the body (e.g. bacterial, food or pollen proteins or complex carbohydrates) which, when introduced into the circulation, stimulates the formation of an antibody

antihistamine – Drug that antagonises the actions of histamine; those that block histamine H_1 receptors are used to treat allergic reactions; those that block H_2 receptors are used to treat peptic ulcers

antihypertensive – Drug, diet or other treatment used to treat hypertension (high blood pressure)

antilipidaemic – Drug, diet or other treatment used to treat hyperlipidaemia by lowering blood lipids

antimetabolite – Compound that inhibits a normal metabolic process, acting as an analogue of a normal metabolite. Some are useful in chemotherapy of cancer; others are naturally occurring toxins in foods, frequently causing vitamin deficiency diseases by inhibiting the normal metabolism of the vitamin

antimotility agents – Drugs used to reduce gastrointestinal motility and hence reduce the discomfort associated with diarrhoea

antimutagen – Compound acting on cells and tissues to decrease initiation of mutation by a mutagen

antioxidant – A substance that retards the oxidative rancidity of fats in stored foods. Many fats, and especially vegetable oils, contain naturally occurring antioxidants, including vitamin E, which protect them against rancidity for some time

antioxidant nutrients – Highly reactive oxygen radicals are formed during normal metabolism and in response to infection and some chemicals. They cause damage to fatty acids in cell membranes, and the products of this damage can then cause damage to proteins and DNA. A number of different mechanisms are involved in protection against, or repair after, oxygen radical damage, including a number of nutrients, especially vitamin E, carotene, vitamin C and selenium. Collectively these are known as antioxidant nutrients

antirachitic – Preventing or curing rickets

antisialagogues – Substances that reduce the flow of saliva

antivitamins – Substances that interfere with the normal metabolism or function of vitamins, or destroy them

apastia – Refusal to take food, as an expression of a psychiatric disturbance

aphagosis – Inability to eat

apo-carotenal – Aldehydes formed by oxidation of carotenes, other than retinaldehyde

apoenzyme – The protein part of an enzyme which requires a coenzyme for activity, and is therefore inactive if the coenzyme is absent

apolipoprotein – The protein of plasma lipoproteins without the associated lipid

aposia – Absence of sensation of thirst

apositia – Aversion to food

arachidonic acid – A long-chain polyunsaturated fatty acid (C20:4 ω6)

arginine – A basic amino acid. Not a dietary essential for adults, but infants may not be able to synthesise enough to meet the high demands of growth

ariboflavinosis – Deficiency of riboflavin (vitamin B_2)

arm, chest, hip index (ACH index) – A method of assessing nutritional status by measuring the arm circumference, chest diameter and hip width

aromatic ring – Stable ring structure with π electrons delocalised around the ring as in benzene

arterial restenosis – Rate of re-occlusion (narrowing) of arteries after artificial (i.e. mechanical) removal of the accumulated plaque coatings. Used as a measure of susceptibility to atherosclerotic disease; it can be followed non-invasively, e.g. by ultrasound measurements

arteriosclerosis – Thickening and calcification of the arterial walls, leading to loss of elasticity, occurring with ageing and especially in hypertension

arthritis – Painful, swollen and/or inflamed joints

ascites – Abnormal accumulation of fluid in the peritoneal cavity, occurring as a complication of cirrhosis of the liver, congestive heart failure, cancer and infectious diseases

ascorbic acid – Vitamin C, chemically L-xyloascorbic acid, to distinguish it from the isomer D-araboascorbic acid (isoascorbic acid or erythorbic acid), which has only slight vitamin C activity

ash – The residue left behind after all organic matter has been burnt off, a measure of the total content of mineral salts in a food

asparagine – A non-essential amino acid; the β-amide of aspartic acid

aspartic acid (aspartate) – A non-essential amino acid

asthma – Chronic inflammatory disease of the airways which renders them prone to narrow too much. The symptoms include paroxysmal coughing, wheezing, tightness and breathlessness. Asthma may be caused by an allergic response or may be induced by non-immunological mechanisms

astringency – The action of unripe fruits and other foods to cause contraction of the epithelial tissues of the tongue, believed to result from a destruction of the lubricant properties of saliva by precipitation by tannins

atheroma – The fatty deposit composed of lipids, complex carbohydrates and fibrous tissue which forms on the inner wall of blood vessels in atherosclerosis

atherosclerosis – Degenerative disease in which there is accumulation of lipids, together with complex carbohydrates and fibrous tissue (atheroma), on the inner wall of arteries. This leads to narrowing of the lumen of the arteries

atrophy – Wasting of normally developed tissue or muscle as a result of disuse, ageing or undernutrition

attrition – Tooth wear caused by grinding

auxotrophe – Mutant strain of microorganism that requires one or more nutrients for growth that are not required by the parent organism. Commonly used for microbiological assay of vitamins, amino acids, etc.

availability – (bioavailability or biological availability). In some foodstuffs, nutrients that can be demonstrated to be present chemically may not be fully available when they are eaten, because the nutrients are chemically bound in a form that is not susceptible to enzymic digestion

avitaminosis – The absence of a vitamin; may be used specifically, as, for example, avitaminosis A, or generally, to mean a vitamin deficiency disease

axial position – Substituent in a 6-membered non-aromatic ring is above or below the average plane of the ring

bacteria – Unicellular microorganisms, ranging from 0.5 to 5 μm in size. They may be classified on the basis of their shape: spherical (coccus), rodlike (bacillus), spiral (spirillum), comma-shaped (vibrio), corkscrew-shaped (spirochaete) or filamentous. Other classifications are based on whether or not they are: stained by Gram's stain; aerobic or anaerobic; and autotrophic or heterotrophic

bacteriophages – Viruses that attack bacteria, commonly known as phages

basal metabolic rate (BMR) – The energy cost of maintaining the metabolic integrity of the body, nerve and muscle tone, respiration and circulation. For children it also includes the energy cost of growth. Experimentally, BMR is measured as the heat output from the body, or the rate of oxygen consumption, under strictly standardised conditions, 12–14 hours after the last meal, completely at rest (but not asleep) and at an environmental temperature of 26–30°C, to ensure thermal neutrality

bdelygmia – An extreme loathing for food

behenic acid – Very-chain saturated fatty acid (C22:0)

beriberi – The result of severe and prolonged deficiency of vitamin B_1, especially where the diet is high in carbohydrate and poor in vitamin B_1

beta linkage (β-linkage) – Bond formed by ring closure of a sugar with the hydroxyl group to the left of the chain in the Fischer projection formula (q.v.)

beta pleat (β pleat) – Common secondary structure in proteins

beta sheet flattened form – Common secondary structure in proteins

bifidogenic – Promoting the growth of (beneficial) bifidobacteria in the intestinal tract

bifidus factor – A carbohydrate in human milk which stimulates the growth of *Lactobacillus bifidus* in the intestine. In turn, this organism lowers the pH of the intestinal contents and suppresses the growth of pathogenic bacteria

bile – Alkaline fluid produced by the liver and stored in the gall bladder before secretion into the small intestine (duodenum) via the bile duct. It contains the bile salts, bile pigments (bilirubin and biliverdin), phospholipids and cholesterol

bile salts (bile acids) – Salts of cholic and deoxycholic acid and their glycine and taurine conjugates, secreted in the bile; they enhance the digestion of fats by emulsifying them

bilirubin, biliverdin – The bile pigments, formed by the degradation of haemoglobin

binge–purge syndrome – A feature of the eating disorder bulimia nervosa, characterised by the ingestion of excessive amounts of food and the excessive use of laxatives

bioassay – Biological assay; measurement of biologically active compounds (e.g. vitamins and essential amino acids) by their ability to support growth of microorganisms or animals

bioavailability – Fraction of an ingested nutrient that is absorbed and used for a defined function in the body (*see* availability)

biocytin – The main form of the vitamin biotin in most foods, bound to the amino acid lysine

bio-electrical impedance (BIE) – A method of measuring the proportion of fat in the body by the difference in the resistance to passage of an electric current between fat and lean tissue

bioflavonoids – *See* flavonoids

biofortification – Food fortification achieved by plant breeding or genetic modification to give a higher content of nutrients

bioinformatics – The application of computational techniques to extract meaning from complex biological data

biological value (BV) – The proportion of absorbed nitrogen that is retained for maintenance and/or growth

biotin – A vitamin, sometimes known as vitamin H, required for the synthesis of fatty acids and glucose, among other reactions, and in the control of gene expression and cell division

birth canal – The bony birth canal comprises the passage through the pelvic bones; there is a soft tissue component to the birth canal in the form of the vagina and its supporting tissues

bisfuran polycyclic compounds – Compounds with several rings including more than two 5-membered oxygen-containing rings

Bitot's spots – Irregularly shaped foam-like plaques on the conjunctiva of the eye, characteristically in vitamin A deficiency, but not considered to be a diagnostic sign without other evidence of deficiency

biuret test – A chemical test for proteins based on the formation of a violet colour when copper sulphate in alkaline solution reacts with a peptide bond

black tongue disease – A sign of niacin deficiency in dogs, the canine equivalent of pellagra

bland diet – A diet that is non-irritating, does not over-stimulate the digestive tract and is soothing to the intestines; generally avoiding alcohol, strong tea or coffee, pickles and spices

blood plasma – The liquid component of blood, accounting for about half its total volume; a solution of nutrients and various proteins. When blood has clotted, the resultant fluid is known as serum

blood sugar – Glucose; normal concentration is about 5 mmol (90 mg)/l, and is maintained in the fasting state by mobilisation of tissue reserves of glycogen and synthesis from amino acids. Only in prolonged starvation does it fall below about 3.5 mmol (60 mg)/l. If it falls to 2 mmol (35 mg)/l there is loss of consciousness (hypoglycaemic coma)

B-lymphocytes – Bursa-equivalent lymphocytes. After maturation into plasma cells they produce antibodies (immunoglobulins) during humoral responses in immunological reactions. They were first discovered in the bursa of Fabricius in the chicken; hence the name

body density – Body fat has a density of 0.90, while the density of fat free body mass is 1.10. Determination of density by weighing in air and in water, or by measuring body volume and weight, permits calculation of the proportions of fat and lean body tissue

body mass index (BMI) – An index of fatness and obesity. The weight (in kg) divided by the square of height (in m). The acceptable (desirable) range is 18–25. Above 25 is overweight, and above 30 is obesity. Also called Quetelet's index

borborygmos – (plural borborygmi); audible abdominal sound produced by excessive intestinal motility

borderline substances – Foods that may have characteristics of medication in certain circumstances, and which may then be prescribed under the National Health Service in the UK

botulism – A rare form of food poisoning caused by the extremely potent neurotoxins produced by *Clostridium botulinum*

bovine somatotrophin (BST) – The natural growth hormone of cattle; biosynthetic BST is used in some dairy herds to increase milk production (approved for use in the USA in 1993, prohibited in the EU)

bovine spongiform encephalopathy (BSE) – A degenerative brain disease in cattle, transmitted by feeding slaughter-house waste from infected animals. Commonly known as 'mad cow disease'. The infective agent is a prion; it can be transmitted to human beings, causing early-onset variant Creutzfeldt–Jakob disease

bradycardia – An unusually slow heartbeat, less than 60 beats/min

bradyphagia – Eating very slowly

bromatology – The science of foods

bronze diabetes – *see* haemochromatosis

brown adipose tissue (brown fat) – Metabolically highly active adipose tissue, which is involved in heat production to maintain body temperature, as opposed to white adipose tissue, which is storage fat and has a low rate of metabolic activity

Brunner's glands – Mucus-secreting glands in the duodenum

buffers – Salts of weak acids and bases that resist a change in the pH when acid or alkali is added

bulimia nervosa – An eating disorder, characterised by powerful and intractable urges to overeat, followed by self-induced vomiting and the excessive use of purgatives

butyric acid – A short-chain saturated fatty acid (C4:0)

cachexia – The condition of extreme emaciation and wasting seen in patients with advanced cancer and AIDS. Due partly to an inadequate intake of food and mainly to the effects of the disease in increasing metabolic rate (hypermetabolism) and the breakdown of tissue protein

cadaverine – Low molecular weight polyamine with biological activity, the decarboxylation product of lysine

caecum – The first part of the large intestine, separated from the small intestine by the ileo-colic sphincter

calcidiol – The 25-hydroxy-derivative of vitamin D, also known as 25-hydroxycholecalciferol, the main storage and circulating form of the vitamin in the body

calciferol – Used at one time as a name for ercalciol (ergocalciferol or vitamin D_2), made by the ultraviolet irradiation of ergosterol. Also used as a general term to include both vitamers of vitamin D (vitamins D_2 and D_3)

calcinosis – Abnormal deposition of calcium salts in tissues. May be due to excessive intake of vitamin D

calciol – The official name for cholecalciferol, the naturally occurring form of vitamin D (vitamin D_3)

calcitriol – The 1,25-dihydroxy-derivative of vitamin D, also known as 1,25-dihydroxycholecalciferol; the active metabolite of the vitamin

calorie – A unit of energy used to express the energy yield of foods and energy expenditure by the body; the amount of heat required to raise the temperature of 1 g of water through 1°C (from 14.5 to 15.5°C). Nutritionally the kilocalorie (1000 calories) is used (the amount of heat required to raise the temperature of 1 kg of water through 1°C), and is abbreviated as either kcal or Cal to avoid confusion with the cal. The calorie is not an SI unit, and correctly the joule is used as the unit of energy, although kcal are widely used. 1 kcal = 4.18 kJ; 1 kJ = 0.24 kcal

calorimeter (bomb calorimeter) – An instrument for measuring the amount of oxidisable energy in a substance, by burning it in oxygen and measuring the heat produced

calorimetry – The measurement of energy expenditure by the body. Direct calorimetry is the measurement of heat output from the body, as an index of energy expenditure, and hence requirements

canbra oil (canola oil) – Oil extracted from selected strains of rapeseed containing not more than 2% erucic acid

cancer – A wide variety of diseases characterised by uncontrolled growth of tissue

canola – A variety of rape which is low in glucosinolates. Canola oil (canbra oil) contains less than 2% erucic acid

canthaxanthin – A red carotenoid pigment which is not a precursor of vitamin A

capric acid – A medium-chain fatty acid (C10:0)

caproic acid – A short-chain fatty acid (C6:0)

caprylic acid – A medium-chain fatty acid (C8:0)

carbohydrate – The major food source of metabolic energy, the sugars and starches. Chemically they are composed of carbon, hydrogen and oxygen in the ratio $C_n:H_{2n}:O_n$

carbohydrate by difference – Historically it was difficult to determine the various carbohydrates present in foods, and an approximation was often made by subtracting the measured protein, fat, ash, and water from the total weight

carboxypeptidase – An enzyme secreted in the pancreatic juice which hydrolyses amino acids from the carboxyl terminal of proteins

carcinogen – A substance that can induce cancer

cardiomyopathy – Any chronic disorder affecting the muscle of the heart. May be associated with alcoholism and vitamin B_1 deficiency

caries – Dental decay caused by attack on the tooth enamel by acids produced by bacteria that are normally present in the mouth

cariogenic – Causing tooth decay (caries) by stimulating the growth of acid-forming bacteria on the teeth; sucrose and other fermentable carbohydrates

cariogenicity – Ability to cause caries

cariostatic – Preventing tooth decay

carnitine – A derivative of the amino acid lysine, required for the transport of fatty acids into mitochondria for oxidation

carnosine – A dipeptide, β-alanyl-histidine, found in the muscle of most animals. Its function is not known

carotenes – The red and orange pigments of plants; all are antioxidant nutrients. Three are important as precursors of vitamin A: α-, β- and γ-carotene

carotenoids – A general term for the wide variety of red and yellow compounds chemically related to carotene that are found in plant foods

carotinaemia – Presence of abnormally large amounts of carotene in blood plasma. Also known as xanthaemia

casein – About 75% of the proteins of milk are classified as caseins; a group of 12–15 different proteins

catabolism – Those pathways of metabolism concerned with the breakdown and oxidation of fuels and hence provision of metabolic energy People who are undernourished or suffering from cachexia are sometimes said to be in a catabolic state, in that they are catabolising their body tissues, without replacing them

catalase – An enzyme that splits hydrogen peroxide to yield oxygen and water; an important part of the body's antioxidant defences

catalyst – An agent that participates in a chemical reaction, speeding the rate, but itself remains unchanged

cathepsins (kathepsins) – A group of intracellular enzymes that hydrolyse proteins. They are involved in the normal turnover of tissue protein, and the softening of meat when game is hung

cation – A positively charged ion

CD4+ cells – Helper T-cells, part of the immune system, recognised by the presence of cluster of differentiation antigen 4 (CD4) on their exterior cell surfaces

CD8+ cells – Suppressor T-cells recognised by the presence of cluster of differentiation antigen 8 (CD8) on their exterior cell surfaces

cellobiose – A disaccharide of glucose-linked β-1,4, which is not hydrolysed by mammalian digestive enzymes; a product of the hydrolysis of cellulose

cellulase – An enzyme that hydrolyses cellulose to glucose and cellobiose. It is present in the digestive juices of some wood-boring insects and in various microorganisms, but not in mammals

cellulose – A polysaccharide of glucose-linked α-1,4 which is not hydrolysed by mammalian digestive enzymes; the main component of plant cell walls

cereal – Any grain or edible seed of the grass family which may be used as food; e.g. wheat, rice, oats, barley, rye, maize and millet. Collectively known as corn in the UK, although in the USA corn is specifically maize

chalasia – Abnormal relaxation of the cardiac sphincter muscle of the stomach so that gastric contents reflux into the oesophagus, leading to regurgitation

cheilosis – Cracking of the edges of the lips, one of the signs of vitamin B_2 (riboflavin) deficiency

chelating agents – Chemicals that combine with metal ions and remove them from their sphere of action, also called sequestrants, e.g. citrates, tartrates, phosphates and EDTA

chemoreceptors – Specialised receptors mainly found in the carotid body, within the carotid arteries of the neck, which are sensitive to changes in the blood concentration of oxygen (PO_2), carbon dioxide (PCO_2) and acidity (pH)

chemotaxis – The movement of phagocytes towards invading bacteria, cell debris or foreign particles

chief cells – Cells in the stomach that secrete pepsinogen, the precursor of the digestive enzyme pepsin (see pepsin)

Chinese restaurant syndrome – Flushing, palpitations, numbness associated at one time with the consumption of monosodium glutamate, and then with histamine, but the cause of these symptoms after eating various foods is not known

chitin – The organic matrix of the exoskeleton of insects and crustaceans, and present in small amounts in mushrooms. It is an insoluble and indigestible non-starch polysaccharide, composed of N-acetylglucosamine. Partial deacetylation results in the formation of chitosans

chitosan – Modified chitin, marketed as a fat binder to reduce fat absorption and aid weight reduction, with little evidence of efficacy

chlorpropamide – Drug used in the treatment of diabetes; it stimulates secretion of insulin. An oral hypoglycaemic agent

cholagogue – A substance that stimulates the secretion of bile from the gall bladder into the duodenum

cholecalciferol – Vitamin D

cholecystokinin – Hormone that stimulates gall bladder and pancreatic secretion

cholestasis – Failure of normal amounts of bile to reach the intestine, resulting in obstructive jaundice. May be caused by bile stones or liver disease

cholesterol – The principal sterol in animal tissues, an essential component of cell membranes and the precursor of the steroid hormones. Not a dietary essential, since it is synthesised in the body

cholestyramine – Drug used to treat hyperlipidaemia by complexing bile salts in the intestinal lumen and increasing their excretion, so increasing their synthesis from cholesterol

choline – A derivative of the amino acid serine; an important component of cell membranes, as the phospholipid phosphatidylcholine (lecithin). It is synthesised in the body, and it is a ubiquitous component of cell membranes and therefore occurs in all foods, so that dietary deficiency is unknown

chromosome – Collection of genes packaged with histone proteins found in the nucleus of cells; humans have 23 pairs (*see* histones)

chronic energy deficiency – A term recently introduced to describe adult malnutrition. Commonly defined by wasting or a low body mass index (*see also* protein–energy malnutrition (PEM))

chylomicrons – Plasma lipoproteins containing newly absorbed fat, assembled in the small intestinal mucosa and secreted into the lymphatic system, circulating in the lymph and bloodstream as a source of fat for tissues. The remnants are cleared by the liver

chyme – The partly digested mass of food in the stomach

chymotrypsin – An enzyme involved in the digestion of proteins; secreted as the inactive precursor chymotrypsinogen in the pancreatic juice

cis – Stereochemistry at a carbon–carbon double bond with both substituents on the same side of the bond

cissa – An unnatural desire for foods; alternative terms are: cittosis, allotriophagy and pica

citrulline – An amino acid formed as a metabolic intermediate, but not involved in proteins, and of no nutritional importance

cittosis – An unnatural desire for foods

coagulation – A process involving the denaturation of proteins, so that they become insoluble; it may be effected by heat, strong acids and alkalis, metals, and other chemicals. The final stage in blood clotting is the precipitation of insoluble fibrin, formed from the soluble plasma protein fibrinogen

cobalamin – Vitamin B_{12}

cocarcinogen – A substance which, alone, does not cause the induction of cancer, but potentiates the action of a carcinogen

Codex Alimentarius – Originally Codex Alimentarius Europaeus; since 1961 part of the United Nations FAO/WHO Commission on Food Standards to simplify and integrate food standards for adoption internationally; website: http://www.codexalimentarius.net

coding sequence (cds) – Region of an mRNA transcript that encodes for protein synthesis (*see* RNA)

codon – Triplet sequence of bases adenine, cytosine, guanine, thymine (A, C, G or T) which encode a specific amino acid used during translation of mRNAs

coeliac disease – Intolerance of the proteins of wheat, rye and barley; specifically, the gliadin fraction of the protein gluten. The villi of the small intestine are severely affected and absorption of food is poor. Stools are bulky and fermenting from unabsorbed carbohydrate, and contain a large amount of unabsorbed fat (steatorrhoea) (*see* gliadin)

coenzymes – Organic compounds required for the activity of some enzymes; most are derived from vitamins

cohort study – Systematic follow-up of a group of people for a defined period of time or until a specified event – also known as longitudinal or prospective study

colectomy – Surgical removal of all or part of the colon, to treat cancer or severe ulcerative colitis

colitis – Inflammation of the large intestine, with pain, diarrhoea and weight loss; there may be ulceration of the large intestine (ulcerative colitis)

collagen – Insoluble protein in connective tissue, bones, tendons and skin of animals and fish; converted into the soluble protein gelatine by moist heat

colloid – Particles (the disperse phase) suspended in a second medium (the dispersion medium); can be solid, liquid or gas suspended in a solid, liquid or gas

colon – Also known as the large intestine or bowel; it terminates at the rectum, where faeces are compacted and stored before voiding

colostomy – Surgical creation of an artificial conduit (a stoma) on the abdominal wall for voiding of intestinal contents following surgical removal of much of the colon and/or rectum

colostrum – The milk produced during the first few days after parturition; it is a valuable source of antibodies for the newborn infant. Animal colostrum is sometimes known as beestings

commercial farming – Agricultural production primarily or exclusively for the market, in contrast to subsistence farming

Committee on Medical Aspects of Food Policy (COMA) – Previous name for the permanent Advisory Committee to the UK Department of Health, now called the Scientific Advisory Committee on Nutrition (SACN)

complementary DNA (cDNA) – A complete or partial copy of a mature mRNA transcript which does not contain intronic sequences (*see* DNA, RNA, intron)

complementation – This term is used with respect to proteins when a relative deficiency of an amino acid in one is compensated by a relative surplus from another protein consumed at the same time. The protein quality is not the average of the separate values, but higher

conjugated linolenic acid – An isomer of linolenic acid in which the double bonds are conjugated, rather than methylene-interrupted

constipation – Difficulty in passing stools or infrequent passage of hard stools

contaminants – Undesirable compounds found in foods, residues of agricultural chemicals (pesticides, fungicides, herbicides, fertilisers, etc.), through the manufacturing process or as a result of pollution

convenience foods – Processed foods in which a considerable amount of the preparation has already been carried out by the manufacturer

coprolith – Mass of hard faeces in colon or rectum due to chronic constipation

coprophagy – Eating of faeces. Since B vitamins are synthesised by intestinal bacteria, animals that eat their faeces can make use of these vitamins, which are not absorbed from the large intestine, the site of bacterial action

corn – (*see* cereal)

corrinoids (corrins) – The basic chemical structure of vitamin B_{12} is the corrin ring; compounds with this structure, whether or not they have vitamin activity, are corrinoids

creatine – A derivative of the amino acids glycine and arginine, important in muscle as a store of phosphate for resynthesis of ATP during muscle contraction and work (*see* ATP)

creatinine – The anhydride of creatine, formed non-enzymically; urinary excretion is relatively constant from day to day, and reflects mainly the amount of muscle tissue in the body, so the amounts of various components of urine are often expressed relative to creatinine

cretinism – Underactivity of the thyroid gland (hypothyroidism) in children, resulting in poor growth, severe mental retardation and deafness

cristal height – A measure of leg length taken from the floor to the summit of the iliac crest. As a proportion of height it increases with age in children, and a reduced rate of increase indicates undernutrition. *See also* anthropometry

critical pH – The pH below which tooth enamel demineralises

Crohn's disease – Chronic inflammatory disease of the bowel, of unknown origin, also known as regional enteritis, since only some regions of the gut are affected

cryptoxanthin – Yellow hydroxylated carotenoid found in a few foods; a vitamin A precursor

cultivar – Horticultural term for a cultivated variety of plant that is distinct and is uniform and stable in its characteristics when propagated

cyanocobalamin – One of the vitamers of vitamin B_{12}

cyanogen(et)ic glycosides – Organic compounds of cyanide found in a variety of plants; chemically cyanhydrins are linked by glycoside linkage to one or more sugars. Toxic through liberation of the cyanide when the plants are cut or chewed

cysteine – A non-essential amino acid, but nutritionally important since it spares the essential amino acid methionine. In addition to its role in protein synthesis, cysteine is important as the precursor of taurine, in formation of coenzyme A from the vitamin pantothenic acid and in formation of the tripeptide glutathione

cystic fibrosis – A genetic disease due to a failure of the normal transport of chloride ions across cell membranes. This results in abnormally viscous mucus, affecting especially the lungs and secretion of pancreatic juice, hence impairing digestion

cystine – The dimer of cysteine produced when its sulphydryl group (–SH) is oxidised forming a disulphide (S–S–) bridge (*see* cysteine)

cytochrome P450 – A family of cytochromes which are involved in the detoxication system of the body (phase I metabolism). They act on a wide variety of (potentially toxic) compounds, both endogenous metabolites and foreign compounds (xenobiotics), rendering them more water-soluble, and more readily conjugated for excretion in the urine

cytochromes – Haem-containing proteins; some cytochromes react with oxygen directly; others are intermediates in the oxidation of reduced coenzymes. Unlike haemoglobin, the iron in the haem of cytochromes undergoes oxidation and reduction

cytokines – Small protein molecules that are the main communication between immune system cells and other tissues. Secreted by immune cells. Both stimulating and suppressing action on lymphocytes and immune response. Include TNF-α, IL-1 and IL-6, which are pro-inflammatory cytokines produced especially by macrophages very early following infection

cytosine – One of the pyrimidine bases of nucleic acids (*see* pyrimidines)

dark adaptation – The time taken to adapt to seeing in dim light; an index of vitamin A status as adaptation is slower and less complete in vitamin A deficiency

deciduous teeth – The first set of 20 teeth that appear during infancy and are lost during childhood and early adolescence as the adult (permanent) teeth erupt. Also known as milk teeth, first teeth

dehydroascorbic acid – Oxidised vitamin C, which is readily reduced back to the active form in the body, and therefore has vitamin activity

dehydrocholesterol – The precursor for the synthesis of vitamin D in the skin

delayed hypersensitivity – An exaggerated immune response that is delayed for a day or more. It is mediated by the response of T-cells to a foreign antigen or allergen

dentate – With natural teeth

dentine – Mineralised tissue beneath tooth enamel

deoxyribonucleic acid (DNA) – The genetic material in the nuclei of all cells. A linear polymer composed of four kinds of deoxyribose nucleotide, adenine, cytosine, guanine and thymidine (A, C, G and T), linked by phosphodiester bonds, that is the carrier of genetic information. In its native state DNA is a double helix

Department of the Environment, Food and Rural Affairs (DEFRA) – website http://www.defra.gov.uk

dermatitis – A lesion or inflammation of the skin; many nutritional deficiency diseases include more or less specific skin lesions, but most cases of dermatitis are not associated with nutritional deficiency, and do not respond to nutritional supplements

designer foods – Alternative name for functional foods

desmosines – The compounds that form the cross-linkage between chains of the connective tissue protein elastin

desmutagen – Compound acting directly on a mutagen to decrease its mutagenicity

dextrins – A mixture of soluble compounds formed by the partial breakdown of starch by heat, acid or amylases

dextrose – Alternative name for glucose. Commercially the term 'glucose' is often used to mean corn syrup (a mixture of glucose with other sugars and dextrins) and pure glucose is called dextrose

diabetes insipidus – A metabolic disorder characterised by extreme thirst, excessive consumption of liquids and excessive urination, due to failure of secretion of the antidiuretic hormone

diabetes mellitus – A metabolic disorder involving impaired metabolism of glucose due to either failure of secretion of the hormone insulin (insulin-dependent or type I diabetes) or impaired responses of tissues to insulin (non-insulin-dependent or type II diabetes)

diarrhoea – Frequent passage of loose watery stools, commonly the result of intestinal infection; rarely as a result of adverse reaction to foods or disaccharide intolerance

dietary fibre – Material mostly derived from plant cell walls which is not digested by human digestive enzymes; a large proportion consists of non-starch polysaccharides

dietary folate equivalents (DFE) – Method for calculating folic acid intake taking into account the lower availability of mixed folates in food compared with synthetic tetrahydrofolate used in food enrichment and supplements. 1 µg DFE = 1 µg food folate or 0.6 µg synthetic folate; total DFE = µg food folate + 1.7 × µg synthetic folate

dietary reference intakes (DRI) – US term for dietary reference values. In addition to average requirement and RDA, include tolerable upper levels (UL) of intake from supplements (*see* dietary reference values)

dietary reference values (DRV) – A set of standards of the amounts of each nutrient needed to maintain good health. People differ in the daily amounts of nutrients they need; for most nutrients the measured average requirement plus 20% (statistically 2 standard deviations) takes care of the needs of nearly everyone and in the UK this is termed reference nutrient intake (RNI), elsewhere known as recommended daily allowances or intakes (RDA or RDI), population reference intake (PRI), or dietary reference intake (DRI). This figure is used to calculate the needs of large groups of people in institutional or community planning. Obviously some people require less than the average (up to 20% or 2 standard deviations less). This lower level is termed the lower reference nutrient intake, LRNI (also known as the minimum safe intake, MSI, or lower threshold intake LTI). This is an intake at or below which it is unlikely that normal health could be maintained. If the diet of an individual indicates an intake of any nutrient at or below LRNI then detailed investigation of his/her nutritional status would be recommended. For energy intake only a single dietary reference value is used, the average requirement, because there is potential harm (of obesity) from ingesting too much

dietetic foods – Foods prepared to meet the particular nutritional needs of people whose assimilation and metabolism of foods are modified, or for whom a particular effect is obtained by a controlled intake of foods or individual nutrients

dietetics – The study or prescription of diets under special circumstances (e.g. metabolic or other illness) and for special physiological needs such as pregnancy, growth, weight reduction

diet-induced thermogenesis – The increase in heat production by the body after eating, due to both the metabolic energy cost of digestion and the energy cost of forming tissue reserves of fat, glycogen and protein. It is approximately 10% of the energy intake but varies with composition of the diet

dietitian (UK), dietician (US) – One who applies the principles of nutrition to the feeding of individuals and groups; plans menus and special diets; supervises the preparation and serving of meals; instructs in the principles of nutrition as applied to selection of foods

differentiation – The process of development of new characters in cells or tissues

digestibility – The proportion of a foodstuff absorbed from the digestive tract into the bloodstream, normally 90–95%. It is measured as the difference between intake and faecal output, with allowance being made for that part of the faeces that is not derived from undigested food residues (shed cells of the intestinal tract, bacteria, residues of digestive juices)

diglycerides (diacylglycerols) – Glycerol esterified with two fatty acids; an intermediate in the digestion of triacylglycerols, and used as emulsifying agents in food manufacture (*see* glycerol)

dipsesis (dipsosis) – Extreme thirst, a craving for abnormal kinds of drink

dipsetic – Tending to produce thirst

dipsogen – A thirst-provoking agent

dipsomania – A morbid craving for alcoholic drinks

disaccharidases – Enzymes that hydrolyse disaccharides to their constituent monosaccharides in the intestinal mucosa: sucrase (also known as invertase) acts on sucrose and isomaltose, lactase on lactose, maltase on maltose, and trehalase on trehalose

disaccharides – Sugars composed of two monosaccharide units; the nutritionally important disaccharides are sucrose, lactose and maltose. *See* carbohydrate

diuresis – Increased formation and excretion of urine; it occurs in diseases such as diabetes, and also in response to diuretics

diuretics – Substances that increase the production and excretion of urine

diverticular disease – Diverticulosis is the presence of pouch-like hernias (diverticula) through the muscle layer of the colon, associated with a low intake of dietary fibre and high intestinal pressure due to straining during defecation. Faecal matter can be trapped in these diverticula, causing them to become inflamed, causing pain and diarrhoea, the condition of diverticulitis

docosahexaenoic acid (DHA) – A long-chain poly-unsaturated fatty acid (C22:6 ω3)

docosanoids – Long-chain polyunsaturated fatty acids with 22 carbon atoms

docosapentaenoic acid – A long-chain polyunsaturated fatty acid (C22:5 ω3 or ω6)

Douglas bag – An inflatable bag for collecting exhaled air to measure the consumption of oxygen and production of carbon dioxide, for the measurement of energy expenditure by indirect calorimetry

duodenum – First part of the small intestine, between the stomach and the jejunum; the major site of digestion

dysgeusia – Distortion of the sense of taste – a common side-effect of some drugs

dyspepsia – Pain or discomfort associated with eating. Dyspepsia may be a symptom of gastritis, peptic ulcer, gall-bladder disease, hiatus hernia, etc.; if there is no structural change in the intestinal tract, it is called 'functional dyspepsia'

dysphagia – Difficulty in swallowing, commonly associated with disorders of the oesophagus

dysphoria – Unpleasant mood characterised by an exaggerated feeling of depression and unrest

ectomorph – Body type characterised by slight bone structure and muscle mass (*see* endomorph, mesomorph)

edentulous – Without natural teeth

eicosanoids – Compounds formed in the body from long-chain polyunsaturated fatty acids (eicosenoic acids, mainly arachidonic acid), formed by cyclooxygenase or lipoxygenase, including the prostaglandins, prostacyclins, thromboxanes and leukotrienes, all of which act as local hormones and are involved in inflammation, platelet aggregation and a variety of other functions

eicosapentaenoic acid (EPA) – A long-chain poly-unsaturated fatty acid (C20:5 ω3)

eicosenoic acids – Long-chain polyunsaturated fatty acids with 20 carbon atoms

electrolytes – Chemically salts that dissociate in solution and will carry an electric current; clinically used to mean the mineral salts of blood plasma and other body fluids, especially sodium and potassium

emaciation – Extreme thinness and wasting, caused by disease or undernutrition

embolism – Blockage of a blood vessel caused by a foreign object (embolus) such as a quantity of air or gas, a piece of tissue or tumour, a blood clot (thrombus) or fatty tissue derived from atheroma, in the circulation

emetic – Substance that causes vomiting

emulsifying agents – Substances that are soluble in both fat and water and enable fat to be uniformly dispersed in water as an emulsion

emulsion – An intimate mixture of two immiscible liquids (for example oil and water), one being dispersed in the other in the form of fine droplets

enamel – Mineralised tissue that forms hard outer surface of tooth

endocrine glands – Ductless glands that produce and secrete hormones. Some respond directly to chemical changes in the bloodstream; others are controlled by hormones secreted by the pituitary gland, under the control of the hypothalamus

endomorph – In relation to body build, means short and stocky. *See* ectomorph; mesomorph

endopeptidases – Enzymes that hydrolyse proteins (i.e. proteinases or peptidases) by cleaving peptide bonds within the protein chain, as opposed to exopeptidases, which remove amino acids from the ends of the chain

endoplasmic (sarcoplasmic) reticulum – Enclosed membranous system with the cytoplasm of cells. It has a number of functions that include acting as an intracellular store for calcium

endothelium – Layer of cells lining blood vessels

endotoxins – Toxins produced by bacteria as an integral part of the cell, so they cannot be separated by filtration

energy – The ability to do work. The SI unit of energy is the joule, and nutritionally relevant amounts of energy are kilojoules (kJ, 1000 J) and megajoules (MJ, 1000000 J)

energy metabolism – The various reactions involved in the oxidation of metabolic fuels (mainly carbohydrates, fats and proteins), to provide energy (linked to the formation of ATP (adenosine triphosphate) from ADP (adenosine diphosphate) and phosphate ions)

enmeshment – A condition where two or more people weave their lives and identities around one another so tightly that it is difficult for any one of them to function independently

enrichment – The addition of nutrients to foods. Although often used interchangeably, the term fortification is used of legally imposed additions, and enrichment means the addition of nutrients beyond the levels originally present

enteral nutrition – Tube feeding with a liquid diet directly into the stomach or small intestine

enteritis – Inflammation of the mucosal lining of the small intestine, usually resulting from infection. Regional enteritis is Crohn's disease

enterocolitis – Inflammation of the mucosal lining of the small and large intestine, usually resulting from infection

enterocytes – The layer of epithelial cells that line the small intestine and are responsible for the absorption of nutrients from the diet

enterogastrone – Hormone secreted by the small intestine which inhibits the activity of the stomach. Its secretion is stimulated by fat; hence, fat in the diet inhibits gastric activity

enterohepatic circulation – Reabsorption from the small intestine of many of the compounds secreted in bile

enterokinase – Obsolete name for enteropeptidase

enteropathy – Any disease or disorder of the intestinal tract

enteropeptidase – An enzyme secreted by the small intestinal mucosa which activates trypsinogen (from the pancreatic juice) to the active proteolytic enzyme

enterotoxin – Substances toxic to the cells of the intestinal mucosa, normally produced by bacteria

enteroviruses – Viruses that multiply mainly in the intestinal tract

entitlements – The amount of food or other necessities that people can command based on their income and assets, given the legal, political, economic, and cultural context in which they live

E-numbers – Within the EU food additives may be listed on labels either by name or by their number in the EU list of permitted additives

enzyme – A protein that catalyses a metabolic reaction, so increasing its rate. Enzymes are specific for both the compounds acted on (the substrates) and the reactions carried out

enzyme activation assays – Used to assess nutritional status with respect to vitamins B_1, B_2 and B_6. A sample of red blood cells in a test-tube is tested for activity of the relevant enzyme before and after adding extra vitamin; enhancement of the enzyme activity beyond a standard level serves as an index of deficiency

enzyme induction – Synthesis of new enzyme protein in response to some stimulus, normally a hormone, but sometimes a metabolic intermediate or other compound

enzyme-linked immunosorbent assay (ELISA) – Extremely sensitive and specific analytical technique using antibodies linked to an enzyme system to amplify sensitivity

enzyme repression – Reduction in synthesis of enzyme protein in response to some stimulus such as a hormone or the presence of large amounts of the end-product of its activity

eosinophil – A white blood cell with granules that can be stained by eosin dyes. Eosinophils participate in allergic and hypersensitivity reactions

eosinophilia myalgia syndrome (EMS) – A syndrome characterised by debilitating muscle pain and high eosinophil count

equatorial position – Bond to a substituent in a 6-membered non-aromatic ring is parallel to one of the bonds in the ring

ergocalciferol – Vitamin D_2

ergosterol – A sterol isolated from yeast; when treated with ultraviolet light, it is converted to ergocalciferol; the main industrial source of vitamin D

erosion – Tooth wear caused by dietary, digestive or environmental acids

erucic acid – A toxic mono-unsaturated fatty acid, (C22:1 ω9) found in rape seed (*Brassica napus*) and mustard seed (*B. junca* and *B. nigra*) oils. Low erucic acid varieties of rape seed (canola) have been developed for food use

eructation – The act of bringing up air from the stomach, with a characteristic sound. Also known as belching

erythorbic acid – The D-isomer of ascorbic acid; used in foods as an antioxidant but has little vitamin activity

erythrocyte – Red blood cell

erythrocyte glutathione reductase activation coefficient (EGRAC) – An index of riboflavin status

erythropoiesis – The formation and development of the red blood cells in the bone marrow

erythropoietin – Hormone that controls erythropoiesis (red blood cell production) in the bone marrow

essential amino acid index (EAA index) – An index of protein quality

essential fatty acids (EFA) – Polyunsaturated fatty acids of the ω6 (linoleic acid) and n-3 (linolenic acid) series, which are essential dietary components because they cannot be synthesised in the (human) body. They are essential components of cell membranes; they are also precursors of prostaglandins, prostacyclins and related hormones and signalling molecules

ester – Compound formed by condensation between an acid and an alcohol, e.g. ethyl alcohol and acetic acid yield the ester ethyl acetate. Fats are esters of the alcohol glycerol and long-chain fatty acids. Many esters are used as synthetic flavours

esterases – Enzymes that hydrolyse esters, i.e. cleave the ester linkage to form free acid and alcohol. Those that hydrolyse the ester linkages of fats are generally known as lipases, and those that hydrolyse phospholipids as phospholipases; *see* ester

estimated average requirement (EAR) – The mean requirement of a group of individuals for a nutrient

ethanol – Systematic chemical name for ethyl alcohol

ethanolamine – One of the water-soluble bases of phospholipids, it is 2-aminoethanol

ethylene diamine tetra-acetic acid (EDTA) – A compound that forms stable chemical complexes with metal ions (i.e. a chelating agent). Also called versene, sequestrol and sequestrene

European Food Safety Authority (EFSA) – website http://www.efsa.ei.int

European Society for Parenteral and Enteral Nutrition (ESPEN) – website http://www.espen.org

eutrophia – Normal nutrition

exchange list – List of portions of foods in which energy, fat, carbohydrate and/or protein content are equivalent, so simplifying meal and diet planning for people with special needs

exclusion diet – A limited diet excluding foods known possibly to cause food intolerance, to which foods are added in turn to test for intolerance (allergy)

exon – Segment of a gene that is represented in the mature mRNA product. Contains the code for producing the gene's protein. Each exon codes for a specific portion of the complete protein, separated by introns that have no apparent function (*see* intron)

exopeptidases – Proteolytic enzymes that hydrolyse the peptide bonds of the terminal amino acids of proteins or peptides (*see* peptides)

exothermic – Chemical reactions that proceed with the output of heat

exotoxins – Toxic substances produced by bacteria which diffuse out of the cells and stimulate the production of antibodies that specifically neutralise them (antitoxins)

extremophiles – Microorganisms that can grow under extreme conditions of heat (thermophiles and extreme thermophiles, some of which live in hot springs at 100°C), or cold (psychrophiles), in high concentrations of salt (halophiles), high pressure, or extremes of acid or alkali

extrinsic factor – Protein secreted in the stomach that is required for the absorption of vitamin B_{12}

F_2-isoprostanes – Oxidation products of lipids which are considered to be useful indices of oxidative damage, e.g. by oxygen free radicals

faeces – Body waste, composed of undigested food residues, remains of digestive secretions that have not been reabsorbed, bacteria from the intestinal tract, cells, cell debris and mucus from the intestinal lining, and substances excreted into the intestinal tract (mainly in the bile)

famine – A catastrophic disruption of the social, economic and institutional systems that provide for food production, distribution and consumption

fasting – Going without food. The metabolic fasting state begins some 4 hours after a meal, when the digestion and absorption of food is complete and body reserves of fat and glycogen begin to be mobilised

fat – Chemically, fats (or lipids) are substances that are insoluble in water but soluble in organic solvents such as ether, chloroform and benzene, and are actual or potential esters of fatty acids. The term includes triacylglycerols (triglycerides), phospholipids, waxes and sterols. In more general use the term 'fats' refers to the neutral fats, which are triacylglycerols, mixed esters of fatty acids with glycerol; *see* fatty acids, glycerol

fat, neutral – Fats that are esters of fatty acids with glycerol, triacylglycerols

fat-replacers – Substances that provide a creamy, fat-like texture used to replace or partly replace the fat in a food. Made from a variety of substances with lower energy content

fatty acids – Organic acids consisting of carbon chains with a carboxyl group at the end. The nutritionally important fatty acids have an even number of carbon atoms. In addition to their accepted names, fatty acids can be named by a shorthand giving the number of carbon atoms in the molecule (e.g. C18), then a colon and the number of double bonds (e.g. C18:2), followed by the position of the first double bond from the methyl end of the molecule as n- or ω (e.g. C18:2 n-6, or C18:2 ω6)

fecundability – *See* fertility

Fenton-type reactions – The formation of hydroxyl radical (OH•) from hydrogen peroxide reacting with iron (II) or copper (I) ions in a process first observed by Fenton in 1894

ferritin – An iron-carrier protein, found in large amounts in liver and spleen, and also at low concentrations in serum, which can be measured as an index of iron stores in the body. However, it is also sensitive to the acute phase reaction: its concentration in serum increases markedly during infection or inflammation; *see* acute phase reaction

fertility – The ability to reproduce, which differs from fecundability, which is the ability of a woman to become pregnant

fibre, crude – The term given to the indigestible part of foods, defined as the residue left after successive extraction under closely specified conditions with petroleum ether, 1.25% sulphuric acid and 1.25% sodium hydroxide, minus ash. No real relation to dietary fibre

fibre, dietary – *See* dietary fibre

fibrin – The blood protein formed from fibrinogen which is responsible for the clotting of blood

Fischer projection formula – Simple method of representing the configuration of stereogenic centres of chemical structures as the intersection of vertical and horizontal lines

flatulence (flatus) – Production of gas by bacteria in the large intestine; hydrogen, carbon dioxide and methane. May be caused by a variety of foods that are incompletely digested in the small intestine

flavin – The group of compounds containing the iso-alloxazine ring structure, as in riboflavin (vitamin B_2), and hence a general term for riboflavin derivatives

flavin adenine dinucleotide (FAD) – One of the coenzymes formed from vitamin B_2 (riboflavin)

flavin mononucleotide (FMN) – (chemically riboflavin phosphate) One of the coenzymes derived from vitamin B_2

flavonoids – Widely found plant pigments; glycosides of flavones; the sugar moiety may be either rhamnose or rhamnoglucose. Some have pharmacological actions, but they are not known to be dietary essentials, although they make a contribution to the total antioxidant intake, and some are phytoestrogens

flavoproteins – Enzymes that contain the vitamin riboflavin, or a derivative such as flavin adenine dinucleotide or riboflavin phosphate, as the prosthetic group. Mainly involved in oxidation reactions in metabolism

fluoroapatite – Crystal incorporating fluoride that forms tooth enamel

fluorosis – Damage to teeth (white to brown mottling of the enamel) and bones caused by an excessive intake of fluoride

foam cells – Macrophages that have accumulated very large amounts of cholesterol as a result of uptake of (chemically modified) low-density lipoprotein. They infiltrate arterial walls and lead to the development of fatty streaks, and eventually atherosclerosis

folinic acid – The 5-formyl derivative of the vitamin folic acid; more stable to oxidation than folic acid itself, and commonly used in pharmaceutical preparations. The synthetic (racemic) compound is known as leucovorin

food, foodstuffs – Any solid or liquid material consumed by a living organism to supply energy, build and replace tissue, or participate in such reactions. Defined by the FAO/WHO Codex Alimentarius Commission as a substance, whether processed, semi-processed or raw, which is intended for human consumption and includes drink, chewing gum and any substance that has been used in the manufacture, preparation or treatment of food but does not include cosmetics, tobacco or substances used only as drugs. Defined in EU directives as products intended for human consumption in an unprocessed, processed or mixed state, with the exception of tobacco products, cosmetics and pharmaceuticals

Food and Agriculture Organization of the United Nations (FAO) – Founded in 1943; headquarters in Rome. Its goal is to achieve freedom from hunger worldwide. According to its constitution the specific objectives are 'raising the levels of nutrition and standards of living … and securing improvements in the efficiency of production and distribution of all food and agricultural products'; website http://www.fao.org

Food and Drug Administration (FDA) – US government regulatory agency; website http://www.fda.gov; website for FDA consumer magazine http://www.fda.gov/fdac

Food and Nutrition Information Center (FNIC) – Located at the National Agricultural Library, part of the US Department of Agriculture; website http://www.nal.usda.gov/fnic

food chain – The chain between green plants (the primary producers of food energy) through a sequence of organisms in which each eats the one below it in the chain and is eaten in turn by the one above. Also used for the chain of events from the original source of a foodstuff (from the sea, the soil or the wild) through all the stages of handling until it reaches the table

food exchange – *See* exchange list

food insecurity – The absence of food security

food poisoning – May be due to (1) contamination with harmful bacteria or other microorganisms; (2) toxic chemicals; (3) adverse reactions to certain proteins or other natural constituents of foods; (4) chemical contamination. The commonest bacterial contamination is due to species of *Salmonella, Staphylococcus, Campylobacter, Listeria, Bacillus cereus* and *Clostridium welchii*. Very rarely, food poisoning is due to *Clostridium botulinum*, botulism

food pyramid – A way of showing a healthy diet graphically, by grouping foods and the amounts of each group that should be eaten each day, based on nutritional recommendations

food science – The study of the basic chemical, physical, biochemical and biophysical properties of foods and their constituents, and of changes that these may undergo during handling, preservation, processing, storage, distribution and preparation for consumption

food security – When all people, at all times, have physical and economic access to sufficient, safe and nutritious food to meet their dietary needs and food preferences for an active and healthy life. Food security requires more than just adequate food availability; it also is a matter of access to the food that is available and appropriate utilisation

Food Standards Agency (FSA) – Permanent advisory body to the UK Parliament through Health Ministers, established in 2000 to protect the public's health and consumer interests in relation to food; website http://www.food.gov.uk

food technology – The application of science and technology to the treatment, processing, preservation and distribution of foods. Hence the term food technologist

Foods for Specified Health Use (FOSHU, Japanese) – Processed foods containing ingredients that aid specific bodily functions, as well as being nutritious (functional foods)

formiminoglutamic acid (FIGLU) test – A test for folate nutritional status, based on excretion of formiminoglutamic acid (FIGLU), a metabolite of the amino acid histidine, which is normally metabolised by a folic-acid-dependent enzyme

formula diet – Composed of simple substances that require little digestion, are readily absorbed and leave a minimum residue in the intestine: glucose, amino acids or peptides, mono- and diacylglycerols rather than starch, proteins and fats

fortification – The deliberate addition of specific nutrients to foods as a means of providing the population with an increased level of intake

fractional test meal – A method of examining the secretion of gastric juices; the stomach contents are sampled at intervals via a stomach tube after a test meal of gruel

free radicals – Highly reactive chemical species with one or more unpaired electrons

free sugars – Mono- and disaccharides added to food, plus sugars in fruit juices, honey and syrup

freeze drying – Also known as lyophilisation. A method of drying in which the material is frozen and subjected to high vacuum. The ice sublimes off as water vapour without melting. Freeze-dried food is very porous, since it occupies the same volume as the original and so rehydrates rapidly. There is less loss of flavour and texture than with most other methods of drying. Controlled heat may be applied to the process without melting the frozen material; this is accelerated freeze drying

fructo-oligosaccharides – Oligosaccharides consisting of fructose

fructosan – A general name for polysaccharides of fructose, such as inulin. Not digested, and hence a part of dietary fibre or non-starch polysaccharides

fructose – Also known as fruit sugar or laevulose. A six-carbon monosaccharide sugar (hexose) differing from glucose in containing a ketone group (on carbon-2) instead of an aldehyde group (on carbon-1)

fruit – The fleshy seed-bearing part of plants (including tomato and cucumber, which are usually called vegetables)

fruitarian – A person who eats only fruits, nuts and seeds; an extreme form of vegetarianism

functional foods – Foods eaten for specified health purposes because of their (rich) content of one or more nutrients or non-nutrient substances which may confer health benefits

galactans – Polysaccharides composed of galactose derivatives

galactose – A six-carbon monosaccharide, differing from glucose only in position of the hydroxyl group on carbon-4

gall-bladder – The organ situated in the liver which stores the bile formed in the liver before its secretion into the small intestine

gallstones (cholclithiasis) – Concretions composed of cholesterol, bile pigments and calcium salts, formed in the bile duct of the gall-bladder when the bile becomes supersaturated

gamma carboxyglutamate (γ-carboxyglutamate) – A derivative of the amino acid glutamate found in prothrombin and other enzymes involved in blood clotting, and the proteins osteocalcin and matrix GLA protein (MGP) in bone, where it has a function in ensuring the correct crystallisation of bone mineral. Its synthesis requires vitamin K

gastric inhibitory peptide (GIP) – A hormone secreted by the mucosa of the duodenum and jejunum in response to absorbed fat and carbohydrate, which stimulates the pancreas to secrete insulin. Also known as glucose-dependent insulinotropic polypeptide

gastrin – Polypeptide hormone secreted by the stomach in response to food, which stimulates gastric and pancreatic secretion

gastritis – Inflammation of the mucosal lining of the stomach; may result from infection or excessive alcohol consumption. Atrophic gastritis is the progressive loss of gastric secretion with increasing age

gastroenteritis – Inflammation of the mucosal lining of the stomach and/or small or large intestine, normally resulting from infection

gastroenterology – The study and treatment of diseases of the gastrointestinal tract

gastroplasty – Surgical alteration of the shape and capacity of the stomach, without removing any part. Has been used as a treatment for severe obesity

gastrostomy feeding – Feeding a liquid diet directly into the stomach through a tube that has been surgically introduced through the abdominal wall. *See also* enteral nutrition; nasogastric tube

gavage – The process of feeding liquids by tube directly into the stomach

gene – Physical and functional unit of heredity. It is the entire DNA sequence necessary for the synthesis of a functional polypeptide or RNA molecule; *see* DNA, RNA

gene expression – Overall process by which information encoded by a gene is converted to an observable phenotype, usually in the form of a protein; *see* phenotype

gene transcription – Conversion of genomic DNA into mRNA; *see* DNA, mRNA

gene translation – The synthesis of protein molecules using the triplet code of mRNA; *see* mRNA

generally regarded as safe (GRAS) – Designation given to food additives when further evidence was required before the substance could be classified more precisely (US usage)

generic descriptor – The name used to cover the different chemical forms of a vitamin that have the same biological activity

genetic polymorphisms – Changes (i.e. variability) in one or more base pairs in the DNA gene sequence encoding a specific protein, which result in the substitution of different amino acids in that protein, which may subtly alter its function. Such polymorphisms, in human populations, are of increasing research interest because in some cases they may alter requirements for certain nutrients

genome – The complete genetic information of an organism; *see* proteome, metabolome

genomics – The study of the structure and function of genes; *see* proteomics, metabolomics

genotype – The entire genetic constitution of an individual cell or organism

ghrelin – A peptide hormone secreted by cells in the gastrointestinal tract that both stimulates the secretion of growth hormone and regulates feeding behaviour and energy balance by acting on the hypothalamus

giardiasis – Intestinal inflammation and diarrhoea caused by infection with the protozoan parasite *Giardia lamblia*

gingivitis – Inflammation of the gums (gingiva)

gliadin – One of the proteins that make up wheat gluten. Allergy to, or intolerance of, gliadin is coeliac disease

globins – Proteins that are rich in the amino acid histidine (and hence basic), relatively deficient in isoleucine, and contain average amounts of arginine and tryptophan. Often found as the protein part of conjugated proteins such as haemoglobin

globulins – Globular (as opposed to fibrous) proteins that are relatively insoluble in water, but soluble in dilute salt solutions

glomerular filtration rate – The rate at which fluid is filtered through the kidney at the renal glomerulus, usually expressed in ml/min. It increases in normal pregnancy and is decreased in renal failure

glossitis – Inflammation of the tongue; may be one of the signs of riboflavin deficiency

glucagon – A hormone secreted by the α-cells of the pancreas which causes an increase in blood glucose by increasing the breakdown of liver glycogen and stimulating gluconeogenesis

glucans – Soluble but undigested complex carbohydrates; found particularly in oats, barley and rye

glucocorticoids – The steroid hormones secreted by the adrenal cortex which regulate carbohydrate metabolism

glucomannan – A polysaccharide consisting of glucose and mannose

gluconeogenesis – The synthesis of glucose from non-carbohydrate precursors, such as glycerol, lactate and a variety of amino acids

gluco-oligosaccharide – A non-digestible oligosaccharide of glucose containing alpha-1,2 and alpha-1,6 glycosidic links; *see* oligosaccharides

glucosan – A general term for polysaccharides of glucose, such as starch, cellulose and glycogen; *see* polysaccharides

glucose – A six-carbon monosaccharide sugar (hexose), with the chemical formula $C_6H_{12}O_6$, occurring free in plant and animal tissues and formed by the hydrolysis of starch and glycogen. Also known as dextrose, grape sugar and blood sugar

glucose polymers – Oligosaccharides of glucose linked with alpha-1,4 and alpha-1,6 glycosidic links

glucose syrup – A type of glucose polymer

glucose tolerance – The ability of the body to deal with a relatively large dose of glucose is used to diagnose diabetes mellitus

glucose tolerance factor (GTF) – An organic complex containing chromium

glucosides – Complexes of substances with glucose. The general name for such complexes with other sugars is glycosides

glucosinolates – Substances occurring widely in plants of the genus *Brassica* (e.g. broccoli, Brussels sprouts, cabbage); broken down by the enzyme myrosinase to yield, among other products, the mustard oils that are responsible for the pungent flavour (especially in mustard and horseradish). There is evidence that the various glucosinolates in vegetables may have useful anti-cancer activity, since they increase the rate at which a variety of potentially toxic and carcinogenic compounds are conjugated and excreted

glucosuria (glycosuria) – Appearance of glucose in the urine, as in diabetes and after the administration of drugs that lower the renal threshold

glucuronides – A variety of compounds are metabolised by conjugation with glucuronic acid to yield water-soluble derivatives for excretion from the body

glutamate – Salts of glutamic acid

glutamic acid – A non-essential amino acid

glutamine – A non-essential amino acid, the amide of glutamic acid

glutathione – A tripeptide (γ-glutamyl-cysteinyl-glycine) which is involved in oxidation-reduction reactions, the conjugation of foreign substances for excretion and the transport of some amino acids into cells; *see* peptides

glutathione peroxidases – A group of selenium-containing enzymes that protect tissues from oxidative damage by removing peroxides resulting from free radical action, linked to oxidation of reduced glutathione; part of the body's anti-oxidant protection; often used as a biochemical index of selenium status

glutathione reductase – Enzyme in red blood cells for which flavin adenine dinucleotide (FAD; derived from vitamin B_2) is the essential cofactor. It converts oxidised to reduced glutathione, with reduced nicotinamide dinucleotide phosphate (NADPH) as co-substrate. Activation of this enzyme in vitro from red cell extracts by added FAD provides a means of assessing vitamin B_2 nutritional status, sometimes known as the erythrocyte glutathione reductase activation coefficient (EGRAC) test

gluten – The protein complex in wheat, and to a lesser extent rye, which gives dough the viscid property that holds gas when it rises. There is none in oats, barley or maize. It is a mixture of two proteins, gliadin and glutelin. Allergy to, or intolerance of, gliadin gluten is coeliac disease

gluten-free foods – Formulated without any wheat or rye protein (although the starch may be used) for people suffering from coeliac disease; *see* coeliac disease

gluten-sensitive enteropathy – Coeliac disease

glycaemic index – The ability of a carbohydrate to increase blood glucose, compared with an equivalent amount of glucose. Glycaemic load is the product of multiplying the amount of carbohydrate in the food by the glycaemic index

glycation – A non-enzymic reaction between glucose and amino groups in proteins, resulting in formation of a glycoprotein; the basis of many of the adverse effects of poor glycaemic control in diabetes

glycerides – Esters of glycerol with fatty acids

glycerol – A trihydric alcohol, (CH_2OH – $CHOH$ – CH_2OH), also known as glycerine. Simple or neutral fats are esters of glycerol with three molecules of fatty acid, i.e. triacylglycerols, sometimes known as triglycerides

glycine – A non-essential amino acid, chemically the simplest of the amino acids, it is amino-acetic acid, CH_2NH_2COOH

glycocholic acid – One of the bile acids

glycogen – The storage carbohydrate in the liver and muscles, a branched polymer of glucose units

glycogenolysis – The breakdown of glycogen to glucose for use as a metabolic fuel and to maintain the normal blood concentration of glucose in the fasting state. Stimulated by the hormones glucagon and adrenaline (epinephrine)

glycolysis – The first sequence of reactions in glucose metabolism, leading to the formation of two molecules of pyruvic acid from each glucose molecule

glycoproteins – Proteins conjugated with carbohydrates such as uronic acids, polymerised glucosamine-mannose, etc., including mucins and mucoids

glycosides – Compounds of a sugar attached to another molecule. When glucose is the sugar, they are called glucosides

glycosidic – Ether-type bond formed by the hydroxyl group of a sugar displacing the hydroxyl group of a second sugar or other molecule

goitre – Enlargement of the thyroid gland, seen as a swelling in the neck; may be hypothyroid, with low production of hormones, euthyroid (normal levels of the hormones) or hyperthyroid

goitrogens – Substances found in foods (especially *Brassica* spp. but including also groundnuts, cassava and soya bean) which interfere with the synthesis of thyroid hormones (glucosinolates) or the uptake of iodide into the thyroid gland (thiocyanates), and hence can cause goitre, especially when the dietary intake of iodide is marginal

Gomez classification – One of the earliest systems for classifying protein–energy malnutrition in children, based on percentage of expected weight for age: over 90% is normal, 76–90% is mild (first degree) malnutrition, 61–75% is moderate (second degree) malnutrition and less than 60% is severe (third degree) malnutrition

gout – Painful disease caused by accumulation of crystals of uric acid in the synovial fluid of joints; may be due to excessive synthesis and metabolism of purines, which are metabolised to uric acid, or to impaired excretion of uric acid

Gram-negative, Gram-positive – A method of classifying bacteria depending on whether or not they retain crystal-violet dye (Gram stain) after staining and decolorising with alcohol

Green Revolution – A process in which cereal crop yields increased as a result of farmer adoption of high-yielding varieties bred at international agricultural research centres and adapted to local conditions at national agricultural research institutions. Planting of these varieties has coincided with expansion of irrigated area and fertiliser use

growth faltering – A term indicating that a child's linear or ponderal growth is falling away from the reference trend. This implies that weight or height has been measured at intervals over a period of time

growth hormone – Somatotrophin, a peptide hormone secreted by the pituitary gland that promotes growth of bone and soft tissues. It also reduces the utilisation of glucose, and increases breakdown of fats to fatty acids; because of this it has been promoted as an aid to weight reduction, with little evidence of efficacy. Sometimes abbreviated to hGH (human growth hormone); growth hormone from other mammals differs in structure and activity

guanine – One of the purines; *see* purines

gum – Substances that can disperse in water to form a viscous mucilaginous mass. They may be extracted from seeds, plant sap and seaweeds, or they may be made from starch or cellulose. Most (apart from dextrins) are not digested and have no food value, although they contribute to the intake of non-starch polysaccharides

haem – The iron-containing pigment which forms the oxygen-binding site of haemoglobin and myoglobin. It is also part of a variety of other proteins, collectively known as haem proteins, including the cytochromes; *see* haemoglobin

haemagglutinins – *See* lectins

haematemesis – Vomiting bright red blood, due to bleeding in the upper gastrointestinal tract

haematinic – General term for those nutrients, including iron, folic acid and vitamin B_{12}, required for the formation and development of blood cells in bone marrow (the process of haematopoiesis), deficiency of which may result in anaemia

haemochromatosis – Iron overload; excessive absorption and storage of iron in the body, commonly the result of a genetic defect. In most cases it is caused by a recessive gene, i.e. it can only be passed on if both parents are carriers of the gene predisposing to the disorder. Around one in seven people in northern Europe are carriers of the recessive gene. Homozygotes are susceptible to iron toxicity from high absorption of dietary iron, which can lead to tissue damage (including liver cancer, heart disease and diabetes) and bronze coloration of the skin. Sometimes called bronze diabetes. The disorder is usually treated by regular venesection, a procedure similar to blood donation, where around 500 ml of blood is removed

haemoglobin – The red haem-containing protein in red blood cells which is responsible for the transport of oxygen and carbon dioxide in the bloodstream

haemorrhoids (or piles) – Varicosity in the lower rectum or anus due to congestion of the veins; caused or exacerbated by a low-fibre diet and consequent straining to defecate

haemosiderin – An iron storage protein

halal – Food conforming to the Islamic (Muslim) dietary laws. Meat from permitted animals (in general grazing animals with cloven hooves, and thus excluding pig meat) and birds (excluding birds of prey). The animals are killed under religious supervision by cutting the throat to allow removal of all blood from the carcass, without prior stunning. Food that is not halal is haram

halophiles (halophilic bacteria) – Bacteria and other microorganisms able to grow in high concentrations of salt

haplotype – Collection of single nucleotide polymorphs (SNPs) which are inherited as a group; *see* SNP

haram – Food forbidden by Islamic law (opposite of halal)

Harvard standard – Tables of height and weight for age used as reference values for the assessment of growth and nutritional status in children, based on data collected in the USA in the 1930s. Now largely replaced by the NCHS (US National Center for Health Statistics) standards

hazard analysis critical control process (HACCP) – The identification of critical process points that must be controlled to produce safe foods

health foods – Substances the consumption of which is advocated by various reform movements, including vegetable foods, whole grain cereals, food processed without chemical additives, food grown on organic compost, supplements such as bees' royal jelly, lecithin, seaweed, etc., and pills and potions. Numerous health claims are made but rarely is there evidence to support these claims

heartburn – A burning sensation in the chest usually caused by reflux (regurgitation) of acid digestive juices from the stomach into the oesophagus. A common form of indigestion, treated by antacids

heat of combustion – Energy released by complete combustion, as, for example, in the bomb calorimeter. Values can be used to predict energy physiologically available from foods only if an allowance is made for material not completely oxidised in the body

hedonic scale – Term used in tasting panels where the judges indicate the extent of their like or dislike for the food

Hegsted score – Method of expressing the lipid content of a diet, calculated as $2.16 \times \%$ energy from saturated fat $-1.65 \times \%$ energy from polyunsaturated fat $-0.0677 \times$ mg cholesterol. *See also* Keys score

Helicobacter pylori – Bacterium commonly infecting the gastric mucosa in patients with ulcers. The underlying cause of ulcers, and implicated in the development of gastric cancer

hemicelluloses – Complex carbohydrates included as dietary fibre, composed of polyuronic acids combined with xylose, glucose, mannose and arabinose. Found together with cellulose and lignin in plant cell walls; most gums and mucilages are hemicelluloses; *see* dietary fibre, cellulose, lignin

hepatitis – Inflammatory liver disease, characterised by jaundice, abdominal pain and anorexia. May be due to bacterial or viral infection, alcohol abuse or various toxins

hepatomegaly – Enlargement of the liver as a result of congestion (e.g. in heart failure), inflammation or fatty infiltration (as in kwashiorkor)

hesperidin – A flavonoid found in the pith of unripe citrus fruits; a complex of glucose and rhamnose with the flavonone hesperin; *see* flavonoids

hexoses – Six-carbon monosaccharides such as glucose or fructose

hiatus hernia – Protrusion of a part of the stomach upwards through the diaphragm. The condition occurs in about 40% of the population, most people suffering no ill-effects; in a small number of people there is reflux of stomach contents into the oesophagus, causing heartburn

histamine – The amine formed by decarboxylation of the amino acid histidine. Excessive release of histamine from mast cells is responsible for many of the symptoms of allergic reactions. It also stimulates secretion of gastric acid, and administration of histamine provides a test for achlorhydria; *see* achlorhydria

histidine – An essential amino acid with a basic side chain

histones – Proteins rich in arginine and lysine that occur mainly in the cell nucleus and are concerned with the regulation of DNA; *see* DNA

hydroxymethylglutaryl CoA (HMG CoA) reductase inhibitors – Drugs that inhibit the enzyme HMG CoA reductase, the controlling enzyme of cholesterol synthesis, used in the treatment of hypercholesterolaemia

holoenzyme – An enzyme protein together with its coenzyme or prosthetic group

homeostasis (homeostatic) – The control of concentration of key components (in blood, etc.) to ensure constancy and physiological normalisation of their concentrations

homocysteine – A sulphur amino acid formed as an intermediate in the metabolism of methionine; it is demethylated methionine. Normally present at only low concentration (e.g. less than $10\ \mu M$ in serum or plasma). High blood concentrations of homocysteine (occurring as a result of poor folic acid, vitamin B_6, and B_{12} status and in certain other dietary and medical situations)

have been implicated in the development of atherosclerosis, heart disease and stroke

homogenisation – Emulsions usually consist of a suspension of globules of varying size. Homogenisation reduces these globules to a smaller and more uniform size

hormones – Compounds produced in the body in endocrine glands, and released into the bloodstream, where they act as chemical messengers to affect other tissues and organs

Human Genome Project – International collaboration of laboratories to decipher the DNA sequence of the entire human genome

human immunodeficiency virus (HIV) – The virus which causes AIDS (acquired immune deficiency syndrome). In many developing countries this virus is acquired by heterosexual intercourse, and may also be acquired 'vertically', either at the time of birth or in breast milk (around 25–30% of all vertical transmission by breastfeeding mothers). The level of access to specific treatment is still much lower in poor countries.

hunger – A condition in which people lack the basic food intake to provide them with the energy and nutrients for fully productive, active lives; it is an outcome of food insecurity

hybridisation – Formation of duplexes by RNA and/or DNA sequences (can be DNA–DNA, RNA–RNA or DNA–RNA) *see* DNA, RNA

hydrogenated oils – Liquid oils hardened by hydrogenation

hydrogenation – Conversion of liquid oils to semi-hard fats by the addition of hydrogen to the unsaturated double bonds

hydrolyse (hydrolysis) – To split a complex compound into its constituent parts by the action of water, either enzymically or catalysed by the addition of acid or alkali

hydroxyapatite – The calcium phosphate complex which is the main mineral of bones and teeth. The crystalline forms make up dental enamel

hydroxylysine – Amino acid found only in connective tissue proteins (collagen and elastin); incorporated into the protein as lysine and then hydroxylated in a vitamin-C-dependent reaction

hydroxyproline – Amino acid found mainly in connective tissue proteins (collagen and elastin); incorporated into the protein as proline and then hydroxylated in a vitamin-C-dependent reaction. Peptides of hydroxyproline are excreted in the urine and the output is increased when collagen turnover is high, as in rapid growth or resorption of tissue

hydroxyproline index – Urinary excretion of hydroxyproline is reduced in children suffering protein–energy malnutrition. The index is the ratio of urinary hydroxyproline to creatinine per kg of body weight, and is low in malnourished children

25-hydroxyvitamin D – The most abundant vitamin D derivative, found mainly in blood serum (plasma), which is usually measured so as to define vitamin D status. It is the precursor of the hormone, 1,25-dihydroxyvitamin D, which is formed in the kidney by an enzyme which is homeostatically controlled so as to liberate the appropriate amount of the hormone that is required for the correct control of calcium transport

hyper- – Prefix meaning above the normal range, or abnormally high

hyperalimentation – Provision of unusually large amounts of energy, either intravenously (parenteral nutrition) or by nasogastric or gastrostomy tube (enteral nutrition)

hypercalcaemia, idiopathic – Elevated plasma concentrations of calcium believed to be due to hypersensitivity of some children to vitamin D toxicity. There is excessive absorption of calcium, with loss of appetite, vomiting, constipation, flabby muscles, and deposition of calcium in the soft tissues and kidneys. It can be fatal in infants

hyperchlorhydria – Excess secretion of hydrochloric acid in the stomach due to secretion of a greater volume of gastric juice rather than to a higher concentration

hypercholesterolaemia – Abnormally high blood concentrations of cholesterol. Generally considered to be a sign of high risk for atherosclerosis and ischaemic heart disease

hyperglycaemia – Elevated plasma concentration of glucose, caused by a failure of the normal hormonal mechanisms of blood glucose control

hyperinsulinism – Excessive secretion of insulin, resulting in hypoglycaemia

hyperkalaemia – Excessively high blood concentration of potassium

hyperkinetic syndrome (hyperkinesis) – Mental disorder of children, characterised by excessive activity and impaired attention and learning ability. Has been attributed to adverse reactions to food additives, but there is little evidence

hyperlipidaemia (hyperlipoproteinaemia) – A variety of conditions in which there are increased concentrations of lipids in plasma: phospholipids, triacylglycerols, free and esterified cholesterol, or unesterified fatty acids

hyperphosphataemia – Excessively high blood concentration of phosphate

hypersalivation – Excessive flow of saliva

hypersensitivity – Heightened responsiveness induced by allergic sensitisation. There are several types of response including that associated with allergy

hypertension – High blood pressure; a risk factor for ischaemic heart disease, stroke and kidney disease. May be due to increased sensitivity to sodium

hypertonic – A solution more concentrated than the body fluids; *see* isotonic, hypotonic

hypervitaminosis – Toxicity due to excessively high intakes of vitamins

hypo- – Prefix meaning below the normal range, or abnormally low

hypocalcaemia – Low blood calcium, leading to vomiting and uncontrollable twitching of muscles if severe; may be due to underactivity of the parathyroid gland, kidney failure or vitamin D deficiency

hypochlorhydria – Partial deficiency of hydrochloric acid secretion in the gastric juice

hypogeusia – Diminished sense of taste. An early sign of marginal zinc deficiency, and potentially useful as an index of zinc status

hypoglycaemia – Abnormally low concentration of plasma glucose; may result in loss of consciousness – hypoglycaemic coma

hypoglycaemic agents – Drugs used to lower blood glucose concentrations in diabetes mellitus

hypokalaemia – Abnormally low plasma potassium

hypophosphataemia – Abnormally low blood concentration of phosphate

hypoplasia (of enamel) – poorly developed, undermineralised enamel

hypoproteinaemia – Abnormally low plasma protein concentration

hypothermia – Low body temperature (normal is around 37°C)

hypothyroidism – Underactivity of the thyroid gland, leading to reduced secretion of thyroid hormones and a reduction in basal metabolic rate. Commonly associated with goitre due to iodine deficiency

hypotonic – A solution more dilute than the body fluids

hypovitaminosis – Vitamin deficiency

iatrogenic – A condition caused by medical intervention or drug treatment; iatrogenic nutrient deficiency is due to drug–nutrient interactions

idiosyncrasy – Unusual and unexpected sensitivity or reaction to a drug or food

ileitis – Inflammation of the ileum

ileostomy – Surgical formation of an opening of the ileum on the abdominal wall, performed to treat severe ulcerative colitis

ileum – Last portion of the small intestine, between the jejunum and the colon (large intestine)

ileus – Obstruction of the intestines

immunoglobulin – A member of a family of proteins from which antibodies are derived. There are five main classes in humans known as IgM, IgG, IgA, IgD and IgE

in vitro – Literally 'in glass'; used to indicate an observation made experimentally in the test-tube, as distinct from the natural living conditions, in vivo

in vivo – In the living state, as distinct from in vitro

inanition – Exhaustion and wasting due to complete lack or non-assimilation of food; a state of starvation

index of nutritional quality (INQ) – An attempt to provide an overall figure for the nutrient content of a food or a diet. It is the ratio between the percentage of the reference intake of each nutrient and the percentage of the average requirement for energy provided by the food

indigestion – Discomfort and distension of the stomach after a meal, also known as dyspepsia, including heartburn

infarction – Death of an area of tissue because its blood supply has been stopped

ingredient – Any substance used in the manufacture or preparation of a foodstuff and still present in the finished product, even if in an altered form. Contaminants and adulterants are not considered to be ingredients

inorganic – Materials of mineral, as distinct from animal or vegetable, origin. Apart from carbonates and cyanides, inorganic chemicals are those that contain no carbon. *See also* organic

inosine monophosphate (IMP) – One of the purine nucleotides; *see* purines, nucleotide

inositol – A carbohydrate derivative, a constituent of phospholipids (phosphatidyl inositols) involved in membrane structure and as part of the signalling mechanism for hormones which act at the cell surface

insulin – Polypeptide hormone that regulates carbohydrate metabolism

insulin resistance – Changes in the biological activity of insulin-sensitive peripheral tissues, which result in reduced disposal of nutrients such as glucose from the plasma for any given concentration of insulin

insulinaemic index – The rise in blood insulin elicited by a test dose of a carbohydrate food compared with that after an equivalent dose of glucose

Interferon – One of a family of naturally occurring proteins produced by the cells of the immune system, attacking viruses, bacteria, tumours and other foreign substances

integrated pest management (IPM) – A flexible approach to pest management that draws upon a range of methods to produce a result that combines the greatest value to the farmer with environmentally acceptable and sustainable outcomes

interleukins (IL) – Soluble polypeptide mediators, produced by activated lymphocytes and other cells during immune and inflammatory response, such as IL1, IL6 (*see* cytokines)

International Network of Food Data Systems (INFOODS) – Created to develop standards and guidelines for collection of food composition data, and standardised terminology and nomenclature; website http://www.fao.org/infoods

International Union of Food Science and Technology (IUFosT) – website http://www.iufost.org

International Union of Nutritional Sciences (IUNS) – website http://www.iuns.org

international units (iu) – Used as a measure of comparative potency of natural substances, such as vitamins, before they were obtained in a sufficiently pure form to measure by weight

intervention study – Comparison of an outcome (e.g. morbidity or mortality) between two groups of people deliberately subjected to different dietary or drug regimes

intestinal flora – Bacteria and other microorganisms that are normally present in the gastrointestinal tract

intestinal juice – Also called succus entericus. Digestive juice secreted by the intestinal glands lining the small intestine, containing a variety of enzymes

intestinal polyposis – Appearance of polyps (growths) on the surface of the intestine, mainly in the rectum and large intestine, which may in some cases be precursors of cancerous growths. Their measurement may be potentially useful as a functional index of pro- versus anti-carcinogenic influences, some of which may be nutrient-sensitive

intestine – The gastrointestinal tract; more specifically the part after the stomach, i.e. the small intestine (duodenum, jejunum and ileum) where the greater part of digestion and absorption takes place, and the large intestine

intrinsic factor – A protein secreted in the gastric juice which is required for the absorption of vitamin B_{12}; impaired secretion results in pernicious anaemia

intron – Segment of a gene that is transcribed but then removed from the primary transcript by splicing and so is not present in the mature mRNA product. Non-coding sequence of DNA between exons; see exon

inulin – Soluble but undigested fructose polymer found in root vegetables. Also called dahlin and alant starch (although it is a non-starch polysaccharide)

inversion – Applied to sucrose, means its hydrolysis to glucose and fructose (invert sugar)

invert sugar – The mixture of glucose and fructose produced by hydrolysis of sucrose, 1.3 times sweeter than sucrose. So called because the optical activity is reversed in the process

invertase – Enzyme that hydrolyses sucrose to glucose and fructose (invert sugar); also called sucrase and saccharase

iodine number (iodine value) – Carbon–carbon double bonds in unsaturated compounds can react with iodine; this provides a means of determining the degree of unsaturation of a fat or other compound by the uptake of iodine

iodised salt – Usually 1 part of iodate in 25000–50000 parts of salt, as a means of ensuring adequate iodine intake in regions where deficiency is a problem

ion – An atom or molecule that has lost or gained one or more electrons, and thus has an electric charge. Positively charged ions are cations, because they migrate towards the cathode (negative pole) in solution, while negatively charged ions (anions) migrate towards the positive pole (anode)

ion-exchange resin – An organic compound that will adsorb ions under some conditions and release them under others

ionisation – The process whereby the positive and negative ions of a salt or other compound separate when dissolved in water. The degree of ionisation of an acid or alkali determines its strength (see pH)

ionising radiation – Electromagnetic radiation that ionises the air or water through which it passes, e.g. X-rays and gamma-rays. Used for the sterilisation of food, etc. by irradiation

irradiation – A method of sterilising and disinfecting foods using ionising radiation (X-rays or gamma-rays) to kill microorganisms and insects. Also used to inhibit sprouting of potatoes

irritable bowel syndrome (IBS) – Also known as spastic colon or mucous colitis. Abnormally increased motility of the large and small intestines, leading to pain and alternating diarrhoea and constipation; often precipitated by emotional stress

ischaemia – Inadequate blood supply to a tissue

ischaemic heart disease or coronary heart disease – Group of syndromes arising from failure of the coronary arteries to supply sufficient blood to heart muscles; associated with atherosclerosis of coronary arteries

islets of Langerhans – The endocrine parts of the pancreas; glucagon is secreted by the α-cells and insulin by the β-cells

isoenzymes – Enzymes that have the same catalytic activity but different structures, properties and/or tissue distribution

isoleucine – An essential amino acid, rarely limiting in food; one of the branched-chain amino acids

isomers – Molecules that have the same empirical formula but differ in position of substituents or functional groups

isotonic – Solutions with the same osmotic pressure; often refers to a solution with the same osmotic pressure as body fluids. Hypertonic and hypotonic refer to solutions that are more and less concentrated

isotopes – Forms of elements with the same chemical properties, differing in atomic mass because of differing numbers of neutrons in the nucleus. Radioactive isotopes are unstable, and decay to stable elements, emitting radiation in the process. Stable isotopes can be detected only by their different atomic mass. Since they emit no radiation, they are safe for use in labelled compounds given to human beings

isozymes – *See* isoenzymes

jejuno-ileostomy – Surgical procedure in which the terminal jejunum or proximal ileum is removed or bypassed. Was formerly used as a treatment for severe obesity

jejunum – Part of the small intestine, between the duodenum and the ileum

joule – The SI (Système Internationale) unit of energy; used to express energy content of foods

keratomalacia – Progressive softening and ulceration of the cornea, due to vitamin A deficiency. Blindness is usually inevitable unless the deficiency is corrected at an early stage

Keshan disease – A disease occurring in parts of China where selenium deficiency is believed to be a problem. The cardiomyopathy of the disease is believed to be of viral origin

ketoacidosis – High concentrations of ketone bodies in the blood

ketogenic diet – A diet poor in carbohydrate (20–30 g) and rich in fat; causes accumulation of ketone bodies in tissue

ketone bodies – Acetoacetate, β-hydroxybutyrate and acetone; acetoacetate and acetone are chemically ketones; although β-hydroxybutyrate is not, it is included in the term ketone bodies because of its metabolic relationship with acetoacetate

ketones – Chemical compounds containing a carbonyl group (C=O), with two alkyl groups attached to the same carbon; the simplest ketone is acetone (dimethylketone, $(CH_3)_2$–C=O)

ketonuria – Excretion of ketone bodies in the urine

ketosis – High concentrations of ketone bodies in the blood

Keys score – Method of expressing the lipid content of a diet, calculated as $1.35 \times (2 \times \%$ energy from saturated fat – % energy from polyunsaturated fat) $+ 1.5 \times \sqrt{}$ (mg cholesterol /1000 kcal)

kGy – Kilogray, a unit of radiation intensity

kilo – As a prefix for units of measurement, one thousand times (i.e. 10^3); symbol k

Kjeldahl determination – Widely used method of determining total nitrogen in a substance by digesting with sulphuric acid and a catalyst; the nitrogen is reduced to ammonia which is then measured. In foodstuffs most of the nitrogen is protein, and the term crude protein is the total 'Kjeldahl nitrogen' multiplied by a factor of 6.25 (since most proteins contain 16% nitrogen)

koilonychia – Development of (brittle) concave finger nails, commonly associated with iron-deficiency anaemia

Korsakoff's psychosis – Failure of recent memory, although events from the past are recalled, with confabulation; associated with vitamin B_1 deficiency, especially in alcoholics

kosher – The selection and preparation of foods in accordance with traditional Jewish ritual and dietary laws. Foods that are not kosher are traife. The only kosher flesh foods are from animals that chew the cud and have cloven hoofs, such as cattle, sheep, goats, and deer; the hindquarters must not be eaten. The only fish permitted are those with fins and scales; birds of prey and scavengers are not kosher. Moreover, the animals must be slaughtered according to ritual, without stunning, before the meat can be considered kosher

Krebs cycle – Or citric acid cycle, a central pathway for the metabolism of fats, carbohydrates and amino acids

kwashiorkor (from the Ga language of West Africa) – A disease which occurs frequently in young (weanling) children in some developing countries where weaning foods are of poor quality, and is characterised by oedema (swelling due to extracellular fluid accumulation), failure to thrive, abnormal hair appearance (dyspigmentation), often enlarged liver and increased mortality risk. Associated especially with poor diets that are low in protein and other nutrients, and also with frequent infections; *see* protein–energy malnutrition

lactase – The enzyme that breaks down lactose (milk sugar) to galactose–glucose in the small intestine

lactation – The process of synthesising and secreting milk from the breasts

lactic acid – The acid produced by the anaerobic fermentation of carbohydrates. Originally discovered in sour milk, it is responsible for the flavour of fermented milk and for the precipitation of the casein curd in cottage cheese

lacto-ovo-vegetarian – One whose diet excludes meat and fish but permits milk and eggs

lactose – The carbohydrate of milk, sometimes called milk sugar, a disaccharide of glucose and galactose

lactulose – A disaccharide of galactose and fructose which does not occur naturally but is formed in heated or stored milk by isomerisation of lactose.

Not hydrolysed by human digestive enzymes but fermented by intestinal bacteria to form lactic and pyruvic acids. Thought to promote the growth of *Lactobacillus bifidus* and so added to some infant formulae; in large amounts it is a laxative

laxative – Or aperient, a substance that helps the expulsion of food residues from the body. If strongly laxative it is termed purgative or cathartic. Dietary fibre and cellulose function because they retain water and add bulk to the contents of the intestine; Epsom salts (magnesium sulphate) also retain water; castor oil and drugs such as aloes, senna, cascara and phenolphthalein irritate the intestinal mucosa. Undigested carbohydrates such as lactulose and sugar alcohols are also laxatives

lecithin – Chemically lecithin is phosphatidyl choline; a phospholipid containing choline. Commercial lecithin is a mixture of phospholipids in which phosphatidyl choline predominates; *see* choline, phospholipids

lectins – Proteins from legumes and other sources which bind to the carbohydrates found at cell surfaces. They therefore cause red blood cells to agglutinate in vitro, hence the old names haemagglutinins and phytoagglutinins

legumes – Members of the family Leguminosae, consumed as dry mature seeds (grain legumes or pulses) or as immature green seeds in the pod. Legumes include the groundnut, *Arachis hypogaea*, and soya bean, *Glycine max*, grown for their oil and protein, the yam bean *Pachyrrhizus erosus*, and African yam bean *Sphenostylis stenocarpa*, grown for their edible tubers as well as seeds

leptin – Hormone secreted by adipose tissue that acts to regulate long-term appetite and energy expenditure by signalling the state of body fat reserves

less-favoured areas – Lands that have low agricultural potential because of limited and uncertain rainfall, poor soils, steep slopes, or other biophysical constraints, as well as lands that may have high agricultural potential but have limited access to infrastructure and markets, low population density, or other socioeconomic constraints

lethal dose 50% (LD50) – An index of toxicity, the amount of the substance that kills 50% of the test population of experimental animals when administered as a single dose

leucine – An essential amino acid; rarely limiting in foods; one of the branched-chain amino acids

leucovorin – The synthetic (racemic) 5-formyl derivative of folic acid; more stable to oxidation than folic acid itself, and commonly used in pharmaceutical preparations. Also known as folinic acid

leukocytes – White blood cells, normally 5000–9000/mm^3; includes polymorphonuclear neutrophils, lymphocytes, monocytes, polymorphonuclear eosinophils, and polymorphonuclear basophils. A 'white cell count' determines the total; a 'differential cell count' estimates the numbers of each type. Fever, haemorrhage, and violent exercise cause an increase (leucocytosis); starvation and debilitating conditions a decrease (leucopenia)

leukocytosis – Increase in the number of leucocytes in the blood

leukopenia – Decrease in the number of leucocytes in the blood

levans – Polymers of fructose (the principal one is inulin) that occur in tubers and some grasses

Lieberkühn, crypts of – Glands lining the small intestine which secrete the intestinal juice

lignans – Naturally occurring compounds in various foods that have both oestrogenic and anti-oestrogenic activity (phytoestrogens)

lignin (lignocellulose) – Indigestible part of the cell wall of plants (a polymer of aromatic alcohols). It is included in measurement of dietary fibre, but not of non-starch polysaccharide

limosis – Abnormal hunger or excessive desire for food

linoleic acid – An essential polyunsaturated fatty acid (C18:2 ω6)

α-linolenic acid – An essential polyunsaturated fatty acid (C18:3 ω3)

γ-linolenic acid – A non-essential polyunsaturated fatty acid (C18:3 ω6)

lipase – Enzyme that hydrolyses fats to glycerol and fatty acids

lipectomy – Surgical removal of subcutaneous fat

lipids – A general term for fats and oils (chemically triacylglycerols), waxes, phospholipids, steroids and terpenes. Their common property is insolubility in water and solubility in hydrocarbons, chloroform and alcohols

lipids, plasma – Triacylglycerols, free and esterified cholesterol and phospholipids, present in lipoproteins in blood plasma. Chylomicrons consist mainly of triacylglycerols and protein;

they are the form in which lipids absorbed in the small intestine enter the bloodstream. Very-low-density lipoproteins (VLDL) are assembled in the liver and exported to other tissues, where they provide a source of lipids. Lipid-depleted VLDL becomes low-density lipoprotein (LDL) in the circulation; it is rich in cholesterol and is normally cleared by the liver. High-density lipoprotein (HDL) contains cholesterol from LDL and tissues that is returned to the liver. *See also* hypercholesterolaemia; hyperlipidaemia

lipodystrophy – Abnormal pattern of subcutaneous fat deposits

lipoedema (lipedema (US)) – Condition in which fat deposits accumulate in the lower extremities, from hips to ankles, with tenderness of the affected parts

lipofuscin – A group of pigments that accumulate in several body tissues, particularly the myocardium, and are associated with the ageing process

lipoic acid – Chemically, dithio-octanoic acid, a coenzyme (together with vitamin B_1) in the metabolism of pyruvate and in the citric acid cycle. Although it is an essential growth factor for various microorganisms, there is no evidence that it is a human dietary requirement

lipolysis – The hydrolysis of fats to glycerol and fatty acids

lipopolysaccharide (LPS) – Bacterial-derived antigenic material that promotes an immune response in animals and humans

liposuction – Procedure for removal of subcutaneous adipose tissue in obese people using a suction pump device

lipotropes (lipotrophic factors) – Compounds such as choline, betaine and methionine that act as methyl donors; deficiency may result in fatty infiltration of the liver

Listeria – A genus of bacteria commonly found in soil of which the commonest is *Listeria monocytogenes*. They can cause food poisoning (listeriosis)

low birthweight (LBW) – Used as shorthand to describe babies born at weight less than 2.5 kg. Average birthweight is close to 3.5 kg (WHO reference mean). LBW can result from delivery before term (preterm) or from intrauterine growth retardation (IUGR) due to many causes including fetal undernutrition

lower reference nutrient intake (LRNI) – Set 2 standard deviations below the EAR for a nutrient. Intakes of nutrients below this point will almost certainly be inadequate for most individuals; *see* reference nutrient intake

lutein – A hydroxylated carotenoid (xanthophyll); not vitamin-A-active

luxus konsumption – An outdated term for diet-induced thermogenesis

lycopene – Red carotenoid, not vitamin-A-active

lymph – The fluid between blood and the tissues in which oxygen and nutrients are transported to the tissues, and waste products back to the blood

lymphatics – Vessels through which the lymph flows, draining from the tissues and entering the bloodstream at the thoracic duct

lysine – An essential amino acid of special nutritional importance, since it is the limiting amino acid in many cereals

lysozyme – An enzyme present in tears and body secretions and fluids that helps in the destruction of bacterial cell walls

macrocytes – Large immature precursors of red blood cells found in the circulation in pernicious anaemia and in folic acid deficiency, due to impairment of the normal maturation of red cells; hence macrocytic anaemia

mad cow disease – Bovine spongiform encephalopathy

Maillard reaction – Non-enzymic reaction between lysine in proteins and sugars, on heating or prolonged storage

malnutrition – Disturbance of form or function arising from deficiency or excess of one or more nutrients

malondialdehyde – An oxidation (degradation) product of unsaturated fatty acids, often used as an index of pro-oxidant action and of potential damage to lipids by pro-oxidant species such as oxygen free radicals

maltase – Enzyme that hydrolyses maltose to yield two molecules of glucose; present in the brush border of the intestinal mucosal cells

maltodextrin – A polymer of glucose made by acid hydrolysis of starch

maltose – Malt sugar, or maltobiose, a disaccharide consisting of two glucose units linked $\alpha1$–4

mannosans – Polysaccharides containing mannose

mannose – A six-carbon (hexose) sugar found in small amounts in legumes, manna and some gums. Also called seminose and carubinose

marasmic kwashiorkor – The most severe form of protein–energy malnutrition in children, with weight for height less than 60% of that expected, and with oedema and other symptoms of kwashiorkor

marasmus – An old term still in common use in Anglophone developing countries. The adjective (marasmic) described abnormally small and thin infants. As noun and adjective the term was later used by nutritionists to define a weight less than 60% of the reference mean weight for age. This definition is still used in resource-poor areas where stature is not measured. Now the term protein–energy malnutrition (PEM) is more commonly used

market – Any context in which the sale and purchase of goods and services takes place. There need be no physical entity corresponding to the market; it might consist of a global telecommunications network on which company shares are traded

market economy – An economic system in which decisions about the allocation of resources and production are made on the basis of prices generated by voluntary exchanges among producers, consumers, workers and owners of the factors of production (i.e. land, labour and capital)

mast cells – Cells found predominantly in connective tissue, although a specialised population of mast cells is found in mucosal sites (e.g. the gut). Following degranulation, mast cells release preformed and newly synthesised mediators of inflammation, including histamine

mastication – Chewing, grinding, and tearing foods with the teeth while it is mixed with saliva

maternal death – Death of a woman whilst pregnant or within 42 days of delivery

MaxEPA – Trade name for a standardised mixture of long-chain marine fatty acids, eicosapentaenoic (EPA, C20:5 ω3) and docosohexaenoic (DHA, C22:6 ω3) acids

medium-chain triacylglycerols – Triacylglycerols containing medium-chain (C:10–12) fatty acids, used in treatment of malabsorption; they are absorbed more rapidly than conventional fats, and the products of their digestion are transported to the liver, rather than in chylomicrons

megavitamin therapy – Treatment of diseases with very high doses of vitamins, many times the reference intakes; little or no evidence for its efficacy; vitamins A, D and B_6 are known to be toxic at high levels of intake

menadione, menaphthone, menaphtholdiacetate – Synthetic compounds with vitamin K

activity; vitamin K_3, sometimes known as menaquinone-0

menaquinones – Bacterial metabolites with vitamin K activity; vitamin K_2

menarche – The initiation of menstruation in adolescent girls, normally occurring between the ages of 11 and 15. The age at menarche has become younger in Western countries, possibly associated with a better general standard of nutrition, and is later in less-developed countries

menhaden – Oily fish, *Brevoortia patronus, B. tyrannus*, from Gulf of Mexico and Atlantic seaboard of the USA, a rich source of fish oils

mesomorph – Description given to a well-covered individual with well-developed muscles. *See also* ectomorph; endomorph

mesophiles – Pathogenic microorganisms that grow best at temperatures between 25 and 40°C; usually will not grow below 5°C

metabolic equivalent (MET) – Unit of measurement of heat production by the body; 1 MET = 50 kcal/hour/m^2 body surface area

metabolic water – Produced in the body by the oxidation of foods; 100 g of fat produces 107.1 g; 100 g of starch 55.1 g; and 100 g of protein 41.3 g of water

metabolic weight – Energy expenditure and basal metabolic rate depend on the amount of metabolically active tissue in the body, rather than total body weight; body weight$^{0.75}$ is generally used to calculate the weight of active tissue

metabolism – The processes of interconversion of chemical compounds in the body. Anabolism is the process of forming larger and more complex compounds, commonly linked to the utilisation of metabolic energy. Catabolism is the process of breaking down larger molecules to smaller ones, commonly oxidation reactions linked to release of energy. There is approximately a 30% variation in the underlying metabolic rate (basal metabolic rate) between different individuals, determined in part by the activity of the thyroid gland

metabolome – The complement of metabolic reactions and metabolic products of an organism

metabolomics – The study of the metabolome

metalloenzyme – An enzyme having a metal (e.g. zinc or copper) as its prosthetic group

metalloproteins – Proteins containing a metal

metaphosphoric acid – A form of phosphoric acid which is used as a preservative for vitamin C (ascorbic acid) because its addition to biological fluids, such as serum or urine, lowers the pH and chelates (i.e. inactivates) the pro-oxidant metal ions such as ferrous and cupric ions

methaemoglobin – Oxidised form of haemoglobin (unlike oxyhaemoglobin, which is a loose and reversible combination with oxygen) which cannot transport oxygen to the tissues. Present in small quantities in normal blood, increased after certain drugs and after smoking; found rarely as a congenital abnormality (methaemoglobinaemia). It can be formed in the blood of babies after consumption of the small amounts of nitrate found naturally in vegetables and in some drinking water, since the lack of acidity in the stomach permits reduction of nitrate to nitrite

methionine – An essential amino acid; one of the three containing sulphur; cystine and cysteine are the other two. Cystine and cysteine are not essential, but can only be made from methionine, and therefore the requirement for methionine is lower if there is an adequate intake of cyst(e)ine

3-methyl-histidine – Derivative of the amino acid histidine, found mainly in the contractile proteins of muscle (myosin and actin)

methylmalonic acid – An intermediate in the metabolic turnover of succinic acid, this substance typically accumulates in conditions of vitamin B_{12} deficiency, and can be measured in serum or urine, as a functional index of vitamin B_{12} status

micelles – Emulsified droplets of partially hydrolysed lipids, small enough to be absorbed across the intestinal mucosa

micro – Prefix for units of measurement, one millionth part (i.e. 10^{-6}); symbol μ (or sometimes mc)

microbiological assay – Method of measuring compounds such as vitamins and amino acids, using microorganisms. The principle is that the organism is inoculated into a medium containing all the growth factors needed except the one under examination; the rate of growth is then proportional to the amount of this nutrient added in the test substance

micronutrients – Vitamins and minerals, which are needed in very small amounts (micrograms or milligrams per day), as distinct from fats, carbohydrates and proteins, which are macronutrients, since they are needed in considerably greater amounts

mid-upper arm circumference (MUAC) – A rapid way of assessing nutritional status, especially applicable to children; *see* anthropometry

migraine – Type of headache, characterised by usually being unilateral and/or accompanied by visual disturbance and nausea

milli – Prefix for units of measurement, one thousandth part (i.e. 10^{-3}); symbol m

mineral salts – The inorganic salts, including sodium, potassium, calcium, chloride, phosphate, sulphate, etc. So called because they are (or originally were) obtained by mining

mineralocorticoids – The steroid hormones secreted by the adrenal cortex which control the excretion of salt and water; *see* steroids

minerals, trace – Those mineral salts present in the body, and required in the diet, in small amounts (parts per million)

minerals, ultra-trace – Those mineral salts present in the body, and required in the diet, in extremely small amounts (parts per thousand million or less); known to be dietary essentials, although rarely if ever a cause for concern since the amounts required are small and they are widely distributed in foods and water

Ministry of Agriculture, Fisheries and Food (MAFF) – Former UK Ministry now replaced by DEFRA and the FSA

miscarriage – Spontaneous loss of a pregnancy before 24 weeks of gestation

mitochondrion – (Plural mitochondria). The subcellular organelles in all cells apart from red blood cells in which the major oxidative reactions of metabolism occur, linked to the formation of ATP from ADP; *see* ADP, ATP

monoamine oxidase – Enzyme that oxidises amines; inhibitors have been used clinically as antidepressant drugs, and consumption of amine-rich foods such as cheese may cause a hypertensive crisis in people taking the inhibitors; *see* amines

monosaccharides – Group name of the simplest sugars, including those composed of three carbon atoms (trioses), four (tetroses), five (pentoses), six (hexoses) and seven (heptoses). The units from which disaccharides, oligosaccharides and polysaccharides are formed

monosodium glutamate (MSG) – The sodium salt of glutamic acid, used to enhance the flavour of savoury dishes and often added to canned meat and soups

mRNA – An RNA copy of genomic DNA containing genes for translation into protein; *see* RNA, DNA, genome

mucilages – Soluble but undigested complexes of the sugars arabinose and xylose found in some seeds and seaweeds

mucin – Viscous mucoprotein secreted in the saliva and throughout the intestinal tract; the main constituent of mucus

mucopolysaccharides – Polysaccharides containing an amino sugar and uronic acid; constituent of the mucoproteins of cartilage, tendons, connective tissue, cornea, heparin and blood-group substances; *see* polysaccharides

mucoproteins – Glycoproteins containing a sugar, usually chondroitin sulphate, combined with amino acids or peptides; occur in mucin; *see* glycoprotein

mucosa – Moist tissue lining, for example, the mouth (buccal mucosa), stomach (gastric mucosa), intestines and respiratory tract

mucous colitis – Irritable bowel syndrome (q.v.)

mucus – Secretion of mucous glands, containing mucin; protects epithelia

mutagen – Compound that causes mutations and may be carcinogenic; *see* mutation

mutation – a permanent structural alteration in DNA

mycoprotein – Name given to mould mycelium used as a food ingredient

mycotoxins – Toxins produced by fungi (moulds), especially *Aspergillus flavus* under tropical conditions and *Penicillium* and *Fusarium* species under temperate conditions

myoglobin – Haemoprotein mainly found in muscle where it serves as an intracellular storage site for oxygen

myristic acid – A medium-chain saturated fatty acid (C14:0)

myxoedema – Low metabolic rate as a result of hypothyroidism, commonly the result of iodine deficiency

nano – Prefix for units of measurement, one thousand-millionth part (i.e. 10^{-9}), symbol n

naphthoquinone – The chemical ring structure of vitamin K; the various vitamers of vitamin K can be referred to as substituted naphthoquinones

nasogastric tube – Fine plastic tube inserted through the nose and thence into the stomach for enteral nutrition

National Center for Health Statistics (NCHS) standards – Tables of height and weight for age used as reference values for the assessment of growth and nutritional status of children, based on data collected by the US National Center for Health Statistics in the 1970s. The most comprehensive such set of data, and used in most countries of the world

National Health and Nutrition Examination Survey (NHANES) – Conducted by the National Center for Health Statistics (NCHS), Centers for Disease Control and Prevention, designed to collect information about the health and diet of people in the United States

natural killer cells (NK) – Specialised T-cells with the continuous task of identifying and eliminating cells recognised as being foreign or non-self

nature-identical – Term applied to food additives that are synthesised in the laboratory and are identical to those that occur in nature

neonatal – Within the first 28 days of life

nephropathy – Diabetic complication that involves the kidney and may lead to chronic renal failure and dialysis

net dietary protein–energy ratio (NDpE) – A way of expressing the protein content of a diet or food taking into account both the amount of protein (relative to total energy intake) and the protein quality. It is protein–energy multiplied by net protein utilisation divided by total energy. If energy is expressed in kcal and the result expressed as a percentage, this is net dietary protein calories per cent, NDpCal%

net protein ratio/retention (NPR) – Weight gain of a test animal plus weight loss of a control animal fed a non-protein diet per gram of protein consumed by the test animal

net protein utilisation (NPU) – The proportion of nitrogen intake that is retained, i.e. the product of biological value (q.v) and digestibility (q.v).

net protein value (NPV) – A way of expressing the amount and quality of the protein in a food; the product of net protein utilisation and protein content per cent

neural tube defect – Congenital malformations of the brain (anencephaly) or spinal cord (spina bifida) caused by failure of closure of the neural tube in early embryonic development

neuropathy – Diabetic complication that involves peripheral and autonomic nervous system

neuropeptide Y – A peptide neurotransmitter believed to be important in the control of appetite and feeding behaviour, especially in response to leptin

niacin – The generic descriptor for two compounds that have the biological activity of the vitamin:

nicotinic acid and its amide, nicotinamide. In the USA niacin is used specifically to mean nicotinic acid, and niacinamide for nicotinamide

niacinamide – US name for nicotinamide, the amide form of the vitamin niacin

niacinogens – Name given to protein–niacin complexes found in cereals; *see* niacytin

niacytin – The bound forms of the vitamin niacin, found in cereals

nicotinamide – One of the vitamers of niacin

nicotinamide adenine dinucleotide and its phosphate (NAD, NADP) – The coenzymes derived from niacin. Involved as hydrogen acceptors in a wide variety of oxidation and reduction reactions; *see* nicotinamide

nicotinic acid – One of the vitamers of niacin

night blindness – Nyctalopia. Inability to see in dim light as a result of vitamin A deficiency

ninhydrin test – For the amino group of amino acids. Pink, purple or blue colour is developed on heating an amino acid or peptide with ninhydrin

nitrogen conversion factor – Factor by which nitrogen content of a foodstuff is multiplied to determine the protein content; it depends on the amino acid composition of the protein. For wheat and most cereals it is 5.8; rice, 5.95; soya, 5.7; most legumes and nuts, 5.3; milk, 6.38; other foods, 6.25. In mixtures of proteins, as in dishes and diets, the factor of 6.25 is used. 'Crude protein' is defined as N × 6.25

N-nitroso compounds – A group of chemicals that occur ubiquitously. They are formed in the environment and can be absorbed from food, water, air and industrial and consumer products, formed within the body from precursors in food, water and air, inhaled from tobacco smoke, and naturally occurring

No Adverse Effect Level (NOAE) – With respect to food additives, equivalent to No Effect Level

No Effect Level (NEL) – With respect to food additives, the maximum dose of an additive that has no detectable adverse effects

Non-digestible oligosaccharide – An oligosaccharide that is not digested (or minimally digested) in the upper gastrointestinal tract

non-esterified fatty acids (NEFA) – Free fatty acids in the blood, as opposed to triacylglycerols

non-starch polysaccharides (NSP) – Those polysaccharides other than starches, found in foods. They are the major part of dietary fibre and can be measured more precisely than total dietary fibre; include cellulose, pectins, glucans, gums, mucilages, inulin and chitin (and exclude lignin); *see* dietary fibre

nor- – Chemical prefix to the name of a compound, indicating: (1) one methyl (CH_3) group has been replaced by hydrogen (e.g. noradrenaline can be considered to be a demethylated derivative of adrenaline); (2) an analogue of a compound containing one fewer methylene (CH_2) groups than the parent compound; (3) an isomer with an unbranched side-chain (e.g. norleucine, norvaline)

noradrenaline (norepinephrine) – Hormone secreted by the adrenal medulla together with adrenaline (epinephrine); also a neurotransmitter. Physiological effects similar to those of adrenaline

norepinephrine – *See* noradrenaline

Northern blotting – Widely used technique for detecting mRNAs by hybridisation with specific probes following transfer of RNA onto a solid support, such as a nylon membrane; *see* mRNA, RNA, hybridisation

Norwalk-like virus – Viral infection similar to that first reported in Norwalk, USA, which causes intestinal illness that occurs in outbreaks

nucleic acids – Polymers of purine and pyrimidine sugar phosphates; two main classes: ribonucleic acid (RNA) and deoxyribonucleic acid (DNA); *see* ribonucleic acid, deoxyribonucleic acid

nucleoproteins – The complex of proteins and nucleic acids found in the cell nucleus

nucleosides – Compounds of purine or pyrimidine bases with a sugar, most commonly ribose. For example, adenine plus ribose forms adenosine. With the addition of phosphate a nucleotide is formed; *see* purines, pyrimidines

nucleotides – Compounds of purine or pyrimidine base with a sugar phosphate

nutraceuticals – Term for compounds in foods that are not nutrients but have (potential) beneficial effects

nutrient density – A way of expressing the nutrient content of a food or diet relative to the energy yield (i.e. /1000 kcal or /MJ) rather than per unit weight

nutrients – Essential dietary factors such as vitamins, minerals, amino acids and fatty acids. Metabolic fuels (sources of energy) are not termed nutrients so that a commonly used phrase is 'energy and nutrients'

nutrification – The addition of nutrients to foods at such a level as to make a major contribution to the diet

nutrition – The process by which living organisms take in and use food for the maintenance of life, growth, and the functioning of organs and tissues; the branch of science that studies these processes

Nutrition Labeling and Education Act (1990) – NLEA, the basis of current US food labelling

nutrition surveillance – Monitoring the state of health, nutrition, eating behaviour and nutrition knowledge of the population for the purpose of planning and evaluating nutrition policy. Especially in developing countries, monitoring may include factors that may give early warning of nutritional emergencies

nutritional genomics (nutrigenomics) – The field encompassing the interactions between nutrients and the genome and gene products, the function of gene products, and the identification and understanding of the genetic basis for individual and population differences in the response to diet

nutritionist – One who applies the science of nutrition to the promotion of health and control of disease, instructs auxiliary medical personnel and participates in surveys

nyctalopia – *See* night blindness

obesity – Excessive accumulation of body fat. A body mass index above 30 is considered to be obese (and above 40 grossly obese)

obstipation – Extreme and persistent constipation caused by obstruction of the intestinal tract

obstructed labour – Failure of descent of the fetal presenting part (usually the head) because of disproportion between the size of the head, which may be unusually large, and the size of the bony birth canal, which may be unusually small. An important cause of maternal and/or fetal death if caesarean section is not available to the labouring woman

oedema – Excess retention of fluid in the body; may be caused by cardiac, renal or hepatic failure or by starvation (famine oedema)

oestrogens – Steroid hormones principally secreted by the ovaries, which maintain female characteristics

Office of Dietary Supplements (ODS) – Office of the US National Institutes of Health; website http://dietary-supplements.info.nih.gov

oleic acid – A mono-unsaturated fatty acid (C18:1 ω9)

oligoallergenic diet – Comprised of very few foods or an elemental diet used to diagnose whether particular symptoms are the result of allergic response to food

oligodipsia – Reduced sense of thirst

oligofructose (or fructo-oligosaccharide) – Polymer of fructose made from sucrose or inulin, a non-digestible oligosaccharide

oligopeptides – Polymers of 4 or more amino acids; more than about 20–50 are termed polypeptides, and more than about 100 are considered to be proteins

oligosaccharides – Carbohydrates composed of 3–10 monosaccharide units (with more than 10 units they are termed polysaccharides). Those composed of fructose, galactose or isomaltose have prebiotic action and encourage the growth of beneficial intestinal bacteria

omophagia – Eating of raw or uncooked food

oncotic pressure – That part of plasma osmotic pressure exerted by proteins

opsomania – Craving for special food

orexigenic – Stimulating appetite

orexins – Two small peptide hormones produced by nerve cells in the lateral hypothalamus, believed to be involved in stimulation of feeding

organic – Chemically, a substance containing carbon in the molecule (with the exception of carbonates and cyanide). Substances of animal and vegetable origin are organic; minerals are inorganic. The term organic foods refers to 'organically grown foods', meaning plants grown without the use of (synthetic) pesticides, fungicides or inorganic fertilisers, and prepared without the use of preservatives

organoleptic – Sensory properties, i.e. those that can be detected by the sense organs. For foods, it is used particularly of the combination of taste, texture and astringency (perceived in the mouth) and aroma (perceived in the nose)

ornithine – An amino acid that occurs as a metabolic intermediate in the synthesis of urea, but is not involved in protein synthesis, so of no nutritional importance

ornithine–arginine cycle – The metabolic pathway for the synthesis of urea

orotic acid – An intermediate in the biosynthesis of pyrimidines; a growth factor for some microorganisms and at one time called vitamin B_{13}. There is no evidence that it is a human dietary requirement; *see* pyrimidines

osmophiles – Microorganisms that can flourish under conditions of high osmotic pressure, e.g. in jams, honey, brine, pickles; especially yeasts (also called xerophilic yeasts)

osmosis – The passage of water through a semi-permeable membrane, from a region of low concentration of solutes to one of higher concentration. Reverse osmosis is the passage of water from a more concentrated to a less concentrated solution through a semi-permeable membrane by the application of pressure

osmotic pressure – The pressure required to prevent the passage of water through a semi-permeable membrane from a region of low concentration of solutes to one of higher concentration, by osmosis

osteocalcin – A calcium-binding protein in bone, essential for the normal mineralisation of bone. Its synthesis requires vitamin K, and is controlled by vitamin D

osteomalacia – The adult equivalent of rickets; a bone disorder due to deficiency of vitamin D, leading to inadequate absorption of calcium and loss of calcium from the bones

osteopenia – Decreased calcification or density of bone

osteoporosis – Degeneration of the bones with advancing age due to loss of bone mineral and protein as a result of decreased secretion of hormones (oestrogens in women and testosterone in men)

oxidases (oxygenases) – Enzymes that oxidise compounds by removing hydrogen and reacting directly with oxygen to form water or hydrogen peroxide

oxidation – The chemical process of removing electrons from an element or compound, frequently together with the removal of hydrogen ions (H^+). The reverse process, the addition of electrons or hydrogen, is reduction

oxycalorimeter – Instrument for measuring the oxygen consumed and carbon dioxide produced when a food is burned, as distinct from the calorimeter, which measures the heat produced

oxyntic cells – Or parietal cells; secretory cells in the stomach that produce the hydrochloric acid and intrinsic factor of the gastric juice

P450 enzymes/proteins – Cytochrome P450 proteins are mainly drug-metabolising enzymes but are also important for metabolising some endogenously derived compounds such as cholesterol, prostacyclin, thromboxane A_2, vitamins A and D, etc. The P450 proteins are categorised into families and subfamilies. In humans there are 18 families and 43 subfamilies. Most drugs are metabolised by three families: CYP1, CYP2 and CYP3. The subfamily CYP3A is the most important and abundant protein, known to metabolise at least 120 drugs

palatinose – Isomaltulose, a disaccharide of glucose and fructose, an isomer of sucrose

palmitic acid – A saturated fatty acid (C16:0)

palmitoleic acid – A mono-unsaturated fatty acid (C16:1 ω9)

pancreas – A gland in the abdomen with two functions: the endocrine pancreas (the islets of Langerhans) secretes the hormones insulin and glucagon; the exocrine pancreas secretes the pancreatic juice

pancreatic juice – The alkaline digestive juice produced by the pancreas and secreted into the duodenum

pancreatin – Preparation made from the pancreas of animals containing the enzymes of pancreatic juice. Used to replace pancreatic enzymes in cystic fibrosis as an aid to digestion

pangamic acid – Chemically the N-di-isopropyl derivative of glucuronic acid. Claimed to be an antioxidant, and to speed recovery from fatigue. Sometimes called vitamin B_{15}, but there is no evidence that it is a dietary essential, nor that it has any metabolic function

panthenol – The biologically active alcohol of pantothenic acid

pantothenic acid – A vitamin of the B complex with no numerical designation

para-aminobenzoic acid (PABA) – Essential growth factor for microorganisms. It forms part of the molecule of folic acid and is therefore required for the synthesis of this vitamin. Mammals cannot synthesise folic acid, and PABA has no other known function; there is no evidence that it is a human dietary requirement. Not normally present in human diets, can be used to validate 24h urine collections, because an oral dose, given at each of three meal-times, is rapidly and quantitatively excreted in the urine

paracellular – Movement of solute between cells

parageusia – Abnormality of the sense of taste

parathormone – Commonly used as an abbreviation for the parathyroid hormone; correctly a trade name for a pharmaceutical preparation of the hormone

parathyroid hormone – The hormone secreted by the parathyroid glands in response to a fall in plasma calcium; it acts on the kidney to increase the formation of the active metabolite of vitamin D (calcitriol)

parenteral nutrition – Slow infusion of solution of nutrients into the veins through a catheter. This may be partial, to supplement food and nutrient intake, or total (TPN, total parenteral nutrition), providing the sole source of energy and nutrients for patients with major intestinal problems

pareve (parve) – Jewish term for dishes containing neither milk nor meat. Orthodox Jewish law prohibits mixing of milk and meat foods or the consumption of milk products for 3 hours after a meat meal

parietal cells – *See* oxyntic cells

PARNUTS – EU term for foods prepared for particular nutritional purposes (intended for people with disturbed metabolism, or in special physiological conditions, or for young children). Also called dietetic foods

parosmia – Any disorder of the sense of smell

passive transport – Movement of solutes across cell membranes from an area of high concentration to an area of lower concentration

pathogens – Disease-causing bacteria, as distinct from those that are harmless

pectin – Plant tissues contain hemicelluloses (polymers of galacturonic acid) known as protopectins, which cement the cell walls together. As fruit ripens, there is maximum protopectin present; thereafter it breaks down to pectin, pectinic acid, and, finally, pectic acid, and the fruit softens as the adhesive between the cells breaks down

pellagra – The disease due to deficiency of the vitamin niacin and the amino acid tryptophan

pentosans – Polysaccharides of five-carbon sugars (pentoses)

pentoses – Monosaccharide sugars with five carbon atoms. The most important is ribose

pentosuria – The excretion of pentose sugars in the urine. Idiopathic pentosuria is an inherited metabolic disorder almost wholly restricted to Ashkenazi (North European) Jews, which has no adverse effects. Consumption of fruits rich in pentoses (e.g. pears) can also lead to (temporary) pentosuria

pepsin – An enzyme in the gastric juice which hydrolyses proteins to give smaller polypeptides; an endopeptidase

peptidases – Enzymes that hydrolyse proteins, and are therefore important in protein digestion

peptide linkage – –CONH linkage formed by reaction of an amine group of one amino acid with the carboxylic acid group of a second amino acid

peptides – Compounds formed when amino acids are linked together through the –CO–NH– (peptide) linkage. Two amino acids so linked form a dipeptide, three a tripeptide, etc.

pescetarian – Vegetarian who will eat fish, but not meat

petechiae (petechial haemorrhages) – Small, pinpoint bleeding under the skin; one of the signs of scurvy

pH – Potential hydrogen, a measure of acidity or alkalinity. Defined as the negative logarithm of the hydrogen-ion concentration. The scale runs from 0, which is very strongly acid, to 14, which is very strongly alkaline. Pure water is pH 7, which is neutral; below 7 is acid, above is alkaline

phagocyte – A blood cell that ingests and destroys foreign particles, bacteria and cell debris

phagomania – Morbid obsession with food; also known as sitomania

phagophobia – Fear of food; also known as sitophobia

pharmafoods – Alternative name for functional foods

phase I metabolism reactions – The first phase of metabolism of foreign compounds (xenobiotics), involving metabolic activation. These reactions occur mainly in the liver but also in the small intestine and lungs and comprise the microsomal or mixed function oxidase system, NADPH-dependent enzymes and cytochrome P450 proteins. Generally regarded as detoxication reactions, but may in fact convert inactive precursors into metabolically active compounds, and be involved in activation of precursors to carcinogens

phase II metabolism reactions – The second phase of the metabolism of foreign compounds, in which the activated derivatives formed in phase I metabolism are conjugated with amino acids, glucuronic acid or glutathione, to yield water-soluble derivatives that are excreted in urine or bile

phenolic hydroxyl group – Hydroxyl group attached to an aromatic ring

phenols – 'Alcohol-like' compounds that have the hydroxyl group bound to a benzene ring

phenotype – The observable characteristics of a cell or organism as distinct from its genotype

phenylalanine – An essential amino acid; in addition to its role in protein synthesis, it is the metabolic precursor of tyrosine (and hence noradrenaline (norepineprhine), adrenaline (epinephrine), and the thyroid hormones)

phlebotomy (venesection) – Removal of blood. This serves as a simple method for reducing body iron levels in people with haemochromatosis

phosphates – Salts of phosphoric acid; the form in which the element phosphorus is normally present in foods and body tissues

phosphatidic acid – Glycerol esterified to two molecules of fatty acid, with the third hydroxyl group esterified to phosphate; chemically diacylglycerol phosphate; intermediate in the metabolism of phospholipids

phospholipids – Glycerol esterified to two molecules of fatty acid, one of which is commonly polyunsaturated. The third hydroxyl group is esterified to phosphate and one of a number of water-soluble compounds, including serine (phosphatidylserine), ethanolamine (phosphatidylethanolamine), choline (phosphatidylcholine, also known as lecithin) and inositol (phosphatidylinositol)

phosphoproteins – Proteins containing phosphate, other than as nucleic acids (nucleoproteins) or phospholipids (lipoproteins), e.g. casein from milk, ovovitellin from egg yolk

phrynoderma – Blocked pores or 'toad-skin' (follicular hyperkeratosis of the skin) often encountered in malnourished people. Originally thought to be due to vitamin A deficiency but possibly due to other deficiencies, and also occurs in adequately nourished people

phylloquinone – Vitamin K

physical activity level (PAL) – Total energy cost of physical activity throughout the day, expressed as a ratio of basal metabolic rate. Calculated from the physical activity ratio for each activity, multiplied by the time spent in that activity

physical activity ratio (PAR) – Energy cost of physical activity expressed as a ratio of basal metabolic rate

phytase – An enzyme (a phosphatase) that hydrolyses phytate to inositol and phosphate

phytate (phytic acid) – Inositol hexaphosphate, present in cereals, particularly in the bran, in dried legumes and some nuts as both water-soluble salts (sodium and potassium) and insoluble salts of calcium and magnesium. Contributes significantly to the daily intake of phosphorus but is also a major inhibitor of the absorption of iron and zinc

phytate inositol polyphosphate – A plant acid which binds divalent metal ions such as ferrous iron, zinc, etc., and makes these ions less bioavailable for intestinal absorption from the food

phytoalexins – Substances, often harmful to humans which increase in plant tissues when they are stressed, as by physical damage, exposure to ultraviolet light, etc.

phytoestrogens (phyto-oestrogens) – Compounds in plant foods, especially soya bean, that have both oestrogenic and anti-oestrogenic action

phytohaemagglutinin – A lectin and mitogen. Capable of promoting a rapid proliferation of immune cells

phytosterol – General name given to sterols occurring in plants, the chief of which is sitosterol

phytotoxin – Any poisonous substance produced by a plant

phytylmenaquinone – Vitamin K

pica – An unnatural desire for foods; alternative words are cissa, cittosis and allotriophagy. Also a perverted appetite (eating of earth, sand, clay, paper, etc.)

pico – Prefix for units of measurement, one million-millionth part (i.e. 10^{-12}); symbol p

plaque – (1) Dental plaque is a layer of bacteria in an organic matrix on the surface of teeth, especially around the neck of each tooth. May lead to development of gingivitis, periodontal disease and caries. (2) Atherosclerotic plaque is the development of fatty streaks in the walls of blood vessels

polycystic ovarian syndrome (PCOS) – Commonly recognised cause of anovulatory infertility which is associated with multiple small ovarian cysts, high androgen levels and insulin resistance

polydipsia – Abnormally intense thirst; a typical symptom of diabetes

polymerase chain reaction (PCR) – A technique for amplifying defined regions of DNA; *see* DNA

polymorphonuclear leucocyte – The most numerous of the white blood cells (also known as neutrophil)

polyols – Sugar alcohols

polypeptides – *See* peptides

polyphagia – Excessive or continuous eating

polyphenols – Common name for several families of complex organic molecules. While many of these molecules are thought to have important functions they also act as major inhibitors of iron absorption; *see* phenols

polysaccharides – Complex carbohydrates formed by the condensation of large numbers of monosaccharide units, e.g. starch, glycogen, cellulose, dextrins, inulin. On hydrolysis the simple sugar is liberated

polyunsaturated fatty acids – Long-chain fatty acids containing two or more double bonds, separated by methylene bridges: $-CH_2-CH= CH-CH_2-CH=CH-CH_2-$

ponderal index – An index of fatness, used as a measure of obesity: the cube root of body weight divided by height. Confusingly, the ponderal index is higher for thin people, and lower for fat people

ponderocrescive – Foods tending to increase weight: easily gaining weight; the opposite of ponderoperditive

ponderoperditive – Stimulating weight loss

postprandial – Occurring after a meal

postprandial lipaemia – The gradual increase in the concentration of blood triacylglycerol following consumption of a meal containing fat

post-translational modification – Alterations to the nascent protein produced by translation

prebiotics – Non-digestible oligosaccharides that support the growth of colonies of potentially beneficial bacteria in the colon

precursors, enzyme – Inactive forms of enzymes, activated after secretion; also called pro-enzymes or zymogens

pre-eclampsia – A complication of pregnancy when high levels of blood pressure are combined with heavy proteinuria; untreated can lead to maternal and/or fetal death

prenylated – Molecule with isoprene (2-methylbutadiene) substituent

prion – The infective agent(s) responsible for Creutzfeldt–Jakob disease, kuru and possibly other degenerative diseases of the brain in humans scrapie in sheep, and bovine spongiform encephalopathy (BSE). They are simple proteins and, unlike viruses, do not contain any nucleic acid. Transmission occurs by ingestion of infected tissue

probiotics – Preparations of live microorganisms added to food (or used as animal feed), claimed to be beneficial to health by restoring microbial balance in the intestine. The organisms commonly involved are lactobacilli, bifidobacteria, streptococci, and some yeasts and moulds, alone or as mixtures

procarcinogen – A compound that is not itself carcinogenic, but undergoes metabolic activation in the body to yield a carcinogen

products of conception – The fetus, placenta, amniotic fluid and fetal membranes

pro-enzymes – Inactive precursors of enzymes, activated after secretion; also called zymogens

progoitrins – Substances found in plant foods which are precursors of goitrogens

proline – A non-essential amino acid

promoter – DNA sequence within a gene that controls the start of transcription for that gene

prosthetic group – Non-protein part of an enzyme molecule; either a coenzyme or a metal ion. Essential for catalytic activity. The enzyme protein without its prosthetic group is the apoenzyme and is catalytically inactive. With the prosthetic group, it is known as the holo-enzyme

proteases – Enzymes that hydrolyse proteins

protein – All living tissues contain proteins; they are polymers of amino acids, joined by peptide bonds. There are 21 main amino acids in proteins, and any one protein may contain several hundred or over a thousand amino acids, so an enormous variety of different proteins occur in nature. Generally a polymer of relatively few amino acids is referred to as a peptide (e.g. di-, tri- and tetrapeptides); oligopeptides contain up to about 50 amino acids; larger molecules are polypeptides or proteins

protein-bound iodine – The thyroid hormones, triiodothyronine and thyroxine, are transported in the bloodstream bound to proteins; measurement of protein-bound iodine, as opposed to total plasma iodine, was used as an index of thyroid gland activity before more specific methods of measuring the hormones were developed

protein, crude – Total nitrogen multiplied by the nitrogen conversion factor = 6.25

protein efficiency ratio (PER) – Weight gain per weight of protein eaten

protein–energy malnutrition (PEM) – A spectrum of disorders, especially in children, due to inadequate feeding. Used to describe children who are wasted or underweight due to insufficient intake of macronutrients. In fact PEM is commonly associated with multiple micronutrient deficiencies. Marasmus is severe wasting and can also occur in adults; it is the result of a food intake inadequate to meet energy expenditure. Kwashiorkor affects only young children and includes severe oedema, fatty infiltration of the liver, and a sooty dermatitis; it is likely that deficiency of antioxidant nutrients and the stress of infection may be involved. Emaciation, similar to that seen in marasmus, occurs in patients with advanced cancer and AIDS; in this case it is known as cachexia; *see* chronic energy deficiency

protein–energy ratio – The protein content of a food or diet expressed as the proportion of the total energy provided by protein (17 kJ, 4 kcal/g). The average requirement for protein is about 7% of total energy intake; average Western diets provide about 14%

protein hydrolysate – Mixture of amino acids and polypeptides prepared by hydrolysis of proteins with acid, alkali or proteases, used in enteral and parenteral nutrition and in supplements

protein induced by vitamin K absence or antagonism (PIVKA) – Under-carboxylated prothrombin, liberated when vitamin K supplies are suboptimal, which is potentially less functionally efficient than the fully carboxylated form in supporting normal blood clotting rates; hence the defect in blood clotting that arises in severe vitamin K deficiency. Assay of PIVKA is a more sensitive index in mild vitamin K deficiency than clotting times are, and it has therefore been used as a vitamin K status index

protein quality – A measure of the usefulness of a dietary protein for growth and maintenance of tissues and, in animals, production of meat, eggs, wool and milk. It is only important if the total intake of protein barely meets the requirement. The quality of individual proteins is unimportant in mixed diets, because of complementation between different proteins

protein retention efficiency (PRE) – The net protein retention converted to a % scale by multiplying by 16, then becoming numerically the same as NPU

protein score – A measure of protein quality based on chemical analysis

proteinases – Enzymes that hydrolyse proteins

proteolysis – The hydrolysis of proteins to their constituent amino acids, catalysed by alkali, acid or enzymes

proteome – The protein complement of a cell, tissue or organism translated from its genomic DNA sequence

proteomics – The study of the proteome

prothrombin – Protein in plasma involved in coagulation of blood. The prothrombin time is an index of the coagulability of blood (and hence of vitamin K nutritional status) based on the time taken for a citrated sample of blood to clot when calcium ions and thromboplastin are added

protoporphyrin – Haem molecule minus iron (i.e. the organic ring-structure without the central metal ion), the accumulation of which, in red cells, indicates either iron deficiency or other situations of impaired iron incorporation into haem, e.g. that caused by lead poisoning. Its quantification in red blood cells can be used as a functional index of iron status

provitamin – A substance that is converted into a vitamin, such as 7-dehydrocholesterol, which is converted into vitamin D, or those carotenes that can be converted to vitamin A

proximate analysis – Analysis of foods and feedingstuffs for nitrogen (for protein), ether extract (for fat), crude fibre and ash (mineral salts), together with soluble carbohydrate calculated by subtracting these values from the total (carbohydrate by difference). Also known as Weende analysis, after the Weende Experimental Station in Germany, which in 1865 outlined the methods of analysis to be used

P/S ratio – The ratio between polyunsaturated and saturated fatty acids. In Western diets the ratio is about 0.6; it is suggested that increasing it to near 1.0 would reduce the risk of atherosclerosis and coronary heart disease

psychrophilic organisms – Bacteria and fungi that tolerate low temperatures. Their preferred temperature range is 15–20°C, but they will grow at or below 0°C; the temperature must be reduced to about −10°C before growth stops, but the organisms are not killed and will regrow when the temperature rises

ptyalin – Obsolete name for salivary amylase

ptyalism – Excessive flow of saliva

pulses – Name given to the dried seeds (matured on the plant) of legumes such as peas, beans and lentils

purines – Nitrogenous compounds (bases) that occur in nucleic acids (adenine and guanine) and their precursors and metabolites; inosine, caffeine and theobromine are also purines

putrescine – Low molecular weight amine with biological activity

pyridoxal phosphate – 5-Phosphate of the aldehyde form of pyridoxine (vitamin B_6): this is the major form of the vitamin in blood and tissues, and is commonly measured as an index of vitamin B_6 status

pyrimidines – Nitrogenous compounds (bases) that occur in nucleic acids: cytosine, thymidine and uracil

pyruvate – Salts of pyruvic acid

pyruvic acid – An intermediate in the metabolism of carbohydrates, formed by the anaerobic metabolism of glucose

QUAC stick – Quaker arm circumference measuring stick. A stick used to measure height which also shows the 80th and 85th centiles of expected mid-upper arm circumference. Developed by a Quaker Service Team in Nigeria in the 1960s as a rapid and simple tool for assessment of nutritional status

quantitative ingredients declaration (QUID) – Obligatory on food labels in the EU since February 2000; previously legislation only required declaration of ingredients in descending order of quantity, not specific declaration of the amount of each ingredient present

Quetelet's index – *See* body mass index

reciprocal ponderal index – An index of adiposity; height divided by cube root of weight

reducing sugars – Sugars that are chemically reducing agents, including glucose, fructose, lactose, pentoses, but not sucrose

reduction – The opposite of oxidation; chemical reactions resulting in a gain of electrons, or hydrogen, or the loss of oxygen

reference intakes (of nutrients) – Amounts of nutrients greater than the requirements of almost all members of the population, determined on the basis of the average requirement plus twice the standard deviation, to allow for individual variation in requirements and thus cover the theoretical needs of 97.5% of the population

reference man, woman – An arbitrary physiological standard; defined as a person aged 25, weighing 65 kg, living in a temperate zone of a mean annual temperature of 10°C. Reference man performs medium work, with an average daily energy requirement of 13.5 MJ (3200 kcal). Reference woman is engaged in general household duties or light industry, with an average daily requirement of 9.7 MJ (2300 kcal)

reference nutrient intake (RNI) – Defined by COMA (Committee on Medical Aspects of Food Policy for the UK Department of Health), most recently in 1991, as being the amount of each nutrient that is sufficient to meet the needs of the majority (mean +2 standard deviations) of healthy people in a defined population, or subgroup of it. Approximately equivalent (in concept, but not necessarily in magnitude) to the US or WHO RDAs (recommended dietary amounts)

reference standards (international reference standard)/growth standards – These refer to databases recording the linear and ponderal growth of healthy children. They include anthropometric data collected on suitably large samples, and analysed with precise specifications to provide a useful basis for reference

relative protein value (RPV) – A measure of protein quality

renal plasma flow – Rate of passage of plasma through the kidneys, directly related to glomerular filtration rate

renal threshold – Concentration of a compound in the blood above which it is not reabsorbed by the kidney, and so is excreted in the urine

respiratory quotient (RQ) – Ratio of the volume of carbon dioxide produced when a substance is oxidised, to the volume of oxygen used. The oxidation of carbohydrate results in an RQ of 1.0; of fat, 0.7; and of protein, 0.8

respirometer – *See* spirometer

restoration – The addition of nutrients to replace those lost in processing, as in milling of cereals. *See also* fortification

reticulocyte – Immature precursor of the red blood cell in which the remains of the nucleus are visible as a reticulum. Very few are seen in normal blood as they are retained in the marrow until mature, but on remission of anaemia, when there is a high rate of production, reticulocytes appear in the bloodstream (reticulocytosis)

retinal (retinaldehyde), retinene, retinoic acid, retinol – Vitamers of vitamin A

retinal maculopathy – Deterioration of the macula (central region of the retina) that occurs progressively in older people, thus irreversibly impairing vision. Thought to be exacerbated by pro-oxidant action such as by oxygen free radicals

retinoids – Compounds chemically related to, or derived from, vitamin A, which display some of the biological activities of the vitamin, but have lower toxicity; they are used for treatment of severe skin disorders and some cancers

retinol-binding protein – A plasma protein which specifically binds retinol (the alcohol form of vitamin A) and prevents it from being excreted. In vitamin A sufficiency, all the RBP is bound to retinol, in a 1:1 complex, but in vitamin A deficiency the protein may become partially desaturated, so that the ratio of protein to retinol then exceeds 1:1 and this can be measured as an index of vitamin A status

retinopathy – Diabetic complication that involves the retina and may lead to blindness

reverse transcriptase – Viral enzyme that catalyses the conversion of mRNA into cDNA; *see* mRNA, cDNA

rexinoids – Compounds chemically related to vitamin A that bind to the retinoid X receptor but not the retinoic acid receptor

rhamnose – A methylated pentose (five-carbon) sugar

rhodopsin – The pigment in the rod cells of the retina of the eye, also known as visual purple, consisting of the protein opsin and retinaldehyde, which is responsible for the visual process. In cone cells of the retina the equivalent protein is iodopsin

riboflavin – Vitamin B_2

ribonucleic acid (RNA) – A linear single-stranded polymer composed of four types of ribose nucleotide, adenine, cytosine, guanine, thymine (A, C, G and U), linked by phosphodiester bonds and formed by the transcription of DNA. The three types of cellular RNA – rRNA, tRNA and mRNA – play different roles in protein synthesis

ribose – A pentose (five-carbon) sugar which occurs as an intermediate in the metabolism of glucose; especially important in the nucleic acids and various coenzymes

rickets – Malformation of the bones in growing children due to deficiency of vitamin D, leading to poor absorption of calcium. In adults the equivalent is osteomalacia. Vitamin-D-resistant rickets does not respond to normal amounts of the vitamin but requires massive doses. Usually a result of a congenital defect in the vitamin D

receptor, or metabolism of the vitamin; it can also be due to poisoning with strontium

risk factor – A factor that can be measured to indicate the statistical or epidemiological probability of an adverse condition, effect or disease. Does not imply that it is a causative factor, nor that reversing the risk factor will reduce the hazard

salatrims – Poorly absorbed fats, used as fat replacers; triacylglycerols containing short- and long-chain fatty acids

saliva – Secretion of the salivary glands in the mouth: 1–1.5 litres secreted daily. A dilute solution of the protein mucin (which lubricates food) and the enzyme amylase (which hydrolyses starch), with small quantities of urea, potassium thiocyanate, sodium chloride and bicarbonate

salivary glands – Three pairs of glands in the mouth, which secrete saliva: parotid, submandibular and submaxillary glands

salt – Usually refers to sodium chloride, common salt or table salt (chemically any product of reaction between an acid and an alkali is a salt). The main sources are either from mines in areas where there are rich deposits of crystalline salt, or deposits left by the evaporation of sea water in shallow pans (known as sea salt)

satiety – The sensation of fullness after a meal

Schilling test – A test of vitamin B_{12} absorption and status

Scientific Advisory Committee on Nutrition (SACN) – providing expert advice to the UK Food Standards Agency and Department of Health

scurvy – Deficiency of vitamin C leading to impaired collagen synthesis, causing capillary fragility, poor wound healing and bone changes

sedoheptulose (sedoheptose) – A seven-carbon sugar which is an intermediate in glucose metabolism by the pentose phosphate pathway

serine – A non-essential amino acid

serum – Clear liquid left after the protein has been clotted; the serum from milk, occasionally referred to as lacto-serum, is whey. Blood serum is blood plasma without the fibrinogen. When blood clots, the fibrinogen is converted to fibrin, which is deposited in strands that trap the red cells and form the clot. The clear liquid that is exuded is the serum

Shigella – Bacteria that grow readily in foods, especially milk, and cause bacterial dysentery

sialagogue – Substance that stimulates the flow of saliva

sialorrhoea – Excessive flow of saliva

siderosis – Accumulation of the iron-storage protein haemosiderin in liver, spleen and bone marrow in cases of excessive red cell destruction and on diets exceptionally rich in iron

single-cell protein – Collective term used for biomass of bacteria, algae and yeast, and also (incorrectly) moulds, of potential use as animal or human food

single nucleotide polymorphism (SNP) – Changes of individual bases in DNA sequences of the same species which account for population variance

sitapophasis – Refusal to eat as expression of mental disorder

sitology – Science of food

sitomania – Mania for eating, morbid obsession with food; also known as phagomania

sitophobia – Fear of food; also known as phagophobia

sitosterol – The main sterol found in vegetable oils

skinfold thickness – Index of subcutaneous fat and hence body fat content. Usually measured at four sites: biceps (midpoint of front upper arm), triceps (midpoint of back upper arm), subscapular (directly below point of shoulder blade at angle of 45°), supra-iliac (directly above iliac crest in mid-axillary line); *see* anthropometry

socially acceptable monitoring instrument (SAMI) – A small heart-rate counting apparatus used to estimate energy expenditure

sol – A colloidal solution, i.e. a suspension of particles intermediate in size between ordinary molecules (as in a solution) and coarse particles (as in a suspension). A jelly-like sol is a gel

solanine – Heat-stable toxic compound (a glycoside of the alkaloid solanidine), found in small amounts in potatoes, and larger and sometimes toxic amounts in sprouted potatoes and when they become green through exposure to light. Causes gastrointestinal disturbances and neurological disorders

somatotrophin – Growth hormone

sorbestrin – Sorbitol ester of fatty acids, developed as a fat replacer

sorbitol (glycitol, glucitol) – A six-carbon sugar alcohol found in some fruits and manufactured from glucose. Although it is metabolised in the body, it is only slowly absorbed from the intestine and is tolerated by diabetics

Southern blotting – Technique for detecting genomic DNA sequences by hybridisation following transfer of DNA onto a solid support, such as a nylon membrane. Named after its inventor, Professor Edwin Southern; *see* DNA, hybridisation

Spanish toxic oil syndrome – Disease that occurred in Spain during 1981/2, with 450 deaths and many people chronically disabled, due to consumption of oil containing aniline-denatured industrial rapeseed oil, sold as olive oil. The precise cause is unknown

specific dynamic action (SDA) – Archaic term for diet-induced thermogenesis

sphygmomanometer – Instrument for measuring blood pressure

spirometer (respirometer) – Apparatus used to measure the amount of oxygen consumed (and in some instances carbon dioxide produced) from which to calculate the energy expended (indirect calorimetry)

sprue – Disease in which the villi of the small intestine are atrophied and food is incompletely absorbed, followed consequently by undernutrition and weight loss

squamous cell carcinoma – Cancer of the flattened (squamous) epithelium

stable isotopes – Atoms with differing numbers of neutrons (and hence differing atomic weights) which are not radioactive, i.e. are not unstable. Molecules that are 'labelled' with relatively rare stable isotopes can be used as metabolic markers for nutrients as they enter the bloodstream and the body stores, and undergo turnover in the body. Measurement is by mass spectrometry

stachyose – Tetrasaccharide sugar composed of two units of galactose and one each of fructose and glucose. Not hydrolysed in the human digestive tract but fermented by intestinal bacteria

stanols – Analogues of cholesterol that inhibit its absorption from the intestinal tract

staple food – The principal food, e.g. wheat, rice, maize, etc., which provides the main energy source for communities

starch – Polysaccharide, a polymer of glucose units; the form in which carbohydrate is stored in the plant; it does not occur in animal tissue

starch blockers – Compounds that inhibit amylase and so reduce the digestion of starch. Used as a slimming aid, with little evidence of efficacy

State Registered Dietitian (SRD) – legal qualification to practise as a dietitian in the UK

statins – A family of related drugs used to treat hypercholesterolaemia. They act by inhibiting hydroxymethylglutaryl CoA reductase (HMG CoA reductase), the first and rate-limiting enzyme of cholesterol synthesis

stearic acid – Saturated fatty acid (C18:0)

steatopygia – Accumulation of larger amounts of fat in the buttocks

steatorrhoea – Excretion of faeces containing a large amount of fat, and generally foul-smelling

steatosis – Fatty infiltration of the liver; occurs in protein–energy malnutrition and alcoholism

stercobilin – One of the brown pigments of the faeces; formed from the bile pigments, which, in turn, are formed as breakdown products of haemoglobin

stercolith – Stone formed of dried compressed faeces

stereo-isomerism – Occurs when compounds have the same molecular and structural formula, but with the atoms arranged differently in space. There are two subdivisions: optical and geometrical isomerism

steroids – Chemically, compounds that contain the cyclopenteno-phenanthrene ring system. All the biologically important steroids are derived metabolically from cholesterol; they include the sex hormones (androgens, oestrogens and progesterone) and the hormones of the adrenal cortex

sterols – Alcohols derived from the steroids; including cholesterol, ergosterol in yeast, sitosterol and stigmasterol in plants, and coprosterol in faeces

stiparogenic – Foods that tend to cause constipation

stiparolytic – Foods that tend to prevent or relieve constipation

strain – Horticultural term for seed-raised plants exhibiting certain desirable characteristics but which are not stable or predictable enough when propagated to be a cultivar

stroke – Also known as cerebrovascular accident (CVA); damage to brain tissue by hypoxia due to blockage of a blood vessel as a result of thrombosis, atherosclerosis or haemorrhage

structural congenital malformations – Abnormalities of the fetus or infant where developmental abnormalities have resulted in malformations of organs of the body

stunting – Reduction in the linear growth of children, leading to lower than expected height for age, generally resulting in lifelong short stature.

A common effect of protein–energy malnutrition, and associated especially with inadequate protein intake

subcostal angle – Angle in degrees subtended by the costal margins in the midline of the body

subsistence farming – Agricultural production exclusively to meet the needs of the farm household, in contrast to commercial farming

substantial equivalence – Term used to denote oil, starch, etc., from genetically modified crops, that does not contain protein or DNA, and cannot be distinguished from the same product from the unmodified crop

substrate – The substance on which an enzyme acts. The medium on which microorganisms grow

sucrase – The enzyme that hydrolyses sucrose to yield glucose and fructose (invert sugar). Also known as invertase or saccharase

sucrose – Cane or beet sugar. A disaccharide composed of glucose and fructose

sugar alcohols – Also called polyols, chemical derivatives of sugars that differ from the parent compounds in having an alcohol group (CH_2OH) instead of the aldehyde group (CHO); thus mannitol from mannose, xylitol from xylose, lacticol from lactulose (also sorbitol, isomalt and hydrogenated glucose syrup). Several occur naturally in fruits, vegetables and cereals. They range in sweetness from equal to sucrose to less than half. They provide bulk in foods such as confectionery (in contrast to intense sweeteners), and so are called bulk sweeteners. They are slowly and incompletely metabolised, and are tolerated by diabetics, and provide less energy than sugars: they are less cariogenic than sucrose

superoxide dismutases – Enzymes which remove potentially harmful (pro-oxidant) superoxide from the body; they require zinc and copper, or manganese, for their enzymatic activity, and their assay can, for instance, be used to measure copper status

surfactants – Surface active agents; compounds that have an affinity for fats (hydrophobic) and water (hydrophilic) and so act as emulsifiers, e.g. soaps and detergents. Used as wetting agents to assist the reconstitution of powders, including dried foods, to clean and peel fruits and vegetables, also in baked goods and comminuted meat products

sweeteners – Four groups of compounds are used to sweeten foods: (1) the sugars, of which the commonest is sucrose (2) bulk sweeteners, including sugar alcohols (3) synthetic non-nutritive sweeteners (intense sweeteners), which are many times sweeter than sucrose (4) various other chemicals such as glycerol and glycine (70% as sweet as sucrose), and certain peptides

synbiotics – Combination nutritional supplements composed of probiotics and prebiotics; *see* prebiotics, probiotics

T_3 – Tri-iodothyronine, one of the thyroid hormones

T_4 – Thyroxine (tetra-iodothyronine), one of the thyroid hormones

tachycardia – Rapid heartbeat, as occurs after exercise; may also occur, without undue exertion, as a result of anxiety, and in anaemia and vitamin B_1 deficiency

tachyphagia – Rapid eating

tagatose – Isomer of fructose (D-lyxo-2-hexulose) obtained by hydrolysis of plant gums and used as a bulk sweetener; 14-times as sweet as sucrose. Not metabolised to any significant extent, so does not raise blood sugar and has zero energy yield

Tanner standard – Tables of height and weight for age used as reference values for the assessment of growth and nutritional status in children, based on data collected in England in the 1960s. Now largely replaced by the NCHS (US National Center for Health Statistics) standards. *See also* anthropometry

tannins – Polyphenol plant constituents which bind divalent metal ions such as ferrous iron, zinc, etc. and make these ions less bioavailable for intestinal absorption from the food. They have an astringent effect in the mouth, precipitate proteins, and are used to clarify beer and wines. Also called tannic acid and gallotannin

Taq DNA polymerase – A thermophilic bacterial enzyme that catalyses the synthesis of double-stranded DNA, utilised in PCR; *see* DNA, PCR

taste – The tongue can distinguish five separate tastes: sweet, salt, sour (or acid), bitter, and savoury (sometimes called umami, from the Japanese word for a savoury flavour), due to stimulation of the taste buds. The overall taste or flavour of foods is due to these tastes, together with astringency in the mouth, texture and aroma

taurine – A derivative of the amino acid cysteine (aminoethane sulphonic acid). Known to be a dietary essential for cats (deficient kittens are blind) and possibly essential for human beings, since the capacity for synthesis is limited, although deficiency has never been observed. In addition to its role in the eye and nervous system it is important for conjugation of the bile salts

T-cells – Thymus-derived lymphocytes or thymocytes. Comprise Th1 and Th2 lymphocytes and natural killer (NK) cells. Th1 lymphocytes are important in cell-mediated immunity and IL-2 and IFN-γ production. Th2 lymphocytes are associated with the promotion of antibody-mediated immunity and production of cytokines IL-4, IL-6, IL-10 and IL-13

teratogen – Substance that deforms the fetus in the womb and so induces birth defects

teratogenesis – Process by which a harmful stimulus, e.g. drugs, can cause structural congenital malformations, almost always active during the period of embryogenesis

tetany – Over-sensitivity of motor nerves to stimuli; particularly affects face, hands and feet. Caused by reduction in the level of ionised calcium in the bloodstream and can accompany severe rickets

tetraenoic acid – Fatty acid with four double bonds, e.g. arachidonic acid

thermic effect of food (TEF) – Alternative term for diet-induced thermogenesis

thermoduric – Bacteria that are heat-resistant but not thermophiles; they survive pasteurisation. Usually not pathogens but indicative of insanitary conditions

thermogenesis – Increased heat-production by the body, either to maintain body temperature (by shivering or non-shivering thermogenesis) or in response to intake of food and stimulants such as coffee, nicotine and certain drugs. *See* diet-induced thermogenesis, brown adipose tissue

thermophiles (thermophilic bacteria) – Bacteria that prefer temperatures above 55°C and can tolerate temperatures up to 75–80°C

thiamin – Vitamin B_1

threonine – An essential amino acid

thrombin – Plasma protein involved in the coagulation of blood

thrombokinase (or thromboplastin) – An enzyme liberated from damaged tissue and blood platelets; it converts prothrombin to thrombin in the coagulation of blood

thrombosis – Formation of blood clots in blood vessels

thymidine, thymine – A pyrimidine; *see* nucleic acids

thyroglobulin – The protein in the thyroid gland which is the precursor for the synthesis of the thyroid hormones. The thyroid-stimulating hormone of the pituitary gland stimulates hydrolysis of thyroglobulin and secretion of the hormones into the bloodstream

thyrotoxicosis – Overactivity of the thyroid gland, leading to excessive secretion of thyroid hormones and resulting in increased basal metabolic rate. Hyperthyroid subjects are lean and have tense nervous activity. Iodine-induced thyrotoxicosis affects mostly older people who have lived for a long time in iodine-deficient areas, have had a long-standing goitre, and then have been given extra iodine. Also known as Jod–Basedow, or Basedow's disease

thyroxine – One of the thyroid hormones

T lymphocytes – Thymus-dependent lymphocytes which, amongst other functions, help B-lymphocytes during immunological responses and provide protection from intracellular microbial infection

tocol, tocopherol, tocotrienol – Vitamers of vitamin E

tocopherols – The chemical descriptor for the most important series of compounds that have vitamin E activity. There are a range of tocopherols, distinguished by different Greek letter prefixes, which differ in their food origins and in their biological activities in the body

tolerable upper intake level (UL) of a nutrient – Maximum intake (from supplements and enriched foods) that is unlikely to pose a risk of adverse effects on health

traife – Foods that do not conform to Jewish dietary laws; the opposite of kosher

trans- – Stereochemistry at a carbon–carbon double bond with the two substituents on opposite sides of the bond; *See cis-*

transaminase – Any enzyme that catalyses the reaction of transamination

transamination – The transfer of the amino group ($-NH_2$) from an amino acid to an acceptor keto- (or oxo-) acid

transcellular – Movement of solutes through cells. This may involve passive and/or active transport

transcription factors – Proteins which influence the activity of genes through modulation of their promoters

transcriptome – The total mRNA complement of cells, tissues or organisms transcribed from the genome; *see* mRNA, genome

transcriptomics – The study of the transcriptome

transferrin receptor – A tissue protein, also found in blood serum, which has a specific recognition-affinity for the iron-transporting protein transferrin. It increases in concentration in conditions of chronic iron deficiency, and is therefore used as an iron status indicator. Unlike most other iron status indices, it is not confounded by the presence of an acute phase reaction (q.v.)

transketolase – Enzyme which inter-converts certain sugar phosphates, and which requires thiamin diphosphate (TPP) as its essential cofactor. Assay of this enzyme in red cell extracts is commonly used as a biochemical index of thiamin status, i.e. by measuring the ratio of the enzyme activity both with and without added TPP

trehalose – Mushroom sugar, also called mycose, a disaccharide of glucose

triacylglycerols – Sometimes called triglycerides; lipids consisting of glycerol esterified to three fatty acids (chemically acyl groups). The major component of dietary and tissue fat. Also known as saponifiable fats, since on reaction with sodium hydroxide they yield glycerol and the sodium salts (or soaps) of the fatty acids

triglycerides – *See* triacylglycerols

tri-iodothyronine – One of the thyroid hormones

trimester – The 40 weeks of pregnancy are divided conventionally into three trimesters: 0–13 weeks, 14–26 weeks and 27 weeks until delivery

Trolox – Trade name for a water-soluble vitamin E analogue

trypsin – A proteolytic enzyme of the pancreatic juice, an endopeptidase

trypsinogen – The inactive precursor of trypsin, secreted in the pancreatic juice

tryptophan – An essential amino acid; the precursor of the neurotransmitter 5-hydroxytryptamine (serotonin) and of niacin

tumour necrosis factor (TNF-α) – *See* cytokines

tyramine – The amine formed by decarboxylation of the amino acid tyrosine

tyrosine – A non-essential amino acid, formed in the body from phenylalanine; the precursor for the synthesis of melanin (the black and brown pigment of skin and hair), and adrenaline (epinephrine) and noradrenaline (norepinephrine)

ubiquinone – Coenzyme in the respiratory (electron transport) chain in mitochondria, also known as coenzyme Q or mitoquinone

umami – Name given to the special taste of monosodium glutamate, protein, certain amino acids and the ribonucleotides (inosinate and guanylate). The Japanese name for a savoury flavour, now considered one of the five basic senses of taste

under-5 – A shorthand term for children under 5 years of age; a period of rapid growth and relatively high nutritional requirements. Mortality in children at this age is a commonly used public health indicator. Clinics targeted at this age group are called under-5 clinics. They traditionally combine nutrition and growth monitoring, immunisation and simple curative treatment

United Nations Children's Fund (UNICEF) – originally the United Nations International Children's Emergency Fund; website http://www.unicef.org

United Nations University (UNU) – web page http://www.unu.edu

unsaturation – Introduction of double bonds

untranslated region (UTR) – Areas of the mRNA transcript that do not encode for protein synthesis but may contain features that control the regulation of gene expression. These are found both proximal (5') and distal (3') to the coding sequence; *see* mRNA

urea – The end-product of nitrogen metabolism, excreted in the urine

uric acid – The end-product of purine metabolism

urticaria – An itchy rash which results from inflammation and leakage of fluid from the blood into the superficial layers of the skin in response to various mediators. Synonyms are 'hives' or 'nettle rash'

US Department of Agriculture (USDA) – Created as an independent department in 1862; website http://www.usda.gov

US Recommended Daily Allowances (USRDA) – Reference intakes used for nutritional labelling of foods in the USA

van der Waals forces – Interaction through space of two non-polar groups

vegans – Those who consume no foods of animal origin. (Vegetarians often consume milk and/or eggs.)

verbascose – A non-digestible tetrasaccharide, galactose-galactose-glucose-fructose, found in legumes; fermented by intestinal bacteria and causes flatulence

villi, intestinal – Small, finger-like processes covering the surface of the small intestine in large numbers (20–40/mm²), projecting some 0.5–1 mm into the lumen. They provide a large surface area (about 300 m²) for absorption in the small intestine

vitafoods – Foods designed to meet the needs of health-conscious consumers which enhance physical or mental quality of life and may increase health status

vitamers – Chemical compounds structurally related to a vitamin, and converted to the same overall active metabolites in the body. They thus possess the same biological activity

vitamin – Thirteen organic substances that are essential in very small amounts in food

vitamin Q – Ubiquinone

vitaminoids – Name given to compounds with 'vitamin-like' activity; considered by some to be vitamins or partially to replace vitamins. Includes flavonoids, inositol, carnitine, choline, lipoic acid and the essential fatty acids. With the exception of the essential fatty acids, there is little evidence that any of them is a dietary essential

waist:hip ratio – Simple method for describing the distribution of subcutaneous and intra-abdominal adipose tissue

wasting/wasted – An old term meaning abnormally thin after weight loss. The term has been used more recently by nutritionists to define weight for height significantly less than the reference range

water activity, a_w – The ratio of the vapour pressure of water in a food to the saturated vapour pressure of water at the same temperature

Waterlow classification – A system for classifying protein–energy malnutrition in children based on wasting (the percentage of expected weight for height) and the degree of stunting (the percentage of expected height for age). *See also* Wellcome classification

weaning foods – Foods specially formulated for infants aged between 3 and 9 months for the transition between breast- or bottlefeeding and normal intake of solid foods

Weende analysis – Proximate analysis; *see* proximate analysis

Weight-control Information Network (WIN) – of the National Institute of Diabetes and Digestive and Kidney Diseases; website http://www.niddk.nih.gov/health/nutrit/nutrit.htm

Wellcome classification – A system for classifying protein–energy malnutrition in children based on percentage of expected weight for age and the presence or absence of oedema. Between 60 and 80% of expected weight is underweight in the absence of oedema, and kwashiorkor if oedema is present; under 60% of expected weight is marasmus in the absence of oedema, and marasmic kwashiorkor if oedema is present

Wernicke–Korsakoff syndrome – The result of damage to the brain as a result of vitamin B_1 deficiency, commonly associated with alcohol abuse. Affected subjects show clear signs of neurological damage (Wernicke's encephalopathy) with psychiatric changes (Korsakoff's psychosis) characterised by loss of recent memory and confabulation (the invention of fabulous stories). *See also* beriberi

wholefoods – Foods that have been minimally refined or processed, and are eaten in their natural state. In general nothing is removed from, or added to, the foodstuffs in preparation. Wholegrain cereal products are made by milling the complete grain

World Cancer Research Fund (WCRF) – Website http://www.wcrf.org

World Food Programme (WFP) – Part of the Food and Agriculture Organization of the United Nations; intended to give international aid in the form of food from countries with a surplus; website http://www.wfp.org

World Health Organization (WHO) – Headquarters in Geneva; website http://www.who.in

xanthelasma – Yellow fatty plaques on the eyelids, due to hypercholesterolaemia

xanthophylls – Yellow-orange hydroxylated carotene derivatives

xanthosis – Yellowing of the skin associated with high blood concentrations of carotene

xenobiotic – Substances foreign to the body, including drugs and some food additives

xerophthalmia – Advanced vitamin A deficiency in which the epithelium of the cornea and conjunctiva of the eye deteriorate because of impairment of the tear glands, resulting in dryness then ulceration, leading to blindness

xylitol - A five-carbon sugar; said to have an effect in suppressing the growth of some of the bacteria associated with dental caries

Xylitol – sugar-alcohol (polyol)

xylose – Pentose (five-carbon) sugar found in plant tissues as complex polysaccharide; 40% as sweet as sucrose. Also known as wood sugar

zymogens – The inactive form in which some enzymes, especially the protein digestive enzymes, are secreted, being activated after secretion. Also called pro-enzymes, or enzyme precursors

Abbreviations

ACE	angiotensin-converting enzyme	CVA	cerebrovascular accident
ACH index	arm chest hip index	DEFRA	Department of the Environment, Food and Rural Affairs (UK)
ACT	antichymotrypsin		
ACTH	adrenocorticotrophin	DEXA	dual-energy X-ray absorptiometry
ADI	acceptable daily intake	DFE	dietary folate equivalents
ADP	adenosine diphosphate	DHA	docosahexaenoic acid
AIDS	acquired immune deficiency syndrome	DHSS	Department of Health and Social Security (UK)
AMC	arm muscle circumference	DIT	diet-induced thermogenesis
AMP	adenosine monophosphate	DMFT	index of decayed, missing and filled permanent teeth
ATP	adenosine triphosphate		
BCAA	branched-chain amino acids (leucine, isoleucine, valine)	Dmft	index of decayed, missing and filled deciduous teeth
BFH	baby friendly hospital	DNA	deoxyribonucleic acid
BIE	bioelectrical impedance	DoH	Department of Health (UK)
BMI	body mass index	DRI	Dietary Reference Intakes (US)
BMR	basal metabolic rate	DRV	dietary reference value (UK)
BSE	bovine spongiform encephalopathy	EAA index	essential amino acid index
		EAR	Estimated Average Daily Requirements (UK)
BSF	biceps skinfold thickness		
BST	bovine somatotrophin	ECF	extracellular fluid
BV	biological value	EDTA	ethylene diamine tetra-acetic acid
cAMP	cyclic adenosine monophosphate	EFA	essential fatty acid
cDNA	complementary DNA	EFSA	European Food Safety Authority
cds	coding sequence	EGRAC	erythrocyte glutathione reductase activation coefficient
CHD	coronary heart disease		
CHI	creatinine-height index	EPA	eicosapentaenoic acid
CMPI	cow's milk protein intolerance	ELISA	enzyme-linked immunosorbent assay
CMV	cytomegalovirus		
COMA	Committee On Medical Aspects of Food Policy	EMS	eosinophilia myalgia syndrome
		ESPEN	European Society for Parenteral and Enteral Nutrition
CoQ	coenzyme Q		
CRP	C-reactive protein	EU	European Union
CSF	cerebrospinal fluid	FA	Fatty acid
CUG	catch-up growth	FABP	FA-binding protein

© 2010 Elsevier Ltd/Inc/BV
DOI: 10.1016/B978-0-7020-3118-2.00035-8

FAD	flavin adenine dinucleotide	K	potassium
FAO	Food and Agriculture Organization	kJ	kilojoule
		LBM	lean body mass
FDA	Food and Drug Administration (US)	LBW	low birthweight
		LCPUFA	long-chain polyunsaturated fatty acid
Fe	iron		
FFA	free fatty acid	LC-TG	long-chain triglycerides
FIGLU	formiminoglutamic acid	LD_{50}	lethal dose 50%
FMN	flavin mononucleotide	LDL	low-density lipoproteins
FNIC	Food & Nutrition Information Center (US)	LPS	lipopolysaccharide
		LRNI	lower reference nutrient intake
FOSHU	Foods for Specified Health Use	LTI	lower threshold intake
FSA	Food Standards Agency	MAC	mid-arm circumference
FTT	failure to thrive	MAFF	Ministry of Agriculture, Fisheries & Food (UK)
GIP	gastric inhibitory peptide		
GLUT-4	glucose transporter protein 4	MCT	medium-chain triglycerides
GRAS	generally regarded as safe	Mg	magnesium
GTF	glucose tolerance factor	MJ	megajoule
H^1	hydrogen ions	MNA	mini nutritional assessment
HACC	Hazard Analysis Critical Control	mRNA	messenger ribonucleic acid
Hb	haemoglobin	MSG	monosodium glutamate
HDL	high-density lipoproteins	MSI	minimum safe intake
HFA	height for age	MUAC	mid-upper arm circumference
HFCS	high-fructose corn syrup	NAD, NADP	nicotinamide adenine dinucleotide and its phosphate
hGH	human growth hormone		
HIV	human immunodeficiency virus	$NaHCO_3$	sodium bicarbonate
HMG	hydroxymethylglutaryl	NCHS	National Center for Health Statistics (US)
HPLC	high-performance or high-pressure liquid chromatography		
		NDNS	National Diet and Nutrition Survey
IBS	irritable bowel syndrome		
IDA	iron-deficiency anaemia	NDpE	net dietary protein – energy ratio
IDDM	insulin-dependent diabetes mellitus	NEFA	non-esterified fatty acids
		NEL	No Effect Level
IDL	intermediate-density lipoproteins	NH_3	ammonia
IFN-γ	interferon-gamma	NHANES	National Health and Nutrition Examination Survey
IHD	ischaemic heart disease		
IL	interleukin	NK	natural killer
IMP	inosine monophosphate	NLEA	Nutrition Labeling and Education ACT (US)
IMTG	intramuscular triacylglycerol		
INFOODS	International Network of Food Data Systems	NOAE	No adverse Effect Level
		NPR	net protein ratio
INQ	index of nutritional quality.	NPU	net protein utilisation
IOC	International Olympic Committee	NSP	non-starch polysaccharides
IOTF	International Obesity Task Force	ODS	Office of Dietary Supplements
IPM	integrated pest management	P	inorganic phosphate
ISC	Indian subcontinent	PABA	para aminobenzoic acid
iu	international units	PAL	physical activity level
IUFOST	International Union of Food Science & Technology	PAR	physical activity ratio
		PARNUTS	Particular Nutrition Purposes (EU)
IUGR	intrauterine growth retardation		
IUNS	International Union of Nutritional Sciences	PBM	peak bone mass
		PCOS	polycystic ovarian syndrome

PCR	polymerase chain reaction		SNP	single nucleotide polymorphism
PEM	protein – energy malnutrition		SOD	superoxide dismutase
PER	protein efficiency ratio		SR	(complex) sarcoplasmic reticulum
PEU	protein – energy undernutrition		SRD	State Registered Dietitian (UK)
PHV	peak height velocity		Taq	thermus aquaticus
PIVKA	protein induced by vitamin K absence or antagonism		TBW	total body water
			TCA-cycle	tricarboxylic acid cycle
PRI	population reference intake (of nutrients)		TEF	thermic effect of food
			TG	triacylglycerol
P/S ratio	polyunsaturated/saturated fatty acid ratio		TK_{ac}	transketolase activation coefficient
PSD	psychosocial deprivation		TLC	total lymphocyte count
PSRL	potential renal solute load		TNF	tumour necrosis factor
PT	preterm		TNF-α	tumour necrosis factor alpha
PUFA	polyunsaturated fatty acids		TOBEC	total body electrical conductivity
Q1–Q3	inter-quartile range		TPN	total parenteral nutrition
QUID	quantitative ingredients declaration		TPP	thiamine diphosphate
			TSF	triceps skinfold thickness
RAST	radioallergosorbent tests for food allergy		UFA	unesterified fatty acid
			UL	upper tolerable intake level
RDA	recommended daily allowance		UNICEF	United Nations Children's Fund
RDI	recommended daily intake		UNU	United Nations University
RE	retinol equivalents		USDA	United States Department of Agriculture
RNA	ribonucleic acid			
RNI	reference nutrient intake (UK)		USRDA	United States Recommended Daily Allowance
RPV	relative protein value, a measure of protein quality			
			UTR	untranslated region
RQ	respiratory quotient		VKDB	vitamin-K-deficiency bleeding
RTF	ready to feed (infant formula)		VLBW	very low birthweight
SACN	Scientific Advisory Committee on Nutrition		VLDL	very-low-density lipoproteins
			$\dot{V}O_{2\,max}$	maximal oxygen uptake
SAMI	Socially Acceptable Monitoring Instrument		WCRF	World Cancer Research Fund
			WFA	weight for age
SCALES	(Sadness; Cholesterol; Albumin; Loss of weight; Eat; Shopping)		WFH	weight for height
			WFP	World Food Programme
			WHO	world Health Organization
SD	standard deviation		WIN	Weight Control Information Network
SDA	Specific dynamic action			
SENECA	Survey in Europe on Nutrition and the Elderly		W_{max}	maximal workload capacity
SGA	small for gestational age		Zn	zinc

Appendix

Dietary reference values

TERMINOLOGY

UNITED KINGDOM (DEPARTMENT OF HEALTH 1991)

Dietary reference values (DRVs) revised in 1991 were previously known as recommended daily amounts (RDAs). The term applies to the range of intakes based on an assessment of the distribution of requirements for each nutrient. DRVs apply to groups of healthy people and are not appropriate for those with disease or metabolic abnormalities. The DRVs for one nutrient presuppose that requirements for energy and all other nutrients are met. For most nutrients, three values are given:

EAR Estimated average requirement, which assumes normal distribution of variability.

LRNI Lower reference nutrient intake, 2 SD below EAR.

RNI Reference nutrient intake, 2 SD above EAR. Where only one value is given in summary tables this is the value chosen.

Other values used include the following:

Safe intakes Some nutrients are known to be important but there are insufficient data on human requirements to set any DRVs. A safe intake is judged to be a level or range of intakes above which there is no risk of deficiency and below a level where there is a risk of undesirable effects.

Individual minimum, individual maximum, population averages These are used for specifying carbohydrates (fibre) and fat needs.

UNITED STATES OF AMERICA

The Recommended Dietary Allowances (RDAs) set in 1998 have been replaced by the Dietary Reference Intakes (DRIs). These comprise four reference values: Estimated Average Requirements (EARs), Recommended Dietary Allowances (RDAs), Adequate Intakes (AIs) and Tolerable Upper Intake Levels (UL). These reference values have been revised and produced by the Food and Nutrition Board, the Institute of Medicine (IOM). The revised values have been put together over the period 1997–2005.

EUROPE EC

European values were revised in 1993. Carbohydrate, fat and non-starch polysaccharide population goals were not included, so those used here are from James (1988).

LTI   Lowest threshold intake
ARI   Average requirement intake
PRI   Population reference intake: mean requirement +2 SD. This is the value chosen for most of the tables in this Appendix
Acceptable range   Range of safe values given where insufficient information is available to be more specific.

FOOD AND AGRICULTURE ORGANIZATION (FAO) AND WORLD HEALTH ORGANIZATION (WHO)

The Joint Food and Agriculture Organization of the United Nations/World Health Organization of the 100 United Nations (FAO/WHO) expert consultation on human vitamin and mineral requirements met in 1998. The RNIs for these nutrients represent the most recent revisions and these are included

© 2010 Elsevier Ltd/Inc/BV
DOI: 10.1016/B978-0-7020-3118-2.00036-X

here. Other nutrient groups have been considered prior to this, as follows: trace elements (1996), carbohydrate, fat, non-starch polysaccharides (1990), energy and protein (1985).

Population requirement safe ranges (1996):

Basal   Lower limit of safe ranges of population mean intakes

Normative   Population mean intake sufficient to meet normative requirements.

This value is used in most of the tables in the Appendix

Maximum   Upper limit of safe ranges of population mean intakes

Recommended intakes (1974) Average requirement augmented by a factor that takes into account inter-individual variability. The amounts are considered sufficient for the maintenance of health in nearly all people.

UNITS

These vary for different nutrients.

ENERGY (KCAL/DAY, KJ/DAY OR MJ/DAY)

All energy values are based on the Schofield equations (FAO/WHO/UNU 1985) and so should be similar for each source. Any variation occurs because the equations are based on weight and activity within broad age bands.

CARBOHYDRATE AND FAT

These are expressed as a percentage of total energy intake including 5% alcohol or as a percentage of food energy, excluding alcohol.

PROTEIN (G/DAY OR G/KG/DAY)

Protein requirements are all based on the FAO/WHO/UNU 1985 Report and, like energy values,

they should be similar from various sources, the only difference being the average weight chosen for each age group.

MOST NUTRIENTS (G/DAY OR MG/DAY OR µG/DAY)

Some exceptions are:

niacin: mg/1000 kcal or mg/MJ

vitamin B_6: mg/g protein

vitamin E: mg/g polyunsaturated fatty acids.

IRON, ZINC

Requirements depend on the bioavailability of the diet which may be low, moderate or high (see Ch. 12). In this Appendix levels were chosen for medium availability from WHO values. The UK and USA values assume Western diets of high availability.

AGE BANDS

The different national and international sources of data have used slightly different age bands in some instances. Where necessary these have been

adjusted to correspond as closely as possible with the most frequently used age bands.

References

Department of Health: *Report on health and social subjects 41. Dietary reference values for food energy and nutrients for the United Kingdom. Committee on Medical Aspects of Food Policy*, London, 1991, HMSO.

EC Scientific Committee for Food Report: *(31st series) Nutrient and energy intakes for the European*

Community, Luxembourg, 1993, Directorate-General, Industry.

FAO/WHO/UNU: *Energy and protein requirements. Report of a joint FAO/WHO/UNU expert consultation. Technical Report Series 724*, Geneva, 1985, World Health Organization (WHO).

Food and Nutrition Board, Institute of Medicine: *Dietary reference intakes for calcium, phosphorus, magnesium, vitamin D and fluoride*, Washington, DC, 1997, National Academy Press.

Food and Nutrition Board, Institute of Medicine: *Dietary reference intakes for thiamin, riboflavin, niacin, vitamin B6, folate, vitamin B12, pantothenic acid, biotin and choline*, Washington, DC, 1998, National Academy Press.

Food and Nutrition Board, Institute of Medicine: *Dietary reference intakes for vitamin C, vitamin E, selenium and carotenoids*, Washington, DC, 2000, National Academy Press.

Food and Nutrition Board, Institute of Medicine: *Dietary reference intakes for vitamin A, vitamin K, arsenic, boron, chromium, copper, iodine, iron manganese, molybdenum, nickel, silicon, vanadium and zinc*, Washington, DC, 2001, National Academy Press.

Food and Nutrition Board, Institute of Medicine: *Dietary reference intakes for energy, carbohydrate, fiber, fat, fatty acids, cholesterol, protein and amino acids micronutrients*, Washington, DC, 2005, National Academy Press.

Food and Nutrition Board, Institute of Medicine: *Dietary reference intakes for energy, carbohydrate, fiber, fat, fatty acids, cholesterol, protein and amino acids (macronutrients)*, Washington, DC, 2005, National Academy Press.

James WPT: *Healthy nutrition. Preventing nutrition-related diseases in Europe.* WHO Regional Publications, European Series No. 24, Copenhagen, 1988, WHO.

WHO: *Diet, nutrition, and the prevention of chronic diseases.* Technical Report Series 797, Geneva, 1990, WHO.

WHO: *Trace elements in human nutrition and health*, Geneva, 1996, WHO, in collaboration with FAO, AEA.

TABLES OF DIETARY REFERENCE VALUES

Table A1a   Dietary reference values for energy for males

AGE	UK AND WHO EAR[1]		USA* AEA[2]		EUROPE	
	(MJ/day)	(kcal/day)	(MJ/day)	(kcal/day)	LOWER[3,4] (MJ/day)	HIGHER[5] (MJ/day)
0–3 months	2.28	545	2.7	650	2.2	
4–6 months	2.89	690	2.7	650	3.0	
7–9 months	3.44	825	3.5	850	3.5	
10–12 months	3.85	920	3.5	850	3.9	
1–3 years	5.15	1230	5.4	1300	5.1	
4–6 years	7.16	1715	7.5	1800	7.1	
7–10 years	8.24	1970	8.3	2000	8.3	
11–14 years	9.27	2220	10.4	2500	9.8	
15–18 years	11.51	2755	12.5	3000	11.8	
19–50 years	10.60	2550	12.1	2900	11.3	12.0
51–59 years	10.60	2550	19.6	2300	11.3	12.0
60–64 years	9.93	2380	9.6	2300	8.5	9.2
65–74 years	9.71	2330	9.6	2300	8.5	9.2
75+	8.77	2100	9.6	2300	7.5	8.5

[1]EAR, estimated average requirement.
[2]AEA, average energy allowance.
[3]No physical activity + desirable body weight for adults.
[4]Children's values are estimated average requirement.
[5]Desirable physical activity + desirable body weight for adults.
*A more recent consideration of energy requirements has led to these being expressed according to age, gender, BM and physical activity level (Food and Nutrition Board, Institute of Medicine 2005).

Table A1b   Dietary reference values for energy for females

AGE	UK AND WHO EAR[1]		USA* AEA[2]		EUROPE	
	(MJ/day)	(kcal/day)	(MJ/day)	(kcal/day)	Lower[3,4] (MJ/day)	Higher[5] (MJ/day)
0–3 months	2.16	515	2.7	650	2.1	
4–6 months	2.69	645	2.7	650	2.8	
7–9 months	3.20	765	3.5	850	3.3	
10–12 months	3.61	865	3.5	850	3.7	
1–3 years	4.86	1165	5.4	1300	4.8	
4–6 years	6.46	1545	7.5	1800	6.7	
7–10 years	7.28	1740	8.3	2000	7.4	
11–14 years	7.92	1845	9.2	2200	8.4	
15–18 years	8.83	2110	9.2	2200	8.9	
19–50 years	8.10	1940	9.2	2200	8.4	9.0
51–59 years	8.00	1900	9.2	2200	8.4	9.0
60–64 years	7.99	1900	9.2	2200	7.2	7.8
65–74 years	7.96	1900	9.2	2200	7.2	7.8
75+	7.61	1810	9.2	2200	6.7	7.6
Pregnancy	+0.80[6]	+200[6]	+1.2	+300	+0.75	
Lactation	+1.9–2.0	+450–480	+2.1	+500	+1.5–1.9	

[1]EAR, estimated average requirement.
[2]AEA, average energy allowance.
[3]No physical activity + desirable body weight for adults.
[4]Children's values are estimated average requirement.
[5]Desirable physical activity + desirable body weight for adults.
[6]Last trimester.
*(As for Table A1.a)

Table A2   Dietary reference values for protein (g/day)

AGE	UK AND WHO		USA RDA/AI	EUROPEAN PRI[3]
	EAR[1]	RNI[1]		
0–3 months	[2]–	12.5[2]	9.1[4]	
4–6 months	10.6	12.7	9.1[4]	14.0
7–9 months	11.0	13.7	11.0	14.5
10–12 months	11.2	14.9	11.0	14.5
1–3 years	11.7	14.5	13	14.7
4–6 years	14.8	19.7	19	19.0
7–10 years	22.8	28.3	19	27.3
Males				
11–14 years	33.8	42.1	34	42.0
15–18 years	46.1	55.2	52	48.5
19–50 years	44.4	55.5	56	56.0
50+ years	42.6	53.3	56	55.0
Females				
11–14 years	33.1	41.2	34	39.7
15–18 years	37.1	45.0	46	51.4
19–50+ years	36.0	45.0	48	47.0
50+ years	37.2	46.5	46	47.0
Pregnancy		+6	71	+10
Lactation		+11	71	+16

RNI, reference nutrient intake; RDA, recommended dietary allowance; AI, adequate intake; PRI, population reference intake.
[1]Based on egg and milk protein; assume complete digestibility.
[2]No WHO value.
[3]Children's values are safe levels.
[4]AI.

Table A3   Dietary reference values for fat and carbohydrate for adults as a percentage of daily total energy intake (percentage food energy)

	UK			USA[2]	WHO (1990)		
	Individual minimum	Population average[1]	Individual maximum		Lower[3]	Upper[3]	European PRI[4] or goal[5]
Saturated fatty acids		10 (11)			0	10	10[4]
Cis-polyunsaturated fatty acids		6 (6.5)	10		3	7	
n-3	0.2			0.6–1.2			0.5[3]
n-6	1.0			5–10			2.0[3]
Cis-monounsaturated fatty acids		12 (13)					
Trans-fatty acids		2 (2)					
Total fatty acids		30 (32.5)					
Total fat		33 (35)		20–35	15	30	20–30[4]
Non-milk extrinsic sugars	0	10 (11)			0	10	10[4]
Intrinsic milk sugars and starch		37 (39)					
Total carbohydrate		47 (50)		45–65	55	75	55–65[4]
Non-starch polysaccharide (g/day)	12	18	24		16	24	30[4]

[1]Total energy intake assumes 5% alcohol; food energy (in parenthesis) excludes alcohol.
[2]Acceptable Macronutrient Distribution Range (adults)
[3]Population nutrient goal.
[4]Population reference intake.
[5]Ultimate goal.

Table A4   Dietary reference values for vitamin A (μg retinol equivalent/day)

AGE	UK			USA RDA/AI	FAO/WHO	EUROPEAN PRI
	LRNI[1]	EAR	RNI			
0–12 months	150	250	350	500[2]	375	
1–3 years	200	300	400	300[2]	400	400
4–6 years	200	300	400	400	450	400
7–10 years	250	350	500	400	500	500
Males						
11–15 years	250	400	600	600	600	600
15–50+ years	300	500	700	900	600	700
Females						
11–50+ years	250	400	600	700	600	600
Pregnancy			+100	770	800	+100
Lactation			+350	1300		+350

[1]LRNI, lower reference nutrient intake.
[2]Adequate intake.

Table A5   Dietary reference values for vitamin D (μg/day)

AGE	UK RNI	USA[2] AI	FAO/WHO	EUROPEAN PRI
Males and females				
0–6 months	8.5	5	5	10–25
7 months–3 years	7.0	5	5	10
4–6 years	0[1]	5	5	0–10
7–10 years	0[1]	5	5	0–10
11–24 years	0[1]	5	5	0–15
25–50+ years	0[1]	5	5	0–10
65+	10	10	15	10
Pregnancy and lactation	10	5	5	10

[1]If exposed to the sun.
[2]In the absence of adequate exposure to sunlight

Table A6   Dietary reference values for vitamin E (mg/day, α-tocopherol)

AGE	UK SAFE INTAKE	USA RDA/AI	WHO/FAO	EUROPEAN PRI
0–6 months	0.4 mg/g PUFA	4[1]	2.7	0.4 mg/g PUFA
7–12 months	0.4 mg/g PUFA	5[1]	2.7	0.4 mg/g PUFA
1–3 years	0.4 mg/g PUFA	6	5	0.4 mg/g PUFA
4–10 years		7	7	
Males				
11–50+ years	>.4	15	10	>.4
Females				
11–50+ years	>.3	15	7.5	>.3
Pregnancy		15	7.5	
Lactation		19		

PUFA, polyunsaturated fatty acid.
[1]AI.

Table A7   Dietary reference values for vitamin K (µg/day)

AGE	UK SAFE INTAKE	USA AI	FAO/WHO	EUROPEAN[1]
0–6 months	10	2.0	5	
7–12 months	10	2.5	10	
1–3 years		30	15	
4–6 years		55	20	
7–10 years		60	25	
Males				
11–14 years	1 µg/kg body weight	60	35–55	1 µg/kg body weight
15–18 years	1 µg/kg body weight	75	35–55	1 µg/kg body weight
19–24 years	1 µg/kg body weight	120	65	1 µg/kg body weight
25+ years	1 µg/kg body weight	120	65	1 µg/kg body weight
Females				
11–14 years	1 µg/kg body weight	60	35–55	1 µg/kg body weight
15–18 years	1 µg/kg body weight	75	35–55	1 µg/kg body weight
19–24 years	1 µg/kg body weight	90	55	1 µg/kg body weight
25+ years	1 µg/kg body weight	90	55	1 µg/kg body weight
Pregnancy	1 µg/kg body weight	90	55	1 µg/kg body weight
Lactation	1 µg/kg body weight	90	55	1 µg/kg body weight

[1]No recommendation, but statement of what appears adequate.

Table A8   Dietary reference values for vitamin C (mg/day)

AGE	UK			USA RDA/AI	FAO/WHO	EUROPEAN PRI
	LRNI	*EAR*	*RNI*			
0–6 months	6	15	25	40[1]	25	
7–12 months	6	15	25	50[1]	30	20
1–3 years	8	20	30	15	30	25
4–6 years	8	20	30	25	30	25
7–10 years	8	20	30	25	35	30
Males						
11–14 years	9	22	35	45	40	35
15–50+ years	10	25	40	90	45	45
Females						
11–14 years	9	22	35	45	40	35
15–50+ years	10	25	40	75	45	40
Pregnancy			+10	85	55	55
Lactation			+30	120	70	70

[1]AI.

Table A9   Dietary reference values for thiamin

AGE	UK				USA RDA/AI (mg/day)	FAO/WHO (mg/day)	EUROPEAN PRI (mg/day)
	LRNI (μg/1000 kcal)	EAR (μg/1000 kcal)	RNI (μg/1000 kcal)	RNI (mg/day)			
0–6 months	0.2	0.23	0.3	0.2	0.2[2]	0.2	
7–12 months	0.2	0.23	0.3	0.3	0.3[2]	0.3	0.3
1–3 years	0.23	0.3	0.4	0.5	0.5	0.5	0.5
4–6 years	0.23	0.3	0.4	0.7	0.6	0.7	0.7
7–10 years	0.23	0.3	0.4	0.7	0.6	0.9	0.8
Males							
11–14 years	0.23	0.3	0.4	0.9	0.9	1.2	1.0
15–50+ years	0.23	0.3	0.4	0.9	1.2	1.2	1.1
Females							
11–14 years	0.23	0.3	0.4	0.7	0.9	1.1	0.9
15–50+ years	0.23	0.3	0.4	0.8	1.1	1.1	0.9
Pregnancy	0.23	0.3	0.4	+0.1[1]	1.4	1.4	1.0
Lactation	0.23	0.3	0.4	+0.2	1.4	1.5	1.1

[1]For last trimester only.
[2]AI.

Table A10   Dietary reference values for riboflavin (mg/day)

AGE	UK			USA RDA/AI	FAO/WHO	EUROPEAN PRI
	LRNI	EAR	RNI			
0–6 months	0.2	0.3	0.4	0.3[1]	0.3	
7–12 months	0.2	0.3	0.4	0.4[1]	0.4	0.4
1–3 years	0.3	0.5	0.6	0.5	0.5	0.8
4–6 years	0.4	0.6	0.8	0.6	0.6	1.0
7–10 years	0.5	0.8	1.0	0.6	0.9	1.2
Males						
11–14 years	0.8	1.0	1.2	0.9	1.3	1.4
15–18 years	0.8	1.0	1.3	1.3	1.3	1.6
19–50 years	0.8	1.0	1.3	1.3	1.3	1.6
50+ years	0.8	1.0	1.3	1.3	1.3	1.6
Females						
11–14 years	0.8	0.9	1.1	0.9	1.0	1.2
15–50+ years	0.8	0.9	1.1	1.1	1.1	1.3
Pregnancy			+0.3	1.4	1.4	1.6
Lactation			+0.5	1.6	1.6	1.7

[1]AI.

Table A11   Dietary reference values for niacin (nicotinic acid equivalent)

AGE	UK				USA RDA/AI (mg/day)	FAO/WHO (mg/day)	EUROPEAN PRI[2] (mg/day)
	LRNI (mg/1000 kcal)	EAR (mg/1000 kcal)	RNI (mg/1000 kcal)	RNI (mg/day)			
0–6 months	4.4	5.5	6.6	3	2[1]	2	
7–12 months	4.4	5.5	6.6	5	4[1]	4	5
1–3 years	4.4	5.5	6.6	8	6	6	9
4–6 years	4.4	5.5	6.6	11	8	8	11
7–10 years	4.4	5.5	6.6	12	8	12	13
Males							
11–14 years	4.4	5.5	6.6	15	12	16	15
15–18 years	4.4	5.5	6.6	18	16	16	18
19–50 years	4.4	5.5	6.6	17	16	16	18
50+ years	4.4	5.5	6.6	16	16	16	18
Females							
11–14 years	4.4	5.5	6.6	12	12	16	14
15–18 years	4.4	5.5	6.6	14	14	16	14
19–50 years	4.4	5.5	6.6	13	14	14	14
50+ years	4.4	5.5	6.6	12	14	14	14
Pregnancy	*	*	*	*	18	18	*
Lactation	*	*	+2.3 mg/day	+2	17	17	+2

*No increment.
[1]AI.
[2]1.6 mg/MJ.

Table A12   Dietary reference values for vitamin B$_6$

AGE	UK				USA RDA/AI (mg/day)	FAO/WHO (mg/day)	EUROPEAN PRI[2] (mg/day)
	LRNI (μg/g protein)	EAR (μg/g protein)	RNI (μg/g protein)	RNI (mg/day)			
0–6 months	3.5	6	8	0.2	0.1[1]	0.1	
7–9 months	6	8	10	0.3	0.3[1]	0.3	0.4
10–12 months	8	10	13	0.4	0.3[1]	0.3	0.4
1–3 years	8	10	13	0.7	0.5	0.5	0.7
4–6 years	8	10	13	0.9	0.6	0.6	0.9
7–10 years	8	10	13	1.0	0.6	1.0	1.1
Males							
11–14 years	11	13	15	1.2	1.0	1.3	1.3
15–18 years	11	13	15	1.5	1.3	1.3	1.5
19–50+ years	11	13	15	1.4	1.7	1.7	1.5
Females							
11–14 years	11	13	15	1.0	1.0	1.2	1.1
15–18 years	11	13	15	1.2	1.2	1.3	1.1
19–50+ years	11	13	15	1.2	1.5	1.5	1.1
Pregnancy	*	*	*	*	1.9	1.9	1.3
Lactation	*	*	*	*	2.0	2.0	1.4

*No increment.
[1]AI.
[2]15 μg/g protein.

Table A13   Dietary reference values for folate (µg/day)

AGE	UK			USA RDA/AI	FAO/WHO	EUROPEAN PRI[2]
	LRNI	EAR	RNI			
0–3 months	30	40	50	65[1]	80	50
4–6 months	30	40	50	65[1]	80	50
7–12 months	30	40	50	80[1]	80	50
1–3 years	35	50	70	150	160	100
4–6 years	50	75	100	200	200	130
7–10 years	75	110	150	200	300	150
Males						
11–14 years	100	150	200	300	400	180
15–50+ years	100	150	200	400	400	200
Females						
11–14 years	100	150	200	300	400	180
15–50+ years	100	150	200	400	400	200
Pregnancy			+100	600	600	400
Lactation			+60	500	500	350

[1]AI.
[2]Assuming bioavailability half that of pure folic acid and 20% coefficient of variation.

Table A14   Dietary reference values for vitamin B$_{12}$ (µg/day)

AGE	UK LRNI	EAR	RNI	USA/AI	FAO/WHO	EUROPEAN PRI
0–6 months	0.1	0.25	0.3	0.4[1]	0.4	
7–12 months	0.25	0.35	0.4	0.5[1]	0.5	0.5
1–3 years	0.3	0.4	0.5	0.9	0.9	0.7
4–6 years	0.5	0.7	0.8	1.2	1.2	0.9
7–10 years	0.6	0.8	1.0	1.2	1.8	1.0
Males						
11–14 years	0.8	1.0	1.2	1.8	2.4	1.3
15–50+ years	1.0	1.25	1.5	2.4	2.4	1.4
Females						
11–14 years	0.8	1.0	1.2	1.8	2.4	1.2
15–50+ years	1.0	1.25	1.5	2.4	2.4	1.4
Pregnancy			*	2.6	2.6	1.6
Lactation			+0.5	2.8	2.8	1.9

*No increment.
[1]AI.

Table A15	Dietary reference values for biotin (μg/day)		
AGE	UK SAFE INTAKE	USA/AI	EUROPEAN ACCEPTABLE RANGE
0–6 months		5	
7–12 months		6	
1–3 years		8	
4–10 years		12–20	
Males and females			
11–50+ years	10–20	30	15–100

Table A16	Dietary reference values for pantothenic acid (mg/day)		
AGE	UK SAFE INTAKE	USA/AI	EUROPEAN ACCEPTABLE RANGE
0–6 months	1.7	1.7	
7–12 months	1.7	1.8	
1–3 years	1.7	2	
4–10 years	3–7	3–4	
Males and females			
11–50+ years	3–7	5	3–12

Table A17	Dietary reference values for calcium (mg/day)					
AGE	UK			USA/AI	FAO/WHO	EUROPEAN PRI
	LRNI	EAR	RNI			
0–6 months	240	400	525	210	300	
6–12 months	240	400	525	270	400	400
1–3 years	200	275	350	500	500	400
4–6 years	275	350	450	800	600	450
7–10 years	325	425	550	800	700	550
Males						
11–14 years	450	750	1000	1300	1300	1000
15–18 years	450	750	1000	1300	1300	1000
19–24 years	400	525	700	1000	1000	700
25–50 years	400	525	700	1000	1000	700
50+ years	400	525	700	1200	1000	700
Females						
11–14 years	480	625	800	1300	1300	800
15–18 years	480	625	800	1300	1300	800
19–24 years	400	525	700	1000	1000	700
25–50 years	400	525	700	1000	1000	700
50+ years	400	525	700	1200	1300	700
Pregnancy	*	*	*	1000	1000	*
Lactation	*	*	*	1000	1000	+500

*No increment.

Table A18   Dietary reference values for phosphorus (mg/day) (No WHO values available)

AGE	UK RNI[1]	USA RDA/AI	EUROPEAN PRI
0–6 months	400	100[2]	
7–12 months	400	275[2]	300
1–3 years	270	460	300
4–10 years	350	500	350–450
Males			
11–18 years	775	1250	775
19–24 years	550	700	550
25–50 years	550	700	550
50+ years	550	700	550
Females			
11–18 years	625	1250	625
19–24 years	550	700	550
25–50+ years	550	700	550
Pregnancy	*	700	550
Lactation	+440	700	+400

*No increment.
[1]Phosphorus RNI is set equal to calcium in molar terms.
[2]AI.

Table A19   Dietary reference values for magnesium (mg/day)

AGE	UK LRNI	UK EAR	UK RNI	USA RDA/AI	FAO/WHO	EUROPEAN ACCEPTABLE RANGE
0–3 months	30	40	55	30[1]	26–36	
4–6 months	40	50	60	30[1]	26–36	
7–9 months	45	60	75	75[1]	53	
10–12 months	45	60	80	75[1]	53	
1–3 years	50	65	85	80	60	
4–6 years	70	90	120	130	73	
7–10 years	115	150	200	130	100	
Males						
11–14 years	180	230	280	240	250	
15–18 years	190	250	280	410	250	
19–50 + years	190	250	300	420	260	150–500
Females						
11–14 years	180	230	280	240	230	
15–18 years	190	250	300	360	230	
19–50 years	190	250	300	320	220	150–500
50 + years	150	200	270	320	220	
Pregnancy	*	*	*	350	270	
Lactation	*	*	*	310	270	

*No increment.
[1]AI.

Table A20   Dietary reference values for sodium (mg/day[1])

AGE	UK		USA AI	WHO POPULATION AVERAGE[2]	EUROPEAN ACCEPTABLE RANGE
	LRNI	RNI			
0–3 months	140	210	120		
4–6 months	140	280	120		
7–9 months	200	320	370		
10–12 months	200	350	370		
1–3 years	200	500	1000		
4–6 years	280	700	1200		575–3500
7–10 years	350	1200	1500		575–3500
Males and females					
11–14 years	460	1600	1500		575–3500
15–50+ years	575	1600	1500	3900	575–3500
Pregnancy	*	*	*		*
Lactation	*	*			*

*No increment.
[1] 1 mmol sodium = 23 mg.
[2] Upper limit.

Table A21   Dietary reference values for potassium (mg/day[1]) (No WHO values available)

AGE	UK		USA AI	EUROPEAN PRI
	LRNI	RNI		
0–3 months	400	800	400	
4–6 months	400	850	400	
7–9 months	400	700	700	800
10–12 months	450	700	700	800
1–3 years	450	800	3000	800
4–6 years	600	1100	3800	1100
7–10 years	950	2200	4500	2000
Males and females				
11–14 years	1600	3100	4700	3100
15–50+ years	2000	3500	4700	3100
Pregnancy	*	*	*	*
Lactation	*	*	5100	*

*No increment.
[1] 1 mmol potassium = 9 mg.

Table A22   Dietary reference values for chloride (mg/day) (No WHO values available)

AGE	UK RNI[1]	USA MINIMUM REQUIREMENT[2]	EUROPEAN ACCEPTABLE RANGE[1]
0–3 months	320	180	
4–6 months	400	180	
7–9 months	500	570	
10–12 months	500	570	
1–3 years	800	1500	
4–6 years	1100	1900	
7–10 years	1100	2300	
Males and females			
11–50+ years	2500	2300	Should match sodium intake
Pregnancy	*	*	*
Lactation	*	*	*

*No increment.
[1]Corresponds to sodium. 1 mmol = 35.5 mg.
[2]No allowance for large losses from the skin through sweat.

Table A23   Dietary reference values for iron[1] (mg/day)

AGE	UK			USA RDA/AI	FAO/WHO[3]	EUROPEAN[4]
	LRNI	EAR	RNI			
0–3 months	0.9	1.3	1.7	0.27[2]	–	
4–6 months	2.3	3.3	4.3	0.27[2]	–	
7–12 months	4.2	6.0	7.8	11	6	6
1–3 years	3.7	5.3	6.9	7	4	4
4–6 years	3.3	4.7	6.1	10	4	4
7–10 years	4.7	6.7	8.7	10	6	6
Males						
11–14 years	6.1	8.7	11.3	8	10	10
15–18 years	6.1	8.7	11.3	11	12	13
19–50+ years	4.7	6.7	8.7	8	9	9
Females						
11–14 years	8.0	11.4	14.8[5]	8	9	18–22[6]
15–50 years	8.0	11.4	14.8[5]	15	22	17–21[6]
50+ years	4.7	6.7	8.7	8	8	8
Pregnancy	*	*	*	27	10	*
Lactation	*	*	*	9	10	10

*No increment.
[1]1 mmol iron = 55.9 mg.
[2]AI.
[3]Median basal requirement on intermediate bioavailability diet.
[4]Bioavailability 15%.
[5]Insufficient for women with high menstrual losses, who may need iron supplements.
[6]Lower value for 90% of population, upper value for 95% of population.

Table A24 Dietary reference values for zinc (mg/day)

AGE	UK			USA RDA/AI	FAO/WHO	EUROPEAN PRI
	LRNI	EAR	RNI			
0–3 months	2.6	3.3	4.0	2.0[1]	2.8	
4–6 months	2.6	3.3	4.0	2.0[1]	2.8	
7–12 months	3.0	3.8	5.0	3	4.1	4.0
1–3 years	3.0	3.8	5.0	3	4.1	4.0
4–6 years	4.0	5.0	6.5	5	5.1	6.0
7–10 years	4.0	5.4	7.0	5	5.6	7.0
Males						
11–14 years	5.3	7.0	9.0	8	9.7	9.0
15–18 years	5.5	7.3	9.5	11	9.7	9.0
19–50+ years	5.5	7.3	9.5	11	7.0	9.5
Females						
11–14 years	5.3	7.0	9.0	8	7.8	9.0
15–18 years	4.0	5.5	7.0	9	7.8	7.0
19–50+ years	4.0	5.5	7.0	8	4.9	7.0
Pregnancy	*	*	*	11	5.5–10	*
Lactation						
0–4 months			+6.0	12.0	9.5	+5.0
4+ months			+2.5	12.0	8.8	+5.0

*No increment.
[1]AI.

Table A25 Dietary reference values for copper[1] (mg/day)

AGE	UK RNI	USA RDA/AI	WHO[3] (1996)	EUROPEAN PRI
0–3 months	0.3	0.2[2]	0.33–0.55[4]	
4–6 months	0.3	0.2[2]	0.37–0.62[4]	
7–12 months	0.3	0.2	0.60	0.3
1–3 years	0.4	0.34	0.56	0.4
4–6 years	0.6	0.44	0.57	0.6
7–10 years	0.7	0.44	0.75	0.7
Males				
11–14 years	0.8	0.7	1.00	0.8
15–18 years	1.0	0.89	1.33	1.0
19–50+ years	1.2	0.90	1.15	1.1
Females				
11–14 years	0.8	0.7	1.00	0.8
15–18 years	1.0	0.89	1.15	1.0
19–50+ years	1.2	0.90	1.15	1.1
Pregnancy		1.0		
Lactation	+0.3	1.3	1.25	+0.3

[1]μmol copper = 63.5 μg.
[2]AI
[3]Normative requirement.
[4]Upper levels should not be habitually exceeded because of risk of toxicity

Table A26   Dietary reference values for selenium (µg/day)[1]

AGE	UK		USA RDA/AI	WHO[2] (1996)	EUROPEAN PRI
	LRNI	RNI			
0–3 months	4	10	15[3]	6	
4–6 months	5	13	15[3]	9	
7–9 months	5	10	20[3]	12	8
10–12 months	6	10	20[3]	12	8
1–3 years	7	15	20	20	10
4–6 years	10	20	30	24	15
7–10 years	16	30	30	25	25
Males					
11–14 years	25	45	40	36	35
15–18 years	40	70	55	40	45
19–50+ years	40	75	55	40	55
Females					
11–14 years	25	45	40	30	35
15–18 years	40	60	55	30	45
19–50+ years	40	60	55	30	55
Pregnancy	*	*	60	35	*
Lactation	115	115	70	40	115

*No increment.
[1] 1 µmol selenium = 79 µg.
[2] Normative requirement.
[3] AI.

Table A27   Dietary reference values for iodine (µg/day)

AGE	UK		USA RDA/AI	WHO (1996)[1]	EUROPEAN PRI
	LRNI	RNI			
0–3 months	40	50	110[2]	50	
4–6 months	40	60	110[2]	50	
7–12 months	40	60	130[2]	50	50
1–3 years	40	70	90	90	70
4–6 years	50	100	90	90	90
7–10 years	55	110	90	120	100
Males and females					
11–14 years	65	130	120	150	120
15–18 years	70	140	150	150	130
19–50+ years	70	140	150	150	130
Pregnancy	*	*	220	200	*
Lactation	*	*	290	200	160

*No increment.
[1] Normative requirement.
[2] AI.

Index